# Evidence-based Oncology

# Evidence-based Oncology

*Edited by*

**Chris Williams**
Cochrane Cancer Network, Institute of Health Sciences,
Oxford, UK

## Associate editors

**Vivien Bramwell**
Tom Baker Cancer Centre, Calgary, Canada

**Xavier Bonfill**
Iberoamerican Cochrane Centre, Hospital de la Santa Creu i
Sant Pau, Barcelona, Spain

**Jack Cuzick**
Imperial Cancer Research Fund, London, UK

**John F Forbes**
Department of Surgical Oncology, Newcastle Mater Hospital,
University of Newcastle, NSW, Australia

**Robin Grant**
Department of Clinical Neurosciences, University of
Edinburgh, UK

**David Guthrie**
Derbyshire Royal Infirmary, Derby, UK

**Malcolm Mason**
Department of Clinical Oncology, Velindre NHS Trust,
Whitechurch, Cardiff, UK

**Peter Simmonds**
Cancer Research UK Oncology Unit, Southampton General
Hospital, UK

**Arun D Singh**
Wills Eye Hospital, Oncology Service, Philadelphia, USA

**Rosalynne Weston**
Cochrane Cancer Network, Oxford, UK

**Hywel C Williams**
Centre of Evidence-Based Dermatology, University of
Nottingham, UK

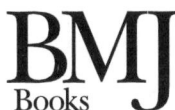

BMJ Books

© BMJ Publishing Group 2003
BMJ Books is an imprint of the BMJ Publishing Group

First published in 2003
by BMJ Books, BMA House, Tavistock Square,
London WC1H 9JR

www.bmjbooks.com

**British Library Cataloguing in Publication Data**
A catalogue record for this book is available from the British Library

ISBN 0 7279 1439 1

Typeset by SIVA Math Setters, Chennai, India
Printed and bound by MPG Books, Bodmin, Cornwall

# Contents

# Contributors

**Jaffer Ajani**
Department of Gastrointestinal Medical Oncology, The University of Texas MD Anderson Cancer Center, Houston, Texas, USA

**Anca Ansink**
Erasmus MC Daniel den Hoed Cancer Center, Rotterdam, The Netherlands

**Ferran Ariza**
Iberoamerican Cochrane Centre, Hospital de la Santa Creu i Sant Pau, Barcelona, Spain

**Wendy Atkin**
Cancer Research UK Colorectal Cancer Unit, St Mark's Hospital, Harrow, UK

**Jim Barber**
Velindre NHS Trust, Cardiff, UK

**Veronique Bataille**
Twin Research Genetic Epidemiology Unit, St Thomas' Hospital, London, UK

**Fiona Bath**
Centre for Evidence-based Dermatology, Queen's Medical Centre, Nottingham, UK

**MJ van den Bent**
Department of Neuro-Oncology, Dr. Daniel den Hoed Cancer Center, Rotterdam, The Netherlands

**William C Black**
Department of Radiology, Dartmouth-Hitchcock Medical Center, Lebanon, New Hampshire, USA

**Xavier Bonfill**
Iberoamerican Cochrane Centre, Hospital de la Santa Creu i Sant Pau, Barcelona, Spain

**Michael Brada**
Neuro-oncology Unit and Academic Unit of Radiotherapy & Oncology, The Institute of Cancer Research and the Royal Marsden NHS Trust, Sutton, UK

**Vivien Bramwell**
Tom Baker Cancer Centre, and University of Calgary, Calgary, Canada

**D Brinkmann**
Gynaecology Oncology Unit, Bart's and The London Queen Mary's School of Medicine and Dentistry, London, UK

**Kathryn Burgon**
Cochrane Unit, Velindre NHS Trust, Whitchurch, Cardiff, UK

**Ian Chau**
Gastrointestinal Unit, Department of Medicine, Royal Marsden Hospital, Sutton, UK

**Chris Coppin**
Medical Oncology, British Columbia Cancer Agency Fraser Valley Centre, Surrey, Canada

**ER Copson**
Cancer Research UK Medical Oncology Unit, The Royal South Hants Hospital, Southampton, UK

**Thomas Crosby**
Velindre Hospital, Whitechurch, Cardiff, UK

**David Cunningham**
Gastrointestinal Unit, Department of Medicine, Royal Marsden Hospital, Sutton, UK

**Jack Cuzick**
Imperial Cancer Research Fund Cancer Research UK, London, UK

**RJ Davies**
Department of General Surgery, Addenbrooke's Hospital, Cambridge, UK

**Lena van Doorn**
University Hospital Utrecht, Utrecht, The Netherlands

**Stephen W Duffy**
Queen Mary University of London, London, UK

**Simon Everett**
Department of Gastroenterology, Leeds General Infirmary, Leeds, UK

**Richard M Fagerstrom**
Biometry Research Group, National Cancer Institute, Bethesda, Maryland, USA

**Rebecca L Faulkner**
Academic Unit of Obstetrics and Gynaecology and Reproductive Health Care, St Mary's Hospital, Manchester, UK

**John F Forbes**
Department of Surgical Oncology, Newcastle Mater Hospital, University of Newcastle, NSW, Australia

**David Forman**
Unit of Epidemiology and Health Services Research, Medical School, University of Leeds, Leeds, UK

**Paula Ghaneh**
Department of Surgery, University of Liverpool, Liverpool, UK

**Julie Glanville**
NHS Centre for Reviews & Dissemination, University of York, UK

**John K Gohagan**
Early Detection Research Group, National Cancer Institute, Bethesda, Maryland, USA

**Robin Grant**
Department of Clinical Neurosciences, University of Edinburgh, UK

**David Guthrie**
Derbyshire Royal Infirmary, Derby, UK

**Santosh G Honavar**
Ocular Oncology Service, LV Prasad Eye Institute, Hyderabad, India

**TJ Iveson**
Cancer Research UK Medical Oncology Unit, The Royal South Hants Hospital, Southampton, UK

**Ian Jacobs**
Unit of Epidemiology and Health Services Research, Medical School, University of Leeds, Leeds, UK

**Philip J Johnson**
Division of Cancer Studies, School of Medicine, University of Birmingham, Birmingham, UK

**Katharine Johnston**
Health Economics Research Centre, Institute of Health Sciences, University of Oxford, UK

**Henry C Kitchener**
Academic Unit of Obstetrics and Gynaecology and Reproductive Health Care, St Mary's Hospital, Manchester, UK

**Barnett S Kramer**
Disease Prevention, National Institutes of Health, Bethesda, Maryland, USA

**Julia Kumpf**
Clinical Economics Group, University Hospital Ulm, Germany

**Howard Kynaston**
Department of Urology, University Hospital of Wales, Cardiff, UK

**Tim Lancaster**
Cochrane Tobacco Addiction Review Group, Institute of Health Sciences, Oxford, UK

**Nannette J Liégeois**
Department of Dermatology, Harvard Medical School, Lahey Clinic, Burlington, MA, USA

**Imogen Locke**
Department of Radiotherapy and Oncology, Royal Marsden Hospital, Sutton, UK

**Conor Magee**
Department of Surgery, University of Liverpool, Liverpool, UK

**Pamela M Marcus**
Biometry Research Group, National Cancer Institute, Bethesda, Maryland, USA

**Malcolm Mason**
Department of Clinical Oncology, Velindre NHS Trust, Whitechurch, Cardiff, UK

**Miquel Mateu**
Thoracic Surgery Service, Hospital Mutua de Terrassa, Barcelona, Spain

**Jane Melia**
Cancer Screening Evaluation Unit, Institute of Cancer Research, Sutton, UK

**Usha Menon**
Gynaecology Oncology Unit, Bart's and The London Queen Mary's School of Medicine and Dentistry, London, UK

**M Michael**
Division of Haematology and Medical Oncology, Peter MacCallum Cancer Institute, Victoria, Australia

**R Miller**
Department of General Surgery, Addenbrooke's Hospital, Cambridge, UK

**Kate Misso**
NHS Centre for Reviews and Dissemination, University of York, UK

**Paul Moayyedi**
Gastroenterology and Health Services Research, University of Birmingham, UK

**Sue Moss**
Cancer Screening Evaluation Unit, Institute of Cancer Research, Sutton, UK

**John P Neoptolemos**
Department of Surgery, University of Liverpool, Liverpool, UK

**Alan Neville**
McMaster University, Hamilton, Canada

**ES Newlands**
Charing Cross Hospitals, London, UK

**Suzanne Olbricht**
Department of Dermatology, Harvard Medical School, Lahey Clinic, Burlington, MA, USA

**Tim Oliver**
Medical Oncology Department, Royal Hospital NHS Trust, St Bartholomews Hospital, London, UK

**William Perkins**
Consultant Dermatologist and Dermatologic Surgeon, University Hospital, Queen's Medical Centre, Nottingham, UK

**Alexandria Phan**
Department of Gastrointestinal Medical Oncology, The University of Texas MD Anderson Cancer Center, Houston, Texas, USA

**Paul F Pinsky**
Early Detection Research Group, National Cancer Institute, Bethesda, Maryland, USA

**Ernst Pöppel**
Institute of Medical Psychology and Human Studies Center, Ludwig Maximilians University Munich, Germany

**Franz Porzsolt**
Clinical Economics Group, University Hospital Ulm, and Evidence Based Health Care, Human Studies Center, Ludwig Maximilians University Munich, Germany

**Philip C Prorok**
Biometry Research Group, National Cancer Institute, Bethesda, Maryland, USA

**Ramón Rami-Porta**
Thoracic Surgery Service, Hospital Mutua de Terrassa, Barcelona, Spain

**Ian G Rennie**
Department of Ophthalmology and Orthoptics, University of Sheffield, Sheffield, UK

**Dafydd Roberts**
Department of Dermatology, Singleton Hospital, Swansea, UK

**Trevor Roberts**
Northern Centre for cancer Treatment, Newcastle General Hospital, Newcastle-upon-Tyne, UK

**Paul A Rundle**
Department of Ophthalmology and Orthoptics, Royal Hallamshire Hospital, Sheffield, UK

**Peter Sasieni**
Cancer Research UK, Department of Epidemiology, Mathematics and Statistics, Wolfson Institute of Preventive Medicine, London, UK

**John H Scholefield**
Division of GI Surgery, University Hospital, Nottingham, UK

**Mireia Serra**
Thoracic Surgery Service, Hospital Mutua de Terrassa, Barcelona, Spain

**Mike Shelley**
Cochrane Prostatic Diseases and Urological Cancers Group, Cochrane Unit, Research Department, Velindre NHS Trust, Cardiff, UK

**Peter Simmonds**
Cancer Research UK Oncology Unit, Southampton General Hospital, UK

**Arun D Singh**
Wills Eye Hospital, Oncology Service, Philadelphia, USA

**Steven Skates**
Department of Medicine, Harvard Medical School and Massachusetts General Hospital, Boston, USA

**Margaret F Spittle**
Meyerstein Institute of Oncology, Middlesex Hospital, London, UK

**Lesley Stewart**
Meta-Analysis Group, MRC Clinical Trials Unit, London, UK

**RP Symonds**
University of Leicester, Leicester Royal Infirmary, Leicester, UK

**Elinor Thompson**
Iberoamerican Cochrane Centre, Hospital de la Santa Creu i Sant Pau, Barcelona, Spain

**Paul A Vasey**
Cancer Research UK Department of Medical Oncology, University of Glasgow, Glasgow, UK

**Jacobus van der Velden**
Academic Medical Center, Amsterdam, The Netherlands

**Charles J Vecht**
Neuro-oncology Unit, Department of Neurology, Medical Center, The Hague, The Netherlands

**Shail Verma**
Ottawa Regional Cancer Centre, Ottawa, Canada

**Rosalynne Weston**
Focus Freelance Writing and Research, Salisbury, and Cochrane Cancer Network, Oxford, UK

**Sean Whittaker**
St John's Institute of Dermatology, Guy's and St Thomas' Hospital, London, UK

**IR Whittle**
University of Edinburgh, Edinburgh, UK

**Nicholas Wilcken**
Department of Medical Oncology, Westmead Hospital, Westmead, Australia

**Chris Williams**
Cochrane Cancer Network, Institute of Health Sciences, Oxford, UK

**Hywel C Williams**
Centre of Evidence-Based Dermatology, University of Nottingham, UK

**JR Zalcberg**
Division of Haematology and Medical Oncology, Peter MacCallum Cancer Institute, Victoria, Australia

# Preface

Cancer has been at the forefront of developments in clinical trials methodology for the past half-century. Some of the earliest randomised controlled trials (RCTs) were in the field of oncology and clinical research has routinely used RCTs to assess new therapies. However, before we congratulate ourselves, perhaps prematurely, we need to look to see how the evidence from RCTs and other clinical studies has been used.

The movement called evidence-based medicine has not suddenly invented the concept of using evidence from clinical experiments – Western medicine has been predicated on this concept for many hundreds of years. However, the tool of the RCT has been honed and we now have the means to synthesise information in a systematic manner that reduces the risk of bias. These developments have come at a time when electronic communication has allowed us for the first time to keep an effective track of clinical research, scientific publications and to bring all of the information together using the methodology of systematic reviews.

In the past, the need for reviews of current knowledge was met by "narrative reviews", usually written by an expert in the field. Such individuals were held to have a thorough grasp of the literature and the ability to interpret it. Readers of reviews need unbiased information and there is consistent evidence (including from cancer) that narrative reviews of healthcare interventions rarely use methods designed to reduce the risk of bias. The fact that narrative reviews are written by experts in the field who have often carried out some of the research that they are reviewing compounds the risk of bias.

Systematic reviews, the bedrock of evidence-based medicine, are designed to reduce the risk of bias. They also bring together all of the pertinent evidence from trials judged to be of good quality. Where appropriate, evidence from these trials can be pooled using the technique of meta-analysis. The result of such a process is to reduce the risk of bias and to maximise the chances of finding a useful outcome, because the intervention is being examined in the largest population possible and not in a few discreet RCTs.

This book uses an evidence-based approach to look at the strength of the underlying evidence used to support some of the key decisions in cancer care. The authors have not been commissioned to carry out systematic reviews to answer each of these questions. Each systematic review is a complex and time-consuming exercise and it would be impractical in a book of this nature. Authors were asked to use systematic searches of the medical literature and to summarise their findings. Where there are systematic reviews these were presented and discussed in the light of the rest of the literature. Where no systematic reviews were available reviewers summarised the available literature with a particular emphasis on RCTs. However, new systematic reviews were usually not carried out.

The conclusions for each review question have been graded according to the strength of the evidence underlying that conclusion. Readers may wish to use these grades in thinking about the believability of the conclusions, but should bear in mind that such grades are a crude approximation. While they provide a summary of the strength of evidence, they are also included to stimulate readers to automatically think about how believable the evidence really is.

Inevitably, in a book of this type there will be many questions that were not included. The limited list of key questions were selected by the authors with the section editor. Often this was driven by those areas where there was known to be RCTs and sometimes systematic reviews. There is an emphasis on questions deemed to be of significance by clinicians because this is where the research has been carried out. Questions of particular importance to patients and their families have often been much less well researched and because of this are even harder to systematically review.

Users of this book should be able to read about the evidence underlying many of the decisions that underpin our current approach to treating the common cancers. Often clear conclusions elude us because there is a paucity of data and some of it is of doubtful quality. In these circumstances systematic reviews are often an essential starting point of new trials.

I hope that readers will find that this book is a useful starting place when looking for evidence for how we currently treat cancer.

**Updates and further information on this book can be found at www.evidbasedoncology.com.**

# Abbreviations

| | |
|---|---|
| 5-FU | 5-fluorouracil |
| AA | anaplastic astrocytoma |
| AD | dissection of axillary nodes |
| AFP | alpha-fetoprotein |
| AIDS | acquired immune deficiency syndrome |
| AJCC | American Joint Committee on Cancer |
| AMED | Allied and Complementary Medicine Database |
| AMS | atypical mole syndrome |
| APC | adenomatous polyposis coli |
| APR | abdominoperineal resection |
| AR | anterior resection |
| ASCO | American Society of Clinical Oncology |
| ATLL | adult T-cell leukaemia lymphoma |
| BCC | basal cell carcinoma |
| BED | biologically effective dose |
| BMI | Body Mass Index |
| BNI | British Nursing Index |
| BP | breast preservation |
| BPH | benign prostatic hyperplasia |
| CBA | cost-benefit analysis |
| CCTR | Cochrane Controlled Trials Register |
| CDSR | Cochrane Database of Systematic Reviews |
| CEA | carcinoembryonic antigen |
| CEA | cost-effectiveness analysis |
| CHART | continuous hyperfractionated accelerated radiotherapy |
| CHRPE | congenital hypertrophy of the retinal pigment epithelium |
| CI | confidence interval |
| CIN | cervical intraepithelial neoplasia |
| CLE | complete local excision of the primary tumour |
| CR | cumulative risk |
| CRC | colorectal cancer |
| CT | computerised tomography |
| CTCL | cutaneous T-cell lymphoma |
| CUA | cost-utility analysis |
| DARE | Database of Abstracts of Reviews of Effects |
| DCIS | duct carcinoma *in situ* |
| DDFS | distant disease-free survival |
| DFS | disease-free survival |
| DPD | dihydropyrimidine dehydrogenase |
| DRE | digital rectal examination |
| DRS | disease-related symptoms |
| DSS | disease-specific survival |
| EBM | evidence-based medicine |
| EBRT | external beam radiotherapy |
| EBT | endobronchial brachytherapy |
| ECG | electrocardiogram |
| ECP | extracorporeal photopheresis |
| ED&C | electrodesiccation and curettage |
| EFS | event-free survival |
| EGFR | epidermal growth factor receptor |

| | |
|---|---|
| ERCP | endoscopic cholangiopancreatography |
| ERM | extended radical mastectomy |
| EUS | endoscopic ultrasound |
| FAMMM | familial atypical multiple mole melanoma |
| FAP | familial adenomatous polyposis |
| FBC | full blood count |
| FNA | fine needle aspiration |
| FOBT | faecal occult blood test |
| GDEPT | gene-directed enzyme prodrug therapy |
| GORD | gastro-oesophageal reflux disease |
| GTD | gestational trophoblastic disease |
| HAART | highly active antiretroviral therapy |
| HAI | hepatic arterial influsional |
| HBV | hepatitis B virus |
| HCC | hepatocellular carcinoma |
| hCG | human chorionic gonadotrophin |
| HCV | hepatitis C virus |
| HGG | high grade glioma |
| HHV8 | human herpes virus 8 |
| HIV | human immunodeficiency virus |
| HNPCC | hereditary non-polyposis colorectal carcinoma |
| HPV | human papillomavirus |
| HTA | Health Technology Assessment |
| HTLV-I | human T-lymphotrophic virus type-1 |
| IARC | International Agency for Research on Cancer |
| ICER | incremental cost-effectiveness ratio |
| IFN$\alpha$ | interferon alfa |
| IGF-1 | insulin-like growth factor 1 |
| IL-2 | interleukin-2 |
| IMH | immunohistochemistry |
| IORT | intraoperative radiotherapy |
| IPD MA | individual patient data meta-analyses |
| IPF | independent prognostic factor |
| IPSID | immunoproliferative small intestinal disease |
| IRA | ileorectal anastomosis |
| KPS | Karnofsky Performance Status |
| KS | Kaposi's sarcoma |
| KSHV | KS-associated herpesvirus |
| LAVH | laparoscopic-assisted vaginal hysterectomy |
| Lev | levamisole |
| LFT | liver function tests |
| LGG | low grade glioma |
| LHRH | luteinising hormone-releasing hormone |
| LINAC | linear accelerator |
| LLETZ/LEEP | large loop excision of the transformation zone |
| LM | lentigo maligna |
| LMM | lentigo maligna melanoma |
| LPA | lysophosphatidic acid |
| LR | local recurrence |
| LSS | limb salvage surgery |
| LV | leucovorin |

| | | | | |
|---|---|---|---|---|
| MALTomas | mucosa-associated lymphoid tissue lymphomas | | QALYs | quality adjusted life-years |
| MeSH | Medical Subject Headings | | QoL | quality of life |
| MF/SS | mycosis fungoides/Sézary syndrome | | Q-TWIST | quality adjusted time without symptoms or toxicity |
| MFH | malignant fibrous histiocytoma | | RCC | renal cell cancer |
| MM | malignant melanomas | | RM | radical mastectomy |
| MMP | matrix metalloproteinase | | RP | radical prostatectomy |
| MMS | Mohs micrographic surgery | | RPC | restorative proctocolectomy |
| MRCP | magnetic resonance cholangiopancreatography | | RR | relative risk |
| MSI | microsatellite instability | | SCC | squamous cell carcinoma |
| MSI-H | microsatellite instability – high | | SCLC | small cell lung cancer |
| NCI | National Cancer Institute | | SD | stable disease |
| NICE | National Institute for Clinical Excellence | | SERM | selective oestrogen receptor modulator |
| NMSC | non-melanomic skin cancer | | SIL | squamous intraepithelial lesions |
| NR | not reported | | SLNB | sentinel lymph node biopsy |
| NSCLC | non-small cell lung cancer | | SR | systematic reviews |
| OMNI | Organising Medical Networked Information | | SRS | stereotactic radiotherapy |
| OR | odds ratio | | SSS | sphincter sparing surgery |
| OS | overall survival | | STS | soft tissue sarcoma |
| OSSN | ocular surface squamous neoplasia | | TACE | transarterial chemoembolisation |
| PA | para-aortic | | Tc-MAA | technetium-99m macroaggregated albumin scan |
| PCI | prophylactic cranial irradiation | | TIMP | tissue inhibitor of matrix metalloproteinase |
| PCNA | proliferating cell nuclear antigen | | TM | total mastectomy |
| PD | progressive disease | | TME | total mesorectal excision |
| PDECGF | platelet derived endothelial cell growth factor | | TNM | Tumour, Node, Metastasis classification |
| PDT | photodynamic therapy | | TP | thymidine phosphorylase |
| PEI | percutaneous alcohol injection | | TRUS | transrectal ultrasound |
| PET | positron emission tomography | | TS | thymidylate synthase |
| PICO/PIOC | population, intervention, comparison and outcome | | TSEB | total skin electron beam therapy |
| PJS | Peutz–Jeghers syndrome | | TUR | transurethral resection |
| PORT | postoperative radiotherapy | | U&E | urea and electrolytes |
| PSA | prostate specific antigen | | VAIN | vaginal intraepithelial neoplasia |
| PSTT | placental site trophoblastic tumours | | VEGF | vascular endothelial growth factor |
| PTC | percutaneous transhepatic cholangiography | | WBRT | whole brain radiotherapy |
| PVI | portal vein infusion | | WW | watchful waiting |
| | | | XRR | external beam radical radiotherapy |
| | | | XRT | external beam radiotherapy |

# Levels of evidence and grades of recommendation used in *Evidence-based Oncology*

Levels of evidence and grades of recommendation appear within the text in the clinical chapters, for example, **Evidence Level Ia** and **Grade A**.

**Levels of evidence**

Ia   Meta-analysis of randomised controlled trials (RCTs)
Ib   At least 1 RCT
IIa  At least 1 non-randomised study
IIb  At least 1 other well designed quasi-experimental study
III  Non-experimental, descriptive studies
IV   Expert committee reports or opinions/experience of respected authorities

**Grades of recommendations**

A   At least one RCT as part of body of literature of overall good quality and consistency addressing recommendation **Evidence levels Ia, Ib**
B   No RCT but well conducted clinical studies available **Evidence levels IIa, IIb, III**
C   Expert committee reports or opinions/experience of respected authorities in the absence of directly applicable good quality clinical studies **Evidence level IV**

From *Clinical Oncology* (2001)**13**:S212
Source of data: MEDLINE, *Proceedings of the American Society of Medical Oncology* (ASCO).

# Section I

## Principles and practice of "critical appraisal"

*Chris Williams, Editor*

# 1 Appraising clinical literature in cancer

*Chris Williams*

We are all of us, whether we are consumers, researchers, or policy makers, inundated with unmanageable and increasing amounts of information on health care. This chapter discusses how we can best appraise and use this information, whether it be from clinical trials or clinical reviews.

Sackett and Haynes[1] have defined evidence-based medicine (EBM) as "the practice [of EBM] is a process of life-long, problem-based learning in which care for our own patients creates the need for evidence about diagnosis, prognosis, therapy and other clinical and health care issues". EBM has been criticised partly because it can be taken to suggest that evidence has just been discovered – it would be more accurate to say that EBM expresses that we can base care on better evidence than we were able to in the past. This is because we have better evidence from trials and better ways of synthesising this evidence. We also now have the technology to transfer large amounts of data easily.

This book is based on the premise that patients and their professional carers need the best available evidence when making clinical decisions.[2] It suggests that we need systematic reviews to efficiently integrate valid information and provide a basis for rational decision making.[3] It is also acknowledged that careful review of the literature is a complicated and time-consuming business and that clinicians are not in a position to carry out systematic reviews on all of the questions that they encounter in clinical practice. As well as understanding how to appraise reports of clinical research, clinicians also need to understand how to appraise systematic reviews. Studies have shown that evidence to support decision making is required more often that most clinicians realise – partly because so many decisions are taken to be routine and the evidence underlying them is not questioned (Covell 1985).[4]

The use of explicit, systematic methods in reviews limits bias (systematic errors) and reduces chance effects by increasing the number of participants, thus providing more reliable results upon which to draw conclusions and make decisions.[5,6] Systematic reviews can establish where effects of health care are consistent and can be applied across populations and in different settings. They can also show where effects may vary significantly.

Meta-analysis, the use of statistical methods to summarise the results of independent studies, can provide more precise estimates of the effects of health care than those derived from the individual studies included in a systematic review.[7–10] Systematic reviews ideally include meta-analysis, but often this is not possible because the questions, trial populations and method of delivering therapy were too variable to allow meaningful pooling of results in a meta-analysis.

Recognition of the key role of reviews in synthesising and disseminating the results of research has prompted people to consider the validity of narrative reviews. Social science and psychology led this field and it was not until the late 1980s that people drew attention to the poor scientific quality of healthcare review articles.[11–13] The first survey of the quality of narrative reviews in cancer was not published until 1997.

This chapter focuses on appraisal of and systematic review of randomised controlled trials (RCTs) because they are likely to provide more reliable information than other sources of evidence on the effectiveness of different therapies.[14] Systematic reviews of other types of evidence can be useful to those wanting to make better decisions about health care, when RCTs are not available. The basic principles of reviewing non-RCT research are the same, although meta-analysis is often not appropriate and care should be taken not to overinterpret the results.

## What is the evidence that RCTs are the best way to test new treatments?

Although it has been long accepted that RCTs are the best way of testing clinical effectiveness, there are few systematic studies testing this hypothesis. The historical data from a variety of conditions supports the contention that randomised trials are more reliable than historically controlled or uncontrolled trials.[15] Sacks *et al.*[16] examined the outcomes in six different clinical questions that had been tested in both RCTs and historically controlled trials (HCTs). Box 1.1 shows that HCTs grossly overestimated the potential benefit of treatment compared with RCTs. Importantly, the differences in outcomes between RCTs and HCTs lay in the outcomes in the control group (where HCT patients fared worse than RCT patients) and not in the experimental arm where the results were similar in HCT and RCT patients.

---

**Box 1.1 A study of comparative results of RCTs and HCTs asking the same question**

- 6 Therapies, 50 RCTs, 56 HCTs
- 44 of 56 HCTs (79%) found the "new" therapy to be significantly better than the control
- 10 of 50 RCTs (20%) found the "new" therapy to be significantly better than the control
- The outcomes for new treatments were similar regardless of whether they were from RCTs or HCTs
- Outcomes were clearly worse for control patients in HCTs when compared with control patients in RCTs

Abbreviations: RCTs, randomised control trials; HCTs, historically controlled trials

---

This might seem academic, but failure to identify effective treatments may delay their use by years and ineffective treatments may be recommended when they are toxic or where there are other genuinely effective therapies. Such misinformation can cause real harm. One of the questions included in the paper by Sacks *et al.* was the use of diethylstilbestrol (DES) in women who have had recurrent miscarriages. Four HCTs were published in the 1960s that appeared to show that DES was highly effective in preventing habitual abortion. However, three RCTs showed that DES had no effect and that the outcome in the control group of the four HCTs was particularly poor (Table 1.1). On the basis of the HCT evidence millions of women worldwide erroneously received DES during pregnancy in an attempt to reduce the chance of miscarriage. Long-term follow up of the RCTs have revealed major toxicity of the DES given during pregnancy when the fetus is vulnerable. The finding of a major excess of vaginal clear cell cancers in the daughters of the DES-treated women was devastating. In addition follow up has shown that the male and female offspring of DES women have an increased incidence of depression and that male offspring are much less likely to form stable long-term relationships.[17–19]

RCTs have become the accepted way of testing therapies because the process of randomisation helps minimise the risk of bias. Where there is doubt that randomisation was adequately concealed, there is strong evidence that the outcome is biased.[20] In this observational study they assessed the methodological quality of 250 controlled trials from 33 meta-analyses (from the Cochrane Pregnancy and Childbirth Database) and then analysed, using multiple logistic regression models, the associations between those assessments and estimated treatment effects. The main outcome measures included associations between estimates of treatment effects and inadequate allocation concealment. Compared with trials in which authors reported adequately concealed treatment allocation, trials in which concealment was either inadequate or unclear (did not report or incompletely reported a concealment approach) yielded larger estimates of treatment effects ($P < 0.001$). Odds ratios were exaggerated by 41% for inadequately concealed trials and by 30% for unclearly concealed trials (adjusted for other aspects of quality). They concluded that there is empirical evidence that inadequate concealment of randomisation is in controlled trials associated with bias.

Although safe randomisation is the key to a reliable RCT, attention also needs to be paid to other features. Among these, sufficient power (number of events) and appropriate endpoints are very important. An individual patient data meta-analysis of 52 RCTs of chemotherapy for non-small cell cancer found fewer than 10 000 patients who had been treated over three decades.[21] During this time period many millions would have died of this disease. None of the trials was powered to answer the questions being asked, the mean size of the treatment arms being less than 100 at a time when only a small benefit was plausible. Although chemotherapy is largely palliative in this setting, there was no usable outcome data on symptom control or quality of life.

Also of paramount importance is the question itself. In addition to the 52 RCTs included in this review a large number of RCTs were identified where the comparison was between two different types of chemotherapy. This was in spite of a lack of evidence that any chemotherapy could provide benefit to patients with advanced non-small cell lung cancer. Clearly, a key to a good RCT is to make the appropriate comparison.

The development of the CONSORT statement and its subsequent iterations will hopefully increase the quality of current and future trials and their reporting.[22] Check lists

---

**Table 1.1** Comparison of the results of RCTs and HCTs testing the ability of diethylstilbestrol to prevent recurrent abortion

| Type of trial | No. of trials | No. of patients | % Live infants DES – treated | Control |
|---|---|---|---|---|
| RCT | 3 | 2175 | 87·3 | 87·6 |
| HCT | 4 | 2358 | 85·3 | 56 |
| HCT [matched] | 1 | 216 | 45 | 8 |

---

**Table 1.2  Items that should be included in reports of randomised trials**

| Heading | Subheading | Descriptor |
|---|---|---|
| Title | | Identify the study as randomised trial |
| Abstract | | Use a structured format |
| Introduction | | State prospectively defined hypothesis, clinical objectives, and planned subgroup or covariate analysis |
| Methods | Protocol | *Describe the:* |
| | | Planned study population, together with inclusion or exclusion criteria |
| | | Planned interventions and their timing |
| | | Primary and secondary outcome measure(s) and the minimum important difference(s), and indicate how the target sample size was projected |
| | | Rationale and methods for statistical analyses, detailing the main comparative analyses and whether they were completed on an intention-to-treat basis |
| | | Prospectively defined stopping rules (if warranted) |
| | | *Describe the:* |
| | Assignment | Unit of randomisation (for example individual, cluster, geographic) |
| | | Method used to generate allocation schedule |
| | | Method of allocation concealment and timing of assignment |
| | | Method to separate the generator from the executor of assignment |
| | Masking (blinding) | *Describe the:* |
| | | Mechanism (for example capsules, tables) |
| | | Similarity of treatment characteristics (for example appearance, taste) |
| | | Allocation schedule control (location of code during trial and when broken) |
| | | Evidence for successful blinding among participants, person doing intervention, outcome assessors, and data analysts |
| Results | Participant flow and follow up | Provide a trial profile summarising participant flow, numbers and timing of randomisation assignment, interventions and measurements for each randomised group |
| | | State estimated effect of intervention on primary and secondary outcome measures, including a point estimate and measure of precision (confidence interval) |
| | Analysis | State results in absolute numbers when feasible (for example 10/20 not 50%) |
| | | Present summary data and appropriate descriptive and interferential statistics in sufficient detail to permit alternative analyses and replication |
| | | Describe prognostic variables by treatment group and any attempt to adjust them |
| | | Describe protocol deviations from the study as planned, together with the reasons |
| Discussion | | State specific interpretation of study findings, including sources of bias and imprecision (internal validity) and discussion of external validity, including appropriate quantitative measures when possible |
| | | State general interpretation of the data in light of the totality of the available evidence |

(Table 1.2) should help improve the quality of published reports of clinical trials and this will aid in synthesising the literature.

In addition to the potential benefit to be gained from improving medical knowledge in general, there is some evidence that inclusion in an RCT is beneficial to patients regardless of the outcome of the trial. Braunholtz *et al.*[23] carried out a systematic review of the literature. They found only 14 research articles (covering more than 21 trials) with relevant primary data. They found that the evidence available was limited in breadth (coming largely from cancer trials) and quality, as well as quantity. There was weak evidence to suggest that clinical trials have a positive effect on the outcome of participants. This does not appear to depend strongly on the trial demonstrating that an experimental treatment is superior. However, benefit to participants is less evident where scope for a "protocol/Hawthorne effect" (benefit from improved routine care within a trial) was apparently limited (because there was no effective routine treatment or because the comparison group also received protocol care). A form of bias, arising if clinicians who tend to recruit to trials also tend to be better clinicians, could also explain these results. They concluded that, while the evidence is not conclusive, it is more likely that clinical trials have a positive rather than a negative effect on the outcome of patients. They found that the effect seems to be larger in trials where an effective treatment already exists and is included in the trial protocol.

Currently very few patients are entered into RCTs. In the UK the current NHS Cancer Plan aims to double recruitment from 3% to 6%. There are complex factors that stop patients being recruited into cancer trials and research into how to improve recruitment is sorely needed.

### Why do we need reviews?

Apart from the need to find time-efficient means of using the literature to help make decisions, there is good evidence that a systematic approach can produce results that change practice. Systematic reviews of therapy for acute myocardial infarction[5] show how careful review of all of the evidence can change thinking (Figure 1.1). Early experience with thrombolytic therapy was largely ignored and narrative reviews and textbooks failed to routinely recommend such treatment for 10–15 years after meta-analysis would have shown these treatments to be effective. Conversely, lidocaine (lignocaine) has been consistently recommended for use in myocardial infarction by narrative reviews and textbooks, when there was no evidence of benefit. Thus, systematic reviews could, in this situation, change practice and help researchers to develop new trials.

Reviews are useful because they:

- are an efficient use of time
- can help support individual patient decisions
- can help in preparing guidelines and treatment protocols
- can help in developing and planning new clinical research.

### What is wrong with narrative reviews?

Reviews are not new, so what is wrong with the classical or narrative review that has been used for many generations? Mulrow[11] was the first to examine the methodological quality of narrative reviews in general medicine. Since then a number of similar studies have examined the methods used in different branches of medicine, including cancer. The findings have been uniformly similar. Bramwell and Williams[24] reported on the methodological quality of reviews published in the *Journal of Clinical Oncology* from its inception in 1983 through to 1995. In the areas that are regarded as key to reducing the risk of bias (data identification, selection of data to be included, assessment of the validity of that data, quantitative synthesis of the data), less than 10% of the reviews used methods designed to reduce bias.

The outcome of this is that narrative reviews may often be unreliable. In the example above,[5] narrative reviews and textbook reviews failed to identify the true situation, as they were often selective in their use of the literature. In order to address this problem the concept of systematic reviews has been developed.

### What are the main elements of a systematic review?

Systematic reviews aim to address the weaknesses identified in narrative reviews by paying careful attention to those areas where bias may be evident in the process of finding, selecting, extracting data from, and synthesising the results of trials asking similar questions. This essentially means writing a protocol setting out how the review is to be carried out in order to minimise bias. The key steps in preparing a systematic review are briefly discussed in the following sections. Users of systematic reviews should be looking to see if the reviewers have done a thorough job in each of these areas.

### Locating and selecting studies

A comprehensive, unbiased search of the literature is one of the key differences between a systematic review and a narrative review. While electronic databases such as

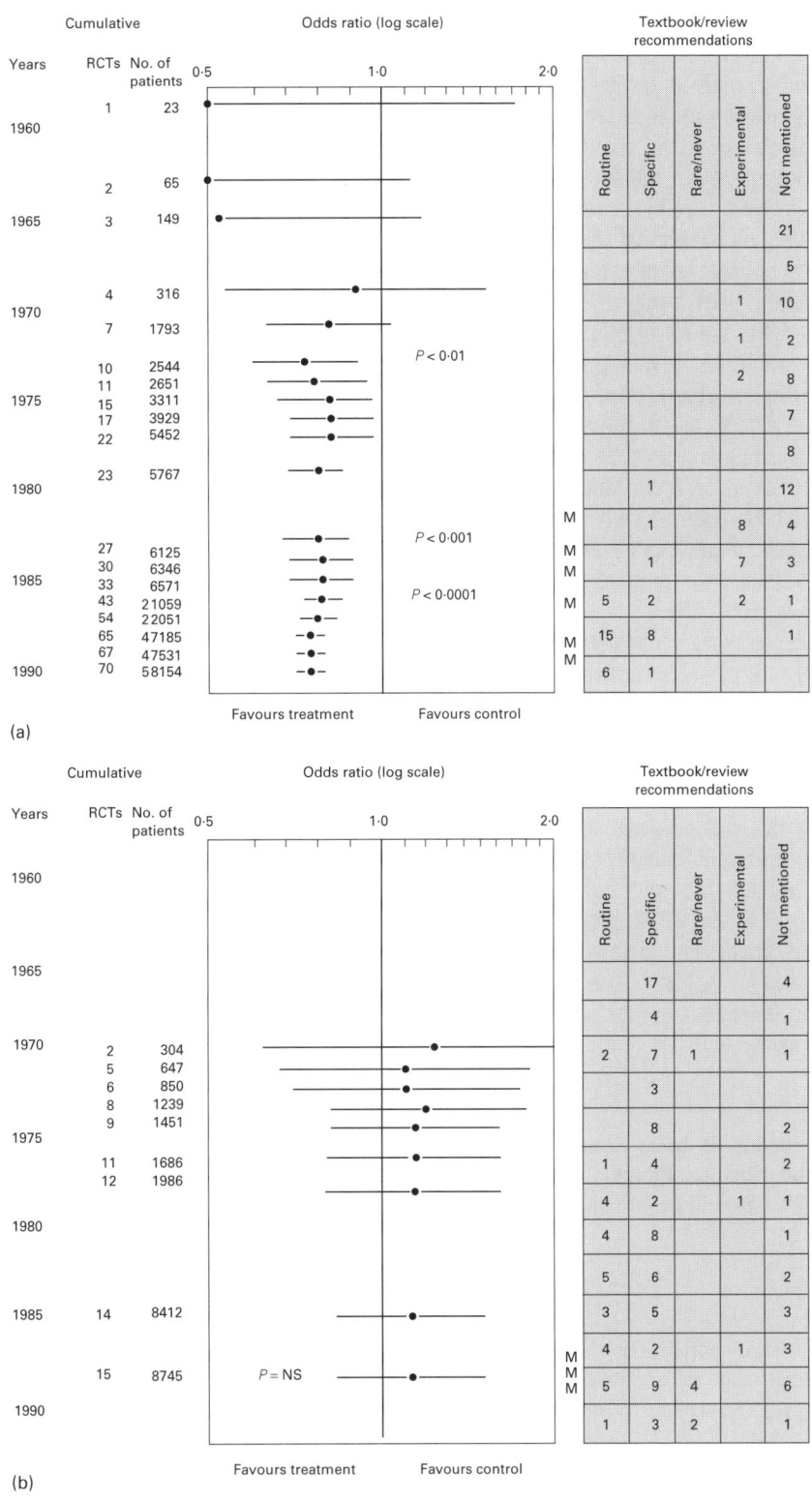

**Figure 1.1** Cumulative meta-analysis of two treatments for acute myocardial infarction compared with treatment recommendations from reviews and textbooks. (a) This summarises the situation for thrombolytic therapy and (b) the use of lidocaine (lignocaine). The meta-analysis for thrombolytic therapy shows that there was good evidence for the use of this treatment from the early 1970s, but it was only in the late 1980s and early 1990s that it was recommended at all or used routinely. In contrast, there has never been any evidence to support the use of lidocaine (if anything, the evidence suggests that it may be harmful), but it was routinely recommended throughout this period. (With permission from *Oxford Textbook of Oncology*)

MEDLINE and Embase are powerful tools, they only include a subset of all biomedical journals. A study by the Cochrane Cancer Network compared the results of hand searching leading cancer journals with an optimal electronic search. The electronic search only found about 50% of the RCTs found by hand searching, even though the journals were in MEDLINE and Embase. If relevant records are in such databases it is still difficult to retrieve them easily. In addition, these databases do not contain the totality of published medical literature and, even if they did, a significant proportion of studies are never published,[25] and abstracts never turned into full peer review publications.[26] Failure to identify all of the available literature would not matter if this failure were a random event. However, there is good evidence that bias is acting and that there is a strong tendency for "positive" trials to be found and "negative" trials to be lost. As well as a bias regarding whether or not a report of a trial is published, there is good evidence that "positive" trials are published several years earlier than those with "negative" results (Box 1.2).[27]

Non-English-language references are underrepresented in MEDLINE and Embase and published articles only are included, so there is the potential for a review to be influenced by publication bias (which means that studies with positive results are selectively published) if one relies on studies identified using MEDLINE and Embase.[25,28–35] There is also some evidence to suggest that there is language bias, with bilingual researchers preferring to publishing "positive" results in English and "negative" results in their own language.[36–38]

In order to reduce the risk of bias it is important to use a variety of sources to identify studies and to have a systematic approach to selecting studies for inclusion in a review. The potential for reference bias (a tendency to preferentially cite studies supporting one's own views) is reduced by using multiple search strategies.[39,40] It should also be remembered that strongly "positive" trials are more likely to be published on multiple occasions, sometimes with different authors and different results.[41]

## Quality assessment of studies

Quality assessment of individual studies summarised in a systematic review is required to:

- limit bias in conducting the systematic review
- gain insight into potential comparisons
- guide interpretation of findings.

This quality assessment should look at those factors related to:

- applicability of the findings (also called external validity or generalisability). This is related to the definition of the key components of the question being addressed. Specifically, whether the findings of the trial are applicable to a particular population, intervention strategy and how the people, interventions and outcomes of interest were defined by these studies and the reviewers;
- validity of individual studies – interpretation of results is dependent upon the validity of the included studies, addressed in more detail in the following sections.

## Validity

When a systematic review (or trial report) is being prepared or read, the validity of an individual study is the extent to which its design and conduct are likely to prevent systematic errors, or bias.[42] An issue that should not be confused with validity is precision.

Precision is a measure of the likelihood of chance effects leading to random errors. It is reflected in the confidence interval around the estimate of effect from each study and the weight given to the results of each study when an overall estimate of effect or weighted average is derived. Thus more precise results are given more weight.

Variation in validity can explain variation in the results of the studies included in a systematic review. More rigorous studies designed to avoid bias should be more likely to yield results that are closer to the "truth". Quantitative analysis of results from studies with varying degrees of validity can result in "false positive" conclusions if the less rigorous studies are biased toward overestimating treatment effectiveness. They can also come to "false negative" conclusions if less rigorous studies are biased towards underestimating an intervention's effect.[43]

It is important to critically appraise all studies in a review, even if there is no variability in either the validity or results

---

**Box 1.2 Publication record of trials submitted to the Royal Prince Alfred Hospital Ethics Committee between 1979 and 1988, correlation with significance outcome**

- 784 Eligible studies
- 520 (70%) Replied to study
- 218 Trials included tests of significance
- Those with positive outcomes were significantly more likely to have been published than negative results (HR, 2·32; 95% CI, 1·47–3.66; $P=0.0003$)
- This result was even stronger for the 130 clinical trials (HR, 3·13; 95% CI, 1·76–5·58; $P=0.0001$)
- Time to publication of the 218 trials was shorter for those with positive outcomes than those with negative results (median 4·8 v 8·0 years)
- The results for time to publication for the 130 clinical trials was similar (median 4·7 v 8·0 years)

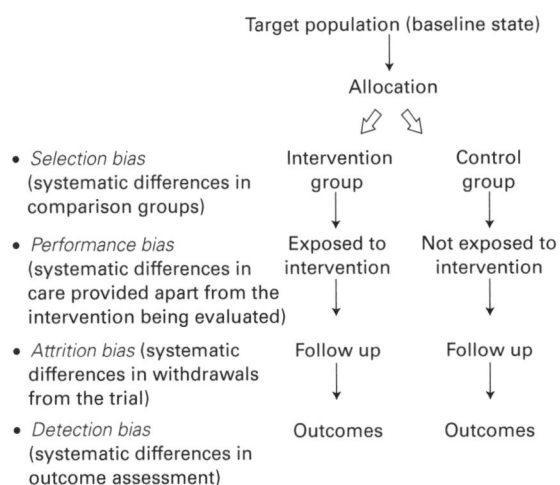

Target population (baseline state)

↓

Allocation

↙  ↘

- *Selection bias*
  (systematic differences in
  comparison groups)

Intervention
group

Control
group

↓

↓

- *Performance bias*
  (systematic differences in
  care provided apart from the
  intervention being evaluated)

Exposed to
intervention

Not exposed to
intervention

↓

↓

- *Attrition bias* (systematic
  differences in withdrawals
  from the trial)

Follow up

Follow up

↓

↓

- *Detection bias*
  (systematic differences in
  outcome assessment)

Outcomes

Outcomes

**Figure 1.2**  Sources of systematic bias

of the included studies. For instance, the results may be consistent among studies, but, if all the studies are flawed, the review's conclusions would not be as strong as in a series of rigorous studies yielding consistent results.

For readers of systematic reviews the key is to look to see if the reviewers made a systematic and prospective attempt to evaluate the validity of included trials.

## Sources of bias in trials of healthcare interventions

There are four sources of systematic bias (Figure 1.2) in trials of health care.

- selection bias
- performance bias
- attrition bias
- detection bias.

Unfortunately, we do not have strong empirical evidence of a relationship between trial outcomes and the risk of these biases,[42,44] but there is a logical basis for suspecting such relationships and good reason to consider these potential biases when assessing studies for a review.[45]

Users of systematic reviews need to ask whether the reviewers have assessed the risk of each of these potential biases when preparing their review.

### Selection bias

The way that comparison groups are assembled may lead to bias.[14]

- *Using an appropriate method to prevent foreknowledge of treatment assignment is crucially important in trial design*

When assessing a potential participant's eligibility for a trial, researchers and participants themselves should remain unaware of the next assignment in the sequence until after the decision about eligibility has been made. The ideal is for the process to be entirely independent of the individuals making the allocation. This is best achieved if assignment is by someone who is not responsible for recruiting subjects, such as someone based in a central trials office or pharmacy.

Concealing assignment should not be confused with "blinding" of patients, researchers, outcome assessors, and analysts. The reason for concealing the assignment schedule is to eliminate selection bias. In contrast, blinding (used after the allocation of the intervention) reduces performance and detection biases (see below).

Empirical research has shown that lack of adequate allocation concealment is clearly associated with bias.[46–48]

- *Concealment has been found to be more important in preventing bias than other components of allocation, such as the generation of the allocation sequence (for example, computer, random number table, alternation)*

The validity of studies can be judged on the method of allocation concealment. The method for assigning participants to interventions should be robust against patient and clinician bias and its description should be clear. The following approaches may be used to ensure adequate concealment schemes. Opaque numbered, sealed envelopes may be less secure that the other methods and a centralised method or pharmacy-controlled randomisation is always preferable (for example, allocation by a central office unaware of subject characteristics) using:

- prenumbered or coded identical containers administered serially to participants;
- on-site computer system combined with allocations kept in a locked unreadable computer file that can be accessed only after the characteristics of an enrolled participant have been entered.

Inadequate approaches to allocation concealment include:

- alternation
- the use of case record numbers (odd or even)
- date of birth or day of the week (odd or even)
- any procedure that is transparent before allocation, such as an open list of random numbers.

When studies do not report any concealment approach, adequacy should be considered unclear. An adequate description of the method of allocation and its concealment is frequently not reported.

### Performance bias

Performance bias refers to systematic differences in the care provided to the participants in the comparison groups other than the intervention under investigation.

To protect against unintended differences in care and placebo effects, those providing and receiving care can be "blinded" so that they do not know the group to which participants have been allocated. Evidence suggests that such blinding is important in protecting against bias.[20,49,50] Studies have shown that contamination (provision of the intervention to the control group) and cointervention (provision of unintended additional care to either comparison group) can affect study results.[51,52]

There is evidence that participants who know their assignment report more symptoms, leading to biased results.[49] For these reasons, readers of trial reports and systematic reviews may want to consider the use of "blinding" as a criterion for validity. The key points are:

- Were the recipients of care unaware of their assigned intervention?
- Were those providing care unaware of the assigned intervention?
- Were those responsible for assessing outcomes unaware of the assigned intervention? This addresses detection bias (see below).

### Attrition bias

Attrition bias refers to systematic differences in loss of participants between the comparison groups in the study. Because of inadequacies in reporting on loss of participants (for example, withdrawals, dropouts, protocol deviations), reviewers should be cautious about implicit accounts of follow up. The approach to handling losses has great potential for biasing the results and reporting inadequacies cloud this problem.

### Detection bias

Detection bias refers to systematic differences between the comparison groups in outcome assessment. Trials that blind the people who will assess outcomes to the intervention allocation should logically be less likely to be biased than trials that do not. Blinding is likely to be particularly important in research with subjective outcome measures such as pain.[20,49,50] Despite this, at least two empirical studies have failed to demonstrate a relationship between blinding of outcome assessment and study results. This may be due to inadequacies in the reporting of studies.[53]

Bias from the selective reporting of results is different from bias in outcome assessment. This source of bias may be important in areas where multiple outcome measures are used.[54] Specification of predefined primary outcomes and analyses by the investigators can be useful indicators of validity.

### Approaches to summarising the validity of studies

Because there is no "gold standard" for the validity of a trial, the possibility of validating any proposed scoring system or scale is limited.[55] While there are a number of scoring systems available, none can be recommended without reservation. They may carry a greater risk of confusing the issue and may not be transparent to readers. For these reasons, it is generally preferable to report how each trial scored on each criterion. Readers should assess whether a review has systematically gathered and reported information on the various aspects of validity discussed above.

### Applying quality assessment criteria

It is preferable that there are multiple reviewers – this may limit bias, minimise errors, and improve reliability of findings. Reviewers should have complementary areas of expertise, such as medical content knowledge and review methodology experience.

Although experts in medical content may have preformed opinions that can bias their assessments,[6] they may also give more consistent assessments of the validity of studies than those without content expertise.[56] Content expertise is important in interpreting the subtleties of the clinical material.

### Limitations of quality assessment

There are two major difficulties when assessing the validity of studies:

- The first is inadequate reporting of trials.[47,57,58,59] Because something was not reported, it does not mean that it was not done. Attempts to obtain additional data from investigators are sometimes necessary, but this may be difficult with no response from the original researchers.
- A second limitation (partly is a consequence of the first) is limited empirical evidence of a relationship between criteria thought to measure validity and actual study outcomes. While there is empirical evidence suggesting that inadequate concealment of allocation and lack of double blinding result in overestimates of the effects of treatment, research is needed to establish which criteria are key determinants of study results. Improved reporting of methods will facilitate such research.

## Summarising effects across studies

An aim of a systematic review is to provide a reliable estimate of the effects of an intervention, based on a weighted average of the results of all the available relevant studies. Typically, the weight given to each study is the inverse of its variance, that is, more precise estimates (from larger studies with more events) are given more weight.[60] It is also possible to give studies more or less weight based on other factors such as their methodological quality, but this is rarely done.[43]

If it makes practical sense to combine the results of a group of studies and the observed differences between the results of the studies are not statistically significant (there is no statistical heterogeneity), it is relatively straightforward to combine the results. Each study is summarised using a measure of effect (such as an odds ratio, a relative risk, or a mean difference) that represents the within study comparison of the intervention and control groups. In this way participants in each study are only compared with other participants in the same study.

It is not the intention of this chapter to summarise current thinking on the methodology of systematic reviews. For those wishing to pursue this, *Systematic Reviews in Health Care: Meta-analysis in Context,*[61] is a useful starting point. Systematic reviews are relatively new and there remains much that is controversial or requiring further work. This includes statistical/methodological issues (such as how to estimate heterogeneity), as well as generic problems, (such as how to review data from non-randomised studies), studies of diagnostic techniques, and prognostic/predictive factors.

Currently methodology for non-randomised trial evidence is a major issue. There is little likelihood that sophisticated methods can make up for what may be deficiencies in the original research methods, but systematic reviews that carefully review the whole literature may help improve future research methods and may identify questions suitable for new research. Not all questions in medicine can be addressed by RCTs and there is a need for better ways of synthesising evidence from unrandomised studies.

## Interpreting results

Although it can be argued that the results of a systematic review should stand on their own, many readers need help interpreting the results. Users of systematic reviews should look for consideration of the following points:

- the strength and reliability of the evidence
- the applicability of the results
- implication of costs and current practice
- clarification of any important trade-offs between the expected benefits and harms.

The primary purpose of a systematic review should be to present information, rather than to offer conclusions. Readers should look to the discussion and conclusions as an aid to understanding the implications of the evidence when making practical decisions.

### Strength of evidence

This should start with a discussion of any important methodological problems in the included trials and the methods used in the review that might affect making practical decisions or future research.

It is often helpful to discuss how the included studies fit into the context of other evidence that is not included in the review. For example, for reviews of drug therapy it may be relevant to refer to dosage studies or non-randomised studies of the risk of adverse events – particularly those that are rare or delayed.

Because conclusions regarding the strength of inferences about the effectiveness of an intervention are essentially causal inferences, readers might want to consider guidelines for assessing the strength of a causal inference, such as those put forward by Hill.[62] In the context of a systematic review of clinical trials, these considerations might include:

- How good is the quality of the included trials?
- How large and significant are the observed effects?
- How consistent are the effects across trials?
- Is there a clear dose–response relationship?
- Is there indirect evidence that supports the inference?
- Have other plausible competing explanations of the observed effects (for example, bias or cointervention) been ruled out?

A variety of approaches to grading strength of evidence is available,[63–67] but none is universally appropriate for a wide range of reviews. Thus grading of evidence (as used in this book) can lack transparency, and should be interpreted with caution, but it may be useful in helping readers think about the reliability of the evidence.

### Applicability

When interpreting evidence from RTCs or systematic reviews, users must decide how applicable the evidence is to their particular question. To do this, they must first decide whether the review provides valid information about potential benefits and harms that are important to them. They then need to decide whether the participants and settings in the included studies are reasonably similar to their own situation. In addition, it is important to consider the characteristics of the interventions and additional care provided during the research. Such consideration requires a difficult extrapolation and Friedman has characterised this as: "A leap of faith is always required when applying any study findings to the population at large ... In making that jump, one must always strike a balance between making justifiable broad generalisations and being too conservative in one's conclusions."[68]

Rather than rigidly applying the inclusion and exclusion criteria of the studies in particular clinical circumstances, it is generally better to ask whether there are compelling reasons why the evidence should not be used in those circumstances.[69] Such reasons, where difference from the original trials might limit applicability of results, include:

- biologic (for example, age, sex, genetic variability)
- cultural variation (local attitudes to disease and its treatment)
- variation in compliance with the therapy
- variation in baseline risk(for example, risk of recurrence in breast cancer).

### Variation in the results of the included studies

As well as identifying limitations of the applicability of results, readers should look for important variation in results within the circumstances to which the results are applicable. Is there predictable variation in the relative effects of the intervention, and are there identifiable factors that may cause effects to vary? These might include:

- patient features, such as age, sex, biochemical markers
- intervention features, such as the timing or intensity of the intervention
- disease features, such as hormone receptor status.

Even in the absence of statistical heterogeneity, these features should be examined by testing whether there is an interaction with treatment and not by subgroup analysis. Differences between subgroups, particularly those that correspond to differences between studies, need to be interpreted cautiously. Chance variation between subgroups is inevitable, so unless there is strong evidence of an interaction then it should be assumed there is none.

### Common errors in reaching conclusions

Common mistakes made in drawing conclusions include:

- confusing "no evidence of effect" with "evidence of no effect";
- describing a positive but statistically non-significant trend as "promising", whereas a "negative" effect of the same magnitude is not commonly described as a "warning sign";

- framing the conclusion in wishful terms, for example "the included studies were too small to detect a reduction in mortality" when the included studies showed a statistically non-significant increase in mortality. (One way of avoiding such errors is to consider the results "blinded"; that is, consider how the conclusions would be presented and framed if you reverse the direction of the results. If the confidence interval for the estimate of the difference in the effects of the interventions overlaps the null value, the analysis is compatible with both a true beneficial effect and a true harmful effect. If one of the possibilities is mentioned in the conclusion, the other possibility should be mentioned as well.);
- reaching conclusions that go beyond the evidence. (Often this is done implicitly, without referring to the additional information or judgements used in reaching the conclusions. Even when conclusions about the implications of a review for practice are supported by additional information and explicit judgements, the additional information that is considered is rarely systematically reviewed.).

Users of reviews need to be alert to the potential that the authors will have fallen into one of these traps.

### Trade-offs

In addition to considering the strength of evidence underlying any conclusions that are drawn, reviewers should be as explicit as possible about any judgements about preferences (the values attached to different outcomes) that they make. Healthcare interventions generally entail costs and risks of harm, as well as expectations of benefit. Drawing conclusions about the practical usefulness of an intervention includes making trade-offs, either implicitly or explicitly, between the estimated benefits and the estimated costs and harms.[2] It is beyond the scope of most systematic reviews to incorporate formal economic analyses – although they might well be used for such analyses.[70,71] However, reviewers should consider all of the potentially important outcomes of an intervention when drawing conclusions, including ones for which there may be no reliable data from the included trials. They should also be cautious about any assumptions that they make about the relative value of the benefits, harms, and costs of an intervention.

### Are all systematic reviews equal?

Systematic reviews, as is all clinical research, are subject to potential bias and poor methodology. The results of a systematic review should be interpreted with caution and require careful assessment of the quality of the methods used and of the strength of the conclusions. Some examples of inconsistent quality of systematic reviews are shown below.

Schwarzer et al.[72] compared the outcomes of Cochrane reviews, said to be of good quality as there is a standard process for producing them, with other systematic reviews. They hand searched volumes 1993–1997 of four general medicine journals (*Annals of Internal Medicine*, *BMJ*, *JAMA*, *Lancet*) and four specialist journals (*American Journal of Cardiology*, *Cancer*, *Circulation*, *Obstetrics and Gynecology*) for meta-analyses based on at least five controlled clinical trials with binary endpoints. The Cochrane Database of Systematic Reviews (Issue 1, 1998) was used to identify Cochrane reviews that reported meta-analyses of at least five trials with binary endpoints. For each journal and Cochrane review, they calculated the combined effect estimates on the odds ratio scale. They then combined pooled estimates from Cochrane and journal meta-analyses in a "meta-meta-analysis" using a random effects model.

Sixty-nine pairs of Cochrane and journal reviews were analysed. Journal meta-analyses reported more beneficial results than Cochrane reviews ($P = 0.007$ by McNemar's test). The pooled odds ratio was 0·72 (95% CI 0·66–0·77) for journal meta-analyses and 0·80 (0·72–0·89) for Cochrane reviews. The trials included in Cochrane meta-analyses tended to be larger than in journal meta-analyses. Methodological quality and reporting quality was clearly superior for Cochrane reviews. They concluded that meta-analyses showing a beneficial effect of the intervention were more likely to be published in journals, whereas inconclusive meta-analyses, or meta-analyses showing adverse effects are more likely to be published electronically on the Cochrane Database of Systematic Reviews. Publication bias at the level of individual trials is well documented, but the potential for publication bias at the level of reviews is a real problem, with some meta-analyses being neither published in print nor electronically.

Similarly, Jüni et al.[73] examined how quality assessment, a key feature of systematic reviews, was performed in meta-analyses of controlled trials published in leading English-language journals. A hand search (1993–1997) of four general medicine journals (*Annals of Internal Medicine*, *BMJ*, *Lancet*, *JAMA*) and four specialist journals (*American Journal of Cardiology*, *Cancer*, *Circulation*, *Obstetrics and Gynecology*) found 133 meta-analyses. They used a standardised questionnaire to extract relevant information and logistic regression for analysis. They found that the quality of trials was assessed in 54 (41%) meta-analyses, 31 (23%) reported on concealment of treatment allocation and blinding, and 25 (19%) performed sensitivity analyses according to quality. Over 40 different approaches were identified, with checklists and quality scales used in similar

proportions. In multivariable analysis quality assessment was less likely to be reported in specialist journals compared to general medicine journals (OR 0·32, 95% CI 0·12–0·87). Affiliation with the Cochrane Collaboration predicted assessment of quality (OR 6·30, 95% CI 1·94–20·4). They concluded that quality assessment of primary studies is relatively uncommon and inconsistent in meta-analyses of controlled trials published in leading medical journals.

Thus, the term "systematic review" does not guarantee the reliability of a review and readers should look to see if the key features required to minimise bias in the review process have been carried out adequately.

## Individual patient data meta-analysis

While systematic review of published reports of trials can make a major contribution to clinical research, synthesis and analysis of the raw data from a series of RCTs can be even more useful. Clarke et al.[74] have reported on the rationale and characterised a series of individual-patient data meta-analyses (IPD MA) and others have commented on the reliability of such meta-analyses.[75,76] They found that IPD MA allowed reviewers to do time-to-event analyses; to define patient subgroups and outcomes consistently, and to conduct standardised checking and correction procedures for each trial. Intention-to-treat analyses and updating of data also become possible. At the time of their report[74] 39 separate IPD MA projects in cancer were identified: 38 of these were investigating the treatment of cancer, others were about mammographic screening for breast cancer. Twenty cancers were included in the treatment projects (acute lymphoblastic leukaemia, acute myeloid leukaemia, bladder, breast, colorectal, chronic lymphocytic leukaemia, chronic myeloid leukaemia, glioma, head and neck, Hodgkin's disease, melanoma, multiple myeloma, non-Hodgkin's lymphoma, non-small cell lung, oesophageal, ovarian, prostate, small cell lung, soft tissue sarcoma and uterine cervix). They concluded that reviewers should consider whether to attempt to include updated and centrally collected individual patient data in their systematic review. They argued that an IPD MA requires more time and resources than other techniques for systematic review, but have proved feasible in cancer and should lead to a more reliable assessment of the treatments under investigation.

## A story of how a systematic review with a meta-analysis can change our thinking

The influence of RCTs, systematic reviews and, in particular, IPD MA is exemplified by the story of ovarian ablation for breast cancer (Clarke et al. 1998).[74] One of the earliest randomised trials of a treatment for cancer was undertaken in the 1950s in Manchester (UK). This was a trial of ovarian irradiation for women with breast cancer; 50 years later, it was included in an Early Breast Cancer Trialists' Collaborative Group (EBCTCG) overview. Clarke *et al.* described the continuing journey along a hierarchy of evidence in health care. The first case report of hormone suppression as a treatment for breast cancer was published in 1896. It was soon followed by several case series and non-randomised comparisons and, between 1948 and 1988, more than a dozen randomised trials took place involving 3500 women. However, none of these trials was large enough to show reliably whether women treated with ovarian ablation were more likely to survive longer than those not treated in this way.

A systematic review was required and the first steps towards this were taken with the formation of the EBCTCG in 1983. This brought together trialists from around the world in an attempt to combine individual patient data from trials of tamoxifen and chemotherapy. In 1995, information was sought on each patient in any randomised trial of ovarian ablation or suppression versus control that began before 1990. Data were obtained for 12 of the 13 studies that assessed ovarian ablation by irradiation or surgery, all of which began before 1980, but not for the four studies that assessed ovarian suppression by drugs, all of which began after 1985. Among 2102 women aged less than 50 when randomised, most of whom would have been premenopausal at diagnosis, 1130 deaths and an additional 153 recurrences were reported; 15-year survival was highly significantly improved among those allocated ovarian ablation (52·4 *v* 46·1% [SD 2·3]; log-rank $2P = 0·001$), as was recurrence-free survival (45·0 *v* 39·0%, $2P = 0·0007$). In the trials of ablation plus cytotoxic chemotherapy versus the same chemotherapy alone, the benefit appeared smaller than in the trials in the absence of chemotherapy. Among 1354 women aged 50 or over when randomised, most of whom would have been perimenopausal or postmenopausal, there was no evidence of a significant improvement in survival and recurrence-free survival.

These RCTs and IPD MAs have shown that adjuvant ovarian ablation in women with breast cancer younger than 50 years improves survival and reduces recurrence. It also highlighted the need for new RCTs of ovarian ablation in these women who also receive adjuvant chemotherapy and clearly shows that older women do not benefit from this treatment. Most importantly it shows how RCTs and systematic reviews can be used in a coordinated way to improve care for individual patients and to design a new generation of RCTs to continue the process.

## Finding systematic reviews

Since systematic reviews are a good starting place when reviewing the literature to answer a specific question, it would be useful to develop a strategy for finding relevant reviews. The key to any search is to be sufficiently sensitive that all or nearly all the appropriate papers are found,[75] while at the same time getting sufficient specificity that not too many inappropriate reports are found.

Shojania and Bero[76] have reported such an optimal search strategy for systematic reviews. Their aim was to develop and evaluate a search strategy for identifying systematic reviews by using a publicly available MEDLINE interface (PubMed). They used the technique of testing what proportion of recognised systematic reviews (indexed in the Cochrane Library's Database of Abstracts of Reviews of Effects [DARE] or in the ACP Journal Club) that were identified by the search strategy. Their PubMed search strategy (see paper for detail) identified 93 of 100 DARE-indexed systematic reviews, a sensitivity of 93% (95% CI 86%–97%). For the sample of 103 systematic reviews drawn from ACP Journal Club, the PubMed strategy achieved a sensitivity of 97% (CI 91%–99%). They concluded that their search strategy identified most systematic reviews without overwhelming users with numerous false positive results. A "single-click" filter based on this strategy is now available as part of the Clinical Queries feature of PubMed.

## Conclusions

This chapter has briefly discussed some of the main features to look for when appraising both clinical trials and reviews. Although this book has used evidence-based methods to assess the literature, the quality of the evidence is often less than optimal and readers should always view any evidence with a questioning mind when appraising a trial or a review. Only by questioning can we hope to improve our understanding of how to care for our patients now – and our ability to do better research in the future.

## References

1  Sackett DL, Haynes RB. On the need for evidence-based medicine. *Evidence-based Med* 1995;**1**:5–6.
2  Eddy DM. Anatomy of a decision. *JAMA* 1990;**263**:4413.
3  Mulrow CD. Rationale for systematic reviews. *BMJ* 1994;**309**:597–9.
4  Covell DG, Uman GC, Manning PR. Information needs in office practice: are they being met? *Ann Intern Med* 1985;**103**:596–9.
5  Antman EM, Lau J, Kupelnick B, Mosteller F, Chalmers TC. A comparison of results of meta-analyses of randomized controlled trials and recommendations of clinical experts. Treatments for myocardial infarction. *JAMA* 1992;**268**:240–8.
6  Oxman AD, Guyatt GH. The science of reviewing research. *Ann NY Acad Sci* 1993;**703**:125–33.
7  Oxman AD, Sackett DL, Guyatt GH. Users' guides to the medical literature. I. How to get started. The Evidence-Based Working Group. *JAMA* 1993;**270**:2093–5.
8  Sacks HS, Berrier J, Reitman D, Ancona-Berk VA, Chalmers TC. Meta-analyses of randomized controlled trials. *N Engl J Med* 1987;**316**: 450–5.

9  L'Abbe KA, Detsky AS, O'Rourke K. Meta-analysis in clinical research. *Ann Intern Med* 1987;**107**:224–33.

10  Thacker SB. Meta-analysis: a quantitative approach to research integration. *JAMA* 1988;**259**:1685–9.

11  Mulrow CD. The medical review article: state of the science. *Ann Intern Med* 1987;**106**:485–8.

12  Yusuf S, Simon R, Ellenberg S (eds). Proceedings of "Methodologic issues in overviews of randomized clinical trials". *Stat Med* 1987;**6**:217–409.

13  Oxman AD, Guyatt GH. Guidelines for reading literature reviews. *Can Med Assoc J* 1988;**138**:697–703.

14  Kunz R, Oxman AD. The unpredictability paradox: review of empirical comparisons of randomised and non-randomised clinical trials. *BMJ* 1998;**317**:1185–90.

15  Kleijnen J, Gotzsche P, Kunz RA, Oxman AD, Chalmers I. So what's so special about randomization? In: Chalmers, I, Maynard A, eds. *Non-Random Reflections on Health Services Research*. London: BMJ, 1997.

16  Sacks HS, Chalmers TC, Smith H. Randomised versus historical controls for clinical trials. *Am J Med*, 1982;**72**:233–40.

17  Beral V, Colwell L. Randomised trials of high doses of stilboestrol and ethisterone therapy in pregnancy: long-term follow up of the children. *J Epidemiol Commun Health* 1981;**35**:155–160.

18  Baird DD, Wilcox AJ, Herbst AL. Self reported allergy, infection and autoimmune disease in women exposed in utero to diethylstilboestrol. *J Clin Epidemiol* 1996;**49**:263–6.

19  Meara J, Vessy M, Fairweather DV. A randomised double-blind controlled trial of diethylstilboestrol in pregnancy: 35 year follow-up in mothers and their offspring. *Br J Obstet Gynaecol* 1989;**96**:620–2.

20  Schulz KF, Chalmers I, Hayes RJ, Altman DG. Empirical evidence of bias: dimensions of methodological quality associated with estimates of treatment effects in controlled trials. *JAMA* 1995;**273**:408–12.

21  Non-small Cell Lung Cancer Collaborative Group. Chemotherapy in non-small cell lung cancer: a meta-analysis using updated data on individual patients from 52 randomised trials. *BMJ* 1995;**311**:899–909.

22  Moher D, Schulz KF, Altman DG. The CONSORT statement: revised recommendations for improving the quality of reports of parallel-group randomized trials *Ann Intern Med* 2001;**134**:657–62.

23  Braunholtz DA, Edwards SJ, Lilford RJ. Are randomized clinical trials good for us (in the short term)? Evidence for a "trial effect". *J Clin Epidemiol* 2001;**54**:217–24.

24  Bramwell VHC, Williams CJ. Do authors of review articles use systematic methods to identify, assess and synthesize information? *Ann Oncol* 1997;**8**:1185–96.

25  Dickersin K, Scherer R, Lefebvre C. Identifying relevant studies for systematic reviews. *BMJ* 1994;**309**:1286–91.

26  Scherer RW, Dickersin K, Langenberg P. Full publication of results initially reported in abstracts: a meta-analysis. *JAMA* 1994;**272**:151–62.

27  Stern JM, Simes RJ. Publication bias: evidence of delayed publication in a cohort study of clinical research projects. *BMJ* 1997;**315**:640–5.

28  Simes RJ. Publication bias: the case for an international registry of clinical trials. *J Clin Oncol* 1986;**4**:1529–41.

29  Dickersin K, Chan S, Chalmers TC, Sacks HS, Smith H. Publication bias and clinical trials. *Controlled Clin Trials* 1987;**8**:343–53.

30  Simes RJ. Confronting publication bias: a cohort design for meta-analysis. *Stat Med* 1987;**6**:11–29.

31  Begg CB, Berlin JA. Publication bias: a problem in interpreting medical data. *J Roy Statist Soc A* 1988;**151**:445–63.

32  Hetherington J, Dickersin K, Chalmers I, Meinert CL. Retrospective and prospective identification of unpublished controlled trials: lessons from a survey of obstetricians and pediatricians. *Pediatrics* 1989;**84**:374–80.

33  Easterbrook PJ, Berlin JA, Gopalan R, Matthews DR. Publication bias in clinical research. *Lancet* 1991;**337**:867–72.

34  Dickersin K, Min YI, Meinert CL. Factors influencing publication of research results: follow-up of applications submitted to two institutional review boards. *JAMA* 1992;**263**:374–8.

35  Dickersin K, Min YI. NIH clinical trials and publication bias. *Online J Curr Clin Trials* [serial online] 1993;Doc No.50.

36  Grégoire G, Derderian F, LeLorier J. Selecting the language of the publications included in a meta-analysis: is there a tower of Babel bias? *J Clin Epidemiol* 1995;**48**:159–63.

37  Moher D, Fortin P, Jadad AR *et al.* Completeness of reporting of trials published in languages other than English: implications for conduct and reporting of systematic reviews. *Lancet* 1996;**347**:363–6.

38  Egger M, Zellweger-Zähner T, Schneider M, Junker C, Lengeler C, Antes G. Language bias in randomised controlled trials published in English and German. *Lancet* 1997;**350**:326–9.

39  Gotzsche PC. Reference bias in reports of drug trials. *BMJ* 1987;**295**:654–6.

40  Ravnskov U. Cholesterol lowering trials in coronary heart disease: frequency of citation and outcome. *BMJ* 1992;**305**:15–19.

41  Tramer MR, Reynolds DJ, Moore RA, McQuay HJ. Impact of covert duplicate publication on meta-analysis: a case study. *BMJ* 1997;**315**:635–40.

42  Moher D, Jadad A, Nichol G, Penman M, Tugwell T, Walsh S. Assessing the quality of randomized controlled trials: an annotated bibliography of scales and checklists. *Controlled Clin Trials* 1995;**16**:62–73.

43  Detsky AS, Naylor CD, O'Rourke K, McGreer AJ, L'Abbe KA. Incorporating variations in the quality of individual randomized trials into meta-analysis. *J Clin Epidemiol* 1992;**45**:255–65.

44  Moher D, Jadad AR, Tugwell P. Assessing the quality of randomized controlled trials: current issues and future directions. *Int J Tech Assess Health Care* 1996;**12**:195–208.

45  Feinstein AR. *Clinical Epidemiology: The Architecture of Clinical Research*. Philadelphia: Saunders, 1985.

46  Chalmers TC, Celano P, Sacks HS, Smith H, Jr. Bias in treatment assignment in controlled clinical trials. *N Engl J Med* 1983;**309**:1358–61.

47  Schulz KF, Chalmers I, Grimes DA, Altman DG. Assessing the quality of randomization from reports of controlled trials published in obstetrics and gynecology journals. *JAMA* 1994;**272**:125–8.

48  Moher D, Pham B, Jones A *et al.* Does quality of reports of randomised trials affect estimates of intervention efficacy reported in meta-analyses? *Lancet* 1998;**352**:609–13.

49  Karlowski TR, Chalmers TC, Frenkel LD, Kapikian AZ, Lewis TL, Lynch JM. Ascorbic acid for the common cold: a prophylactic and therapeutic trial. *JAMA* 1975;**231**:1038–42.

50  Colditz GA, Miller JN, Mosteller F. How study design affects outcomes in comparisons of therapy. I: medical. *Stat Med* 1989;**8**:441–54.

51  The Canadian Cooperative Study Group (CCSG). The Canadian trial of aspirin and sulfinpyrazone in threatened stroke. *N Engl J Med* 1978;**299**:53–9.

52  Sackett DL. Bias in analytic research. *J Chronic Dis* 1979;**32**:51–63.

53  Reitman D, Chalmers TC, Nagalingam R, Sacks H. Can efficacy of blinding be documented by meta-analysis? Presented to the Society for Clinical Trials, San Diego, 23–26 May, 1988.

54  Gotzsche PC. Methodology and overt and hidden bias in reports of 196 double-blind trials of nonsteroidal antiinflammatory drugs in rheumatoid arthritis. *Controlled Clin Trials* 1989;**10**:3–56.

55  Jüni P, Witschi A, Bloch R, Egger M. The hazards of scoring the quality of clinical trials for meta-analysis. *JAMA* 1999;**282**:1054–60.

56  Jadad AR, Moore RA, Carroll D *et al.* Assessing the quality of reports of randomized clinical trials: Is blinding necessary? *Controlled Clin Trials* 1996;**17**:1–12.

57  SORT – The Standards of Reporting Trials Group. A proposal for structured reporting of randomized controlled trials. *JAMA* 1994;**272**:1926–31.

58  WGRR – Working Group on Recommendations for Reporting of Clinical Trials in the Biomedical Literature. Call for comments on a proposal to improve reporting of clinical trials in the biomedical literature. *Ann Intern Med* 1994;**121**:894–5.

59  Begg CB, Cho M, Eastwood S *et al.* Improving the quality of reporting of randomized controlled trials. The CONSORT statement. *JAMA* 1996;**276**:637–9.

60  Laird NM, Mosteller F. Some statistical methods for combining experimental results. *Int J Tech Assess Health Care* 1990;**6**:5–30.

61  Egger M, Davey Smith G, Altman DG, eds. *Systematic Reviews in Health Care: Meta-analysis in Context*. London: BMJ Books, 2001.

62  Hill AB. *Principles of Medical Statistics. 9th edn.* London: Lancet, 1971.

63  CTFPHE – Canadian Task Force on the Periodic Health Examination. The periodic health examination. *Can Med Assoc J* 1979;**121**: 1193–254.

64  Cook DJ, Guyatt GH, Laupacis A, Sackett DL. Rules of evidence and clinical recommendations on the use of antithrombotic agents. Antithrombotic Therapy Consensus Conference. *Chest* 1992;**102**: 305S–311S.

65  Gyorkos TW, Tannenbaum TN, Abrahamowicz M *et al.* An approach to the development of practice guidelines for community health interventions. *Can J Public Health* 1994;**85**(Suppl. 1):S8–S13.

66  Guyatt GH, Sackett DL, Sinclair JC, Hayward R, Cook DJ, Cook RJ, for the Evidence-Based Medicine Working Group. *JAMA* 1995;**274**: 1800–4.

67  US Preventive Services Task Force. *Guide to Clinical Preventive Services, 2nd edn.* Baltimore: Williams & Wilkins, 1996.

68  Friedman LM, Furberg CD, DeMets DL. *Fundamentals of Clinical Trials, 2nd edn.* Littleton, MA: John Wright PSG Inc, 1985.

69  Guyatt GH, Sackett DL, Cook DJ, for the Evidence-Based Medicine Working Group. Users' guides to the medical literature, II: how to use an article about therapy or prevention, B: what were the results and will they help me in caring for my patients? *JAMA* 1994;**271**:59–63.

70  Mugford M, Kingston J, Chalmers I. Reducing the incidence of infection after caesarean section: implications of prophylaxis with antibiotics for hospital resources. *BMJ* 1989;**299**:1003–6.

71  Mugford M, Piercy J, Chalmers I. Cost implications of different approaches to the prevention of respiratory distress syndrome. *Arch Dis Child* 1991;**66**:757–64.

72  Schwarzer G, Antes G, Tallon D, Egger M. Review publication bias? Matched comparative study of Cochrane and journal meta-analyses. 9th Annual Cochrane Colloquium Abstracts, October 2001, Lyon.

73  Jüni P, Tallon D, Egger M. "Garbage in – garbage out"? Assessment of the quality of controlled trials in meta-analyses published in leading journals. 3rd Symposium on *Systematic Reviews: Beyond the Basics*, July 2000, Oxford.

74  Clarke M, Stewart L, Pignon JP, Bijnens L. Individual patient data meta-analysis in cancer. *Br J Cancer* 1998;**77**:2036–44.

75  Hunt DL, Haynes RB, Browman GP. Search the medical literature for the best evidence to solve clinical questions. *Ann Oncol* 1998;**9**:377–83.

75  Parmar MKB, Stewart LA, Altman DG. Meta-analysis of randomised trials: when the whole is more than just the sum of the parts. *Br J Cancer* 1996;**74**:496–501.

76  Shojania KG, Bero LA. Taking advantage of the explosion of systematic reviews: an efficient MEDLINE search strategy. *Effect Clin Pract* 2001;**4**:157–62.

## Further reading

Bero L, Grilli R, Grimshaw J, Mowatt G, Oxman A, Zwarenstein M, eds. Effective Practice and Organisation of Care Module. In: The Cochrane Library, Issue 2, 1999. Oxford: Update Software.

Horton R, Smith R. Time to register randomised trials. *BMJ* 1999;**319**: 864–5.

Straus SE, Sackett DL. Review on evidence-based cancer medicine. Applying evidence to the individual patient. *Ann Onco* 1999;**10**: 29–32.

Stewart LA, Parmar MKB. Meta-analysis of the literature or individual patient data: is there a difference? *Lancet* 1993;**341**:418–22.

# 2 Finding the "best evidence" for cancer care

*Kate Misso, Julie Glanville*

This chapter describes how to define a search question, how to construct a search and the key resources for identifying best evidence for cancer care.

Finding the best evidence for cancer care usually involves searching databases in which research evidence is recorded. These databases tend to be very large because of the volume of research being published. MEDLINE, the best-known and most widely used biomedical database, contains over 11 million records. Even more focused collections of research, such as the *Cochrane Library*, contain hundreds of thousands of records. It can be time consuming and frustrating to search databases if searches produce hundreds of results, many of which may not be deemed relevant by the searcher. It can also be difficult to focus on the best quality research information when large databases are being searched. These frustrations can be reduced by a structured approach to search strategy design, by searching the most appropriate resources and by seeking assistance from information professionals, such as librarians, who are skilled in searching.

## Defining a clear search question

The search process involves:

1. defining the question – what is the object of the search?
2. building the strategy – translate the clinical question into a searchable strategy
3. identifying appropriate resources to search
4. searching.

The first step in planning a literature search is to define a question. A focused question should be structured and should clearly capture the problem to be resolved. Clinical questions can be constructed using an approach known as PIOC or PICO.[1,2] This approach breaks a question into four "facets" or aspects: population, intervention, comparison, and outcome. Alternatively, asking questions such as "Who?", "What?", "What else?" and "What happens?" (Box 2.1) can clarify the question being asked. Clear questions are essential to structuring an effective search.

---

**Box 2.1 Components of a clinical question**

**Population**

- Disease, condition, sex, age, race?
- Who is the question about?

**Intervention**

- Treatment, exposure, risk factors or specific cause.
- What is happening to/being done to "P"?

**Comparison**

- Alternatives? Another treatment or placebo?
- What could be done instead of "I"?

**Outcome**

- What outcomes are of interest?
- How is effectiveness defined?
- Mortality, morbidity, adverse effects, cost-effectiveness, quality of life?
- What happens to "P" as a result of "I"?

---

Although the PIOC framework is a helpful guide to question definition and strategy development, not all the PIOC components are always required for every search: appropriate selection is another key to effective search construction.

Structuring searches based on PIOC can maximise the relevance of the records retrieved. If required, additional "facets" can be added to focus further. For example, animal studies or specific publication types can be included or excluded as desired, and date limits can be applied.

The examples in Box 2.2 show how the PIOC principle can be applied to real research questions examined as part of the NHS Cancer Guidance Projects for Breast Cancer and Haematological Malignancies.

Other questions can be answered by adapting this approach appropriately. For example, if the search is very focused, say for a named new drug or a specific intervention, a comparison or outcome facet may not be needed.

---

**Box 2.2 How to develop a search strategy using the PIOC framework**

**Question 1**

- Is there evidence that better detection of bone lesions by MRI improves patient outcomes (for example fracture morbidity) for patients with myeloma?

Break the question down into "facets":

| | |
|---|---|
| *Population* | People with myeloma |
| *Intervention* | MRI |
| *Condition* | Bone lesions |
| *Outcome* | Fracture morbidity |

**Question 2**

- How effective are different treatment options for the management of lymphoedema in breast cancer?

Break the question down into "facets":

| | |
|---|---|
| *Population* | People with breast cancer + lymphoedema |
| *Intervention* | Compression bandages/sleeves |
| *Comparison* | Liposuction |

---

## Term generation

It is important to think about the different terminology used to describe each concept of interest. This is helpful both when asking an intermediary, such as a librarian, to carry out a search, and when conducting searches personally. Synonyms and related terms are important because researchers rarely describe conditions, treatments, and outcomes in the same words. Searches have to try to capture those variations in description. For example, cancers may also be referred to as neoplasms, tumours or malignancies and, if only one of these words is used in a search, there is a risk of missing other relevant research.

Lists of relevant terms can be developed using the following approaches.

- Consider how another clinician or health professional might describe the topic in question.
- Are there commonly used abbreviations or acronyms?
- Are there variations in US and UK terminology and spelling?
- Use dictionaries and thesauri to identify synonyms.
- Check terms in the titles and abstracts of relevant references already identified.
- Use specific cancer resources to generate synonyms: CancerBACUP, NCI PDQ patient information web pages, and ICD-10 codes for additional terms.[3–5]
- Use the National Cancer Institute Types of Cancer service.[6]

---

**Box 2.3 Identifying synonyms and related terms**

**Question 1**

- Is there evidence that better detection of bone lesions by MRI improves patient outcomes (for example, fracture morbidity) for patients with myeloma?

For the Intervention facet, the following terms may be used to describe MRI:

| *Text terms* | MEDLINE Subject Headings |
|---|---|
| *MRI* | Magnetic-Resonance-Imaging |
| *Contrast enhanced* | Nuclear-Magnetic- |
| *magnetic resonance* | Resonance |
| *Dynamic magnetic* | |
| *resonance* | |
| *Roentgenography* | |
| *Skeletal survey* | |

**Question 2**

- How effective are different treatment options for the management of lymphoedema in breast cancer?

For the Population facet, the following terms may be used to describe breast cancer:

| *Text terms* | MEDLINE Subject Headings |
|---|---|
| *Breast cancer* | Breast-Neoplasms |
| *Breast tumor* | Mammary-Neoplasms |
| *Breast tumour* | |
| *Breast carcinoma* | |
| *Breast neoplasm* | |
| *Breast malignancy* | |
| *Lymphoedema* | Lymphedema |
| *Lymphedema* | |

---

Examples of synonyms and related terms are given in Box 2.3.

As well as using related terms and synonyms many databases offer options to speed up searching and to cope with spelling variations. Wildcard symbols (such as ?) allow the searcher to find variations of the same word. For example, "organi?ation" will find "organisation" and "organization". When searching international databases such as MEDLINE, wildcards allow for UK/US variations in spelling such as "leuk?emia", "p?ediatric", "h?emorrhage", and "tumo?r".

Databases may also offer truncation options. The symbol differs with each database (it may be $, * or ?) and in some cases truncation may be applied automatically. Truncation allows the searcher to find variations of the same word. For example, "child$" will find references containing child, children, and children's. It is important to be aware of the possible word variations that truncation might retrieve. When searching for "study" or "studies" it is tempting to use truncation. However, "stud$" will retrieve not only study and studies, but also student, studio, studious, and studfarm.

Anticipating variations in terminology will minimise the chances of missing relevant research. For example, when searching for tumours of the breast, it is usually best to include both variants of the word: "tumor" and "tumour". Omission of the alternative spelling could bias the results of the search.

The more terms used in the search the more results will be identified. However, for some searches, extensive synonym identification may not be required. A quick scoping search, for example, will be served by a less exhaustive search strategy than searches for research evidence to inform systematic reviews.

In addition to thinking of synonyms, consideration should also be given to using any thesaurus terms offered by the databases. A thesaurus is a controlled vocabulary that is used to index each record on a database. A thesaurus tries to control for variations in description by giving all records about the same topic the same index term. In MEDLINE for example all research about breast cancer should receive the Medical Subject Heading (MeSH) BREAST NEOPLASMS (see Box 2.2). MeSH is probably the best known medical thesaurus and is used not only in MEDLINE, but also in CANCERLIT, DARE, and other databases. MeSH compensates for variability in the terminology used by authors.

Although MeSH contains subject terms for particular cancers, it is not possible to specify cancer staging. So when searching for cancer stages it is advisable to include text words (from the title and abstract) in combination with MeSH terms. The following example is for the OVID interface:

Breast neoplasms/and (primary or local or advanced). ti,ab.

Other databases use their own thesauri: EMBASE, for example, is indexed using the EMTREE thesaurus. Because different thesauri may use different controlled vocabulary for the same concepts, when you are transferring a MEDLINE strategy to another database the MeSH has to be "translated" to the correct terminology for that database. For example:

MEDLINE uses Urologic-Neoplasms
EMBASE uses Urinary-Tract-Cancer

## Constructing the search

Once the search facets, search terms, and synonyms have been identified, the search can be constructed. The usual approach is to link similar terms within facets together with

---

**Box 2.4 Converting a search topic into a strategy**

**The question**

● What are the optimum surgical margins to avoid recurrence of cancer?

Break the question down into "facets"

*Population*     Any invasive/*in situ* cancer
*Intervention*    Surgical margins
*Comparison*    Complete excision
*Outcome*     Recurrence/relapse

Identify variations in terminology and synonyms for each facet, for example the following alternatives may be useful when searching for the Intervention facet: surgical margin, surgical cavity, excision margin, tumour margin, tumour perimeter, margin status, histological margin, negative margin, positive margin, optimum margin

● Sample search (SilverPlatter interface to MEDLINE)

explode "Neoplasms"/all subheadings
(cancer* or neoplas* or malignan* or tumor* or tumour* or carcinoma* or adenocarcinoma*) in ti,ab,mesh
(dcis or cis) in ti,ab
carcinoma* insitu
carcinoma* in-situ
"carcinomas in situ" or "carcinoma in situ"
#1 or #2 or #3 or #4 or #5 or #6
surgical margin*
surgical cavity or surgical cavities or excision cavity or excision cavities
tumo?r* margin* or excision margin*
tumo?r* perimeter*
margin* status
histolog* margin*
negative* margin*
positive* margin*
margin* size*
margin* width*
margin* depth
margin* circumference*
(optimum* margin*) or (optimal* margin*)
(optimum* excis*) or (optimal* excis*)
(optimum* resect*) or (optimal* resect*)
patholog* near2 margin*
#8 or #9 or #10 or #11 or #12 or #13 or #14 or #15 or #16 or #17 or #18 or #19 or #20 or #21 or #22 or #23
((complete or success* or total*) near2 (excis* or resect* or remov*)) or (residual tumo?r*)
(incomplete or unsuccess* or partial*) near2 (excis* or resect* or remov*)
#25 or #26
"Recurrence"/ all subheadings
"Neoplasm-Recurrence-Local"/ all subheadings
recur* or relaps*
#28 or #29 or #30
#7 and #24 and #27 and #31

*(Continued)*

---

**Box 2.4** *(Continued)*

**Note**

- Set 7 has all the records that capture the concept of "cancer".
- Set 24 has records that capture concepts around surgical margins. This concept might be described in many ways.
- Set 27 captures the comparison concept of "complete or incomplete excision".
- Set 31 captures the concept of "recurrence".
- These result sets are then combined using the AND operator to focus on just those records that contain *all* four concepts.

---

**Box 2.5 Searching summary**

**Prepare the search**

1  Break the search into facets or concepts (for example population, intervention, condition).
2  Identify search terms and synonyms for each concept.
3  Link similar terms within concepts using OR.
4  Combine different concepts using AND.
5  Consider using relevant limits for example publication date or language.
6  Select relevant databases or resources for example Cochrane Library, DARE.

---

a logical operator called OR. Facets are then combined using the AND operator, which is the option that focuses the search. OR makes searches broader, AND produces focus. Box 2.4 gives an example of search construction.

Box 2.5 summarises the most important points when searching.

## Hierarchy of evidence

Once the search topic is clearly conceptualised, the search for reliable evidence can begin. The searcher should consider the research methodology most likely to answer the question. Underpinning evidence-based health care is the concept of different types of research providing different levels or hierarchies of evidence (Box 2.6).

When searching for information on the effectiveness of interventions, the best approach is to concentrate on the top of the hierarchy of evidence and to identify systematic reviews (Box 2.7). If no relevant systematic reviews are identified, then the search could progress to well-conducted randomised controlled trials.

---

**Box 2.6 Levels of evidence (based on Bandolier, 1994 and CEBM hierarchy, 1998)[7,8]**

- At least one well-conducted systematic review
- At least one well-designed randomised controlled trial of appropriate size
- Well-designed non-randomised trials
- Well-designed non-experimental studies from more than one source
- Opinions of respected authorities

Further reading on levels of evidence:

- National Cancer Institute. *Levels of evidence for cancer treatment studies: definition and use*[9]
- New York Online Access to Health. *Ask NOAH about: Evidence Based Medicine*[10]
- WISDOM. *Evidence-Based Practice Resources*[11]

---

**Box 2.7 Systematic reviews and randomised controlled trials**

**Systematic reviews (SRs)**

A systematic review seeks to identify and synthesise as much relevant research as possible on a given topic, including unpublished material and research in languages other than English. A systematic review should include an extensive literature search and describe clearly how studies were chosen and how data were extracted from studies and synthesised. Systematic reviews offer a scientific rather than a subjective summary of the great volume of biomedical research.

Suggestions for further reading:

- CRD guidelines (2001),[12] Chalmers and Altman (1995),[13] Egger *et al.* (2001)[14]

**Randomised controlled trials (RCTs)**

A randomised controlled trial is a planned study in which one intervention, such as a drug, is compared to another intervention. For example, Drug A might be compared to Drug B, or a placebo. The allocation between Drugs A and B must be effectively randomised to reduce the opportunity for assignment to be influenced by researchers or patients.

Suggestions for further reading:

- Duley and Farrell (2002),[15] Jadad (1998),[16] Matthews (2000)[17]

---

## Finding systematic reviews and evidence-based summaries and guidance

### Systematic reviews (SRs)

The best single source of well-conducted systematic reviews is the *Cochrane Library*.[18] The *Cochrane Library* contains the Cochrane Database of Systematic Reviews (CDSR), which is a collection of completed and ongoing systematic reviews compiled by researchers in the Cochrane Collaboration according to clear methodological guidelines. The *Cochrane Library* can be accessed in many ways (see Box 2.8) and for several countries, including the UK and Northern Ireland, is free to all healthcare professionals. An important aspect of Cochrane reviews is that they are continuously updated as new relevant research is identified.

The *Cochrane Library* also contains the Database of Abstracts of Reviews of Effects (DARE). This database is produced by the NHS Centre for Reviews and Dissemination and offers critical appraisals of published systematic reviews. It is the end product of a huge identification and quality sifting process and is intended to save healthcare professionals time and effort. The Health Technology Assessment (HTA) database, also on the *Cochrane Library*, is a collection of completed and ongoing technology assessments being undertaken by major research teams around the world. Many of these projects involve systematic reviews.

When searching the *Cochrane Library*, it is best to search using words in the title and abstract as well as Medical Subject Headings (see above) because not all records in the databases have MeSH.

As well as Cochrane reviews and reviews recorded on DARE, the output of the UK NHS R&D programme including NICE (National Institute for Clinical Excellence) appraisals should also be searched as sources of high level evidence (Box 2.9). US reviews can be identified from HSTAT (see Box 2.8). Collections of evidence-based guidance are available, including the NHS Cancer Guidance publications and the US National Guideline Clearing House collection (Box 2.9). Many of the search options for these resources are simple, which means that complicated searches such as the one described in Box 2.3 may not be possible. Some resources also lack thesauri. This means that the most practical way to search databases with simple search interfaces may be to focus on one facet of the PIOC model, for example the Intervention, and search using a range of synonyms for that facet.

Searching resources individually is the most comprehensive way to ensure that relevant effectiveness publications are not missed. However, if time is pressing, these resources can be searched via the TRIP index (http://www.tripdatabase.com/). A search of TRIP may suffer from small publication lags (the lag caused by the time taken for TRIP to add new records to its database) and differences in the amount of information being searched. However, it is a very useful index for the busy health professional once these issues are appreciated.

## Finding trials

If searches of systematic review collections do not provide answers to an effectiveness question, it may be necessary

---

### Box 2.8 Accessing systematic reviews and summaries of research evidence

The *Cochrane Library*, containing CDSR, DARE and the HTA database, is available via:

- National electronic Library for Health (NeLH). Free of charge to NHS staff: http://www.nelh.nhs.uk/cochrane.asp
- subscription (CD Rom/internet access): http://www.update-software.com/cochrane/
- TRIP (Turning Research into Practice) : http://www.tripdatabase.com/
- OVID Evidence-Based Medline Reviews: http://www.ovid.com/products/clinical/ebmr.cfm
- The *Cochrane Cancer Library* provides access to the subset of cancer Cochrane reviews, plus additional research around cancer care: http://www.update-software.com/cancer/

**DARE** and the HTA database are also available from a free website:

http://nhscrd.york.ac.uk/welcome.htm

**UK R&D Health Technology Assessment** programme publications and ongoing projects:

http://www.hta.nhsweb.nhs.uk/

**Health Services Technology/Assessment Text (HSTAT)**, a US collection of full-text clinical practice guidelines and technology assessments:

http://hstat.nlm.nih.gov/

---

to search larger databases to locate reports of trials (see Box 2.10). The best starting point for randomised controlled trials and controlled trials is the Cochrane Central Register of Controlled Trials (CCTR).[19] CCTR is part of the *Cochrane Library* and is the single best source for finding controlled trials in health care, with 336 092 records at January 2002 (*Cochrane Library*, Issue 1:2002). It is best to search the database using both text words (in the title and abstract) and MeSH and EMTREE terms. This is because CCTR contains records culled from MEDLINE, EMBASE, and hand searches of thousands of journals, and is not indexed by any single thesaurus.

For a searcher focusing on trials, CCTR saves time and effort searching and sifting several large databases. It also contains records of research that would never be found on other databases. However, there is a gap between the time a record is published on MEDLINE, for example, and the time it reaches CCTR. So to be comprehensive, a search of CCTR should be followed by a search of the last two years of CancerLit, MEDLINE, and EMBASE to identify very recent records of trials. Using a methodological search filter

---

**Box 2.9 Evidence-based guidance**

**NHS Cancer Guidance publications**

● Guidance on commissioning cancer services. Completed publications *(Improving Outcomes in Colorectal Cancer, Gynaecological Cancers, Lung Cancer and Upper Gastro-intestinal Cancers)* available at: http://www.doh.gov.uk/cancer/

Work is currently ongoing in the areas of:

● update of the previous breast cancer guidance
● update of the previous colorectal cancer guidance
● haematological malignancies
● urological cancers
● head and neck cancers.

**US National Guideline Clearinghouse**

● Collection and index to US guidelines with links to full text of guidelines where available: http://www.guideline.gov/index.asp

**National Institute for Clinical Excellence (NICE)**

● Publications and ongoing projects: recent topics have included: capecitabine, trastuzumab and vinorelbine for breast cancer, capecitabine, tegafur uracil, irinotecan, oxaliplatin and raltitrexed for colorectal cancer, and rituximab for lymphoma: http://www.nice.org.uk

---

**Box 2.10 Finding trials**

**Cochrane Controlled Trials Register[19]**

● Part of the *Cochrane Library* (see Box 2.8).

**CancerLit**

● Available online, and in CD Rom and internet formats, with free access provided from the National Cancer Institute website: http://www.cancer.gov/search/cancer_literature/

**MEDLINE**

● The OMNI website (Organising Medical Networked Information)[20] lists free MEDLINE options: http://omni.ac.uk/medline/
● The National Library of Medicine's own free route to MEDLINE is PubMed: http://www.ncbi.nlm.nih.gov/entrez/query.fcgi

**EMBASE**

● EMBASE is a database of over 8 million records of the international literature on biomedicine, specialising in drug-related information and pharmaceuticals. It has a strong European focus and is available on subscription: http://www.elsevier.nl/homepage/sah/spd/site/locate_embase.html

**Registers of trials giving access to completed and ongoing clinical trials**

● National Research Register (NRR), for the UK: http://www.update-software.com/National/
● ClinicalTrials.gov for the USA: http://www.clinicaltrials.gov/
● Controlled-trials.com has a database of trials and links to many other registers: http://www.controlled-trials.com/

---

with MEDLINE or EMBASE will reduce the number of irrelevant records. Search filters are described in more detail below.

CancerLit contains a subset of MEDLINE, but it also has unique information, including records of conference proceedings such as the ASCO series. Searching CancerLit rather than MEDLINE may be a useful way of incorporating focus into a search. All CancerLit records are indexed using the MeSH thesaurus.

## Search filters

A search filter is a collection of search terms designed to capture a study design or study focus such as diagnosis. Details of some typical filters are given in Box 2.11. When searching for trials or reviews in large databases such as CancerLit or MEDLINE, the search filter can be added to the search and acts like an additional facet in the PIOC structure. Limiting a search by methodology using a filter can help to focus the search. Search filter design is rapidly evolving and filters should be subjected to the same critical appraisal as other research tools.[21–24]

Methodological filters are sometimes referred to as "quality filters". This is misleading because filters just retrieve records by methodology or topic and do not guarantee the quality of the records retrieved. To determine the methodological quality of studies, a critical appraisal of the research should also be undertaken. There are many guides to critical appraisal (Box 2.12).

Many questions will go beyond issues of effectiveness and other databases may be useful sources of evidence. There are many specialist databases covering particular aspects of care or with a focus on types of research (Box 2.13). Some databases offer sophisticated searching options and others offer more basic search facilities that may force a selective use of the PIOC elements.

**Box 2.11 Methodological search filters**

Further information and examples of search filters designed to find study designs can be found in Phase 3 – Identification of research in Stage II: Conducting the review, which is published in *Undertaking systematic reviews of research on effectiveness:*[12] http://www. york.ac.uk/inst/crd/report4.htm

**CASPfew filters**

http://www.phru.org.UK/~casp/caspfew/filters/index.htm

**NHS Centre for Reviews and Dissemination**

Search strategies to identify reviews and meta-analyses in MEDLINE and CINAHL: http://www.york.ac.uk/inst/crd/search.htm

**Centre for Evidence-Based Medicine, Oxford**

Introduction to filters and when to use them: http://minerva.minervation.com/cebm/

**PubMed**

This free MEDLINE interface now has a "Clinical Queries" option to focus a search by limiting to therapy, diagnosis, aetiology, or prognosis. http://www.ncbi.nlm.nih.gov/entrez/query/static/clinical.html

**Box 2.12 Selected critical appraisal resources**

- CASP (Critical Appraisal Skills Programme): http://www.phru.org.uk/~casp/resources/index.htm
- Crombie IK. *Pocket guide to critical appraisal: a handbook for healthcare professionals.* London: BMJ Publishing Group, 1996.
- Greenhalgh T. *How to read a paper: the basics of evidence-based medicine.* London: BMJ Publishing Group, 1997.
- Guyatt G, Rennie D eds. *Users guide to the medical literature: essentials of evidence-based clinical practice.* Chicago: AMA Press, 2001.
- JAMA series: *Users' Guides to the Medical Literature:* http://www.shef.ac.uk/~scharr/ir/userg.html

**Box 2.13 Looking beyond therapy questions**

- AMED (Allied and Alternative Medicine): http://www.bl.uk/services/information/amed.html
- British Nursing Index (BNI): http://www.silverplatter.com/catalog/brni.htm
- CancerBACUP: http://www.cancerbacup.org.uk/
- CINAHL (Cumulative Index of Nursing and Allied Health Literature): http://www.cinahl.com/
- Cochrane Cancer Network: http://www.canet.org/
- Department of Health cancer pages (includes NHS Cancer Guidance publications): http://www.doh.gov.uk/cancer/
- Health Evidence Bulletins Wales: http://hebw.uwcm.ac.uk/
- Health Development Agency Evidence Base: http://194.83.94.80/hda/docs/evidence/eb2000/corehtml/intro.htm
- Health Management Information Consortium (HMIC): http://www.silverplatter.com/catalog/hmic.htm
- HealthPromis: http://healthpromis.hda-online.org.uk/
- LILACS (Latin American and Caribbean Health Sciences Literature): http://www.bireme.br/iah2/homepagei.htm
- OMNI (Organising Medical Networked Information): http://omni.ac.uk/
- PsycINFO: http://www.apa.org/psycinfo/
- National Cancer Institute (NCI): http://www.cancer.gov/cancer_information/
- National electronic Library for Cancers (NeLC): http://www.nelc.org.uk/
- NHS Centre for Reviews and Dissemination Effective Health Care bulletins on cancer topics (summarising the NHS Cancer Guidance series): http://www.york.ac.uk/inst/crd/ehcb.htm
- ASCO's Conference Proceedings: http://www.asco.org/ac/1,1003,_12-002095,00.asp/

Allied and Alternative Medicine (AMED) records research on alternative and complementary medicine and aspects of palliative care. Nursing questions merit searches of nursing-specific databases such as CINAHL and the British Nursing Index (BNI) as well as MEDLINE and EMBASE. Information on cancer prevention can be found in Health Evidence Bulletins Wales, the Health Development Agency Database, and HealthPromis, along with EMBASE, MEDLINE, and PsycINFO. PsycINFO is the major database recording psychological publications.

OMNI (Organising Medical Networked Information) is a database of evaluated internet resources in health and medicine. All those resources have been appraised against structured evaluation guidelines.

To identify non-English language research may require wider searching in resources such as LILACS. LILACS is a free biomedical database of Latin American and Caribbean health sciences literature.

Information specifically aimed at people with cancer can be found via cancer support groups such as CancerBACUP and research funders such as the National Cancer Institute. Research around service delivery and service organisation is particularly difficult to capture in searches because of the widely different ways service delivery is described and the generally weak indexing of service delivery concepts. Key resources for information on service delivery are the UK Cancer Guidance documents (see Box 2.13), Effective Health Care bulletins, and the HMIC database, as well as MEDLINE and EMBASE.

## Looking for current research

Most of the databases described above focus on published research. However, research can take time to reach publication and some research may never be formally published. Conference proceedings can offer intelligence on current and recent research. Many conferences now put their abstracts and proceedings on the internet, and key among these is the American Society of Clinical Oncology (ASCO). The proceedings are on the internet (see Box 2.13) and until recently have been recorded on CancerLit.

Ongoing projects and trials can be identified from the growing range of trials registers described in Box 2.10.

## Summary

When searching for research evidence, taking time to plan the search will produce more effective searches. Defining the question, planning the strategy, and identifying the most appropriate resources to search will help to focus on the most relevant research. Identifying tools, such as search filters, that can focus searches may save time and effort. Searchers should consider the type of evidence required to answer the question and the amount of time and resources available to carry out the search. Information professionals such as librarians are skilled in searching and can advise on strategies and resources.

## References

1 Counsell C. Formulating the questions and locating the studies for inclusion in systematic reviews. In: Mulrow C, Cook D eds. *Systematic reviews. Synthesis of best evidence for health care decisions.* Philadelphia: American College of Physicians, 1998.
2 Golder S, Ritchie G. Focusing the question: presentation at the BMA Finding the Evidence Course October 22, 2002 [online], 2002. Available from: http://www.bma.org.uk/ap.nsf/Content/LIBFinding the Evidence Courses
3 CancerBACUP (2002) CancerBACUP website [online]. Available from: http://www.cancerbacup.org.uk/
4 National Cancer Institute. *Cancer information* [online]. Available from: http://www.cancer.gov/cancer_information/
5 World Health Organization. *ICD-10. International statistical classification of diseases and related health problems.* 10th revision. 2 volumes. Geneva: World Health Organization; 1992.
6 National Cancer Institute. *Types of cancer* [online]. Available from: http://www.cancer.gov/cancer_information/cancer_type/
7 Bandolier. *Assessment Criteria: Type & Strength of Evidence* [online]. Bandolier 1994 6–5. Available from: http://www.jr2.ox.ac.uk/bandolier/band6/b6-5.html
8 Centre for Evidence-Based Medicine. *Levels of evidence and grades of recommendations* [online]. Oxford: Centre for Evidence-Based Medicine, 1998. Available from: http://minerva.minervation.com/cebm/
9 National Cancer Institute. *Levels of Evidence for Cancer Treatment Studies: Definition and Use (PDQ®)* [online]. National Cancer Institute, 2001. Available from: http://www.cancer.gov/cancer_information/doc.aspx?viewid=2B9AC8C6-7202-4728-9DD0-77CA57170044
10 New York Online Access to Health. *Ask NOAH About: Evidence Based Medicine* [online]. New York: NOAH; 2001. Available from: http://www.noah-health.org/english/ebhc/ebhc.html
11 WISDOM. Wisdom Resource Database [online]. Sheffield: WISDOM Centre. Available from: http://www.wisdomnet.co.uk/seminar.asp#EBP
12 NHS Centre for Reviews and Dissemination. *Undertaking Systematic Reviews of Research on Effectiveness: CRD's Guidance for Carrying Out or Commissioning Reviews* [online]. CRD Report 4 2nd edn. York: NHS CRD, 2001. Available from: http://www.york.ac.uk/inst/crd/report4.htm
13 Chalmers I, Altman DG, eds. *Systematic reviews.* London: BMJ Publishing Group, 1995.
14 Egger M, Davey Smith G, Altman DG eds. *Systematic reviews in health care: meta analysis in context.* London: BMJ Publishing, 2001.
15 Duley L, Farrell B eds. *Clinical trials.* London: BMJ Books, 2002.
16 Jadad A. *Randomised controlled trials: a user's guide.* London: BMJ Books, 1998.
17 Matthews JNS. *An introduction to randomized controlled clinical trials.* London: Arnold, 2000.
18 The *Cochrane Library.* Oxford: Update Software;, 2002.
19 Cochrane Controlled Clinical Trials Register (CCTR). In: *Cochrane Library.* Oxford: Update Software, 2002.
20 Organising Medical Networked Information (OMNI). *Internet Medline service web page* [online]. Nottingham: OMNI, 2001. Available from: http://omni.ac.uk/medline/
21 Haynes RB, Wilczynski N, McKibbon KA, Walker CJ, Sinclair JC. Developing optimal search strategies for detecting clinically sound studies in MEDLINE. *J Am Med Informatics Ass* 1994;1:447–58.
22 McKibbon A. *Evidence-based principles and practice.* London: BC Decker Inc, 1999.
23 Boynton J, Glanville J, McDaid D, Lefebvre C. Identifying systematic reviews in Medline: developing an objective approach to search strategy design. *J Inform Sci* 1998;24:137–57.
24 White VJ, Glanville JM, Lefebvre C, Sheldon TA. A statistical approach to designing search filters to find systematic reviews: objectivity enhances accuracy. *J Inform Sci* 2001;27:357–70.

# 3 Understanding the concepts behind health economics

*Katharine Johnston*

Economics is the study of how individuals and societies choose to allocate resources (such as labour and capital) between alternative uses. The decision to devote scarce resources to one activity has an opportunity cost associated with it, that is, benefits are forgone by not allowing resources to be employed in alternative and competing uses. Economists use the concept of efficiency as the primary criterion for determining how to maximise total benefit from scarce resources. Efficiency is not about cost cutting, but about making choices that derive the maximum total benefit from finite resources available.

All healthcare systems have a limited budget and hence choices have to be made about the allocation of healthcare resources. No healthcare system can provide all the technically feasible, or even all potentially beneficial, treatments. As the gap between what is technically feasible and what is economically feasible widens, the demand for evidence on how to allocate healthcare resources increases. New drugs and treatments regularly emerge, increasing the number of alternative treatments. Yet even if the evidence base suggests the new drug or treatment to be more effective than the alternative, economic evidence is required in order to judge whether it might represent an efficient and equitable use of resources.

Health economics is a subdiscipline of economics with foundations in microeconomics. Current research in health economics addresses a wide range of issues including financing of health care as well as the demand for and supply of health care. One area of health economics research that has increased in recent years is economic evaluation in health care. A number of economic evaluation techniques have been developed to help identify the most efficient allocation of resources. This chapter focuses on this economic evaluation in health care rather than health economics in general because this area of health economics has particular relevance to oncology.

## Key concepts in health economics

### Opportunity cost

Healthcare resources are scarce and choices have to be exercised about which healthcare treatments to adopt as well as which ones not to adopt. If resources are used in this way, there is an opportunity forgone of using the resources in some other way to obtain benefits.[1] The opportunities forgone represent the opportunity cost. Opportunity cost ensures that the implications of alternative uses of resources are considered. The concept also encourages consideration of costs with no monetary value. For example, the time of an unpaid carer may not have a market price but there is an opportunity cost of the carer's time since the carer's time has alternative uses. The concept of opportunity cost lies at the heart of health economics.

### Efficiency

Economists use the concept of efficiency as the primary criterion for determining how to maximise total benefit from scarce resources. There are two types of efficiency: technical and allocative. For technical efficiency to be attained there are two requirements. The first is that for any given amount of output, the amount of inputs (such as labour and capital) used to produce it should be minimised.[2] If this condition were not met it would be possible either to release some of the resources to alternative uses without sacrificing any current output or it would be possible to obtain more output from a different configuration of resources. The second requirement for technical efficiency is that inputs be combined so as to minimise the cost of any given output. This second requirement takes into account the relative cost of different inputs.

In addition to the requirements for technical efficiency, allocative efficiency requires that resources be used to produce the types and amounts of outputs that best satisfy people's wants, that is, the outputs which people value most highly. By necessity, statements about allocative efficiency involve value judgements about the criteria to be used to judge whether a particular resource allocation best satisfies people's wants. The standard criterion used states that allocative efficiency is attained when it is not possible to reallocate resources to make any one person better off without making at least one other person worse off.[3]

## Equity

In addition to efficiency, the concept of equity also determines how healthcare resources should be allocated. Broadly speaking, equity represents a concern that healthcare resources and benefits should be distributed in some fair or just way. It is recognised, however, that there is a trade-off between equity and efficiency and that this trade-off is inevitable precisely because resources are scarce.[4] If an efficient allocation of healthcare resources were to be redistributed according to some equity criteria, then some groups in society would lose healthcare resources whilst others would gain. The fact that it may be possible for some groups to lose means that equity objectives should be made as explicit as possible. Although in principle, equity considerations can be taken into account in considering the allocation of healthcare resources, in practice, most studies focus on efficiency.[5]

## Discounting

As an economy it is possible to defer consumption and undertake investment so that a higher level of future consumption can be enjoyed. Thus the opportunity cost of current consumption is some higher level of future consumption. Discounting is a formal recognition of this opportunity cost.[6]

Different types of healthcare treatment will incur costs and accrue outcomes in differing time periods. For example, a cancer-screening programme involves high set-up costs in the short term but the benefits accrue in the long term. In order to compare the costs and outcomes of different healthcare treatments, their costs and outcomes must be related to the same point in time. Hence future costs and outcomes are discounted to their present value. Discounting is based on the premise that, generally, individuals prefer to receive a benefit today rather than in the future and to incur a cost later rather than sooner. The concept of discounting is important, since discounting practice plays a central role in determining the relative value for money of healthcare treatments.[7]

## Introduction to economic evaluation in health care

### Overview

Opportunity cost, efficiency, equity, and discounting are key concepts that underlie economic evaluation. Economic evaluation is concerned with evaluating alternative uses of resources in terms of both their costs and outcomes. An important point to highlight about economic evaluation is that it is comparative, that is, it always compares at least two alternatives. In oncology, for example, this would involve comparing an existing drug treatment with a new drug treatment and then estimating and comparing the costs and outcomes associated with each.

The precise methods used to identify, measure and value costs and outcomes will depend on the context and the particular economic question being posed. A number of general principles exist that govern the way costs and outcomes are measured and valued and these are set out in detail in a number of texts.[8,9] There are a number of types of economic evaluation and the following sections highlight these as well as some of key issues in the measurement and valuation of costs and outcomes.

### Types of economic evaluation

There are a number of different types of economic evaluation[8,9] and they differ according to the way the outcomes are measured. The three most commonly used are summarised in Table 3.1 and are now discussed.

The first is cost-effectiveness analysis (CEA) where costs of alternative treatments are compared to a summary measure of the outcomes, or effect, of the alternative treatment. Outcomes may be measured in terms of natural units such as cancers detected or life-years. The incremental costs and effects of a treatment are then presented in terms of an incremental cost-effectiveness ratio, such as the incremental cost per additional case detected or incremental cost per life year gained. CEA addresses technical efficiency, for example, which drug is the more efficient for treating advanced breast cancer.

Table 3.1 Summary of types of economic evaluation in health care

| Type of economic evaluation | Measurement of outcomes | Type of efficiency |
| --- | --- | --- |
| Cost-effectiveness analysis | Cancers detected<br>Life years | Technical |
| Cost-utility analysis | Quality adjusted life-years | Technical<br>Allocative within health sector if cost per QALY league table approach adopted |
| Cost-benefit analysis | Outcomes valued in monetary terms | Allocative across public sector |

The second is cost-utility analysis (CUA) where the costs of alternative treatments are compared to the outcomes, or effects, of alternative treatments but where the outcomes are measured in terms of quality adjusted life-years (QALYs). QALYs incorporate both the treatment's impact on survival as well as health-related quality of life (QALYs are explained in more detail below). The additional costs and effects of a treatment are then presented in terms of an incremental cost-utility ratio, such as the additional cost per QALY gained. Cost-utility analysis is useful for addressing the most efficient way of treating a particular condition, that is, technical efficiency. More controversially, QALYs can also be used in cost per QALY league tables to assess allocative efficiency and assist in judging relative priorities across different healthcare programmes[8] (this is discussed in more detail below). CUA is the type of economic evaluation used most often in oncology.[10]

The third is cost-benefit analysis (CBA) where the costs of alternative treatments are compared to the benefits, which themselves are valued in monetary terms. Methods to obtain monetary outcome values exist; such as "willingness to pay",[11] although to date there are few examples in oncology (although see[12] for one example). Despite the common use of the term "cost-benefit analysis", in practice true cost-benefit studies are rarely undertaken because of the practical and ethical issues associated with putting a monetary value on life. The results of CBA are presented as a net monetary benefit. CBA addresses allocative efficiency in the public sector as it prioritises treatments and programmes with the greatest net monetary benefit.

## Perspective of economic evaluation

Irrespective of the type of economic evaluation adopted, an economic evaluation may be conducted from a number of perspectives. The two most common perspectives are a health service perspective and a societal perspective. Adoption of a health service perspective means that only health service costs and health-related quality-of-life outcomes are included. Adoption of a societal perspective means that a much broader set of costs and outcomes are included. Societal costs will include, for example, non-health service costs, such as productivity costs (discussed further below), and societal outcomes such as impacts on groups other than the individual being treated.

## Frameworks for economic evaluation

Economic evaluation requires evidence on the clinical effectiveness of treatments to estimate the outcomes required for CEA and CUA. The two most common sources of evidence of clinical effectiveness are clinical trials and modelling.

In recent years, a notable trend in the economic evaluation of healthcare treatments is the number that have been conducted alongside, or as part of, clinical trials.[13,14] One of the main advantages of using clinical trials as a framework for economic evaluation is that they provide the opportunity to collect and analyse patient-specific data on costs and outcomes. There are also disadvantages with clinical trials, however – for example, the limited generalisability of costs and outcomes and limited ability to capture the full extent of costs and outcomes because of a restricted time horizon in the clinical trial.

An alternative to using clinical trials as a framework for economic evaluation is to adopt a modelling approach.[15] This may be appropriate where a clinical trial is not feasible or where it is not practical to incorporate an economic evaluation into a clinical trial. Instead, modelling techniques can be used to synthesise data from a number of sources in order to estimate overall costs and outcomes for the treatment and its alternative. Data required for the model will be cost and probabilities for events within the model, and can be obtained from the literature.[16] For example, in a model of the cost-effectiveness of a breast cancer drug, the costs would be the cost of the drug and the cost of day in hospital and the probabilities would be, for example, the probability of a breast cancer recurrence. There are a number of different modelling approaches including decision tree models and Markov models.[15] Decision trees represent chance events and decision over time. A limitation of decision trees is that they are not well suited to representing multiple outcomes events that occur over time. Markov models represent a more efficient representation of treatments involving recurring events.[17] In Markov models, the disease process is split into a series of states each representing a phase of the disease.

In most economic evaluations, the choice is not a simple assessment of whether a clinical trial or a modelling approach should be adopted, since in many clinical trials modelling is required to augment clinical trial data so that some of the disadvantages of clinical trials can be overcome. For example, modelling may be required to generalise the results to extrapolate from short-term to long-term outcomes.

## Costs in economic evaluation

### Overview

In economic evaluation, cost is the product of two factors, the quantity of resources consumed (such as days in hospital) and the valuation of the resources (such as unit cost per hospital day). In clinical trials, the quantity of resource use is measured on a patient-specific basis but the valuation of resources (unit cost) is the same per patient. Clearly, it is only by valuing the resource use, that is, by

**Table 3.2   Types of cost in economic evaluation**

| Health service costs | Non-health service costs |
|---|---|
| Direct costs of the whole treatment | Costs incurred by other public sector budgets |
| General illness costs | Informal care costs |
| Trial costs | Patients' travel and time costs incurred in receiving treatment |
| Future costs | Other out of pocket expenses incurred by the patient |
| | Productivity costs |
| | Future costs (for example food and accommodation costs) |

applying unit costs to resource use, that a total cost is estimated. There are a number of different types of resource use (and cost) that can be included in an economic evaluation. In the past, costs were classified into two types: direct and indirect. Recently, however, partly as a result of the confusion regarding the interpretation of indirect costs, there has been a move away from this classification.[8,9] Instead, a more useful approach is to classify costs into two different types: health service costs and non-health service costs.[18] The categories of cost that fall into these two types are now discussed and summarised in Table 3.2. In some cases it may not be necessary to include all categories of cost in an economic evaluation and the decision as to inclusion can be based on a number of factors such as relative quantitative importance of the cost as well as attribution to the treatment.[18] In general, it is useful to consider explicitly whether a cost is related or unrelated to the treatment. Related costs only need be included in the final analysis as they are attributable to the treatment.

## Health service costs

Health service costs include the direct costs of the whole treatment such as inpatient and outpatient costs as well as broader costs arising from the treatment such as the costs of complications and side effects. They also include the use of buildings, other capital and equipment, and overheads, such as heating and lighting, arising from the health service treatment. The term "whole treatment" is used to stress the fact that the costs of the treatment should include broader health service costs.

General illness costs are the costs of being treated for illnesses whilst being treated for the treatment being evaluated. For example, attendance at a cancer screening clinic may identify an illness, for example depression, for which treatment may be required and a cost incurred. If the illness is related to the treatment, then the cost should be included.

Trial costs are the costs of procedures in the trial protocol that are required solely for the purposes of the trial rather than the costs of doing the research. These costs may arise because patients are more closely monitored in the trial or

because of the necessity to preserve blinding.[19] The more pragmatic the trial design, the more the costs are likely to reflect actual practice and the less of an issue trial costs become. Trial costs should only be ignored if the resource use they represent could not affect outcome.

Future health service costs are the costs of treatment for diseases arising in years of life lived anyway or in life-years gained.[9,20] These costs can be further classified by whether they are related or unrelated to the treatment.[9,20] Related costs in years of life lived anyway are the costs of treating the disease that would be incurred without the treatment. Unrelated costs in years of life lived anyway are the costs of treating other diseases that would be incurred without the treatment. Related costs in life-years gained are the costs of treating the disease arising in the life-years gained from the treatment. Future costs in years of life gained occur commonly in prevention and cancer screening treatments if individuals gain life-years as a result of the treatment. Unrelated costs in life-years gained are the costs of treating other diseases arising in the life-years gained from the treatment. There is no consensus in the literature as to whether all types of future cost should be included. There is particular disagreement about whether unrelated future costs in life years gained should be included.

Box 3.1 presents an applied example of the different types of health service cost.

## Non-health service costs

Non-health service costs are the costs incurred by other public sector budgets (such as social services)[21] as well as informal care costs. They also include costs incurred by patients and productivity costs incurred by society as result of a patient's treatment. For costs incurred by other public sector budgets, it is important to recognise that the sector incurring costs may change as the budgetary arrangements change. For example, health service costs may be shifted to social care.

Informal care costs are the costs incurred by family or friends in caring for patients, usually unpaid. These costs include the financial outlays incurred by the carer but also

---

<table>
<tr><td style="vertical-align:top; width:50%; border:1px solid; padding:8px;">

**Box 3.1 Illustrative example of types of health service cost**

**Study context**

A randomised trial of a taxane drug for breast cancer aims to improve quality of life and reduce cancer mortality. Examples of the different types of health service cost measured in this context are:

*Direct costs of the whole treatment*

- Drug regimens
- Outpatient visits at breast clinic
- Inpatient stays
- Costs of side effects, toxicities, and palliative care costs (broader health service costs)

*General illness costs*

- Costs of treating illnesses related to the treatment: for example, where a follow up visit to a breast clinic identifies depression as a side effect of the drug for which treatment is required.
- Costs of treating illnesses unrelated to the treatment: for example, inpatient costs for an unrelated accident.

*Trial costs*

- Costs of any tests undertaken only for the purposes of the trial, for example extra visits to breast clinic.

*Future costs*

- Related costs arising in years of life lived anyway: the costs associated with treatment of breast cancer episodes without the treatment.
- Related costs arising in life-years gained: the costs of treating all breast cancer episodes in the life-years gained from the treatment.
- Unrelated costs arising in years of life lived anyway: the costs of treating non-breast cancer in life-years lived without the treatment.
- Unrelated costs arising in life years gained: the costs of treating non-cancer events in the life-years gained. For example, costs of treatment for cardiovascular disease.

</td><td style="vertical-align:top; width:50%; border:1px solid; padding:8px;">

**Box 3.2 Illustrative example of types of non-health service cost**

**Study context**

A randomised trial of a taxane drug for breast cancer aims to improve quality of life and reduce cancer mortality. Examples of the different types of non-health service cost measured in this context are:

*Costs incurred by other public sector budgets*

- Costs of meals-on-wheels by social services

*Informal care costs*

- Costs incurred by family and friends in caring for patient at home

*Patient travel and time costs*

- Travel costs incurred by patient in attending breast clinic
- Time costs associated with travel to and time spent at the breast clinic

*Productivity costs*

- Costs, in terms of lost production, resulting from absence from work because of treatment

</td></tr>
</table>

Productivity costs may be incurred by society and these include the costs, in terms of time and lost production, associated with the patient taking time off work. Productivity costs may be separated into two phases: treatment and morbidity (incurred as a result of patients being ill).[23]

Box 3.2 presents an applied example of the different types of non-health service cost.

## Analysis of costs

If resource use has been collected on a patient-specific basis, as is the case in a clinical trial, then total cost per patient is calculated by multiplying patient-specific resource use data by the unit cost of the resource and summing over all categories of cost.[8] At its simplest, a mean total cost per patient per treatment is then constructed by summing each patient's total cost across all patients and then dividing by the number of patients receiving each treatment. A mean cost difference between alternative treatments is calculated by subtracting one mean cost from the other. An indication of variability in mean costs should be reported, such as a standard deviation around a mean cost. This is particularly important since it is often the case that cost data are skewed as a result of a few patients having a high cost event such as inpatient stay.[24] Certain features of the data, such as missing or censored data, complicate the calculation of mean cost and may need to be addressed.[24]

the time spent by the informal carer in providing care. The potential for shifting costs onto carers should be considered when deciding whether to include informal care costs.

Patients may incur non-health service costs including travel costs and other out of pocket expenses associated with receiving treatment or attending for screening. The opportunity cost of patients' time associated with receiving treatment is a further type of non-health service cost. These types of cost may be quantitatively important in cancer screening and oncology treatment programmes.[22]

If costs have been identified from the literature and used as inputs into a model, then a patient-specific analysis of costs is not possible and the model will produce mean total cost for each treatment being compared.

For both trials and models, the costs will need to be discounted to reflect the fact that the costs may be occurring at different time periods. In the UK, the recommended discount rate for discounting is 6%.[25] Discounting is an important part of the methodology that many oncology studies have neglected.[10]

In analysing cost data in both trials and models, it is also useful to conduct sensitivity analysis in order to explore the impact on the results of using different estimates, such as alternative unit costs.[8] (There are some good examples of cost-analysis in oncology studies.[26,27])

## Outcome measures in economic evaluation

### Overview of outcome measures

Economic evaluation is not only about alternatives and costs it is also about outcomes (as well as about the relationship between costs and outcomes). There is increasing demand for, and growing evidence of, outcome measures that incorporate patient preferences and quality of life. Considering quality-of-life effects is particularly important in oncology where many treatments obtain modest improvements in response or survival at the expense of toxicity.

In CUA, quality of life is assessed by incorporating utilities into the analysis. Utilities reflect the fact that individuals with similar ability or disability to function may regard that level of functioning differently. Life-years are then weighted by utilities in order to estimate quality adjusted life-years (QALYs) in CEA.[8,9] A simplification of the QALY method, sometimes adopted in oncology studies, is the Q-TWIST (quality adjusted time without symptoms or toxicity) where utilities are set at 0·5.[28]

In CBA, quality of life can be incorporated by asking patients their willingness to pay for a treatment with the quality-of-life effects of the treatment described in the valuation process. The willingness to pay for the treatment is then compared to the costs of the treatment. Although the willingness to pay approach has been used in oncology,[12] CUA remains the most common approach.[10] The remainder of this section will therefore focus on estimation of utilities and QALYs.

### Utilities

Utility reflects the preferences of individuals or society and, in the context of economic evaluation, refers to the relative value placed on a specific health. The quality of life associated with a health state is measured on a scale of zero to one, where death is assigned a value of zero and full health is assigned a value of one. It is also possible to have utilities of less than zero reflecting the fact that a severe health state may be considered worse than death. There are two approaches to estimating utilities: direct and indirect.

Direct approaches require patients (or the general public) to value described health states using one of three techniques (visual analogue, time trade-off method and standard gamble).[8] The described health state includes a series of statements referring to the quality-of-life effects. The visual analogue technique is a thermometer-like scale marked out with one at the top and zero at the bottom. Patients are asked to rate the described health state on the visual analogue scale in order to represent how good or bad they perceive the described health state to be. The point marked on the scale is then the utility for that state. The time trade-off technique requires patients to consider the number of years of good health that are equivalent to a longer period of time in the described health state (which is less than good health). The number of equivalent years is then divided by the total number of years to give a utility for the health state. The standard gamble technique requires patients to choose between the described health state with certainty and a gamble between good health and death. The probabilities are varied between zero and one until the patient is indifferent to the two alternatives. The utility value for the described state is then the value at which the patient is indifferent.[8]

Indirect approaches involve asking patients to complete a health-related quality-of-life questionnaire that describes quality of life across a range of dimensions and asks the patient to complete the questionnaire indicating how their health is affected on each dimension. The results are then converted into utilities by using equations that have been estimated elsewhere. The most common indirect approach is the EQ-5D (sometimes known as EuroQol).[29] The EQ-5D asks patients to consider their health status in five dimensions (mobility, self-care, usual activities, pain/discomfort and anxiety/depression). Each dimension has three levels and the patient selects a level for each dimension to represent how they are affected on each. The result of this process is then a five-digit code that can be converted into a utility using an equation that has been derived from a survey of the general population in the UK.[30]

The indirect approach to estimating utilities, specifically the EQ-5D, is increasingly being used, particularly in clinical trials where patients are asked to complete the EQ-5D at various time points throughout the trial. In modelling studies, utilities for health states are likely to be derived from add-on studies using direct methods or utility estimates published in the literature.[31]

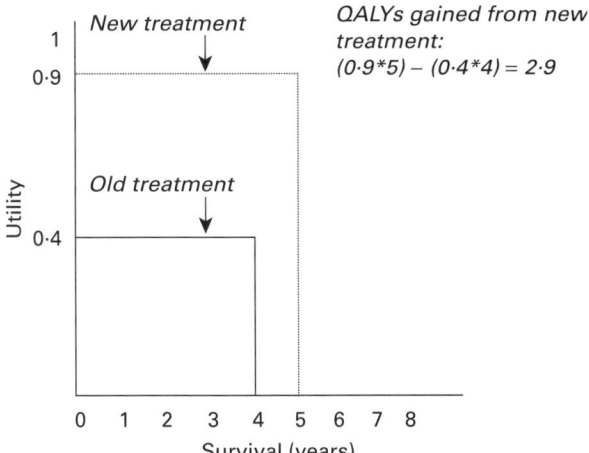

**Figure 3.1**  Illustration of QALY calculation

## QALYs

Once utilities have been estimated, QALYs are calculated by weighting the length of time (duration) in each health state by its utility value. Figure 3.1 illustrates this calculation. It shows the QALYs for two treatments: a new treatment and an old treatment. The utility value associated with the new treatment is 0·9 and the duration (survival) is 5 years. Multiplying one by the other gives 4·5 QALYs for the new treatment. The utility associated with the old treatment is 0·4 and the duration (survival) is 4 years. Multiplying the utility by the duration gives 1·6 QALYs. The QALYs gained from the new treatment is then the difference between the two (2·9 QALYs).

## Analysis of outcomes

As with cost analysis, QALYs should be discounted to reflect the fact that they are occurring in the future. In the UK, the recommended discount rate for discounting QALYs is 1·5%.[25] As with costs, the discounting of outcomes is an important part of the methodology that many oncology studies have neglected.[10]

In analysing outcome data, it is also useful to conduct sensitivity analysis in order to explore the impact on the results of using different estimates, such as utilities. (There are good review articles on QALY estimation in oncology studies.[10,32])

## Combining costs and outcomes in economic evaluation

The results of CEA and CUA are presented as a ratio of cost to outcomes where in CEA, the outcomes are cases of

cancer prevented or life years and in CUA the outcomes are QALYs. Both CEA and CUA involve calculating incremental cost-effectiveness ratios (ICERs) by dividing the incremental costs between the comparators by the incremental outcomes between old and new treatments. By contrast, the results from CBA are presented as a net monetary amount (benefits minus costs).

Table 3.3 presents an example of the estimation of ICERs from a study comparing two treatments (tamoxifen versus tamoxifen with chemotherapy) for node-positive early breast cancer.[33] The table summarises the methods adopted by the study as well as its findings. The study adopted both a CEA and a CUA approach and so two ICERs are presented: an incremental cost per life-year gained of £2389 (CEA) and an incremental cost per QALY of £3502 (CUA). It is important to note that these ratios are point estimates and that there is uncertainty associated with them.[32]

Do these ICERs provide evidence that tamoxifen and chemotherapy is cost-effective relative to tamoxifen alone? The relative cost-effectiveness of alternative treatment can be represented on the cost-effectiveness plane (Figure 3.2). The example falls into the top right quadrant where the new treatment (tamoxifen with chemotherapy) is more costly but also more effective than the alternative (tamoxifen). In situations such as this, there is uncertainty as to the threshold below which a treatment can be considered cost-effective. Figure 3.2 illustrates a maximum acceptable ICER ratio to reflect this threshold. If, for example, policy-makers set the maximum acceptable cost-effectiveness ratio to be £30 000 per QALY gained, then all treatments with an incremental cost per QALY of less than this amount would be considered cost-effective. In the example, tamoxifen with chemotherapy would therefore be considered cost-effective because it has a cost per QALY of £3502. In the UK, however, there is no numerical value for the threshold value and therefore for treatments in the top right quadrant of the cost-effectiveness plane there is an element of subjectivity and it is left to decision makers to judge the treatment's cost-effectiveness. The cost-effectiveness plane can also represent other situations, such as where a new treatment costs less but is more effective than the old treatment. In such a situation, adoption of the new treatment would be recommended.

In the past, ratios from CUA have been ranked in terms of increasing magnitude in order to help judge relative priorities across the healthcare sector in order to inform allocative efficiency. Treatments are ranked in a table according to their incremental (additional) cost per QALY gained and, in the context of a fixed budget for health care, those treatments offering additional QALYs at lowest additional cost per QALY should be given priority. Such tables are known as cost per QALY league tables.

**Table 3.3    Illustrative example of the methods and results of the cost effectiveness of treatments for breast cancer***

| Method | Approach adopted |
|---|---|
| Comparators | Tamoxifen versus tamoxifen plus chemotherapy in postmenopausal women with node-positive early breast cancer |
| Type of economic evaluation | CEA and CUA |
| Perspective | Health service |
| Framework | Model with seven states (disease-free interval, soft tissue metastases, bone metastases, visceral metastases, locoregional relapse, remission, dead)[†] |
| Health service costs | Costs of tamoxifen, chemotherapy, toxicities, metastases, locoregional relapse are included and are attached to states in the model |
| Non-health service costs | Excluded |
| Discounting of costs | Costs are discounted at 6% |
| Utilities | Utilities of chemotherapy, toxicities, metastases, locoregional relapse are based on estimates from the literature and attached to states in the model |
| Life-years | Life-years are estimated by the model by inputting probabilities of transitions between states into the model |
| QALYs | QALYs are estimated by the model by inputting probabilities of transitions between states into the model and by attaching utilities to those states |
| Discounting of life years and QALYs | Life-years and QALYs are discounted at 1·5% |
| *Results* | *Findings* |
| Incremental costs | Average total cost of tamoxifen £7115<br>Average total cost of tamoxifen plus chemotherapy £9146<br>Incremental cost £2031 (£9146 minus £7115) |
| Incremental life-years | Average total life-years of tamoxifen 15·16<br>Average total life-years of tamoxifen plus chemotherapy 16·01<br>Incremental life-years 0.85 (16·01 minus 15·16) |
| Incremental QALYs | Average total QALYs of tamoxifen 11·56<br>Average total QALYs of tamoxifen plus chemotherapy 12·14<br>Incremental QALYs 0.58 (12·14 minus 11·56) |
| ICER (CEA) | Incremental cost per life-year gained £2389<br>(£2031 divided by 0·85) |
| ICER (CUA) | Incremental cost per QALY gained £3502<br>(£2031 divided by 0·58) |

*Source: adapted from Karnon and Brown[33]
†Details of structure of model are given in reference 33.

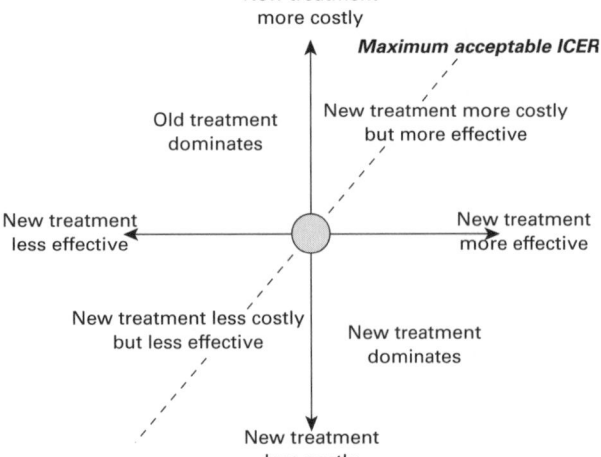

**Figure 3.2**    The cost-effectiveness plane

Reservations have also been expressed about these tables since they inevitably involve summarising a large amount of information into one figure per evaluation.[8] In particular, it is often argued that cost per QALY tables do not perform incremental analysis on disaggregated costs and outcomes. Furthermore caution is necessary in that it is difficult to transfer results from the table to another geographic area if, for example, the incidence and prevalence of the disease differs between two areas. Despite this, it has to be recognised that resource allocation decisions are made in the healthcare sector and are often not explicit. QALYs can be used to aid resource allocation decisions and assist in making those decisions more explicit, but they should be viewed as being indicative rather than determinate.

## Conclusions

In oncology, new drugs and treatments regularly emerge, increasing the number of alternative treatments. Even if the evidence base suggests the new drug or treatment to be more effective than an alternative, judgement is required as to whether it is cost effective to provide the new drug or treatment at all. Health economics, and economic evaluation in particular, can help to illuminate such a decision through a rigorous consideration of the costs and outcomes of alternative treatments.

## References

1 Mooney G. *Economics, medicine and health care, 2nd edn.* Hertfordshire: Harvester Wheatsheaf, 1992.
2 Folland S, Goodman AC, Stano M. *The economics of health and health care, 2nd edn.* New Jersey: Prentice Hall, 1997.
3 Boadway R, Bruce N. *Welfare economics.* Oxford: Basil Blackwell, 1984.
4 Donaldson C, Gerard K. *Economics of health care financing: the visible hand.* London: Macmillan, 1993.
5 Sassi F, Archard L, Le Grand J. Equity and the economic evaluation of healthcare. *Health Technol Assess* 2001;**5**:3.
6 Cairns J, van der Pol M, Eliciting time preferences for health. In Stevens A *et al.*, eds. *The advanced handbook of methods in evidence based healthcare.* London: Sage, 2001.
7 Cairns J. Discounting in economic evaluation. In Drummond M, McGuire A, eds. *Economic evaluation in health care: Merging theory with practice.* Oxford: Oxford University Press, 2001.
8 Drummond MF, O'Brien B, Stoddart GL, Torrance GW. *Methods for the economic evaluation of health care programmes, 2nd edn.* Oxford: Oxford University Press, 1997.
9 Gold M, Siegel J, Russell L, Weinstein M. *Cost effectiveness in health and medicine.* New York: Oxford University Press, 1996.
10 Earle CC, Chapman RH, Baker CS *et al.* Systematic overview of cost-utility assessments in oncology. *J Clin Oncol* 2000;**18**:3302–17.
11 Pauly MV. Valuing health care benefits in money terms. In Sloan FA, ed. *Valuing health care: cost, benefits and effectiveness of pharmaceuticals and other medical technologies.* New York: Cambridge University Press, 1995.
12 Frew, E, Wolstenholme JL, Whynes DK. Willingness-to-pay for colorectal cancer screening. *Eur J Cancer* 2001;**37**:1746–51.
13 Bonsel GJ, Rutten FFH, Uyl-deGroot CA. Economic evaluation alongside cancer trials: Methodological and practical aspects. *Eur J Cancer* 1993;**29A**:S10–S14.
14 van Agthoven M, Vellenga E, Fibbe WE, Kingma T, Uyl-de Groot CA. Cost analysis and quality-of-life assessment comparing patients undergoing autologous peripheral blood stem cell transplantation or autologous bone marrow transplantation for refractory or relapsed non-Hodgkin's lymphoma or Hodgkin's disease: a prospective randomised trial. *Eur J Cancer* 2001;**37**:1781–9.
15 Petitti DB. *Meta-analysis, decision analysis and cost effectiveness analysis: Methods for quantitative synthesis in medicine, 2nd edn.* New York: Oxford University Press, 2000.
16 Mandelblatt J, Fryback, DG, Weinstein MC, Russell LB, Gold MR and members of the Panel on Cost-Effectiveness in Health and Medicine. Assessing the effectiveness of health interventions for cost-effectiveness analysis. *J Gen Intern Med* 1997;**12**:551–8.
17 Kuntz K, Weinstein M. Modelling in economic evaluation. In Drummond M, McGuire A, eds. *Economic evaluation in health care: merging theory with practice.* Oxford: Oxford University Press, 2001.
18 Johnston K, Buxton MJ, Jones DR, Fitzpatrick R. Assessing the costs of health care technologies in clinical trials. *Health Technol Assess* 1999;**3**:6.
19 Coyle D, Davies L, Drummond M. Trials and tribulations: Emerging issues in designing economic evaluations alongside clinical trials. *Int J Technol Assess Health Care* 1998;**14**:135–44.
20 Meltzer, D. Accounting for future costs in medical cost-effectiveness analysis. *J Health Econom* 1997;**16**:33–64.
21 Donaldson C, Shackley P. Economic evaluation. In Detels R *et al.*, eds. *Oxford textbook on public health.* Oxford: Oxford University Press, 1997.
22 Seckler-Walker RH, Vacek PM, Hooper GJ, Plante DA, Detsky AS. Screening for breast cancer: Time, travel, and out of pocket expenses. *J Natl Cancer Inst* 1999;**91**:702–8.
23 Sculpher M. The role and estimation of productivity costs in economic evaluation. In: Drummond M, McGuire A, eds. *Economic evaluation in health care: merging theory with practice.* Oxford: Oxford University Press, 2001.
24 Heyse J, Cook J, Carides G. Statistical considerations in analysing health care resource utilization and cost data. In: Drummond M, McGuire A, eds. *Economic evaluation in health care: merging theory with practice.* Oxford: Oxford University Press, 2001.
25 National Institute for Clinical Excellence. Interim guidance for manufacturers and sponsors [www.nice.org.uk] 2000.
26 Wolstenholme JL, Whynes DK. The hospital costs of treating lung cancer in the United Kingdom. *Br J Cancer* 1999;**80**:215–18.
27 Coyle D, Small N, Ashworth A *et al.* Costs of palliative care in the community, in hospitals and in hospices in the UK. *Crit Rev Oncol Hematol* 1999;**32**:71–85.
28 Gelber RD, Goldhirsch A, Cole BF *et al.* A quality adjusted time without symptoms or toxicity (Q-TWIST) analysis of adjuvant radiation therapy and chemotherapy for resectable rectal cancer. *J Natl Cancer Inst* 1996;**88**:1039–45.
29 Brooks R. EuroQol: the current state of play. *Health Policy* 1996;**37**: 53–72.
30 Dolan P, Gudex C, Kind P, Williams A. A social tariff for EuroQol: results from a UK general population survey. Centre for Health Economics, Discussion Paper 138, York: University of York.
31 Tengs TO, Wallace A. One thousand health-related quality of life estimates. *Med Care* 2000;**38**:583–637.
32 Brown J, Sculpher M. Benefit valuation in economic evaluation of cancer therapies: A systematic review of the published literature. *Pharmacoeconomics* 1999;**16**:17–31.
33 Karnon J, Brown J. Tamoxifen plus chemotherapy versus tamoxifen alone as adjuvant therapies for node-positive postmenopausal women with early breast cancer: A stochastic economic evaluation. *Pharmacoeconomics* 2002;**20**:119–37.

# 4 Stringent application of epidemiological criteria changes the interpretation of the effects of immunotherapy in advanced renal cell cancer

*Franz Porzsolt, Julia Kumpf, Chris Coppin, Ernst Pöppel*

Renal cell cancer (RCC) accounts for 1–2% of all malignancies with increasing incidence. At diagnosis 25–30% of all patients suffer from metastatic disease.[1] The course of the disease is variable. There are spontaneous remissions as well as cases which are refractory to various types of treatment. The median survival for advanced renal cell cancer is about 9 months. As the results of chemotherapies are not too promising, major expectations are put on cytokine therapies using interleukin-2 (IL-2) or interferon alfa (IFN$\alpha$).

As the results of these cytokine studies look promising but are based on either non-controlled studies or small randomised trials with restricted power we prepared, together with Canadian colleagues, a review on immunotherapy for advanced renal cell cancer now published in the Cochrane database of systematic reviews.[2] The specific hypotheses were as follows.

- High dose IL-2, the approved treatment option in the USA, results in better survival than other options.
- IFN$\alpha$, the most frequently used option in other countries, produces longer survival than other options.

The review was prepared according to standard criteria for systematic reviews as outlined in the handbook of the Cochrane Collaboration.

A total of 98 randomised trials were included, of which 42, involving a total of 4216 patients, fulfilled the inclusion criteria for acceptance in the meta-analysis. Based on the remission rates from 42 studies and the survival data from 26 studies, we were able to demonstrate that IFN$\alpha$ significantly reduced the 1-year mortality as compared to controls who received no immunotherapy. The odds ratio of this successful treatment was 0·67 (95% CI 0·50–0·89). This effect corresponds to an increase in survival by 2·6 months.

Reconsidering the interpretation of the data, we detect reasons that might question our previous interpretation. Today we question that IFN$\alpha$ is the cause of prolonged survival. There is no doubt that the observed effect is true and is associated with interferon but we are no longer confident that this effect was really caused by IFN$\alpha$.

As this topic will need a more profound discussion if our assumption is correct, we want to present our concerns and offer a possibility to explain the observed effect.

## Method

The re-interpretation of the data is based on a semiquantitative analysis of the criteria, which may support a causal relationship of an intervention and an observed effect.[3] The criteria described by available data and included in this analysis are the quality of the single studies that were accepted for the review, the specificity of the effect including its possible misinterpretation, the biologic plausibility, and the dose–response relationship.

## Results

### Quality of single studies accepted for systematic reviews

The quality of a systematic review depends on the quality of the identified studies and their reporting of methodological details. We applied quality parameters such as randomisation, concealed allocation, intention to treat analysis, blinding, and independent blinded outcome evaluation. Details are described in our Cochrane Review.[2]

Unfortunately, these criteria could not be applied to all studies because of the lack of published information. Only few studies were in fact declared as blinded and many trials were rather small (average 39 patients per study arm). The conclusions drawn from a meta-analysis based on individual patient data would be a lot stronger than a meta-analysis – like ours – based on published trials.

Clinical epidemiologists listed the established pros and cons to either support or reject the assumption of a causal effect.[3] The argument for a causal effect is strengthened, for example, by demonstrating specificity, biologic plausibility, and the existence of a dose–response relationship, in the order of increasing importance. These three criteria were analysed rigorously to see if they would rather support or reject the assumption of a causal relationship between immunotherapies and survival.

## Specificity

In our review it was difficult to demonstrate specificity. Considering the two studies, which compared the effects of IL-2 and of IFNα on survival, no significant differences could be demonstrated.[4,5] A second example for the lack of specificity is described in the study by Gleave *et al.*,[6] which described no survival difference following treatment with IFNγ or placebo.

Other studies which compared IL-2 with any other therapy are lacking; for example, there are no randomised studies comparing high dose IL-2 and non-immunotherapies.

When IFNα was compared with non-immunotherapies, a significant survival advantage of the groups treated by IFNα could be shown. However, this observation does not answer the question whether only IFNα or any immunotherapy can mediate this effect. Additional studies investigating the effect of immunotherapies other than IFNα are necessary to solve this problem.

## Possible misinterpretation of the specificity of the effect

The only exception to the last mentioned observation were the results of IFNγ. When IFNγ was tested against placebo there was no difference, either in the response rate or in survival. This result suggests that IFNγ may be considered as a control that produces similar results like placebo.

There are several other studies that seem to confirm this conclusion. In the study of DeMulder *et al.*,[7] there was no significant difference between a combination of IFNα plus IFNγ compared with single agent IFNα suggesting that the addition of IFNγ did not produce any additional effect.

A similar result was observed in another three-armed study, which compared IFNα versus IFNγ with the combination of both types of interferon. There were no differences in outcomes.[8] The surprising observation in this study was the lack of a difference between IFNα and IFNγ!

This surprising observation was confirmed by the study of Lummen *et al.* who did not see any survival difference when comparing the combination of IL-2 and IFNα with IFNγ. This observation – that the two active substances, IFNα and IL-2 seem to be no more active than IFNγ, which probably does not mediate any specific effect – induces serious concerns about the specificity of the two drugs considered to be active.

If we accept that IFNγ produces a placebo effect,[6] based on the results of Foon[8] and Lummen,[9] we have also to consider that IFNα has possibly no other effect on survival than a placebo. As there were no other corresponding placebo-controlled trials in advanced RCC, we lack formal information to demonstrate that other immunotherapies produce longer survival than placebo.

We probably induced a "pseudospecificity", that is, the assumption of specific effects just by imprecise discussion. In our review we thought to compare immunotherapy against non-immunotherapy but in fact compared only IFNα against non-immunotherapy. Other immunotherapies than IFNα were investigated only in studies that did not address exactly the critical problem.

An example is the experiment by Henriksson *et al.*[10] Instead of comparing IFNα against IL-2 against tamoxifen in their three armed study, they compared combinations of tamoxifen plus a cytokine with tamoxifen alone. As the combinations were not better than tamoxifen alone, it is possible that neither IL-2 nor IFNα had an effect in addition to tamoxifen.

## Biologic plausibility

Given the available data, it is difficult to postulate biologic plausibility for a specific effect of IFNα in advanced RCC, unless it is assumed that different pharmacological mechanisms would produce the same result. In this case one would expect that the combination of immunotherapies would produce additive or synergistic effects. However, there are no data to support this expectation, as the results summarised in the meta-analysis demonstrated that IL-2 plus IFNα versus IL-2 produced a non-significant Peto odds ratio of 0·87 (95% CI 0·58–1·29) in four studies.[4,5,11,12]

## Dose–response relationship

We were not able in our review to establish the optimum type, route, dose, schedule, and duration of IFNα treatment on survival. It was stated that the dose–response relationship seems to be relatively weak. These studies used only the reduction of tumour size but not survival as the endpoint. With large dose ratios of 3:1 or 10:1 examined in three studies,[13–16] the Peto odds ratio for response can be calculated as being 1·85 (0·76–4·54). Data on dose-specific effects on survival are not available.

## Discussion and conclusion

In our review published in the Cochrane library we concluded that IFNα significantly prolongs survival.[2] We do not want to question the size of the described effect but its interpretation. The weighted average median improvement in survival of 2·6 months is probably true but not the interpretation that this is caused by IFNα.

There are too few epidemiological criteria completed to conclude a causal relationship between IFNα treatment and prolongation of survival in advanced RCC.

The observed effect is not specific, there is no convincing biologic plausibility, and data supporting a possible dose–response relationship between IFNα and survival are missing.

To demonstrate specificity an experiment should compare IFNα versus other immunotherapies versus non-immunotherapy and show that only IFNα but not the other immunotherapies prolong survival as compared to non-immunotherapies. This experiment, however, is missing.

The lack of methodological quality and the epidemiological weakness was recognised in our Cochrane review but not consequently respected enough. This led to the conventional interpretation of the results concluding that IFNα prolongs survival in patients with advanced RCC. Considering the epidemiological problems discussed above, we came to the conclusion that IFNα is associated with prolonged survival but not necessarily the cause of this effect. Unfortunately, we have to state that our initial interpretation of the results was biased.

A different interpretation of the results could be that IFNα, like any other immunotherapy, is more promising to the physician and induces more hope and a more favourable perspective to the patient than any non-immune therapy. In our internal discussion we use the term "knowledge framing" to describe these desired effects avoiding the negative connotation that might be associated with the term "placebo". We consider the concepts but not the effects of "knowledge framing" and of "placebo" to be different and this may be expressed in four assumptions.

1  A placebo effect is considered to be an "as-if" effect, while the effect of knowledge framing is accepted as one of several components in the overall effect of a healthcare intervention.
2  Placebo is not thought of as a specific physical effect; knowledge framing is considered a specific effect of the information provided. There are indeed data to support the view that placebo effects – not the placebo itself – are

organ-specific,[17] which is in agreement with our concept of knowledge framing.
3  The placebo effect is thought to lie below the threshold of standard therapy, while the effect of knowledge framing is assumed to lie above that threshold.
4  The use of placebos is limited to clinical trials, whereas knowledge framing is not; knowledge framing is part of any doctor–patient encounter.

Our interpretation may not be accepted by others who think that there is no justification for placebos.[18] However, even these colleagues consider the possibility of placebo effects if they are psychologically mediated, which fits the concept of "knowledge framing".

Neurologists recently used positron emission tomography (PET) to estimate dopamine activity in the brains of patients with Parkinson's disease following injection of either inactive saline or apomorphine.[19] There was no difference in the dopamine release indicating that both the pharmacologically active drug and the placebo (in combination with the right information) induce the release of dopamine. This result demonstrates that we begin to understand the pathways by which placebos might work: the information to the patient is probably the critical component.

Very recently, Kirsch *et al.*[20] analysed the data submitted to the US Food and Drug Administration for approval of the six most widely prescribed antidepressants between 1987 and 1999. They found that approximately 80% of the response to medication was duplicated in placebo control groups, and the mean difference between drug and placebo was approximately 2 points on the 50-point and 62-point Hamilton Depression Scale. Improvement at the highest doses of medication was no different from improvement at the lowest doses.

Finally, the criteria requested by epidemiologists to increase the chance of a causal relationship between an intervention and an observed outcome should be applied more rigorously to avoid misleading interpretations.

## Summary

In this chapter we reconsider the interpretation of our data which was published in the Cochrane Database of Systematic Reviews 2000 entitled *Immunotherapy for Advanced Renal Cell Cancer*. In the published review we concluded that the moderate extension of survival (2·6 months) was caused by interferon alfa. In this revised version of the interpretation we applied the criteria of clinical epidemiology in a more stringent way and came up with the conclusion that a psychological effect called "knowledge framing" may have caused the observed outcome.

Additional data will be necessary to find out which of the interpretations is more adequate. The considerations discussed in this chapter may trigger the development of new approaches in the design and analysis of clinical trials.

## References

1  Young RC. Metastatic renal-cell carcinoma: what causes occasional dramatic regressions? *N Engl J Med* 1998;**338**:1305–6.
2  Coppin C, Porzsolt F, Kumpf J, Coldman A, Wilt T. Immunotherapy for advanced renal cell cancer (Cochrane Review). In: *Cochrane Library*, Issue 1, 2000. Oxford: Update Software.
3  Fletcher RH, Fletcher SW, Wagner EH. *Clinical Epidemiology. The Essentials, 2nd edn.* Baltimore: Williams & Wilkins, 1996.
4  Boccardo F, Rubagotti A, Canobbio L *et al.* Interleukin-2, interferon-α and interleukin-2 plus interferon-α in renal cell carcinoma. A randomized Phase II trial. *Tumori* 1998;**84**:534–9.
5  Negrier S, Escudier B, Lasset C *et al.* Recombinant human interleukin-2, recombinant human interferon alfa-2α, or both in metastatic renal-cell carcinoma. *Groupe Français d'Immunotherapie. N Engl J Med* 1998;**338**:1272–8.
6  Gleave ME, Elhilali M, Fradet Y *et al.* Interferon gamma-1β compared with placebo in metastatic renal-cell carcinoma. Canadian Urologic Oncology Group. *N Engl J Med* 1998;**338**:1265–71.
7  De Mulder PH, Oosterhof G, Bouffioux C, van Oosterom AT, Vermeylen K, Sylvester R. EORTC (30885) randomised phase III study with recombinant interferon alpha and recombinant interferon alpha and gamma in patients with advanced renal cell carcinoma. The EORTC Genitourinary Group. *Br J Cancer* 1995;**71**:371–5.
8  Foon K, Doroshow J, Bonnem E *et al.* A prospective randomized trial of alpha 2b- interferon/gamma-interferon or the combination in advanced metastatic renal cell carcinoma. *J Biolog Resp Modifiers* 1988;**7**:540–5.
9  Lummen G, Goepel M, Mollhoff S, Hinke A, Otto T, Rubben H. Phase II study of interferon-gamma versus interleukin-2 and interferon-alpha 2b in metastatic renal cell carcinoma. *J Urol* 1996;**155**:455–8.
10  Henriksson R, Nilsson S, Colleen S *et al.* Survival in renal cell carcinoma – a randomized evaluation of tamoxifen vs interleukin 2, alpha-interferon (leucocyte) and tamoxifen. *Br J Cancer* 1998;**77**:1311–17.
11  Jayson GC, Middleton M, Lee SM, Ashcroft L, Thatcher N. A randomized phase II trial of interleukin 2 and interleukin 2-interferon alpha in advanced renal cancer. *Br J Cancer* 1998;**78**:366–9.
12  Lissoni P, Barni S, Ardizzoia A *et al.* A randomized study of low-dose interleukin-2 subcutaneous immunotherapy versus interleukin-2 plus interferon-alpha as first line therapy for metastatic renal cell carcinoma. *Tumori* 1993;**79**:397–400.
13  Fujita T, Inagaki J, Asano H *et al.* Effects of low-dose interferon-alpha (Hlbi) following nephrectomy in metastatic renal cell carcinoma (Mrcc). (Meeting Abstract). *Proc Ann Mtg Am Soc Clin Oncol* 1992;**11**:A685.
14  Kirkwood JM, Harris JE, Vera R *et al.* A randomized study of low and high dose of leukocyte αinterferon in metastatic renal cell carcinoma: the American Cancer Society collaborative trial. *Cancer Res* 1985;**45**:863–71.
15  Quesada JR, Rios A, Swanson D, Trown P, Gutterman JU. Antitumor activity of recombinant-derived interferon alpha in metastatic renal cell carcinoma. *J Clin Oncol* 1985;**3**:1522–8.
16  Muss HB, Constanzi JJ, Leavitt R *et al.* Recombitant alfa interferon in renal cell carcinoma: a randomised trial of two routes of administration. *J Clin Oncol* 1987;**5**:285–91.
17  Meissner K. Gibt es organspezifische Placeboeffekte? Placeboeffekte an physiologischen Parametern und ihre mögliche Vermittlung über kortikale Organrepräsentationen. Aachen: Shaker, 2000.
18  Hróbjartsson A, Goetzsche PC. Is the placebo powerless? An analysis of clinical trials comparing placebo with no treatment. *N Engl J Med* 2001;**344**:1594–602.
19  de La Fuente-Fernandez R, Lim AS, Sossi V *et al.* Apomorphine-induced changes in synaptic dopamine levels: positron emission tomography evidence for presynaptic inhibition. *J Cereb Blood Flow Metab* 2001;**10**:1151–9.
20  Kirsch I, Moore TJ, Soboria A, Nicholls SS. The emperor's new drugs: an analysis of antidepressant medication data submitted to the U.S. Food and Drug Administration. *Prevent Treatment* 2002;**5**: Article 23.

# Section II

## Cancer prevention

*Rosalynne Weston, Editor*

# Preface

*Rosalynne Weston*

The chapters in this prevention section outline the current evidence for risk reduction strategies (primary, secondary, and tertiary prevention) for specific cancers. Such evidence may be integral, that is, chapters earlier or later than in this section may include prevention evidence for a specific cancer (for example, breast cancer). Readers are encouraged to cross-reference prevention evidence within and across all chapters. Currently, health professionals are required to develop seamless care pathways for all patients, to improve the quality and efficiency of medical care, quality of life, and convalescence. Hence, prevention rightly becomes part of such care pathways and specific chapters echo this development. The chapters in this prevention section are generally agreed to be key elements of cancer care pathways but also major public health issues ensuring the continued reduction of specific cancers, especially those related to health and lifestyle behaviour.

## Quality of primary and secondary evidence

Evidence of effectiveness is not the only measure of successful risk reduction. Acknowledging the fact that anyone can develop cancer no matter how healthy their lifestyle, how effectively they have followed risk reduction guidelines, or how expertly treatment has been delivered is an important aspect in communicating cancer prevention messages. Exercising caution in the interpretation of primary and secondary evidence, even when there is reasonable confidence about statistical reliability, for example data from meta-analysis based on clinical trials or randomised controlled trials, is necessary to avoid victim blaming. The evidence in this section is based on the best available at this point in time. It is important not to overestimate risk reduction possibilities as this may inadvertently raise patient expectation (that a healthy lifestyle will ensure cancer does not develop). Following surgery and treatment (radiotherapy and chemotherapy) it may be necessary to encourage patients to change their lifestyle as a tertiary prevention measure with the intention of preventing recurrence and such advice needs to be realistic.

## Behaviour change

Successful risk reduction interventions depend on personal behaviour change and compliance as much as they do on

evidence. As well as prevention evidence, effectiveness depends on other less measurable factors: communication strategies, personal social support, the patient's relationship with their GP, primary care team, and their hospital team; and belief in the intervention, maintenance strategies, and support offered by the primary care team and others. These remain important confounding variables in many risk reduction intervention studies particularly for primary prevention.

## Definitions

The chapters in the prevention section discuss primary, secondary, and sometimes tertiary (that following treatment) prevention. It is necessary to define the meaning of these terms as they are used in this section.

### Primary prevention

The intervention that is in place and/or undertaken to prevent the onset of disease as in lifestyle programmes including tobacco and healthy eating interventions. These interventions rely, for successful outcomes, on individual, and/or community behaviour change to reduce risk. Professionals are involved in communicating risk and risk factors and explaining ways in which behaviour change can be implemented or maintained: for example, skin protection in the sun at an individual level and shaded school playgrounds or beaches at the community level. For healthy eating, the individual may be encouraged to reduce fat or increase fruit and vegetables in their diet. At the community level it is necessary to make low fat foods and fruit and vegetables available at reasonably low prices. A policy about commercially prepared foods that include high levels of fat and sugar is needed, especially in relation to illness risk relating to obesity. How the intervention is planned, delivered, evaluated and communicated may make a difference to the received outcome and ultimately to the achievement of outcome objectives.

Evidence of effectiveness for some primary risk reduction interventions is not wholly reliable because the studies from which it is drawn have internal and external validity problems as well as many confounding influences. In the chapters in this section the quality of the original studies and outcome data are discussed to enable practitioners to realistically assess the potential of such interventions.

## Secondary prevention

This refers to risk reduction interventions that improve the availability and effectiveness of early diagnosis or early intervention: for example, screening programmes or interventions that encourage patients to present with symptoms as early as possible: after 10–12 days of onset of symptoms.

### *Tertiary prevention*

Risk reduction interventions that are encouraged after surgery or treatment to reduce the risk of reoccurrence or advancement of the disease.

## Acknowledgement

Dr Rosalynne Weston's research was originally funded by the Health Education Authority. The views expressed in these chapters are not the views of the Health Education Authority (currently The Health Development Agency).

## Further reading

Scott D, Weston R. *Evaluating Health Promotion*. Cheltenham: Nelson Thornes, 1988.

# 5 Which interventions help individuals to stop smoking?

*Tim Lancaster*

## Background

Smoking is the most important preventable risk factor for cancer. In addition to its well known relationship with lung cancer, smoking increases the risk for cancers of the oropharynx, oesophagus, bladder and cervix. Abnormal cervical smears are more likely to revert to normal if women give up smoking. Smoking also contributes significantly to morbidity and mortality from conditions other than cancer, particularly vascular and respiratory disease. These illnesses are among the commonest causes of death in the developing world. Increasing tobacco consumption in developing countries means that smoking-related mortality is on the rise in many of these areas. Peto has estimated that current patterns of cigarette smoking will cause about 450 million deaths worldwide in the next 50 years. A reduction of 50% in the number of current smokers would avoid about 20 to 30 million premature deaths in the first quarter of the century and about 150 million in the second quarter.[1] Preventing young people from starting smoking will also reduce tobacco-related mortality but the effects will not be seen until after 2050.

Quitting by current smokers is therefore the only way in which tobacco-related mortality can be reduced in the medium term. Although many ex-smokers report that they quit without formal help, there is evidence that an increasing number of successful quit attempts have been achieved using some form of behavioural, psychological, pharmacological, or complementary treatment.[2] The aim of this chapter is to summarise what is known about the effectiveness of the available interventions.

## Evidence

The conclusions of this review are based on meta-analyses of randomised controlled trials. Where there are insufficient trials for meta-analysis, we report the findings of individual randomised trials. The meta-analyses are based on work conducted by The Cochrane Tobacco Addiction Review group,[3] which seeks to identify and summarise the evidence for interventions to reduce and prevent tobacco use. The group produces and maintains systematic reviews to inform policymakers, clinicians and individuals wishing to stop smoking. Over 20 systematic reviews have been published in the *Cochrane Library*. They have contributed to the evidence base for smoking cessation guidelines in the United Kingdom and elsewhere.[4–5]

Details of the methods and results of each review are available in the *Cochrane Library* abstracts.[6] The reviews summarise results from randomised controlled trials with at least 6 months follow up. Trials must report data on smoking status, and not just the effects of treatment on withdrawal symptoms. Where possible, we report estimates of treatment effect based on meta-analysis, expressed as Peto odds ratios (OR)[7] with 95% confidence intervals (CI). An OR greater than 1 indicates more quitters in the intervention group. Although the absolute risk difference and number needed to treat are easier measures to interpret, they cannot be calculated reliably from the available data because of variations in baseline quit rates in different populations. There is evidence that the relative effects of treatment are constant, but the actual number of quitters achieved depends on the population offered the treatment. Treatment usually produces more quitters in populations with a higher baseline stopping rate (for example, motivated patients attending a specialist smoking clinic) and fewer when the baseline rate is lower (for example, all smoking patients attending a general practitioner).[8]

## Interventions

### Interventions from doctors and nurses

The effect of simple advice from doctors during routine clinical care has been studied in 31 trials including over 26 000 smokers. The studies were conducted in a variety of settings including primary care, hospital wards, outpatient clinics and industrial clinics.[9] The Cochrane review found that simple advice increased the quit rate (OR 1·69 [95% CI 1·45–1·98]). More intensive advice was slightly more effective. There is some evidence that the main effect of advice is to motivate a quit attempt, rather than to increase the chances of a success.[10] A recent Cochrane review found that interventions from nurses also increased quit rates.[11] Most of the studies included in this review assessed the impact of nurses providing specialised counselling rather than giving advice as part of routine clinical care. Studies of advice from nurses as part of general health promotion have not shown a similar effect.

## Behavioural and psychological interventions

Motivated smokers may seek further help from specialist smoking cessation counsellors or clinics. Treatment may be delivered one-to-one, or in a group. Both individual counselling and group therapy increase the chances of quitting.[12,13] Nine of 11 studies of individual counselling included in the Cochrane review compared counselling to brief advice or usual care.[13] The combined results favoured counselling (OR 1·55 [95% CI 1·27–1·90]). In 22 trials, group therapy programmes were more effective than self-help materials, but not consistently better than other interventions involving personal contact.[12] There was no difference between group and individual therapy in the two trials that included both. Groups are theoretically more cost-effective, but their usefulness may be limited by difficulties in recruiting and retaining participants.[14]

In the trials, the therapists were usually clinical psychologists, but the interventions drew on a variety of psychological techniques rather than a distinctive theoretical model. There is therefore little evidence about the relative effectiveness of different psychological approaches. The exception is aversion therapy, which pairs the pleasurable stimulus of smoking to an unpleasant stimulus with the goal of extinguishing the urge to smoke. The Cochrane review of 24, mainly small, trials of aversion therapy failed to detect an effect of non-specific aversive stimuli (for example, focusing on negative aspects of cigarettes while smoking). However, there was some evidence that rapid smoking (inhaling rapidly to induce nausea) increased the likelihood of quitting.[15] Silver acetate is a pharmacological method of aversive stimulation. It produces an unpleasant metallic taste when combined with cigarettes and is analogous to the use of disulfiram for alcoholism. Two studies with 6-month or greater follow up failed to detect a benefit with silver acetate, although confidence intervals were wide (OR 1·05 [95% CI 0·63–1·73]).[16]

## Self-help

The approaches used in one-to-one or group counselling can be delivered through written materials, audiotapes, videotapes or computer programmes. Self-help materials have the potential to reach many more people than therapist-delivered interventions. Many forms of self-help materials are available ranging from brief leaflets to complex manuals. They may be given as an adjunct to brief advice or without any personal contact.[17] The Cochrane review found that self-help materials had no additional benefit over brief personal advice. However, in 12 trials with no face-to-face contact, there was a small effect of self-help materials compared to no intervention (OR 1·23 [95% CI 1·02–1·49]).

More recent approaches have concentrated on ways of making self-help materials appropriate for the needs of individual smokers who differ in their reasons for smoking, level of addiction and motivation to quit. After collection of baseline information, smokers receive materials matched to their readiness to change,[18] or to other factors such as self-efficacy and motivation. In eight trials that compared individually tailored materials to standard or stage based materials, there was a benefit of the personalised intervention (OR 1·41 [95% CI 1·14–1·75]). There was no evidence that materials tailored solely to group characteristics (such as age, gender, or race) were better than standard materials.

Telephone contact may be an economical way of adding some personal contact to self-help materials. In 10 trials that compared proactive telephone counselling to a minimal intervention control, three showed a significant benefit, four showed a trend towards a benefit, and three showed non-significantly lower quit rates. Four trials provided telephone support following a face-to-face intervention, and did not show that this significantly improved long-term quit rates. Four trials that compared telephone support to use of nicotine replacement therapy alone failed to show an additional benefit of the counselling. Providing access to a hotline showed a significant benefit in one trial and was associated with lower quit rates in another. Varying the type of counselling provided did not affect outcome.[19]

Increasingly self-help materials are available on computer or through the internet, although there is as yet little evidence of whether the method of delivery affects the effectiveness of the materials.

## Nicotine replacement therapy (NRT)

The aim of NRT is to replace nicotine from cigarettes, thus reducing withdrawal symptoms associated with stopping smoking. NRT is available as chewing gum, transdermal patch, nasal spray, inhaler, sublingual tablet and lozenge. Over 90 trials of NRT have been reported. Although there is some evidence of publication bias (negative trials not published), the Cochrane review found that NRT does help people to stop smoking.[8] Overall, NRT increased the chances of quitting about 1·5- to 2-fold (OR 1·71 [95% CI 1·60–1·85]), whatever the level of additional support and encouragement. The quit rate was higher in

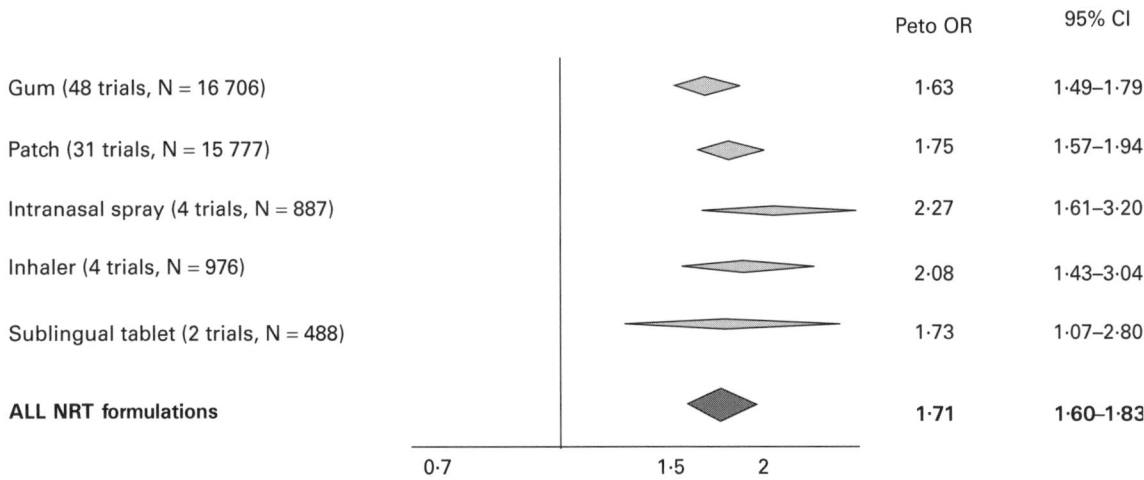

| | Peto OR | 95% CI |
|---|---|---|
| Gum (48 trials, N = 16 706) | 1·63 | 1·49–1·79 |
| Patch (31 trials, N = 15 777) | 1·75 | 1·57–1·94 |
| Intranasal spray (4 trials, N = 887) | 2·27 | 1·61–3·20 |
| Inhaler (4 trials, N = 976) | 2·08 | 1·43–3·04 |
| Sublingual tablet (2 trials, N = 488) | 1·73 | 1·07–2·80 |
| **ALL NRT** formulations | 1·71 | 1·60–1·83 |

**Figure 5.1**  Meta-analysis of the effect of nicotine replacement therapy trials on smoking cessation[5]

both placebo and NRT arms of trials that included intensive support, so the effect of NRT seems to be to increase the rate from whatever baseline is set by other interventions. Since all the trials of NRT reported so far have included at least some form of brief advice, this is the minimum that should be offered in order to ensure its effectiveness. Most studies of NRT have involved smokers with evidence of nicotine dependence. Its usefulness for less heavily dependent smokers is uncertain.

There is little direct evidence that any NRT product is more effective than another (Figure 5.1). Thus the decision about which to use should be guided by individual preferences. The nicotine patch delivers a steady level of nicotine throughout the day, and can be worn unobtrusively. The main side effect is skin irritation. Wearing the patch only during waking hours (16 hours a day) is as effective as wearing it for 24 hours a day. Eight weeks of patch therapy is as effective as longer courses and there is no evidence that tapered therapy is better than abrupt withdrawal. The nicotine inhaler resembles a cigarette and may be useful for individuals who want a substitute for the act of smoking. The nasal spray delivers nicotine more rapidly and may be suitable for satisfying surges of craving. Gum, spray, inhaler and lozenges may all cause local irritation in the nose or mouth. There is evidence that, for highly dependent smokers, a 4 mg dose of nicotine gum is more effective than a 2 mg dose.

Some clinicians recommend combinations of nicotine products (for example, providing a background nicotine level with patches, and controlling cravings with faster acting preparations such as gum or spray). There have been too few trials to provide clear evidence about the effectiveness of patch and gum combinations,[20,21] but one trial has shown significantly greater efficacy for nasal spray and patch than patch alone.[22]

### Antidepressants

There is both scientific and commercial interest in the neurochemical and genetic basis of tobacco dependence and its implications for therapy. Anxiolytics are not effective, but there is growing evidence that some antidepressants increase the likelihood of a quit attempt being successful.[23] Bupropion is an atypical antidepressant that is thought to inhibit neuronal uptake of noradrenaline and dopamine. A slow-release form is licensed for smoking cessation in many countries. There is evidence from six published trials and three unpublished studies that it increases the chances of quitting (OR 2·54 [95% CI 1·90–3·41]). These trials recruited heavier smokers who were also offered behavioural support. One trial found that bupropion alone or combined with a nicotine patch was more effective than nicotine patch alone.[24] On its own this finding is insufficient to define the relative efficacy of the two drugs.[25] Bupropion can cause dry mouth and insomnia, but serious side effects were rare in the trials. The manufacturers report a 0·1% risk of seizures using sustained-release bupropion up to 300 mg per day, and this is approximately the level at which they have been observed in practice.[26] Three trials have shown a benefit from the tricyclic antidepressant nortriptyline (OR 2·77 [95% CI 1·73–4·44]). Various other antidepressants have been tested for smoking cessation, but there is insufficient evidence to determine whether they are effective.[27]

It is unclear how antidepressant drugs aid smoking cessation. Smoking and depression are known to be linked, but whether this reflects a common genetic predisposition or neurochemical effects of nicotine is uncertain.[28] In the trials they were effective irrespective of whether depression was present. Whether efficacy for smoking cessation is drug-specific, or shared by classes of antidepressant drugs, is unresolved.

## Other pharmacological therapies

Although licensed primarily as an antihypertensive, clonidine shares some pharmacological effects with bupropion and tricyclic antidepressants. The Cochrane review of six clinical trials has shown evidence of efficacy (OR 1·89 [95% CI 1·30–2·74]), but its usefulness is limited by a significant incidence of sedation and postural hypotension.[29] The nicotine antagonist mecamylamine (used in the past for blood pressure reduction) has been investigated as a cessation aid in combination with nicotine replacement, but is not licensed for this use. The evidence from two studies suggests that there is an effect of mecamylamine, which begins precessation and continues postcessation, in aiding smoking cessation.[30] It is not clear whether this effect is significantly greater than that of nicotine replacement alone. The studies also suggest that the combination of mecamylamine with nicotine replacement, started before cessation, may increase the rates of cessation beyond those achieved with nicotine alone.

Lobeline is an alkaloid derived from the leaves of an Indian tobacco plant (*Lobelia inflata*). It was recognised in the early 1900s as a partial nicotinic agonist. The first reported use for smoking cessation was in the 1930s, and it has been used in proprietary smoking remedies. The Food and Drug Administration no longer permits it to be marketed in the United States, although Health Canada has recently licensed a quit aid containing lobeline. The Cochrane review identified no trials that met the inclusion criteria of 6 months follow up. An unpublished multicentre study of a sublingual tablet found no evidence of efficacy at 6 weeks.[31]

The possibility that release of endogenous opioids may play some part in the rewarding effects of nicotine has led to interest in opioid antagonists for smoking cessation. Two trials of naltrexone reported long-term cessation data. Both trials failed to detect a significant difference in quit rates between naltrexone and placebo. Meta-analysis failed to detect a significant effect of naltrexone on long-term abstinence, though confidence intervals were wide (OR 1·34 [95% CI 0·49–3·63]). No trials of naloxone reported long-term follow up.[32]

## Complementary therapies

The Cochrane review of 20 trials found no benefit of acupuncture compared to sham acupuncture. Acupuncture may be better than doing nothing, at least in the short term, but this may be a placebo effect.[33]

The Cochrane review of hypnotherapy found it no more effective than other behavioural interventions.[34] The nine trials identified were small and of variable quality. Hypnotherapy is particularly difficult to evaluate in the absence of a sham procedure that can control for non-specific effects.

A number of herbal preparations are advocated for smoking cessation, but none has been formally evaluated.

## Conclusions

Social attitudes, legislation and public health measures influence changes in tobacco use.[35] Against this background, many smokers give up without clinical intervention. Nevertheless, most health professionals believe that they have an obligation to offer help to individuals seeking to stop.[36] Current evidence shows that there is an increasing number of effective strategies available to individuals seeking to stop smoking and the health professionals who advise them. There are relatively few studies that have directly compared the available treatments, so it is difficult to recommend one approach over another. Many people who smoke make multiple attempts to quit, and will benefit from the availability of a number of different aids to help them.

## Acknowledgements

The Cochrane Tobacco Addiction Review Group is supported by a grant from the National Health Service and by the Imperial Cancer Research Fund.

---

**Summary box: effective strategies for stopping smoking**

- Brief advice from a physician
- Structured intervention from a nurse
- Individual counselling
- Group counselling
- Self-help materials (effectiveness limited unless individually tailored)
- Nicotine replacement therapy
- Bupropion
- Nortriptyline
- Clonidine

## References

1 Peto R, Lopez AD. The future world-wide health effects of current smoking patterns. In: Everett Koop C, Pearson CE, Schwarz MR eds. *Global Health in the 21st Century*. New York: Jossey-Bass (in press).

2 Hughes JR. Four beliefs that may impede progress in the treatment of smoking. *Tobacco Control* 1999;**8**:323–6.

3 Cochrane Tobacco Addiction Review group: http://www.dphpc.ox.ac. uk/cochrane_tobacco/

4 Raw M, McNeill A, West R. Smoking cessation guidelines for health professionals – a guide to effective smoking cessation interventions for the health care system. *Thorax* 1998;**53**:S1–S19.

5 Raw M, McNeill A, West R. Smoking cessation: evidence based recommendations for the healthcare system. *BMJ* 1999;**318**:182–5.

6 Cochrane Library abstracts: http://www.update-software.com/ccweb/ cochrane/revabstr/g160index.htm

7 Yusuf S, Peto R, Lewis J, Collins R, Sleight P. Beta blockade during and after myocardial infarction: an overview of the randomized trials. *Prog Cardiovasc Dis* 1985;**27**:335–71.

8 Silagy C, Mant D, Fowler G, Lancaster T. Nicotine replacement therapy for smoking cessation (Cochrane Review). In: *Cochrane Library*. Issue 1. Oxford: Update Software, 2001.

9 Silagy C. Physician Advice for smoking cessation (Cochrane Review). In: *Cochrane Library*. Issue 1. Oxford: Update Software, 2002.

10 Hughes JR, Goldstein MG, Hurt RD, Shiffman S. Recent advances in the pharmacotherapy of smoking. *JAMA* 1999;**281**:72–6.

11 Rice VH, Stead LF. Nursing interventions for smoking cessation (Cochrane Review). In: *Cochrane Library*. Issue 1. Oxford: Update Software, 2002.

12 Stead LF, Lancaster T. Group behaviour therapy programmes for smoking cessation (Cochrane Review). In: *Cochrane Library*. Issue 1. Oxford: Update Software, 2002.

13 Lancaster T, Stead LF. Individual behavioural counselling for smoking cessation (Cochrane Review). In: *Cochrane Library*. Issue 1. Oxford: Update Software, 2002.

14 Hollis JF, Lichtenstein E, Vogt TM, Stevens VJ, Biglan A. Nurse-assisted counseling for smokers in primary care. *Ann Intern Med* 1993;**118**: 521–5.

15 Hajek P, Stead LF. Aversive smoking for smoking cessation (Cochrane Review). In: *Cochrane Library*. Issue 1. Oxford: Update Software, 2002.

16 Lancaster T, Stead LF. Silver acetate for smoking cessation (Cochrane Review). In: *Cochrane Library*. Issue 1. Oxford: Update Software, 2000.

17 Lancaster T, Stead LF. Self-help interventions for smoking cessation (Cochrane Review). In: *Cochrane Library*. Issue 1. Oxford: Update Software, 2002.

18 Prochaska JO, Velicer WF. The transtheoretical model of health behavior change. *Am J Health Promot* 1997;**12**:38–48.

19 Lancaster T, Stead LF. Telephone counselling for smoking cessation (Cochrane Review). In: *Cochrane Library*. Issue 1. Oxford, Update Software, 2002.

20 Kornitzer M, Boutsen M, Dramaix M, Thijs J, Gustavsson G. Combined use of nicotine patch and gum in smoking cessation: a placebo-controlled clinical-trial. *Prev Med* 1995;**24**:41–7.

21 Puska P, Vartiainen E, Korhonen HJ, Urjanheimo EL, Gustavsson G, Westin A. Combined use of nicotine patch and gum compared with gum alone in smoking cessation: a clinical trial in North Karelia. *Tobacco Control* 1995;**4**:231–5.

22 Blondal T, Gudmundsson LJ, Olafsdottir I, Gustavsson G, Westin A. Nicotine nasal spray with nicotine patch for smoking cessation: randomised trial with six year follow up. *BMJ* 1999;**318**:285–8.

23 Hughes JR, Stead LF, Lancaster T,. Antidepressants for smoking cessation (Cochrane Review). In: *Cochrane Library*. Issue 1. Oxford: Update Software, 2002.

24 Jorenby DE, Leischow SJ, Nides MA *et al.* A controlled trial of sustained-release bupropion, a nicotine patch, or both for smoking cessation. *N Engl J Med* 1999;**340**:685–91.

25 Hughes JR. Smoking cessation. *N Engl J Med* 1999;**341**:610–11.

26 Glaxo Wellcome Inc. Zyban (bupropion hydrocholride) Sustained-Release Tablets Product Information. April 1999.

27 Niaura R, Spring B, Keuthen NJ *et al.* Fluoxetine for smoking cessation: A multicenter randomized double blind dose response study. *Ann Behav Med* 1997;**19**:S042.

28 Benowitz NL. Treating tobacco addiction – nicotine or no nicotine? *N Engl J Med* 1997;**337**:1230–1.

29 Gourlay SG, Stead LF, Benowitz NL. Clonidine for smoking cessation (Cochrane Review). In: *Cochrane Library*. Issue 1. Oxford: Update Software, 2002.

30 Lancaster T, Stead LF. Mecamylamine for smoking cessation (Cochrane Review). In: *Cochrane Library*. Issue 1. Oxford: Update Software, 2002.

31 Stead LF, Hughes JR. Lobeline for smoking cessation (Cochrane Review). In: *Cochrane Library*. Issue 1. Oxford: Update Software, 2002.

32 David S, Lancaster T, Stead LF. Opioid antagonist for smoking cessation (Cochrane Review). In: *Cochrane Library*. Issue 1. Oxford: Update Software, 2002.

33 White AR, Rampes H, Ernst E. Acupuncture for smoking cessation (Cochrane Review). In: *Cochrane Library*. Issue 1. Oxford: Update Software, 2002.

34 Abbot NC, Stead LF, White AR, Barnes J, Ernst E. Hypnotherapy for smoking cessation (Cochrane Review). In: *Cochrane Library*. Issue 1. Oxford: Update Software, 2002.

35 Chapman S. Unravelling gossamer with boxing gloves: problems in explaining the decline in smoking. *BMJ* 1993;**307**:429–32.

36 McAvoy BH, Kaner EF, Lock CA, Heather N, Gilvarry E. Our Healthier Nation: are general practitioners willing and able to deliver? A survey of attitudes to and involvement in health promotion and lifestyle counselling. *Br J Gen Pract* 1999;**49**:187–90.

# 6 Breast cancer prevention trials

*Jack Cuzick*

Following the observation that tamoxifen reduced the incidence of contralateral breast cancer when used in the adjuvant setting and had a low toxicity profile,[1,2] it was suggested[3] that prevention of breast cancer in high risk women might also be possible with this drug. A pilot study was initiated in 1986 under the auspices of the United Kingdom Coordinating Committee for Cancer Research (UKCCCR) at the Royal Marsden Hospital (RMH). As a result of the favourable compliance data and lack of unexpected toxicities in the RMH trial, the UKCCCR launched its main trial, the International Breast Cancer Intervention Study (IBIS-I) in 1992. Similar trials were initiated in the USA in 1992 under the auspices of the National Surgical Adjuvant Breast Project (NSABP) and in Italy. All trials were placebo-controlled studies of 5 years of tamoxifen administration.

These four trials have now reported on the use of tamoxifen as prophylaxis to prevent breast cancer. Relevant information is also available on side effects and new contralateral cancers from the overview of 11 adjuvant trials, which assessed the efficacy and safety of 3 or more years of tamoxifen treatment. The related selective oestrogen receptor modulator (SERM), raloxifene, has also been investigated in one trial.

A secondary prevention trial using the synthetic retinoid fenretinide to prevent contralateral tumours in women with low risk primary breast cancer has also been conducted.

Currently the STAR trial is comparing tamoxifen to raloxifene in 22 000 postmenopausal women at increased risk of breast cancer, and the IBIS II trial is comparing anastrozole to placebo in 6000 high risk postmenopausal women, and anastrozole to tamoxifen in 4000 postmenopausal women with completely locally excised DCIS. Pilot studies of the oestrogen agonist goserelin plus raloxifene versus placebo (IBIS RAZOR) are also being carried out among high risk premenopausal women.[4]

The main results of the tamoxifen trials have recently been overviewed and combined estimates of the main effects computed,[5] and this report relies heavily on that source. Data from the Multiple Outcome Raloxifene Evaluation (MORE) trial are also presented.

## Trials

Data from the International Breast Cancer Intervention Study I (IBIS-I), National Surgical Adjuvant Breast and Bowel Project P-1 Study (NSABP-P1), and MORE trial are based on material published in the original trial reports,[6–8] whereas those from the Royal Marsden Hospital and Italian studies were provided specifically for the meta-analysis report[5] and update published reports.[9,10,11] The adjuvant-trial data are taken from the 2000 overview and update a previous report.[2] Follow up was made up to January 2002 for the IBIS-I and the Royal Marsden trials, and up to February 2001 for the Italian trial, and about January 2000 for the adjuvant trials. No further follow up data are available for NSABP-P1 after March 31 1998, or for the MORE trial after November 1999.

Entry criteria for these trials varied and are shown in Table 6.1. Briefly, the Marsden trial focused more on younger women with very strong family histories; the P-1 and IBIS trials were similar, and the Italian trial entered only hysterectomised women, but did not require women to be at increased risk. The MORE trial was primarily a trial of osteoporosis treatment, and breast cancer was a secondary endpoint. All women were postmenopausal and substantially older on average than for the other trials. The tamoxifen adjuvant overview and fenretinide trials evaluated new contralateral cancers in women with early breast cancer. Specifically the fenretinide trial looked at the prevention of contralateral breast tumours in 2972 postmenopausal women with invasive cancer or DCIS. Fenretinide was used at a daily dose of 200 mg for 5 years and compared with placebo.[12,13]

## Results

### Breast cancer reduction

The incidence data are shown in Table 6.2. The combined data from the prevention trials supported a reduction in breast cancer incidence of 30–40% with tamoxifen (Figure 6.1). When analysed by a fixed-effect model, the reduction was 38% (95% CI 28–46; $P < 0.0001$) and all studies were

**Table 6.1    Breast cancer prevention trials which have reported efficacy results**

| Trial (entry dates) | Population | Number randomised | Agents (*v* placebo) and daily dose | Intended duration of treatment |
|---|---|---|---|---|
| Royal Marsden (1986–1996) | High risk Family history | 2471 | Tamoxifen 20 mg | 5–8 years |
| NSABP-P1 (1992–1997) | >1·6% 5 years risk | 13 388 | Tamoxifen 20 mg | 5 years |
| Italian (1992–1997) | Normal risk Hysterectomy | 5408 | Tamoxifen 20 mg | 5 years |
| IBIS-I (1992–2001) | >2-fold relative risk | 7139 | Tamoxifen 20 mg | 5 years |
| MORE (1994–1999) | Normal risk Postmenopausal women with osteoporosis | 7705 | Raloxifene 60 or 120 mg (3 arm) | 4 years |
| Adjuvant Overview (1976–1995) | Women with ER+ operable breast cancer in 11 trials | 14170 | Tamoxifen 20–40 mg with or without chemotherapy in both arms | 3 years or more (average ~5 years) |

**Table 6.2    Number of patients and breast cancer detected (by receptor status) in the prevention trials**

| | Royal Marsden | NSABP-P1 | Italian | IBIS-I | All tamoxifen prevention trials | Adjuvant (5 years tamoxifen) | MORE (raloxifene *v* placebo) | Fenretinide |
|---|---|---|---|---|---|---|---|---|
| Number randomised | 1238 *v* 1233 | 6681 *v* 6707 | 2700 *v* 2708 | 3573 *v* 3566 | 14 192 *v* 14 214 | 7 085 *v* 7 085 | 2 557 + 2 572 *v* 2 576 | 1496 *v* 1476 |
| *Breast cancers* | | | | | | | | |
| Total | 62 *v* 75 | 124 *v* 244 | 34 *v* 45 | 69 *v* 101 | 289 *v* 465 | 105 *v* 192 | 31/2 *v* 43 | 65 *v* 71 |
| Invasive | 54 *v* 64 | 89 *v* 175 | 28 *v* 40 | 64 *v* 85 | 235 *v* 364 | 105 *v* 192 | 22/2 *v* 39 | NA |
| DCIS | 7 *v* 7 | 35 *v* 69 | 5 *v* 4 | 5 *v* 16 | 52 *v* 96 | NA | 9/2 *v* 4 | NA |
| Unknown | 1 *v* 4 | | 1 *v* 1 | | 2 *v* 5 | | | NA |
| *ER status (Invasive only)* | | | | | | | | |
| Positive | 31 *v* 44 | 41 *v* 130 | 19 *v* 30 | 44 *v* 63 | 135 *v* 267 | NA | 10/2 *v* 31 | NA |
| Negative | 17 *v* 10 | 38 *v* 31 | 14 *v* 12 | 19 *v* 19 | 88 *v* 72 | NA | 9/2 *v* 4 | NA |

NA, not available

compatible with this result. When analysed by a random effects model, the reduction was 34% (95% CI 16–48; $P = 0.0007$). The adjuvant studies showed a slightly greater reduction of 46% (95% CI 31–57; $P < 0.0001$). An even larger reduction of 64% (95% CI 44–78) was found in the raloxifene trial. There was no significant heterogeneity among the tamoxifen trials ($P = 0.09$). However, the results of the MORE trial clearly differed, with the 95% CI not reaching the overall estimate of the tamoxifen prevention trials, leading to significant overall heterogeneity ($P = 0.03$).

There was no reduction in the incidence of ER-negative breast cancers (hazard ratio 1·22 [0·89–1·67]; Figure 6.2), but the incidence of ER-positive cancers was reduced by 48% (36–58) in the tamoxifen prevention trials and an even larger difference was seen for raloxifene (Figure 6.2). Age had no apparent effect on the degree of breast-cancer reduction ($P = 0.96$; hazard ratio 0·66 [0·52–0·85] for age < 50 years and 0·63 [0·51–0·77] for age ≥ 50 years).

In the fenretinide study there was no significant difference overall in contralateral tumours (65 fenretinide

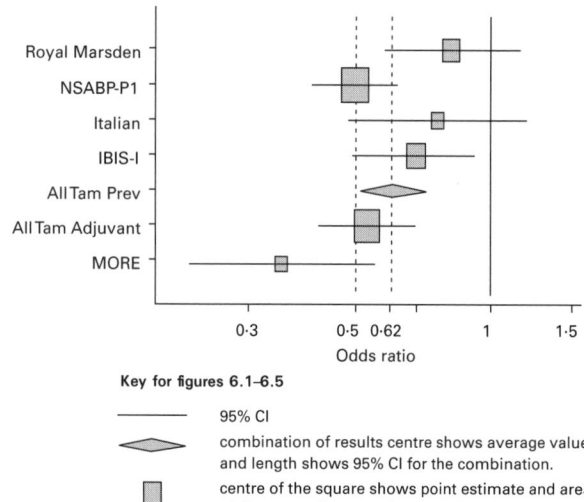

Key for figures 6.1–6.5

——————  95% CI

◆  combination of results centre shows average value and length shows 95% CI for the combination.

▨  centre of the square shows point estimate and area of the square is proportional to size of the trial.

**Figure 6.1**  Overview of all breast cancer, including DCIS, except adjuvant. Tam, tamoxifen; Prev, prevention.

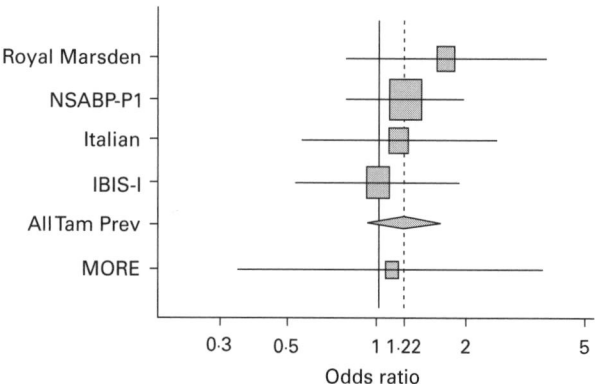

**Figure 6.2**  Overview of ER-negative invasive breast cancer. Tam, tamoxifen; Prev, prevention.

patients *v* 71 controls, *P* = 0·6) or ipsilateral recurrences (100 fenretinide *v* 121 placebo *P* = 0·17). However, there was some non-significant evidence for an effect in premenopausal women, where the hazard ratio for contralateral tumours was 0·66 (95% CI 0·41–1·07).

## Side effects

### *Endometrial cancer*

Rates of endometrial cancer were increased with tamoxifen in all prevention trials; the consensus relative risk was 2·4 (RR 1·5–4·0; *P* < 0·001; Figure 6.4). So far no increase in endometrial cancer has been observed with raloxifene. A larger risk was seen in the adjuvant studies

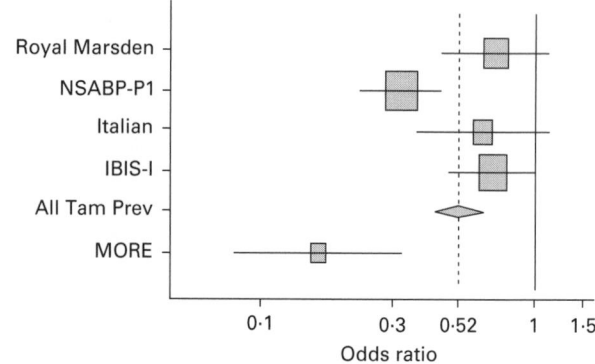

**Figure 6.3**  Overview of ER-positive invasive breast cancer. Tam, tamoxifen; Prev, prevention.

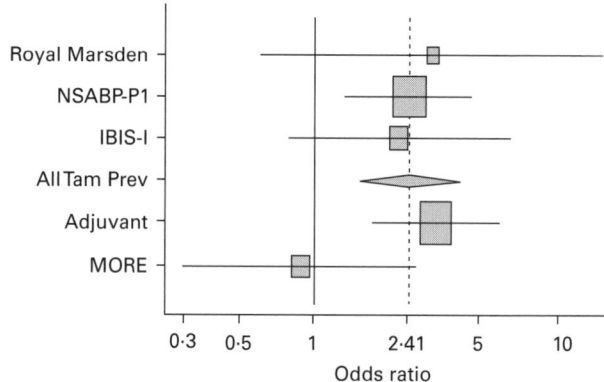

**Figure 6.4**  Overview of endometrial cancer. Tam, tamoxifen; Prev, prevention.

(hazard ratio 3·4 [1·8–6·4]; *P* < 0·001). Most of the excess risk is seen in women aged 50 years or older.

## Venous thromboembolic events

Venous thromboembolic events were increased in all studies; a relative risk of 2·0 (1·4–2·6; *P* < 0·001) was seen in the tamoxifen prevention trials, and similar results were observed in the MORE trial (Figure 6.5). The available data suggest that the relative risk is similar in women under and over age 50 at entry, although the absolute risk is higher in older women.

### *Other side effects*

Tamoxifen is also associated with a range of other side effects mostly related to oestrogen deprivation. These are mostly vasomotor and gynaecologic symptoms such as hot

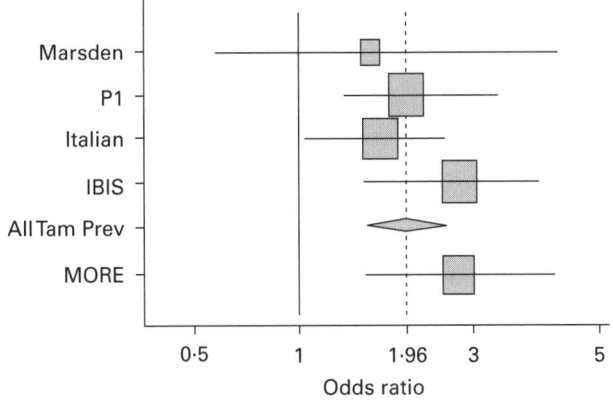

**Figure 6.5** Overview of thromboembolic events. Tam, tamoxifen; Prev, prevention.

not currently clear as to whether strokes are increased by this drug, although there are some data to suggest this.[7,14]

For the fenretinide trial, the most common adverse events were diminished dark adaptation (cumulative incidence, 19·0%) and dermatologic disorders (18·6%). Less common events were gastrointestinal symptoms (13·0%) and disorders of the ocular surface (10·9%). In comparison, incidence figures in the control arm were 2·9% for diminished dark adaptation, 2·9% for dermatologic disorders, 5·4% for gastrointestinal symptoms, and 3·2% for disorders of the ocular surface.

### Mortality

It is too soon to see a difference in breast cancer mortality in the trials. With the early closure of the P1 study, there may never be clear results, but this must still be monitored closely, as it is the most important endpoint, and the differential effect of tamoxifen on receptor-positive cancers makes it difficult to be sure that the effects on incidence will translate into mortality reductions. Other causes of death are similar except for a small increase in pulmonary embolism and a possible increase in endometrial cancer deaths.

flushes, vaginal discharge, and menstrual irregularities. A recent comprehensive summary has been published for the IBIS I trial (Table 6.3).[6] Cancers other than breast and endometrial appear to be unaffected by tamoxifen and it is

**Table 6.3 Side effects reported at any time or severity according to allocated treatment[6]**

| Side effect | Placebo n = 3567 | Tamoxifen n = 3573 | P value |
|---|---|---|---|
| Gynaecological/vasomotor | 2346 | 2880 | <0·001 |
| Headaches & migraines | 1060 | 988 | 0·12 |
| All gastrointestinal | 719 | 687 | 0·41 |
| All musculoskeletal (excluding fractures) | 474 | 453 | 0·51 |
| All osteoporotic fractures | 89 | 80 | 0·54 |
| Non-osteoporotic fractures | 60 | 51 | 0·45 |
| General symptoms | 416 | 379 | 0·2 |
| Breast complaints | 463 | 370 | 0·001 |
| Dermatological (excluding nails & hair) | 242 | 250 | 0·75 |
| Nail changes | 65 | 108 | 0·001 |
| Hair changes | 53 | 60 | 0·86 |
| All cardiovascular | 273 | 305 | 0·2 |
| Eye (excluding cataracts) | 248 | 237 | 0·65 |
| Cataracts | 26 | 30 | 0·69 |
| Urology & renal | 153 | 149 | 0·86 |
| All respiratory | 95 | 106 | 0·48 |
| Ear/nose/throat | 83 | 76 | 0·63 |
| Thyroid | 68 | 68 | 1 |
| Depressive illness | 22 | 38 | 0·05 |
| Other psychiatric | 24 | 30 | 0·5 |
| Haematological | 52 | 60 | 0·51 |
| Diabetes | 31 | 30 | 1 |
| Accidents | 24 | 16 | 0·27 |
| Dental | 18 | 13 | 0·47 |

## Current trials

New trials in postmenopausal women are focusing on evaluating the SERM raloxifene and the aromatase inhibitors.

The STAR trial is comparing raloxifene versus tamoxifen in 22 000 postmenopausal women at increased risk of breast cancer. The IBIS II trial is comparing the aromatase inhibitor anastrozole against placebo in 6000 postmenopausal women at increased risk, and against tamoxifen in a further 4000 postmenopausal women with locally excised DCIS. An NSABP trial is also comparing anastrozole versus tamoxifen in 3000 women with DCIS. A prevention trial of the steroidal aromatase inhibitor exemestane is also planned.

The options are more difficult for premenopausal women, where aromatase inhibitors are unlikely to be effective. However, the same approach of reducing oestrogen levels with a GnRH agonist is being studied in pilot studies. In the UK, goserelin with raloxifene as an add-back is being compared with placebo in very high risk premenopausal women (IBIS-RAZOR), and in Germany goserelin with a bisphosphonate add-back is being compared with placebo. Both these studies are in the pilot phase, and early indications are that it may be difficult to attract women to join these studies.[15]

## Current strength of evidence

The box below shows current strength of evidence for the various treatments discussed.

---

**Box 6.1 Strengths of evidence**

*Tamoxifen*

- Effective for preventing ER-positive tumours – Level Ia
- Ineffective for preventing ER-negative tumours – Level Ia

*Raloxifene*

- Effective for preventing ER positive tumours – Level Ib
- Ineffective for preventing ER negative tumours – Level Ib

*Anastrozole*

- Effective for preventing breast cancer – Level IIa

*Other aromatases*

- Inhibitors: no information
- GnRH agonists: indirect evidence based on ovarian ablation – effective at preventing breast cancer – Level IIa

---

## References

1  Cuzick J, Baum M. Tamoxifen and contralateral breast cancer (letter). *Lancet* 1985;**ii**:282.
2  Early Breast Cancer Trialists' Collaborative Group. Tamoxifen for early breast cancer: an overview of the randomised trials. *Lancet* 1998; **351**:1451–67.
3  Cuzick J, Wang DY, Bulbrook RD. The prevention of breast cancer. *Lancet* 1986;**ii**:83–86.
4  Cuzick J. A brief review of the current breast cancer prevention trials and proposals for future trials. *Eur J Cancer* 2000;**36**:1298–302.
5  Cuzick J, Powles T, Veronesi U *et al.* Overview of the main outcomes in breast-cancer prevention trials. *Lancet* 2003;**361**:269–300.
6  IBIS investigators. First results from the International Breast Cancer Intervention Study (IBIS-1): a randomised prevention trial. *Lancet* 2002;**360**:817–24.
7  Fisher B, Costantino JP, Wickerham DL *et al.* Tamoxifen for prevention of breast cancer: Repost of the National Surgical Adjuvant Breast and Bowel Project P-1 Study. *J Natl Cancer Inst* 1998;**90**: 1371–87.
8  Cauley JA, Norton L, Lippman ME *et al.* Continued breast cancer risk reduction in postmenopausal women treated with raloxifene: 4-year results from the MORE trial. *Breast Cancer Res Treat* 2001;**65**: 125–34.
9  Powles TJ, Eeles R, Ashley S *et al.* Interim analysis of the incidence of breast cancer in the Royal Marsden Hospital tamoxifen randomised chemoprevention trial. *Lancet* 1998;**352**:98–101.
10  Veronesi U, Maisonneuve P, Costa A *et al.* Prevention of breast cancer with tamoxifen: preliminary findings from the Italian randomised trial among hysterectomised women. *Lancet* 1998;**352**:93–7.
11  Veronesi U, Maisonneuve P, Sacchini V *et al.* Tamoxifen for breast cancer among hysterectomised women. *Lancet* 2002;**359**:1122–24.
12  Veronesi U, De Palo G, Marubini E *et al.* Randomized trial of fenretinide to prevent second breast malignancy in women with early breast cancer. *J Natl Cancer Inst* 1999;**91**:1847–56.
13  Camerini T, Mariani L, de Palo G *et al.* Safety of the synthetic retinoid fenretinide: long-term results from a controlled clinical trial for the prevention of contralateral breast cancer. *J Clin Oncol* 2001;**19**: 1664–70.
14  The ATAC (Arimidex, Tamoxifen Alone or in Combination) Trialists' Group. Anastrozole alone or in combination with tamoxifen versus tamoxifen alone for adjuvant treatment of post-menopausal women with early breast cancer: first results of the ATAC randomised trial. *Lancet* 2002;**359**:2131–9.
15  Evans D, Lalloo F, Shenton A, Boggis C, Howell A. Uptake of screening and prevention in women at very high risk of breast cancer. *Lancet* 2001;**358**:889–90.

# 7 Is cancer risk reduced by a health-enhancing diet?

*Rosalynne Weston*

## Background

Sir Richard Doll, in his Royal Society Lecture in 1986, first proposed that cancer risk might be reduced by dietary change; that modification of diet might reduce the incidence of specific cancers by up to a third. Animal studies showed that diet could influence the incidence of cancer in many different ways: by introducing into the body carcinogens, or substances from which carcinogens are formed *in vivo*, by affecting the metabolism of carcinogens and the body's reaction to them. He also speculated that diet might hold the key to the control of some cancers, especially three of the four major cancers: breast, stomach and large bowel.

Assessing the evidence from animal studies and patient case–control studies he concluded that there could be no increased preventative and beneficial effects from additional intake of vitamin A. For vitamin E, beta-carotene and selenium the evidence from case–control and cohort studies was sufficiently strong to suggest the desirability of increasing the consumption of fruit, green vegetables and fibre.[1]

Diet and cancer studies demonstrate that generally vegetables and fruit, dietary fibre and certain specific nutrients seem to protect against cancer. It is hard, however, to demonstrate how this mechanism works, to prove conclusively that specific foods actually reduce the risk of cancer at specific sites. Research demonstrates the hypothetical relationship between excessive fat, calories, and alcohol and increased cancer risk. Chemoprevention research is closely linked to diet and represents a logical research progression. Epidemiological dietary studies have helped to identify many naturally occurring chemopreventative agents and randomised controlled studies are ongoing and specifically targeted at the prevention of breast, colorectal, lung and prostate cancer.[2]

Epidemiological studies, animal and *in vitro* studies suggest that there is a relationship between dietary constituents and the risk of cancer at some specific sites. Vegetables, fruits, dietary fibre, and certain specific micronutrients appear to protect against cancer. Data, however, are not consistent across studies. Food is a complex mixture of nutrients and non-nutritive substances that are difficult to unravel and measure accurately. Individual differences, including genetic susceptibility, also constitute a risk.[3]

The Working Group on Diet and Cancer of the Committee on Medical Aspects of Food and Nutrition (COMA Committee, DH, England) and other international government health and cancer voluntary agencies have reviewed the evidence for the cancer protective potential of diet as have the International Agency for Research on Cancer who recently published three meta-analyses on specific vitamins A, carotenoids and retinoids.[4-6] As a result many statutory and non-statutory agencies have issued healthy eating guidelines encouraging individuals to change their behaviour, to eat a health-enhancing diet in order to reduce their risk of specific cancers and other major degenerative diseases (Box 7.1). The evidence is less consistent for specific foods or micronutrients.

The committee also assessed the evidence for the cancer-related risk from obesity and physical exercise and the International Agency for Research on Cancer recently published a meta-analysis on weight control and physical activity. There is evidence of an exponential risk for weight and body mass increase, especially obesity, for some cancers. These require a chapter in their own right and are not specifically addressed in this chapter. Weight control and physical exercise, however, remain necessary components of any public cancer education and prevention programme.[7]

## Diet as a primary prevention strategy to reduce the incidence of specific cancers – a summary of the evidence

### Dietary fat and cancer

Epidemiological evidence suggests a direct relationship between total fat intake, the consumption of animal fat, and increased risk at several sites, including postmenopausal breast, colorectal and prostate cancers.[8-10] Migrant studies demonstrate that a change from a low fat high fibre Eastern diet toward a high fat low fibre Western diet results in a

**Box 7.1 Healthy eating guidelines**

These are consistent in their advice about dietary change and can be summarised as:

- Consume a life-long, varied diet rich in plant foods including fruit and whole grains
- Include fruit and vegetables in every meal
- Use fruits and vegetables as snacks
- Substitute beans for meat
- Select whole grain products
- Include high fibre foods in the diet
- Intake of fatty foods should be restricted
- Meat portions should be small relative to plant servings
- Meat should be trimmed of fat
- Fish and poultry should be preferred to meat
- Limit intake of food fried in fats and oils
- Limit additions of fats and oils to prepared foods
- Alcoholic beverages should be limited or avoided
- Foods should be stored and prepared in ways that reduce microbial and fungal contamination
- Fresh foods should be properly cleaned before storage
- Perishable foods should be refrigerated
- Limit consumption of salted, nitrate treated, smoked and pickled foods
- Avoid charred foods
- Reduce the use of added salt during food preparation and eating
- Dietary intake and energy expenditure should be balanced. Avoid increases in weight and obesity and extreme low weight
- Eat small portions of high calorie foods
- Exercise to maintain weight
- Supplementary vitamins and minerals should not be relied upon for a balanced and adequate diet
- Maximise intake of essential nutrients by including vitamin- and mineral-rich foods
- Use supplements only for needs not adequately provided for in the diet

rise of breast cancer incidence: 1·6 times higher for Asian–American women born in the West than those from the East.[6] Case–control and cohort studies have not found a significant association between fat intake and breast cancer incidence and a meta-analysis of 23 studies reports an RR of 1·21 for case–control and 1·01 for cohort studies. This is concordant with the results from a recent meta-analysis of cohort studies with an RR of 1·05.[9,11]

Several factors may account for such inconclusive evidence between fat and breast cancer risk: diet before adulthood, the methodology used in individual studies, inaccurate estimates of dietary assessment and genetic susceptibility, as well as breast cancer heterogeneity within

specific populations. International correlation studies show strong associations between colorectal incidence and intake of red meat or animal fats.[5,12] Case–control and cohort studies, including those using adenomatous polyps as markers of risk, support this association with red meat.

The data on fat are less consistent.[6,13] Cross-cultural and migrant studies support the suggestion that a Western diet is associated with increased disease risk for prostate cancer.[14] A review of epidemiological studies found that numerous case–control and cohort studies indicate a consistent relationship between prostate cancer and consumption of either fat or high fat foods, especially red meat.[5] A multi-ethnic study in the USA and Canada reported a significant direct association with fat with the highest risk for Asian–Americans. Different saturated fat intake accounted for only approximately 10% of Black/White difference and 15% Asian/American/White differences in prostate cancer incidence indicating that there may be an aetiological role for other environmental factors or genetically determined variations.[5]

Type of fat appears to be important in cancer development. Data for international correlations in case–control studies link animal fat and red meat to colon cancer risk.[6,11,15] For prostate cancer, some data suggest that alinoleic acid appears to increase risk (RR = 3·43). Saturated fat (RR = 0·95), monosaturated fat (RR = 1·58) and linoleic acid (RR = 0·64) show no significant association with risk. The relationship between breast cancer and type of fat is unclear. Saturated and omega-6 polyunsaturated fat has been correlated with breast cancer risk.[11] In a recent study saturated fat showed no association (RR = 0·95), whereas total polyunsaturated fatty acids (RR = 0·70), oleic acid (RR = 0·81) and monosaturated fatty acid showed an inverse relationship with breast cancer risk. Consumption of olive oil (of which oleic acid is a major constituent) appears to reduce cancer risk (R = 0·87).[16]

International correlation studies show highly unsaturated omega-3 fatty acids, found in fish oils, are not associated with increased breast cancer risk but that these have been hypothesised to be protective.[17]

The COMA committee found that there was weak evidence to support risk reduction of breast cancer by reducing red and fried meat consumption. The evidence that greater adiposity, particularly central adiposity and weight gain during adulthood, increases the risk of postmenopausal breast cancer is strong. Greater height and earlier menarche are both influenced by diet and are associated with higher risk of breast cancer. Lifetime exposure to circulating oestrogens may account for the effects of obesity and early menarche. Epidemiological data show moderately consistent evidence of a relationship between high red and fried meat consumption and a higher risk of breast cancer.

For lung cancer there is weakly consistent evidence for a weak association between high consumption of red meat and increased risk of lung cancer. Smoking remains the main risk factor for lung cancer. There was weak evidence to support red meat consumption with increased risk for colorectal cancer. For prostate cancer the association was weak and for preserved meats and gastric cancer there was insufficient evidence to suggest an association between risk reduction and intake. The evidence is weak for the risk reducing potential of reduced red meat intake for pancreatic cancer.

For total intake of fat COMA found that there was moderate evidence to support the hypothesis that total fat intake in adult life does not influence the risk of breast cancer independently of BMI (Body Mass Index). There was weak evidence to support the hypothesis that total fat intake did influence the risk of colorectal cancer. There was not enough evidence to conclude that total fat intake influences the risk of prostate cancer.[18]

## Vegetables, fruits and whole grains

Epidemiological data provide strong evidence that high intakes of vegetables, fruits and whole grains are associated with reduced cancer risk. Reviews of case–control and prospective cohort studies found a relationship between high vegetable and fruit intake and reduced cancer risk, which appears strongest for cancers of the alimentary canal and respiratory tract, colon, lung, oesophagus and oral cavity, and weakest for hormone-related cancers such as breast, ovary, cervix, endometrium and prostate.[19] Reduced cancer risk has been linked to the consumption of raw vegetables and fresh fruit (citrus, carrots, green leafy vegetables and cruciferous vegetables) soy products and whole grain wheat products.[17,20] It is not clear whether such beneficial effects are related to these individual foods or combinations, including the interrelationship with fibre, micronutrients and phytochemicals. Studies on micronutrients, nutrients and non-nutrients are difficult to assess because of the problems of separating these substances.

The COMA committee found that there was weak evidence to suggest that high consumption of fruits and vegetables does reduce the risk of breast cancer. Higher intakes of fruit and vegetables do not mitigate the overwhelming effects of smoking to reduce the risk of lung cancer. Higher intakes do not reduce the risk of colorectal cancer but there was moderate evidence to suggest that higher intakes of fruits and vegetables could reduce the risk of gastric cancer but that these would not reduce the risk of oesophageal cancer. They did, however, recommend increasing the overall intake of fruits and vegetables.[18]

## Dietary fibre

This is usually defined as a group of endogenous compounds in plant foods that are resistant to digestive enzymes but that may play a beneficial, though not clearly defined role, in reducing the risk of cancer. Epidemiological studies generally support the hypothesis that fibre has cancer-protective properties and some demonstrate that fibre may modulate the risk-enhancing effects of dietary fat.[21,22] There was a lower incidence of colon cancer risk in Finland than in Denmark or New York. Finland has an average intake of high dietary fibre, twice that of the other two, even though all three had high dietary intake (34–37%).[23,24] The type of fibre may be important to cancer risk reduction. Wheat bran appears to inhibit colon cancer in animals more effectively than other sources of bran.[25] Current clinical studies are focusing on the difference and the possible protective mechanisms of various fibre types at different subsites within the colon.[26]

Some epidemiological studies suggest an inverse relationship between fibre and fibre-rich foods and breast cancer risk. The overall influence of fibre on breast cancer risk relative to other foods is far from clear.[27,28] The risk for breast cancer may (as well as other hormone-dependent cancers) be influenced by the modulating effects of fibre metabolism or actions at cellular level.[26] Dietary fibre may influence oestrogens primarily associated with breast cancer aetiology through the alteration of the microbial population and enzymes in oestrogens, and so the amount available for reabsorption. Phyto-oestrogens, which appear to compete with oestrogens for receptor-binding sites, may potentially reduce breast cancer risk and are produced in the intestine from fibre-related precursors.

The COMA committee found that there was not enough evidence to draw conclusions on the relationship between dietary fibre and the risk of breast cancer, but there is moderate evidence to suggest that diets rich in fibre reduce the risk of colorectal cancer.[18]

## Micronutrients

Epidemiological studies have demonstrated cancer preventative properties for foods high in antioxidants such as vitamin C, beta-carotene, vitamin E and selenium, as well as the micronutrients vitamin A, calcium and folate. There has been consistent support for the preventative effect of vitamin C for cancers of the stomach, oesophagus, and oral cavity, and moderate protective effects for cancers of the cervix, rectum, breast and lung. Recently data from clinical trials suggest a possible preventative effect for vitamin E in colorectal and prostate cancer and many epidemiological studies support the role of dietary calcium in colon cancer.[29]

The COMA committee found that for vitamins A, C, E and beta-carotene there was not enough evidence to conclude that the intake of vitamins A, C and E modulates the risk of breast cancer. The evidence from intervention trials provides moderate evidence that beta-carotene supplements do not mitigate the risk of lung cancer, and that these may indeed have adverse effects. There is not enough evidence to draw conclusions on vitamin E specifically and the risk of lung cancer. Neither is there evidence to conclude that these vitamins modulate the risk of colorectal cancer, prostate or gastric, cervical, or oesophageal cancer.[18]

## Phytochemicals

Fruit and vegetables contain a variety of phytochemicals, for example terpenes, organosulphides, isothiocyanates, indoles, dithiolthiones, polyphenols, flavones, tannins, protease inhibitors, non-vitamin A-active carotenoids, that have hypothetical potential cancer preventative effect. Common fruits and vegetables contain about 50 carotenoids, compounds that exhibit antioxidant activity. Lutein (found in yellow and orange fruits and vegetables) and lycopene especially abundant in tomatoes and tomato-based foods have very strong antioxidant activity. A large prospective epidemiological study reported that an increased intake of lycopene and tomato-based foods might be associated with reduced cancer risk.[1]

The mechanisms of possible cancer prevention effects are not clear and may be varied. It is thought that brassinin, found in cabbage, might block carcinogenic action by activating and inducing phase 11 enzymes involved in xenobiotic detoxification. Curcumin, a compound in tumeric, may inhibit colon tumourgenesis by modulating arachidonic acid metabolism. Separation and understanding the actions of such phytochemicals may prove very difficult and thus conclusive evidence may remain impossible.[30]

## Alcohol

Epidemiological data suggest that associations between alcohol consumption and cancer vary by site and type of alcoholic beverage. Alcohol intake is reported to be directly associated with cancers of the oral cavity, pharynx, oesophagus and larynx, where alcohol is synergistically active with smoking and thus increases risk. A meta-analysis of studies linking alcohol consumption and breast cancer incidence reports an estimated 25% increase in risk for daily alcohol intake equivalent to two drinks, as well as a dose–response relationship.[31] Analysis of data from the Health Professionals Follow-Up Study showed that men who drank more than two drinks daily, for example 30 g of alcohol, had twice the risk of developing colon cancer, especially of the distal colon, as men who drank less than

one quarter of a drink daily. Inadequate intake of folate and methionine increases alcohol-associated risk for cancer of the distal colon approximately seven-fold, even after adjustment for age, history of polyps/endoscopy, smoking, level of physical activity, body mass index, intakes of red meat and total energy, as well as multivitamin use.[32,33]

Two major population trials are testing the efficacy of low fat, high fibre, high fruit and vegetable intake for the protective effect for major degenerative disease including cancer.

### *Ongoing research: the Polyp Prevention Trial*

This was a multicentre randomised controlled dietary intervention examining the effect of a low fat (20% of calories from fat), high fibre (18g/1000 calories), high vegetable and fruit (five to eight servings per day combined) dietary pattern on the occurrence of adenomatous polyps of the large bowel. As polyps are precursors of most colorectal cancers, an intervention reporting a reduction in polyp occurrence would suggest that the same intervention would be successful in reducing cancer incidence. The trial provided 90% power to detect a reduction of 24% in the annual adenoma recurrence rate. A total of 1905 randomised subjects (91·6%) completed the study. Of the 958 intervention group subjects and the 947 control subjects who completed the study, 39·7% and 39·5% respectively had a least one recurrent adenoma: unadjusted risk ratio 1·00 (95% CI 0·90–1·12). Among subjects with recurrent adenomas the mean (± SE) number of such lesions was $1·85 \pm 0·07$ in the control group. The rate of recurrence of large adenomas (maximal diameter of at least 1 cm or at least 25% villous elements or evidence of high dysplasia, including carcinoma) did not differ significantly between the two groups.

The authors conclude that adopting a diet that is low in fat and high in fibre, fruits and vegetables does not influence the risk of colorectal adenomas.[33]

### *The Women's Health Initiative*

This is a 10-year study due to report in 2003. It is a multidisciplinary trial including dietary and chemopreventative interventions intended to examine the effectiveness of a low fat eating pattern (20% calories from fat), high fruit, vegetable and fibre intake, hormone replacement therapy, and calcium and vitamin D supplementation for cancer preventative effects, cardiovascular disease and osteoporosis prevention in 63 000 postmenopausal women of all races and socioeconomic status. It includes a prospective surveillance of a further 100 000 women for aetiological factors and predictors of illness. Community-based intervention studies are an integral part of this intervention intended to provide information on effective ways to promote cancer, cardiovascular and osteoporosis preventative behaviours.

## Conclusions

Current evidence suggests that a health-enhancing diet can reduce the risk of specific cancers at some sites. Such a diet includes the control of body mass index and obesity and therefore includes regular moderate exercise. These are integral elements for planned interventions for improving healthy eating in populations.

Many food interactions *in vitro* are extremely complex and conclusive evidence of the risk reduction potential of specific foods, and their protective mechanisms, is not yet available, and so general population messages are still the main primary intervention strategy for most individuals. High risk individuals, by definition of phenotype, genetic disposition, familial patterns, and lifestyle behaviour may require specific dietary interventions to reduce risk, instigated and monitored by primary care practitioners.

Such interventions require long-term behaviour change and this has implications for primary care. Behaviour change interventions require effective maintenance strategies to ensure behaviour change becomes a long-term habit. Smoking cessation effectiveness evidence has demonstrated the benefits of such approaches. Healthy eating interventions should now learn from smoking cessation interventions and implement similar strategies especially for high risk individuals.[5,34]

Research for such primary prevention interventions needs to concentrate on the development of effective interventions and long-term evaluation of such. This has two purposes: to provide evidence of effectiveness that in turn feeds into the intervention planning cycles with the express purpose of improving interventions.[34]

Research continues on specific foods and their risk reduction potential for cancer at specific sites, as well as for their hypothesised general protective effects. The results from long-term clinical trials will provide data on the role of diet in the prevention of chronic diseases.[35] The results will guide future research and intervention planning. Future research could be enhanced by combining chemoprevention approaches with modifications in eating behaviour, especially for those with high risk. More effective methods for identifying individuals at high risk are increasingly important. Primary care practitioners are an important focal point for identifying these individuals and for developing and monitoring tailored interventions for them. Identifying subtypes of disease (for example different tumour types) for those at high risk may result in specific site cancers being viewed as heterogeneous diseases, therefore encouraging a variety of preventative approaches. Finding effective

prevention strategies is important to be able to make further progress against this complex disease. As development is also complex, over 20 years or more, we need to be able to find interventions that are effective in preventing initiation or, at the very least, halt early development of the disease. This remains a priority.[35]

In the meantime the consistent advice for statutory health agencies and for non-government agencies, especially those dealing with cancer, is for general population interventions using a health-enhancing diet as described in Box 7.1.

## References

1 Doll R. *Possibilities for the Prevention of Cancer*. Lecture for the Royal Society of London, 13th November 1986.
2 Greenwold P, McDonald S. National Cancer Institute (NCI). Maryland: Scientific Consulting Group Address, 2001.
3 Kosary CL, Ries LAG, Miller BA *et al*, eds. *Tables and Graphs, SEER Cancer Statistics Review*. Maryland: NCI, 1995.
4 National Academy of Sciences, National Research Council, Commission of Life Sciences, Food and Nutrition Board. *Diet and health: Implications for reducing chronic disease risk*. Washington DC: National Academy Press, 1989.
5 US Department of Health and Human Services. *The Surgeon General's Report on Nutrition and Health*. National Institute of Health (NIH) Publications No. 8850210. Washington DC: Public Health Service Office, 1988.
6 Rose DP, Boyer AP, Wynder EL. International comparisons of mortality rates for cancer of the breast, ovary, prostate and colon and per capita food consumption. *Cancer* 1986;**58**:2363–71.
7 Nomura AM, Kolonel LN. Prostate cancer, a current perspective. *Epidemiol Rev* 1991;**13**:200–27.
8 Roberts-Thompson I, Ryan P, Khoo K. Diet, acetylator phenotype and risk of colorectal neoplasia. *Lancet* 1996;**347**:1372–4.
9 Boyd NF, Martin JJ, Noffel M. A meta-analysis of studies of dietary fat and breast cancer risk. *Br J Cancer* 1993;**68**:627–36.
10 Hunter DJ, Spiegelman D, Adami HO. Cohort studies of fat intake and the risk of breast cancer- a pooled analysis. *N Engl J Med* 1996;**334**:356–61.
11 Hursting SD, Thornquist M, Henderson MM. Types of dietary fat and the incidence of five cancer sites. *Prev Med* 1990;**19**:242–53.
12 Giovannucci E, Rimm EB, Stampfer MJ. Intake of fat, meat and fibre in relation to colon cancer in men. *Cancer Res* 1994;**54**:2390–7.
13 Giovannucci E, Willett WC. Dietary factors and risk of colon cancer. *Ann Med* 1994;**26**:443–52.
14 Whittemore AS, Kolonel LN, Wu AH. Prostate cancer in relation to diet, physical activity and body size in blacks, whites and Asians in the USA and Canada. *J Natl Cancer Inst* 1995;**87**:652–61.
15 Potter JD, Slattery ML, Bostick RM. Colon cancer, a review of the epidemiology. *Epidemiol Rev* 1993;**15**:499–545.
16 Giovannucci E, Rimm EB, Colditz GA *et al.* A prospective study of dietary fat and risk of prostate cancer. *J Natl Cancer Inst* 1993;**85**:1571–9.
17 La Vecchia C, Negri E, Franceschi S. Olive oil, other dietary fats and the risk of breast cancer (Italy). *Cancer Causes Control* 1995;**6**:545–50.
18 Nutritional Aspects of the Development of Cancer. *Report of the Working Group on Diet and Cancer of the Committee on Medical Aspects of Food and Nutrition Policy, No. 48*. Department of Health, UK. London: The Stationery Office, 1998.
19 Steinmetz KA, Potter JD. Vegetables, fruit and cancer prevention, a review of the epidemiological evidence. *Cancer Causes Control* 1991;**2**:325–57.
20 Negri E, La Vecchia CL, Franceschi S. Vegetable and fruit consumption and cancer risk. *Int J Cancer* 1991;**48**:350–4.

21  Jacobs Jr DR, Slavin J, Marquart L. Whole grain intake and cancer, a review of the literature. *Nutr Cancer* 1995;**24**:221–9.

22  Kritchevsky D, ed. *Evaluation of Publicly Available Scientific Evidence Regarding Certain Nutrient Disease Relationships, 5. Dietary Fibre and Cancer. Food Safety and Applied Nutrition.* FDA, DHHS. Washington, DC: Life Sciences Research Office, 1991.

23  Reddy B, Hedges A, Laasko K. Metabolic epidemiology of large bowel cancer, fecal bulk and constituents of high risk. North American and low risk Finnish populations. *Cancer* 1978;**42**:2832–8.

24  Jenson OM, MacLennon R, Wahrendorf J. Diet, bowel function, fecal characteristics and large bowel cancer in Denmark and Finland. *Nutr Cancer* 1982;**4**:519.

25  Folino M, McIntyre A, Young GP. Dietary fibres differ in their effects on large bowel epithelial proliferation and fecal formation, dependent events in rats. *J Nutr* 1995;**125**:1521–8.

26  Zhang J, Lupton JR. Dietary fibres stimulate colonic cell proliferation by different mechanisms at different sites. *Nutr Cancer* 1994;**22**: 267–76.

27  Lipworth L. Epidemiology of breast cancer. *Eur J Cancer Prev* 1995;**4**:730.

28  Byers T, Guerrero N. Epidemiological evidence for beta-carotene and cancer prevention. *Am J Clin Nutr* 1995;**62**:1385–92.

29  The Alpha-Tocopherol Beta-Carotene Cancer Prevention Study Group. The effect of vitamin E and beta-carotene on the incidence of lung cancer and other cancers in male smokers. *N Engl Med J* 1994;**330**:1029–35.

30  Rao CV, Rivenson A, Simi B. Chemoprevention of colon cancer by dietary curcumin, a naturally occurring plant phenolic compound. *Cancer Res* 1995;**55**:259–66.

31  Giovannucci E, Rimm EB, Ascherio A *et al.* Alcohol, low methionine, low folate diets and risk of colon cancer in men. *J Natl Cancer Inst* 1995;**87**:265–273.

32  Kato I, Nomura AM. Alcohol in the aetiology of upper areodigestive tract cancer. *Eur J Cancer* 1994;**30B**:7581.

33  Schatzkin A, Lanza E, Corle D *et al.* Lack of effect of a low fat, high fibre diet on the recurrence of colorectal adenomas, Polyp Prevention Trial Study Group. *N Engl J Med* 2000;**342**:1149–55.

34  Lancaster T. Which interventions help individuals to stop smoking?. In: Williams C, ed. *Evidence-Based Oncology,* London: BMJ Books, 2003.

35  Scott D, Weston R. *Evaluating Health Promotion.* Cheltenham: Nelson Thorne, 1998.

# 8 Is cancer risk reduced by the intake or supplementation of retinoids and carotenoids?

*Rosalynne Weston*

## Background

The International Union of Cancer, the World Health Organization's research programme in the International Agency for Research on Cancer, the National Cancer Institute, and the UK COMA report have reviewed the role of specific micronutrients for their cancer risk reducing potential at specific sites.[1–4] These meta-analyses were located by a standard search on Medline and PubMed. Isolating specific substances in the diet of individuals/ populations remains problematic because of the complexity of cultural and individual preferences, food availability, cultivation practices, climate, processing and preservation practices, and food diaries as reliable records of intake.[1] Research is continuing because micronutrients and chemoprevention remain possible cancer risk reducing agents. Evidence for their preventative effect is not consistent and often contradictory.

The toxicity of vitamin A at high doses limits its use as a preventative agent. Toxic effects are seen in various organs, skin, circulation (hypertriglyceridaemia), liver, nervous system and bones. The developing embryo may be affected by vitamin A supplements. This has led to the development of thousands of synthetic retinoids designed to have better specific properties but with lower toxicity. The therapeutic index relationship has been considered for these agents for all included studies.[1]

Vitamin A and retinyl esters are hypothesised as possible effective agents for certain preneoplastic lesions. Vitamin A and its metabolite action is understood to be due to the action of retinoid receptors (of which six isoforms are known). Each receptor mediates a set of unique biological functions in certain cells or tissue types, and retinoids with varying receptor profiles have consistently been associated with inhibition of cell growth, cell differentiation, and cell death: apoptosis and prevention of angiogenesis. Vitamin A is used as the generic name for preformed vitamin A (all transretinol and its esters) and some of the carotenoids.[1]

## Carotenoids

Beta-carotene is the best characterised of a large group of carotenoid pigments that are widely distributed in vegetables and fruit, and the normal constituents of blood and tissues of humans, birds, fish and cattle. The seven predominant carotenoids in humans are beta-carotene, lycopene, lutein, alpha-carotene, alpha-cryptoxanthin, beta-cryptoxanthin, and zeaxanthin. Epidemiological evidence supports the hypothesis that high intakes and high serum levels are associated with lower incidence of cancers but the chemoprevention trials using beta-carotene have been unable to prove this hypothesis and have provided some evidence for detriment in smokers and asbestos high risk individuals. A meta-analysis using case–control and prospective blood studies found that beta-carotene provided no benefit and could be harmful in high doses, and there is little evidence that the protective effects of diets rich in carotene-containing fruits and vegetables are due to any individual carotenoid.[5]

## Specific confounding problems with food intake research

One of the problems with the research on dietary intake and specific food substances such as vitamin A, carotenoids, and retinoids is that studies have been performed at very different levels of vitamin A nutritive status. Vitamin A deficient status would be unethical for humans, hence the proliferation of animal studies. Vitamin A studies have mostly been measured by relative dose–response tests and have been case–control studies. Case–control studies provide limited evidence for causal relationships with vitamin A intake. The results may not be accurate if the controls are not representative of the population (selection bias). Obtaining accurate and reliable data about food intake from both case and controls remains problematic, and recall bias may also be a confounding variable, especially if there has been recent publicity or health education initiatives: individuals are more likely to give expected favourable answers. For patients who are very ill and for those who have died, information by proxy, for example from a spouse, may be all that is available. These biases are very important when searching for small effects. The differences between highest and lowest categories of intake can be obscured by minor degrees of bias.

The major advantage of cohort studies (prospective or follow up studies) is the assessment of diet before the onset of disease. Selection bias is not such a problem as the comparison group for the cases is explicit (non-cases in the cohort). The major limitation is that a large group of subjects need to be enrolled and followed for many years to provide sufficient cancer diagnosis to achieve statistical power. For rare cancer types, or sites, a prospective study may never accrue enough cases. They are also limited to exposure data collected at the beginning of the study, unless blood samples have been taken and stored. Most investigators record information using food frequency questionnaires. In the main these are useful, but they are imperfect research instruments. Willett *et al.*[6] showed that a correlation between total vitamin A intakes, estimated from a 61-item food frequency questionnaire, compared with 4 weeks of diet records, in a population of women in the USA, was $r-0.5$ ($P < 0.05$).

Case–control studies are problematic for other reasons: cancer and cancer treatment usually reduce retinol levels from pretreatment values. Consequently case–control studies that relied solely on blood retinol levels were omitted from the review. A further confounding problem is fat-saturated foods that are high in preformed vitamin A, such as dairy products. There may be an artefactual positive association with preformed vitamin A at sites where cancer has a positive relation with saturated fat. This may be the case whenever total vitamin A intakes reflect intake of provitamin-rich vegetables; confounding by other potentially anticarcinogenic nutrients in these vegetables is a problem. If vitamin supplements were used, the details of these were given only if they were evaluated. The limited observational studies on supplement use for cancer risk were not included in the IARC meta-analysis.[1]

The COMA report reviewed the evidence on dietary links (carcinogenic and protective) for a number of cancers including micronutrients from epidemiological studies, intervention trials (randomised controlled trials), case–control studies, prospective cohort studies, nested case–control studies, observational studies, and ecological and migrant studies. The summary evidence for carcinogenic risk and risk reduction is mainly from prospective cohort and case–control studies and is therefore open to interpretation, cultural bias and over generalisation.[3]

## Evidence for cancer risk reduction potential of retinols for specific cancer sites

### Lung cancer

The largest body of evidence for the cancer-preventative effects of vitamin A exists for lung cancer. Case–control studies reported an inverse association between total vitamin A intake and lung cancer although there were exceptions.[1] Two studies reported that an increased consumption of fruit and vegetables was associated with significantly decreased risk, but the association was strongest for vegetables that are poor sources of vitamin A.[1]

Generally the studies that examined preformed vitamin A and carotenoid intake separately showed no association, or only a weak association of intake of preformed vitamin A and reduced cancer risk. Most of these studies have observed an inverse association with increased carotenoid consumption.[1] One study reported follow up data on another from an extended cohort (168 cases) and observed a relative risk (RR) of 0.5 for high versus low intake of vitamin A. This inverse association was mostly attributable to the intake of carrots and other vegetables, with some additional contribution from milk. This study reported a more consistent beneficial effect of carotenoid sources of vitamin A than for preformed vitamin A.[7] Preformed vitamin A was reported independently after 19 years follow up (in 2107 men, 33 cases occurred) in one study and was found to be weakly positively associated with disease risk. A strong inverse association was observed for carotenoid intake, which was similar in magnitude for smokers and non-smokers.[8] One study observed little protective effect of total vitamin A or preformed vitamin A, but a moderate decrease in lung cancer risk, in both men and women, in the upper tertile of carotenoid intake, and another observed a weak positive relationship with preformed vitamin A among smokers; yet another observed little evidence of any association with total vitamin A (24-hour recall estimates of dietary intake) and an RR of 1.3 for high versus low intake of preformed vitamin A.[9,10]

Blood retinols were found to be poor indicators of preformed vitamin A intake but blood carotenoids did reflect carotenoid intake. A protective effect of being in the highest category of blood beta-carotene level or total carotenoid intake was a remarkably consistent finding in the nested case–control studies. None, however, observed a significant association with blood retinol levels. Observational studies (including case–control and prospective) support the effect of higher intakes of foods containing carotenoids on the risk of lung cancer but suggest that it is possible that other components of carotenoid-rich foods may be responsible for the apparent effect of carotenoids. This requires further research. The data support the conclusion that dietary intake of preformed vitamin A does not influence cancer risk.

## Cancers of the aerodigestive tract

Two studies found direct associations significant in males. This included the largest investigation on this topic, 831 cases and 979 controls which yielded RRs of 1·6 in men ($P$ trend = 0·007) and 1·4 ($P$ trend = 0·27) in women in the highest quartile of intake, with another finding a significantly reduced risk for the highest tertile for vitamin A intake.[11,12] Eight case–control studies evaluated the relationship between retinol intake and cancer of the oesophagus and approximately two-fold elevated RRs were reported in four investigations, the largest from Calvados in France with one study reporting adjustment for total energy intake.[13] No studies reported risk reduction in individuals reporting a high retinol intake.

For cancer of the larynx three case–control studies suggested either an elevated risk after allowance for total energy intake, one reporting little or no effect on risk reduction.[14] For cancer of the hypolarynx, risk was elevated, with an RR of 0·6 observed in the highest quartile for preformed vitamin A. A prospective study of postmenopausal women in USA reported RRs of 0·9 (95% CI 0·4–2·2) based on 33 cases of cancer of the oral cavity, pharynx and oesophagus.[15,16]

Mean levels of retinol and total retinoids were very similar in cancer cases and 138 controls in a cohort of 6832 American men of Japanese ancestry. Serum levels were measured 6 years before diagnosis of cancer of the oral cavity and larynx (16 cases), oesophagus (28 cases) or larynx (23 cases).[17] Four studies reported RRs for intake of vitamin A supplements and or multivitamin preparations. These reported systematically below unity reporting RRs of 0·4 (95% CI 0·2–0·8) for 10 or more years of vitamin A supplement use. This was seen consistently in men and women and after adjustment for vitamin E intake (the strongest protective factor) became 0·6 (95% CI 0·3–1·4).[11,18]

## Gastric cancer

Most evidence for gastric cancer is from case–control studies that observed a positive association between total vitamin A intake, as reported by next of kin, and gastric cancer risk. One study observed a strong inverse association with beta-carotene but not preformed vitamin A.[19] Five studies reported an inverse association with beta-carotene but not for retinol, with yet another reporting a strong positive association with preformed vitamin A intake and a significant inverse association with beta-carotene.[20–24] No association of preformed vitamin A with cancer risk was

reported in one study, with another observing no relationship between serum retinol levels and the subsequent risk of gastric cancer but a modest inverse trend with beta-carotene levels.[25,26] Substantial data suggest that components of carotenoid-rich vegetables are protective against gastric cancer but no data suggest that preformed vitamin A has such an influence.[1]

## Colon cancer

Evidence for colon cancer comes mostly from case–control and cohort studies that report a weak positive relationship between preformed vitamin A intake and colon cancer mortality ($r = 0·27$) after adjustment for animal fat and cereal fibre intake. There was essentially no association with reduced risk and the intake of vegetables and fruits (the main source of carotenoids).[27,28] No substantial protective association of preformed vitamin A or carotenoids among either men or women was found in one study, with another observing no overall relationship. In a sex-specific analysis of this study, a modest protective association with total vitamin A intake among women was observed, adjusted for age and energy only.[29,30] One study, however, observed a significant inverse association with higher intake of beta-carotene after adjusting for age, obesity, crude fibre, and energy intake; no significant association was observed for total vitamin A, and one study found no protective effect.[31] High retinol intake was inversely associated with colon cancer (RR in highest $v$ lowest intake quintile, 0·7; 95% CI, 0·5–0·9) in one study, although this was not the case for rectal cancer risk (corresponding RR, 0·8; 95% CI, 0·6–1·1).[32]

One large case–control study of the colon and rectum between 1992 and 1996, in six areas of Italy, using more detailed validated food frequency questionnaires and food consumption tables, found that retinol was not associated with either colon or rectal cancer.[33] No substantial protective effects of either preformed vitamin A, provitamin A, or carotenoids were found in another. One study observed a modest non-significant inverse association between higher intake of total vitamin A and both colon and rectal cancer; (RR, 0·7; $P$ trend = 0·1) and (RR, 0·8; $P$ trend = 0·4) respectively, with a similar inverse association being observed between preformed vitamin A intake for colon (RR, 0·7; $P$ trend = 0·2) but not for rectal cancer (RR, 1·0; $P$ trend = 0·8). Subjects in the upper quintile of serum retinol were at reduced risk of colon cancer (RR, 0·3; 95% CI, 0·1–0·8) after up to 9 years of follow up. These results should be treated with caution because of the limitations of serum retinol levels.[34,35] One other study observed higher median levels of retinol but lower levels of beta-carotene among men who subsequently developed colon cancer compared with controls.[36] There is little evidence from these studies to suggest that vitamin A is protective against colon cancer as data are sparse and inconsistent. Animal fat and fibre may be important determinants of colon cancer and more studies that carefully control for these are needed.[1]

## Skin cancer

One case–control study for both squamous cell carcinoma (SCC) and basal cell carcinoma (BCC), three cohort studies (for BCC and SCC, and one for BCC only), and one prospective blood study of which three were conducted with Caucasian populations reported a wide range of disease risk and no effect of vitamin A intake on cancer risk. The risk estimates in individual studies were generally greater than unity and in each instance the 95% CI included 1·0.[36–38] Two prospective studies have reported on the relationship between prediagnostic levels of retinol and melanoma; both reported no significant association (30 and 10 cases) with reduced risk or incidence.[9,38] This is consistent with the findings of a case–control study of melanoma and dietary intake of preformed vitamin A. There is insufficient evidence to suggest that vitamin A or preformed vitamin A reduces the risk of skin cancer either for basal cell carcinoma or squamous cell carcinoma.[40]

## Breast cancer

Six case–control studies consistently reported an inverse association between intake and risk for total vitamin A. Four case–control studies reporting on preformed vitamin A observed modest decreases in risk with higher intake.[41–44] A further seven studies found no association. A meta-analysis of 12 case–control studies showed that the RR in the highest quintile for total vitamin A intake was 0·9 ($P = 0.04$), for beta-carotene 0·9 ($P = 0.0007$), and for preformed vitamin A 1·0 ($P = 0.52$). The RR comparing the highest tertile of total vitamin A intake with lowest tertile was 0·8 ($P > 0.05$); for preformed vitamin A the risk was 0·7 ($P > 0.05$).[45] A further follow up study reported (89 494 nurses) an RR of 0·8 (95% CI, 0·7–1·0) for women in the highest quintile of total vitamin A intake compared with lowest. The comparable relative risk for preformed vitamin A was 0·8 (95% CI, 0·7–1·0). The association for total vitamin A was slightly stronger among premenopausal women (RR, 0·8) than postmenopausal (RR, 0·9).[46] One study observed evidence suggestive of an inverse association for both total vitamin A and preformed vitamin A, but others with postmenopausal women observed no relationship with disease risk for either total vitamin A or preformed vitamin A.[47–50] Studies of blood retinol and breast cancer risk were limited with one study reporting a non-significant lower risk associated with higher retinol levels at baseline. Case–control data for breast cancer are compatible with modest inverse associations with higher intakes of vitamin A as for lung cancer; this association is somewhat stronger for total vitamin A than for preformed vitamin A.[51]

## Prostate cancer

There is little consistency in the data from a range of studies for the protective effect of vitamin A. One case–control study observed a positive association between higher intakes of total vitamin A and risk of prostate cancer and a case–control study of Black men observed a positive association, statistically significant in the subgroup of men aged 30–49 years. Another reported a significantly elevated relative risk for consumption of high levels of total vitamin A but not preformed vitamin A among men aged 70 and older in Hawaii. The findings were essentially null for men aged < 70 years. In a further evaluation of this study the excess risk was found to be almost entirely attributable to increased consumption of papaya (which is very high in carotenoids but not retinol) among cases. Most other studies have not confirmed this increased risk. No elevated risk was observed for beta-carotene from other food sources.[52]

One study in Japan observed an inverse association for beta-carotene concordant with studies for African–Americans (the relation was null in White populations) and Canadian men,[53,54] and another observed an elevation in risk with higher intake of vitamin A for men aged 68 years or older, but not among younger men.[55] One study observed no association of vitamin A intake with cancer risk (RR in highest $v$ lowest tertile 1·1, 95% CI, 0·8–1·6).[56] In another study, a direct association emerged for men aged 70 years or more (RR, 2·2 95% CI, 1·1–4·2) with yet another observing a weak positive association between retinol intake and prostate cancer. A significant trend of decreasing risk of prostate cancer with increasing intake of preformed vitamin A was reported in another study.[57–59]

There were very little prospective data on which to base conclusions with one study reporting an elevated risk for men in the highest tertile of total vitamin A mainly attributable to an increased supplement of vitamin A. In a 20-year follow up study of 17 633 White men, no overall association between vitamin A intake and risk of prostate cancer was observed, but in another there was an elevated risk for men aged less than 75 years balanced by an inverse association for men aged 75 years or older. A significant positive association with retinol intake, stronger for men over 70 years of age, was reported in another study. There is no consistent evidence that dietary vitamin A protects against prostate cancer. Initial studies suggesting adverse effects have not been consistently confirmed. The possibility that higher intakes may increase risk requires further investigation. As most preformed vitamin A is derived from foods of animal origin, it is possible that other factors in animal foods may be associated with increased risk of prostate cancer, or there may be other confounding factors associated with incidence or development of prostate disease.[46,60,61]

## Bladder cancer

There have been few observational studies on the relationship of vitamin A and bladder cancer. One large hospital case–control study reported a lower risk associated with higher levels of total vitamin A intake; the measures included vitamin A in plant and animal sources.[55] Four population-based case–control studies found no association with vitamin A, with another in the USA finding a lower risk for those in the highest quintile of preformed vitamin A.[56,62–65] These studies do not support the hypothetical association between dietary preformed vitamin A intake and the risk of bladder cancer.

## Cervical cancer

A large case–control study found no association between vitamin A and cervical cancer (sources: meat and milk) with another three reporting little association between preformed vitamin A intake and cancer risk.[66] Three studies found little or no association with retinol intake and cervical cancer and one reported that the point estimates for high versus low intake of vitamin A were less than unity, but the effect was relatively small, 10–20% reduction and not statistically significant. A re-evaluation of one of these studies analysed serum retinol levels and found a weak positive association for serum retinol and a weak inverse relationship with beta-carotene.

The available data suggest there is no relationship between preformed vitamin A intake and risk of cervical cancer.[67–70]

## Large scale primary prevention intervention studies: cancer as endpoint

These large-scale phase III clinical trials are considered the best means available to test whether dietary or chemopreventative interventions reduce cancer risk. These aimed to determine the cancer-preventative effectiveness of the intervention and identify and validate potential biomarkers as surrogate endpoints for cancer.

There is no consistent evidence from six population trials (The Linxian Trials [The National Cancer Institute, USA and North China], the completed Beta-Carotene Trials, the Wittenoom Trial, and The South-West Skin Cancer Prevention Studies 1 and 2 [Arizona, USA 1984–88]).

The CARET study showed there was a significantly elevated risk in the retinol and beta-carotene supplement group compared to the placebo group, except for subjects who had stopped smoking. The risk of carcinoma of the lung among asbestos miners with lung cancer was less common in the retinol group than in the beta-carotene group but the difference was not statistically significant. It is possible that retinol may be less harmful than beta-carotene or have no effect.

In the CARET trial (crocidolite-exposed workers in Australia), retinol appeared to lead to a reduction in incidence of mesothelioma, whereas in the CARET study retinol in combination with beta-carotene reported no such reduction. Further studies on the effect of retinol on mesothelioma are needed. The two Lixian studies did not support the benefit of retinol even in a nutrient deficient population. In the Skin Trial no benefit was found with respect to basal cell carcimoma of the skin. For squamous cell carcinoma, a risk reduction of about 25% in moderate risk individuals is difficult to reconcile with the lack of benefit in high risk individuals but the endpoint details have still not been published for this study.[70,71]

## Systemic biomarker studies

Studies, using biomarkers as intermediate endpoints, have been performed in relation to oral leukoplakia and oesphageal dysplasia. Of the premalignant lesions leukoplakia is the best studied. Studies in developing countries have shown the best results, but how far these should be extrapolated to other populations remains unclear.

### Reversal of oral premalignancy

In cancer prevention trials and other studies the efficacy of agents (retinoids, retinol, or beta-carotene) in reversing oral leukoplakia has been demonstrated. These studies show that retinol seems to be active in oral leukaplakia. Occurrences after treatment suggest that it is difficult to be certain that these results can be extrapolated to other oral cancers. Owing to trial designs it is difficult to assess the benefits of high doses of vitamins.[72,73]

### Skin

The National Co-operative Group Trial with early stage cutaneous melanoma thicker than 0·75 mm tested whether vitamin A (100 000 IU orally and daily for 18 months) increased disease-free or overall survival: 248 patients were randomised to vitamin A (N = 121) with eight late stage exclusions. Median follow up exceeded 8 years. No differences emerged between the two groups (RR, 1·1; $P = 0·71$) for survival and (RR, 1·2; $P = 0·41$), for disease-free survival. These results were upheld after subset analysis by sex, type of therapy, and Breslow thickness. Overall 12% of patients who received vitamin A experienced severe toxicity. An Indian trial (second primaries of head and neck) involved 11 of 56 patients in the vitamin A group who had locoregional recurrence compared with 5 of 50 and 10% in the placebo group who showed a non-significant difference.[1]

## Lung

One randomised placebo-controlled trial using beta-carotene and retinol to reduce the incidence of sputum atypia showed no significant reduction in sputum atypia after treatment with 50 mg beta-carotene per day and 25 000 IU of retinol per day on alternate days. This resulted in significant increases in serum concentrations of both with no significant toxicity. No significant reduction in sputum atypia was observed after treatment compared with placebo.[74]

## Cervical dysplasia

Trials comparing serum levels of vitamin A and carotene in patients with cervical intraepithelial neoplasia (CIN) reported no significant evidence of vitamin A deficiency. Two studies found that high plasma levels of retinol were related to the regression of CIN while another found that mean plasma levels of carotenoids and α-tocopherol were significantly lower in women with CIN and cervical cancer.[75]

## Larynx

One trial for laryngeal squamous cell hyperplasia using retinyl palmitate at 30 000 IU daily and increasing for resistant lesions with a maintenance dose at 150 000 IU daily, reported 15 out of 20 cases showing complete response, and in five more a partial response.[76]

## Pharyngeal

A nested case–control study in the USA investigated the possible relationship between dietary intake and risk of second primary tumours in a cohort of 1090 oral and pharyngeal cancer patients. Individuals in the highest risk intake quartile showed RRs of 1·6 of developing a second primary compared with the lowest quartile (*P* value of chi square for trend, 0·09). Only one of these randomised studies showed a significant benefit from supplementation

(that is, a significant delay in new primary tumours after resection of the lung cancer).[77]

## Oesophagus and stomach

A randomised double-blind intervention trial in China (using retinol, riboflavin, and zinc), designed to test whether these supplements could lower the prevalence of precancerous lesions, reported a significantly lower number of lesions in those where retinol increased over the years. It is hypothesised that improvement of vitamin A status may reduce inflammatory lesions in the oesophagus. These findings were subjected to logistical regression analysis combining all data.[78,79]

## Colorectal

Two case–control studies and one Spanish study provide limited evidence that previtamin A (RR, 0·7; 95% CI, 0·4–1·1 for highest tertile) compounds in fruit and vegetables are protective but no association for retinol was found. This limited evidence would support a protective role for previtamin A compounds in fruit and vegetables but no significant association for retinol in colorectal adenomas.[80]

## Prevention of second primary cancers

After epidemiological studies of vitamin A and cancer began to be published in the 1970s, several clinical trials tested the efficacy of retinoids and, less frequently, vitamin A as adjuvant therapy in patients in relation to different malignancies. In one study of adjuvant therapy of high doses of vitamin A in 307 patients with Stage 1 non-small cell lung cancer in Milan, Italy, the onset of second primaries was significantly delayed in the treatment group ($P = 0·045$ log-rank test). There were no significant differences in overall survival.[81]

A chemoprevention study in curatively treated patients with oral laryngeal cancer and lung cancer (EUROSCAN) started in June 1988. Treatment was aqueous emulsified retinyl palmitate (300 000 IU per day for a year, and half this dose during a second year, or both drugs or neither in a $2 \times 2$ factorial design) 2595 patients from 81 institutes in 14 countries were enrolled and, of these, 1566 (60·4%) had head and neck cancer and 1029 had lung cancer. Of those receiving palmitate, 10% stopped because of side effects but no other complications were observed.[82]

One study compared the efficacy of two multiple vitamin regimes (RDA doses *v* high doses) in diminishing recurrences of transitional cell carcinoma of the skin. Sixty-five patients (11 women) were randomised to receive, in addition to other vitamins, B1, B2, B3, B5, B6, B12, C, D3, E, folic acid, and zinc (either 5000 [N = 30] or 4000 IU [N = 35]) of retinyl acetate daily. After 12 months of treatment there were 11 recurrences (37%) in the RDA group and three (9%) in the high dose group (HDG) ($P = 0 \cdot 008$ Fisher's exact test). Overall recurrence rates were 80% (24/30) and 40% (14/35) and survival rates were similar (75% RDA $v$ 76% HDG).[82]

## Beta-carotene

Results of epidemiological studies, viewed in aggregate, do not support the notion that beta-carotene has generalised cancer prevention effects. Observational data suggest that cancer prevention effects are not consistent for lung, oral, or pharyngeal cancers, the incidences of which tend to be inversely related to beta-carotene (or provitamin A carotenoid) intake or blood concentrations. Beta-carotene may only be a marker of the intake of other beneficial substances in fruits and vegetables or perhaps lifestyle habits. No clinical trial of beta-carotene as a single agent has shown a reduction in the risk of cancer at any specific site, and there is evidence of an increased risk for lung cancer among smokers and asbestos workers receiving beta-carotene supplements at high doses, which resulted in blood concentration levels on average 10–15 times higher than normal. Information from these controlled trials is based on 12 years of intervention and there are no data available for effects for longer intervention. There is no information available on beta-carotene supplementation early in the carcinogenic process and doses in intervention trials greatly exceed normal daily intakes. There is only limited inconsistent information on carotenoids other than beta-carotene.[5]

## Conclusions

For some sites there is limited evidence for the cancer-preventative effect of vitamin A in animals and there is even less evidence for such an effect in humans. There is little evidence of the cancer-preventative effect for preformed vitamin A for cancers of the upper aerodigestive tract, lung, breast (among postmenopausal women), colorectal, bladder, prostate and stomach. Studies have demonstrated that there is inadequate evidence for the possible cancer-preventative activity of preformed vitamin A at all other sites and for second primary cancers of the lung. Furthermore there is little evidence to support the hypothesis that, within a wide range of doses taking into account deficiency and toxicity, modulating preformed vitamin A intake will have any substantial cancer-preventative effect. There is, however, evidence suggesting a lack of cancer prevention activity of

beta-carotene when used as a supplement at high doses, but there is inadequate evidence for the cancer-preventative effect of beta-carotene at usual dietary levels. There is inadequate evidence for the possible cancer-preventative effect of other individual carotenoids.

Research continues to enable clarification of dose–response relationships for the possible protective effect and toxic effects of micronutrients. Until there is strong conclusive evidence, the implications for practice in primary care and health promotion (the health community) are to promote a health-enhancing diet to populations that includes BMI and weight control through moderate regular exercise. High-risk individuals may require specialist interventions and primary care specialists remain critical to their identification. Behaviour change is main intervention aim especially for long-term maintenance of healthy eating. There is a need for longitudinal randomised trials that include outcome measures for behaviour change relating to healthy eating, weight control and excercise. The results of these are important if health professionals more easily instigate and support such change.

## References

1  IARC. Vitamin A, Vol. 3. Lyon, France: IARC Press, 1988.
2  National Cancer Institute Diet and Nutrition Programme. Bethesda, MD, 1998.
3  International Union of Cancer. *Health Enhancing Diet*. Geneva: UICC, 2001.
4  Department of Health. Working Group on Diet and Cancer of the Committee on Medical Aspects of Food and Nutrition Policy. *Nutritional Aspects of the Development of Cancer*. Report 48. The Stationery Office: London.
5  IARC. Carotenoids, Vol. 2. Lyon, France: IARC Press, 1988.
6  Willet WC, Sampson L, Stampfer MJ *et al*. Reproducibility and validity of a semi-quantitative food frequency questionnaire. *Am J Epidemiol* 1985;**122**:51–65.
7  Kvale G, Bjelke E, Gart JJ. Dietary habits and lung cancer risk. *Int J Cancer* 1983;**31**;397–405.
8  Shekelle RB, Lepper M, Liu S *et al*. Dietary vitamin A and risk of cancer in the Western Electric Study. *Lancet* 1981;**2**:1185–90.
9  Paganini-Hill A, Choa A, Ross RK. Vitamin A, beta-carotene and the risk of cancer: a prospective study. *J Natl Cancer Inst* 1987;**79**:443–8.
10  Knekt P, Jarvinen R, Seppanen R *et al*. Dietary anti-oxidants and the risk of lung cancer. *Am J Epidemiol* 1991;**134**:471–9.
11  McLaughlin JK, Gridley G, Block G *et al*. Dietary factors in oral and pharyngeal cancer. *J Natl Cancer Inst* 1988;**80**:1237–43.
12  Gridley G, McLaughlin JK, Block G, Blot WJ, Winn DM, Greenberg RS. Vitamin supplement use and reduced risk of oral and pharyngeal cancer. *Am J Epidemiol* 1990;**135**:1083–92.
13  Graham S, Marshall J, Mettlin C, Rzepka T, Nemoto T, Byers T. Nutritional epidemiology of cancer of the oesophagus. *Am J Epidemiol* 1990;**131**:454–67.
14  Freudenheim JL, Graham S, Byers TE *et al*. Diet, smoking and alcohol in cancer of the larynx: a case-control study. *Nutr Cancer* 1992;**17**:33–45.
15  MacKerras D, Buffler PA, Randall DE, Nichaman MZ, Pickle LW, Mason TJ. Carotene intake and the risk of laryngeal cancer in coastal Texas. *Am J Epidemiol* 1988;**128**:980–8.
16  Esteve J, Riboli E, Pequignot G, Terracini B, Merletti E, Crosignani P. Diet and cancers of the larynx and hypopharynx: the IARC

multi-centre study in southwestern Europe. *Cancer Causes Control* 1996;**7**:240–52.

17 Nomura AM, Stemmermann GN, Ziegler RG, Chyou PH, Craft NE. Serum micronutrients and upper aerodigestive tract cancer. *Cancer Epidemiol Biomarker Prev* 1997;**6**:407–12.

18 Gridley G, MacLaughlin JK, Block G *et al.* Diet, oral cancer and pharyngeal cancer among blacks. *Nutr Cancer* 1990;**14**:219–25.

19 Stehr PA, Gloninger MF, Kuller LH, Marsh GM, Radford EP, Weinberg GB. Dietary vitamin A deficiencies and stomach cancer. *Am J Epidemiol* 1985;**121**:65–70.

20 Risch HA, Jain M, Choi NW *et al.* Dietary factors and the incidence of cancer of the stomach. *Am J Epidemiol* 1985;**122**:947–59.

21 La Vecchia C, Negri E, Decarli A, D'Avanzo B, Franceshi S. A case-control study of diet and gastric cancer in northern Italy. *Int J Cancer* 1987;**40**:484–9.

22 You WC, Blot WJ, Chang YS *et al.* Diet and high risk of stomach cancer in Shandong, China. *Cancer Res* 1988;**48**:3518–23.

23 Buiatti E, Palli D. Decarli A *et al.* A case-control study of gastric cancer and diet in Italy: II Association with nutrients. *Int J Cancer* 1990;**45**:896–901.

24 Gonzalez CA, Riboli E, Badosa J *et al.* Nutritional factors and gastric cancer in Spain. *Am J Epidemiol* 1994;**139**:466–73.

25 Graham V, Surwit ES, Weiner S, Meyskens FLJ *et al.* Phase II trial of beta-all-trans-retinoic acid for cervical intraepithelial neoplasia delivered by a collagen sponge and cervical cap. *West J Med* 1986;**145**:192–5.

26 Nomura AM, Stemmermann GN, Chyou PH *et al.* Gastric cancer among Japenese in Hawaii. *Jap J Cancer Res* 1995;**86**:916–23.

27 McKeowen-Eyssen GE, Bright-See E. Dietary factors in colon cancer: international relationships. *Nutr Cancer* 1994;**6**:160–70.

28 Potter JD, McMichael AJ. Diet and cancer of the colon rectum: a case-control study. *J Natl Cancer Inst* 1986;**76**:557–69.

29 Lyon JI, Mahoney AW, West DW *et al.* Energy intake: its relationship to colon cancer risk. *J Natl Cancer Inst* 1988;**78**:853-61.

30 West DW, Slattery, ML, Robison LM *et al.* Dietary intake and colon cancer: sex-and anatomic site-specific associations. *Am J Epidemiol* 1989;**130**:883–94.

31 Grahm S, Marshall J, Haughey B *et al.* Dietary epidemiology of cancer of the colon in western New York. *Am J Epidemiol* 1988;**128**:490–503.

32 Ferraroni M, La Vecchia C, D'Avanz, B, Negri E, Franceshi S, Decarli A. Selected micronutrient intake and the risk of colorectal cancer. *Br J Cancer* 1994;**70**:1150–5.

33 La Vecchia C, Bragag C, Negri E *et al.* Intake of selected micronutrients and risk of colorectal cancer. *Int J Cancer* 1997;**73**:525–30.

34 Heibrun LK, Nomura A, Hankin JH, Stemmermann GN. Diet and colorectal cancer with special reference to fibre intake. *Int J Cancer* 1989;**44**:1–6.

35 Nomura AM, Stemmermann GN. Serum vitamin levels and the risk of cancer of specific sites in men of Japanese ancestry in Hawaii. *Cancer Res* 1985;**45**:2369–72.

36 Hunter DJ, Colditz GA, Stampfer MJ, Rosner B, Willett WC, Speizer FE *et al.* Diet and risk of basal cell carcinoma of the skin in a prospective cohort of women. *Ann Epidemiol* 1992;**2**:231–9.

37 Middleton B, Byers T, Marshall J, Graham S *et al.* Dietary vitamin A and cancer: a multi-site case-control study. *Nutr Cancer* 1986;**8**:107–16.

38 Kune GA, Bannerman S, Field B *et al.* Diet, alcohol, smoking, serum beta-carotene and vitamin A in male non melanocytic skin cancer patients and controls. *Nutr Cancer* 1992;**18**:237–44.

39 Breslow RA, Alberg AJ. Serological precursors of cancer: malignant melanoma, basal and squamous cell skin cancer, and pre-diagnostic levels of retinal, beta-carotene, lycopene, a-tocopherol and selenium. *Cancer Epidemiol Biomarkers Prev* 1995;**4**:837–42.

40 Kirkpatrick CS, White E, Lee JA *et al.* Case-control study of malignant melanoma in Washington State, II Diet, alcohol, and obesity. *Am J Epidemiol* 1994;**139**:869–80.

41 Katsonyanni K, Willet W, Trichopoulos D *et al.* Risk of breast cancer among Greek women in relation to nutrient intake. *Cancer* 1988;**61**:181–5.

42 Marubini E, Decarli A, Costa A *et al.* The relationship of dietary intake and serum levels of retinal and beta-carotene with breast cancer. Results of a case-control study. *Cancer* 1988;**61**:173–80.

43 Zaridze D, Lifanova Y, Maximovitch D, Day NE, Duffy SW. Diet, alcohol consumption and reproductive factors in a case-control study of breast cancer in Moscow. *Int J Cancer* 1991;**48**:493–501.

44 Longnecker MP, Newcomb PA, Mittendorf R, Greenberg ER, Willett WC. Intake of carrots, spinach, and supplements containing vitamin A in relation to risk of breast cancer. *Cancer Epidemiol Biomarker Prev* 1997;**6**:887–92.

45 Howe GR, Hirohata T, Hislop TG *et al.* Dietary factors and risk of breast cancer: combined analysis of 12 case-control studies. *J Natl Cancer Inst* 1990;**82**:561–9.

46 Paganini-Hill A, Chao A, Ross RK, Henderson BE. Vitamin A, beta-carotene and the risk of cancer: a prospective study. *J Natl Cancer Inst* 1987;**79**:443–8.

47 Rohan TE, Howe GR. Dietary fibre, vitamin A, C and E, and risk of breast cancer: a cohort study. *Cancer Causes Control* 1993;**4**:29–37.

48 Graham S, Zielezny M, Marshall J. Diet in the epidemiology of postmenopausal breast cancer in the New York State Cohort. *Am J Epidemiol* 1992;**136**:1327–37.

49 Kushi LH, Fee RM, Sellers TA, Zheng W, Folsom AR. Intake of vitamins A, C and E and postmenopausal breast cancer. The Iowa Women's Health Study. *Am J Epidemiol* 1996;**144**:165–74.

50 Verhoeven DT, Assen N, Goldbohm RA *et al.* Vitamins C and E retinal, beta-carotene and dietary fibre in relation to breast cancer risk: a prospective cohort study. *Br J Cancer* 1997;**75**:149–55.

51 Knekt P, Aromaa A, Maatela J *et al.* Serum vitamin A and subsequent risk of cancer: cancer incidence follow-up of the Finnish Mobile Health Clinic Health examination survey. *Am J Epidemiol* 1990;**132**:857–70.

52 Graham S, Haughey B, Marshall J *et al.* Diet in the epidemiology of carcinoma of the prostate gland. *J Natl Cancer Inst* 1983;**70**:687–92.

53 Heshmat MY, Kaul L, Kovi J *et al.* Nutrition and prostate cancer: a case-control study. *Prostate* 1985;**6**:7–17.

54 Kolonel LN, Yoshizawa CN, Hankin JH. Diet and prostate cancer: a case-control study in Hawaii. *Am J Epidemiol* 1988;**127**:999–1012.

55 Mettlin C, Graham S, Natarajan N, Huben R. Vitamin A and lung cancer. *J Natl Cancer Inst* 1979;**62**:1435–8.

56 Nomura M, Kolonel LN, Hankin JH, Yoshizawa CN. Dietary factors in cancer of the lower urinary tract. *Int J Cancer* 1991;**48**:199–205.

57 Ohno Y, Yoshida O, Oishi K, Okada K, Yamabe H, Schroeder FH. Dietary b-carotene and cancer of the prostate: a case-control study in Kyoto. *Jap Cancer Res* 1988;**48**:1331–6.

58 Mettlin C, Selenskas S, Natarajan N, Huben R. Beta-carotene and animal fats and their relationship to prostate cancer risk. A case-control study. *Cancer* 1989;**54**:605–12.

59 Rohan TE, Howe GR, Burch JD, Jain M. Dietary factors and risk of prostate cancer: a case-control study in Ontario, Canada. *Cancer Control* 1995;**6**:145–54.

60 Hsing AW, McLaughlin JK, Schuman LM *et al.* Diet, tobacco use, and fatal prostate cancer: results from the Lutheran Brotherhood Cohort Study. *Cancer Res* 1990;**50**:6836–40.

61 Giovannucci E, Ascherio A, Rimm EB *et al.* Intake of carotenoids and retinol in relation to risk of prostate cancer. *J Natl Cancer Inst* 1995;**87**:1767–76.

62 Riboli E, Gonzalez CA, Lopez Abente G *et al.* Diet and bladder cancer in Spain: a multi-centre case-control study. *Int J Cancer* 1991;**49**:214–19.

63 Risch AA, Burch JD, Miller AB, Hill GB, Steele R, Howe GR. Dietary factors and the incidence of cancer of the stomach. *Am J Epidemiol* 1988;**122**:947–59.

64 Bruemmer B, White E, Vaughan TL, Cheney CL. Nutrient intake in relation to bladder cancer among middle-aged men and women. *Am J Epidemiol* 1996;**144**:485–95.

65 Marshall J, Graham S, Mettlin C, Shedd D, Swanson M. Diet and smoking in the epidemiology of oral cancer. *Nutr Cancer* 1982;**3**:145–9.

66 Brock KE, Berry G, Mock PA, MacLennan R, Truswell AS, Brinton LA. Nutrients in diet and plasma and risk of in situ cervical cancer. *J Natl Cancer Inst* 1988;**80**:580–5.

67  Verreault R, Chu J, Manelson M, Shy K. A case-control study of diet and invasive cervical cancer. *Int J Cancer* 1989;**43**:1050–4.

68  Herrero R, Potischman N, Brinton LA *et al.* A case-control study of nutrient status and invasive cervical cancer. I. Dietary indicators. *Am J Epidemiol* 1991;**134**:1335–46.

69  La Vecchia C, Declarli A, Fasoli M *et al.* Dietary vitamin A and the risk of intraepithelial and invasive cervical neoplasia. *Gynecol Oncol* 1988;**30**:187–95.

70  Slattery ML, Abbott TM, Overall JC *et al.* Dietary vitamins A, C and E and selenium as risk factors for cervical cancer. *Epidemiology* 1990;**1**:8–15.

71  Ziegler RG, Brinton LA, Hammam RE *et al.* Diet and the risk of invasive cervical cancer among white women in the USA. *Am J Epidemiol* 1990;**132**:432–45.

72  Potischman N, McCulloch CE, Byers T *et al.* Breast cancer and dietary and plasma concentrations of carotenoids and vitamin A. *Am J Clin Nutr* 1990;**52**:909–15.

73  Greenwald MD, McDonald MS. *The Roles of Diet and Chemoprevention.* Bethesda. MD: NCI, 2001.

74  Stitch HF, Stitch W, Parida BB. Elevated frequency of micronucleated cells in the buccal mucosa of individuals at high risk for oral cancer: betel quid chewers. *Cancer Lett* 1982;**17**:125–34.

75  Meyskens FL, Liu PY, Tuthill RJ *et al.* Randomised trial of vitamin A versus observation as adjuvant therapy in high-risk primary malignant melanoma: a Southwest Oncology Group study. *J Clin Oncol* 1994;**12**:2060–5.

76  McLarty JW, Holiday DB, Girad WM, Yanagihara RH, Kummet T, Greenberg SD. Beta-carotene, vitamin A, and lung cancer chemoprevention: results of an intermediate end-point study. *Am J Clin Nutr* 1995;**62**:1431S–8S.

77  Lambert B, Brisson G, Bielmann P *et al.* Plasma vitamin A and cancerous lesions of cervix uteri: a preliminary report. *Gynecol Oncol* 1981;**11**:136–9.

78  Issing WJ, Struck R, Naumann A. Positive impact of retinyl palmitate in leuloplakia of the larynx. *Eur Arch Otorhinolarayngol* (Suppl.) 1997;**254**:S105–S109.

79  Munoz N, Wahrendorf J, Bang LJ *et al.* No effect of riboflavin, retinol, and zinc on prevalence of pre-cancerous lesions of the oesophagus. Randomised double-blind intervention study in high-risk population in China. *Lancet* 1985;**2**:111–14.

80  Wahrendorf J, Munoz N, Lu JB, Thurnham DI, Crespi M, Bosch FX. Blood, retinal and zinc riboflavin status in relation to pre-cancerous lesions of the oesophagus: findings from a vitamin intervention trial in the People's Republic of China. *Cancer Res* 1988;**48**:2280–3.

81  Olsen JA, Kronborg O, Lyngaard J, Ewertz M *et al.* Dietary risk factors for cancer and adenomas of the large intestine. A case-control study within a screening trial in Denmark. *Eur J Cancer* 1994;**30A**:53–60.

82  Pastorino U, Infante M, Maioli M *et al.* Safety of high dose vitamin A. Randomised controlled trial on lung cancer chemoprevention. *Oncology* 1993;**48**:131–7.

# 9 Do primary and secondary prevention interventions for sun protection reduce the risk of skin cancers?

*Rosalynne Weston*

## Background

### Incidence

Skin cancer is more common than any other type of cancer and the estimated age-standardised rates of cutaneous melanoma in several countries are given in Figure 9.1.[1]

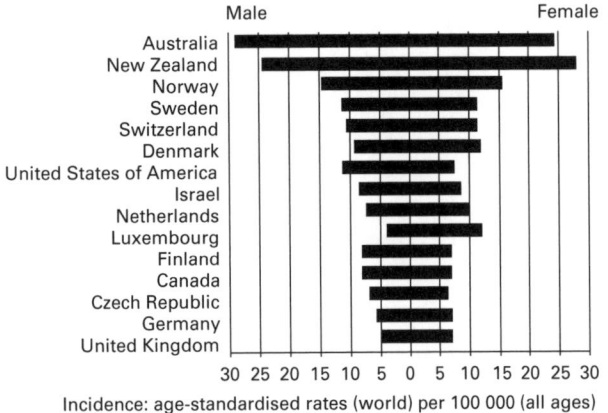

**Figure 9.1** Estimated age-standardised rates for cutaneous melanoma of the skin in 15 countries in 1990

### Mortality and morbidity

It is estimated that about 106 000 people around the world were diagnosed with cutaneous melanoma in 1990. Since melanoma can be a fatal disease if diagnosed at a late stage these represent many lost potential life years as well as direct costs to health services. It is estimated that at least 2 750 000 people were diagnosed with non-melanocytic cancers (basal and squamous cell carcinomas) of the skin in 1985. These represent more than 30% of newly diagnosed cancers.[2] Mortality from melanoma increased after the 1970s especially in White men possibly as a result of increased recreational exposure to sunlight.[3,4] During the next few years about 51 400 individuals are expected to develop melanoma and almost 7800 to die of melanoma. Incidence increased 126% between 1973 and 1995 at a rate of approximately 6% per year. Non-melanocytic skin cancers are not usually considered life-threatening but they represent a huge toll on health service budgets as well as days lost at the workplace and therefore employer and insurance costs. In Australia and increasingly in the USA, UK and Europe, rising incidence rates are causing further increased direct health costs as well as individual morbidity and mortality. Incidence continues to rise particularly in males compared to females.[5] Caucasian populations are currently experiencing a reduction in incidence and mortality in some target groups such as young people with at least one population showing reduced incidence for basal cell carcinoma but not for squamous cell carcinoma. Reduced incidence has also been reported for melanoma in areas where health promotion interventions have encouraged people to reduce their sun exposure.[3]

### Risk factors

Epidemiological evidence suggests that skin cancers, non-melanomic skin cancers (NMSCs) and melanoma are caused in the main by exposure to UV radiation and repeated episodes of sunburn (erythema) in childhood and adulthood. Genetic susceptibility or phenotype, including the number of naevi on the skin, may have a role in the development of skin cancers for some populations and individuals. Exposure to UVR and susceptibility (phenotype) are risk factors associated with the incidence of sunburn, solar keratoses, and precancerous lesions. The type of exposure (high intensity intermittent *v* chronic) and pattern of exposure (continuous *v* intermittent) may differ among the three main types of cancer.[6,7] The incidence of melanoma rises rapidly in Caucasians after the age of 20. Fair-skinned individuals exposed to the sun are at higher risk. The best risk reduction strategy is protection from UV light. Individuals with certain types of pigmented lesions (dysplastic or atypical naevus), with several large non-dysplastic naevi, with many small naevi, or with moderate freckling, have a two-fold to three-fold risk of developing melanoma. Individuals with familial dysplastic naevus syndrome or with several dysplastic or atypical naevi are at high risk (over five-fold) risk of developing melanoma.[7,8] Evidence for the relationship between total exposure to the sun and melanoma remains to be proved. Further evidence that UVR causes skin cancer has been provided from observations that people with the rare genetic condition xeroderma pigmentosum have a very high risk for skin cancer. Some studies show that individuals who have occupational sun exposure have a lower risk for melanoma than those with less exposure.[8–10]

Mutation of the *p53* gene appears to be an important step in the development of skin cancers. Exposure to sunlight causes a number of chemical changes in DNA. If this is not repaired then mutation begins. DNA damage can produce signature mutations in DNA and these are hypothesised as being linked definitively to carcinogenesis. Signature mutations have been found on the tumour suppresser *p53* gene in normal skin cells and their presence has been correlated with extent of exposure. They have also been found often in the *p53* gene in basal and squamous cell carcinomas of the skin whereas they are rare in this gene in other types of cancer. In the general population there is conflicting evidence about excision repair of DNA and the risk for basal cell carcinoma.[11–13]

## Aims for primary prevention

Primary prevention refers to the interventions designed to prevent skin cancer from occurring for the first time. Interventions for primary sun protection aim to change risk behaviour to reduce new skin cancers. Studies that evaluate such interventions usually use behaviour change as a surrogate for decrease in melanoma incidence, because of the difficulties in following up very large populations over decades in order to document such incident tumours. Proxy measures such as knowledge and attitudes can also be used. The main sun-protection strategies are the wearing of wide-brimmed hats, staying out of the sun between 11.00 and 15.00 hours, and the use of shade. Sunscreens are a popular prevention strategy and the evidence of their effectiveness in reducing the risk of skin cancers is considered in Chapter 10.

## Aims for secondary prevention

Interventions for secondary prevention aim to encourage people to recognise skin changes and seek early diagnosis and treatment as well as improving effective diagnosis.

## Search strategy

The studies for this review were found by searching PubMed (the original search for these chapters was carried out in 1998 using Medline) combining the following study types as keywords: meta-analysis, randomised controlled trials, case–control, and direct observation studies with the following cancer terms: melanoma, basal cell carcinoma, rodent ulcer, squamous cell carcinoma, non-melanoma skin cancers. The Cochrane database and the following health promotion journals (*Health Education Research*, *Health Education*) were searched for appropriate studies with the additional keywords: health promotion interventions. One unpublished meta-analysis (Girgis A *et al.* University of Newcastle, New South Wales, Australia, 1998) was submitted. Very few randomised controlled trials were found for primary prevention, although there were more for chemoprevention and secondary prevention. Most studies used direct observation. Randomised population surveys were located for Australia and the USA where there have been concerted year-on-year campaigns aimed at changing population behaviour in the sun.

## Review of evidence

Few randomised controlled trials were located and those found had already been included in an unpublished review of 11 intervention studies, which also included randomised pretest and post-test studies. This review suggested that little work has been undertaken to identify the most effective strategies for disseminating interventions, particularly in schools, the community and workplaces, where effective interventions have been identified. The analysis indicated a low prevalence of sun-protection behaviours, particularly for the use of hats (randomised observational study) and protective clothing, although the use of shade was increasing in a number of target groups. In a randomised observation study of beach behaviour in Australia, 17% used hats, 15% used shade, and recommended shorts and shirts were used by 15%. Outdoor market traders did not use such clothing.[14–16]

## Comments

The review suggests that primary prevention interventions need to be multistrategic across all health, education and leisure/travel settings. Such interventions should include strategies for motivating individual behaviour change through effective sun-protection policies that include the development of shaded areas, low-cost clothing, and sunscreens. Media dissemination is an important vehicle for reinforcing sun-protection messages through education, public media campaigns and healthcare providers. There is a need for randomised controlled trials or controlled studies with multiple outcome measures for prevention aimed at increasing public awareness of UV radiation reduction as an effective method of solar protection. Such studies should have specific outcome measures for each component, that is, hats, clothes and shade. It is imperative that research continues into the relationship between sun exposure and new skin cancers and precancerous lesions such as solar keratoses, to establish a dose–response curve for the protective effect of shade and appropriate protective clothing and hats. We have little direct evidence of population knowledge, attitudes and behaviour regarding their use.

## Primary prevention

### Campaigns: Australian Awareness Weeks (1988–97)

Publicity campaigns such as the Australian Awareness Weeks (randomised surveys) have concentrated on primary prevention and early detection. In 1997 90% of Australians had heard the term melanoma and more than 95% believed that skin cancer could be dangerous. There has been a reduction in the desire for a suntan with 65% of people surveyed by telephone saying they did not like to be suntanned in 1995 compared to 39% in 1988. In 1995 20% stated they wore a wide-brimmed hat between 11·00 and 15·00 hours when outdoors compared with 19% in 1998. The proportion of people, following weekend activities, with sunburn dropped between surveys in 1988 and 1995. For men the rates dropped from 15% to 9% and for women from 9% to 5% (to date 9000 have taken part in these surveys).[17]

### Comment

The Australian community does show a substantial improvement in sun-protection behaviours over the years with women showing greater improvement than men and with little or few social class differences. Further improvements will be harder to achieve as the campaigns move from initiation stage to action and maintenance of change, and researchers will require a longer intervention cycle to bring about health gains for more of the population (Girgis A. *Review of sun protection studies*. Faculty of Behavioural Health Science, University of Newcastle, New South Wales, 1998 [unpublished]). Future intervention planners need to continue frequent reminders for protection and argue for structural change (policy development) that makes it easier for people to embrace protective behaviour. There is a need to develop long-term strategies and interventions making behaviour change habitual particularly

in young people. In primary care settings there is a need to encourage general practitioners to offer opportunistic advice on sun protection as well as early diagnosis opportunities.

An Australian cohort analysis for melanoma incidence demonstrates a levelling off in younger groups and even slight reduction compared with older cohorts in which incidence continues to rise. This could be due to the effect of publicity campaigns. Mortality is also reducing in younger groups as well as in younger women. This is likely to be the effect of early diagnosis and treatment rather than the single effect of the primary prevention campaigns, and health promoters and policy-makers cannot afford to be complacent. Such campaigns are expensive and it is necessary to have specific outcome objectives for each specific sun-protection strategy.

### Education

Several groups have conducted studies, few randomised, to learn more about the possible intervention strategies for the reduction of exposure to UV radiation and the development and implementation of sun-protection policies. Many of these studies had knowledge rather than behaviour as their main outcome measure and so have not been included here. The included studies show that education seems to be the most appropriate way to help populations understand the risks associated with sun exposure, sunburn and sun-protection strategies. Long-term reminders may have some impact on reducing sun exposure in individuals who have been treated for non-melanoma skin cancer, but it seems to be the educational intervention at the time of treatment that had the greatest impact.[17-19]

### Comments

Two studies suggest that educational messages about sun-protection behaviour change are more effective when the damage is done. In this high risk group few were able to sustain their sun-protection behaviour in the long term despite their experience. Maintenance of long-term behaviour change continues to be problematic in other lifestyle change behaviours, such as smoking, alcohol, healthy eating and weight control, and in the recreational use of drugs.[20] Health promoters need to consider designing long-term randomised studies with specific behaviour outcome measures for each element of the intervention. Research on the role of knowledge in behaviour change has shown that knowledge alone does not necessarily lead to behaviour change. The relationship is complex and too many studies rely on a hypothesised link between the two, particularly when knowledge is stated as an outcome measure, thus weakening any evidence accruing from the intervention.

## Public health policy implementation and effectiveness

No randomised studies reported on the effectiveness of sun-protection policies in schools and communities. Only two direct observation studies and one survey were located even though public health policy is deemed the appropriate context for the promotion of individual behaviour change for sun protection, for example the development of shaded areas in communities, on beaches, in school playgrounds and outside spaces. Schofield *et al.* reported on the dissemination of sun-protection polices in schools and their impact. The schools were randomised but the evidence regarding use of protective clothes, hat wearing and shade was from direct observational studies.[21]

Horsley *et al.* carried out a survey for the Department of Health in the UK[22] (1295 primary, 59 middle and 216 secondary schools: 10% sample of schools). In 1995 The Health Education Authority in partnership with the Department of Health and the British Association of Dermatologists introduced Sun Awareness Guidelines to schools. Seven items from the guidelines, that is, education, uniform, shade, outdoor activities, sunscreens, staff awareness, and parent and governor alliances were chosen as outcome measures. The results showed that most schools had taken at least one of the seven actions (mean, 2·67; SD 0·88). Of the schools that had addressed sun protection the majority had done so after the release of the guidelines in 1995. The proportion of schools beginning to take action was greater than those who began in the previous year. Teaching in the curriculum was the most frequent action and was information giving. Brimmed hats and long sleeves were rarely part of summer school wear. Most schools had less than 25% of their outside break in shade but action was being taken to increase this. Sports days were usually scheduled for the afternoon. Sunscreen was allowed in over 80% of schools but its application caused problems for teachers. Few staff manuals included sun-awareness issues, few staff attended in service training on the issue, but two-thirds of head teachers would support staff attending such training. The researchers concluded that more support, government guidelines, funding, materials and courses were required if sun awareness is to be improved.

### Comment

It is too early to report the effectiveness of such policies. Where such policies have been implemented skin cancer reduction is only one element of the policy and other lifestyle issues attract rather more funding. There is a need to evaluate how the implementation of sun-protection policy/ies influences behaviour in community settings. Such studies need to be long-term randomised population studies that include specific outcome measures for each element of the policy in relation to specific target groups. Research so far shows that they have had a very limited effect in two populations and only for one or two outcome measures. Public health policy was intended to be the driver for more effective interventions and funding. To date it is difficult to assess how effective they have been. Australia has used them most effectively to reduce taxes on sun-protection clothing and sunscreens.

## Secondary prevention

### Chemoprevention for skin cancer

The International Agency for Research on Cancer (WHO) recently produced three separate meta-analyses of vitamin A intake,[23] carotenoids,[24] and retinoids[25] and their effect on cancers including skin. They concluded that no association was found between the dietary intake of retinol and the risk of skin cancer in a small number of observational studies (one case–control and three cohort studies). These studies were conducted among Caucasian populations with a wide range of disease risk. The risk estimates in the individual studies were generally greater than unity, in every instance the 95% CI included 1·0. In two prospective studies reporting on prediagnostic levels of retinol and melanoma[23] both reported no significant association on the basis of 30 and 10 cases. This is consistent with the findings of a case–control study of melanoma and dietary intake of preformed vitamin A.[22]

For carotenoids there is evidence suggesting a lack of cancer-preventative effects for beta-carotene when used as a supplement at high doses. There is inadequate evidence with regard to the cancer-preventative effect of beta-carotene at usual dietary levels. There is inadequate evidence with respect to the possible cancer-preventative activity of other individual carotenoids. This is in contrast to some results from animal studies.

In the field of chemoprevention a number of randomised studies have evaluated the efficacy of chemoprevention agents, such as isotretinoin and beta-carotene for individuals at increased risk of developing NMSC. High dose isotretinoin was found to prevent new skin cancers in individuals with xeroderma pigmentosum. A randomised clinical trial of long-term treatment with isotretinoin in individuals previously treated for basal cell carcinoma showed that such treatment did not prevent reoccurrence of new basal cell carcinoma and did produce side effects characteristics of isotretinoin treatment.[23]

A randomised clinical trial on long-term treatment with beta-carotene in individuals treated for non-melanoma skin cancer showed no benefit for the occurrence of new NMSCs concordant with the IARC meta-analysis results.[26] For both these trials it is not known if treatment would benefit individuals at high risk (sun-damaged skin) who have not yet developed skin cancer or if longer follow up would show a long-term effect in the prevention of subsequent skin cancers.

A multicentre double blind randomised placebo controlled trial of 1312 patients with a history of basal cell or squamous cell skin cancer and a mean follow up of 6·4 years showed that 200 micrograms selenium (in brewer's yeast tablets) did not have a significant effect on the primary endpoint of the development of basal cell or squamous cell carcinoma of the skin.[27]

A case–control study on the use of oral contraceptives and an increased risk of melanoma found that a significant two-fold increase in risk of melanoma (RR = 2·0; 95% CI 1·2–3·4) was observed among current users with 10 or more years of use (RR = 3·4; 95% CI 1·7–7·0). Risk did not appear elevated among past oral contraceptive users even among those with longer duration of use, and risk did not decline linearly with time since last use. Risk of premenopausal melanoma may be increased among those with longer duration of use, and further research is needed to determine whether low-dosage oestrogen pills in particular are associated with an increase in risk and to describe possible interactions between oral contraceptive use and sun exposure or other risk factors for melanoma.[28]

### Comment

The evidence from randomised controlled trials for vitamin A and beta-carotene suggests that these are not effective chemopreventative agents for the prevention of skin cancers. The evidence for the effect of isotretinoin is equivocal and there is no evidence that brewer's yeast tablets have a preventative effect for NMSCs. There is some evidence from one case–control study that long-term use of oral contraceptives may be associated with increased risk of melanoma.

### Early diagnosis and treatment

Early detection and diagnosis are generally accepted as the most effective secondary prevention intervention likely to reduce the morbidity and mortality for skin cancer. Melanoma survival rates are linked to early diagnosis and treatment and especially to the thickness of the tumour (Breslow thickness). Patients with thin tumours (< 1·5 mm) have a 5-year survival rate in excess of 90% compared with a survival rate of 68% for tumours greater than 3 mm in thickness. The major determinant of delay in excising such tumours is delay in seeking advice.[29]

Self-examination for skin pigmentary characteristics associated with melanoma such as freckling may be a useful way to identify individuals at increased risk of developing melanoma. Skin type, the propensity to burn after sun exposure and tanning ability alone or with other physical characteristics such as hair colour has been used as a measure of sun sensitivity in epidemiological studies.[30,31]

Other interventions for early detection and diagnosis involve primary care practitioners and dermatology clinics and an early study revealed the problems with such a policy. The work overload on dermatology clinics in particular was a major outcome of the seven-centre study: The Cancer Research Campaign's Mole Watcher Study.[30] This has implications for policy planners. A recent study in the UK looked at the feasibility of targeted early detection for melanoma using a postal questionnaire and an invitation to screening by a consultant dermatologist (a population cross-sectional study with 1600 participants aged 25–69 years and stratified by a social deprivation score of wards within one general practice). These were randomly selected from a population of 8000: 1227 (77%) returned the questionnaire and 896 (56%) attended the screening clinic. Uptake was lower for men (P < 0·001) and skin types 3 and 4 (men only, P < 0·001); 20% of women and 10% of men felt nervous about attending the clinic but only 4% were worried by the questionnaire. The level of agreement between self and the dermatologist's assessment of risk factors was best for hair colour (Kappa = 0·67; sensitivity, 73%; and specificity, 98%). People tended to underreport their level of risk. Over 95% knew about at least one major sign of skin cancer with 54% reporting incorrect signs of melanoma.[31–38]

A recent study in Leicestershire, UK, examined the effect of the introduction of a pigmented lesion clinic on the referral interval between patients with melanoma presenting to their general practitioner.[37] There was a significant initial reduction in the mean referral interval following the introduction of the clinic from 27·9 days (SEM −6·6) in 1984 to 11·3 (23) days in 1987 (P < 0·01). This was not maintained over the following seven years and rose to a mean of 20·4 (4·4) days in 1994. This was not significantly better than the 1985/1986 level. The rise was due to melanomas being directly referred to other clinics. By 1994 only 48% of melanomas were being referred to the pigmented lesion clinics compared to 70% in 1987 with more than 50% of melanomas correctly diagnosed by general practitioners.

### Comment

The evidence for the effectiveness of targeted early detection by screening clinics and dermatologists is inconclusive. The limited evidence suggests that targeted screening for melanoma in the UK will be hampered by difficulties in accurately identifying the target population. Strategies to improve skin self-awareness rather than screening should be developed and evaluated.

## Dermatoscopic diagnosis

A Danish meta-analyses reviewed dermatoscopic diagnosis of cutaneous melanoma as distinguishing malignant melanoma from benign naevus and found that this is often difficult. The macroscopic clinical ABCD rule and the Glasgow seven-point checklist are helpful but often inaccurate yielding many false-positive and false-negative diagnoses. Dermatoscopy performed by a trained physician has increased the diagnostic accuracy to a sensitivity of 80% (in a meta-analysis of 11 studies).[39]

Similarly a French meta-analyses on dermatoscopy compared dermatoscopy to diagnosis by the naked eye. Eight of the 672 studies retrieved to specific criteria were included in this meta-analysis. The selected studies represented 328 melanomas mostly less than 0·76 mm thick and 1865 mostly melanocytic benign pigmented lesions. For dermatoscopic diagnosis of melanoma, the sensitivity and specificity ranges were 0·75–0·96 and 0·79–0·98 respectively. Dermatoscopy had significantly higher discriminating power than clinical examination with respective estimated odds ratios of 76 (95% CI, 25–223) and 16 (95% CI, 9–31) ($P = 0·88$), and respective estimated positive likelihood ratios of 9 (95%CI, 5·6–19·0) and 3·7 (95% CI, 2·8–5·3).[40]

A further study to test the effectiveness of dermatoscope diagnosis used patients referred to a pigmented lesion clinic by their general practitioner. These patients had melanocytic lesions requiring excision (using dermatological criteria). A set of 74 sequentially observed lesions, 37 melanomas, and 37 melanocytic naevi made up the initial set. A second set of 52 lesions: 32 melanomas and 20 melanocytic naevi was used to validate conclusions drawn from the original set. The clinical features studied were: appearance, history and dermatoscopic features. Following pathological examination both sets of lesions showed that the most powerful identifying effect of the lesion was the presence of three or more colours seen on examination by dermatoscopy. In the initial set the age of the patient and the irregular edge and largest diameter of the lesion also contributed to diagnosis. In the second set these were less useful. The sensitivity and specificity of the three-colour dermatoscopy test for melanoma versus naevus was 92% and 51% respectively with the potential to reduce minor surgical work and patient morbidity.[41]

## Comment

The roles of the number of lesions analysed, the percentage of melanoma lesions, the instrument used, and

dermatoscopic criteria used in each study could not be proved. This limited evidence suggests that for experienced users dermatoscopy was more accurate than clinical examination for the diagnosis of melanoma pigmented skin lesions. This hypothesis needs further testing in a multicentre study.

## Postgraduate training in early detection

An Australian randomised controlled trial evaluated the effectiveness of postgraduate skin cancer training programme for improving doctors' knowledge and clinical practice in skin examinations and diagnosis; 41 out of 59 family doctors gave their consent and 69% enrolled on the training programme. Half were allocated to the intervention group and others were allocated to the waiting list status control group. Pre- and post-test data were collected to assess doctors' change in knowledge, perceived confidence and clinical practice. The training programme involved three sessions including information and education, a practical session at the local melanoma clinic, and a practical surgical procedure.[42-44]

## Comment

There were significant improvements in accurate diagnosis when lesions were presented on colour slides with accompanying case history and the correct management was identified. Doctors felt very or extremely confident in their ability to advise patients on screening frequency, to advise on signs of skin cancer, and to decide whether changes in lesions were malignant. Significant improvements in clinical practice were found by recording pathology request forms. The study suggested that it was easy to bring about improvement in knowledge through training but more difficult to change clinical practice. This was essentially a pilot study and could be a useful marker for training in general practice.

## Implications for practice

The major implication for health promotion practice and research for solar protection interventions resulting from this summary is the need for randomised controlled long-term community trials using multistrategic primary and secondary interventions across targeted populations within communities. Such trials should use partnership or health alliance models including partners from health, education and workplace settings, or use existing partnerships where these are already operational. These trials should include training and education in general practice as well as early detection and diagnosis outcomes. Interventions targeted at high risk groups could be a discrete element of the trial, especially identification of high risk patients.

To date there is a problematic time lag in research, and researchers and policy-planners have not capitalised on the results from successful early pilot or short-term sun-protection interventions to develop such long-term trials.

It is necessary to include behaviour change outcome measures for each specific element of the trial as well as at least one other outcome measure, for example knowledge, for primary prevention interventions. Further research is needed to establish the link between knowledge and behaviour in the process of long-term behaviour change. For secondary prevention such trials should include behaviour change outcome measures for populations as well as for clinical practice where appropriate. As global warming continues there is an urgent need for more individuals to make long-term behaviour (maintained) change. Primary care practitioners need to be convinced that they have a role in primary as well as secondary prevention of skin cancers, as well as identifying high risk individuals. Such improvements and the research required to substantiate them will require considerable funding.

## Conclusions

- There is limited evidence from systematic reviews of population; epidemiological, randomised, observational and case–control studies that primary prevention interventions have had some impact on sun-related behaviour in the short term. This is substantially weakened by the research study designs and the lack of published long-term randomised controlled trials. This suggests both lack of funding and commitment to long-term multistrategy outcome measure studies within communities.

- There is no evidence that the development and implementation of public health policy for sun protection has improved intervention design or improved the implementation of long-term trials following effective pilot or short-term studies.

- There is no evidence that funding followed this development either. Australia has used public policy to reduce tax on clothing, hats, and sunscreens but there is only very limited evidence that this has changed behaviour, that is, use of these protectors.

- There is a need for policies to be reviewed and a further consideration of how they can drive intervention development in the long term. There needs to be multimethodological evaluation of such policy implementation and effect.

- There is some evidence from case–control, observational and epidemiological population studies that primary and secondary prevention programmes may be associated with reduced incidence of skin cancers in specific populations and age groups.

- There is some evidence (weakened by study design and short-term studies) that protective clothing messages are successful in encouraging reduced solar exposure in specific populations and target groups: particularly women and children (by definition of carers' actions and role-modelling).

- There is some evidence from surveys that schools have begun to address solar protection education and information giving, but little evidence of behaviour change for solar protection from the sustained use of clothing, especially hats, and from shaded areas.

- There is some evidence that information about skin self-examination (signs of change in the skin) is an effective strategy for encouraging specific target groups to seek early diagnosis (more women seek early diagnosis than men). There is no convincing evidence that routine screening is a cost-effective strategy for reducing the incidence of skin cancers or melanomas.

- There is no evidence that regular screening for skin cancer in general practice settings is a cost-effective prevention strategy for melanoma and NMSCs.

- There is very limited evidence that dermatoscopy is a more effective diagnostic tool than naked eye diagnosis for melanoma and skin cancers.

## References

1 Parkin DM, Pisai P, Farley J. Estimates of the world-wide incidence of 25 major cancers in 1990. *Int J Cancer* 1999;**80**:827–41.
2 Hall HI, Miller DR, Rogers JD *et al.* Update of the incidence and mortality from melanoma in USA. *J Am Acad Dermatol* 1999;**40**:35–42.
3 Wingo PA, Ries LA *et al.* Cancer incidence and mortality 1973–1995: A Report Card for US. *Cancer* 1998;**82**:1197–207.
4 Hall HI, Miller DR, Rogers JD *et al.* Update on the incidence and mortality for melanoma in USA. *J Am Acad Dermatol* 1998;**40**:35–42.
5 Mathers C, Penm R, Sanson-Fisher R, Campbell E. *Health System Costs of Cancer in Australia 1993–94.* Canberra: Australian Institute of Health and Welfare,1998.
6 Baron JA. Prevention of non-melanoma skin cancer. *Arch Dermatol* 2000;**136**:200–45.
7 Armstrong BK. Melanoma: Childhood or lifelong sun exposure. In: Grob JJ, Stern RS, MacKie RM, Weinstock WA, eds. *Epidemiology, Causes and Prevention of Skin Diseases.* Oxford: Blackwell Science, 1997.
8 Tucker MA, Halpen A, Holly EA *et al.* Clinically recognized dysplastic nevi: a central risk factor for cutaneous melanoma: *JAMA* 1996;**277**: 1439–44.
9 Elwood JM, Jobson J. Melanoma and sun exposure: an overview of published studies. *Int J Cancer* 1997;**73**:198–203.
10 Severi G, Giles, GG, Robertson C, Boyle , Autier P. Mortality from cutaneous melanoma: evidence for contrasting trends between populations. *Br J Cancer* 2000;**82**:1887–91.
11 Whiteman DC, Whiteman CA, Green AC. Childhood sun exposure as a risk factor for melanoma a systematic review of epidemiological studies. *Cancer Causes Control* 2001;**12**:69–82.

12  Zeigler A, Jonason A, Simon J, Leffell D, Brash DE. Tumour suppressor gene mutations and photocarcinogenesis. *Photochem Photobiol* 1996;**63**:432–5.

13  Ouhtit A, Ueda M, Nakazawa H *et al.* Quantitative detection of ultra-violet light-specific p53 mutations in normal skin from Japanese patients. *Cancer Epidimiol Biomarkers Prev* 1997;**6**:433–8.

14  Girgis A, Sanson-Fisher RW, Tripodi DA, Golding T. Evaluation of interventions to improve solar protection in primary schools. *Health Educ Q* 1993;**20**:275–87.

15  Girgis A, Campbell EM, Redman S, Sanson-Fisher RW. Screening for melanoma: a community survey of prevalence and predictors. *Med J Australia* 1991;**154**:338–43.

16  Girgis A, Sanson-Fisher RW, Watson A. A workplace intervention for increasing outdoor workers' use of solar protection. *Am J Publ Hlth* 1994;**84**:77–81.

17  Marks R, Hill D. Primary prevention of skin cancer: where to now in reducing sunlight exposure? *Med J Aust* 1997;**167**:515–16.

18  Robinson JK. Compensation strategies in sun protection behaviours by a population with non-melanoma skin cancer. *Prev Med* 1992;**21**:754–65.

19  Scott D, Weston R. *Evaluating Health Promotion*. Cheltenham: Nelson Thornes, 1998.

20  Berwick M, Fine JA *et al.* Sun exposure and sunscreen use following a community skin cancer screening *Prev Med* 1992;**21**:302–10.

21  Schofield MJ, Edwards K, Pearce R. Effectiveness of two sun protection policy disseminations strategies in New South Wales primary and secondary schools. *Aust NZ J Publ Health* 1997;**21**:743–50.

22  Horsley L, Charlton A, Wiggett C. Current action for skin cancer risk reduction in English schools: a report on a survey carried out for the Department of Health. *Health Educ Res* 2000;**15**:249–59.

23  IARC. *Handbooks on Cancer Prevention. Vitamin A.* 1998; Vol. 3. Lyon, France: IARC Press.

24  IARC. *Handbooks on Cancer Prevention. Retinoids.* 1998; Vol. 4. Lyon, France: IARC Press.

25  The Isotretinoin-Basal Cell Carcinoma Study Group. Long-term therapy with low dose isotretinoin for prevention of basal cell carcinoma: a multi-centre clinical trial. *J Natl Cancer Inst* 1993;**84**:328–32.

26  The Skin Cancer Prevention Study Group. A clinical trial of beta-carotene to prevent basal cell and squamous cell cancers of the skin. *N Engl J Med* 1990;**323**:789–95.

27  Clark LC, Combs GF, Turnbull BW *et al.* Effects of selenium supplementation for cancer prevention in patients with carcinoma of the skin: a randomized controlled trial. *JAMA* 1996;**276**:1957–63.

28  Feskanich D, Hunter DJ, Willet WC *et al.* Oral contraceptive use and risk of melanoma in premenopausal women. *Br J Cancer* 1999;**81**:918–23.

29  Blois MS, Sagebiel RW, Abarnanel RM *et al.* Malignant melanoma of the skin: the association of tumour depth and type, and patient sex, age and site with survival. *Cancer* 1999;**52**:1330–41.

30  Friedman RJ, Rigel DS, Kopf AW. Early detection of malignant melanoma: the role of the physician examination and self examination of the skin CA. *Cancer J Clin* 1985;**35**:130–51.

31  MacKie RM, Hole D. Audit of public education campaign to encourage earlier detection of malignant melanoma. *BMJ* 1992;**304**: 1012–15.

32  Melia J, Moss S, Graham-Brown R *et al.* The relation between mortality from malignant melanoma and early detection in the Cancer research Campaign Mole Watcher Study. *Br J Cancer* 2001;**85**:803–7.

33  Farmer ER, Gonin R, Hanna MP. Discordance in the histopathologic diagnosis of melanoma and melanocytic nevi between expert pathologists. *Human Pathol* 1996;**27**:528–31.

34  Berwick M, Begg CB, Fine JA. Screening for cutaneous melanoma by skin self-examination. *J Natl Cancer Inst* 1996;**88**:17–23.

35  Ferrini RL, Perlman M, Hill L. *Screening for Skin Cancer.* American College of Preventive Medicine: Practice Policy Statement, 2001.

36  Asri GD, Clarke WH Jr, Guerry DVI *et al.* Screening and surveillance of patients at high risk for malignant melanoma result in the detection of earlier disease. *J Am Acad Dermatol* 1990;**22**:1042–8.

37  Melia J, Harland C, Moss S, Eiser JS, Pendry L. Feasibility of targeted early detection for melanoma: a population-based screening study. *Br J Cancer* 2000;**82**:1605–9.

38  Altman JF, Oliveria SA, Christos PJ, Halpern AC. A survey of skin cancer screening in the primary care setting: a comparison with other cancer screenings *Arch Fam Med* 2000;**9**:1022–7.

39  Lorentzen HF, Weismann K. Dermatoscopic diagnosis of cutaneous melanoma. Secondary Prophylaxis. Ugeskr Laeger, June 5. 2000;**162**: 3312–16.

40  Bafounta ML, Beauchet A, Aegerter P, Saiag P. Is dermoscopy useful for the diagnosis of melanoma? Results of a meta-analysis using techniques adapted to the evaluation of diagnostic tests *Arch Dermatol* 2001;**137**:1343–50.

41  MacKie RM, Fleming C *et al. Br J Dermatol* 2002;**146**:481–4.

42  Schofield MJ, Walsh RA, Sanson-Fisher RW. Training medical students in behavioural and cognitive strategies. *Behav Change* 1994;**11**:6–18.

43  Girgis A, Sanson-Fisher RW. Postgraduate training for family physicians: evaluation of a skin cancer training programme (unpublished grey literature) University of Newcastle, NSW, Australia, 1994.

44  Sanson-Fisher RW, Redman S, Walsh R. Training medical practitioners in information transfer skills: the new challenge in Medical Education (unpublished) Department of Behavioural Science in Medicine, University of Newcastle, NSW, Australia 1991.

# 10 Do sunscreens reduce the incidence of skin cancers?

*Rosalynne Weston*

## Background

### Historical development and sun protection factor (SPF)

Sunscreens were first used in1928 and became popular with those intentionally trying to gain a suntan. They mainly filter out the wavelengths responsible for sunburn (UVB, 280–315 nm). Following evidence that longer wavelengths of sunlight (UVA, 315–400 nm) are involved in the sunburn reaction and photocarcinogenesis, UVA absorbers have been added to most sunscreens to widen their absorption spectra. There is concordant evidence that sunscreens undoubtedly protect against sunburn, but evidence for a role in the prevention of skin cancers is still somewhat equivocal.[1,2] The concept of a sunscreen effectiveness index (ratio) is attributed to Schulze and Greiter, who proposed the specific term "sun protection factor" (SPF), and the associated method for assessing SPF.[3] SPF activity is the ratio of the least amount of UV energy required to produce erythema (reddening of the skin) on sunscreen-protected skin to the amount of energy to produce the same effect on unprotected skin.

### Testing and regulation of sunscreens

Topical sunscreens applied to the skin act by absorbing and/or scattering incident UV radiation (UVR). The shape of the absorption spectrum is the fundamental attribute of a topical sunscreen. It is expressed as the extinction coefficient: the measure of the degree to which the sunscreen absorbs individual wavelengths across the terrestrial UVR spectrum (290–400 nm). Absorption is the product of the extinction coefficient, the concentration of the active ingredient, and the effective thickness of application on exposed parts of the body.

Sunscreens are regulated for specific formulations in most countries. In the EU, Japan, and South Africa they are regulated as cosmetics and in other countries (Australia, Canada and New Zealand) as drugs. Testing for toxic effects is mandatory in each country. Control in Europe is by a directive of the European Commission (2000). This mandates that labelling should include a full list of ingredients in decreasing order of concentration, and that this should be displayed on the containers of all cosmetics that include sunscreen formulations.[4-7] Sunscreens are now readily available in most countries during all seasons. In Australia the availability of sunscreens has been maximised through sales tax exemptions and they are now available in workplaces and schools; their use by children is actively promoted.[8-10]

### Paradoxical findings: problems with use of sunscreen as a primary prevention aim

Protecting against sun damage and reducing the risk of sunburn and skin cancers involves behavioural choices. Studies demonstrate that increased use of sunscreens often means a reduction in other photo-protective methods: wearing of hats and protective clothing and the use of shade (Figure 10.1), thus increasing net sun exposure. Most sunscreens are made to prevent against sunburn and most sunburn, in both children and adults, occurs during intentional exposure to the sun.[11-14] The use of sunscreens,

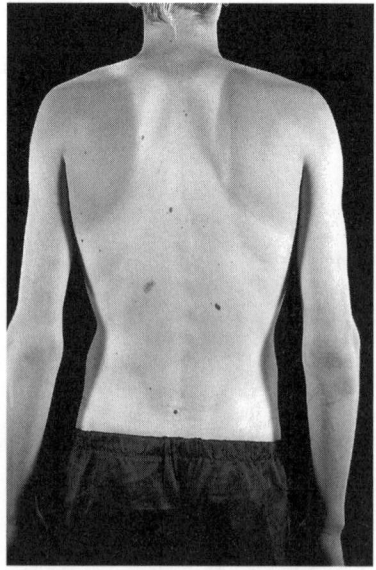

**Figure 10.1** Patient with sunburn and dysplastic naevus syndrome

including those with high SPFs, during intentional exposure has been found to have little effect on the occurrence of sunburn.[15–17] This is concordant with the results from surveys of beachgoers which suggest that increased overreliance on sunscreens reduces the use of other protective measures. Individuals seem to balance protective behaviours according to personal motivation and characteristics and the desire for a suntan.[18–24]

## Intended and actual sun protection from sunscreens

There is some evidence that the numerical measure of protection indicated on the product pack is generally higher than that achieved in practice. The photo-protection of sunscreens (the SPF) is measured by photo-testing *in vivo* at internationally agreed levels of thickness of application – 2 mg cm$^{-2}$. To receive the SPF quoted on sunscreen packaging, an individual would need to use 35 ml of sunscreen for total body surface protection. Studies have demonstrated that individuals are more likely to use 0·5–1·5 mg cm$^{-2}$ and that most users get, in protective terms, the benefit of between one-quarter and one-half of the product.[25] Individuals get sunburnt because they use too little sunscreen, spread it unevenly, miss parts of the body surface exposed to the sun and because sunscreen is rubbed or washed off. Thus, individuals' use of a sunscreen makes a difference in how effective sunscreens are in the prevention of sunburn and explains why sunburn still occurs even with higher SPF sunscreens. If individuals want to be supine in the sun for long periods of time (hours) then it is recommended that SPFs of 20–30 or higher are necessary. Sunscreens need to be applied evenly 30 minutes before going out in the sun. They need to be reapplied at regular intervals as much is washed off by swimming and other water sports and by any abrasive action particularly from sand on the beach.[25]

## Possible drawbacks of sunscreens

No published studies have demonstrated toxic effects of sunscreens in humans. Case reports suggest there is an increase in the frequency of photocontact dermatitis among patients who are frequent sunscreen users and who have photodermatoses such as polymorphic light eruption. There is no evidence that sunscreen use affects vitamin D levels.[25] Using sunscreen does not cause adverse effects on reproduction or fetal development, although some effects have been seen with high oral doses of sunscreen ingredients in animal models. In some experimental conditions topically applied sunscreen (in the absence of UVR) affects the immune system but most toxicity studies have shown that the active ingredients in sunscreens are safe when applied topically at recommended concentrations. DNA damage has been reported in one study.[25]

## Search strategies

Searches of Medline, PubMed and the *Cochrane Library* was carried out using "sunscreen" as a key word and searching for appropriate meta-analyses and randomised controlled trials (RCTs). Health education and promotion journals were also searched. This search located the International Agency for Research on Cancer (IARC) meta-analysis of sunscreen use.[25]

## Outcome measures

Ideally, the main outcome measure of studies addressing sunscreen use and cancer risk would be numbers of incident cancers in those using sunscreens compared with those not using sunscreens. However, this is unrealistic because of the long latency period for a skin cancer to develop and the relative rarity of such events. Surrogate outcome measures such as reported protective behaviour are therefore often used in studies. Intermediate outcomes such as incidence of actinic keratoses or reduction in naevi are also used as short-term surrogates for longer term skin cancer risk. All of these surrogate measures have their problems. There are many confounding factors when assessing sunscreen use. Many studies use behaviour (for example, reported use of sunscreen or sun avoidance) as the outcome measure. The data may still be unreliable as recall of use is not necessarily accurate and other protective measures are confounding factors. Lack of specificity of outcome measures remains problematic.

## Can the use of sunscreen prevent cutaneous melanoma?

### Efficacy

There are no reported RCTs or cohort studies on the use of sunscreens and the risk for cutaneous melanoma. There are a total of 15 case–control studies[26–40] (Table 10.1). In attempting to assess the evidence from these it is important to note that these studies use very different populations and different cultural groups. This analysis does not compare like with like: each uses a different study design, has different terms of reference and uses different methods for data collection. The term sunscreen is variously described and does not refer to one category. Sun lotion, sun-tanning oil and sun protection factor are used throughout these studies. This makes it particularly difficult to assess the reported results unless these terms were clearly defined to study participants, or confounding factors accounted for, as part of the data analysis process. Overall, however, these studies showed a low prevalence of sunscreen use (Table 10.1).

Klepp and Magnus (1979),[26] Graham *et al.* (1985)[27] and Herzfeld *et al.* (1985)[28] reported an increased risk between sunscreen use and melanoma with Graham *et al.* reporting

**Table 10.1  Case–control studies of sunscreen use and risk for cutaneous melanoma**

| Population place/date | Type of cases/ controls | No. of cases/ controls | Exposure | RR[a] (95% CI) | Comments | Reference |
|---|---|---|---|---|---|---|
| Norway 1974–75 | Hospital cases Other cancer controls | 78 cases 131 controls | Sometimes, often or almost always use sun lotion/oil | M 2·8[b] (1·2–6·7) F 1·0[b] (0·42–2·5) T 2·3[b] (1·3–4·1) | Elevated risks among males only Sunscreens not differentiated from "sun lotions" | Klepp and Magnus (1979)[26] |
| USA 1974–80 | Hospital cases Other cancer controls | 404 cases 521 controls | Used sunscreen Used suntan lotion | M 2·2[b] (1·2–4·1) M 1·7 (1·1–2·7) F "no added risk" | Elevated risks among males only | Graham *et al.* (1985)[27] |
| USA 1977–79 | Population cases and controls | 324 male trunk melanoma cases 415 controls | Always used "suntan lotion" | 2·6[b] (1·4–4·7) Not significant after control for "tendency to sunburn and water sports" | "Suntan lotions" and "sunscreens" not differentiated in questionnaire | Herzfeld *et al.*[28] (1993) |
| Sweden 1978–83 | Hospital cases Population controls | 523 cases 505 controls | Often used sun protection agents | 1·8[b] (1·2–2·7) | | Beitner *et al.*[29] (1990) |
| Canada 1979–81 | Population cases and controls | 369 trunk and lower limb melanomas 369 controls | Used sunscreen almost always | 1·1 (0·75–1·6) | Highest risk in those using sunscreen "only for first few hours" RR1·62 (1·04–2·52) | Elwood and Gallagher[30] (1999) |
| Australia 1980–81 | Population cases and controls | 507 cases 507 controls | Used sunscreens ≤ 10 years | 1·1 (0·71–1·6) | | Holman *et al.*[31] (1986) |
| USA 1981–86 | Population cases and controls | 452 cases 930 controls | Always used sunscreens | All cutaneous melanoma 0·62[b] (0·49–0·83) Superficial spreading melanoma (SSM) 0·43 (CI not available) | Study involved only women aged 25–59 at diagnosis. CI estimated. RR for SSM adjusted for host factors and sun exposure | Holly *et al.*[32] (1995) |
| Denmark 1982–85 | Population cases and controls | 474 cases 926 controls | Always used sunscreens | 1·1[b] (0·8–1·5) | | Osterlind *et al.* (1997)[33] |
| Australia 1987–94 | Population cases Controls from same school | 50 cases 156 controls All children < 15 | Always used sunscreens on holidays 0·7 (0·1–6·0) at school | 2·2 (0·4–12) on holidays 0·7 (0·1–6·0) at school | | Whiteman *et al.* (1997)[34] |
| Sweden 1988–90 | Population cases and controls | 400 cases 640 controls | Almost always used sunscreens | Trunk 1·4 (0·6–3·2) Other sites 2·0 (1·1–3·7) | No information on duration of use | Westerdahl *et al.* (1995)[35] |
| Spain 1989–93 | Hospital cases Hospital visitors | 105 cases 138 controls | Always used sunscreens | 0·2 (0·04–0·79) | | Rodenas *et al.* (1996)[36] |
| Spain 1990–94 | Hospital cases and controls | 116 cases 235 controls | Used sunscreen | 0·48 (0·34–0·71) | Inadequate description of measurement of sunscreen use | Espinoza-Arranz *et al.* (1991)[37] |

*(Continued)*

**Table 10.1** *(Continued)*

| Population place/date | Type of cases/ controls | No. cases/ controls | Exposure | RR[a] (95% CI) | Comments | Reference |
|---|---|---|---|---|---|---|
| Europe 1991–92 | Hospital cases Neighbourhood controls | 418 controls 438 controls | Ever use psoralen sunscreens Ever use sunscreen | 2·3 (1·3–4·0) 1·5 (1·1–2·1) M 1·8 (1·1–2·7) F 1·3 (0·87–2·0) | Highest risk for sun-sensitive subjects using sunscreens to tan: RR 3·7 (1·0–7·6) | Autier *et al.* (1995, 1997b)[38] |
| Austria 1993–94 | Hospital cases and controls | 193 cases 319 controls | Often used sunscreen | 3·5 (1·8–6·6) | | Wolf *et al.* (1998)[39] |
| Sweden 1995–97 | Population cases and controls | 571 cases 913 controls | Always used sunscreen Used sunscreens to spend more time sunbathing | 1·8 (1·1–2·9) 8·7 (1·0–76) | | Westerdahl *et al.* (2000)[40] |

[a] Relative risk estimates adjusted for phenotype and sun-related factors where possible.
[b] Crude relative risk ratio available only.
Reproduced from Vainio H and Bianchini F, *IARC Handbooks of Cancer Prevention. Vol. 5 Sunscreens.* Lyon: IARC Publications 2001: 71–72, with permission.

an increased risk particularly in men. Beitner *et al.* (1990)[29] reported increased risk for those who used sunscreens "often" or "very often". This study controlled for age, sex and hair colouring. Elwood and Gallagher (1999)[30] assessed the relationship between phenotype, history of sun-tanning and sunburn, exposure to sunlight and the risk for melanoma in four Western provinces of Canada. Analysis of a subset of cases of melanoma on intermittently exposed sites (trunk and lower limbs) and controls provided information about the use of sunscreens on these sites during outdoor activity. Risk for those reporting sunscreen "almost always used" was very similar to that of those using sunscreen "sometimes". Those using sunscreen only in the first few hours had increased risk after adjustment for hair, eye and skin colouring and propensity to burn.

Holman *et al.* (1986)[31] found that those who had used sunscreens for less than 10 years did not have a reduced risk for cutaneous melanoma: risk was not reduced for those who had used sunscreens for 10–15 years. Frequency of use did not appear to be related to risk. This study did find a positive relationship between the use of sunscreen and the risk for cutaneous melanoma but in the absence of control for pigmentary traits and sun sensitivity. Sunscreens were not available in Australia when the subjects in this study were younger and therefore they were unable to use them at a time when they may have given protection.

Holly *et al.* (1995)[32] found that women who reported "almost always" using sunscreens had a lower risk for cutaneous melanoma than those who reported that they "never" used sunscreens. After controlling for superficial spread of melanoma, sun sensitivity and sunburn history before the age of 12 years the risk for women "almost always" using was lower than for those "never" using. The

authors concluded that sunscreen use was strongly protective against melanoma. This study showed that the highest level of risk was for women with the least exposure after controlling for sun sensitivity.

Osterlind *et al.* (1988)[33] found that compared to those who "never" used sunscreens, a small non-significant increase in risk was seen for those who had used them for less than 10 years, or for those using for more than 10 years. Frequency of use was not associated with the risk of melanoma among those "always using" against those who "hardly ever used" or "never used". Effective sunscreens were not available to the study group in their youth.

Whiteman *et al.* (1997)[34] found, after controlling for tanning ability, freckling and number of naevi, those who had "always" used sunscreens while on holiday had a non-significant elevated risk for cutaneous melanoma compared to those not using sunscreens. The use of sunscreens at school was associated with a non-significant reduced risk. The RRs have very wide confidence intervals in this study (only 11 "always" used on holiday and only two reported sunscreen use at school).

Westerdahl *et al.* (1995)[35] found, after controlling for history of sunburn; history of sunbathing; number of raised naevi; freckling and hair colour, those "almost always" using sunscreen had similar risk estimates to those "never" using in both men and women. Risk for use before age 15, at ages 15–19 and at age 19 years reported elevated odds ratios at each stage similar to those of people "always using" sunscreens. Risk for melanomas of the trunk were similar to that found for melanomas of the extremities, and head and neck, after adjustment for sunburns, frequent sunbathing, freckling and naevi.

Rodenas *et al.* (1996)[36] reported that the use of sunscreen appeared to protect against melanoma and that risk was strongly associated with the sensitivity of the skin to the sun (relative risk of 2·0) for those who always burned. This study failed to give a description of how sunscreen use was measured. Espinoza-Arranz *et al.* (1999) found similar results.[37]

Autier *et al.* (1995 and 1997)[38] found that those who had "never" used psoralen-containing sunscreens had an increased risk for cutaneous melanoma after controlling for age, sex, hair colouring, and number of weeks spent in sunny climes each year. An elevated risk was found particularly among those who reported no history of sunburn. Use of psoralen-containing sunscreens, however, was not common. Those "ever" using these sunscreens (psoralen) also had increased risk after adjustment for some factors compared to those "never" using. Increased risk was reported for those using sunscreens and those having light or dark hair. Sensitive and sun-insensitive participants showed an increased risk with the use of sunscreens. The authors concluded that use of sunscreen tended to be associated with higher risk for cutaneous melanoma among sunbathers. Highest risk was for those using sunscreen and who had no history of sunburn after age 14 years. The use of clothing, rather than sunscreen, appeared protective. It was the use of sunscreen, particularly in UVA as well as UVB light, that was found to be associated with increased risk.

Wolf *et al.* (1998)[39] reported "often used" sunscreen had a significant higher risk for melanoma compared to "never used" (study controlled for skin colouring, sunbathing and history of sunburn). The authors concluded that use of sunscreen did not prevent melanoma.

Westerdahl *et al.* (2000)[40] reported a significantly increased risk for melanoma for regular use (always used) of sunscreen after adjustment for hair colour, history of sunburns, frequency and duration of sunbathing. Risk was significantly increased among those using sunscreens with an SPF less than 10 compared with those who did not use sunscreens and for those with no history of sunburn when they used sunscreens. The risk was even higher for those using sunscreen to increase sunbathing time (deliberate exposure). In an analysis of subsites, risk was significantly increased only for melanoma of the trunk.

The following studies could be assessed as supporting a positive association between sunscreen use and risk of cutaneous melanoma but this tentative conclusion should be viewed cautiously.[26–29,38–40] Confounding factors such as: sunscreen use, sun exposure, sun sensitivity, a history of sun-related neoplasia and sun-protective behaviour such as the use of protective clothing, staying indoors or seeking shade were problematic in these studies. There was idiosyncratic reporting of these confounding factors casting doubt on the significance of the results.

Three studies[30,31,33] reported no increased risk for use of sunscreen and cutaneous melanoma with non-significant

increase being reported in one study.[34] Three studies reported sunscreen as protective against cutaneous melanoma.[34,36]

## Studies that have assessed naevus count as an indicator of melanoma risk

One study using naevi count as an intermediate endpoint showed that the median number of new naevi in Caucasian children was reduced in the sunscreen users. Sunscreen was more effective in preventing naevi in children who freckled than in those who did not.[41] Difference in exposure time was not a significant variable. One cohort study[42] showed increasing naevi development with sunscreen use. Further analysis showed that this was because children who used sunscreen had longer cumulative exposure time but no data were available to support this conclusion. The cross-sectional study[43] reported that the use of summer sunscreen reduced the number of sunburns but was not associated with annual sun exposure or with naevi number or density. This study was criticised for not reporting all data.

Studies using naevus count as an outcome do not provide any conclusive evidence about the relationship between the use of sunscreen and reduced naevi and thus reduced risk for cutaneous melanoma. In all studies the confounding variables and lack of reported data were problematic. A consistent finding of all these studies was the link between cumulative exposure and risk.

## Comment on sunscreen use and melanoma risk

Some studies demonstrate a positive association between sunscreen use and risk for cutaneous melanoma whereas others do not. Many confounding factors prevented any firm conclusions as to the possible protective or harmful effect on the use of sunscreens. The most likely reason for an apparently increased risk is that individuals who use sunscreen stay in the sun longer because they falsely believe that sunscreen protects them. This needs further research, particularly to clarify knowledge and attitudes to suntanning, sunscreen use and knowledge of skin cancer. It would seem that individuals intent on gaining a suntan use sunscreens to give themselves more time in the sun without sunburn. Reducing their risk of cancer is a secondary motive. Risk is also related to phenotype and history of sun exposure and sunburn. There is equivocal evidence about the use of sunscreen and the use of other photo-protective measures. Further research is needed to assess these factors in long-term randomised studies with specific target groups. Such research needs to include a formative stage that seeks to explore knowledge and attitude to sunscreen use and other photo-protective measures. This information will enable specific outcome objectives to be developed for each aspect of the study, thus reducing confounding factors. There is a need for an agreed definition of "sunscreen use" and specific definition and description of such use: how, when and what SPF is used in specific situations.

## Can the use of sunscreen reduce the risk of basal cell carcinoma (BCC) and squamous cell carcinoma (SCC)?

The Nambour Skin Cancer Prevention Trial (a randomised study exploring risk of both SCC and BCC) demonstrated that sunscreen use could be significant in reducing the risk of SCC.[44] This was a complex trial including 1850 residents aged 20–69. They were invited to use a daily application of SPF 16 sunscreen and use 30 mg of beta-carotene supplement in the prevention of skin cancer; 1647 attended baseline assessment that included a cancer risk factor assessment and a full skin examination by a dermatologist. Any detected skin cancers were removed at the start of the study. Out of these 1647 residents, 1621 agreed to take part in the study. They were randomised to one of four study groups, sunscreen and beta-carotene; sunscreen and placebo; no sunscreen and beta-carotene; and no sunscreen and placebo. The participants attended a clinic every 3 months to receive new sunscreen and beta-carotene. The weight of the sunscreen returned to these clinics every three months was recorded. A random subgroup of sunscreen users kept a seven-day diary on three occasions to record their frequency of sunscreen application and sun exposure. Dermatologist examinations were given at these visits and any cancers removed and recorded. No protective effect for prevention of SCC was found in the beta-carotene group. Sunscreen use was analysed for all groups, regardless of beta-carotene use as no interaction was seen between the two interventions (sunscreen and beta-carotene). A total of 28 new SCCs were detected in the group given sunscreen and 46 in those not given sunscreen (RR 0·61; 95% CI 0·50–1·6) a statistically significant difference. The authors concluded that sunscreen use could be of significant benefit in protecting against SCC. No placebo sunscreen was used and the results need to be interpreted with caution because the comparison group was not ideal, reducing the power of the study to detect an effect of daily sunscreen use. Green *et al.* (1999)[45] subsequently reported that solar exposure of those given sunscreen did not differ from those not given sunscreen. The prevalence of sunburn was lower for those receiving sunscreen to those not receiving it (tested on a random sample of participants wearing photosensitive badges). The findings suggest that the reduction of incidence of SCC seen in the group using sunscreens was probably due to the attenuation [*sic* thinning] of the UVR by the sunscreen rather than in behaviour change (reducing time in the sun). Higher factor sunscreen use, especially for older people, may not result in them spending longer time in the sun.

A cohort study by Grodestein *et al.* (1995)[46] reported that sunscreens used over a 2-year period by women who spent 8 or more hours per week in the sun was not protective by comparison with no use of such agents (RR 1·1; 95% CI 0·83–1·7).

Timing of exposure to UVR was a significant risk factor for SCC in a case–control study by Pogoda and Preston-Martin (1996).[47] There is little evidence that sunscreen use protects against BCC. Some patients may have been advised to use sunscreens following diagnosis, which may have confounded results. Following diagnosis of SCC, use of sunscreen was examined retrospectively in three age groups: 8–14, 15–19 and 20–24 years. Those in the 8–14 group who had used sunscreens seemed to have a slightly reduced risk of SCC (RR 0·61; 95% CI 0·82–4·4) not statistically significant. Those using sunscreen in the 15–19 age group had a relative risk of 1·9 (95% CI 0·82–4·4) and those in the 20–24 group had a risk of 0·99 (95% CI 0·44–2·2). No strong protective effect of sunscreens was found.

One cohort, Hunter *et al.* (1990)[48] and one case–control study by Kricker *et al.* (1995)[49] reported increased risks for BCC in sunscreen users. No significant association between sunscreen use and cancer risk was observed in one cohort and one case–control study of SCC,[50] one of SCC and BCC of the skin or one case–control study of SCC of the vermilion border of the lip.[47] Confounding of sun sensitivity and exposure were present in these studies, as in previously described studies.

Kricker *et al.*[49] found that subjects who had used sunscreens for at least half the time spent in the sun 1–9 years prior to diagnosis had a higher relative risk for BCC than those who had never used sunscreens or had used them less than half the time (RR 1·8; 95% CI 1·1–2·9). This risk persisted after adjustment for age, sex, ability to tan and site of lesion. No change in RR was found for those who had used sunscreens more than half the time in the 1–9 years, prior to diagnosis (RR 1·1; 95% CI 0·69–1·7) in comparison to those who had not used sunscreens or who had used them for half the time. Few subjects had access to sunscreens 11–30 years before diagnosis.

## Studies that have used intermediate endpoints such as incidence of solar keratoses as markers for BCC and SCC risk

Actinic (solar) keratoses are a risk factor for BCC and a precursor lesion for SCC. They are related to solar exposure and phenotype. The rate of development for SCC is low and many regress spontaneously, especially when exposure to UVR is reduced. These lesions have therefore been used as an intermediate endpoint in studies on the use of sunscreens in the prevention of SCC.[47,51] The Maryborough Trial in Australia[51] assessed whether the daily use of sunscreen had any effect in reducing the development of actinic keratoses in those already having these. This was a short-term study using a placebo and included body site examination and diaries to record the time of day patients applied sunscreen. Those using placebo had greater mean increase in the number of keratoses during the study $(1 \cdot 0 \pm 0 \cdot 3$ SE) than those given sunscreen $(0 \cdot 6 \pm 0 \cdot 3$; RR $1 \cdot 5$; 95% CI $0 \cdot 81 - 2 \cdot 2$). Fewer new keratoses were found in the sunscreen group $(1 \cdot 6 \ v \ 2 \cdot 3$ lesions per subject; RR $0 \cdot 62$; 95% CI $0 \cdot 54 - 0 \cdot 71$). After controlling for sex and sun sensitivity, the likely remission of keratoses (those with keratoses at the start of study) was greater for the sunscreen group (25% $v$ 18% initial lesions regressing: RR $1 \cdot 5$; 95% CI $1 \cdot 3 - 1 \cdot 8$).[51]

## Comment on sunscreen use and BCC and SCC

There is no conclusive evidence that sunscreen protects against either SCC or BCC and there is some limited evidence to suggest that risk may increase with sunscreen use. However, these non-randomised studies had confounding variables that make it difficult to be conclusive about such evidence.

Although the Maryborough acitinic keratoses trial[51] was a short-term trial, the confounding factors were well accounted for. The study suggests that sunscreen can prevent the development of new actinic keratoses. Further research is required to provide conclusive evidence.

## Do multistrategy interventions increase intention to use sunscreens as a protective measure for reducing the risk of melanoma and non-melanocytic skin cancers?

A number of studies have assessed the effectiveness of targeted sun protection interventions combined with sunscreen use.[52–79] Sunscreen use is only one of many outcome measures in these multistrategic interventions targeted at specific groups or to communities in general but was reported separately. Seven studies[54,55,60,61,68,71,72] were conducted in schools; four at beaches[52,57,63,64]; two at pools[52,75]; and three in other recreational settings.[62,65,67]; There were two studies in the workplace[69,72]; and two in clinical/medical settings.[58,61] There was one study in the tourist industry[53] and four multicomponent community studies.[56,66,70,73] Most studies were short term and aimed at improving sun-protection behaviour among specific high-risk groups, including children, young people, beachgoers, outdoor workers and patients with non-melanoma skin cancers.

In the main the studies used interactive educational presentations and communication strategies including peer-led programmes, role modelling, parental activities and materials aimed at increasing knowledge, including specific recommendations for sunscreen use. Interventions to enable policy change such as developing social and physical environments (shaded areas) for sun protection were the focus of three interventions.[52,60,73] Parental activities[62] and home activities[63] were the focus of two interventions. Medical interventions mainly used information giving to raise awareness of primary and secondary prevention of skin cancer.[56,58,60] More complex community interventions used incentives for beach guards, booklets,[52,56,61] primary and secondary prevention information and education,[66,73–76,79] and in schools.[54,55,67,71,73]

Twenty-two studies, quasirandomised and longitudinal studies reported on at least one outcome measure with regard to sunscreen use; proxy measures for behaviour were used in some studies (for example, the intention to use sunscreen). Eleven out of sixteen targeted interventions were successful in increasing knowledge and behaviour[52,54,56,59,61–64] and six were successful in increasing solar potection, either the use of shade, staying out of the sun or the use of clothing[52–59,62,64,68,73] and increased sunscreen use.[52,54,56–58,62,64,66–89] The duration and intensity of the intervention affected the success of the intervention. Successful interventions were longer, had multiple components or were supported by broader community initiatives.

Other reported successful educational intervention strategies were those intended to increase the perception of risk for developing skin cancer. Strategies that involved showing young people computer photoimages of their own faces with superimposed ageing and images of skin lesions were successful in improving both the frequency of sunscreen use and the application of sunscreen.[65]

An intervention for outdoor workers increased the use of sun protection but the use of sunscreen was not reported separately.[69] The impact of an intervention at swimming pools in which clients were given incentives and exposed to role modelling of lifeguards is unclear, although the authors reported that the sun-protection score was improved when two or more sun-protection measures were taken together, with no change in the mean quantity of free sunscreen used at pools.[52]

There have been six reported community interventions aimed at improving knowledge of skin cancer, encouraging the use of protective clothing and sunscreen use[74–79] Experience suggests that they require long-term funding, commitment and evaluation. Cross-sectional population surveys included the "Slip, Slap, Slop" and "SunSmart" campaigns in Australia[74,75]; "Sun Awareness" in Canada[76]; UVR index forecasting in the US[71]; the Melanoma and Skin Cancer Detection and Prevention Programme in the US[72]; and the Falmouth Safe Skin Programme in the US.[77] These were aimed at improving community knowledge about skin cancer and sun protection, and included mass media components, distribution of educational leaflets, the development of school curriculum for sun protection and sometimes partnership working in locality settings. Five of these large-scale community interventions had a positive impact on sunscreen use at population level.[74–79] The UVR index study reported no effect on sunscreen use but sunscreen use was associated with increased awareness of weather forecasts.[71,72]

## Comment on multifacet strategies to increase sunscreen use and sun protective behaviour

These multistrategic interventions are the most difficult to interpret collectively because of the plethora of outcome objectives. They remain difficult to design and require substantive formative research to appropriately determine specific behavioural outcome measures for each target group and for the selection of educational strategies for delivering the intervention. Those reporting indicate that interactive educational strategies are the most effective for increasing solar protection scores. Campaigns over time have the best outcome for increasing knowledge about skin cancer and use of sunscreens.

## Implications for clinical practice

- There is little good evidence that sunscreens reduce the risk of cutaneous melanoma.
- There is some evidence that sunscreen use may inadvertently increase risk because it may encourage longer periods in the sun.
- There is no clear evidence that sunscreen use decreases the incidence of BCC.
- There is some evidence that sunscreen use can decrease the incidence of actinic keratoses and SCC.

Educational messages are needed to ensure:

- that sunscreens are not used as the first or only choice for skin cancer prevention
- that sunscreens are not used as a means of extending total sun exposure (that is, sunbathing and suntanning).
- that sunscreens are not used as a substitute for clothes on body sites that are not usually exposed, such as the trunk and buttocks.
- the daily use of sunscreen with a high SPF ($> 15$) on areas of the body that are not usually exposed is recommended for those in areas of high isolation who work outdoors or undertake regular outdoor leisure pursuits
- daily use of a sunscreen can reduce actinic keratoses and SCC.

In addition:

- Protecting children against solar exposure during childhood is more important than at any time in life.
- Using photo-protective clothing, hats and shade is essential. Parents, carers, schools and leisure organisations need to encourage and promote knowledge about sun-protective behaviour.
- Primary prevention interventions should first and foremost promote hats with as wide a brim as possible to protect the head, neck and face (see Chapter 9).
- Shade should be promoted as protective whenever possible, including avoiding outdoor activities between 11·00 and 15·00 hours.

## Recommendations for future research

- Future research should seek to understand the role of sunscreens in the prevention of skin cancers and the role of UVR in the causation of these diseases, the dose–response relationship, the dose rate and pattern of delivery on risk and the action spectrum for each effect.
- RCTs should be conducted in adults to evaluate whether a reduction in late-stage exposure to UVR can reduce the incidence of cutaneous melanoma and precursor lesions such as clinically atypical naevi.
- In children, studies are needed to evaluate whether a reduction in early-stage exposure to UVR can reduce the prevalence of acquired naevi, the precursor of cutaneous melanoma and SCC.
- Trials should ideally include a quantitative assessment of solar exposure and an evaluation of the various methods for reducing solar exposure – sunscreens, clothing and sun avoidance.
- As sunscreens are increasingly used on children, an evaluation of their safety for long-term use is needed.
- There is a need to evaluate whether the qualitative rating of the potential function of sunscreens against UVR, such as low, medium, high and ultra-high, rather than SPF, would promote appropriate use of sunscreens.
- There is a need to understand better the role of the mechanisms of skin cancer aetiology and how sunscreens might affect this. Intermediate endpoints (for example, naevi and biochemical markers of carcinogenesis such as DNA damage and *p53* mutations) could be studied to assess their relationship to sunscreen use.
- Researchers in health promotion need to develop qualitative and quantitative methods for measuring sunscreen use in order to identify major confounding variables such as sun sensitivity and sun exposure.

- There is a need to be able to measure, in the field, how much protection is provided by sunscreens at various sites on the skin.
- There is a need to understand how efficiently individuals use sunscreen. This would enable manufacturers to develop sunscreens that achieve adequate protection against UVR when in common use.

## Conclusions

In the past 20 years, promoting the use of sunscreens has been the main focus of primary prevention for skin cancer together with photo-protective clothing and shaded areas. This summary demonstrates that health promoters across all settings, including primary care and hospital settings, need to re-think their sun protection promotion.

There is inadequate evidence in humans as to whether topical use of sunscreen has a preventative effect against cutaneous malignant melanoma and BCC of the skin and there is limited evidence for a protective effect against SCC of the skin. There is, however, good evidence that sunscreen prevents SCC of the skin induced in mice by solar-simulated radiation.

The review supports the hypothesis that the topical use of sunscreens reduces the risk of sunburn in humans and probably prevents SCC of the skin when used during intentional sunbathing. There is inconclusive evidence about the cancer-preventive effects of topical use of sunscreens against BCC and cutaneous melanoma. It seems that sunscreen can extend intentional sun exposure (sunbathing and suntanning) and that this increased exposure may subsequently increase the risk for cutaneous melanoma.

It is essential that the main educational message promoting long-term changes to attitude and behaviour in the sun should focus on the use of photo-protective clothing and shade; sunscreens should be promoted as an extra protective measure, after the use of clothing and shade. There should be very positive messages about the use of sunscreen including application and re-application at regular intervals. This will prevent individuals from having a false sense of security engendered by the use of sunscreens, particularly for intentional suntanning behaviour.

Promoting the use of photo-protective clothing and shade remains the most effective way to prevent against unintentional exposure. It is imperative that policy includes the development of shaded areas in communities and on beaches, even in temperate climes. Sunscreens may give a false sense of security about protection, putting individuals at increased risk for sun exposure and thus for cutaneous skin cancers.

Communication and appropriate efficacious delivery of messages intended to change behaviour remain the main goal point of long-term randomised studies across communities. This is very important as we face the threat of continued global warming. This will be a challenge for all in public health and health promotion.

## References

1 Shaath NA. Evolution of modern sunscreen chemicals. In: Lowe NJ, Shaath NA, Pathak MA, eds. *Sunscreens, Development, Evaluation and Regulatory Aspects. 2nd edn. Cosmetic Science and Technology Series* 1997;**15**:3–33.

2 Bestak R, Barneston RS, Neath MR, Halliday GM. Sunscreen protection of contact hypersensitivity responses from chronic solar-simulated ultra irradiation correlates with the absorption spectrum of the sunscreen. *J Invest Dermatol* 1995;**105**:345–51.

3 Schulze R. Some tests and remarks regarding the problem of sunscreens that are found on the market (in German). *Parfum Kosmet* 1956;**37**:310–16.

4 Quinn AG, Diffey BL *et al.* Definition of the minimal erythema dose used for diagnostic phototesting. *Br J Dermatol* 1994;**131**:56–9.

5 Lock-Anderson J, Wulf HC Threshold level for measurement of UV sensitivity: Reproducibility of phototest. *Photodermatol Photoimmunol Photomed* 1996;**12**:154–61.

6 Janousek A. *Regulatory aspects of sunscreens in Europe.* In: Lowe NJ, Shaath NA, Pathak MA, eds. *Sunscreens, development, evaluation and regulatory aspects. 2nd edn: Cosmetic Science and Technology Series* 1997;215–25.

7 Fukuda M, Takata S. The evolution of recent sunscreens. In: Altmeyer P, Hoffmann K, Stuker M, eds. *Skin Cancer and UV Radiation.* Berlin: Springer-Verlag 1997:265–76.

8 Australian/New Zealand Standards. *Sunscreen products – Evaluation and Classification.* Homebush Standards, Australia; Wellington Standards; New Zealand, 1998.

9 Health Canada. *Regulatory Strategy for Pharmaceutical Products with Photo- Co-carcinogneic Potential.* Ottawa: Therapeutic Products Programme, 1999.

10 European Commission. Directive 76/78 Guidelines for testing of cosmetic ingredients (SCCMF), 1976.

11 Hill D, White V, Marks R *et al.* Melanoma prevention: Behavioural and non-behavioural factors in sunburn among an Australian urban population. *Prev Med* 1992;**21**:654–69.

12 McGee R, Williams S, Cox B, Elwood M, Bulliard JL. A community survey of sun exposure, sunburn and sun protection. *NZ Med J* 1995;**108**:508–10.

13 Melia J, Bulman A. Sunburn and tanning in a British population. *J Public Hlth Med* 1995;**17**:223–9.

14 Autier P, Dore AU JF, Cattaruzza MS *et al.* Sunscreen use, wearing clothes, and number of nevi in 6–7 year old European children. *J Natl Cancer Inst* 1998;**90**:1873–80.

15 Wulf HC, Stender IM, Lock-Andersen J. Sunscreens used at the beach do not protect against erythema: A new definition of SPF is proposed. *Photoderm Photoimmunol Photomed* 1997;**13**:129–32.

16 Autier P, Dore JF, Negrier S *et al.* Sunscreen use and duration of sun exposure: A double blind randomised trial. *J Natl Cancer Inst* 1999;**91**:1304–9.

17 McCarthy EM, Ethridge KP, Wagner JF Jr. Beach holiday sunburn: The sunscreen paradox and gender differences. *Cutis* 1999;**64**:37–42.

18 Hill D, White V, Marks R, Borland R. Changes in sun-related attitudes and behaviours, and reduced sunburn prevalence in a population at high risk of melanoma. *Eur J Can Prev* 1993;**2**:447–56.

19 Baade PD, Balanda KP, Lowe JB. Changes in sun protection behaviours, attitudes and sunburn in a population with the highest incidence of skin cancer in the world. *Cancer Detect Prev* 1996;**20**:566–75.

20 Rivers JK, Gallagher RP. Public education projects in skin cancer: Experience of the Canadian Dermatology Association. *Cancer* 1995;**75**(Suppl.):661–6.

21  Miller RW, Rabkin CS. Merkel cell carcinoma and melanoma: Etiological similarities and differences. *Cancer Epidemiol Biomark Prev* 1999;**8**:153–8.

22  Lombard D, Neubauer TE, Canfield D, Winett RA. Behavioural community intervention to reduce risk of skin cancer. *J Appl Behav* 1991;**24**:677–86.

23  Gooderham MJ, Guenther L. Sun and the skin: Evaluation of a sun awareness program for elementary school students. *J Cutan Med Surg* 1999;**3**:230–5.

24  Cockburn J, Thompson S, Marks R, Jolley D, Schofield D, Hill D. Behavioural dynamics of a clinical trial of sunscreens for reducing solar keratoses in Victoria, Australia. *J Epidemiol Community Hlth* 1997;**51**:716–21.

25  IARC 2001 *Handbooks of Cancer Prevention. Vol. 5 Sunscreens.* Lyon, France: IARC Press.

26  Klepp O, Magnus K. Some environmental and bodily characteristics of melanoma patients. A case-control study. *Int J Cancer* 1979;**23**: 482–6.

27  Graham S, Marshall J, Haughey B *et al.* An inquiry into the epidemiology of melanoma. *Am J Epidemiol* 1985;**122**:606–19.

28  Herzfeld PM, Fitzgerald EF, Hwang SA, Stark A. A case-control study of malignant melanoma of the trunk among white males in upstate New York. *Cancer Detect Prev* 1993;**17**:601–8.

29  Beitner H, Norell SE, Ringborg U, Wennersten G, Mattson B. Malignant melanoma: Aetiological importance of individual pigmentation and sun exposure. *Br J Dermatol* 1990;**122**:43–51.

30  Elwood M, Gallagher RP. More about: Sunscreen use, wearing clothes and number of nevi in 6–7 year old European children. *J Natl Cancer Inst* 1999;**91**:1164–6.

31  Holman CDJ, Armstrong BK, Heenan PJ. Relationship of cutaneous melanoma to individual sunlight exposure habits. *J Natl Cancer Inst* 1986;**76**:403–14.

32  Holly EA, Kelly JW, Shpall SN, Chiu SH. Number of melanocytic nevi as a major risk factor for malignant melanoma. *J Am Acad Dermatol* 1987;**17**:459–68.

33  Osterlind A, Tucker MA, Stone BJ, Jenson OM. The Danish case-control study of cutaneous maligant melanoma. II. Importance of UV-light exposure *Int J Cancer* 1988;**42**:319–24.

34  Whiteman DC, Valery P, McWhirter W, Green AC. Risk factors for childhood melanoma in Queensland, Australia. *Int J Cancer* 1997;**70**:26–31.

35  Westerdahl J, Olsson H, Masback A, Ingvar C, Jonsson N. Is the use of sunscreens a risk factor for malignant melanoma? *Melanoma Res* 1995;**5**:59–65.

36  Rodenas JM, Delgado-Rodriguez M, Herranz M, Tercedor J, Serrano S. Sun exposure, pigmentary traits, and risk of cutaneous malignant melanoma: A case control study in a Mediterranean population. *Cancer Causes Control* 1996;**7**:275–83.

37  Espinoza-Arranz J, Sanchez-Hernandez JJ, Bravo Fernandez P, Gonzalez-Baron M, Zamora Aunon P. Cutaneous maligant melanoma and sun exposure in Spain. *Melanoma Res* 1999;**9**:199–205.

38  Autier P, Dore JF, Sciffers E *et al.* Melanoma and use of sunscreens: An EORTC case-control study in Germany, Belgium and France. *Int J Cancer* 1995;**61**:749–55.

39  Wolf P, Quehenberger F, Mulleger R, Stranz B, Kerl H. Phenotypic markers, sunlight-related factors and sunscreen use in patients with cutaneous melanoma: An Austrain case-control study. *Melanoma Res* 1998;**8**:370–8.

40  Westerdahl J, Ingvar C, Masback A, Olsson H. Sunscreen use and malignant melanoma. *Int J Cancer* 2000;**87**:145–50.

41  Elwood M *et al.* More about: Sunscreen use, wearing clothes, and number of nevi in 6–7 year old European children. *J Natl Cancer Inst* 1999;**91**:1164–6.

42  Luther H, Altmeyer P, Garbe C, Ellwanger U, Jahn S, Hoffmann K, Sergerling M. Increase of melanocytic nevus counts in children during 5 years of follow up and analysis of associated factors. *Arch Dermatol* 1996;**132**:1473–8.

43  Pope DJ, Sorahan T, Marsden JR, Ball PM, Grimely RP, Peck LM. Benign pigmented nevi in children. *Arch Dermatol* 1992;**128**:1201–6.

44  Green A, Williams G, Nelae R *et al.* Daily sunscreen application and beta-carotene supplementation in prevention of basal cell and squamous cell carcinomas of the skin: A randomised controlled trial. *Lancet* 1999;**354**:723–9.

45  Green A, Williams G, Neale R, Battistutta D. Beta-carotene and sunscreen use. (Author's reply). *Lancet* 1999;**354**:2163–4.

46  Grodestein F. Speizer FE, and Hunter DJ. A prospective study of incident squamous cell carcinoma of the skin in the nurses' health study. *J Natl Cancer Inst* 1995;**87**:1061–6.

47  Pogoda JM, Preston-Martin S. Solar radiation lip protection and lip cancer risk in Los Angeles Country women. *Cancer Causes Control* 1996;**7**:458–63.

48  Hunter DJ, Colditz GA, Strampfer MJ, Rosner B, Willett WC, Speizer FE. Risk factors for basal-cell carcinoma in a prospective cohort of women. *Ann Epidemiol* 1990;**1**:13–23.

49  Kricker A, Armstrong BK, English DR, Heenana PJ. Does intermittent sun exposure cause basal-cell carcinoma? A case control study in Western Australia. *Int J Cancer* 1995;**60**:489–94.

50  English DR, Armstrong BK, Kricker A, Winter MG, Heenana PJ, Randell PL. Demographic characteristics, pigmentary and cutaneous risk factors for squamous cell carcinoma of the skin: A case control study. *Int J Cancer* 1998;**76**:628–34.

51  Thompson SC, Jolley D, Marks R. Reduction in solar keratoses by regular sunscreen use. *N Engl J Med* 1999;**329**:1147–51.

52  Dobinson S, Borland R, Anderson M. Sponsorship and sun protection practices in lifesavers. *Health Prom Int* 1999;**14**:167–75.

53  Segan CJ, Borland R, Hill DJ. Development and evaluation of a brochure on sun protection and sun exposure for tourists. *Health Educ J* 1999;**58**:177–91.

54  Gooderham MJ, Guenther L. Sun and the skin: Evaluation of a sun awareness program for elementary school students. *J Cutan Med Surg* 1999;**3**:230–5.

55  Hughes BR, Altman DG, Newton JA. Melanoma and skin cancer: Evaluation of a health education programme for secondary schools. *Br J Dermatol* 1993;**128**:412–17.

56  Putman GL, Yanagisako KL. Skin cancer comic book: Evaluation of a public education vehicle. *Cancer Detect Prev* 1982;**5**:349–56.

57  Robinson JK, Rademarker AW. Sun protection by families at the beach. *Arch Pediatr Adolescent Med* 1995;**152**:466–70.

58  Robinson JK, Rademaker AW. Skin cancer risk and sun protection learning by helpers of patients with non-melanoma skin cancer. *Prev Med* 1995;**24**:333–41.

59  Lombard D, Neubauer TE, Canfiled D, Winett RA. Behavioural community intervention to reduce the risk of skin cancer. *J Appl Behav* 1991;**24**:677–86.

60  Memelstein RJ, Riesenberg LA. Changing knowledge and attitudes about skin cancer risk factors in adolescents. *Health Psychol* 1992; **11**:371–6.

61  Buller DB, Callister M, Reichert T. Skin cancer prevention by parents of young children: Health information sources, skin cancer knowledge, and sun protection practices *Oncol Nurs Forum* 1995;**22**:1559–6.

62  Glanz K, Chang L, Song V, Silverio R, Munecka L. Skin cancer prevention for children, parents, and caregivers: A field test of Hawaii's SunSmart program. *J Am Acad Dermatol* 1998;**384**:13–17.

63  Detweiler JB, Bedell BT, Salovey P, Pronin E, Rothman AJ. Message framing and sunscreen use: Gain-framed messages motivate beachgoers. *Health Psychol* 1999;**18**:189–96.

64  Weinstock MA, Rossi JS, Redding CA, Maddock JE. Randomised trial of intervention for sun protection among beachgoers. *J Invest Dermatol* 1992;**110**:589.

65  Novick M. To burn or not to burn: Use of computer-enhanced stimuli to encourage application of sunscreens. *Cutis* 1997;**60**:105–8.

66  Dietrich AJ, Olson AL, Sox CH, Stevens M, Tosteson TD, Ahles TA. Community based randomised trial encouraging sun protection for children. *Paediatrics* 1998;**102**:E64–E71.

67  Parrot R, Duggan A, Cremo J, Eckles A, Jones K, Steiner C. Commuicating about youth's sun exposure risk to soccer coaches and parents: A pilot study in Georgia. *Hlth Educ Behav* 1993;**26**:385–95.

68  Girgis A, Sanson-Fisher RW, Tripodi DA, Golding T. Evaluation of interventions to improve solar protection in primary schools. *Health Ed Q* 1993;**20**:275–87.

69  Girgis A, Sanson-Fisher RW, Watson A. A workplace intervention for increasing outdoor workers' use of solar protection. *Am J Public Health* 1994;**84**:77–81.

70  Lawler PE. Be sensible; Steps towards safety in the sun- An information handout. *Oncol Nurs Forum* 1989;**16**:424–7.

71  Reding DJ, Fischer V, Gunderson P, Lapper K. Skin cancer prevention: A peer education model. *Wisconsin Med J* 1995;**94**:77–81.

72  Friedman LC, Webb JA, Bruse S, Weinberg AD, Cooper HP. Skin cancer prevention and early detection intentions and behaviour. *Am J Prev Med* 1995;**11**:59–65.

73  Grant-Peterson J, Dietrich AJ, Sox CH, Winchell CW, Stevens MM. Promoting sun protection in elementary schools and child care settings. The Sunsafe project. *School Health* 1999;**69**:100–7.

74  Hill D, White V, Marks R, Borland R. Changes in sun-related attitudes and behaviours, and reduced sunburn prevalence in a population at high risk of melanoma. *Eur J Cancer Prev* 1993;**2**:447–56.

75  Borland R, Hill D, Noy S. Being Sun Smart: Changes in community awareness and reported behaviour following a primary prevention programe for skin cancer control. *Behav Changes* 1990;**7**:126–35.

76  Rivers JK, Gallagher RP. Public education projects in skin cancer: Experience of the Canadian Dermatology Association. *Cancer* 1995;**75**(Suppl.):661–6.

77  Miller RW, Rabkin CS. Merkel cell carcinoma and melanoma: Etiological similarities and differences. *Cancer Epidemiol Biomark Prev* 1999;**8**:153–8.

78  Geller AC, Hufford D *et al.* Evalutation of the ultraviolet index: Media reactions and public response. *J Am Acad Dermatol* 1997;**37**:935–41.

79  Robinson JK, Rigel DS, Ammonete RA. Trends in sun exposure knowledge, attitudes and behaviours: 1986–1996. *J Am Acad Dermatol* 1997;**37**:179–86.

# 11 Can lifestyle behaviour change reduce the risk and incidence of urological cancers?

*Mike Shelley, Kathryn Burgon, Malcolm Mason*

Cancers of the bladder, prostate, kidney and testis account for approximately 9% of all new cancers and represent a major health problem worldwide. The number of new cases per year for all urological cancers in the USA is estimated to be 275 000 compared to 158 000 in Europe.[1,2] Although chemotherapy for testicular cancer is very effective, new treatments are needed to improve on mortality rates for bladder, prostate and renal cancers. One potential way to address this is to direct research towards the prevention of urological cancers. The protracted natural history of bladder and prostate cancers makes these diseases amenable to preventive intervention; however, in order to implement prevention trials, epidemiological studies need to identify risk factors that can then direct prevention strategies. The following sections present the evidence for the major risk factors for urological cancers, and describe relevant chemoprevention trials and preventive opportunities to reduce the risk of these diseases.

Opportunities for prevention of urological cancers are discussed in the final paragraph of the Testicular Cancer section.

## Bladder cancer

### Background

Cancer of the urinary bladder is the eleventh most common cancer in the world and causes considerable mortality and morbidity. The World Health Organization reported that 300 000 cases of bladder cancer were diagnosed in 1996 accounting for approximately 3% of all cancers worldwide.[3] The incidence rate is higher in developing countries such as North America and Europe. It is more common in men – for example, the incidence rate per 100 000 in England and Wales in 1997 was 33·2 for men compared to 13·4 for women.[4] The majority of patients present with early stage disease confined to the urothelium or lamina propria (Ta and T1), but approximately 20% will have invasive disease.

### Aetiology

The aetiology of bladder cancer is poorly understood but a number of causative agents have been identified.

### Smoking

Many epidemiological studies have identified smoking as a risk factor in the development of bladder cancer. Approximately 50% of all male bladder cancers and 30% of all female bladder cancers might be attributable to smoking.[5] Although the incidence of bladder cancer is greater in men, the risk may be significantly higher ($P = 0·01$) in women who have smoked comparable amounts of cigarettes.[6] A recent systematic review and meta-analysis has quantified different smoking characteristics based on data from 43 case–control and cohort studies.[7] Current cigarette smokers have approximately three times the risk of developing urinary tract cancer compared to non-smokers (odds ratio [OR] 3·18; 95% CI, 2·35–4·29). The risk is positively associated with the number of cigarettes smoked per day (OR 2·66; 95% CI, 2·06–3·42 for men) and the duration of smoking (for example more than 20 years OR 2·59; 95% CI, 1·83–3·67). Men who stopped smoking for fewer than 10 years had higher risks compared to those who had stopped for longer than 10 years (OR 1·23; 95% CI, 0·80–1·87). Furthermore, starting smoking at a young age, for example at younger than 20 years, tended to be associated with a higher risk (OR 1·25; 95% CI, 1·07–1·47).

The mechanism by which smoking may induce bladder cancer is unknown, but many carcinogenic metabolites from tobacco are excreted by the kidneys and stored in the bladder, allowing direct exposure to the urothelium and the potential for cancer development. 2-Naphthylamine, 4-aminobiphenol, and several nitrosamines in tobacco smoke are suspected as the major causative agents for bladder cancer.[8] N-acetylation, regulated by the enzyme N-acetyltransferase, can detoxify tobacco carcinogens and, owing to the lack of two functional alleles, two distinct phenotypes – "fast" and "slow" acetylators – exist. A meta-analysis of 16 bladder cancer studies, has suggested that the relationship of smoking and bladder cancer is strongest among "slow" acetylators (OR 1·3; 95% CI, 1·0–1·6).[9] An overview of 21 case–control studies, with considerable overlap with the previous report, suggested that the "slow" acetylation phenotype may be associated with a small increase in bladder cancer risk (OR 1·41) but, owing to possible publication bias, could not provide definitive evidence.[10] Another meta-analysis indicated a modest increase in risk of bladder cancer with "slow" acetylation, but there was heterogeneity between the included studies.[11] There is suggestive evidence of a link between smoking and genetic abnormalities, such as chromosome 9 defects[12] and *p53* mutations[13] in the aetiology of bladder cancer.

Based on the available data, there is strong evidence that smoking is a major preventable factor in the development of urinary tract cancer. Patients who continue to smoke after diagnosis of bladder cancer may have worse disease-associated outcomes.[14] Encouraging patients to stop or reduce cigarette consumption could therefore be used as a tertiary prevention strategy.

## Occupational exposure

Exposure to carcinogenic chemicals in the workplace increases the risk of developing bladder cancer by 21% to 25%.[15] Exposure to aromatic amines is associated with the highest risk and these have been used extensively in paint, plastic, and dye industries, and are now found in diesel fumes. A large population-based study reported that employment in the production of organic chemicals was associated with a 1·3-fold increased risk among men (95% CI, 0·8–1·2), which increased with the duration of employment (OR 2·4, $P = 0.06$).[16] There was an increased risk associated within the plastic and rubber industry, particularly in procedures that produced dust (OR 4·6; 95% CI, 1·0–20·4). The use of pesticides was also associated with an increased risk of developing bladder cancer (OR 2·3; 95% CI, 0·6–8·20). Others have identified elevated relative risks (RR) of 1·5 for painters (95% CI, 1·2–2·0), of 1·3 for truck drivers (95% CI, 1·1–1·4), and of 1·4 for drill press operators (95% CI, 0·9–2·1).[15] A pooled analysis of 11 case–control studies reported a statistically significant increased risk for bladder cancer for European women in the following occupations: metal workers (OR 2·0; 95% CI, 1·1–3·6), tobacco workers (OR 3·1; 95% CI, 1·1–9·3), agricultural workers (OR 1·8; 95% CI, 1·0–3·1), saleswomen (OR 2·6; 95% CI, 1·0–6·9), dressmakers (OR 1·4; 95% CI, 1·0–2·1), and mail-sorting clerks (OR 4·4; 95% CI, 1·0–19·5).[17] Systematic reviews have associated a higher risk of developing bladder cancer in

workers exposed to metalworking fluids[18] and diesel fumes (RR 1·44; 95% CI, 1·18–1·76).[19] Exposure to carbon black in longshoremen has been recently identified as a potential risk factor for bladder cancer and steps have now been taken to eliminate the risk in handling this compound.[20]

## Schistosomiasis and bladder irritation

Several epidemiological studies have suggested that urinary schistosomiasis (*Schistosomiasis haematobium*) has a role in the multistage process of bladder carcinogenesis.[21–23] The evidence is mainly derived from a geographical correlation between the two conditions, particularly in countries such as Egypt, where bladder cancer rates are high and infestation is common. Further evidence is based on a positive history of urinary schistosomiasis in patients with bladder cancer, the average duration of infection before bladder cancer being 12 years, and the identification of *Schistosomiasis haematobium* ova in tumour tissue. It has been estimated that 16% of bladder cancers in endemic areas may be explained by a history of urinary schistosomiasis.[24] Mechanistic studies have examined the generation of carcinogenic nitrosamines by bacteria commonly associated with schistosomiasis infection.[25] Others have shown a reduced ATPase activity in tumour cells associated with schistosomiasis possibly rendering them more susceptible to the carcinogenic action of environmental alkylating agents.[26]

Other forms of bladder irritation and infection have been suggested as risk factors in the aetiology of bladder cancer. In a large epidemiological study of 2982 bladder carcinoma patients and 5782 controls from 10 geographical areas of the USA, a history of three or more urinary tract infections was associated with a significantly elevated risk (RR 2·0). The occurrence of bladder stones was also associated with a higher risk (RR 1·8) for bladder cancer.[27]

## Diet and nutrition

Many studies have suggested that diet may have a causal and preventive action in the development of bladder cancer. In a cohort study of 8000 men, after adjustment for smoking, fruit consumption was inversely related to bladder cancer risk (RR 0·6; $P = 0.38$) but no relationship with fat intake was found.[28]

Evidence from a prospective study suggests that fried vegetables consumed at least five times per week is associated with a relative risk for bladder cancer of 2·6 (95% CI, 0·6–10·4) compared with once per week or less.[28] Two case–control studies report an increased risk of bladder cancer with fried meat, eggs, potatoes and gravy (OR 2·4; 95% CI, 1·4–4·2)[29] and fried foods more than twice per week compared to none (OR 2·2; 95% CI, 1·3–4·0).[30]

Heterocyclic amines are possible candidates since they are produced in meats cooked at high temperatures[31] and induce bladder tumours in animals.[32]

Other studies have associated high consumption of animal fat with an increased risk of bladder cancer. A recent meta-analysis, using a search of MEDLINE and CancerLit, identified 38 case–control and cohort studies linking six dietary factors to bladder cancer.[33] Elevated relative risks were found for diets high in fat intake (RR 1·37; 95% CI, 1·16–1·62) and low in fruit intake (RR 1·40; 95% CI, 1·08–1·83), but not for diets with a low intake of vegetables, retinol, beta-carotene, or a high intake of meat. In a prospective study of 120 825 subjects followed for 6·3 years, a number of specific vegetables were identified as having a significant inverse association, such as cauliflower (RR 0·77; 95% CI, 0·61–0·98), cooked carrots (RR 0·66; 95% CI, 0·47–0·96), and mandarins (RR 0·63; 95% CI, 0·42–0·96).[34] The results suggest that diets high in fruit and vegetables and low in fat may have a beneficial effect, but the role of individual constituents remains unknown.

## Fluid intake, coffee, tea, artificial sweeteners and alcohol consumption

Fluid loading and bladder distention has been reported to increase the incidence of chemically-induced bladder tumours in rats.[35] The mechanism may involve flattening of the urothelium leading to a greater exposure of urine-borne carcinogens. This has led to a number of studies examining total fluid intake and the risk associated with bladder cancer. Three case–control studies indicate an increased risk with higher fluid intake, with an OR (95% CI) of 3·3 (1·4–7·40) for men consuming 4 litres/day compared with 1 litre/day[36]; 4·9 (2·0–12·3) for 3 litres/day, compared with < 2·00[37] and 1·43 (1·23–1·67) when 2 litres per day are compared with < 1 litre per day.[38] Two prospective studies[39,40] and four case–control studies[41–44] reported no significant relationships with total fluid intake and bladder cancer. In addition, in a prospective study of 47 909 participants followed for 10 years, a high fluid intake was associated with a decreased risk of bladder cancer in men.[45] The evidence from these studies is conflicting and does not allow discrimination between fluid intake *per se* and its constituents. As a result, no firm conclusion can be made.

The relationship between coffee consumption and the risk of bladder cancer has been investigated in a large series of studies, although the quality and power of many are limited, owing to confounding factors such as smoking. A critical review and statistical summary reported on 35 case–control studies published between 1971 and 1992.[46] The summary data from eight studies that met the inclusion criteria showed no evidence for an increased risk of lower urinary tract cancer with coffee drinking in men or women after the adjustment for smoking (OR 1·07; 95% CI, 1·00–1·14 for men; OR 0·91; 0·81–1·03 for women). The evidence from a more recent review of six prospective and 36 case–control studies of coffee consumption and bladder cancer, suggests a slight increase in risk with higher intake of over five cups per day.[47]

A number of cohort and case–control studies of bladder cancer have examined the association with black tea consumption. The available evidence suggests no strong or consistent link with an increased risk of bladder cancer.[47]

Experimental studies in animals, suggesting that high doses of saccharin initiated the development of bladder tumours, led to concerns that a similar effect may occur in humans. In 1977, a Canadian case–control study of 480 men and 152 women reported a positive association between the use of artificial sweeteners and the risk of bladder cancer, with a risk ratio of 1–6.[48] Saccharin and cyclamates are found in many foods, typically in ratios of 1:1, which confounds their individual extent of risk. Over 30 epidemiological studies have now been published on saccharin and cyclamates, either individually or combined, concerning daily intakes, dietetic food, beverages, and the frequency and duration of consumption. A comprehensive review of the literature suggests that consumption of saccharin at concentrations found in the normal diet is not related to bladder cancer risk.[47] The limited data on the more recently used cyclamates also suggest no relationship.

A recent review of two prospective and 19 case–control studies reported that high alcohol intake has no relationship with the risk of bladder cancer.[47] However, evidence from a meta-analysis of 16 studies published up to 1999 indicates a slightly increased risk from alcohol consumption for men (OR 1·3; 95% CI, 0·9–2·0).[49]

## Vitamin C, A (retinol), E and carotenoids

Four case–control studies[29,42,50,51] and one cohort study[52] reported no relationship between daily intake of vitamin C and the risk of developing bladder cancer. However, moderate protection was reported in two additional studies with ORs of 0·5 (95% CI, 0·3–0·9)[30] and 0·6 (95% CI, 0·2–1·4).[53] There appears to be a reduced risk with vitamin supplementation (RR 0·6; 95% CI, 0·5–1·7).[52] A strong protective effect was associated with an intake of 502 mg/day (OR 0·4: 95% CI, 0·2–0·8).[30] Two other studies report a weak reduced risk with vitamin C supplementation.[29,53]

Data on retinol intake and the risk of bladder cancer are inconsistent. Four case–control studies show no significant association,[29,42,50,51] one study reports an increased risk in men[53] whilst others indicate a significant protective effect with ORs of 0·4–0·5.[30,54]

Two prospective studies have shown no association of vitamin E and bladder cancer,[52,55] whilst two others report a non-significant protective effect with ORs of 0·7 in both studies.[30,50]

The data for carotenoids intake and bladder cancer risk are conflicting. Four case–control studies report no association.[29,41–51] One further study suggests a weak relationship (OR 0·5 men and 0·7 women)[51] and two indicate a protective effect with ORs of 0·5–0·7.[53] One cohort study reports a non-significant relative risk of 1·3.[53] The available evidence suggests a preventive role for carotenoids but more data are needed to make a firm statement.

## Pharmaceuticals

A number of drugs have been implicated as risk factors for bladder cancer. Heavy acetaminophen exposure may have a small, non-significant increased risk with odds ratios of 1·9 (95% CI, 0·6–2·8)[56] and 1·43 (95% CI, 0·87–2·35).[57] Patients with rheumatoid arthritis treated with oral cyclophosphamide are at an increased risk of bladder cancer.[58] Cancer patients receiving cyclophosphamide may be at risk of developing secondary bladder cancer.[59,60]

## Chemoprevention trials

The developmental cascade of superficial bladder cancer is characterised by a long latent period which may last as long as 30 years. This makes it amenable to intervention with preventive agents, such as vitamins, which are readily available and generally well tolerated.

Twenty patients with refractory and recurring bladder tumours showed no response to oral 13-*cis*-retinoic acid.[61] In a double-blind clinical trial of 30 patients with Ta/T1, G1–2 superficial bladder cancer, the synthetic retinoid, etretinate, significantly reduced tumour recurrence compare to placebo from 87% to 60% ($P = 0·01$).[62] Etretinate activity was confirmed in a subsequent placebo controlled, randomised trial.[63]

Vitamin B6 (pyridoxine) ameliorates the abnormal tryptophan metabolism, thought to occur in bladder cancer, which would otherwise lead to potentially carcinogenic metabolites. In a randomised trial, tumour recurrence was reported in 60% of control patients (placebo), 46% receiving pyridoxine and 47% receiving intravesical thiotepa.[64] An EORTC double-blind randomised trial failed to confirm the efficacy of pyridoxine compared to placebo.[65]

The efficacy of a normal daily intake of vitamins compared to a mega-dose vitamin combination (A, B6, C, E) was evaluated in a double-blind randomised trial.[66] The 5-year estimates of tumour recurrence were 91% in the normal daily intake group compared to 41% in the

mega-dose group ($P = 0·004$). These data suggest that further studies are warranted.

## References

1 Woolam GL. Cancer statistics, 2000: a benchmark for the new century. *CA Cancer J Clin* 2000;**50**:6–33.
2 Jensen OM, Esteve J, Moller H, Renard H. Cancer in the European Community and its member states. *Eur J Cancer* 1990;**26**:1167–256.
3 WHO. *The world health report: Geneva.* Geneva: World Health Organization, 1997.
4 Office for National Statistics. *Mortality statistics – cause, England and Wales, 1999.* London: The Stationery Office, 2000.
5 Hartge P, Silverman D, Hoover R *et al.* Changing cigarette habits and bladder cancer risk: a case–control study. *J Natl Cancer Inst* 1987;**78**: 1119–25.
6 Castelao JE, Yuan JM, Skipper PL *et al.* Gender- and smoking-related bladder cancer risk. *J Natl Cancer Inst* 2001;**93**:538–45.
7 Zeegers MP, Tan FE, Dorant E, van Den Brandt PA. The impact of characteristics of cigarette smoking on urinary tract cancer risk: a meta-analysis of epidemiologic studies. *Cancer* 2000;**89**:630–9.
8 Ross RK, Jones PA, Yu MC. Bladder cancer epidemiology and pathogenesis. *Semin Oncol* 1996;**23**:536–45.
9 Marcus PM, Hayes RB, Vineis P *et al.* Cigarette smoking, N-acetyltransferase 2 acetylation status, and bladder cancer risk: a case-series meta-analysis of a gene-environment interaction. *Cancer Epidemiol Biomarker Prevent* 2000;**9**:461–7.
10 Green J, Banks E, Berrington A, Darby S, Deo H, Newton R. N-acetyltransferase 2 and bladder cancer: an overview and consideration of the evidence for gene-environment interaction. *Br J Cancer* 2000;**83**:412–17.
11 Johns LE, Houlston RS. N-acetyl transferase-2 and bladder cancer risk: a meta-analysis. *Environ Molecular Mutagenesis* 2000;**36**:221–7.
12 Zhang ZF, Shu XM, Cordon-Cardo C *et al.* Cigarette smoking and chromosome 9 alterations in bladder cancer. *Cancer Epidemiol Biomarker Prevent* 1997;**6**:321–6.
13 Zhang ZF, Sarkis AS, Cordon-Cardo C *et al.* Tobacco smoking, occupation, and p53 nuclear overexpression in early stage bladder cancer. *Cancer Epidemiol Biomarker Prevent* 1994;**3**:19–24.
14 Fleshner N, Garland J, Moadel A *et al.* Influence of smoking status on the disease-related outcomes of patients with tobacco-associated superficial transitional cell carcinoma of the bladder. *Cancer* 1999;**86**:2337–45.
15 Silverman DT, Levin LI, Hoover RN, Hartge P. Occupational risks of bladder cancer in the United States: I. White men. *J Natl Cancer Inst* 1989;**81**(19):1472–80.
16 Zahm SH, Hartge P, Hoover R. The National Bladder Cancer Study: employment in the chemical industry. *J Natl Cancer Inst* 1987;**79**: 217–22.
17 Mannetje A, Kogevinas M, Chang-Claude J *et al.* Occupation and bladder cancer in European women. *Cancer Causes Control* 1999;**10**:209–17.
18 Calvert GM, Ward E, Schnorr TM, Fine LJ. Cancer risks among workers exposed to metalworking fluids: a systematic review. *Am J Industrial Med* 1998;**33**:282–92.
19 Boffetta P, Silverman DT. A meta-analysis of bladder cancer and diesel exhaust exposure. *Epidemiology* 2001;**12**:125–30.
20 Puntoni R, Ceppi M, Reggiardo G, Merlo F. Occupational exposure to carbon black and risk of bladder cancer. *Lancet* 2001;**358**:562.
21 Mustacchi P SM. Cancer of the bladder and infection with schistosoma hematobium. *J Natl Cancer Inst* 1958;**20**:825–42.
22 Gelfand M, Weinberg RW, Castle WM. Relation between carcinoma of the bladder and infestation with *Schistosoma haematobium. Lancet* 1967;**1**:1249–51.
23 Bedwani R, Renganathan E, El Kwhsky F *et al.* Schistosomiasis and the risk of bladder cancer in Alexandria, Egypt. *Br J Cancer* 1998;**77**:1186–9.

24  Bedwani R, el-Khwsky F, La Vecchia C, Boffetta P, Levi F. Descriptive epidemiology of bladder cancer in Egypt. *Int J Cancer* 1993;**55**:351–2.

25  El-Merzabani MM, El-Aaser AA, Zakhary NI. A study on the aetiological factors of bilharzial bladder cancer in Egypt–1 Nitrosamines and their precursors in urine. *Eur J Cancer* 1979;**15**:287–91.

26  Badawi AF, Cooper DP, Mostafa MH *et al*. O6-alkylguanine-DNA alkyltransferase activity in schistosomiasis-associated human bladder cancer. *Eur J Cancer* 1994;**30A**:1314–19.

27  Kantor AF, Hartge P, Hoover RN, Narayana AS, Sullivan JW, Fraumeni JF. Urinary tract infection and risk of bladder cancer. *Am J Epidemiol* 1984;**119**:510–15.

28  Chyou PH, Nomura AM, Stemmermann GN. A prospective study of diet, smoking, and lower urinary tract cancer. *Ann Epidemiol* 1993;**3**:211–16.

29  Steineck G, Hagman U, Gerhardsson M, Norell SE. Vitamin A supplements, fried foods, fat and urothelial cancer. A case-reference study in Stockholm in 1985–87. *Int J Cancer* 1990;**45**:1006–11.

30  Bruemmer B, White E, Vaughan TL, Cheney CL. Nutrient intake in relation to bladder cancer among middle-aged men and women. *Am J Epidemiol* 1996;**144**:485–95.

31  Sinha R, Rothman N, Brown ED *et al*. Pan-fried meat containing high levels of heterocyclic aromatic amines but low levels of polycyclic aromatic hydrocarbons induces cytochrome P4501A2 activity in humans. *Cancer Res* 1994;**54**:6154–9.

32  Takahashi M, Toyoda K, Aze Y, Furuta K, Mitsumori K, Hayashi Y. The rat urinary bladder as a new target of heterocyclic amine carcinogenicity: tumor induction by 3-amino-1-methyl-5H-pyrido[4,3-b]indole acetate. *Jap J Cancer Res* 1993;**84**:852–8.

33  Steinmaus CM, Nunez S, Smith AH. Diet and bladder cancer: a meta-analysis of six dietary variables. *Am J Epidemiol* 2000;**151**:693–702.

34  Zeegers MPA GA, van den Brandt PA. Consumption of vegetables and fruit and urothelial cancer incidence: A prospective study. *Cancer Epidemiol Biomarker Prevent* 2001;**10**:1121–8.

35  Shibata MA, Nakanishi K, Shibata M, Masui T, Miyata Y, Ito N. Promoting effect of sodium chloride in 2-stage urinary bladder carcinogenesis in rats initiated by N-butyl-N-(4-hydroxybutyl)nitrosamine. *Urol Res* 1986;**14**:201–6.

36  Jensen OM, Wahrendorf J, Knudsen JB, Sorensen BL. The Copenhagen case–control study of bladder cancer. II. Effect of coffee and other beverages. *Int J Cancer* 1986;**37**:651–7.

37  Kunze E, Chang-Claude J, Frentzel-Beyme R. Life style and occupational risk factors for bladder cancer in Germany: A case–control study. *Cancer* 1992;**69**:1776–90.

38  Cantor KP, Hoover R, Hartge P *et al*. Bladder cancer, drinking water source, and tap water consumption: a case–control study. *J Natl Cancer Inst* 1987;**79**:1269–79.

39  Mills PK, Beeson WL, Phillips RL, Fraser GE. Bladder cancer in a low risk population: results from the Adventist Health Study. *Am J Epidemiol* 1991;**133**:230–9.

40  Zeegers MP, Dorant E, Goldbohm RA, van den Brandt PA. Are coffee, tea, and total fluid consumption associated with bladder cancer risk? Results from the Netherlands Cohort Study. *Cancer Causes Control* 2001;**12**:231–8.

41  Slattery ML, West DW, Robison LM. Fluid intake and bladder cancer in Utah. *Int J Cancer* 1988;**42**:17–22.

42  Risch HA, Burch JD, Miller AB, Hill GB, Steele R, Howe GR. Dietary factors and the incidence of cancer of the urinary bladder. *Am J Epidemiol* 1988;**127**:1179–91.

43  Dunham LJ, Rabson AS, Stewart HL, Frank AS, Young JL. Rates, interview, and pathology study of cancer of the urinary bladder in New Orleans, Louisiana. *J Natl Cancer Inst* 1968;**41**:683–709.

44  Geoffroy-Perez B, Cordier S. Fluid consumption and the risk of bladder cancer: results of a multicenter case–control study. *Int J Cancer* 2001;**93**:880–7.

45  Michaud DS, Spiegelman D, Clinton SK *et al*. Fluid intake and the risk of bladder cancer in men. *N Engl J Med* 1999;**340**:1390–7.

46  Viscoli CM, Lachs MS, Horwitz RI. Bladder cancer and coffee drinking: a summary of case–control research. *Lancet* 1993;**341**:1432–7.

47  American Institute for Cancer Research and World Cancer Research Fund. Bladder. In: *Food nutrition and the prevention of cancer: A global perspective*. Washinton DC: AICR, 1997.

48  Howe GR, Burch JD, Miller AB *et al*. Artificial sweeteners and human bladder cancer. *Lancet* 1977;**2**:578–81.

49  Zeegers MP, Tan FE, Verhagen AP, Weijenberg MP, van den Brandt PA. Elevated risk of cancer of the urinary tract for alcohol drinkers: a meta-analysis. *Cancer Causes Control* 1999;**10**:445–51.

50  Riboli E, Gonzalez CA, Lopez-Abente G *et al*. Diet and bladder cancer in Spain: a multi-centre case–control study. *Int J Cancer* 1991;**49**:214–19.

51  Vena JE, Graham S, Freudenheim J *et al*. Diet in the epidemiology of bladder cancer in western New York. *Nutr Cancer* 1992;**18**:255–64.

52  Shibata A, Paganini-Hill A, Ross RK, Henderson BE. Intake of vegetables, fruit, beta-carotene, vitamin C and vitamin supplements and cancer incidence among the elderly: a prospective study. *Br J Cancer* 1992;**66**:637–79.

53  Nomura AM, Kolonel LN, Hankin JH, Yoshizawa CN. Dietary factors in cancer of the lower urinary tract. *Int J Cancer* 1991;**48**:199–205.

54  La Vecchia C, Negri E, Decarli A, D'Avanzo B, Liberati C, Franceschi S. Dietary factors in the risk of bladder cancer. *Nutr Cancer* 1989;**12**:93–101.

55  Helzlsouer KJ, Comstock GW, Morris JS. Selenium, lycopene, alpha-tocopherol, beta-carotene, retinol, and subsequent bladder cancer. *Cancer Res* 1989;**49**:6144–8.

56  Derby LE, Jick H. Acetaminophen and renal and bladder cancer. *Epidemiology* 1996;**7**:358–62.

57  Castelao JE, Yuan JM, Gago-Dominguez M, Yu MC, Ross RK. Non-steroidal anti-inflammatory drugs and bladder cancer prevention. *Br J Cancer* 2000;**82**:1364–9.

58  Radis CD, Kahl LE, Baker GL *et al*. Effects of cyclophosphamide on the development of malignancy and on long-term survival of patients with rheumatoid arthritis. A 20-year follow-up study. *Arthritis Rheum* 1995;**38**:1120–7.

59  Levine LA, Richie JP. Urological complications of cyclophosphamide. *J Urol* 1989;**141**:1063–9.

60  Silverman DT MA, Devesa SS. Bladder cancer. In: Scottenfeld DFJ, ed. *Cancer Epidemiology and Prevention*. New York: Oxford University Press; 1996.

61  Prout GR, Barton BA. 13-cis-retinoic acid in chemoprevention of superficial bladder cancer. The National Bladder Cancer Group. *J Cell Biochem* 1992;**16I**(Suppl.):148–52.

62  Alfthan O, Tarkkanen J, Grohn P, Heinonen E, Pyrhonen S, Saila K. Tigason (etretinate) in prevention of recurrence of superficial bladder tumors. A double-blind clinical trial. *Eur Urol* 1983;**9**:6–9.

63  Studer UE, Jenzer S, Biedermann C *et al*. Adjuvant treatment with a vitamin A analogue (etretinate) after transurethral resection of superficial bladder tumors. Final analysis of a prospective, randomized multicenter trial in Switzerland. *Eur Urol* 1995;**28**:284–90.

64  Byar D, Blackard C. Comparisons of placebo, pyridoxine, and topical thiotepa in preventing recurrence of stage I bladder cancer. *Urology* 1977;**10**:556–61.

65  Newling DW, Robinson MR, Smith PH *et al*. Tryptophan metabolites, pyridoxine (vitamin B6) and their influence on the recurrence rate of superficial bladder cancer. Results of a prospective, randomised phase III study performed by the EORTC GU Group. EORTC Genito-Urinary Tract Cancer Cooperative Group. *Eur Urol* 1995;**27**:110–16.

66  Lamm DL, Riggs DR, Shriver JS, van Gilder PF, Rach JF, DeHaven JI. Megadose vitamins in bladder cancer: a double-blind clinical trial. *J Urol* 1994;**151**:21–6.

## Acknowledgements

The authors are grateful to Mrs Bernadette Coles MSc for designing and implementing the search strategy for this study.

# Kidney cancer

## Background

Kidney cancer is rare and accounts for only 2% of cancers worldwide, although the incidence rate is increasing by about 3% per year.[1] This cancer generally affects those over 40 years of age and is more common in men than women. The aetiology is unknown but chemoprevention may be of value in those at high risk of this disease, in particular patients with von Hippel–Lindau disease, since 10–25% will develop kidney cancer.[2] A number of systematic reviews have addressed the issue of risk factors for kidney cancer and the subsequent implications for prevention.

## Aetiology

### Smoking

Smoking tobacco is an established cause of kidney cancer. A systematic review of 10 case–control studies and one cohort study reported odds ratios ranging from 1·3 to 9·3.[3] In another systematic review, a dose–response relationship was reported for tobacco use and kidney cancer with relative risks in the range 1·5–2·2.[2] The risk declines by about 30% after 10–15 years of cessation. It has been estimated that 25% of all kidney cancers are attributable to smoking.[1]

### Analgesics

Phenacetin use has been reported to increase the risk of kidney cancer in a number of case–control studies.[4–6] However, other studies report no association.[7,8] Acetaminophen, a metabolite of phenacetin, significantly increased the risk in heavy users of this drug in case–control studies,[6,9] but this was not confirmed by others.[5]

### Obesity

The association between obesity and kidney cancer has been reported in two cohort studies and 12 case–control studies and presented in two systematic reviews.[3,10] The two cohort studies indicated a 2·0–2·7-fold increased risk of dying from kidney cancer in obese cases. Eleven of the 12 case–control studies reported an increased risk, with odds ratios of 1·3–2·4 for men and 1·0–3·8 for women. The underlying mechanism relating obesity to kidney cancer is unknown but hormonal changes and altered lipid metabolism may be involved.

## Diet

A recent, comprehensive study reviewed dietary components and the risk associated with kidney cancer.[10] Data from two ecological studies indicated a strong correlation between dietary fat intake and kidney cancer incidence ($r = 0.7–0.8$); however, further data are required to make any firm judgement. Similarly, no conclusions could be reached with regard to the intake of saturated, polyunsaturated fats and cholesterol. Eight case–control studies evaluated the risk associated with dietary meat. Three reported a significant increased risk with increased consumption, with odds ratios (OR) of 1·5–4·0. The relationships between kidney cancer and the intake of beta-carotene,[11,12] vitamin C,[11] and retinol,[11,12] are unclear and require further studies. Three out of five case–control studies found a statistically significant protective association for at least one vegetable or fruit with ORs ranging from 0·3 to 0·6.[11]

Six case–control studies showed no association between alcohol consumption and kidney cancer.[10]

## Occupational exposure

Asbestos exposure has been strongly linked to mesothelioma but the evidence from numerous studies for a link with kidney cancer is unclear. A meta-analysis of 37 cohort studies evaluated the associated risk of asbestos exposure and kidney cancer.[13] The pooled, standardised mortality ratio for kidney cancer was 1·1 (95% CI, 0·9–1·3). The authors conclude that low exposure of asbestos has minimal risk for kidney cancer but may have a slight risk at high levels.

Workers in the steel industry, in particular coke-plant workers (RR 7·5) exposed to high levels of polycyclic aromatic hydrocarbons, are reported to be at increased risk for kidney cancer.[14–16] The data from a 30-year follow up study confirmed an elevated risk for coke-oven workers for kidney cancer with a relative risk of 1·93.[17]

A cohort study of over 9000 workers in the petroleum refining industry indicates a significant increased risk of kidney cancer for those with at least 5 years' employment.[18] However, a meta-analysis of nearly 100 reports did not confirm this.[19] Other workers regularly exposed to carcinogens and reported to be at increased risk include firefighters (RR 4·89; 95% CI, 2·47–8·93),[20] painters (RR 1·79; 95% CI, 1·31–3·44),[20] and textile workers (OR 6·2; 95% CI, 1·1–33·7).[21]

## References

1 McLaughlin JK, Lipworth L. Epidemiologic aspects of renal cell cancer. *Semin Oncol* 2000;**27**:115–23.
2 Dayal H, Kinman J. Epidemiology of kidney cancer. *Semin Oncol* 1983;**10**:366–77.

3  Dhote R, Pellicer-Coeuret M, Thiounn N, Debre B, Vidal-Trecan G. Risk factors for adult renal cell carcinoma: a systematic review and implications for prevention. *Br J Urol Int* 2000;**86**:20–7.

4  McCredie M, Stewart JH, Day NE. Different roles for phenacetin and paracetamol in cancer of the kidney and renal pelvis. *Int J Cancer* 1993;**53**:245–9.

5  Kreiger N, Marrett LD, Dodds L, Hilditch S, Darlington GA. Risk factors for renal cell carcinoma: results of a population-based case–control study. *Cancer Causes Control* 1993;**4**:101–10.

6  Gago-Dominguez M, Yuan JM, Castelao JE, Ross RK, Yu MC. Regular use of analgesics is a risk factor for renal cell carcinoma. *Br J Cancer* 1999;**81**:542–8.

7  Mellemgaard A, Niwa S, Mehl ES, Engholm G, McLaughlin JK, Olsen JH. Risk factors for renal cell carcinoma in Denmark: role of medication and medical history. *Int J Epidemiol* 1994;**23**:923–30.

8  McCredie M, Pommer W, McLaughlin JK *et al.* International renal-cell cancer study. II. Analgesics. *Int J Cancer* 1995;**60**:345–9.

9  Derby LE, Jick H. Acetaminophen and renal and bladder cancer. *Epidemiology* 1996;**7**:358–62.

10  American Institute for Cancer Research and World Cancer Research Fund. Kidney. In: *Food nutrition and the prevention of cancer: A global perspective.* Washington DC: AICR, 1997.

11  McLaughlin JK, Mandel JS, Blot WJ, Schuman LM, Mehl ES, Fraumeni JF. A population-based case–control study of renal cell carcinoma. *J Natl Cancer Inst* 1984;**72**:275–84.

12  Maclure M, Willett W. A case–control study of diet and risk of renal adenocarcinoma. *Epidemiology* 1990;**1**:430–40.

13  Sali D, Boffetta P. Kidney cancer and occupational exposure to asbestos: a meta-analysis of occupational cohort studies. *Cancer Causes Control* 2000;**11**:37–47.

14  Schlehofer B, Heuer C, Blettner M, Niehoff D, Wahrendorf J. Occupation, smoking and demographic factors, and renal cell carcinoma in Germany. *Int J Epidemiol* 1995;**24**:51–7.

15  Mandel JS, McLaughlin JK, Schlehofer B *et al.* International renal-cell cancer study. IV. Occupation. *Int J Cancer* 1995;**61**:601–5.

16  Redmond CK, Ciocco A, Lloyd JW, Rush HW. Long-term mortality study of steelworkers. VI. Mortality from malignant neoplasms among coke oven workers. *J Occup Med* 1972;**14**:621–9.

17  Costantino JP, Redmond CK, Bearden A. Occupationally related cancer risk among coke oven workers: 30 years of follow-up. *J Occup Environ Med* 1995;**37**:597–604.

18  Pukkala E. Cancer incidence among Finnish oil refinery workers, 1971–1994. *J Occup Environ Med* 1998;**40**:675–9.

19  Wong O, Raabe GK. Critical review of cancer epidemiology in petroleum industry employees, with a quantitative meta-analysis by cancer site. *Am J Indust Med* 1989;**15**:283–310.

20  Delahunt B, Bethwaite PB, Nacey JN. Occupational risk for renal cell carcinoma. A case–control study based on the New Zealand Cancer Registry. *Br J Urol* 1995;**75**:578–82.

21  Auperin A, Benhamou S, Ory-Paoletti C, Flamant R. Occupational risk factors for renal cell carcinoma: a case–control study. *Occup Environ Med* 1994;**51**:426–8.

# Prostate cancer

## Background

Prostate cancer is the ninth most common cancer globally and the fourth most common cancer in men.[1] There is considerable variation in the incidence of prostate cancer worldwide, with a particularly high rate (per 100 000) in African–Americans of 100, compared to 25 for Western European men and 10 for Asians.[2] The high incidence of this disease results in a substantial financial and social burden, which has led to an increased interest in primary disease prevention, the success of which depends on the identification of definitive risk factors for prostate cancer development.

## Aetiology

### Dietary fat

A systematic review and meta-analysis of dietary fat and prostate cancer risk reported that eight of the 10 studies indicated a high risk with high consumption of total dietary fat (RR 1·3; 95% CI, 1·11–1·51).[3] However, the authors emphasise caution in interpreting the pooled data due to possible publication bias.

Additional studies not included in the above review have evaluated the role of dietary fat in the aetiology of prostate cancer. A study of 207 cases and 207 controls, based in Canada, found no clear association with total fat intake and prostate cancer risk.[4] However, several other case–control studies report a non-significant positive correlation.[5–7]

Further studies report a significant association with total fat intake and prostate cancer including a case–control study of 1655 Black, White, Chinese, and Japanese Americans (OR 1·4; 95% CI, 1·1–1·8),[8] and a cohort study of 20 316 men followed for up to 14 years (RR 1·6; 95% CI, 1·0–2·4).[9] In addition, a strong correlation between total fat intake per capita from over 20 countries and the mortality of prostate cancer ($r = 0·69$) has been reported in three epidemiological studies.[10–12]

A number of studies have differentiated between the influence of dietary saturated and unsaturated fats with prostate cancer mortality. Two cohort studies show no association with saturated fat,[13,14] and two a slight increased risk.[9,15] Several case–control studies report a significant association with saturated fat with odds ratios of 1·7 to 3·2.[8,16,17] The data for monounsaturated fats are inconsistent. One case–control study[17] and one cohort study[13] indicate an increased risk, the former being statistically significant (OR 3·6; 95% CI, 1·3–9·7), whereas two other studies report no association.[4,8] The intake of

α-linolenic acid was reported to be a significant risk factor for prostate cancer in one cohort study (RR 3·4)[13] and two case–control studies with odds ratios of 2·7[17] and 3·91,[18] whilst others report no association.[4,8]

No negative associations have been reported and, although the data are not consistent, the overall trend indicates that high fat intake appears to be associated with a higher risk of prostate cancer.

Total energy intake has been distinguished from fat intake in six reports. Three studies report no association between total energy intake and prostate cancer,[13,14,19] whilst three report a non-significant increased risk.[4,8,17] The data are, at present, insufficient to make a statement on energy intake and the risk of prostate cancer.

### Vegetables

A systematic review and meta-analysis found no association between the consumption of green vegetables and prostate cancer (OR 0·93; 95% CI, 0·73–1·18).[3] A more comprehensive systematic review reported no association with green vegetables in four studies, a weak protective effect of vegetables in five studies and of dried fruit in four studies, and a slight increased risk with vegetables in two other studies.[20] In a large cohort study of 58 279 men followed for 6·3 years, the association between 21 vegetables and 8 fruits and prostate cancer risk was assessed.[21] The non-significant relative risk for total, prepared, and raw vegetables ranged from 0·8 to 0·96, and for total fruit was 1·3. In a multi-ethnic case–control study (1619 cases), an inverse relationship was observed for prostate cancer risk and the intake of total legumes, yellow-orange vegetables, and cruciferous vegetables with respective ORs (95% CI) of 0·62 (0·49–0·80), 0·67 (0·48–0·94), and 0·61 (0·42–0·88).[22] A negative correlation ($r = -0·38$) has been reported between prostate cancer death and total vegetable supply per capita for 30 countries.[10]

There has been recent interest in the antioxidant properties of lycopene, a carotenoid found in tomatoes. A systematic review reported an inverse relationship with the consumption of tomatoes or tomato-based products and prostate cancer in nine of 10 studies, six of which were significant (RR 0·5–0·99).[23] A more recent report indicates no relationship.[22] The evidence for a protective effect of vegetables on prostate cancer is weak and inconsistent, but it cannot be ruled out that certain vegetables may decrease the risk.

### Beta-carotene and vitamin A

The risk of prostate cancer associated with dietary beta-carotene was presented in a meta-analysis of seven studies and reported a summary relative risk for carotene intake of 0·99 (95% CI, 0·85–1·16).[3] Two additional studies confirm no association.[4,24] Serum levels of beta-carotene were reported to have no association with prostate cancer risk[25,26] or an increased risk with elevated levels.[27]

Several studies have reported on prostate cancer risk and vitamin A or retinol intake. The data are confusing with some trials reporting an increased risk,[5,15] which may be restricted to men over 70 years of age[16,24,28] or younger than 70,[25] whereas others report no association[29] or a weak reduced risk.[4,6,17] A case–control study indicated that the mean serum level of retinol was significantly lower ($P = 0.05$) in prostate cancer patients than controls,[26] whereas cohort studies report that elevated levels are associated with a reduced risk[25,30] or no association.[27]

Based on these data, it is unlikely that dietary beta-carotene provides a benefit against the risk of prostate cancer, although no clear picture has yet emerged for vitamin A.

## Smoking

Several studies have evaluated the role of smoking in relation to the risk of prostate cancer. In a meta-analysis of data on current smokers or ex-smokers versus non-smokers, 10 out of 20 studies indicated an increased risk with smoking.[3] A statistically significant summary odds ratio of 1·16 was reported, but no confidence intervals were stated. The result should be interpreted with caution since some of the negative studies were not included in the summary, because the confidence intervals were not published. The risk associated with cigarette smoking may also be confounded by the effect on sex hormones, which are known to influence the growth of prostatic tissue.[31]

## Vasectomy

Vasectomy is a common form of contraception that has been suggested as a risk factor for prostate cancer since vasectomised men have higher levels of circulating testosterone.[32] A systematic review reported on 221 826 patients from 14 original studies (1985–1996) addressing the association between vasectomy and prostate cancer.[33] Relative risks ranged from 0·44–6·7 with an overall risk of 1·23 (95% CI, 1·01–1·49), although the data may be subject to trial design and publication bias. The authors conclude that vasectomised men are not at an increased risk of prostate cancer.

## Familial genetics/race

A systematic review evaluated 10 case–control studies reporting the incidence of prostate cancer in the families of men with this disease.[34] The relative risk ranged from 1·7 to 8·7 for first-degree relatives of men with prostate cancer. This has been confirmed by more recent case–control studies.[35,36] It is also well reported that prostate cancer is more common in Blacks than Whites or Asians, which cannot be completely accounted for by ethnic diet or lifestyle, and may imply a genetic predisposition.[37]

## Infection/sexual activity

A systematic review and meta-analysis of 10 case–control studies has reported on sexual behaviour and risks factors for prostate cancer.[3] Both age at first intercourse (RR 1·31; 95% CI, 1·06–1·61) and the number of partners (RR 1·24; 95% CI, 1·00–1·54) were weakly related to prostate cancer. A recent population-based study of 918 cases and 1315 controls indicated a significantly increased risk where there was a history of gonorrhoea or syphilis (OR 1·6; 95% CI, 1·2–2·1).[38]

## Occupational exposure

Certain occupations have been associated with an increased incidence of prostate cancer such as farmers,[39–42] electrical workers,[43,44] and metal workers.[41] A significant increased risk for prostate cancer has been reported for men exposed to cadmium,[45,46] certain radionuclides, such as tritium, $^{51}$Cr, $^{59}$Fe, $^{60}$Co, or $^{65}$Zn (RR 5·32; 95% CI, 1·87–17·24),[47] and diesel fumes (OR 3·7; 95% CI, 1·4–9·8).[48]

## Chemoprevention trials

The Alpha-Tocopherol (a form of vitamin E), Beta-carotene Cancer Prevention study (ATBC) was originally designed to investigate the effect these agents had on the prevention of lung cancer, hence the participants were all smokers. A total of 29 133 men were enrolled and randomised to receive either α-tocopherol (50 mg), beta-carotene (20 mg), both agents, or placebo daily for 5–8 years.[49] During the follow up period, 246 new cases and 62 deaths from prostate cancer were identified. A 32% decrease in incidence was seen in the α-tocopherol group compared to those not receiving it. Mortality was 41% lower in the former group. The incidence was 23% higher in the beta-carotene group compared to those not receiving it. In a follow up study of smokers and non-smokers, the risk of metastatic prostate cancer was lower for smokers, and those who had quit smoking, who consumed at least 100 IU vitamin E per day, but there was no effect in non-smokers.[50] These data suggest that further trials with α-tocopherol are warranted.

Various animal and ecological studies report an inverse association between low dietary selenium intake and risk of various types of cancer, suggesting that selenium supplementation may have a preventative role.[51] The effect of selenium and vitamin E in reducing prostate cancer is being evaluated in a randomised, prospective, double-blind, placebo-controlled trial (SELECT study).[52] A total of 32 400 healthy men will be randomised to receive selenium plus placebo, vitamin E plus placebo, selenium plus vitamin E, or placebo plus placebo. The primary endpoint will be the clinical incidence of prostate cancer. Recruitment began in 2001 and results will be available in 2013.

The growth of prostatic tissue, from benign hyperplasia to most carcinomas, is stimulated by circulating androgens, suggesting that early androgen deprivation may be beneficial in terms of prevention. Finasteride, a steroidal analogue of testosterone that competitively inhibits 5-$\alpha$-reductase and reduces circulating testosterone, is being evaluated in the Prostate Cancer Prevention Trial.[53] Over 18 000 men have been randomised to placebo or finasteride and will be followed for 7 years for the development of prostate cancer.

A small randomised trial investigated the effects of lycopene supplementation in men with newly diagnosed prostate cancer.[54] Interventions were given 3 weeks before prostatectomy. Those receiving daily lycopene (15 mg) had less surgical margin involvement ($P = 0.02$) and a greater frequency of tumours less than 4 cm (84% $v$ 45%). The data suggest that lycopene may decrease the growth of prostate cancer.

Other randomised trials on prostate cancer prevention, at an early stage of recruitment at the NCI, include chemoprevention with eflornithine, and diets low in fat and high in soy, fruits, vegetables, green tea, vitamin E and fibre.

## References

1 WHO. *The world health report: Geneva*. Geneva: World Health Organization, 1997.

2 Greenlee RT, Murray T, Bolden S, Wingo PA. Cancer statistics, 2000. *CA Cancer J Clin* 2000;**50**:7–33.

3 Key T. Risk factors for prostate cancer. *Cancer Surv* 1995;**23**:63–77.

4 Rohan TE, Howe GR, Burch JD, Jain M. Dietary factors and risk of prostate cancer: a case–control study in Ontario, Canada. *Cancer Causes Control* 1995;**6**:145–54.

5 Heshmat MY, Kaul L, Kovi J *et al*. Nutrition and prostate cancer: a case–control study. *Prostate* 1985;**6**:7–17.

6 Mettlin C, Selenskas S, Natarajan N, Huben R. Beta-carotene and animal fats and their relationship to prostate cancer risk. A case–control study. *Cancer* 1989;**64**:605–12.

7 Hayes RB, Ziegler RG, Gridley G *et al*. Dietary factors and risks for prostate cancer among blacks and whites in the United States. *Cancer Epidemiol Biomarker Prevent* 1999;**8**:25–34.

8 Whittemore AS, Kolonel LN, Wu AHJ *et al*. Prostate cancer in relation to diet, physical activity, and body size in blacks, whites, and Asians in the United States and Canada. *J Natl Cancer Inst* 1995;**87**:652–61.

9 Le Marchand L, Kolonel LN, Wilkens LR, Myers BC, Hirohata T. Animal fat consumption and prostate cancer: a prospective study in Hawaii. *Epidemiology* 1994;**5**:276–82.

10 Rose DP, Boyar AP, Wynder EL. International comparisons of mortality rates for cancer of the breast, ovary, prostate, and colon, and per capita food consumption. *Cancer* 1986;**58**:2363–71.

11 Armstrong B, Doll R. Environmental factors and cancer incidence and mortality in different countries, with special reference to dietary practices. *Int J Cancer* 1975;**15**:617–31.

12 Hursting SD, Thornquist M, Henderson MM. Types of dietary fat and the incidence of cancer at five sites. *Prevent Med* 1990;**19**:242–53.

13 Giovannucci E, Rimm EB, Colditz GA *et al*. A prospective study of dietary fat and risk of prostate cancer. *J Natl Cancer Inst* 1993;**85**:1571–9.

14 Severson RK, Nomura AM, Grove JS, Stemmermann GN. A prospective study of demographics, diet, and prostate cancer among men of Japanese ancestry in Hawaii. *Cancer Res* 1989;**49**:1857–60.

15 Mills PK, Beeson WL, Phillips RL, Fraser GE. Cohort study of diet, lifestyle, and prostate cancer in Adventist men. *Cancer* 1989;**64**:598–604.

16 Graham S, Haughey B, Marshall J *et al*. Diet in the epidemiology of carcinoma of the prostate gland. *J Natl Cancer Inst* 1983;**70**:687–92.

17 West DW, Slattery ML, Robison LM, French TK, Mahoney AW. Adult dietary intake and prostate cancer risk in Utah: a case–control study with special emphasis on aggressive tumors. *Cancer Causes Control* 1991;**2**:85–94.

18 De Stefani E D-PH, Boffetta P, Ronco A, Mendilaharsu M. α-Linolenic acid and risk of prostate cancer: a case control study in Uruguay. *Cancer Epidemiol Biomarker Prevent* 2000;**9**:335–8.

19 Ghadirian P, Lacroix A, Maisonneuve P *et al*. Nutritional factors and prostate cancer: a case–control study of French Canadians in Montreal, Canada. *Cancer Causes Control* 1996;**7**:428–36.

20 American Institute for Cancer Research and World Cancer Research Fund. Prostate. In: *Food nutrition and the prevention of cancer: A global perspective*. Washington DC: AICR, 1997.

21 Schuurman AG, Goldbohm RA, Dorant E, van den Brandt PA. Vegetable and fruit consumption and prostate cancer risk: a cohort study in The Netherlands. *Cancer Epidemiol Biomarker Prevent* 1998;**7**:673–80.

22 Kolonel LN, Hankin JH, Whittemore AS *et al*. Vegetables, fruits, legumes and prostate cancer: a multiethnic case–control study. *Cancer Epidemiol Biomarker Prevent* 2000;**9**:795–804.

23 Giovannucci E. Tomatoes, tomato-based products, lycopene, and cancer: review of the epidemiologic literature. *J Natl Cancer Inst* 1999;**91**:317–31.

24 Giovannucci E, Ascherio A, Rimm EB, Stampfer MJ, Colditz GA, Willett WC. Intake of carotenoids and retinol in relation to risk of prostate cancer. *J Natl Cancer Inst* 1995;**87**:1767–76.

25 Hsing AW, Comstock GW, Abbey H, Polk BF. Serologic precursors of cancer. Retinol, carotenoids, and tocopherol and risk of prostate cancer. *J Natl Cancer Inst* 1990;**82**:941–6.

26 Hayes RB, Bogdanovicz JF, Schroeder FH *et al*. Serum retinol and prostate cancer. *Cancer* 1988;**62**:2021–6.

27 Knekt P, Aromaa A, Maatela J. Serum vitamin A and subsequent risk of cancer: cancer incidence follow-up of the Finnish Mobile Clinic Health Examination Survey. *Am J Epidemiol* 1990;**132**:857–70.

28 Kolonel LN, Yoshizawa CN, Hankin JH. Diet and prostatic cancer: a case–control study in Hawaii. *Am J Epidemiol* 1988;**127**:999–1012.

29 Middleton B, Byers T, Marshall J, Graham S. Dietary vitamin A and cancer – a multi-site case–control study. *Nutr Cancer* 1986;**8**:107–16.

30 Reichman ME, Hayes RB, Ziegler RG *et al*. Serum vitamin A and subsequent development of prostate cancer in the first National Health and Nutrition Examination Survey Epidemiologic Follow-up Study. *Cancer Res* 1990;**50**:2311–15.

31 Dai WS, Gutai JP, Kuller LH, Cauley JA. Cigarette smoking and serum sex hormones in men. *Am J Epidemiol* 1988;**128**:796–805.

32 Honda GD, Bernstein L, Ross RK, Greenland S, Gerkins V, Henderson BE. Vasectomy, cigarette smoking, and age at first sexual intercourse as risk factors for prostate cancer in middle-aged men. *Br J Cancer* 1988;**57**:326–31.

33 Bernal-Delgado E, Latour-Perez J, Pradas-Arnal F, Gomez-Lopez LI. The association between vasectomy and prostate cancer: a systematic review of the literature. *Fertil Steril* 1998;**70**:191–200.

34  McLellan DL, Norman RW. Hereditary aspects of prostate cancer. *Can Med Assoc J* 1995;**153**:895–900.

35  Cerhan JR, Parker AS, Putnam SD *et al.* Family history and prostate cancer risk in a population-based cohort of Iowa men. *Cancer Epidemiol Biomarker Prevent* 1999;**8**:53–60.

36  Ghadirian P, Howe GR, Hislop TG, Maisonneuve P. Family history of prostate cancer: a multi-center case–control study in Canada. *Int J Cancer* 1997;**70**:679–81.

37  Shibata A, Whittemore AS. Genetic predisposition to prostate cancer: possible explanations for ethnic differences in risk. *Prostate* 1997;**32**:65–72.

38  Hayes RB, Pottern LM, Strickler H *et al.* Sexual behaviour, STDs and risks for prostate cancer. *Br J Cancer* 2000;**82**:718–25.

39  Sharma-Wagner S, Chokkalingam AP, Malker HS, Stone BJ, McLaughlin JK, Hsing AW. Occupation and prostate cancer risk in Sweden. *J Occup Environ Med* 2000;**42**:517–25.

40  Krstev S, Baris D, Stewart P *et al.* Occupational risk factors and prostate cancer in U.S. blacks and whites. *Am J Industrial Med* 1998;**34**:421–30.

41  van der Gulden JW, Kolk JJ, Verbeek AL. Prostate cancer and work environment. *J Occup Med* 1992;**34**:402–9.

42  Parker AS, Cerhan JR, Putnam SD, Cantor KP, Lynch CF. A cohort study of farming and risk of prostate cancer in Iowa. *Epidemiology* 1999;**10**:452–5.

43  Robinson CF, Petersen M, Palu S. Mortality patterns among electrical workers employed in the U.S. construction industry, 1982–1987. *Am J Industrial Med* 1999;**36**:630–7.

44  Aronson KJ, Siemiatycki J, Dewar R, Gerin M. Occupational risk factors for prostate cancer: results from a case–control study in Montreal, Quebec, Canada. *Am J Epidemiol* 1996;**143**:363–73.

45  Kipling MWJ. Cadmium and prostate carcinoma. *Lancet* 1967;**1**:730–1.

46  Elghany NA, Schumacher MC, Slattery ML, West DW, Lee JS. Occupation, cadmium exposure, and prostate cancer. *Epidemiology* 1990;**1**:107–15.

47  Rooney C, Beral V, Maconochie N, Fraser P, Davies G. Case–control study of prostatic cancer in employees of the United Kingdom Atomic Energy Authority. *BMJ* 1993;**307**:1391–7.

48  Seidler A, Heiskel H, Bickeboller R, Elsner G. Association between diesel exposure at work and prostate cancer. *Scand J Work Environ Health* 1998;**24**:486–94.

49  Heinonen OP, Albanes D, Virtamo J *et al.* Prostate cancer and supplementation with alpha-tocopherol and beta-carotene: incidence and mortality in a controlled trial. *J Natl Cancer Inst* 1998;**90**:440–6.

50  Chan JM, Stampfer MJ, Ma J, Rimm EB, Willett WC, Giovannucci EL. Supplemental vitamin E intake and prostate cancer risk in a large cohort of men in the United States. *Cancer Epidemiol Biomarker Prevent* 1999;**8**:893–9.

51  Yoshizawa K, Willett WC, Morris SJ *et al.* Study of prediagnostic selenium level in toenails and the risk of advanced prostate cancer. *J Natl Cancer Inst* 1998;**90**:1219–24.

52  Klein EA TI, Lippman SM, Goodman PJ, Albanes D, Taylor PR, Coltman C. SELECT; The next prostate cancer prevention trial. *J Urol* 2001;**166**:1311–15.

53  Thompson IM, Coltman CA, Crowley J. Chemoprevention of prostate cancer: the Prostate Cancer Prevention Trial. *Prostate* 1997;**33**:217–21.

54  Kucuk O, Sarkar FH, Sakr W *et al.* Phase II randomized clinical trial of lycopene supplementation before radical prostatectomy. *Cancer Epidemiol Biomarker Prevent* 2001;**10**:861–8.

# Testicular cancer

## Background

Testicular cancer is a relatively rare malignancy; however, it remains the most commonly occurring cancer in young men aged between 15 and 35 years.[1] The prevalence of testicular cancer has increased over the past 20 years; the reasons for this increase are unclear, however, because of effective treatment regimens, death rates have decreased. There is evidence to suggest a correlation between the incidence of testicular tumours and several predisposing factors such as age, histology, social class, ethnicity and geographical location.[2] The incidence is higher in White males compared with Black or Oriental males, with the highest recorded incidence in northern European countries and North America and the lowest in Asian and African countries.[3]

## Aetiology

### Cryptorchidism

A number of studies report a positive association between cryptorchidism and pure seminoma.[4–6] Recent research by the American Cancer Society 2001, indicates that approximately 14% of testicular malignancies occur in men with a history of cryptorchidism. A study by the UK Testicular Cancer Study Group reported that an undescended testis was associated with a slightly higher risk of seminoma when compared with other tumour types.[4] Inguinal hernias and congenital anomalies of the genitourinary tract are also suggested anatomical risk factors.[7] The mechanism is unclear but orchipexy before puberty, to correct the positioning of the testicles, may assist with reducing risk factors in later life.

### Family history

Family history has been identified in several studies as a risk factor for testicular cancer and was observed most frequently in combination with cryptorchidism.[3,8] Knowledge of family history, particularly in immediate family members, is a vital component in primary and secondary prevention and is essential in the promotion of awareness among young men.

### Diet

Very few studies have addressed links between diet and testicular cancer. One study found that increased total daily calories, saturated fat, and cholesterol consumption was associated with an increased risk of non-seminoma testicular cancer.[9] Seminoma increased slightly with increasing total and saturated fat, and total fat consumption was also marginally related to an increase in mixed germ cell tumours.[9] Another study correlated dietary practices with incidence and mortality rates of testicular and prostatic cancers in 42 countries.[10] Cheese was found to be most closely correlated with incidence of testicular cancer in men aged 20–39, followed by animal fats and milk. Maternal or prepubertal consumption of cheese was also considered a possible risk factor. Further comprehensive studies are required to determine accurately the extent of links between diet and testicular cancer.

### Height and body mass

In a study of approximately 500 000 Norwegian men, testicular cancer was found to be inversely related to body mass index and positively associated with increasing height.[11] The effect of obesity on hormone levels and subsequent effects on tumour growth was inconclusive.

### Exercise

No conclusive evidence can be determined from the literature addressing testicular cancer risk or prevention in relation to exercise. One study reports that frequent, moderate, or strenuous recreational activity or occupational demands, have an adverse effect on testicular cancer risk.[12] Another study indicated that high levels of physical activity were associated inversely with testicular cancer risk.[5] However, no correlation was found in a study of 53 000 Norwegian men, regardless of physical activity at work or during recreation.[13] Trauma and injury to the scrotum and testicles caused during participation in sport, such as cycling and equestrian activities, have been associated with an increased risk of developing testicular cancer, although there is insufficient evidence to support this.[7]

### Microlithiasis

Intratesticular microlithiasis is considered a predominant risk factor in confirmed cases of testicular cancer or testicular mass.[14]

### Environmental risk factors

A small study of 250 men, indicated that exposure to extreme high and low temperatures in the workplace, elevated the risk of developing testicular cancer.[15] Certain occupational groups appear to have higher than average incidence rates of testicular cancer, for example oil and gas workers, leather workers, and utility workers, the majority of whom are exposed to potential carcinogens in the workplace.[3] Testicular cancer has been associated with occupational use of herbicides and chlorophenols.[16] Childhood exposure to nitrates and fertilizers has also been associated with an increase in tumour development.[17,18] Fetal or childhood exposure to oestrogenic, or other hormonally active environmental chemicals, is also associated with an increased risk of reproductive defects and testicular cancer.[19] Maternal use of hormones has also been tentatively associated with testicular cancer development in male offspring. Men whose mothers took the synthetic oestrogen diethylstilbestrol during pregnancy have been historically associated with an increased risk of reproductive dysfunction, although it is uncertain whether this is also related to incidences of testicular malignancy. Further investigation is essential in order to gain a clearer understanding of the role of these modifiable risk factors in possible testicular cancer development.

## Infection

Viral infections such as mumps and the associated atrophy of the testicles, can be correlated with a subsequent risk of malignancy.[7] Encouraging vaccination is an important step in reducing the incidence of the mumps virus.

There is some inconclusive evidence that men with the human immunodeficiency virus (HIV) and particularly those with AIDS are at increased risk of tumour development in the testis.[10]

## Opportunities for prevention of urological cancers

The accumulated evidence of risk factors for urological cancers, suggests that there is considerable ground for prevention. However, it is important to develop health messages that reflect the best available evidence on urological cancers that can be related to primary care clinicians and the public.

There is overwhelming evidence that tobacco use is the single most preventable cause of death from bladder and kidney cancers and, to a lesser extent, prostate cancers. There are a number of strategies that are aimed at smoking prevention and cessation. The young are a major target population for prevention of smoking, and school-based interventions using trained staff, teachers, and student peer leaders are encouraging.[20] Other effective approaches aimed at the young include mass media campaigns, community-wide programmes structured to discourage young people from starting to smoke, and restriction on the sale of cigarettes to minors.[21] Advice from health professionals, in particular primary care physicians, reduces the number of smokers by 2%, which can be further improved when training is given (OR 1·48; 95% CI, 1·20–1·83).[22] In addition, combining primary care advice with nicotine

replacement therapy, such as patches, can reduce smoking by 12% in motivated cases.[23] Other areas aimed at reducing smoking include restrictive smoking at work, a reduction in tobacco advertising and increasing the price of tobacco, although the effectiveness of these measures is unclear.[21]

Apart from smoking, epidemiological evidence strongly indicates an association between urinary schistosomiasis and bladder cancer, particularly in Egypt, although a direct causal effect has yet to be proven. However, there is a need for more education, improvements in irrigation and farming methods, in addition to better detection and treatment of urinary schistosomiasis, to prevent the possible development of bladder cancer. If preventive measures were successful in controlling urinary schistosomiasis, and concurrently, in reducing smoking, then bladder cancer would be a rare neoplasm in Egypt.[24]

The available evidence suggests that diets low in fat and high in vegetables and possibly fruit may have a beneficial effect in preventing bladder, prostate and kidney cancers. Maintenance of a healthy weight would also be a positive preventive measure for kidney cancer. This message of a healthy lifestyle is promoted by many primary health campaigns and should be emphasised for groups that are at risk of developing urological cancers.

High-risk groups, such as those with familial clustering of prostate cancer, increase the potential to identify causes of this disease and develop effective prevention strategies. Early detection should be implemented in men with one or more first degree relatives with prostate cancer, in particular American Blacks, to offer the possibility of useful early intervention. This approach also applies to testicular cancer where testicular self-examination should not only be promoted in the general male population but emphasised to those with a family history of this disease or cryptorchidism. Health professionals and school teachers, particularly those involved in sport, are in an ideal position to educate young men.[25]

It is clear that some occupations are at higher risk of developing urological cancers such as those exposed to diesel fumes and aromatic amines. Action should also be taken to reduce the exposure to carcinogens in the workplace and environment. The identification of occupations that expose workers to a high level of carcinogenic agents will allow preventative measures, such as new legislation on minimum exposure limits and a change in working practices to be implemented, and potentially reduce the incidence of bladder and kidney cancers.

Communication is a major component of prevention strategies and the internet is an ideal tool to educate people, especially the young. With this in mind, the Cancer Research Foundation of America developed an educational CD Rom for 8–12-year-olds (*Dr. Health'nstein's Body Fun*) which is structured as a "road to life" along which the player must pass. During the journey, decisions must be made about food and exercise that reflect the players' health rating or score. In addition, this game allows children to see the effect of diet, fitness, cigarettes and drugs on various organs. This example is a positive move to educate the young and instil a healthy lifestyle that may impact on the incidence of urological cancers in the decades to come. At the other end of the age spectrum, life expectancy is increasing, particularly in developed countries, and urological cancers in the elderly are an escalating burden. Although more attention is now being directed towards the causes and prevention of these diseases, prevention studies are complex and protracted, and it will be some time yet before we know whether antismoking campaigns and dietary interventions have an impact on the incidence of urological cancers.

## References

1  Woolam GL. Cancer statistics, 2000: a benchmark for the new century. *CA Cancer J Clin* 2000;**50**:6–33.

2  Peate I. Testicular cancer: the importance of effective health education. *Br J Nurs* 1997;**6**:311–16.

3  American Cancer Society AC. *Testicular Cancer Prevention and Early Detection*, 2001. http://www.cancer.org (accessed Feb 2002).

4  Coupland CA CC, Davey G *et al.* Risk factors for testicular germ cell tumours by histological tumour type. *Br J Cancer* 1999;**80**:1859–63.

5  Gallagher RP, Huchcroft S, Phillips N *et al.* Physical activity, medical history, and risk of testicular cancer (Alberta and British Columbia, Canada). *Cancer Causes Control* 1995;**6**:398–406.

6  Giwercman A, Grindsted J, Hansen B, Jensen OM, Skakkebaek NE. Testicular cancer risk in boys with maldescended testis: a cohort study. *J Urol* 1987;**138**:1214–16.

7  Frank-Stromborg M, Rohan K. Nursing's involvement in the primary and secondary prevention of cancer. *Nat Internat Cancer Nurs* 1992;**15**:79–108.

8  Ondrus D, Kuba D, Chrenova S, Matoska J. Familial testicular cancer and developmental anomalies. *Neoplasma* 1997;**44**:59–61.

9  Sigurdson AJ, Chang S, Annegers JF *et al.* A case–control study of diet and testicular carcinoma. *Nutr Cancer* 1999;**34**:20–6.

10  Ganmaa d, Li XM, Wang J. Incidence and mortality of testicular and prostatic cancers in relation to world dietary practices. *Am J Cancer* 2002;**98**:262–7.

11  Akre O, Ekbom A, Sparen P, Tretli S. Body size and testicular cancer. *J Natl Cancer Inst* 2000;**92**:1093–6.

12  Srivastava A, Kreiger N. Relation of physical activity to risk of testicular cancer. *Am J Epidemiol* 2000;**151**:78–87.

13  Thune I, Lund E. Physical activity and the risk of prostate and testicular cancer: a cohort study of 53,000 Norwegian men. *Cancer Causes Control* 1994;**5**:549–56.

14  Bach AM, Hann LE, Hadar O *et al.* Testicular microlithiasis: what is its association with testicular cancer? *Radiology* 2001;**220**:70–5.

15  Zhang ZF, Vena JE, Zielezny M *et al.* Occupational exposure to extreme temperature and risk of testicular cancer. *Arch Environ Health* 1995;**50**:13–18.

16  Saracci R, Kogevinas M, Bertazzi PA *et al.* Cancer mortality in workers exposed to chlorophenoxy herbicides and chlorophenols. *Lancet* 1991;**338**:1027–32.

17  Moller H. Work in agriculture, childhood residence, nitrate exposure, and testicular cancer risk: a case–control study in Denmark. *Cancer Epidemiol Biomarker Prevent* 1997;**6**:141–4.

18  Kristensen P, Andersen A, Irgens LM, Bye AS, Vagstad N. Testicular cancer and parental use of fertilizers in agriculture. *Cancer Epidemiol Biomarker Prevent* 1996;**5**:3–9.

19  Toppari J, Larsen JC, Christiansen P *et al.* Male reproductive health and environmental xenoestrogens. *Environ Health Perspectives* 1996;**104**(Suppl. 4):741–803.

20  US Department of Health and Human Services. *Preventing tobacco use among young people. A report of the Surgeon General.* Atlanta, Georgia: Centers for Disease Control and Prevention, 1994.

21  NHS Executive. *Guidance on Commissioning Cancer Services: Improving Outcome in Lung Cancer: The Research Evidence.* London: NICE, 1998.

22  Lancaster T, Silagy CGF. Training health professionals in smoking cessation. In: *Cochrane Library.* Oxford: Update Software, 1998.

23  Law M, Ling Tang J. An analysis of the effectiveness of interventions intended to help people stop smoking. *Arch Intern Med* 1995;**155**: 1933–41.

24  Bedwani R, el-khwsky F, La Vecchia C, Boffetta P, Levi F. Descriptive epidemiology of bladder cancer in Egypt. *Int J Cancer* 1993;**55**:351–2.

25  Wohl RE, Kane WM. Teachers' beliefs concerning teaching about testicular cancer and testicular self-examination. *J School Health* 1997;**67**:106–11.

# 12 What is the role of prophylactic surgery in the prevention of colorectal cancer?

*RJ Davies, R Miller*

Colorectal cancer (CRC) is the second commonest malignancy worldwide, with 945 000 new cases and 492 000 deaths attributed to the disease each year.[1] In the United Kingdom alone there were over 32 000 new cases diagnosed in 1995 and the incidence continues to rise.[2] Surgical resection remains the most effective treatment option for CRC, and is usually reserved for those cases where the disease has already been diagnosed. However, in some circumstances, including inherited polyposis syndromes and dysplasia in ulcerative colitis, there is a role for prophylactic surgery.

A search of the MEDLINE, PubMed, and Embase databases, and the *Cochrane Library* was undertaken to identify relevant English language publications. The reference lists of identified papers were scanned manually. Based on these findings, we describe in this chapter the rationale for a prophylactic surgical approach in the prevention of CRC.

## Inherited polyposis syndromes

### Familial adenomatous polyposis

Familial adenomatous polyposis (FAP)[3] is an autosomal dominant disease accounting for up to 1% of all CRCs. It is characterised by the development of numerous adenomas in the colon and rectum (Figure 12.1), often over 1000, and various other extracolonic manifestations.[4] These include adenomas in the upper gastrointestinal tract, desmoid tumours, osteomas and congenital hypertrophy of the retinal pigment epithelium (CHRPE). The disease is due to a mutation in the adenomatous polyposis coli (*APC*) gene, which is situated on chromosome 5.[5,6] The majority of those with FAP will develop colorectal adenomas in their second and third decade of life, and without prophylactic surgery virtually all will develop CRC by the age of 50.[4,7]

Some individuals have an attenuated form of FAP due to mutations of the *APC* gene, which are distinct from those causing the classical disease.[8] In these cases, there are usually fewer polyps in the colon and rectum, with the average age at CRC diagnosis some 15 years later than for

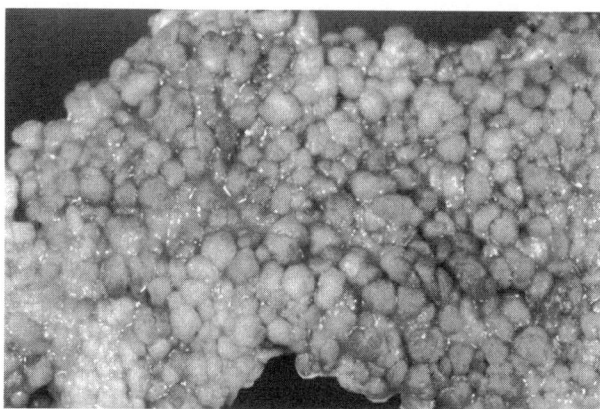

(a)

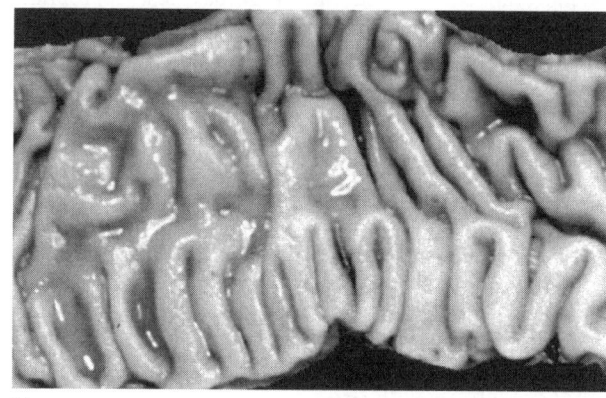

(b)

**Figure 12.1** An example of numerous polyps in (a) the colonic resection specimen of a patient with FAP, (b) with normal colon shown at the same magnification for comparison

those with the classical form.[9] Diagnosis of classical and attenuated FAP now commonly relies on DNA testing (identification and characterisation of the *APC* mutation by single-strand conformational analysis).[10] through a single blood test in children and siblings of FAP-affected individuals, as well as those newly diagnosed during clinical and endoscopic investigations. It is important, however, that any genetic analysis should be carried out in the setting of a multidisciplinary genetic counselling clinic, and only following informed consent from the patient involved.

Despite attempts at chemoprevention with celecoxib,[11] a cyclo-oxygenase-2 inhibitor, and sulindac,[12,13] another non-steroidal anti-inflammatory drug, prophylactic surgical resection remains the treatment of choice in FAP. Three main surgical options, namely proctocolectomy, total colectomy with ileorectal anastomosis (IRA), and restorative proctocolectomy (RPC) with ileo-anal pouch formation, are generally considered in the treatment of these patients. Owing to the need for a permanent ileostomy when performing proctocolectomy, IRA and RPC are the procedures most commonly performed today.

It has previously been recommended that young people (perhaps less than 30 years of age), those with large numbers of rectal polyps, and those who will not comply with follow up following IRA are more suitable candidates for RPC. However, in those teenagers with relatively few rectal polyps, it is possible to offer colectomy with IRA as an initial treatment, with conversion to a RPC with ileo-anal pouch at a later stage, should the rectum develop further numerous adenomas. Otherwise, in deciding between the two procedures, no formal guidelines exist in the decision-making process.[14] Molecular genetic tests, particularly mutational analysis, have been applied in the context of surgical management in FAP,[15] but there is now evidence to suggest that IRA may be most appropriate in patients with attenuated FAP or in those with few or no rectal adenomas.[16,17] Restorative proctocolectomy is the procedure of choice in virtually all other cases and, to be most effective in CRC prevention, should be considered in patients between the ages of 10 and 19 years.[18]

Proctocolectomy with end-ileostomy is only indicated in the rare instance of a low rectal carcinoma at initial presentation requiring sacrifice of the anal sphincter complex, in those who decide against a restorative procedure, and in those patients with poor anal sphincter function.

### Total colectomy with IRA

Total colectomy with IRA is a relatively simple, single-stage procedure associated with low morbidity and mortality.[19–21] Pelvic dissection is not required during this operation, so the risks of sexual and urinary dysfunction are minimised, and patients often report good outcomes in terms of bowel function, with high levels of satisfaction and quality of life.[22] However, the rectum will require regular, lifelong endoscopic surveillance, as the risk of further adenoma and even carcinoma development in the rectal stump remains, and is mainly related to increased patient age.[23] The risk of subsequent rectal excision after total

colectomy with IRA does exist,[24] not only because of the possibility of development of rectal cancer but also of multiple large adenomas, dysplasia, stricture formation and incontinence.

### Restorative proctocolectomy with ileo-anal pouch formation

This procedure involves surgical excision of the entire colon and rectum. An ileal pouch is then formed, and is anastomosed to the anus to restore bowel continuity. The procedure can be carried out successfully in teenagers with FAP.[25] It is usually performed as a two stage procedure: the RPC with ileo-anal pouch is performed with the anastomosis protected temporarily with a loop ileostomy, requiring closure at a second operation. Some surgeons do not routinely use a covering ileostomy, and perform the RPC as a single stage procedure with acceptable results.[26] In general, RPC has a higher complication rate than IRA,[27] including those complications associated with pelvic dissection, and may require pouch excision at a later time owing to complications or pouch malfunction.

Two techniques are commonly used in the operation of RPC:

- a double-stapled anastomosis between the pouch (often a J-pouch) and the anal canal at the level of the anorectal junction, and
- a hand-sewn ileo-anal anastomosis at the level of the dentate line following mucosectomy to ensure radical removal of the rectal mucosa.

The former technique is considered technically simpler, but has the disadvantage of leaving a possible 1–2 cm cuff of rectal mucosa, which requires regular endoscopic surveillance in order to detect further adenoma[28] or carcinoma[29] development. However, there have been reports of adenoma[30] and carcinoma[31] formation in the ileo-anal pouch following hand-sewn anastomosis to the dentate line with complete mucosectomy. On this basis, some groups offer anastomotic and pouch surveillance following RPC, whilst others are less convinced of its benefits.

Overall, prophylactic colectomy in FAP has decreased the incidence of CRC such that duodenal malignancy and desmoid tumours are now the leading causes of death.[32] Therefore, duodenal surveillance via oesophagogastroduod-enoscopy is recommended every 1–5 years,[33] dependent on the stage of duodenal polyposis.[34]

### Hereditary non-polyposis colorectal cancer

Hereditary non-polyposis colorectal cancer (HNPCC) is an inherited, autosomal dominant condition characterised by early onset of colorectal tumours, particularly those proximal to the splenic flexure. It arises from mutations in mismatch repair genes, whose normal function is to repair mistakes made during DNA replication. Mismatch repair genes implicated in the development of HNPCC include *hMLH1*, *hMSH2*, *hMSH6*, *hPMS1*, *hPMS2* and *hPMS3*, with mutations in these genes leading to instability in the length of microsatellite sequences in the DNA (microsatellite instability or MSI[35,36]) from HNPCC tumours. As well as a predisposition for the right side of the colon, CRC in patients with HNPCC is more likely to be multiple in nature (both synchronous and metachronous tumours), mucinous, poorly differentiated, and to have a lymphocytic infiltrate. Like FAP, HNPCC is associated with extracolonic tumour development, including carcinomas of the endometrium, ovary, breast, stomach, small bowel, pancreas, hepatobiliary tract, ureter, renal pelvis and skin.[37]

The lifetime risk of CRC development in HNPCC is 80–85%,[38,39] and genetic testing is available for those patients in whom the suspicion of HNPCC is raised. This can take the form of germline genetic testing via a blood sample (similar to FAP) or immunohistochemical analysis of colonic tissue following biopsy or surgical resection. As with FAP, any genetic analysis should only be carried out in the setting of a genetic counselling clinic.

As approximately 20% of individuals carrying the HNPCC mutations will not develop CRC, the question of prophylactic colectomy is less clear in this condition. The options available include colonoscopic surveillance among gene carriers every 1–2 years, starting age 20–25 years, increasing to annually after age 35,[40] or prophylactic colectomy. There are recommendations both for[41,42] and against[43–45] prophylactic colectomy in the absence of CRC in HNPCC. For the question to be answered more accurately, a case–control study would be needed to compare prophylactic colectomy versus colonoscopic surveillance in germline mutation carriers,[40] but ethical considerations may preclude such a study from ever being undertaken because of reports of interval cancers occurring 1–5 years after colonoscopy.[46] Therefore, when the option of prophylactic surgery in HNPCC germline mutation carriers is under discussion, the patient's age, family history of CRC, comorbidity, bowel function, anal sphincter function, and compliance with colonoscopic surveillance[41] should all be taken into account.

If prophylactic surgery is considered appropriate, then total colectomy with IRA (see section on FAP) would normally be the procedure of choice, although endoscopic surveillance of the remaining rectal mucosa would be necessary as its cancer risk is approximately 1% per year.[47] In women, consider also prophylactic bilateral oophorectomy and hysterectomy,[42,48–51] particularly in those who are postmenopausal.

In the end, the final decision regarding prophylactic surgery in HNPCC will depend on the level of risk that an otherwise well patient is willing to put themselves through, and the level of risk a multidisciplinary team is willing to impose on a patient in recommending such an operation.[52]

## Other inherited polyposis syndromes

Other forms of inherited polyposis include Peutz–Jeghers syndrome (multiple gastrointestinal hamartomatous polyps associated with mucocutaneous pigmentation), juvenile polyposis (an autosomal dominant condition with multiple hamartomatous juvenile polyps), Cowden disease (inherited risk of gastrointestinal polyps and cancers, with increased risk of breast, uterine, thyroid, and cervical cancer), and multiple hyperplastic polyps. There is currently no strong evidence to advise prophylactic surgery in these conditions, but close colonoscopic surveillance, every 1–2 years, should be mandatory. Based on these colonoscopic findings, prophylactic colectomy may prove appropriate in individual cases.

## Dysplasia in ulcerative colitis

In those patients with total or extensive ulcerative colitis, there is an increased risk of CRC. This risk increases with time, but is thought to be in the region of 5–15%[53,54] after 10 years disease duration. On this basis, colonoscopic surveillance with biopsies[55,56] is currently recommended every 2 years in patients with a 10-year history of extensive disease, with the aim of detecting dysplastic changes in the colon and thereby enabling prophylactic colectomy (usually a RPC with ileo-anal pouch – see the FAP section above) to be performed before frank malignancy has developed. The evidence for this approach is not, however, conclusive.

The diagnosis of dysplasia in ulcerative colitis is controversial for several reasons:

- interobserver agreement amongst pathologists is generally poor,[57,58] leading Greenson to suggest that diagnosing dysplasia is "a highly subjective art rather than a science"[59]
- dysplastic changes may be very localised and therefore colonoscopy may find the area of dysplasia only by chance through random biopsy; and
- associated carcinomas may still be present once dysplasia has been diagnosed.[60]

It is generally accepted[61] that colectomy is appropriate in the setting of high grade dysplasia (Figure 12.2) or dysplasia-associated lesions or masses (DALM).[62] The rationale for

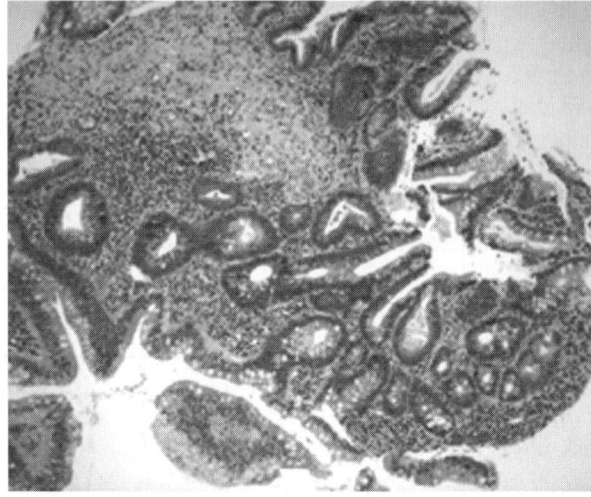

(a)

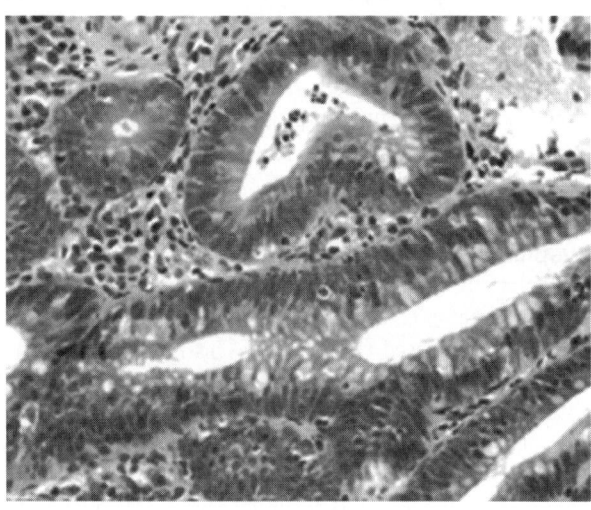

(b)

**Figure 12.2**  Haematoxylin and eosin stain at low (a) and high (b) magnification confirming dysplasia in a colonic biopsy from a patient with ulcerative colitis. Other histological features of ulcerative colitis evident in this biopsy include Paneth cell metaplasia and goblet cell depletion

this approach is based on a 32% likelihood of CRC in high grade dysplasia and 43% in DALM.[60] Some authors also recommend colectomy in the presence of low grade dysplasia,[60,63] while others do not agree with this strategy.[61] However, if colectomy is not performed in the presence of low grade dysplasia, a repeat colonoscopy within 6 months would, in the authors' opinion, be a minimum requirement.

An alternative approach to surveillance colonoscopy is prophylactic colectomy[64,65] in those patients with extensive ulcerative colitis for at least 10 years. We know that quality of life after RPC with ileo-anal pouch compares favourably with that of patients with medically treated colitis,[66] but no studies

have been carried out to assess how many cancers would be prevented by this more aggressive approach. Without such data, prophylactic colectomy in the absence of any pathological abnormality would be difficult to recommend. Thus, any decision regarding prophylactic colectomy is once again likely to involve a flexible approach to individual cases.

## Summary

Other than in FAP, controversy persists in the role of prophylactic surgery as a method of preventing CRC. In the absence of definitive evidence, a close colonoscopic surveillance programme is likely to be the favoured approach in many cases. A more aggressive approach involving a colectomy may be appropriate in selected patients after discussion in a multidisciplinary environment, and patients need to be very well informed of the potential risks and benefits of all the considered treatment options.

## References

1   Maxwell Parkin D. Global cancer statistics in the year 2000. *Lancet Oncology* 2001;**2**:533–43.

2   CRC. *Cancer Stats: Large Bowel – UK, 1999.* London: Cancer Research Campaign, 1999.

3   Spigelman AD, Thomson JPS, Philips RKS. Nomenclature: familial adenomatous polyposis (Bussey–Gardner polyposis). In: Philips RKS, Spigelman AD, Thomson JPS, eds. *Familial adenomatous polyposis.* London: Edward Arnold, 1994.

4   Bussey HJ. *Familial polyposis coli.* Baltimore: Johns Hopkins University Press, 1975.

5   Kinzler KW, Nilbert MC, Su LK *et al.* Identification of FAP locus genes from chromosome 5q21. *Science* 1991;**253**:661–5.

6   Groden J, Thliveris A, Samowitz W *et al.* Identification and characterization of the familial adenomatous polyposis coli gene. *Cell* 1991;**66**:589–600.

7   Giardiello FM. Genetic testing in hereditary colorectal cancer. *JAMA* 1997;**278**:1278–81.

8   Spirio L, Olschwang S, Groden J *et al.* Alleles of the APC gene: an attenuated form of familial polyposis. *Cell* 1993;**75**:951–7.

9   Ivanovich JL, Read TE, Ciske DJ, Kodner IJ, Whelan AJ. A practical approach to familial and hereditary colorectal cancer. *Am J Med* 1999;**107**:68–77.

10  Orita M, Iwahana H, Kanazawa H, Hayashi K, Sekiya T. Detection of polymorphisms of human DNA by gel electrophoresis as single-strand conformation polymorphisms. *Proc Natl Acad Sci USA* 1989;**86**:2766–70.

11  Steinbach G, Lynch PM, Philips RKS *et al.* The effect of celecoxib, a cyclooxygenase-2 inhibitor, in familial adenomatous polyposis. *N Engl J Med* 2000;**342**:1946–52.

12  Giardiello FM, Yang VW, Hylind LM *et al.* Primary chemoprevention of familial adenomatous polyposis with sulindac. *N Engl J Med* 2002;**246**:1054–9.

13  Cruz-Correa M, Hylind LM, Romans KE, Booker SV, Giardiello FM. Long-term treatment with sulindac in familial adenomatous polyposis: A prospective cohort study. *Gastroenterology* 2002;**122**:641–65.

14  Vasen HFA, Bulow S, and The Leeds Castle Polyposis Group. Guidelines for the surveillance and management of familial adenomatous polyposis (FAP): a worldwide survey among 41 registries. *Colorectal Dis* 1999;**1**:214–21.

15  Vasen HFA, van der Luijt RB, Slors JFM *et al*. Molecular genetic tests as a guide to surgical management of familial adenomatous polyposis. *Lancet* 1996;**348**:433–5.

16  Bulow C, Vasen H, Jarvinen H, Bjork J, Bisgaard ML, Bulow S. Ileorectal anastomosis is appropriate for a subset of patients with familial adenomatous polyposis. *Gastroenterology* 2000;**119**:1454–60.

17  Vasen HFA, van Duijvendijk P, Buskens E *et al*. Decision analysis in the surgical treatment of patients with familial adenomatous polyposis: a Dutch-Scandinavian collaborative study including 659 patients. *Gut* 2001;**49**:231–5.

18  Miltenburg DM, Conklin L, Sastri S. The role of genetic screening and prophylactic surgery in surgical oncology. *J Am Coll Surg* 2000;**190**:619–28.

19  Jagelman DG. Choice of operation in familial adenomatous polyposis. *World J Surg* 1991;**15**:47–9.

20  Madden MV, Neale KF, Nicholls RJ *et al*. Comparison of morbidity and function after colectomy with ileorectal anastomosis or restorative proctocolectomy for familial adenomatous polyposis. *Br J Surg* 1991;**78**:789–92.

21  Ambroze WL Jr, Dozios RR, Pemberton JH, Beart RW Jr, Ilstrup DM. Familial adenomatous polyposis: results following ileal pouch-anal anastomosis and ileorectostomy. *Dis Colon Rectum* 1992;**35**:12–15.

22  Church JM, Fazio VW, Lavery IC, Oakley JR, Milsom J, McGannon E. Quality of life after prophylactic colectomy with ileorectal anastomosis in patients with familial adenomatous polyposis. *Dis Colon Rectum* 1996;**39**:1404–8.

23  Setti-Carraro P, Nicholls RJ. Choice of prophylactic surgery for the large bowel component of familial adenomatous polyposis. *Br J Surg* 1996;**83**:885–92.

24  DeCosse JJ, Bulow S, Neale K, and the Leeds Castle Polyposis Group. Rectal cancer risk in patients treated for familial adenomatous polyposis. The Leeds Castle Polyposis Group. *Br J Surg* 1992;**79**:1372–5.

25  Parc YR, Moslein G, Dozios RR, Pemberton JH, Wolff BG, King JE. Familial adenomatous polyposis: Results after ileal pouch-anal anastomosis in teenagers. *Dis Colon Rectum* 2000;**43**:893–902.

26  Sugerman HJ, Sugerman EL, Meador JG, Newsome HH, Kellum JM, DeMaria EJ. Ileal pouch anal anastomosis without ileal diversion. *Ann Surg* 2000;**232**:530–41.

27  Setti-Carraro P, Ritchie JK, Wilkinson KH, Nicholls RJ, Hawley PR. The first 10 years' experience of restorative proctocolectomy for ulcerative colitis. *Gut* 1994;**35**:1070–5.

28  van Duijvendijk P, Vasen HF, Bertario L *et al*. Cumulative risk of developing polyps or malignancy at the ileal pouch-anal anastomosis in patients with familial adenomatous polyposis. *J Gastrointest Surg* 1999;**3**:325–30.

29  Vuilleumier H, Halkic N, Ksontini R, Gillet M. Columnar cuff cancer after restorative proctocolectomy for familial adenomatous polyposis. *Gut* 2000;**47**:732–4.

30  Parc YR, Olschwang S, Desaint B, Schmitt G, Parc RG, Tiret E. Familial adenomatous polyposis: Prevalence of adenomas in the ileal pouch after restorative proctocolectomy. *Ann Surg* 2000;**233**:360–4.

31  von Herbay A, Stern J, Herfcath C. Pouch-anal cancer after restorative proctocolectomy for familial adenomatous polyposis. *Am J Surg Path* 1996;**20**:995–9.

32  Jagelman DG, DeCosse JJ, Bussey HJ. Upper gastrointestinal cancer in familial adenomatous polyposis. *Lancet* 1988;**1**:1149–51.

33  Groves CJ, Saunders B, Spigelman AD, Phillips RKS. Duodenal cancer in patients with familial adenomatous polyposis (FAP): results of a 10 year prospective study. *Gut* 2002;**50**:636–41.

34  Spigelman AD, Williams CB, Talbot IC *et al*. Upper gastrointestinal cancer in patients with familial adenomatous polyposis. *Lancet* 1989;**2**:783–5.

35  Thibodeau SN, Bren G, Schaid D. Microsatellite instability in cancer of the proximal colon. *Science* 1993;**260**:816–19.

36  Frayling IM. Microsatellite instability. *Gut* 1999;**45**:1–4.

37  Lynch HT, de la Chapelle A. Genetic susceptibility to non-polyposis colorectal cancer. *J Med Genet* 1999;**36**:801–18.

38  Vasen HF, Wijnen JT, Menko FH *et al*. Cancer risk in families with hereditary nonpolyposis colorectal cancer diagnosed by mutational analysis. *Gastroenterology* 1996;**110**:1020–7 (erratum in: *Gastroenterology* 1996;**111**:1402).

39  Aarnio M, Mustonen H, Mecklin JP, Jarvinen HJ. Prognosis of colorectal cancer varies in different high risk conditions. *Ann Med* 1998;**30**:75–80.

40  Lynch HT. Is there a role for prophylactic subtotal colectomy among hereditary nonpolyposis colorectal cancer germline mutation carriers? *Dis Colon Rectum* 1996;**39**:109–10.

41  Church JM. Prophylactic colectomy in patients with hereditary nonpolyposis colorectal cancer. *Ann Med* 1996;**28**:479–82.

42  Lynch HT, Lynch J. Lynch syndrome: genetics, natural history, genetic counselling, and prevention. *J Clin Oncol* 2000;**18**:19S–31S.

43  DeCosse JJ. Surgical prophylaxsis of familial colon cancer: Prevention of death from familial colorectal cancer. *Monogr Natl Cancer Inst* 1995;**17**:31–2.

44  Rodriguez-Bigas MA. Prophylactic colectomy for gene carriers in hereditary nonpolyposis colorectal cancer. Has the time come? *Cancer* 1996;**78**:199–201.

45  Syngal S, Weeks JC, Schrag D, Garber JE, Kuntz KM. Benefits of colonoscopic surveillance and prophylactic colectomy in patients with hereditary nonpolyposis colorectal cancer mutations. *Ann Intern Med* 1998;**129**:787–96.

46  Lanspa SJ, Jenkins JX, Cavalieri RJ *et al*. Surveillance in Lynch syndrome: how aggressive? *Am J Gastroenterol* 1994;**89**:1978–80.

47  Rodriguez-Bigas MA, Vasen HFA, Mecklin JP *et al*. Rectal cancer risk in hereditary nonpolyposis colorectal cancer after abdominal colectomy. *Ann Surg* 1997;**225**:202–7.

48  Lynch HT, Smyrk TC, Watson P *et al*. Genetics, natural history, tumor spectrum, and pathology of hereditary nonpolyposis colorectal cancer: An updated review. *Gastroenterology* 1993;**104**:1535–49.

49  Lynch HT, Smyrk T. Hereditary nonpolyposis colorectal cancer (Lynch syndrome): An updated review. *Cancer* 1996;**78**:1149–67.

50  Lynch HT, Smyrk T, Lynch J. An update on HNPCC (Lynch syndrome). *Cancer Genet Cytogenet* 1997;**93**:84–99.

51  Lynch HT, Smyrk T. An update on Lynch syndrome. *Curr Opin Oncol* 1998;**10**:349–56.

52  Bilimoria MM. Prophylactic surgery in hereditary cancer syndromes: An ounce of prevention may be the only cure. *J Surg Oncol* 2002;**79**:131–3.

53  Butt JH, Price AB, Williams CB. Dysplasia and cancer in ulcerative colitis. In: Allan RN, Keighley MRB, Alexander Williams J, Hawkins C, eds. *Inflammatory bowel disease*. Edinburgh: Churchill Livingstone, 1996.

54  Lennard Jones JE, Melville DM, Morsom BC, Ritchie JK, Williams CB. Pre-cancer and cancer in extensive ulcerative colitis: findings among 401 patients over 22 years. *Gut* 1990;**31**:800–6.

55  Dickinson RJ, Dixon MF, Axon ATR. Colonoscopy and the detection of dysplasia in patients with longstanding ulcerative colitis. *Lancet* 1980;**2**:620–2.

56  Cello JP, Schneiderman JP. Ulcerative colitis. In: Sleisinger MH, Fordtran JS, eds. *Gastrointestinal disease: pathophysiology, diagnosis, management, 4th edn*. Philadelphia: WB Saunders, 1989.

57  Melville DM, Jass JR, Morson BC *et al*. Observer study of the grading of dysplasia in ulcerative colitis; comparison with clinical outcome. *Hum Pathol* 1989;**20**:1008–14.

58  Dixon MF, Brown IJ, Gilmour HM *et al*. Observer variation in the assessment of dysplasia in ulcerative colitis. *Histopathology* 1988;**13**:385–97.

59  Greenson JK. Dysplasia in inflammatory bowel disease. *Semin Diagn Pathol* 2002;**19**:31–7.

60  Bernstein CB, Shanahan F, Weinstein WF. Are we telling patients the truth about dysplasia surveillance in ulcerative colitis? *Lancet* 1994;**343**:71–4.

61  Axon T. Management of dysplasia in ulcerative colitis: Is prophylactic colectomy the preferred strategy? *J Gastrointest Surg* 1998;**2**:322–4.

62  Blackstone MO, Riddell RH, Gerald Rogers BH, Levin B. Dysplasia-associated lesion or mass (DALM) detected by colonoscopy in long-standing ulcerative colitis: an indication for colectomy. *Gastroenterology* 1981;**80**:366–74.

63  Riddell RH. Grading of dysplasia. *Eur J Cancer* 1995;**31A**:1169–70.

64 Macdougall I. The cancer risk in ulcerative colitis. *Lancet* 1964;**ii**:65–8.

65 Crowson TD, Ferrante WF, Gathright JB Jr. Colonoscopy: inefficacy for early carcinoma detection in patients with ulcerative colitis. *JAMA* 1976;**236**:2651–2.

66 Sagar PM, Lewis W, Holdsworth PJ, Johnston D, Mitchell C, Macfie J. Quality of life after a restorative proctocolectomy compares favourably with that of patients with medically treated colitis. *Dis Colon Rectum* 1993;**36**:584–92.

## Acknowledgement

We are very grateful to Dr Mark Arends for providing the clinical photographs used in this chapter.

# Section III

## Screening for cancers

*Jack Cuzick, Editor*

# 13 Screening for breast cancer

*Stephen W Duffy*

## How important is the cancer in public health terms?

Breast cancer is the commonest female cancer in the developed countries and either the commonest or second most common in the developing world. It is a significant contributor to female mortality from around age 40 onwards. Incidence rates vary considerably among countries, but in the USA and Western Europe, rates typically rise from zero in childhood to approximately 2 per 1000 per year at around the time of menopause. Rates plateau briefly around the age of menopause and continue to rise at a slower pace thereafter.[1] Figure 13.1 shows the incidence by age in England and Wales in 1988, before the inception of the breast screening programme (so that incidence patterns are not distorted by extra anticipated cases in the age groups screened).

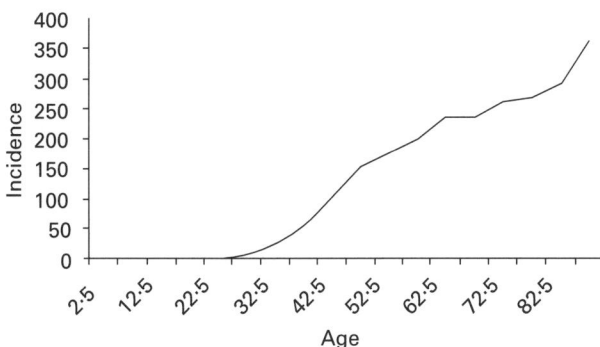

**Figure 13.1** Age-specific incidence of breast cancer in England and Wales, 1998

The principle of screening for cancer is to detect tumours at a stage of development in which they are more amenable to treatment. This is intended to have a dual benefit, a reduction in deaths from disease and a move towards less aggressive therapy. In recent decades, survival from breast cancer has generally improved,[2] incidence has increased and mortality has declined. The reduction in mortality from breast cancer is due partly to changes in therapy, and partly to earlier stage at presentation, which in turn is due to both increased awareness and the advent of mammographic screening.[2,3]

## How much is known about the natural history of the disease and the potential value of early intervention?

It has long been known that there is a strong gradient in breast cancer prognosis with stage at presentation, as represented by tumour size or regional lymph node status. As an example, see Figure 13.2, which shows survival of 2294 invasive breast cancer cases by maximum diameter of the primary tumour.[4] Clearly the smaller tumours have considerably better survival than the larger and the differences in survival are greater than one could hope for from variations in therapy. Observations of this kind gave rise to the idea of screening for the disease in order to diagnose it while it is more amenable to therapy and therefore less likely to prove fatal.

The fact that early stage tumours are associated with much better survival than late stage does not in itself indicate that screening will be effective in reducing deaths from the disease. The screening tools available may not be sufficiently sensitive to advance the diagnosis to a more successfully treatable phase, the screening may simply extend length of life with the disease without changing the time of death (lead time bias) or may selectively detect only the less rapidly fatal cases (length bias), or even detect cases which would never have come to clinical attention in the absence of screening (overdiagnosis). For these reasons, evaluation of the efficacy of screening is best carried out by randomised trial, with mortality from the disease in question as the primary endpoint. Mortality in this context means the deaths from the disease offset by the numbers of healthy persons enrolled in the study, not by the number of disease cases. The latter is case fatality and is susceptible to the biases above.

Before reliable imaging techniques for breast tissue were available, the most obvious potential screening modalities were self-examination and clinical examination of the breasts by a trained health professional. In the late twentieth century, high quality $x$ ray imaging of the breast (mammography) became possible.

## What are the appropriate age groups and intervals?

### Basic screening results

The first randomised trial of breast cancer screening was the Health Insurance Plan of Greater New York (HIP)

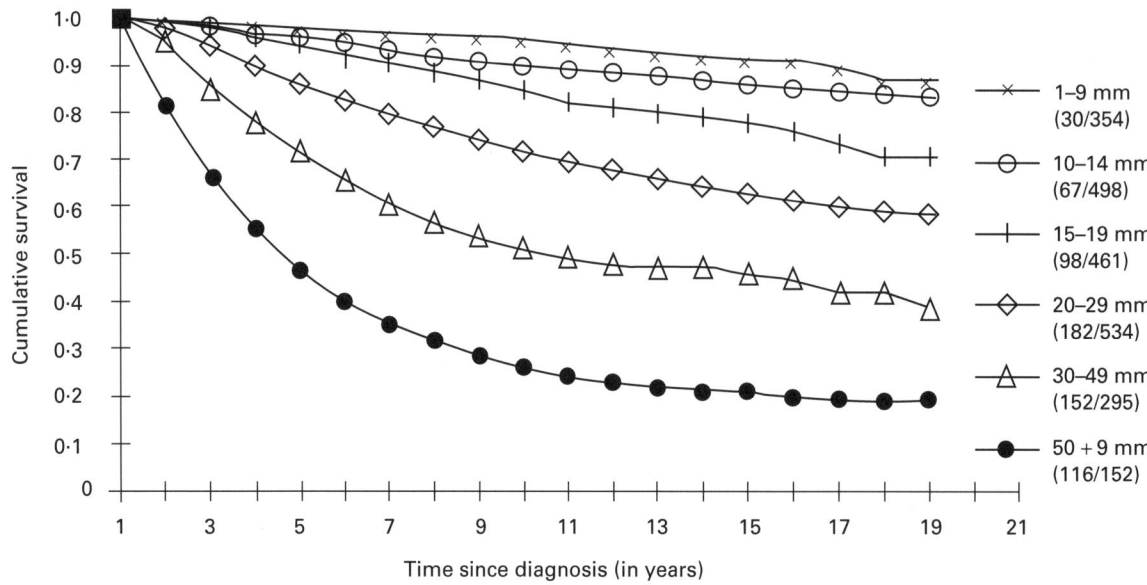

**Figure 13.2** Survival of 2294 breast cancer cases by tumour size

Study,[5] set up in 1963. To those randomised to screening, the trial offered annual two-view (craniocaudal and mediolateral oblique) mammography and physical breast examination. The study found a significant 20–30% reduction in breast cancer mortality in the study group at both short and long-term follow up.[5–7]

The HIP study was followed by the Swedish Two-County Trial of breast cancer screening, set up in late 1977, the first breast cancer screening trial to use modern, screen-film mammography. The Two-County Trial offered single-view mammography every 2 years to women aged 40–49 at randomisation and every 33 months to women aged 50–74. The first results on mortality were published in 1985, showing a significant 30% reduction in breast cancer mortality in the study group.[8] This has been maintained after 20 years of follow up.[9]

Other randomised trials followed, in Sweden,[10–12] Canada,[13,14] and the UK.[15] All used mammography, the UK and Canada trials also using physical examination. The Canadian National Breast Screening Study-2 (NBSS-2) among women aged 50–59 compared invitation to mammography and physical examination in the study group with physical examination alone in the control group.

Table 13.1 summarises the age groups, interventions and most recent results of the randomised trials. Overall, there is a significant 24% reduction in breast cancer mortality in the mammography groups. Non-randomised prospective studies, with temporal or geographical controls, tend to find similar results.[3,17–19] It should be noted that this is the "intention to treat" result, that is, it pertains to invitation to screening, rather than actually to receiving screening. Since there will be women in the invited group who do not attend and those in control group who arrange to be screened in any case, one might suspect that the true benefit of actually being screened is higher. In terms of the screening regime used, two-view mammography with screening every 24–36 months in women aged 50 or over and every 12–18 months in women under age 50 (see below) would be expected to achieve a mortality reduction at least as large as that observed in the trials.

Case–control evaluations obtain similar,[20] or more positive,[21] results. In the case–control approach, cases are deaths from breast cancer, with women alive at the time of death of the cases as controls, usually matched for age. The cases and controls are then compared with respect to history of breast cancer screening. The case–control approach has disadvantages, in particular the fact that those who opt to accept screening are often healthier *a priori* than those who do not, which biases the result in favour of screening.[22] There are, however, methods of addressing this issue in analysis, including matching or adjusting for a measure of socioeconomic status, as this is the major

**Table 13.1** Age ranges, interventions offered and mortality reductions observed in the randomised trials of breast cancer screening worldwide

| Study | Age range | Study group intervention | Control group intervention | % Mortality reduction (95% CI) |
|---|---|---|---|---|
| HIP[7] | 40–64 | 2-view mammography + PE* | Normal care | 24 (7, 38) |
| Malmö[10] | 45–69 | 2-view mammography | Normal care | 19 (−8, 39) |
| Two-County, Sweden[9] | 40–74 | 1-view mammography | Normal care | 32 (20–41) |
| Edinburgh[15] | 45–64 | 2 or 1-view mammography + PE | Normal care | 21 (−2,40) |
| Stockholm[11] | 40–64 | 1-view mammography | Normal care | 26 (−10, 50) |
| Canada NBSS-1[13] | 40–49 | 2-view mammography + PE | Normal care | −14 (−56, 17) |
| Canada NBSS-2[14] | 50–59 | 2-view mammography + PE | PE | −2 (−33, 22) |
| Gothenburg[16] | 39–59[†] | 2-view mammography | Normal care | 16 (−39, 49) |
| All trials combined | 39–74 | Mammography with or without PE | Normal care with or without PE | 24 (18, 30) |

*PE, physical examination
[†]There are more recent publications from the Gothenburg trial but they refer only to the under 50 age group.

confounder of attendance and survival,[23] or correcting for the disproportionate mortality in non-attenders observed in the randomised trials of screening.[24]

Thus the evidence clearly supports a reduction in mortality from mammographic screening. Methodological criticism of the trials that provide much of this evidence[25] has itself been shown to be methodologically questionable.[26] There is now a consensus that mammographic screening reduces deaths from breast cancer. The unresolved or partially resolved issues that remain are age-specific effects of screening on mortality, the role of screening in women at high risk of breast cancer, and possible alternative modalities of screening.

## Age subgroups

Throughout the 1990s, there was considerable controversy over the lower age limit for mammographic screening.[27] The debate was polarised essentially over whether to start at age 40 or at age 50, with the latter age point being treated as an approximate surrogate for menopausal status. Breast tissue is radiologically denser in premenopausal women,[28] potentially reducing the sensitivity of mammography. In addition, there is evidence that the disease progresses more rapidly through the preclinical screen-detectable period in younger women, so that screening has a lesser opportunity to advance the time of diagnosis.[29]

A recent meta-analysis of the randomised trials accepting only women aged 40–49 gives a significant 18% reduction in breast cancer mortality (95% CI 5–29%) with invitation to screening, compared to the 27% (95% CI 16–37%) observed in women aged 50 or more. Thus there appears to be a benefit of screening in women aged 40–49, albeit a lesser one

than in women aged 50–74. It should be noted that the meta-analysis result is based on a combination of trials with around 40% single-view and 60% two-view mammography, an average interscreening interval of around 22 months, and average attendance rate of around 75%. It is anticipated that in this age group, uniform use of two-view mammography and an 18-month interval would yield a mortality reduction comparable to that observed in the older women.[30,31]

It is clear that screening women aged 50 or over is effective and, consequently, many national screening programmes have been instituted aimed at this age group. From the above, it is evident that screening women under 50 involves a considerable outlay of resources in a group with a relatively low incidence of breast cancer. There will probably never be a universal consensus on mammographic screening in this age group. Whether the expenditure is justified by the benefit will always be a matter of judgement, depending on the age-specific incidence in the particular population, considered societal attitude and the availability of resources and expertise.

## Screening in high risk groups

The most commonly identified high risk group is women with a family history of breast cancer. A woman who presents at genetic clinics with a family history of breast cancer strong enough to indicate risk significantly elevated above the population level, but not strong enough to raise a serious suspicion of a high risk gene mutation, is often referred for mammographic surveillance more frequently and at an earlier age than is the policy in the general population.[32] While this seems a prudent policy and small studies do suggest that it is likely to be effective,[33,34] it has not been fully evaluated. At the time of writing, a major evaluation project is planned.[32]

For women under 40 years who have such a strong familial risk that there is a serious probability of having a high risk gene mutation, mammography may not be appropriate as a surveillance strategy. This is firstly because, at ages under 40, there is greater sensitivity of the subjects to radiation, secondly because at these ages, the mammographic appearance is particularly dense and difficult to read, and thirdly because women with high risk gene mutations tend to have high grade, rapidly developing tumours[35] for which the window of opportunity for early detection by mammography may be too short (see other modalities, below).

Another high risk group which is being increasingly identified since the advent of population mammography screening programmes is that of women with dense mammographic patterns. Dense patterns confer a substantial increase in risk. The relative risk associated with dense patterns varies from around 2 to 5, depending on the density classification system used and the definition of the baseline category.[36] In addition to an increased risk of breast cancer, dense mammographic patterns also impair the sensitivity of mammographic screening. This raises the possibility of individual screening regimens – women with dense patterns invited to more frequent screening or to screening with additional views, readers, or other investigations.

## What are the possible treatment options following screening?

The preferred primary treatment for breast cancer is surgery to excise the tumour. This may take the form of wide local excision, mastectomy, or either of these accompanied by axillary lymph node dissection. Thereafter, depending on the stage of disease, extent of surgery, histological grade and type of tumour, and hormone receptor status, there may be adjuvant radiotherapy, cytotoxic chemotherapy, or hormonal chemotherapy. The same criteria for choice of treatment are applied to screen-detected tumours as to clinically detected, although there may be more scope for less radical treatment in tumours diagnosed at an early stage as a result of screening. This is dealt with in more detail in the next section.

## How effective are screening/treatment options in terms of morbidity and mortality?

### Mammography, mortality, and treatment

Screening is clearly effective in reducing mortality from breast cancer, as can be seen from Table 13.1 and the preceding section. Table 13.1 indicates a 24% mortality reduction associated with invitation to screening in a series of trials with intervals ranging from 12 to 33 months, compliance rates ranging from 60% to almost 90%, and various numbers of views and readers. Recent research indicates that for women actually receiving regular, high quality screening, the mortality reduction can be in excess of 50%.[3]

Although long considered a potential benefit of screening, perhaps less attention has been paid to the quantification of the reduction in need for more radical therapy with earlier detection.[37] This reduction is potentially two-fold: firstly, smaller tumours may be more amenable to local excision than to mastectomy; secondly, early detection may obviate the necessity for adjuvant treatments such as cytotoxic chemotherapy, which has unpleasant side effects and incurs undesirable potential future risks (see the section below on *What side effects are associated with treatment?*). There is some evidence from one of the trials of less use of cytotoxic chemotherapy in screen-detected tumours than in interval cancers or unscreened controls, although this dates from largely before the epoch of widespread adjuvant chemotherapy for breast cancer.[38] It is, however, clear that the epoch of mammography has seen a considerable reduction in the rates of mastectomy.[39]

## Other screening modalities

Other possible screening tools include education in breast self-examination, professional clinical breast examination, and other imaging techniques. Randomised trial evidence on breast self-examination is not encouraging, with both major trials failing to show any benefit.[40,41] Table 13.2 shows the results of the two randomised trials.

There is very little evidence on clinical breast examination as a screening modality. The only evidence is circumstantial, a lack of a significant difference between the mammography arm and the physical examination arm in the Canadian NBSS-2.[14] However, the quality of the mammography and the random allocation of subjects have both been questioned in this trial.[42,43] The idea of physical examination as a screening strategy in developing countries is an attractive one, as it requires a relatively small outlay of financial resources and no expensive technology for the front-line screening tool. The arguments against it are that there is no serious evidence of any benefit over routine health care and that, in countries for which mammography is not an option, the infrastructure and public attitudes to diagnosis and treatment are often not conducive to any modality of screening. For example, in the trial of breast cancer screening by physical examination in the Philippines, intervention was discontinued due to non-compliance of women recalled for further assessment of suspicious lumps.[44]

**Table 13.2  Mortality results from the two randomised trials of breast self-examination**

| Trial | Breast cancer deaths/population | | RR (95% CI) |
|---|---|---|---|
| | Study group | Control group | |
| Shanghai[40] | 25/133 375 | 25/133 665 | 1·00 (0·57–1·75) |
| St Petersburg[41] | 157/57 712 | 164/64 759 | 1·07 (0·86–1·33) |

Other breast imaging techniques that arguably may have a role in front-line screening include ultrasound and magnetic resonance imaging.[45] While ultrasound is an essential component of diagnostic work-up of abnormalities observed on mammography or clinical examination, it is not at present suitable as a first-line screening tool. Magnetic resonance imaging has great potential, but is too expensive for use in general population screening. It has a role, however, in surveillance of young women at high genetic or familial risk.[46]

At the moment therefore the only established screening tool is mammography. Technical improvements to this are ongoing, including digital mammography, with or without computer-aided identification of suspicious abnormalities.[45] The early twenty-first century, however, is a period of rapid technological improvement in many imaging methods and it may be that the next decade or so sees the development of an alternative to mammographic screening.

**How acceptable is the screening method?**

One should first consider the barriers to acceptability, that is the human costs to the subjects screened. There are three inevitable human costs to all those who attend for mammographic screening: anxiety associated with being tested for a serious illness, the discomfort of compression of the breasts for *x* ray, and exposure to radiation. Subjects invited to screening should be reassured that only a small minority of screens result in a suspicious lesion that requires further assessment and indeed that the majority of referrals for assessment result in a benign diagnosis. Pain from compression can be minimised by well-trained radiographic staff.[47] The communication and interpersonal skills of the radiographic staff are important here. The subject should be reassured that not only is compression essential to the effectiveness of the screen, it also reduces the radiation absorbed by the breast. The radiation dose involved in modern mammography is relatively small and poses no more than a theoretical risk in women aged over 40 years.[48]

The dose may be associated with real hazards of radiation-induced tumours in women under age 40.

Other human costs are related to assessment of mammographically suspicious lesions. Anxiety on the part of women referred to assessment is a major concern, and many assessment clinics have a nurse counsellor on the staff. Diagnostic work-up of lesions which are ultimately found not to be malignant incur both financial and human costs. This indicates the importance of good image quality of the initial mammogram, so that only those women with a clearly suspicious feature on a high quality mammogram are called for assessment. Good positioning and image quality also reduce the numbers of women given repeat examinations because of inadequate images.

For those who are recalled for assessment, there are a variety of further tests, of varying degrees of invasion. Clearly, the fewer invasive procedures used on women whose abnormality subsequently proves to be benign, the better. There are conflicting pressures here. On the one hand it is desirable to minimise the numbers of both percutaneous and surgical biopsies. On the other hand, since surgical biopsy is the more traumatic, the assessment process is usually required to diagnose the majority of cancers by percutaneous biopsy before referral to surgery. This necessarily means that a large number of percutaneous biopsies must take place, many of which will have a non-malignant result. It is estimated that around 1% of women screened in the UK National Breast Screening Programme are subject to percutaneous biopsy.[49]

Table 13.3 shows selected minimum standards for screening and assessment from the UK's National Breast Screening Programme.[49] Screening centres would be expected to aim at exceeding these standards, in some cases considerably so. For example the limits of 10% and 5% on women called for assessment at first and subsequent screens respectively seem high, since in the age group targeted in the UK, 50–64 years, the incidence is roughly 2·3 per 1000 per year. In fact, good results have been obtained by programmes referring around half these percentages.[4] The limits on the numbers of surgical biopsies represent around

**Table 13.3  Extract from minimum standards for the UK National Breast Screening Programme**

| Criterion | Minimum standard |
| --- | --- |
| Attendance | At least 70% |
| Radiation dose | At most 2 mGy |
| Number of repeat examinations | No more than 3% of total examinations |
| Number called for assessment (first screen) | Less than 10% of those screened |
| Number called for assessment (subsequent screens) | Less than 5% of those screened |
| Number of cancers with preoperative diagnosis | At least 70% of cancers |
| Number of benign surgical biopsies (first screen) | Less than 3·6/1000 screened |
| Number of benign surgical biopsies (subsequent screens) | Less than 2·0/1000 screened |
| Number of women sent their result within 2 weeks | At least 90% of those screened |
| Assessment within one week of decision to assess | At least 90% of those assessed |

50% of surgery cases arising from the screening. In fact, with the advent of percutaneous biopsy, levels of 10% have been reported.[50]

Finally a potential harm of screening for disease is overdiagnosis, that is the diagnosis of cases that would never have come to clinical attention had screening not taken place. While there is no evidence of overdiagnosed cases of invasive carcinoma of the breast in mammographic screening, it is likely that there are overdiagnosed cases of ductal carcinoma *in situ*, particularly in premenopausal women.[27] This is difficult to quantify, but detection rates of ductal carcinoma *in situ* are too high to be explained as stage shifting by early detection of cases that would otherwise have been invasive. Programmes in which more than 20% of screen-detected cases are non-invasive may be seriously overdiagnosing ductal carcinoma *in situ* or missing small invasive tumours.[4]

Having listed the barriers to acceptability, it has to be said that in organised mammography programmes, the acceptance rates tend to be high. Rates of 60–90% were observed in the randomised trials.[4,5,10–15] Rates of 70–85% are typically observed more recently in service screening programmes.[3,17,18] Repeat screens seem to be well attended, suggesting that women attending a first screen are not dissuaded from attending subsequent screens by negative aspects of the experience.

**What side effects are associated with treatment?**

The side effects of surgery are two-fold: the psychological damage incurred by loss of a breast or a substantial part of a breast, and the physical side effects of axillary surgery and/or radiotherapy. While almost all women will experience the former, the range of severity of the psychological effect is difficult to assess. It is inevitable, but there is the compensatory psychological effect of the knowledge that the tumour has been excised. As for the physical symptoms of axillary surgery, these are essentially sensory changes, arm swelling, weakness in the arm or shoulder, and arm stiffness.[51] Sensory changes take place in the majority of patients having axillary surgery, although for the most part the symptoms are very mild. Around 25% of patients experience stiffness and the same proportion experience arm swelling (although the figure for serious arm swelling which requires intervention is closer to 10%). Around 10% experience stiffness of the arm. Radiation to the axilla considerably increases the risk of arm swelling.

Adjuvant (cytotoxic) chemotherapy has a wide range of immediate unpleasant side effects and confers long-term risk of non-solid tumours.[52] The immediate effects include hair loss, fatigue, nausea, diarrhoea, irritation of the eyes, mouth and digestive tract, and climacteric symptoms. Almost all women given cytotoxic therapy experience the first three of these. The side effects may be palliated by further therapies, but these in turn may have side effects. Adjuvant hormonal therapies are less unpleasant, the main problems being climacteric symptoms and a predisposition to blood clots, but they need to be tolerated for longer. A course of cytotoxic chemotherapy usually lasts for 4–6 months, whereas a course of tamoxifen typically lasts for 5 years.

The general effect of screening in terms of side effects of treatment is positive. The earlier a tumour is diagnosed, the less likely it is that radical and aggressive therapies are required (see section above on *How effective are screening/treatment options in terms of morbidity and mortality?*).

**What is the cost-effectiveness of screening?**

Cost-effectiveness in terms of screening is usually quoted in terms of cost per year of life saved. Before considering cost-effectiveness, one should note that this will vary between programmes depending partly on variation in labour and equipment costs in different countries, but mainly on variation in the quality of the programme. Higher quality in terms of sensitivity will mean a larger number of deaths prevented, and hence a lower cost per year of life saved. It will also mean earlier stage at presentation and may therefore cause a saving on treatment costs. Higher quality in terms of specificity will mean fewer unnecessary recalls and therefore lower expenditure on diagnostic procedures. A variety of cost-effectiveness figures have been reported but before citing these, we should consider the process of monitoring the screening quality.

The results of the randomised trials in Table 13.1 show that mammographic screening can reduce deaths from breast cancer in principle. Delivering the mortality reduction in a service screening setting entails achieving at least the same quality of screening and diagnostic activity as in the trials. To do so, while minimising the financial costs and the human costs (described in section above on *How acceptable is the screening method?*), great attention has to be paid to quality at every stage of the procedure. Good positioning of the subject at *x* ray, high quality film and processing are necessary for a good and complete image. Sensitivity and specificity of film reading are crucial. Thus, training of both radiological and technological staff is of great importance.[4] For those recalled for further assessment, a multidisciplinary approach to diagnosis and treatment is of great benefit.[53]

Some measures of quality, with suggested minimum standards are shown in Table 13.4. These have been adapted from Day *et al.*[54] Monitoring of the criteria should be augmented by technical and radiological quality control, with intercentre assessment of image quality, audit of previous "normal" mammograms of breast cancer cases, and other evaluations of technique.

Note that an important indicator of screening quality is the rate at which cancers occur symptomatically after a negative screen. The exact limits to put on the rate are debatable (for example, one might pose a separate limit for the first and second years after a negative screen), but clearly a high rate of interval cancers would raise concerns about screening sensitivity. A high rate of detection of tumours at screening is not sufficient to demonstrate good sensitivity, since detection rates are potentially affected by length bias. The latter refers to the case where screening is more effective in detection of indolent than of aggressive tumours.

In relation to this, another standard, suggested by Tabar *et al.*[4] is of interest. A low proportion of advanced stage tumours detected at screening is no guarantee of efficacy since this too may be a product of length bias. However, Tabar and colleagues suggested that the proportion of histological grade 3 screen-detected tumours diagnosed while small would be a useful measure. They suggested that at least 30% of screen-detected grade 3 tumours should be less than 15 mm in maximum diameter. The advantage of this measure is that grade 3 tumours are fast-growing aggressive cancers and typically present at considerably larger sizes in the clinical setting. They cannot be considered as indolent or "length bias" cases. Therefore, an indication that screen detection is advancing the diagnosis of these tumours should be a reliable indicator of effectiveness. This provides a potential early (usable once a single screen is complete) measure of the programme's likely effect.

Failure to achieve the standards in Table 13.4 would be a strong indicator that the programme is not on target to deliver the required mortality reduction, and remedial action should be taken. Satisfying the standards, however, is not an absolute guarantee of a substantial mortality reduction, although such an outcome would be likely. To fully evaluate the effect of a screening programme on mortality, one would wish to link the targeted clinical endpoint, death from breast cancer or not, to individual history of exposure or non-exposure to screening.

Tabar *et al.*[3] addressed this issue by identifying all deaths from breast cancer in a 29-year period, and linking this with history of mammographic screening in both the women who died of breast cancer and the population at risk. This was a substantial informatic task, and it is desirable to seek more rapid means of evaluation. One possibility is the case–control design, where women who have died of breast

**Table 13.4  Selected quality standards for monitoring a mammographic screening programme**

| Criterion | Minimum standard |
| --- | --- |
| Prevalence at first screen | At least 3 times annual incidence |
| Interval cancer rate – first two years after negative screen | At most 25% of 2 years' incidence |
| Interval cancer rate – third year after negative screen | At most 60% of annual incidence |
| Stage II or worse cancers at first screen | At most 40% of cancers detected |
| Stage II or worse cancers at subsequent screens | At most 30% of cancers detected |
| Incidence of stage II or worse cancers in the programme (regardless of mode of diagnosis), after 7 years of the programme | At most 70% of the incidence of stage II or worse cancers before screening |

cancer (cases) are compared to women who were alive at the cases' dates of death (controls) with respect to history of exposure to screening.[20] As described above, although prone to biases, there are methods available for dealing with the biases.[23,24]

After the publication of the first results of the Swedish Two-County Trial,[8] healthcare providers in various countries began to consider the possibilities of mass screening programmes and their likely costs. The costs and effects depend on the screening regime, typical stage at presentation in the absence of screening, screening quality, and the incidence of breast cancer in the population served (and therefore the age group screened). Early estimates of the cost per year of life saved were in the region of US $5000.[55] More recently, estimates have ranged from as little as US $2500 to US $18 000 or more.[56,57] If quality is carefully monitored as described and remedial action taken where necessary to provide a high quality of screening as seen in some of the randomised trials, the costs per year of life saved will be in the lower area of this range. In any case, at the mid-point of the range, around US $10 000 per year of life saved, screening is cost-effective in comparison with other preventive measures.

Mammographic screening has therefore been demonstrated to be both effective and cost-effective. It has moved on from an era where trials were necessary to demonstrate its efficacy to one when screening programmes should be implemented where the circumstances permit. Many mass screening programmes have been implemented and more are likely to be initiated in the immediate future. The monitoring and evaluation of these programmes is a crucial task for research and audit in the future.

## References

1   Parkin DM, Whelan SL, Ferlay J, Raymond L, Young J, eds. *Cancer Incidence in Five Continents Volume VII*. Lyon, France: International Agency for Research on Cancer, 1997.

2   Peto R, Boreham J, Clarke M, Davies C, Beral V. UK and USA breast cancer deaths down 25% in year 2000 at ages 20–69 years. *Lancet* 2000;**355**:1822.

3   Tabar L, Vitak B, Chen HHT, Yen MF, Duffy SW, Smith RA. Beyond randomised controlled trials: Organized mammographic screening substantially reduces breast carcinoma mortality. *Cancer* 2001;**91**:1724–31.

4   Tabar L, Fagerberg G, Duffy SW, Day NE, Gad A, Gröntoft O. Update of the Swedish two-county program of mammographic screening for breast cancer. *Radiol Clin N Am* 1992;**30**:187–210.

5   Shapiro S, Strax P, Venet L. Periodic breast cancer screening in reducing mortality from breast cancer. *JAMA* 1971;**215**:1777–85.

6   Shapiro S, Venet W, Strax P, Venet L, Roeser R. Ten- to fourteen-year effect of breast cancer screening on mortality. *J Natl Cancer Inst* 1982;**69**:349–55.

7   Shapiro S. Periodic screening for breast cancer: the HIP randomized controlled trial. *Monogr Natl Cancer Inst* 1997;**22**:27–30.

8   Tabar L, Fagerberg CJG, Gad A *et al.* Reduction in mortality from breast cancer after mass screening with mammography. *Lancet* 1985;**i**:829–32.

9   Tabar L, Vitak B, Chen HH *et al.* The Swedish Two-County Trial twenty years later: updated mortality results and new insights from long-term follow-up. *Radiol Clin N Am* 2001;**38**:625–51.

10   Andersson I, Nyström L, Mammography screening. *J Natl Cancer Inst* 1995;**87**:1263–4.

11   Frisell J, Lidbrink E, Hellstrom L, Rutqvist LE. Follow-up after 11 years-update of mortality results in the Stockholm mammographic screening trial. *Breast Cancer Res Treat* 1997;**45**:263–70.

12   Bjurstam N, Björneld L, Duffy SW *et al.* The Gothenburg Breast Screening Trial: first results on mortality, incidence and mode of detection for women ages 39–49 years at randomization. *Cancer* 1997;**80**:2091–9.

13   Miller AB, To T, Baines CJ, Wall C. The Canadian National Breast Screening Study – update on breast cancer mortality. *Monogr Natl Cancer Inst* 1997;**22**:37–41.

14   Miller AB, To T, Baines CJ, Wall C. Canadian National Breast Screening Study-2: 13-year results of a randomized trial in women aged 50–59 years. *J Natl Cancer Inst* 2000;**92**:1490–9.

15   Alexander FE, Anderson TJ, Brown HK *et al.* 14 years of follow-up from the Edinburgh randomised trial of breast-cancer screening. *Lancet* 1999;**353**:1903–8.

16   Nyström L, Rutqvist LE, Wall S *et al.* Breast cancer screening with mammography: overview of Swedish randomised trials. *Lancet* 1993;**341**:973–8.

17   Hakama M, Pukkala E, Heikkila M, Kallio M. Effectiveness of the public health policy for breast cancer screening in Finland: population-based cohort study. *BMJ* 1997;**314**:864–7.

18   McCann J, Duffy S, Day N. Predicted long-term mortality reduction associated with the second round of breast screening in East Anglia. *Br J Cancer* 2001;**84**:423–8.

19   UK Trial of Early Detection of Breast Cancer Group. 16-year mortality from breast cancer in the UK Trial of Early Detection of Breast Cancer. *Lancet* 1999;**353**:1909–14.

20   Palli D, Rosselli del Turco M *et al.* A case–control study of the efficacy of a non-randomized breast cancer screening program in Florence (Italy). *Int J Cancer* 1986;**38**:501–4.

21   Collette HJ, Day NE, Rombach JJ, de Waard F. Evaluation of screening for breast cancer in a non-randomised study (the DOM project) by means of a case–control study. *Lancet* 1984;**i**:1224–6.

22   Moss SM. Case–control studies of screening. In: Miller AB, Chamberlain J, Day NE, Hakama M, Prorok PC, eds. *Cancer Screening*. Cambridge: Cambridge University Press, 1991.

23   Sasieni PD, Cuzick J, Lynch-Farmery E. Estimating the efficiency of screening by auditing smear histories of women with and without cervical cancer. *Br J Cancer* 1996;**73**:1001–5.

24   Duffy SW, Cuzick J, Tabar L *et al.* Correcting for non-compliance bias in case–control studies to evaluate cancer screening programmes. *Appl Statist* 2002;**51**:235–43.

25   Gøtzsche PC, Olsen O. Is screening for breast cancer with mammography justifiable? *Lancet* 2000;**355**:129–34.

26   Duffy SW. Interpretation of the breast screening trials: a commentary on the recent paper by Gøtzsche and Olsen. *Breast* 2001;**10**:209–12.

27   Fletcher SW. Breast Cancer Screening among women in their forties: an overview of the issues. *Monogr Natl Cancer Inst* 1997;**22**:5–9.

28   De Stavola BL, Gravelle IH, Wang DY *et al.* Relationship of mammographic parenchymal patterns with breast cancer risk factors and risk of breast cancer in a prospective study. *Int J Epidemiol* 1990;**19**:247–54.

29   Chen HH, Duffy SW, Tabar L, Day NE. Markov chain models for progression of breast cancer. Part 1. Tumour attributes and the preclinical detectable phase. *J Epidemiol Biostat* 1997;**2**:9–23.

30   Organizing Committee and Collaborators, Falun Meeting. Breast cancer screening with mammography in women aged 40–49 years. *Int J Cancer* 1996;**68**:693–9.

31   Tabar L, Duffy SW, Vitak B, Chen HH, Prevost TC. The natural history of breast carcinoma: what have we learned from screening? *Cancer* 1999;**86**:449–62.

32   Mackay J, Roger C, Fielder H *et al.* Development of a protocol for evaluation of mammographic surveillance services in women under 50 with a family history of breast cancer. *J Epidemiol Biostat* 2001;**6**:365–9.

33 Nixon RM, Pharoah P, Tabar L *et al.* Mammographic screening in women with a family history of breast cancer: some results from the Swedish Two-County Trial. *Rev Epidemiol Sante Publ* 2000;**48**: 325–31.

34 Kollias J, Sibbering DM, Blamey RW *et al.* Screening women aged less than 50 years with a family history of breast cancer. *Eur J Cancer* 1998;**34**:878–83.

35 Armes JE, Egan AJ, Southey MC *et al.* The histologic phenotypes of breast carcinoma occurring before age 40 years in women with and without BRCA1 or BRCA2 germline mutations: a population-based study. *Cancer* 1998;**83**:2335–45.

36 Warner E, Lockwood G, Tritchler D, Boyd NF. The risk of breast cancer associated with mammographic parenchymal patterns: a meta-analysis of the published literature to examine the effect of method of classification. *Cancer Detect Prevent* 1992;**16**:67–72.

37 Tabar L, Fagerberg G, Day NE, Duffy SW, Kitchin RM. Breast cancer treatment and natural history: New insights from the results of screening. *Lancet* 1992;**339**:412–14.

38 Tabar L, Chen HHT, Duffy SW, Krusemo UB. Primary and adjuvant therapy, prognostic factors and survival in 1053 breast cancers diagnosed in a trial of mammography screening. *Jpn J Clin Oncol* 1999;**29**:608–16.

39 Wingo PA, Guest JL, McGinnis L *et al.* Patterns of inpatient surgeries for the top four cancers in the United States, National Hospital Discharge Survey, 1988–95. *Cancer Causes Control* 2000;**11**: 497–512.

40 Thomas DB, Gao DL, Self SG *et al.* Randomized trial of breast self-examination in Shanghai: methodology and preliminary results. *J Natl Cancer Inst* 1997;**89**:339–40.

41 Semiglazov VF, Moiseyenko VM, Manikhas AG *et al.* Role of breast self-examination in early detection of breast cancer: Russia/WHO prospective randomized trial in St Petersburg. *Cancer Strategy* 1999;**1**:145–51.

42 Kopans DB. Breast cancer detection in an institution: is mammography detrimental? *Cancer* 1993;**72**:1457–60.

43 Boyd NF. The review of randomization in the Canadian National Breast Screening Study. Is the debate over? *Can Med Assoc J* 1997;**156**:207–9.

44 International Agency for Research on Cancer. *Biennial Report 1998–99.* Lyon, France: IARC, 2000.

45 Jochelson M. Breast cancer imaging: the future. *Semin Oncol* 2001;**28**:221–8.

46 UK MRI Breast Screening Study Advisory Group. Magnetic resonance imaging screening in women at genetic risk of breast cancer: imaging and analysis protocol for the UK multicentre study. *Magn Reson Imaging* 2000;**18**:765–76.

47 Eklund GW, Cardenosa G. The art of mammographic positioning. *Radiol Clin N Am* 1992;**30**:21–53.

48 Feig SA, Ehrlich SM. Estimation of radiation risk from screening mammography: recent trends and comparison with expected benefits. *Radiology* 1990;**174**:638–47.

49 Wilson R, Asbury D, Cooke J, Michell M, Patnick J, eds *Clinical Guidelines for Breast Cancer Screening Assessment.* Sheffield: NHS Cancer Screening Programmes, 2001.

50 Warren R. Team learning and breast cancer screening. *Lancet* 1991;**338**:514.

51 Mansel R. Local treatment and reconstruction. In: Souhami RL, Tannock I, Hohenberger P, Horiot JC, eds. *Oxford Textbook of Oncology.* Oxford: Oxford University Press, 2002.

52 Goldhirsch A, Senn HJ. Adjuvant therapy for breast cancer. In: Souhami RL, Tannock I, Hohenberger P, Horiot JC, eds. *Oxford Textbook of Oncology.* Oxford: Oxford University Press, 2002.

53 Tabar L, Dean PB, Kaufman CS, Duffy SW, Chen HH. A new era in the diagnosis of breast cancer. *Surg Oncol Clin N Am* 2000;**9**:233–77.

54 Day NE, Williams DRR, Khaw KT. Breast cancer screening programmes: the development of a monitoring and evaluation system. *Br J Cancer* 1989;**59**:954–8.

55 Department of Health and Social Security. *Breast Cancer Screening: Report to the Health Ministers of England, Wales, Scotland and Northern Ireland.* London: HMSO, 1986.

56 Rosenquist CJ, Lindfors KK. Screening mammography beginning at age 40 yeas: a reappraisal of cost-effectiveness. *Cancer* 1998;**82**: 2235–40.

57 De Koning HJ. Breast cancer screening; cost-effective in practice? *Eur J Radiol* 2000;**33**:32–7.

# 14 Cervical screening

*Peter Sasieni*

## The public health importance of cervical cancer

Worldwide, there are an estimated half a million new cases of cervical cancer each year, accounting for about 10% of all female cancers.[1] The cumulative rate of incidence up to the age of 74 ranges from over 5% in parts of Latin America (and probably sub-Saharan Africa) to around 0·5% in parts of the Middle East and in Finland. In most European countries it is under 2%.[2] Rates of cervical cancer also vary considerably between different ethnic populations within a given geographic area. Thus for instance, the Maori population of New Zealand have nearly three times the risk of the non-Maori and, in Los Angeles, Hispanic women have more than twice the risk of non-Hispanic White women who in turn have nearly twice the risk of Japanese Americans (Table 14.1).

Incidence of cervical cancer in most countries has decreased substantially since the 1960s.[3] In the UK, mortality from cervical cancer has been declining since 1950 except in young women (aged 20–39) in whom rates more than doubled between 1970 and the mid 1980s.[4] The incidence rates of cervical cancer show strong birth cohort effects.[5] It is estimated that, in the absence of screening, the cumulative risk of cervical cancer up to the age of 74 in women born during the 1960s is likely to be around 4–5%.[6] That would make cervical cancer third in importance after breast and lung in women, and underlines the need for a successful screening programme.

After adjusting for cohort effects, the incidence rates of cervical cancer, in most countries, rise steeply between the ages of 25 and 39 and are then fairly constant for a further 40 years. Hence, cervical cancer can result in the death of middle-aged women with devastating effects on families.

**Table 14.1** Cumulative incidence of cancer of the cervix in different populations, 1988–1992[2]

| Population | Cumulative incidence (age 0–74) per 1000 women |
|---|---|
| New Zealand | |
| Maori | 34 |
| Non-Maori | 12 |
| Los Angeles | |
| Hispanic | 18 |
| Black | 12 |
| White (non-Hispanic) | 8 |
| Japanese | 4 |
| Harare* | |
| African | 67 |
| European | 10 |
| Israel | |
| Jews | 5 |
| Non-Jews | 3 |
| Singapore | |
| Chinese | 18 |
| Malay | 12 |
| Indian | 9 |
| Europe | |
| Denmark | 16 |
| Finland | 4 |
| Eastern Germany | 21 |
| The Netherlands | 7 |
| Sweden | 8 |
| UK | 13 |

*The rates for Harare are the age-standardised incidence per 100 000.

## Natural history

Few studies have directly observed the natural history of cervical cancer development because of the ethical difficulties in not treating precancerous cervical disease. The situation is further complicated by the possibility that the process of taking a biopsy, required for definitive diagnosis of disease, may affect the natural history by stimulating regression.[7] Most of what is known about the natural history of cervical precancer is derived from the follow up of women with cytological abnormalities and the study of the incidence and prevalence of cervical lesions.

For well over 90% of cervical cancers, the first step is exposure to one of the oncogenic human papillomaviruses (HPV).[8] The time from infection to the development of invasive cancer is thought to be many years, typically 5–50. Longitudinal studies on young women show that the majority of HPV infections are transient,[9,10] and that the virus is indeed sexually transmitted.[11,12] Persistence of infection has been shown to be associated with the development of cervical lesions.[13–15] It is generally believed that one of the key steps in the development of cancer is integration of the viral DNA in the host genome,[16] although some carcinomas only have episomal viral DNA.[17]

Cervical neoplasia appears to constitute a disease continuum ranging from cervical intraepithelial neoplasia (CIN) grades I to III (often specified as 1 to 3 in more recent literature), to microinvasive and frank invasive cancer. However, CIN I is frequently not associated with HPV infection and may not therefore be part of the continuum.[18]

Follow up studies of women with CIN have found that about 60% of CIN I regresses compared with about 33% of CIN III; 11% and 22% of CIN I and II, respectively, progressed to CIN III.[19] Others claim that regression is more common in younger women and that three-quarters of CIN in women under 35 years of age will regress.[20] They estimate the mean duration of CIN to be 12 years and that the time from HPV infection to CIN is between 1 and 10 years. Although the details of progression and regression are largely speculative, it is clear that at most about a third of high grade CIN will progress to cancer over about 15 years and that the majority of CIN I will regress.

CIN III is very rare in women under the age of 20.[21] The rates rise rapidly peaking at about age 30 and fall again rather more slowly, reaching around half their peak by age 40 and just 10–20% of their maximum by age 50. It is not completely clear to what extent published CIN III rates reflect prevalence of an untreated condition and to what extent they mirror incidence.

## Who should be screened and how often?

Cervical screening aims to detect and treat precancerous lesions, thereby preventing cervical cancer. Since the treatment does not depend on the severity of the precursor lesion and many lesions regress spontaneously, theory dictates that screening should be offered to all those at an appreciable risk of disease at the latest possible opportunity. Waiting as long as is practically possible should result in fewer women being treated unnecessarily for lesions that would spontaneously regress and avoid excessive screening in young women whose risk of cervical cancer is small. Screening intervals will be determined by available resources, but should take into account the rate of interval cancers as a function of time since last screened. Once the interval cancer rate reaches an appreciable fraction of the cancer rate of unscreened women, it is clearly time to screen again, but considerably shorter intervals may be chosen in order to bring down cervical cancer rates as far as possible.

## Should the screening interval be risk-factor dependent?

There is limited evidence to suggest that cervical lesions may progress more rapidly in smokers,[22,23] but this accelerated natural history is not generally considered to warrant more frequent screening. Women who are immune-suppressed, by contrast, are at high risk of not only HPV infection, but also of HPV persistence and, in all likelihood, more rapid progression to cancer.[24–27] There are many who believe that such women should be screened annually. With the advent of highly active antiretroviral therapy (HAART) for management of HIV infection, the life expectancy of HIV-positive women has increased considerably. Clinical guidelines for cervical screening HIV-positive women are still emerging, but most would agree that such women should be screened more intensely that the general population. There is no evidence to support more frequent screening in women with other factors associated with increased risk of cervical cancer such as multiple sexual partners, oral contraceptive use, or other sexually transmitted diseases.

## When should screening start?

Although some researchers have suggested that cervical screening be introduced a certain number of years after first sexual intercourse, such a rule is not practical for the running of an invitation-based screening programme. Most cervical screening programmes start in women aged between 20 and 30 years. Those who start earlier will have been persuaded by the argument that high grade abnormality rates (and HPV infection rates) are very high even a few years after coitarche and are greatest after about 10 years. Those that start later are more influenced by the low rates of cervical cancer under the age of 30 and extremely low rates under the age of 25. Additionally, the rates of low grade abnormalities fall considerably in women between the ages of 20 and 30, so that screening women in their 20s results in substantial numbers being recalled or referred with minor lesions that do not require treatment. Although decisions as to when to start screening should be based on relevant age-specific cancer incidence rates, one should be aware of the influence of previous screening on the rates in young women.

## When should screening stop?

In some countries there is no upper age limit on cervical screening but, in many, screening ceases after the age of 60 or 65 years. The reasons for not continuing to screen older women are:

- the rate of high grade lesions detected on screening in women over the age of 50 is low compared to the rates in younger women;

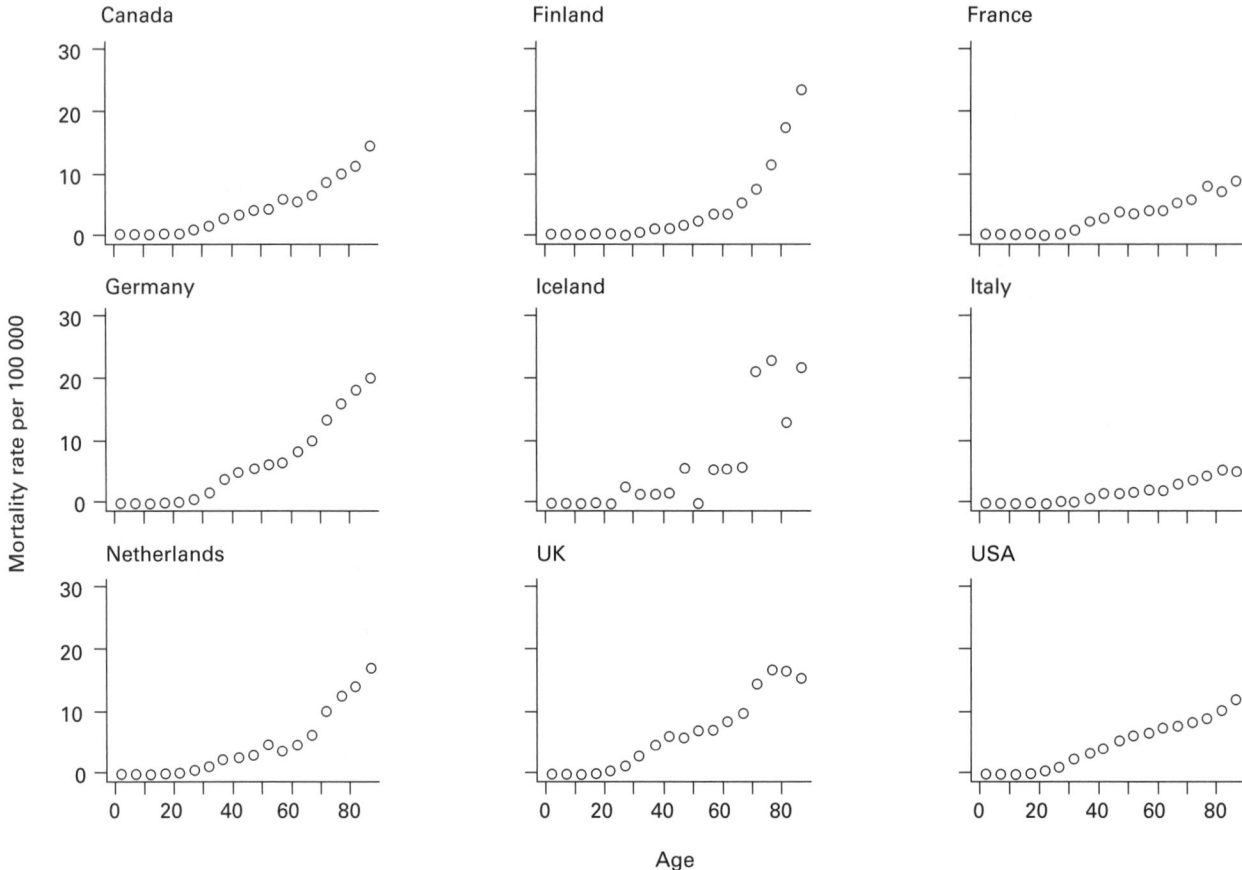

**Figure 14.1** Cervical cancer mortality as a function of age in various countries. (Data from www.depdb.iarc.fr/who/menu.htm are for 1993–1997, except for Iceland: 1990–1996)

- cervical screening is more uncomfortable in older women and the gain in terms of added years of cancer-free life decreases with increasing age;
- it is believed that almost all cervical cancer in older women results from HPV infection under the age of 35, so that older women who have had two or three recent negative screens are at extremely low risk of developing cancer in the future.

Indeed it has been argued that screening could cease at age 50 in women who have been previously well screened,[28] based on the extremely rare finding of incident high grade disease in such women.

Those who argue for continued screening of older women would point to the sharply increasing mortality rates over the age of 65 observed in many countries (Figure 14.1).

### Screening interval

There have been no randomised studies comparing the efficacy of cytological screening at different intervals and so

decisions need to be made based on observational studies and external factors such as political considerations. The resource implications of screening at different intervals are not difficult to estimate, but the effects of screening at different intervals, primarily the effect on cervical cancer incidence, are harder to estimate.

Cytological screening has variously been carried out at intervals of 5, 3 and 1 years. Annual screening is the norm in the USA and Germany, whereas 5-year screening is recommended in countries such as the Netherlands and Finland with a public health-based screening programme. Most European countries aim at 3-year screening starting at age 20–30 and continuing until age 59–65. Although there are certain overheads associated with running a screening programme that are independent of the amount of screening undertaken, these are small and the major determinant of cost is the number of smears taken each year. The latter is determined by the number of smears offered per woman in her lifetime and the compliance (both coverage and "overscreening") with the programme policy. Although there is some evidence that the rate of high grade abnormality per

Table 14.2 Percentage reduction in cervical cancer in women screened at various intervals as estimated by IARC[30] and Sasieni *et al.*[31] Two additional columns show the effect of sensitivity on the effectiveness of different screening intervals. The illustrations are for tests with 75% or 60% sensitivity relative to the IARC test

| Screening interval (years) | | Reduced sensitivity | | |
|---|---|---|---|---|
| | IARC | 75% | 60% | UK audit (%) |
| 1 | 93·5 | 92·5 | 90·6 | 82 |
| 3 | 90·8 | 84·7 | 77·4 | 75 |
| 5 | 83·6 | 71·0 | 60·8 | 65 |
| 10 | 64·1 | 48·0 | 38·4 | 35 |

screen increases with the screening interval, the per screen rate of low grade abnormality would appear to be independent of the screening interval.[29] Thus roughly speaking, annual screening is three times as expensive as 3-year screening which in turn is 66% more expensive than 5-year screening.

For many years, the meta-analysis conducted by the International Agency for Research on Cancer (IARC),[30] provided the best estimates of the relative effectiveness of cytological screening at different intervals (Table 14.2) and provides the "input parameters" for many of the models looking at the effectiveness of different screening policies. That paper suggested that whereas annual screening could prevent 93·5% of cervical cancer, 3-year screening was almost as good (90·8%), whilst 5-year screening was slightly less effective (83·6%) (Table 14.2). Based on these figures, most people were agreed that annual screening was excessive, but the choice between 3- and 5-year screening was less straightforward. On the one hand, 3-year screening would be 66% more expensive, but would only prevent 8·6% (7·2/83·6) more cancer. On the other hand the risk of cancer with 5-year screening is 78% greater than with 3-year screening (7·2/[100−90·8]). Thus on purely economic grounds, 3-year screening would not seem to be good value for money, but considering we are talking about a cancer that affects middle-aged women often with fatal consequences, it is difficult not to want to provide the additional protection afforded by 3-year screening.

Two more recent studies from the UK also provide estimates of the relative benefit of different screening intervals. A UK-based audit included the screening histories of 348 women with invasive cervical cancer in a case–control study,[31] and Herbert *et al.*[32] studied the screening histories of 83 women with invasive cancer and compared them to known performance indicators of the local screening programme. Both studies found a substantial difference in the risk of cancer associated with 3- and 5-year screening. Sasieni *et al.*[31] considered both time since last negative smear and also time since last smear (regardless of result), but

excluding all smears taken within 6 months of diagnosis. In both analyses, the relative risk 5 years after screening compared to no screening is around 65%, whereas the relative risk after 3 years is around 30–35%. Thus it would appear that even the marginal cost of 3-year screening compared to 5-year screening is justified by the marginal benefit. Herbert *et al.*[32] also found that the benefit of 5-year screening (compared to no screening) was less than in the IARC[30] overview and that the relative benefit of 3- compared to 5-year screening was greater. Whether or not they excluded screen-detected cancers, they found the relative benefit of 3- compared to 5-year screening to be similar to the relative benefit of 5-year screening compared to no screening.

In Table 14.3, we compare the "effectiveness" of screening at different intervals as estimated from the IARC study and from the UK audit. The table includes the effect of imperfect sensitivity on the results from the IARC study. Assuming the relative rates obtained from the IARC study apply to a test with 100% sensitivity, we also look at what the results would be for a test with either 75% or 60% sensitivity. Such sensitivities seem reasonable when cytology is compared to other screening tests such as HPV testing. The effect of taking into account imperfect sensitivity is to reduce the effectiveness of screening (at any interval) and to increase the relative benefit of more frequent screening (assuming the results of cytology taken at different times in a given woman are conditionally independent, given her true disease status).

## Who need not be screened?

Women whose cervix has been removed during a hysterectomy need not be screened. If the hysterectomy was done because of a high grade cervical lesion, vault smears should be taken as part of post-treatment surveillance.

Women who have never been sexually active do not need to be screened, but not having been active since the last

**Table 14.3 Approximate costs of various components of cervical screening**

| Procedure | Cost (£) |
| --- | --- |
| Screening smear | 20 |
| Colposcopy | 200 |
| Management of low-grade CIN | 800 |
| Management of HIGH-grade CIN | 1 150 |
| Treatment of microinvasive cancer | 3 000 |
| Treatment of frank invasive cancer | 6 000 |
| Care for advanced disease | 10 000 |

screening test is not considered to be adequate reason for not being screened. There is evidence to suggest that lesbian women are at risk of HPV infection and cervical cancer and should be screened regardless of their sexual history with men.[33] It is likely that a woman who has had two negative tests for high risk HPV since last having sexual intercourse does not require further screening, but there is no empirical evidence as to the risk of cervical cancer in such women.

Multiple sexual partners, smoking and oral contraceptive use have been associated with an increased risk of cervical cancer, but monogamous non-smoking women not taking the pill are at sufficiently high risk of cervical cancer to warrant screening.

Treatment of cervical lesions during pregnancy runs the risk of significant morbidity.[34] For this reason, routine screening is generally avoided during pregnancy.

## Treatment options following screening

High grade CIN or squamous intraepithelial lesions (SIL) should be removed surgically in order to minimise the risk of progression to invasive cancer. Conservative surgical techniques can be divided into those that excise the lesion (knife cone biopsy, laser conisation, large loop excision of the transformation zone (LLETZ or LEEP) and those that destroy it (laser ablation, cryocautery, cold coagulation and radical diathermy). A Cochrane review of 28 randomised trials concluded that no one treatment is obviously superior to any other.[35] However, others have found that the rate of clearance of CIN III by cryocautery is poor.[36,37] Excisional techniques have the advantage of providing adequate biopsy material for histology (including assessing the margins) and are therefore preferred. LLETZ is the preferred treatment of most gynaecological oncologists. Ablative techniques should only be used if the entire transformation zone is visualised and there is no evidence of glandular disease. Hysterectomy is also used to treat high grade lesions. Although hysterectomy is not usually necessary, recurrence

rates after hysterectomy are significantly lower than after other treatments.[38,39]

Treated women should be followed annually for a number of years (at least 5 years for CIN III, and probably 10) because of the risk of recurrence, but the incidence of invasive cervical cancer following treatment is low. In a UK study, the cumulative rate of invasive cancer 8 years after conservative treatment of CIN was 5·8 per 1000 women treated.[40] Even lower rates were reported in a study linking registrations of carcinoma *in situ* to later registrations of invasive cervical cancer in the same women in Sweden.[41]

## Effectiveness of cytological screening

Having demonstrated that smear tests could be used to detect CIN[42] and that microinvasive cervical tumours were often adjacent to areas of CIN, doctors offered cervical screening to women well before its effectiveness had been shown. By the time people considered the possibility of evaluating cervical screening in a randomised controlled clinical trial, the indirect evidence of the benefits of such screening made a trial in which some women were deprived of screening unethical. Randomised trials of different screening intervals or of variants in screening technique, with cancer incidence as their primary endpoint, would need to be extremely large and none have been undertaken. Thus estimates of the effectiveness of cervical screening are based on observational studies or computer simulations using models of the natural history of disease and the sensitivity and specificity of the screening test. As we have seen, details of the natural history are largely unknown and the models must therefore be interpreted with extreme caution.

The earliest evidence of the effectiveness of cervical screening came from monitoring trends in the incidence of and mortality from cervical cancer after the introduction of screening. Perhaps the most persuasive evidence of this type came from the Nordic countries.[43] Finland, Iceland and Sweden all had organised screening programmes in place by the early 1970s; only 5% of women in Norway were covered by organised screening; and the situation in Denmark was variable with only a minority of counties having organised screening. Cytological smears taken outside of organised screening were common in all Nordic countries with the exception of Iceland. There was a strong correlation between the extent of organised screening and changes in the incidence of invasive cervical cancer between the late 1960s and the mid 1980s (Figure 14.2). The relative reduction was greatest in Finland (65% fall) and least in Norway (20%). The result is even more impressive since these two countries had almost identical rates of cervical cancer in the early 1960s. In women aged 40–49 years the

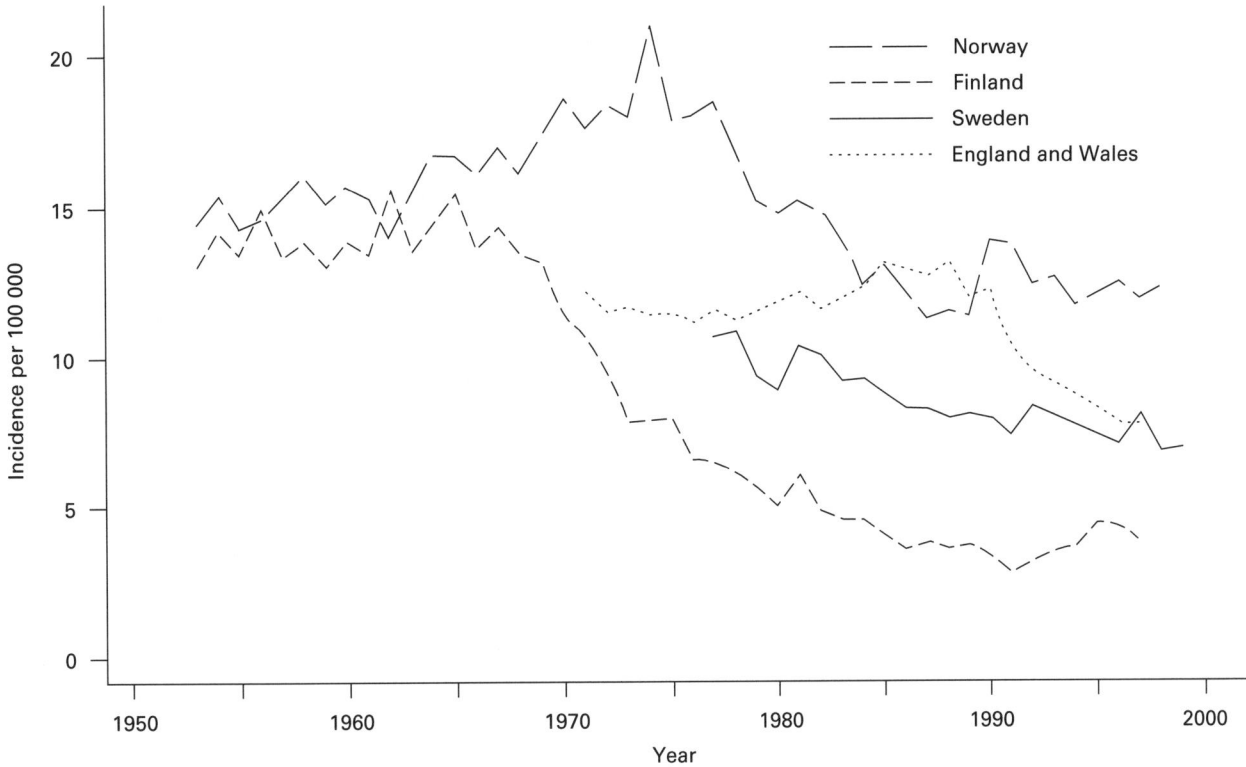

**Figure 14.2** Trends in the age-standardised incidence of cervical cancer in Nordic countries and England and Wales for 1950–1999. (Data obtained from websites of the cancer registries)

reduction was 80% in Finland and 50% in Norway. Rates in women aged 60–64 fell less and there was an increase in incidence in women aged 20–24. Trends in mortality were similar. Further, plotting trends by birth cohort imply that the effect of screening in older women may carry over for 10 or even 15 years after they were last screened. Incidence and mortality data from Iceland are extremely variable owing to the small population, but an increase in microinvasive cancers following the introduction of screening in the late 1960s was clearly visible. The rates of microinvasive cancers fell again once women started to attend for their second screen 2 to 3 years later. The numbers of smears taken per woman in Finland, where screening was offered 5-year between the ages of 30 and 55, and in Norway were similar. This emphasises the importance of *organised* screening which is able to achieve high population coverage.

Although similar trends were seen in other populations in which screening was introduced, one never knows what would have happened in the absence of screening. The substantial fall in mortality (around 35%) in women aged over 65 in England and Wales between 1950 and 1970 serves as a warning about unpredictability of trend data.

However, once one takes into account the substantial effects of birth cohort on cervical cancer rates, the data from England and Wales are supportive of a beneficial effect of cervical screening mostly since the late 1980s and particularly in women aged 25 to 44.

In the absence of randomised trials, researchers sought evidence from studies that looked at screening at the individual level rather than in populations (Table 14.4). These have mostly been carried out as case–control studies, comparing the screening experience of women diagnosed with or dying from cervical cancer with that of healthy women. The fact that women with cervical cancer are less likely to have been screened than healthy women could be confounded by socioeconomic status and attitudes to healthy lifestyles. Women who do not attend for screening may be at greater risk than those who attend, even if screening is useless, simply because they are more likely to smoke, to have a poor diet and to be exposed to oncogenic HPVs. However, considering both case–control and population trend studies, one sees a picture in which overall cancer rates are falling and women who have been screened are less likely to develop cancer than those who have not.

**Table 14.4** Summary of the epidemiological studies looking at the effectiveness of cervical screening at an individual level

| First author, year | Area | Type of study | Years of diagnosis | No. invasive cancers | Choice of comparison group | Notes | Summary of results |
|---|---|---|---|---|---|---|---|
| Aristizabal 1984[44] | Colombia | Case–control Interview | 1977–81 | 204 | 2 controls/case: 1 health centre, 1 neighbourhood | Only 22% of potential cases participated Analysis biased for screen-detected cases (in favour of screening) | 4% of cases screened 12–72 months prior to diagnosis, 52% of health centre controls, 31% of neighbourhood controls |
| La Vecchia 1984[45] | Milan | Case–control Interview | 1981–83 | 191 | 191 hospital controls | 98% participation 61% stage I | Relative protection decreased with time since last -ve, and was greater with 2+ -ve |
| Berrino 1986[46] | Milan | Case–control Clinical records | 1978 | 121 | 3 controls/case | Hospital controls | Risk within 24 months of -ve smear ~15% of that in those with no such smear |
| Choi 1986[47] | Manitoba | Cohort | 1968–75 | 86 | Historical cohort | Cases had negative smear between 1963 and 1972 | Incidence decreased with no. of -ve smears, but did not increase with time since -ve |
| Clarke 1986[48] | Toronto | Case–control Interview | 1973–76 | 156 | 5 controls/case | Squamous, stage IB+ 67% of potential cases consented | Relative protection decreased with time since last -ve, and lasted up to 48 months |
| Geirsson 1986[49] | Iceland | Case–control Clinical records | 1969–84 | 101 | 5 controls/case | Cases (59% screen-detected) and controls screened at least once | Relative protection decreased with time since last -ve, was substantial and lasted up to 119 months |
| Lynge 1986[50] | Denmark | Cohort | 1966–82 | 53 | Historical cohort | | Relative protection decreased with time since last -ve, and was greater with 2+ -ve |
| Macgregor 1986[51] | Aberdeen | Case–control Clinical records | 1968–83 | 85 | 5 controls/case | Cases (59% screen-detected) and controls screened at least once | Relative protection decreased with time since last -ve, and was greater with 2+ -ve |
| Magnus 1986[52] | Norway | Cohort | 1959–82 | 73 | Neighbouring counties | Cases had negative smear | No clear effect of -ve smears |
| Pettersson 1986[53] | Sweden | Cohort | 1967–80 | 446 | Historical cohort | Only recorded organised screening | Incidence increases with time since last -ve, up to 5 years Risk less after two -ve |

*(Continued)*

**Table 14.4** *(Continued)*

| First author, year | Area | Type of study | Years of diagnosis | No. of invasive cancers | Choice of comparison group | Notes | Summary of results |
|---|---|---|---|---|---|---|---|
| Raymond 1986[54] | Geneva | Case–control | 1970–76 | 186 | 1 control/case | | Relative protection greatest within 12 months of -ve smear |
| van Oortmarssen 1986[55] | British Columbia | Cohort | 1949–69 | 68 | Unscreened part of population | Cases had negative smear | No clear trend in incidence with time since last -ve |
| Wangsuphachart 1987[56] | Thailand | Case–control Interview | 1979–83 | 189 | 1023 controls | Hospital controls | Relative protection ~4 for annual screening, ~2·5 for 2–5 yearly |
| Olesen 1988[57] | Denmark | Case–control GP questionnaire | 1983 | 428 | 1 control/case GP matched | 82% of potential cases enrolled | Relative protection ~4 with 1 previous smear, ~6 with 2+ |
| Sobue 1988[58] | Japan | Case–control Clinical records | 1965–87 | 28 | 10 controls/case | Controls matched for screening in year of diagnosis  Paper also reports on deaths | Risk greatest in those with no -ve, and least in those with -ve within 4 years  2 smears better than 1 |
| van der Graaf 1988[59] | Netherlands | Case–control Interview | 1979–85 | 36 | 6 controls/case | Stage IB+  30% of potential cases did not survive (or too ill) to interview  Control response rate 55% | Protection greatest 2–5 years after smear, but still 3-fold after 5 years |
| Klassen 1989[60] | Maryland | Case–control Interview | 1982–84 | 101 | 396 controls | 16% of potential cases did not survive (or too ill) to interview  Telephoned controls  73% response | Relative protection decreased with time since last smear, and lasted 5–10 years |
| Herrero 1992[61] | Latin America | Case–control Interview | 1986–87 | 759 | 2 controls/case | Hospital and community controls  Participation >96% | Protection greatest within 4 years of smear, but last for 10 years |
| Cohen 1993[62] | Manitoba | Case–control Clinical records | 1981–84 | 341 | 27164 controls | 5% of cases could not be linked to screening databases, 18% had <5 years "follow up"  Smears taken in year prior to diagnosis ignored | Relative risk for smear 2–5 years prior to diagnosis ~0·5 overall  Effect least in women aged 25–34 |

*(Continued)*

**Table 14.4** *(Continued)*

| First author, year | Area | Type of study | Years of diagnosis | No. of invasive cancers | Choice of comparison group | Notes | Summary of results |
|---|---|---|---|---|---|---|---|
| Macgregor 1994[63] | Aberdeen | Case–control Clinical records | 1982–91 | 282 | 2 controls/case | 22% of cases were screen-detected | Risk greatest when last -ve smear was over 9 years ago (or never) Risk greater if within 3 years than 3–9 years |
| Makino 1995[64] | Japan | Case–control Clinical records and questionnaire | 1984–89 | 198 | 2 controls/case | 65% of cases were screen-detected | Relative protection decreased with time since last -ve, and was greatest within 2 years |
| Mitchell 1996[65] | Australia | Case–Cohort | 1993 | 233 | Cohort negatively screened 1990–93 | Includes all diagnoses | Very low rates of cancer within 3 years of a – ve |
| Herbert 1996[32] | England | Cohort | 1991–93 | 83 | Cohort (116 022) | 72% of cases, stage I Used proportion of cohort screened within 3·5 and 5·5 years | Incidence greatest in those never screened and least in those screened within 3.5 years |
| Sasieni 1996[31] | UK | Case–control Clinical records | 1992 | 348 | 2 controls/case | 26% microinvasive analysed separately | Relative protection decreased with time since last -ve |
| Hernandez-Avila 1998[66] | Mexico | Case–control Interview | 1990–92 | 397 | 1005 controls | Participation 95% (cases) 85% (controls) Recorded gynaecological symptoms | Risk least in those screened at least every 4 years and least in those never screened |
| Jimenez-Perez 1999[67] | Mexico | Case–control Interview | 1991–94 | 143 | 311 controls | Health centre controls Response 94% | Risk greatest in those never screened and least in those screened within 5 years Proportion screened less in advanced cancers |
| Nieminen 1999[68] | Helsinki | Case–control Questionnaire | 1987–94 | 179 | 1507 controls | Cases had to survive until 1994 Response 87% (cases), 76% (controls) | No data on screening interval Organised screening more protective than spontaneous screening |
| Viikki 1999[69] | Finland | Cohort | 1971–94 | 48 | Cohort (N = 45 572) with normal smear in 1971–76 | | Relative protection of screening 23 |

*(Continued)*

**Table 14.4** *(Continued)*

| First author, year | Area | Type of study | Years of diagnosis | No. of invasive cancers | Choice of comparison group | Notes | Summary of results |
|---|---|---|---|---|---|---|---|
| Andersson-Ellstrom 2000[70] | Sweden | Case–control Clinical records | 1990–97 | 112 | 112 controls | 61% stage I | 50% cases and 55% of controls (but 69% of stage I and 9% of stage III–IV) screened within 3 years |
| Kinney 2001[71] | California | Case–control Clinical records | 1983–95 | 482 | 2 controls/case | Abstract only | Risk within 18 months of −ve half that within 19–42 months |

A meta-analysis of 10 studies carried out in eight countries demonstrated that cervical screening could be effective in identifying women at increased risk of developing cervical cancer.[30] The study found that:

- women with two or more negative smear results were less likely to develop cervical cancer than women with just one previous negative smear;
- compared to women who had never been screened, women with two or more negative smears were 15 times less likely to develop cervical cancer within a year of having a negative test, eight times less likely 24–35 months later, five times 36–47 months later, three times 48–59 months later and three times 60–71 months later;
- there was no evidence of risk of cervical cancer being any lower 10 years after a negative smear than in women who had never been screened;
- there was no evidence of age influencing the sensitivity of screening or the sojourn time of disease.

The fact that having two negative smears was associated with lower risk than having one suggests that smear tests are not 100% reproducible: a woman who has a single negative test might have a positive test were the smear to be repeated. The chance of having two such "false negative" smear results in a row is quite small.

The lower risk of cervical cancer following a negative smear is due to the test being able to identify those who will develop cancer. It is only through treating precursor lesions that cancer is prevented. The reduction in risk associated with a recent negative smear result would only translate to a similar reduction in cancer incidence, if every woman with a non-negative smear result, who does not already have cancer, is successfully treated. Unfortunately, we know that this is not the case. Whether because of mismanagement or unsuccessful treatment, a substantial minority of cervical cancer in the UK is now being diagnosed in women who have a past history of positive cytology.[31] Thus the IARC estimates that 3- and 5-year screening could reduce cervical cancer incidence by 91% and 84% respectively are likely to be overly optimistic.

The extent to which these findings are likely to overestimate the benefits of screening can be judged by a more recent UK study in which 8% of cancers in women under 70 had been preceded by a smear history requiring referral to colposcopy at least 6 months prior to diagnosis.[31] That paper also estimated the protective effect of participating in screening by studying the risk of cancer within 3 years of a screening test. This risk was about 50% greater than the risk within 3 years of a negative smear.

Trend data from England and Wales also point towards a beneficial effect of screening once the substantial birth cohort effects have been taken into account.[72] The age-specific time trends in mortality (Figure 14.3) fit well with well-organised screening replacing poorly organised screening in 1989. Although one might expect the benefits of screening on mortality to take between 5 and 20 years to materialise, early benefits might result from the detection of occult cancers. Further, screening had been in place for many years and had been slowly improving during the 1980s. Prior to 1989 coverage was poor in older women and this is perhaps reflected by the more modest time trends in women aged 55–69. Similar analyses of trends in cancer incidence lead to similar conclusions.[6] Although staging was not always recorded by the cancer registries, it is generally agreed that there has been an increase in stage I cancers and a substantial decrease in stage III and IV cancers in keeping with screening leading to earlier detection of invasive cancers.

## Acceptability of screening

Cytological screening is widely accepted in many countries. Coverage is often measured in terms of the proportion of women (in the target age group) who have been screened at least once in the past 3 or 5 years. Coverage rates of over 75% and as high as 93% have been achieved in many Western countries.[73–75] Coverage is considerably lower in some ethnic groups and a variety of measures can be used to make screening more acceptable. In particular, many women prefer to have the smear taken by another woman. Additionally, providing appropriate information about screening in a format and language that can be understood by the intended audience can help to dispel myths.

The high coverage rate reflects the fact that most women tolerate the discomfort of having a smear taken and are willing to attend for even very frequent screening. Although there are no physical side effects, anxiety caused by the results of screening is common. Women should be properly informed about screening in advanced so as to minimise the anxiety associated with an abnormal, positive, or even inadequate result. The psychosocial impact of abnormal cervical smears has been reviewed by Posner.[76]

Little is known about the acceptability of routine screening using HPV testing, but in numerous research studies the test has been found to be as acceptable as cytology despite initial fears about the difficulties in reporting the presence of a sexually transmitted viral infection.

Nevertheless, great care is needed in communicating the results of an HPV test so as to avoid anxiety and confusion about the significance of the result, not only in terms of the woman's health, but also in terms of the fidelity of a long-term monogamous relationship.

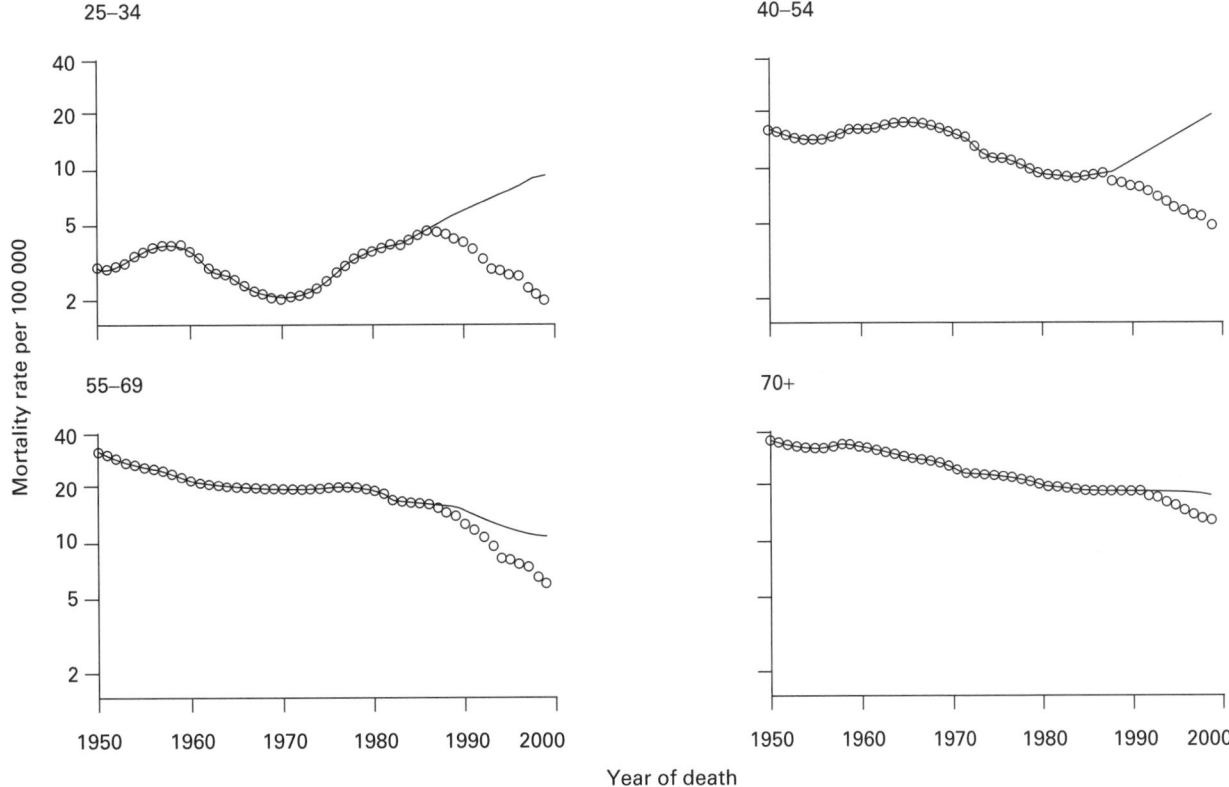

**Figure 14.3** Actual (circles) and predicted (lines) mortality rates in England and Wales, 1950–1999. Predictions are based on the product of an age-specific rate multiplied by a different factor depending on the year of birth (a cohort effect). The rates are plotted on a logarithmic scale. The predictions fit very well between 1950 and 1985. Deviations between the actual and the predicted rates thereafter may be attributed to screening

## Complications of treatment

All conservative treatments for CIN are considered to be safe with few complications. Some bleeding and a watery discharge are common following all forms of treatment other than cryocautery, but only rarely warrant further intervention. It is not uncommon for women to be extremely anxious about having CIN and for this anxiety to have psychosexual consequences. However, the anxiety is generally greatest prior to treatment,[76] transient in nature,[77] and can be reduced by providing information and counselling prior to treatment. Long-term psychosexual morbidity is very rare. Some degree of cervical stenosis is common with some forms of treatment, but serious long-term complications are very rare.

Primary haemorrhage is the most common complication of treatment, particularly in women with cervicitis, but in the vast majority of patients it can be easily controlled. Secondary haemorrhage occurs in about 2% of patients, but will usually respond to rest and antibiotics and is only very rarely severe enough to necessitate a blood transfusion.[78]

Morbidity rates of 2–4% have been reported for loop diathermy,[79] but long-term effects on menstruation and fertility are minimal.[80] Older treatments are associated with higher rates of complications. Luesley *et al.*[81] reported on 915 women treated by cone biopsy: 13% had primary or secondary haemorrhage and 17% had cervical stenosis.

## Costs involved in screening

There is considerable variation in the costs ascribed to various procedures associated with cervical screening. The smear test for instance has been said to cost as little as $10,[82] and as much as $50.[83] The estimated cost of treating CIN varies to an even greater extent. According to its web site (in 2001) the annual cost of the NHS Cervical Screening Programme in England is £132 million or about £34 per woman screened. A detailed estimate of the costs of screening (excluding treatment) in Tayside, Scotland in 1991 has been published by Waugh *et al.*[84] The cost of treatment was estimated by van Ballegooijen *et al.* in 1997.[20] Table 14.3 provides one set of costs based on these papers.

## Cost-effectiveness

The cost-effectiveness of cervical screening depends critically on the efficiency of the screening offered.[73] Most would agree that, no matter how the benefit is measured, the cost in terms of unit benefit increases substantially with the frequency of screening, so that, in particular, annual screening is almost three times as expensive than 3-year screening. The relative effectiveness of 3- and 5-year screening is less well determined.[30–32] A crude estimate of the cost per cancer prevented can be obtained from the English programme. It is estimated that between 1100 and 3900 cancers are prevented each year in England,[31] yielding costs of around £70 000 per cancer prevented. With just over half as many lives saved at an average age of about 45 years, that works out at about £4000 per year of life saved. The effectiveness of screening and therefore the cost-effectiveness, depends not only on coverage, but also on the quality of screening. Effective cytological screening is an interdisciplinary collaboration that requires commitment to training and quality assurance.

## References

1 Parkin DM. Global cancer statistics in the year 2000. *Lancet Oncology* 2001;**2**:533–43.

2 World Health Organization. Age-specific and standardized incidence rates. In: Parkin DM, Muir CS, Whelan SL *et al.* eds. *Cancer Incidence in Five Continents, Vol VII* (IARC Scientific Publications No. 143). Lyon: International Agency for Research on Cancer, 1997.

3 World Health Organization. Trends in cancer incidence and mortality. In: Coleman MP, Esteve J, Damiecki P *et al.* eds. (IARC Scientific Publications No. 121). Lyon: International Agency for Research on Cancer, 1993.

4 Sasieni P. Trends in cervical cancer mortality [letter] [see comments]. *Lancet* 1991;**338**:818–19.

5 Beral V. Cancer of the cervix: a sexually transmitted infection? *Lancet* 1974;**1**:1037–40.

6 Sasieni PD, Adams J. Analysis of cervical cancer mortality and incidence data from England and Wales: evidence of a beneficial effect of screening. *J Roy Stat Soc [A]* 2000;**163**:191–209.

7 Campion MJ, McCance DJ, Cuzick J, Singer A. Progressive potential of mild cervical atypia: prospective cytological, colposcopic, and virological study. *Lancet* 1986;**2**:237–40.

8 Walboomers JM, Jacobs MV, Manos MM *et al.* Human papillomavirus is a necessary cause of invasive cervical cancer worldwide. *J Pathol* 1999;**189**:12–19.

9 Wheeler CM, Greer CE, Becker TM, Hunt WC, Anderson SM, Manos MM. Short-term fluctuations in the detection of cervical human papillomavirus DNA. *Obstet Gynecol* 1996;**88**:261–8.

10 Hildesheim A, Schiffman MH, Gravitt PE *et al.* Persistence of type-specific human papillomavirus infection among cytologically normal women. *J Infect Dis.* 1994;**169**:235–40.

11 Burk RD, Ho GY, Beardsley L, Lempa M, Peters M, Bierman R. Sexual behavior and partner characteristics are the predominant risk factors for genital human papillomavirus infection in young women. *J Infect Dis* 1996;**174**:679–89.

12 Dillner J, Kallings I, Brihmer C *et al.* Seropositivities to human papillomavirus types 16, 18, or 33 capsids and to *Chlamydia*

*trachomatis* are markers of sexual behavior. *J Infect Dis* 1996;**173**:1394–8.

13 Koutsky LA, Holmes KK, Critchlow CW *et al.* A cohort study of the risk of cervical intraepithelial neoplasia grade 2 or 3 in relation to papillomavirus infection. *N Engl J Med* 1992;**327**:1272–8.

14 Remmink AJ, Walboomers JM, Helmerhorst TJ *et al.* The presence of persistent high-risk HPV genotypes in dysplastic cervical lesions is associated with progressive disease: natural history up to 36 months. *Int J Cancer* 1995;**61**:306–11.

15 Ho GY, Burk RD, Klein S *et al.* Persistent genital human papillomavirus infection as a risk factor for persistent cervical dysplasia. *J Natl Cancer Inst* 1995;**87**:1365–71.

16 Cullen AP, Reid R, Campion M, Lorincz AT. Analysis of the physical state of different human papillomavirus DNAs in intraepithelial and invasive cervical neoplasm. *J Virol* 1991;**65**:606–12.

17 Das BC, Sharma JK, Gopalakrishna V, Luthra UK. Analysis by polymerase chain reaction of the physical state of human papillomavirus type 16 DNA in cervical preneoplastic and neoplastic lesions. *J Gen Virol* 1992;**73**:2327–36.

18 Kiviat NB, Critchlow CW, Kurman RJ. Reassessment of the morphological continuum of cervical intraepithelial lesions: does it reflect different stages in the progression to cervical carcinoma? *IARC Sci Publ* 1992;(**119**):59–66.

19 Ostor AG. Natural history of cervical intraepithelial neoplasia: a critical review. *Int J Gynecol Pathol* 1993;**12**:186–92.

20 van Ballegooijen M, van den Akker-van Marle ME, Warmerdam PG, Meijer CJ, Walboomers JM, Habbema JD. Present evidence on the value of HPV testing for cervical cancer screening: a model-based exploration of the (cost-)effectiveness. *Br J Cancer* 1997;**76**:651–7.

21 Evans J, Redburn J, Roche M. *Cervical Cancer in Berkshire, Buckinghamshire, Northamptonshire and Oxfordshire.* Oxford: Oxford Cancer Intelligence Unit, 1997.

22 Luesley D, Blomfield P, Dunn J, Shafi M, Chenoy R, Buxton J. Cigarette smoking and histological outcome in women with mildly dyskaryotic cervical smears. *Br J Obstet Gynaecol* 1994;**101**:49–52.

23 Szarewski A, Jarvis MJ, Sasieni P *et al.* Effect of smoking cessation on cervical lesion size. *Lancet* 1996;**347**:941–3.

24 Alloub MI, Barr BB, McLaren KM, Smith IW, Bunney MH, Smart GE. Human papillomavirus infection and cervical intraepithelial neoplasia in women with renal allografts. *BMJ* 1989;**298**:153–6.

25 Petry KU, Scheffel D, Bode U *et al.* Cellular immunodeficiency enhances the progression of human papillomavirus-associated cervical lesions. *Int J Cancer* 1994;**57**:836–40.

26 Sun XW, Kuhn L, Ellerbrock TV, Chiasson MA, Bush TJ, Wright TC Jr. Human papillomavirus infection in women infected with the human immunodeficiency virus. *N Engl J Med* 1997;**337**:1343–9.

27 Sasadeusz J, Kelly H, Szer J, Schwarer AP, Mitchell H, Grigg A. Abnormal cervical cytology in bone marrow transplant recipients. *Bone Marrow Transplant* 2001;**28**:393–7.

28 Van Wijngaarden WJ, Duncan ID. Rationale for stopping cervical screening in women over 50. *BMJ* 1993;**306**:967–71.

29 Sigurdsson K, Adalsteinsson S. Risk variables affecting high-grade Pap smears at second visit: effects of screening interval, year, age and low-grade smears. *Int J Cancer* 2001;**94**:884–9.

30 IARC Working Group on evaluation of cervical cancer screening programmes. Screening for squamous cervical cancer: duration of low risk after negative results of cervical cytology and its implication for screening policies. *BMJ* 1986;**293**:659–64.

31 Sasieni PD, Cuzick J, Lynch-Farmery E. Estimating the efficacy of screening by auditing smear histories of women with and without cervical cancer. The National Co-ordinating Network for Cervical Screening Working Group. *Br J Cancer* 1996;**73**:1001–5.

32 Herbert A, Stein K, Bryant TN, Breen C, Old P. Relation between the incidence of invasive cervical cancer and the screening interval: is a five year interval too long? *J Med Screen* 1996;**3**:140–5.

33 Marrazzo JM, Koutsky LA, Kiviat NB, Kuypers JM, Stine K. Papanicolaou test screening and prevalence of genital human

papillomavirus among women who have sex with women. *Am J Public Health* 2001;**91**:947–52.

34 Robinson WR, Webb S, Tirpack J, Degefu S, O'Quinn AG. Management of cervical intraepithelial neoplasia during pregnancy with LOOP excision. *Gynecol Oncol* 1997;**64**:153–5.

35 Martin-Hirsch PL, Paraskevaidis E, Kitchener H. Surgery for cervical intraepithelial neoplasia. *Cochrane Database Syst Rev* 2000;(**2**): CD001318.

36 Ostergard DR. Cryosurgical treatment of cervical intraepithelial neoplasia. *Obstet Gynecol* 1980;**56**:231–3.

37 Walton LA, Edelman DA, Fowler WC Jr, Photopulos GJ. Cryosurgery for the treatment of cervical intraepithelial neoplasia during the reproductive years. *Obstet Gynecol* 1980;**55**:353–7.

38 Mettlin C, Mikutra JJ, Natarajan N, Priore R, Murphy GP. Treatment and follow-up study of squamous cell carcinoma *in situ* of the cervix uteri. *Surg Gynecol Obstet* 1982;**155**:481–8.

39 Robertson JH, Woodend BE, Crozier EH, Patterson A. Risk of recurrence after treatment of severe intraepithelial neoplasia of the cervix. A follow-up of 896 patients. *Ulster Med J* 1987;**56**:90–4.

40 Soutter WP, de Barros Lopes A, Fletcher A *et al.* Invasive cervical cancer after conservative therapy for cervical intraepithelial neoplasia. *Lancet* 1997;**349**:978–80.

41 Pettersson F, Malker B. Invasive carcinoma of the uterine cervix following diagnosis and treatment of *in situ* carcinoma. Record linkage study within a National Cancer Registry. *Radiother Oncol* 1989;**16**: 115–20.

42 Papanicolaou GN. New cancer diagnosis. In: Proceedings of the Third Race Betterment Conference. Battle Creek, Michi: Race Betterment Foundation; 1928:528–34.

43 Laara E, Day NE, Hakama M. Trends in mortality from cervical cancer in the Nordic countries: association with organised screening programmes. *Lancet* 1987;**1**:1247–9.

44 Aristizabal N, Cuello C, Correa P, Collazos T, Haenszel W. The impact of vaginal cytology on cervical cancer risks in Cali, Colombia. *Int J Cancer* 1984;**34**:5–9.

45 La Vecchia C, Franceschi S, Decarli A, Fasoli M, Gentile A, Tognoni G. 'Pap' smear and the risk of cervical neoplasia: quantitative estimates from a case-control study. *Lancet* 1984;**2**:779–82.

46 Berrino F, Gatta G, d'Alto M, Crosignani P, Riboli E. Efficacy of screening in preventing invasive cervical cancer: a case-control study in Milan, Italy. *IARC Sci Publ* 1986;(**76**):111–23.

47 Choi NW, Nelson NA. Results from a cervical cancer screening programme in Manitoba, Canada. *IARC Sci Publ* 1986;(**76**):61–7.

48 Clarke EA, Hilditch S, Anderson TW. Optimal frequency of screening for cervical cancer: a Toronto case-control study. *IARC Sci Publ* 1986;(**76**):125–31.

49 Geirsson G, Kristiansdottir R, Sigurdsson K, Moss S, Tulinius H. Cervical cancer screening in Iceland: a case-control study. *IARC Sci Publ* 1986;(76):37–41.

50 Lynge E, Poll P. Risk of cervical cancer following negative smears in Maribo County, Denmark, 1966–1982. *IARC Sci Publ* 1986;(**76**): 69–86.

51 Macgregor JE, Moss S, Parkin DM, Day NE. Cervical cancer screening in north-east Scotland. *IARC Sci Publ* 1986;(**76**):25–36.

52 Magnus K, Langmark F. Cytological mass screening in Ostfold County, Norway. *IARC Sci Publ* 1986;(**76**):87–90.

53 Pettersson F, Naslund I, Malker B. Evaluation of the effect of Papanicolaou screening in Sweden: record linkage between a central screening registry and the National Cancer Registry. *IARC Sci Publ* 1986;(**76**):91–105.

54 Raymond L, Obradovic M, Riotton G. Additional results on relative protection of cervical cancer screening according to stage of tumour from the Geneva case-control study. *IARC Sci Publ* 1986;(**76**): 107–10.

55 van Oortmarssen GJ, Habbema JD. Cervical cancer screening data from two cohorts in British Columbia. *IARC Sci Publ* 1986;(76): 47–60.

56 Wangsuphachart V, Thomas DB, Koetsawang A, Riotton G. Risk factors for invasive cervical cancer and reduction of risk by 'Pap' smears in Thai women. *Int J Epidemiol* 1987;**16**:362–6.

57 Olesen F. A case-control study of cervical cytology before diagnosis of cervical cancer in Denmark. *Int J Epidemiol* 1988;**17**:501–8.

58 Sobue T, Suzuki T, Hashimoto S, Yokoi N, Fujimoto I. A case-control study of the effectiveness of cervical cancer screening in Osaka, Japan. *Jpn J Cancer Res* 1988;**79**:1269–75.

59 van der Graaf Y, Zielhuis GA, Peer PG, Vooijs PG. The effectiveness of cervical screening: a population-based case-control study. *J Clin Epidemiol* 1988;**41**:21–6.

60 Klassen AC, Celentano DD, Brookmeyer R. Variation in the duration of protection given by screening using the Pap test for cervical cancer. *J Clin Epidemiol* 1989;**42**:1003–11.

61 Herrero R, Brinton LA, Reeves WC *et al.* Screening for cervical cancer in Latin America: a case-control study. *Int J Epidemiol* 1992;**21**: 1050–6.

62 Cohen MM. Using administrative data for case-control studies: the case of the Papanicolaou smear. *Ann Epidemiol* 1993;**3**:93–8.

63 Macgregor JE, Campbell MK, Mann EM, Swanson KY. Screening for cervical intraepithelial neoplasia in north east Scotland shows fall in incidence and mortality from invasive cancer with concomitant rise in preinvasive disease. *BMJ* 1994;**308**: 1407–11.

64 Makino H, Sato S, Yajima A, Komatsu S, Fukao A. Evaluation of the effectiveness of cervical cancer screening: a case-control study in Miyagi, Japan. *Tohoku J Exp Med* 1995;**175**:171–8.

65 Mitchell HS, Giles GG. Cancer diagnosis after a report of negative cervical cytology. *Med J Aust* 1996;**164**:270–3.

66 Hernandez-Avila M, Lazcano-Ponce EC, de Ruiz PA, Romieu I. Evaluation of the cervical cancer screening programme in Mexico: a population-based case-control study. *Int J Epidemiol* 1998;**27**:370–6.

67 Jimenez-Perez M, Thomas DB. Has the use of pap smears reduced the risk of invasive cervical cancer in Guadalajara, Mexico? *Int J Cancer* 1999;**82**:804–9.

68 Nieminen P, Kallio M, Anttila A, Hakama M. Organised vs. spontaneous Pap-smear screening for cervical cancer: A case-control study. *Int J Cancer* 1999;**83**:55–8.

69 Viikki M, Pukkala E, Hakama M. Risk of cervical cancer after a negative Pap smear. *J Med Screen* 1999;**6**:103–7.

70 Andersson-Ellstrom A, Seidal T, Grannas M, Hagmar B. The pap-smear history of women with invasive cervical squamous carcinoma. A case-control study from Sweden. *Acta Obstet Gynecol Scand* 2000;**79**:221–6.

71 Kinney WK, Miller M, Sung H, Sawaya GF, Kearney KA, Hiatt RA. Risk of invasive squamous carcinoma of the cervix associated with screening intervals of 1, 2, and 3 years: a case-control study. *Obstet Gynecol* 2001;**97**(Suppl. 1):S3.

72 Sasieni P, Adams J. Effect of screening on cervical cancer mortality in England and Wales: analysis of trends with an age period cohort model. *BMJ* 1999;**318**:1244–5.

73 van Ballegooijen M, van den Akker-van Marle E, Patnick J *et al.* Overview of important cervical cancer screening process values in European Union (EU) countries, and tentative predictions of the corresponding effectiveness and cost-effectiveness. *Eur J Cancer* 2000;**36**:2177–88.

74 Saraiya M, Lee NC, Blackman D, Smith MJ, Morrow B, McKenna MA. Self-reported Papanicolaou smears and hysterectomies among women in the United States. *Obstet Gynecol* 2001;**98**:269–78.

75 Department of Health. Cervical screening programme, England 2000–2001. *Statist Bull* 2001/2. [Available at www.doh.gov.uk/public/sb0122.htm]

76 Posner TN. The psychosocial impact of cervical intra-epithelial neoplasia and its management. In Luesley DM, Barrasso R. eds. *Cancer and pre-cancer of the cervix*. London: Chapman & Hall, 1998.

77 Gath DH, Hallam N, Mynors-Wallis L, Day A, Bond SA. Emotional reactions in women attending a UK colposcopy clinic. *J Epidemiol Community Health* 1995;**4**:79–83.

78 Luesley DM, Barrasso R.The diagnosis and treatment of cervical intra-epithelial neoplasia and its management. In Luesley DM, Barrasso R. eds. *Cancer and pre-cancer of the cervix*. London: Chapman & Hall, 1998.

79 Murdoch JB, Grimshaw RN, Monaghan JM. Loop diathermy excision of the abnormal cervical transformation zone. *Int Gynecol Cancer* 1991;**1**:105–111.

80 Bigrigg A, Haffenden DK, Sheehan AL, Codling BW, Read MD. Efficacy and safety of large-loop excision of the transformation zone. *Lancet* 1994;**343**:32–4.

81 Luesley DM, McCrum A, Terry PB *et al.* Complications of cone biopsy related to the dimensions of the cone and the influence of prior colposcopic assessment. *Br J Obstet Gynaecol* 1985;**92**:158–64.

82 Hristova L, Hakama M. Effect of screening for cancer in the Nordic countries on deaths, cost and quality of life up to the year 2017 *Acta Oncol* 1997;**36**:1–60.

83 Chesebro MJ, Everett WD. A cost-benefit analysis of colposcopy for cervical squamous intraepithelial lesions found on Papanicolaou smear. *Arch Fam Med* 1996;**5**:576–81.

84 Waugh N, Smith I, Robertson A, Reid GS, Halkerston R, Grant A. Costs and benefits of cervical screening. I. The costs of the cervical screening programme. *Cytopathology* 1996;**7**:231–40.

# 15 Screening for prostate cancer

*Jane Melia, Sue Moss*

## How important is prostate cancer in public health terms?

Prostate cancer is one of the most frequently diagnosed cancers in Western men, with the highest incidence rates being reported in the USA. In 1998 more than 184 000 cases of prostate cancer were expected in the USA.[1] In 1988–92 the annual incidence rate, age-adjusted to the world standard, was 100·8 per 100 000 in US Whites and 137 per 100 000 in US Blacks, using SEER data.[2] The lowest rate of 2·3 per 100 000 was reported in Shanghai, China. Genetic factors may explain some of the large differences in incidence between different countries and ethnic groups.

The incidence rate has been rising in most countries, including those with low rates such as China (Table 15.1). Between 1973–77 and 1988–92 the increases were most striking in the USA, Canada, Australia, France and the Asian countries.[2] The percentage increases ranged from 25% to 114%, 24% to 55%, and 15% to 104% in countries with high, medium, and low initial incidences, respectively.

The rise in incidence in Western countries in the 1980s can, in part, be attributed to the increased use of transurethral resection of the prostate for benign hyperplasia and associated increased examination of pathological specimens. During the late 1980s and 1990s testing of prostate specific antigen (PSA) increased initially in the USA and then in other Western countries both for diagnostic purposes in men with symptoms and in asymptomatic men as a screening test. This will also have been associated with increased examination of biopsy tissue.[3] A true rise in incidence may also have occurred because of changing exposure to environmental factors.

Prostate cancer is also a major cause of cancer death in men in many countries. In the USA in 1998 there were over 39 000 deaths from prostate cancer.[4] In 1988–92 the mortality rate age-adjusted to the world standard ranged from 2·8 per 100 000 person-years in Hong Kong to 20·8 per 100 000 person-years in Sweden and 34·3 per 100 000 person-years in US Blacks.[2]

**Table 15.1    Age-adjusted incidence rates\* of prostate cancer in 10 countries, 1973–77 and 1988–92[†]**

| Countries | 1973–77 incidence* | 1988–92 incidence* | % changes[†] |
|---|---|---|---|
| *High risk* | | | |
| US Black, SEER[‡] | 79·9 | 137·0 | 71·5 |
| US Whites, SEER | 47·9 | 100·8 | 110·4 |
| Canada, BC[¶] | 39·8 | 84·9 | 113·3 |
| Sweden | 44·4 | 55·3 | 24·5 |
| Australia, NSW[§] | 28·4 | 53·5 | 88·4 |
| France, Bas-Rhine | 23·0 | 48·1 | 109·1 |
| *Medium risk* | | | |
| England, S. Thames** | 20·1 | 29·3 | 45·8 |
| Italy, Varese | 22·8 | 28·2 | 23·7 |
| *Low risk* | | | |
| Japan, Miyagi | 4·9 | 9·0 | 83·7 |
| Hong Kong | 5·1 | 7·9 | 54·9 |
| China, Shanghai | 1·6 | 2·3 | 43·8 |

\*Per 100 000 person-years, age-adjusted using the world standard.
[†]Per cent change from 1973–77 to 1988–92.
[‡]Surveillance, Epidemiology and End Results program; [¶]Canada, British Columbia; [§]Australia, New South Wales; **United Kingdom, England, South Thames.

**Table 15.2  Age-adjusted mortality rates\* of prostate cancer in nine countries, 1973–77 and 1988–92**

| Countries | 1973–77 mortality\* | 1988–92 mortality\* | % change[†] |
|---|---|---|---|
| *High risk* | | | |
| US Blacks | 27·6 | 34·3 | 24·3 |
| US Whites | 13·4 | 15·7 | 17·2 |
| Canada | 14·3 | 17·0 | 18·9 |
| Sweden | 21·6 | 20·8 | –3·7 |
| Australia | 15·6 | 17·9 | 14·7 |
| France | 15·0 | 17·1 | 14·0 |
| *Medium risk* | | | |
| England and Wales | 12·1 | 16·8 | 38·8 |
| Italy | 10·5 | 11·5 | 9·5 |
| *Low risk* | | | |
| Japan | 2·4 | 3·8 | 58·3 |
| Hong Kong | 2·1 | 2·8 | 33·3 |

\*Per 100 000 person-years, age-adjusted to the world standard.
[†]Per cent change from 1973–77 to 1988–92.

Mortality has risen less than incidence, but the greatest percentage increase in mortality has been seen in Asian countries (Table 15.2). Between 1973–77 and 1988–92, the percentage changes ranged from –3·7% in Sweden to 95 % in Singapore. Since 1991/2 a decline in prostate cancer mortality has been reported in the USA, and more recently to a lesser extent in England and Wales.[5–7] The cause of the changing mortality rates is likely to be complex. It has been suggested that one factor is increased use of the PSA test for screening.[8] However, the changes in mortality seem to have occurred too soon after the start of PSA testing, and in the UK there has been a decline in mortality without the huge increase in PSA testing as seen in the USA. Survival may have increased as a result of improved treatment of advanced disease, for example by anti-androgen therapies, which can delay disease progression by 2–3 years such that men die of other causes.[9]

Other factors related to the decrease in mortality from prostate cancer include changes in death certification. Prostate cancer may be increasingly recorded as the cause of death because of increasing diagnosis and awareness of the disease,[10] and changes in coding of deaths could have contributed to temporal changes.

## How much is known about the natural history of the disease and the potential value of early intervention?

The fact that a far higher proportion of men die with, rather than from, prostate cancer suggests that screening

may detect a large number of cases that would otherwise remain undiagnosed. One UK autopsy study showed that about 38% of men aged over 50 who died of causes other than prostate cancer had unsuspected disease.[11] Scardino *et al.*[12] reported a similar proportion (30% in men aged over 50) and compared it with 10% of men diagnosed with the disease in their life-time, and 3% who died from prostate cancer. Two international autopsy studies of men who had not been diagnosed with prostate cancer have shown a greater proportion of men with latent prostate cancer in those from Western countries, such as Sweden and the USA, than those from Eastern countries, such as Japan,[13,14] reflecting the differences in incidence and mortality rates.

Afro-Caribbeans and men with a family history of prostate cancer are at high risk from developing the disease. High levels of 5-α reductase activity as well as environmental and cultural factors may explain this difference.[15] Familial risk of prostate cancer could account for up to 10% of cases, the proportion being much higher at young ages: 43% in men aged 55 or less.[16] The risk of prostate cancer increases with the number of first- or second-degree affected relatives, from about 2·0 with a single first-degree relative to 8·8 with both a first- and second-degree relative. Several genes are involved and it will be some time before known genes and specific alleles can be used to screen patients for risk of prostate cancer.[17,18]

The exact level of overdiagnosis, and overtreatment associated with screening is unknown, but has major implications for the economic and human costs of screening.

**Table 15.3** Summary of stage and grade of cancers detected in randomised controlled trials

| Country | Screening round | Stage: clinically local | Grade (WHO) | | |
|---|---|---|---|---|---|
| | | | Grade 1 | Grade 2 | Grade 3 |
| Finland[20,21] | Prevalent round | 85% 100/118 | 42% 49/118 | 50% 59/118 | 8% 10/118 |
| Rotterdam[22] | Prevalent round | 78% 358/459 | Clinical grade well differentiated: 58·6% 269/459 Gleason* grade 4: 3·5% | Clinical grade moderately differentiated: 31·6% 145/459 Gleason grade 5–7 85% | Clinical grade poorly differentiated: 9·8% 45/459 Gleason grade 8–10 11·5% |
| Canada[23,24†] | Prevalent round | 66% 212/322 | Well differentiated: 22% 72/322 | Moderately differentiated: 63% 204/322 | Poorly differentiated: 10% 31/322 |
| | Up to 6 annual screens | 83% 97/117 | 32% 37/117 | 56% 65/117 | 3% 4/117 |

*Gleason 2–4 low, 5–7 medium, 8–10 high grade.
†Low compliance rate of 23%.

Screening will increase the detection of non-palpable cancers (T1). In one study of tumours diagnosed by needle biopsy following PSA (T1c), a third showed a degree of capsular penetration with a Gleason sum of 7 or more. This proportion is intermediate between undiagnosed T1a and T2 tumours.[19] The stage and grade of cancers detected in the randomised controlled trials of screening are summarised in Table 15.3.

The rate of progression is not known precisely. The progression of prostate cancer from undiagnosed, asymptomatic to clinically symptomatic disease may be a slow, unrelenting progression[25] or multiple genetic hits resulting in variable progression.[26] A mean lead-time of 7 years from an increased PSA (> 3 ng ml$^{-1}$) to clinical diagnosis was estimated in a study using a serum bank stored from a cohort of 658 men with no previously known prostate cancer.[27] The rate of progression for local stage prostate cancer may be slow, for example in a cohort of patients followed for 15 years, only 10% of deaths were associated with the cancer.[28]

The prognostic factors most important and useful in clinical patient management are preoperative PSA, TNM staging, histologic grade using the Gleason score, and surgical margin.[29] The TNM system[30] is favoured in Europe whereas the Whitmore–Jewett (WJ) system is more commonly used in the USA to stage prostate cancer. Categorisation of the primary tumour in both systems is based on the method of tumour detection. Five-year survival rates are strongly associated with stage: > 95% for localised and regional stages, and 32% for distant stages.[31] The Gleason grading score is the sum of the grades for the primary (dominant) and secondary (other) patterns. If only one pattern is present the score is doubled. The Gleason score (2–4, low grade; 5–7, medium and 8–10, high grade) is a good predictor of prognosis.[32] In a pooled analysis of 828 cases from six non-randomised studies,[33] the progression rate to death was similar for grade 1 and grade 2 disease (13%, WHO grading) and much greater for grade 3 disease (66%) at 10 years, whereas progression to metastases increased with increasing grade (19%, 42% and 74% in grades 1, 2 and 3, respectively).

Efforts to identify and define precursors of prostatic cancer have been hampered with difficulties associated with not being able to perform repeat biopsies at the same sites within the prostate. There are two possible morphological precursors of prostate cancer: prostatic intraepithelial neoplasia (PIN) and atypical adenomatous hyperplasia (AAH). PIN exhibits cytological atypia with nuclear pleomorphism and nucleolar prominence, similar to that seen in prostate cancer. High grade PIN is associated with prostate cancer more frequently in the peripheral zone than in the transitional zone. The biological significance of AAH is less certain than for PIN. AAH has histological and cytological features intermediate between benign prostatic hyperplasia (BPH) and low grade cancer. It may be a precursor to cancer in the transitional zone. Intraductal carcinoma has been found in one small study to be associated with more aggressive cancers than PIN.[34] Research into genetic markers may help our understanding of the relationship between these various lesions.

## What are the appropriate groups and age intervals to offer screening (age, risk factors)?

Age is a strong determinant of prostate cancer risk. In the USA, 83% of incident cases occur in men aged 65 or more.[35] In countries with lower rates of PSA testing such as the UK, the age at diagnosis is older: 88% of cases occur in men aged 65 or more in 1993.[36] Mortality is highest in even older age groups with over 97% of prostate cancer deaths in the USA,[35] and 93% of these in England and Wales occurring at ages 65 or over.[37] Because of the duration of asymptomatic disease phase and probable need for radical treatment, screening is most likely to benefit men with a life expectancy of 10 or more years, and the optimum age for which there is interest in screening is 55–69 years, below the age of peak incidence.

Prostate cancer may progress faster in high risk groups than in the general population, but results need to be adjusted for age, stage, and grade at diagnosis.[38,39] If screening by PSA is conducted in high risk groups, it may need to take into account the younger age distribution of the disease.[40]

## What are the possible treatment options following screening?

One commonly expressed concern about screening for prostate cancer is the lack of definitive evidence on appropriate treatment for early screen-detected disease. As yet, no randomised controlled trial to compare the three main choices of treatment for early stage disease has been completed. For men with localised disease the alternatives are watchful waiting (WW), radical prostatectomy (RP), or external beam radical radiotherapy (XRR). WW has developed into "active surveillance" involving the delay of radical or systemic treatment until signs of progression appear, usually while the man is still asymptomatic, so treatment becomes active management. RP involves nerve sparing (leading to less complications) or non-sparing removal of the prostate gland. Early hormonal therapies may be combined with radical treatments with the aim of improving local control, although further research is needed to confirm improved survival. Neoadjuvant androgen deprivation such as combined androgen blockade and adjuvant therapy such as luteinising hormone-releasing hormone agonists may be used in association with RP or XRR.

The staging and grading of prostate cancer, volume and lymph node status are used to help decide who is most likely to benefit from the more invasive treatments of RP and XRR, and to decide if the patient is suitable for nerve sparing or non-sparing RP.[41] One of the difficulties in the decision about treatment is the inaccuracy of clinical staging. The most accurate staging and grading can only occur following surgery. In the USA, of those men clinically staged by sextant biopsy as unilateral cancer,[42] 16–27% of men undergoing RP are upstaged to spread beyond the capsule. A small proportion of cancers, < 10%, are pathologically downstaged.[43]

Results from clinical series of patients suggest that radical prostatectomy may be the most effective treatment for men with organ-confined disease who have no comorbidities and a life expectancy of 10 or more years. However, these results are potentially biased because of the selection of patients to different treatments. One study analysed survival rates for locally confined cancers according to intention-to-treat. Both intention-to-treat and treatment-received analyses showed similar results with higher survival after radical prostatectomy than after the other treatments. However, 10-year disease-specific survival after prostatectomy was lower by intention-to-treat (83%) than by treatment-received (89%).

Further developments in radiotherapy which are currently under evaluation include conformal techniques[44] and brachytherapy.[45] A randomised controlled trial of treatment of localised prostate cancer is also underway, funded by the NHS Health Technology Assessment programme (http://www.hta.nhsweb.nhs.uk/).

## The choice of screening tests, and their performance

Three screening tests for prostate cancer are the measurement of serum prostate specific antigen (PSA), digital rectal examination (DRE) and transrectal ultrasound (TRUS). It is now generally agreed that PSA is the most acceptable test. DRE has been shown to have poor sensitivity in men with PSA levels < 4 ng ml$^{-1}$.[46,47] The addition of DRE is therefore unlikely to increase sensitivity substantially and is likely to reduce compliance and increase costs.[48] TRUS is the most expensive, requiring specialised equipment, and is less accessible; it is mainly used for further diagnostic tests. It is also less good at detecting hypoechoic areas of the prostate.

PSA is a serine protease produced primarily by the epithelial cells lining the acini and ducts of the prostate gland. Its main biological function is liquefaction of the seminal coagulum post-ejaculation. A small proportion of PSA is absorbed into the blood stream where it is mostly bound to

**Table 15.4   Effects of strategies for PSA testing on screening sensitivity and specificity compared with using total PSA > 4 ng ml⁻¹**

| Approach | Effect on sensitivity | Effect on specificity | Implications for this screening trial |
|---|---|---|---|
| Cut-off point lowered from 4 ng ml⁻¹ to 3 ng ml⁻¹ | Increased (fewer false negatives) | Decreased (more false positives) | Proportion of test-positive men increased to 20%, increasing costs and decreasing acceptability |
| Use of age-related reference ranges | Slightly increased (fewer false negatives) | Decreased (more false positives) | Insufficient evidence to suggest a benefit in age range recommended for screening |
| Measurement of total PSA and, where total PSA between 4 and 10 ng ml⁻¹, measurement of free PSA and calculation of the free:total ratio | Decreased (more false negatives) | Increased (fewer false positives in the total PSA range 4–10 ng ml⁻¹) | Increased cost of testing as two tests required (only where total PSA between 4 and 10 ng ml⁻¹) More rigorous specimen handling required if free PSA measured |
| Measurement of total PSA and, where total PSA 2.5–4 ng ml⁻¹, measurement of free PSA and calculation of the free:total ratio | Decreased (more false negatives) | Increased (fewer false positives in the total PSA range 2·5–4 ng ml⁻¹) | Increased cost of testing as two tests required (only where total PSA 2·5–4 ng ml⁻¹) More rigorous specimen handling required if free PSA measured |
| Measurement of complexed and total PSA and, where total PSA between 4 and 10 ng ml⁻¹ calculation of the complexed:total ratio | Decreased (more false negatives) | Increased (fewer false positives in the total PSA range 4–10 ng ml⁻¹) | Increased cost of testing as two tests required (only where total PSA between 4 and 10 ng ml⁻¹) |

either antichymotrypsin or alpha macroglobulin. A small proportion remains free, uncomplexed PSA. The total level of serum PSA levels is normally very low in healthy men but is frequently elevated (> 4 ng ml⁻¹) in those with prostatic disease (benign prostatic hyperplasia [BPH], prostatic cancer, or prostatitis). As total PSA levels rise above 10 ng ml⁻¹ the probability of prostatic cancer becomes increasingly higher. A low proportion of free PSA expressed as a percentage of the total PSA is also associated with the presence of cancer.

A major challenge in any screening programme for prostatic cancer is detecting as many clinically significant cancers as possible (that is, maximising sensitivity) while controlling the number of unnecessary biopsies carried out in healthy men (that is, maximising specificity). Several approaches to the use of PSA have been investigated. Current American Cancer Society recommendations are that 4 ng ml⁻¹ should be the cut-off point above which men should be referred for further diagnostic tests (the decision limit for prostatic cancer screening).[49] This is estimated to result in detection rates at prevalence screen of between 2·2% and 4·0%, with specificity ranging from 93% to 97%.[50] Sensitivity may be 70–80%.[51] The detection rate at rescreening is not known and will depend on the choice of screening interval. The optimum interval is thought to be biennial screening[52] but this will be informed by results of randomised controlled trials.

Other measures of PSA include a lower cut-off level of 3 ng ml⁻¹, percentage of free PSA, age-specific levels and complexed PSA. The cut-off level of 3 ng ml⁻¹ will increase sensitivity but reduce specificity.[27] In Finland, in the European Randomized Study of Prostate Cancer (ERSPC) screening,[20] 106 cancers were detected using a cut-off level of 4 ng ml⁻¹, and a further nine cancers in the range 3–3·9 ng ml⁻¹ in 5053 men screened in the prevalent round. All of the latter group were moderately differentiated (WHO grades 1 or 2) compared with 90% in the former group.

Free PSA could be used in combination with total PSA in certain ranges (Table 15.4). The overall effect would be to increase sensitivity but decrease specificity.[53,54] However, in a case–control study using data from four prospective screening studies,[55] there was only a slight increase in sensitivity from 95% to 97%. Given that an additional assay would increase the cost of screening, and there may be problems keeping free PSA stable between time of testing and assay, the use of free PSA does not seem promising. The level of PSA depends on the men's activities, the time from taking the blood sample to analysis, and the performance of the laboratory. The effects of different testing strategies on screening performance are summarised in Table 15.4.

Age-specific cut-off levels of total PSA have been investigated but only seem to improve sensitivity and specificity in men below the age of 55, who might be considered for screening if there is a family history of disease.[56]

Complexed PSA, which represents the major proportion of measurable serum PSA, could be an alternative to free PSA although the two tests do not detect the same population of cancers.[57] PSA velocity is not yet recommended but, measured over a 2-month period following a negative biopsy, it may improve specificity by 17% in those patients with a PSA $4–10$ ng ml$^{-1}$.[58]

Other potential screening tests include insulin-like growth factor 1 (IGF-1), which is raised in prostate cancer patients because of its association with suppressing apoptosis. However, in a screening trial,[59] serum IGF-1 did not improve the detection of cancer in men with PSA $\geq 4$ ng ml$^{-1}$, and was associated with enlargement of the prostate gland.

## How effective are screening/treatment options in terms of mortality and morbidity reduction?

No randomised controlled trial has yet reported on the effects of screening on mortality from prostate cancer. Trials are in progress in Europe[51,60,61] and in the USA, both designed to have adequate statistical power to analyse mortality after 10 years follow up.

The trial in Europe (ERSPC)[61] has seven centres currently participating (Belgium, the Netherlands, Italy, Portugal, Finland, Spain, and Sweden)[51,61,62] (Table 15.5). The number of men it is intended to recruit to the trial is 185 946; the overall age range is 50–74, with the core being 55–69. The central aim of the ERSPC trial is to compare prostate cancer mortality in men randomised to be offered screening with that in a control group. There are differences in protocol between centres. Some of these concern methods of recruitment (general population with preconsent randomisation or a selected population who have given consent), the number of screening modalities offered (some centres do or have in the past included DRE and transrectal ultrasound alongside PSA testing), the interval between routine rescreens and the criteria for biopsy recommendation (although a PSA level $\geq 4$ ng ml$^{-1}$ has led to this in all centres at all times).

The Prostate, Lung, Colon and Ovary (PLCO) trial[64] in the USA aims to recruit 74 000 men aged 55–74 randomised to two equal groups. Those in the intervention arm will be offered four annual screens by PSA and DRE. In the pilot study, which included approximately 10 000 men, methods of recruitment led to a selected population, with a large percentage of men in the control arm having had a recent PSA test, and recruitment methods have now been altered to attempt to recruit a more suitable population. The

ERSPC and PLCO have agreed to coordinate their work to facilitate combined (overview) analysis.[65]

One "randomised trial" in Quebec has recently reported a 69% prostate cancer mortality reduction in men screened.[23] Unfortunately, the results are at present uninterpretable[66] because of the low compliance rate (23%), and invalid analytical procedures aimed at overcoming this.

Results of a geographical comparison of prostate cancer mortality in Tyrol, Austria (PSA testing encouraged and available without charge from 1993) with the rest of Austria are emerging[67] and the authors suggest that PSA screening may lead to an marked reduction in prostate cancer mortality over 5 years of follow up. However, another study comparing Seattle, which adopted early detection and aggressive treatment early in the 1990s, and Connecticut, which did not, has not found a difference in prostate cancer mortality.[68]

## How acceptable is the screening method? In particular, what levels of test acceptance have been achieved?

The uptake rate of screening will be affected by the type of screening tests being used, the method of invitation to arrange an appointment, and the method of informed consent. In the ERSPC,[20] a higher uptake rate (69%) was obtained in Finland, where only PSA was used, than in Rotterdam (43%), where a combination of PSA, DRE and TRUS were used. An intermediate uptake rate of 58% was obtained in the UK when men attended for screening by PSA and DRE at one general practice in Bristol.[69] This study also showed that the highest response rate of 78% was achieved when the men were given an appointment for screening, rather than being left to make their own appointment. Similarly indirect invitation through the media may result in a low response: in Austria only 30% of men responded to a call for screening during a 1-year period.[70]

## What side effects are associated with the diagnostic procedures and treatment, and how common and severe are they?

Men with a false-positive screening test (that is, those with a positive PSA who are not found to have prostate cancer) will be subject to unnecessary further investigation including biopsy. Although there is a risk of infection following biopsy, the rate of severe complications is low.[71] Transrectal ultrasound guided prostate biopsy (six needles) is associated with pain and haematochezia (10%), and haematospermia (71%).[72] Prophylactic antibiotics are routinely administered to prevent infection.

**Table 15.5  Summary of randomised controlled trials methodology – modified from Auvinen et al.[63]**

| Item | Belgium | Canada, nationwide | Canada, Quebec | Finland | Italy | Rotterdam, NL | Nijmegen, NL | Portugal | Sweden | USA |
|---|---|---|---|---|---|---|---|---|---|---|
| | | | | | | Country | | | | |
| Death from prostate cancer | Yes | Yes | Yes | Yes | Yes | Yes | Yes | Yes | Yes | Yes |
| Quality of life | Possibly | Yes | Pending | Yes | Yes | Yes | Yes | Yes | Yes | Planning |
| Cost effectiveness | Possibly | Yes | Yes | Yes | Yes | Yes | Yes | No | Yes | Planning |
| Type of trial | Population based | Efficacy | Population based | Population based | Population based | Population based | Population based | Efficacy | Population based | Efficacy |
| *Recruitment* | | | | | | | | | | |
| Mechanism | Pop Reg | Pop Reg, GPs, mass media | Electoral registry | Pop Reg | Military lists | Pop Reg | Pop Reg | GPs | Pop Reg | Mail, mass media |
| Randomisation | After consent | After consent | After consent | Before consent | After consent | After consent | After consent | After consent | Before consent | After consent |
| Period | 1991–98 | 1996–2000 | 1988– | 1996–99 | Not defined | 1992–98 | 1996–99 | 1994–99 | 1995–96 | 1993–97 |
| Age at entry (years) | 55–74 | 55–74 | 45–80 | 55–67 | 50–69 | 55–74 | 55–70 | 50–65 | 50–65 | (55–) 60–74 |
| *Exclusion criteria* | | | | | | | | | | |
| Prevalent prostate cancer | Yes | Yes | Yes | Yes | Yes | Yes | Yes | Yes | Yes | Yes |
| Benign hyperplasia | No | Yes | No | No | No | No | No | No | No | No |
| Prior PSA | No | Yes | No | No | No | No | No | No | No | Yes |
| *Target sample size* | | | | | | | | | | |
| Screening group | 8750 | 36 000 | 8032* | 22 500 | 27 500 | 20 000 | 10 000 | 7500 | 16 200 | 37 000 |
| Control group | 8750 | 36 000 | 20 000 | 45 000 | 27 500 | 20 000 | 10 000 | 7500 | 16 200 | 37 000 |
| *Screening test†* | | | | | | | | | | |
| PSA (ng ml⁻¹) | 4·0 | 4·0 | 3·0 | 2·0/4·0 | 4·0 | 4·0 | 4·0 | 4·0 | 3·0 | 4·0 |
| DRE | All | PSA >2·0 | All | PSA driven | All | All | PSA driven | All | No | All |
| TRUS | All | No | PSA >3·0 and/or DRE+ | No | No | All | PSA driven | No | No | No |
| Screening interval (years) | 4 | 2 | 1 | 4 | 4 | 4 | 4 | 1 | 2 | 1 |
| *Source of follow up information* | | | | | | | | | | |
| Incidences‡ | No | Ca Reg | Ca Reg | Ca Reg | Local hospitals | Ca Reg | Ca Reg | Active | Ca Reg | Active |
| Mortality¶ | Pop Reg | Pop Reg | Pop Reg | Pop Reg | Pop Reg | Pop Reg | Pop Reg | Pop Reg | Pop Reg | Active |
| Death certificate§ | All | All | All | All | All | All | All | All | All | All |

Abbreviations: Ca Reg, cancer registry; Pop Reg, population registry; PSA, prostate specific antigen; DRE, digital rectal examination; TRUS, transrectal ultrasound
*Number of men enrolled so far.
†The cut-off level for PSA, criteria for application of other screening test.
‡The source of incidence data.
¶The source of mortality data.
§Availability of death certificates: All, all death certificates.

All three main options for treatment of early stage disease will result in complications. There will also be psychosocial effects associated with the physical and social impact of the complications, and the uncertainty of the success of treatment. Ideally quality-of-life measures should be compared between the three choices of patient management in a randomised controlled trial of treatment to avoid the biases associated with the selection of healthier, younger patients for radical prostatectomy.

Radical prostatectomy after treatment will cause severe incontinence in about 22% men, impotence in 22% and < 1% of men may die from the operation. The severity of incontinence and impotence can lessen with time. By 12–18 months[73,74] the percentage of patients with urinary incontinence was reduced by about one-third and those with impotence by about a half. Radical radiotherapy in the first few months is associated with incontinence in up to 20%, impotence in 38% and bowel problems in over 30%. The long-term complications rates are not fully known, although one study showed greater deterioration in sexual function for patients receiving RR than in those receiving RP.[75] Watchful waiting or conservative management does not initially cause complications, but these will develop in association with progression of the disease, and will vary according to the success with which progression is arrested and treated while the disease remains organ confined.

Psychosocial factors include those associated with the treatment itself (that is, uncertainty of immediate outcome and disease progression, complications of the treatment), and the impact of these factors on close family. In one study,[76] men treated by WW had significantly more emotional problems, after adjusting for age and comorbidity, than men receiving more active treatment. However, there has since been considerable development of the WW approach to more active management.

The percentage of men affected by complications and resulting psychosocial factors will depend in part on the levels of expertise of the surgeon or radiologist performing the procedures. In the USA the rates of serious complications are lower in hospitals with a high volume of procedures than hospitals with lower volumes.[77]

Future developments in treatment could help to reduce the rate of complications and psychosocial damage. For radical prostatectomy, more accurate clinical staging of the disease would reduce the percentage of men upstaged following the operation.[41] Neoadjuvant therapies may also reduce the size of the cancer, and reduce the frequency of positive margins.[78] For radiotherapy, new techniques such as conformal radiotherapy[44] will reduce the complication rates, and this may be further enhanced by neoadjuvant therapy.

Further investigation is needed into other effects such as fatigue, anxiety, and depression in both the men and their families at different stages of the screening process and subsequent diagnosis and treatment. For example, in the study by Monga[79] 11% of patients diagnosed through screening were subsequently dissatisfied with treatment received, although this was not significantly different between the different treatment groups.[80] In the study of men who had volunteered to be screened in the USA[81] after 6 years, most men were not bothered by their current urinary function, but the majority were bothered by their current sexual function.

## What are the costs of screening and subsequent work-up?

The costs of screening will include those associated with the screening test itself, including both taking of a blood sample and the PSA assay, and those associated with further investigation and biopsy of those screened positive. Cost of the PSA assay will increase if free PSA as well as total PSA is measured. There will also be pathology costs associated with the examination of biopsy specimens. Coley *et al.*[82] used cost estimates from the 1992 Medicare fee schedule in a cost-effectiveness analysis, and quoted costs of US $45 for a PSA test and $633 for subsequent work-up for suspicious results, including biopsy guided by transrectal ultrasonography. Holmberg *et al.*[83] presented data from a Swedish study in 1996 prices, and quoted the cost of a PSA test as 131 SEK (approx. US $20) and of a fine-needle aspiration biopsy as 1104 SEK (approx. US $166). A pilot study at a general practice in the UK in 1991 estimated the cost of the screening test (including both PSA and DRE) as £21 ($34).[69]

This considerable variation in estimated costs will reflect both differences in healthcare setting, different procedures used, and whether items such as capital equipment etc., are included in the cost estimates. Estimates of the cost per cancer detected vary from £1654 ($2679) in the UK study in 1991[69] to 18 600 SEK ($2797) in Sweden in 1996.

However, screening for prostate cancer will also increase treatment costs by increasing the number of men receiving radical treatment, although this needs to be balanced against any reduction in the costs of treating advanced disease. Again, there is a considerable variation in cost estimates; Coley *et al.*[82] quote $8084 for a medical prostatectomy (Medicare 1992) whilst Holmberg *et al.*[83] estimate 138 400 SEK ($20 000) for management of localised disease with curative treatment.

## What is the cost-effectiveness of screening?

The cost-effectiveness of screening for prostate cancer cannot be determined until the screening trials have reported on mortality. Analyses of cost-effectiveness need to take into account not only years of life gained but also increased morbidity as a result of earlier radical treatment. Costs of screening and further investigations need to be considered together with changes in costs of treatment. There have been several modelling studies, mostly in the USA, but the results are difficult to compare because different models and data have been used.[82–88] Different assumptions have been made about the type and frequency of screen, treatment efficacy, utilities, disease progression and disease staging.

Krahn *et al.* 1994[85] used decision analysis to compare the cost-effectiveness, in terms of cost per life-year and quality adjusted life-years (QALYs), between four screening options and a no-screening strategy, based on only a single (prevalent) round of screening. All options resulted in a net increase in costs. Screening by PSA and DRE resulted in an increase in life expectancy, but when the morbidity of radical prostatectomy was considered there was a net loss in terms of quality-adjusted life expectancy. The cost per life-year estimates ranged from $113 000–$189 000 for screening by PSA alone. Some have criticised the results for being unrealistic.[89]

Coley *et al.*[89] evaluated the cost-effectiveness of a one-time PSA and DRE prevalence screen. Their model predicted the cost per life-year saved as a result of a prevalence screen to be $12 491 (age 50–59), $18 769 (age 60–69) and $65 909 (age 70–79).

Key factors affecting the balance of cost-effectiveness are the level of over (unnecessary) diagnosis, and the rate of complications associated with treatment. Prostate cancer screening is at present very likely to be less cost-effective than breast cancer screening, but the level of effectiveness remains unknown.

## Conclusions

Prostate cancer is one of the major cancers causing death in men. As there is no obvious method for primary prevention and the choice of treatment for early stage disease is uncertain, there is increasing demand for screening. This is enhanced by the fact that screening by the PSA test is easy and inexpensive to carry out. However, there are two important reasons why screening should not yet be made available as part of routine health care to men who are asymptomatic. First, there are no reliable markers of progression with which to distinguish between fast-growing and slow-growing cancer. As many men die with the disease, rather than from it, there is a risk that a large proportion of men will receive unnecessary treatment. Second, the optimum treatment for early stage prostate cancer is not known, and the choices range from watchful waiting, to radical surgery, or radiotherapy with immediate complications, such as incontinence and impotence. Until results become available from the randomised controlled trials of screening, the public and their medical practitioners should have available all the necessary information with which to make a fully informed choice about whether to screen or not.

## References

1 Landis SH, Murray T, Bolden S, Wingo PA. Cancer statistics, 1998 [published errata appear in *CA Cancer J Clin* 1998;**8**:192; 1998;**48**:329]. *CA Cancer J Clin* 1998;**48**:6–29.

2 Hsing AW, Tsao L, Devesa SS. International trends and patterns of prostate cancer incidence and mortality. *Int J Cancer* 2000;**85**:60–7.

3 Skarsgard D, Tonita J. Prostate cancer in Saskatchewan Canada, before and during the PSA era. *Cancer Causes Control* 2000;**11**: 79–88.

4 American Cancer Society. Cancer facts and figures. ACS, 1998 [http://www.cancer.org/].

5 Hankey BF, Feuer EJ, Clegg LX *et al.* Cancer surveillance series: interpreting trends in prostate cancer – Part I: Evidence of the effects of screening in recent prostate cancer incidence, mortality, and survival rates. *J Natl Cancer Inst* 1999;**91**:1017–24.

6 Stephenson RA, Huntsman JM. Population-based trends in the United States before and after widespread use of PSA of screening and detection of prostate cancer. In: Sanila R, ed. *Monograph on Evaluation and Monitoring of Screening Programmes.* Lyon, France: IARC, 2000.

7 Oliver SE, Gunnell D, Donovan JL. Comparison of trends in prostate-cancer mortality in England and Wales and the USA. *Lancet* 2000;**355**:1788–9.

8 Etzioni R, Cha R, Feuer EJ, Davidov O. Asymptomatic incidence and duration of prostate cancer. *Am J Epidemiol* 1998;**148**:775–85.

9 Dearnaley DP, Melia J. Early prostate cancer – to treat or not to treat? *Lancet* 1997;**349**:892–3.

10 Newschaffer CJ, Otani K, McDonald K, Penberthy LT. Causes of death in elderly prostate cancer patients and in a comparison nonprostate cancer cohort. *J Natl Cancer Inst* 2000;**92**:613–21.

11 Franks LM. Latent carcinoma of the prostate. *J Pathol Bacteriol* 1954;**68**:603–16.

12 Scardino PT, Weaver R, Hudson MA. Early detection of prostate cancer. *Hum Pathol* 1992;**23**:211–22.

13 Yatani R, Chigusa I, Akazaki K, Stemmermann GN, Welsh RA, Correa P. Geographic pathology of latent prostatic carcinoma. *Int J Cancer* 1982;**29**:611–61.

14 Breslow N, Chan CW, Dhom G *et al.* Latent carcinoma of prostate at autopsy in seven areas. Collaborative study organized by the International Agency for Research on Cancer, Lyons, France. *Int J Cancer* 1977;**20**:680–8.

15 Ross RK, Bernstein L, Lobo RA *et al.* 5 alpha reductase activity and the risk of prostate cancer among Japanese and US white and black males. *Lancet* 1992;**339**:887–9.

16 Carter BS, Bova GS, Beaty TH *et al.* Hereditary prostate cancer: epidemiologic and clinical features. *J Urol* 1993;**150**:797–802.

17 Carter BS, Ewing CM, Ward WS *et al.* Allelic loss of chromosomes 16q and 10q in human prostate cancer. *Proc Natl Acad Sci USA* 1990;**87**:8751–5.

18 Smith JR, Frieje D, Carpten JD *et al.* Major susceptibility locus for prostate cancer on chromosome 1 suggested by a genome-wide search. *Science* 1996;**274**:1371–4.

19 Epstein JI, Walsh PC, Brendler CB. Radical prostatectomy for impalpable prostate cancer: the Johns Hopkins experience with tumors found on transurethral resection (stages T1A and T1B) and on needle biopsy (stage T1C). *J Urol* 1994;**152**:1721–9.

20  Maattanen L, Auvinen A, Stenman UH *et al.* European randomized study of prostate cancer screening: first year results of the Finnish trial. *Br J Cancer* 1999;**79**:1210–14.

21  Auvinen A, Tammela T, Stenman UH *et al.* Screening for prostate cancer using serum prostate-specific antigen: A randomised, population-based pilot study in Finland. *Br J Cancer* 1996;**74**:568–72.

22  Rietbergen JBW, Hoedemaeker RF, Kruger AEB, Kirkels WJ, Schroder FH. The changing pattern of prostate cancer at the time of diagnosis. Characteristics of screen detected prostate cancer in a population based screening study. *J Urol* 1999;**161**:1192.

23  Labrie F, Candes B, Dupont A *et al.* Screening Decreases Prostate Cancer Deaths: First Results of the 1988 Quebec Prospective Randomised Controlled Trial. *Prostate* 1999;**38**:83–91.

24  Labrie F, Candas B, Cusan L *et al.* Diagnosis of advanced or noncurable prostate cancer can be practically eliminated by prostate-specific antigen. *Urology* 1996;**47**:212–17.

25  Stamey TA. Cancer of the prostate. An analysis of some important contributions and dilemmas. *Monogr Urol* 1982;**3**:67–94.

26  Carter HB, Piantadosi S, Isaacs JT. Clinical evidence for and implications of the multistep development of prostate cancer. *J Urol* 1990;**143**:742–6.

27  Hugosson J, Aus G, Becker C *et al.* Would prostate cancer detected by screening with prostate-specific antigen develop into clinical cancer if left undiagnosed? A comparison of two population-based studies in Sweden [In Process Citation]. *BJU Int* 2000;**85**:1078–84.

28  Johansson J-E, Adami H-O, Andersson S-O, Bergstrom R, Holmberg L, Krusemo UB. High 10-year survival rate in patients with early, untreated prostatic cancer. *JAMA* 1992;**267**:2191–6.

29  Bostwick DG, Grignon DJ, Hammond ME *et al.* Prognostic factors in prostate cancer. College of American Pathologists Consensus Statement 1999. *Arch Pathol Lab Med* 2000;**124**:995–1000.

30  The British Association of Urological Surgeons TNM Subcommittee. The TNM classification of prostate cancer: a discussion of the 1992 classification. *Br J Urol* 1995;**76**:279–85.

31  Greenlee RT, Murray T, Bolden S, Wingo PA. Cancer statistics, 2000. *CA Cancer J Clin* 2000;**50**:7–33.

32  Gleason DF. Histologic grading of prostate cancer: a perspective. *Hum Pathol* 1992;**23**:273–9.

33  Chodak GW, Thisted RA, Gerber GS *et al.* Results of conservative management of clinically localised prostate cancer. *N Engl J Med* 1994;**330**:242–8.

34  Cohen RJ, McNeal JE, Baillie T. Patterns of differentiation and proliferation in intraductal carcinoma of the prostate: significance for cancer progression. *Prostate* 2000;**43**:11–19.

35  SEER. Cancer Statistics Review 1973–1999. *SEER* 1999 [http://seer.cancer.gov/csr/1973_1999/].

36  Office for National Statistics. *1993 Cancer statistics registrations. England and Wales. Series MB1 no. 26.* London: The Stationery Office, 1999.

37  Office for National Statistics. *Mortality Statistics – Cause.* Series DH2 No. 23 London: The Stationery Office, 1996.

38  Gronberg H, Isaacs SD, Smith JR *et al.* Characteristics of prostate cancer in families potentially linked to the hereditary prostate cancer 1 (HPC1) locus. *JAMA* 1997;**278**:1251–5.

39  Kupelian PA, Kupelian VA, Witte JS, Macklis R, Klein EA. Family history of prostate cancer in patients with localized prostate cancer: an independent predictor of treatment outcomes. *J Clin Oncol* 1997;**15**:1478–80.

40  Powell IJ, Banerjee M, Sakr W *et al.* Should African-American men be tested for prostate carcinoma at an earlier age than white men? *Cancer* 1999;**85**:472–7.

41  Graefen M, Hammerer P, Michl U *et al.* Incidence of positive surgical margins after biopsy-selected nerve-sparing radical prostatectomy. *Urology* 1998;**51**:437–42.

42  Witjes WP, Schulman CC, Debruyne FM. Preliminary results of a prospective randomized study comparing radical prostatectomy versus radical prostatectomy associated with neoadjuvant hormonal combination therapy in T2–3 N0 M0 prostatic carcinoma. The European Study Group on Neoadjuvant Treatment of Prostate Cancer. *Urology* 1997;**49**:65–9.

43  Lu-Yao GL, Yao SL. Population-based study of long-term survival in patients with clinically localised prostate cancer. *Lancet* 1997;**349**:906–10.

44  Dearnaley DP, Khoo VS, Norman AR *et al.* Comparison of radiation side-effects of conformal and conventional radiotherapy in prostate cancer: a randomised trial. *Lancet* 1999;**353**:267–72.

45  Kwon ED, Loening SA, Hawtrey CE. Radical prostatectomy and adjuvant radioactive gold seed placement: results of treatment at 5 and 10 years for clinical stages A2, B1 and B2 cancer of the prostate. *J Urol* 1991;**145**:524–31.

46  Lodding P, Aus G, Bergdahl S *et al.* Characteristics of screening detected prostate cancer in men 50 to 66 years old with 3 to 4 ng/ml prostate specific antigen. *J Urol* 1998;**159**:899–903.

47  Schroder FH, van der Maas P, Beemsterboer P *et al.* Evaluation of the digital rectal examination as a screening test for prostate cancer. *J Natl Cancer Inst* 1998;**90**:1817–23.

48  Beemsterboer PM, Kranse R, De Koning HJ, Habbema JD, Schroder FH. Changing role of 3 screening modalities in the European randomized study of screening for prostate cancer (Rotterdam). *Int J Cancer* 1999;**84**:437–41.

49  American Urological Association. Prostate-Specific Antigen (PSA) Best Practice Policy. *Oncology* 2000;**14**:267–86.

50  Labrie F, Dupont A, Suburu R *et al.* Serum prostate specific antigen as pre-screening test for prostate cancer. *J Urol* 1992;**147**:846–52.

51  Schroder FH, Bangma CH. The European Randomized Study of Screening for Prostate Cancer (ERSPC). *Br J Urol* 1997;**79**:68–71.

52  Ross KS, Carter HB, Pearson JD, Guess HA. Comparative efficiency of prostate-specific antigen screening strategies for prostate cancer detection. *JAMA* 2000;**284**:1399–405.

53  Djavan B, Zlotta A, Kratzik C *et al.* PSA, PSA density, PSA density of transition zone, free/total PSA ratio, and PSA velocity for early detection of prostate cancer in men with serum PSA 2.5 to 4.0 ng/ml. *Urology* 1999;**54**:517–22.

54  Bangma CH, Rietbergen JBW, Kranse R, Blijenberg BG, Petterson K, Schroder FH. The free-to-total prostate specific antigen ratio improves the specificity of prostate specific antigen in screening for prostate cancer in the general population. *J Urol* 1997;**157**:2191–6.

55  Wald NJ, Watt HC, George L, Knekt P, Helzlsouer KJ, Tuomilehto J. Adding free to total prostate-specific antigen levels in trials of prostate cancer screening. *Br J Cancer* 2000;**82**:731–6.

56  Gustafsson O, Mansour E, Norming U, Carlsson A, Tornblom M, Nyman CR. Prostate-specific antigen (PSA), PSA density and age-adjusted PSA reference values in screening for prostate cancer – a study of randomly selected population of 2,400 men. *Scand J Urol Nephrol* 1998;**32**:373–7.

57  Brawer MK, Cheli CD, Neaman IE *et al.* Complexed prostate specific antigen provides significant enhancement of specificity compared with total prostate specific antigen for detecting prostate cancer. *J Urol* 2000;**163**:1476–80.

58  Lynn NN, Collins GN, O'Reilly PH. The short-term prostate-specific antigen velocity before biopsy can be used to predict prostatic histology. *Br J Urol Int* 2000;**85**:847–50.

59  Finne P, Auvinen A, Koistinen H *et al.* Insulin-like growth factor I is not a useful marker of prostate cancer in men with elevated levels of prostate-specific antigen. *J Clin Endocrinol Metab* 2000;**85**:2744–7.

60  Schroder FH, Bangma CH. The European randomized study of screening for prostate cancer (ERSPC). *Br J Urol* 1997;**79**:68–71.

61  Auvinen A, Rietbergen JBW, Denis LJ, Schroder FH, Prorok PC, for the International Prostate Cancer Screening Trial Evaluation Group. Prospective evaluation plan for randomised trials of prostate cancer screening. *J Med Screen* 1996;**3**:97–104.

62  Schroder FH, Denis LJ, Kirkels W, de Koning HJ, Standaert B. European randomized study of screening for prostate cancer. Progress report of Antwerp and Rotterdam Pilot Studies. *Cancer* 1995;**76**:129–34.

63  Auvinen A, Rietbergen JB, Denis LJ, Schroder FH, Prorok PC. Prospective evaluation plan for randomised trials of prostate cancer screening. The International Prostate Cancer Screening Trial Evaluation Group. *J Med Screen* 1996;**3**:97–104.

64  Gohagan JK, Prorok PC, Kramer BS, Hayes RB, Cornett JE. The Prostate, Lung, Colorectal, and Ovarian Cancer Screening Trial of the National Cancer Institute. *Cancer* 1995;**75**:1869–73.

65  International Prostate Screening Evaluation Group (IPSTEG). Rationale for Randomised Trials of Prostate Cancer Screening. *Eur J Cancer* 1999;**3S**:262–71.

66  Alexander FE, Prescott R. Screening decreases prostate cancer deaths. Reply to Labrie *et al.* (letter). *Prostate* 1999;**40**:135–6.

67  Bartsch G, Horninger W, Klocker H *et al.*, Tyrol Prostate Cancer Screening Group. Prostate cancer mortality after introduction of prostate-specific antigen mass screening in the Federal State of Tyrol, Austria. *Urology* 2001;**58**:417–24.

68  Reynolds T. Prostate cancer: numbers may not tell the whole story. *J Natl Cancer Inst* 2000;**92**:1873–6.

69  Chadwick DJ, Kemple T, Astley JP *et al.* Pilot study of screening for prostate cancer in general practice. *Lancet* 1991;**338**:613–16.

70  Reissigl A, Bartsch G. Prostate-specific antigen as a screening test. The Austrian experience. *Urol Clin N Am* 1997;**24**:315–21.

71  Rietbergen JB, Kruger AE, Kranse R, Schroder FH. Complications of transrectal ultrasound-guided systematic sextant biopsies of the prostate: evaluation of complication rates and risk factors within a population-based screening program. *Urology* 1997;**49**:875–80.

72  Naughton CK, Ornstein DK, Smith DS, Catalona WJ. Pain and morbidity of transrectal ultrasound guided prostate biopsy: a prospective randomized trial of 6 versus 12 cores. *J Urol* 2000;**163**: 168–71.

73  Benoit RM, Naslund MJ, Cohen JK. Complications after radical retropubic prostatectomy in the medicare population. *Urology* 2000;**56**:116–20.

74  Walsh PC. Radical prostatectomy for localized prostate cancer provides durable cancer control with excellent quality of life: a structured debate. *J Urol* 2000;**163**:1802–7.

75  Litwin MS, Flanders SC, Pasta DJ, Stoddard ML, Lubeck DP, Henning JM. Sexual function and bother after radical prostatectomy or radiation for prostate cancer: multivariate quality-of-life analysis from CaPSURE. Cancer of the Prostate Strategic Urologic Research Endeavor. *Urology* 1999;**54**:503–8.

76  Litwin MS, Hays RD, Fink A *et al.* Quality of life outcomes in men treated for localized prostate cancer. *JAMA* 1995;**273**:129–35.

77  Yao S-L, Lu-Yao G. Population-based study of relationships between hospital volume of prostatectomies, patient outcomes, and length of hospital stay. *J Natl Cancer Inst* 1999;**91**:1950–6.

78  Hugosson J, Abrahamsson P-A, Ahlgren G *et al.* The risk of malignancy in the surgical margin at radical prostatectomy reduced almost three-fold in patients given neo-adjuvant hormone treatment. *Eur Urol* 1996;**29**:413–19.

79  Monga U, Kerrigan AJ, Thornby J, Monga TN. Prospective study of fatigue in localized prostate cancer patients undergoing radiotherapy. *Radiat Oncol Invest* 1999;**7**:178–85.

80  Carvalhal GF, Smith DS, Ramos C *et al.* Correlates of dissatisfaction with treatment in patients with prostate cancer diagnosed through screening. *J Urol* 1999;**162**:113–18.

81  Smith DS, Carvalhal GF, Schneider K, Krygiel J, Yan Y, Catalona WJ. Quality-of-life outcomes for men with prostate carcinoma detected by screening. *Cancer* 2000;**88**:1454–63.

82  Coley CM, Barry MJ, Fleming C, Fahs MC, Mulley AG. Early detection of prostate cancer. Part II: Estimating the risks, benefits, and costs. *Ann Intern Med* 1997;**126**:468–79.

83  Holmberg L, Carlsson P, Lofman O, Varenhorst E. Economic evaluation of screening for prostate cancer: A randomized population based programme during a 10-year period in Sweden. *Health Policy* 1998;**45**:133–47.

84  Fleming C, Wasson JH, Albertsen PC, Barry MJ, Wennberg JE. A decision analysis of alternative treatment strategies for clinically localized prostate cancer. Prostate Patient Outcomes Research Team. *JAMA* 1993;**269**:2650–8.

85  Krahn MD, Mahoney JE, Eckman MH, Trachtenberg J, Pauker SG, Detsky AS. Screening for prostate cancer: a decision analytic view. *JAMA* 1994;**272**:773–80.

86  Optenberg SA, Thompson IM. Economics of screening for carcinoma of the prostate. *Urol Clin N Am* 1990;**17**:719–37.

87  Office of Technology Assessment. *Costs and effectiveness of prostate cancer screening in elderly men.* Washington DC: OTA, 1995.

88  Cantor SB, Spann SJ, Volk RJ, Cardenas MP, Warren MM. Prostate cancer screening: a decision analysis. *J Fam Pract* 1995;**41**:33–41.

89  Benoit RM, Naslund MJ. The socioeconomic implications of prostate-specific antigen screening. *Urol Clin N Am* 1997;**24**:451–8.

# 16 Screening for ovarian cancer

*Usha Menon, D Brinkmann, Steven Skates, Ian Jacobs*

Among women in the UK, ovarian cancer is the sixth commonest cancer. However, it is the fourth commonest cause of death from cancer, after breast, colon and lung.[1] The cancer is typically associated with vague, non-specific symptoms and over 75% of women have Stage III or IV disease at diagnosis. The high mortality is believed to be a direct result of the advanced stage, as early stage disease is associated with a 5-year survival of over 90%.[2] The link between stage and mortality suggests that screening for ovarian cancer may have an impact on disease mortality and this has led to efforts to develop an effective screening strategy.

## Precursor lesions

A central principle of cancer screening is detection of a preinvasive or early invasive cancer, thereby reducing disease mortality and morbidity of treatment.[3,4] Many solid cancers have a preinvasive or intraepithelial phase. The cervical cancer model best represents this. About 30% of cervical high grade intraepithelial lesions may progress to invasive disease if left untreated.[5] Other cancers associated with detectable premalignant conditions include oesophagus, large bowel, endometrium and vulva.

The hallmark of these preinvasive lesions is the presence of an intraepithelial lesion with the histological features of cancer but the absence of destructive stromal invasion. Borderline ovarian tumours, otherwise called ovarian neoplasms of low malignant potential or ovarian intraepithelial neoplasms, fulfil the histological criteria of preinvasive lesions. However, there is increasing evidence that suggests that borderline tumours are different from ovarian cancers. Although they can occasionally be multifocal at presentation, in a manner suggestive of metastatic disease, recent studies have shown that while the majority of metastatic invasive ovarian cancers are in fact clonal in nature, metastatic borderline tumours are truly multifocal and not from the same clone.[6] In addition borderline and invasive ovarian cancers do not share similar genetic events. The tumour suppressor gene *tp53* is mutated in ovarian cancers in up to 75% of cases while it is rarely mutated in borderline tumours. *K-ras* mutations occur relatively frequently in borderline tumours and uncommonly in ovarian cancers, the exception being mucinous cystadenocarcinoma.[7–10] Borderline tumours are rarely aneuploid whilst cancer is typically so.[11] So, although borderline tumours resemble intraepithelial neoplastic lesions, they are probably not the precursor lesions for the majority of ovarian cancers. Borderline tumours, however, increase the false-positive rate of screening programmes as they are phenotypically similar to ovarian cancers, making it almost impossible on imaging to differentiate the two.

The other lesion that has been considered as a possible precursor lesion for ovarian cancer is benign ovarian neoplasm. If a large proportion of ovarian cancers arose in this way, removal of benign cysts in a screening programme would impact on future ovarian cancer incidence. Crayford *et al.* analysed data from a cohort of 5479 self-referred, asymptomatic women who participated in an ovarian cancer screening trial and who had been followed up for an average of 15 years: 202 women had bilateral salpingo-oophorectomies as a result of findings on ultrasound screening. The removal of persistent ovarian cysts was not associated with a decrease in the proportion of expected deaths from ovarian cancer. The main limitation of this study were the use of ovarian cancer mortality rather than incidence as the endpoint, the absence of a control group, and the fact that 59% of the lesions removed were physiological or simple cysts rather than benign neoplasms.[12] More recently, Hartge *et al.*[13] assessed whether asymptomatic complex ovarian cysts detected on ultrasonography in postmenopausal women were precursors to ovarian cancer. In 20 000 postmenopausal women enrolled in an ongoing randomised cancer screening trial, they compared the risk factor profile of women with complex ovarian cysts to the established risk factors for ovarian cancer. The women with complex ovarian cysts did not share the same risk factor profile as ovarian cancer, suggesting that majority of the complex cysts and other clinically suspicious abnormalities detected on ultrasonography were not immediate precursors of ovarian cancer. Thus, a true precursor lesion for ovarian cancer has yet to be identified, limiting the goal of screening to detection of asymptomatic, preclinical low volume disease.

**Table 16.1    Prospective ovarian cancer screening studies in the general population using the multimodal strategy**

| Study | Main features | Screening strategy | No. screened | No. of invasive epithelial ovarian cancers detected[a] | No. of positive screens | No. of operations/ cancer detected |
|---|---|---|---|---|---|---|
| *CA125 only* | | | | | | |
| Einhorn *et al.* 1992 | Age ≥ 40 years | Serum CA125 | 5550 | 6 2 stage I | 175[a] | 29[b] |
| *Multimodal approach CA125 (level 1 screen), then USS (level II screen)* | | | | | | |
| Jacobs *et al.* 1988[15] 1993[16] 1996[17], | Age ≥ 45 years (median 56) Postmenopausal | Serum CA125 TAS, if CA125↑ | 22 000 | 11 4 stage I | 41 | 3·7 |
| Jacobs *et al.* 1999[18] | Age ≥ 45 years (median 56) Postmenopausal | RCT Serum CA125 TAS/TVS, if CA125↑ 3 screens | 10 958 | 6 3 stage I | 29 | 4·8 |
| Grover *et al.* 1995[19] | Age ≥ 40 years (median 51) or with family history (3%) | Serum CA125 TAS/TVS, if CA125↑ | 2550 | 1 0 stage I | 16 | 16 |
| Adonakis *et al.* 1996[20] | Age ≥ 45 years (mean 58) | Serum CA125 TVS, if CA125↑ | 2000 | 1(1) 1 stage I | 15 | 15 |
| Total | | | | 19(1) | 101 | 5·3 |

[a]Primary invasive epithelial ovarian cancers. The borderline/granulosa tumours detected are shown in parenthesis.
[b]Not all of these women underwent surgical investigation as the study design involved intensive surveillance rather than surgical intervention.

## Target populations

### High risk population

Hereditary syndromes account for approximately 5% of ovarian cancers. First-degree female relatives of affected members from ovarian or breast and ovarian, or bowel and ovarian cancer families have a greater than 15% lifetime risk of developing ovarian cancer. Women with documented mutations in *BRCA1* may have as high as a 40% lifetime risk of developing ovarian cancer while the lifetime risk associated with *BRCA2* mutations maybe as high as 26%. Screening for ovarian cancer from the age of 35 has been recommended in this group, although its effectiveness remains unknown. Such women may also benefit from prophylactic salpingo-oophorectomy in their forties after completion of their families.

### General population

The majority of ovarian cancers are sporadic and occur in the general population. The greatest risk factor in this group is age. Trials are usually limited to women over 50 years of age. Other risk factors for targeting women at increased risk within the general population are menopausal status, years of oral contraceptive use and parity. Various groups are investigating the role of single nucleotide polymorphisms, in certain low penetrance genes. It may be possible to identify women with increased susceptibility for sporadic ovarian cancer by virtue of their genetic profile.

## Screening tests

Serum CA125 continues to be the tumour marker most extensively used in ovarian cancer screening (Table 16.1). Sensitivity and specificity has been improved as a result of developing a more sophisticated approach to interpretation of CA125 results in place of cut-off levels. It has been observed that elevated CA125 levels in women without ovarian cancer are static or decrease with time, while levels associated with malignancy tend to rise. This has led to the formulation of separate complex change-point statistical models of the behaviour of serial preclinical CA125 levels for cases and controls. These models take into account a woman's age related risk of ovarian cancer and her CA125 profile with time. The risk of the individual having ovarian cancer is calculated using a computerised algorithm based on Bayes' theorem that compares each individual's serial CA125 levels to the pattern in cases compared to controls. The closer the CA125 profile to the CA125 behaviour of known cases of ovarian cancer, the greater the risk of ovarian cancer. The final result is presented as the individual's estimated risk of having ovarian cancer so that a risk of 2% implies a risk of 1 in 50.[21] This approach is now incorporated into the multimodal screening strategy used by Jacobs *et al.* in their ongoing pilot randomised controlled trial of ovarian cancer screening (Randomised trial of screening for ovarian cancer [protocol]: Ovarian Cancer Screening Unit, The Royal Hospitals Trust, 1996), and forms part of the strategy in the UK Collaborative Trial of Ovarian Cancer Screening. (UK Collaborative Trial of Ovarian Cancer Screening [protocol]; Gynaecological Oncology Unit, Bart's and the London Queen Mary's School of Medicine and Dentistry, London, United Kingdom, 2000 [http://www.mds. qmw.ac.uk/gynaeonc/UKCTOCS/design. htm]).

Among the newly described tumour markers, plasma lysophosphatidic acid (LPA), a bioactive phospholipid with mitogenic and growth factor-like activities may have a potential role in ovarian cancer screening. LPA levels were detected in nine of 10 patients with stage I ovarian cancer and all 24 patients with stage II, III, and IV ovarian cancer. In comparison, only 28 of 47 had elevated CA125 levels, including two of nine patients with stage I disease.[22] A larger study involving 1600 women is underway to clarify the role of LPA in primary screening.

Transvaginal ultrasonography is used in all screening strategies. The aim is to detect the early architectural changes in the ovary that accompany carcinogenesis. Persistence of ultrasound features on serial scanning is used to reduce false-positive rates. The lack of physiological changes in ovarian volume in postmenopausal women improves the specificity in this group compared to premenopausal women. Most screening protocols use a weighted scoring system or morphological index based on ovarian volume, outline, presence of papillary projections, and cyst complexity (that is, number of locules, wall structure, thickness of septae and echogenecity of fluid). Based on gross anatomic changes at the time of surgery, papillary projections have the highest, and simple cysts and septal thickness the lowest correlation with a diagnosis of ovarian malignancy.[23]

As data regarding outcome accumulates with long-term follow up of the participants of the early screening trials, it has been possible to further define risk of ovarian cancer associated with various ultrasound findings. Postmenopausal women from the general population with an elevated serum CA125 level but normal ovarian morphology on ultrasound were found to have a cumulative risk (CR) of ovarian cancer during 6·8 years of median follow up similar to that of the entire population. In contrast, postmenopausal women with an elevated serum CA125 level with abnormal ovarian morphology on ultrasound had a significantly increased relative risk.[24] The use of ovarian morphology to interpret pelvic ultrasound may increase sensitivity and use of complex ovarian morphology may increase the positive predictive value of a multimodal screening strategy.[25] Similar follow up of participants of the largest ultrasound-based ovarian cancer screening trial has established that unilocular ovarian cysts < 10 cm in diameter are found in 3·3% of asymptomatic postmenopausal women aged ≥ 50 years and are associated with a minimal risk for ovarian cancer. In contrast, complex ovarian cysts with wall abnormalities or solid areas are associated with a significant risk for malignancy.[26]

Such data are invaluable in interpreting ultrasound findings and determining operative intervention in screening trials. It may be possible to decrease the false-positive rate further through use of three-dimensional ultrasound and power Doppler as second-line tests.[27,28] One of the other limiting factors with ultrasound is its subjectivity. Applying self-teaching computer models such as neural networks may help to overcome this to some extent and make results more reproducible.[29–38]

## Screening interval

Most trials to date have empirically chosen annual screening. If the screening interval is too short this will lead to higher false-positive rates with its resultant cost and morbidity. If, however, the screening interval is too long, then one may miss the opportunity of detecting women with early stage disease. Based on an analysis of follow up data from screening trials, Skates *et al.* (unpublished data) have estimated the preclinical phase of the disease in the general population to be about 1·9 years. Studies are underway to determine optimal screening intervals in patients at high risk.

## Screening strategies

Two distinct screening strategies have emerged, one ultrasound based with transvaginal scanning as the primary test and the other blood based with measurement of the serum tumour marker CA125 as the primary test and ultrasound as the secondary test (multimodal screening).

**Table 16.2    Prospective ovarian cancer screening studies using ultrasound as the primary test in the general population**

| Study | Main features | Screening strategy | No. screened | No. of invasive epithelial ovarian cancers detected[a] | No. of positive screens | No. of positive screens/ cancer detected |
|---|---|---|---|---|---|---|
| *USS only approach* | | | | | | |
| *USS (level I screen), then repeat USS (level II screen)* | | | | | | |
| van Nagell *et al.* 2000[40] | | | | | | |
| De Priest *et al.* 1997[41] | Age ≥ 50 years and postmenopausal | TVS Annual screens | 14 469 | 11 (6) 5 stage I | 180 | 16·3 |
| van Nagell *et al.* 1995[42] | or ≥ 30 with family history | Mean 4 screens/ woman | | | | |
| Sato S *et al.* 2000[43] | Part of general screening programme Retrospective | TVS | 51 550 | 22 17 stage I | 324 | 14·7 |
| Hayashi *et al.* 1999[44] | Age ≥ 50 years | TVS | 23 451 | 3 (3) | 258 | [b] |
| Tabor *et al.* 1994[45] | Aged 46–65 years | TVS | 435 | 0 | 9 | – |
| Campbell *et al.* 1989[46] | Age ≥ 45 years (mean 53) or with family history (4%) | TAS 3 screens at 18-month intervals | 5479 | 2 (3) 2 stage I | 326 | 163 |
| Millo *et al.* 1989[47] | Age ≥ 45 years Or postmenopausal (mean 54) | USS (not specified) | 500 | 0 | 11 | – |
| Goswamy *et al.* 1983[48] | Age 39–78 Postmenopausal | TAS | 1084 | 1 1 stage I` | | |
| *USS and CDI (level I screen)* | | | | | | |
| Kurjak *et al.* 1995[49] | Aged 40–71 years (mean 45) | TVS and CDI | 5013 | 4 4 stage I | 38 | 9·5 |
| Vuento *et al.* 1995[50] | Aged 50–61 years (mean 59) | TVS and CDI | 1364 | (1) | 5 | – |
| *USS (level I) and other test (level II screen)* | | | | | | |
| Parkes *et al.* 1994[51] | Aged 50–64 | TVS then CDI if TVS positive | 2953 | 1 1 stage I | 15[c] | 15 |
| Holbert *et al.* 1994[52] | Postmenopausal Aged 30–89 years | TVS then CA125 if TVS positive | 478 | 1 1 stage I | 33[d] | 33 |
| Schincaglia *et al.* 1994[53] | Aged 50–69 | TAS, then aspiration/ biopsy | 3541 | 2 0 stage I | 98 | 9·5 |
| Total | | | 110 317 | 47 (30) | 1297 | 27·6 |

Abbreviations: RCT, randomised controlled trial; TAS, transabdominal ultrasound; TVS, transvaginal ultrasound
[a]Primary invasive epithelial ovarian cancers. The borderline/granulosa tumours detected are shown in parenthesis.
[b]Only 95 women consented to surgery and there are no follow up details of the remaining.
[c]86 women had abnormal USS prior to CDI.
[d]Only 11 of these women underwent surgery.

Overall the data from the large prospective studies of screening for ovarian cancer in the general population (Tables 16.1 and 16.2) suggest that sequential multimodal screening has superior specificity and positive predictive value compared to strategies based on transvaginal ultrasound alone. However, ultrasound as a first-line test

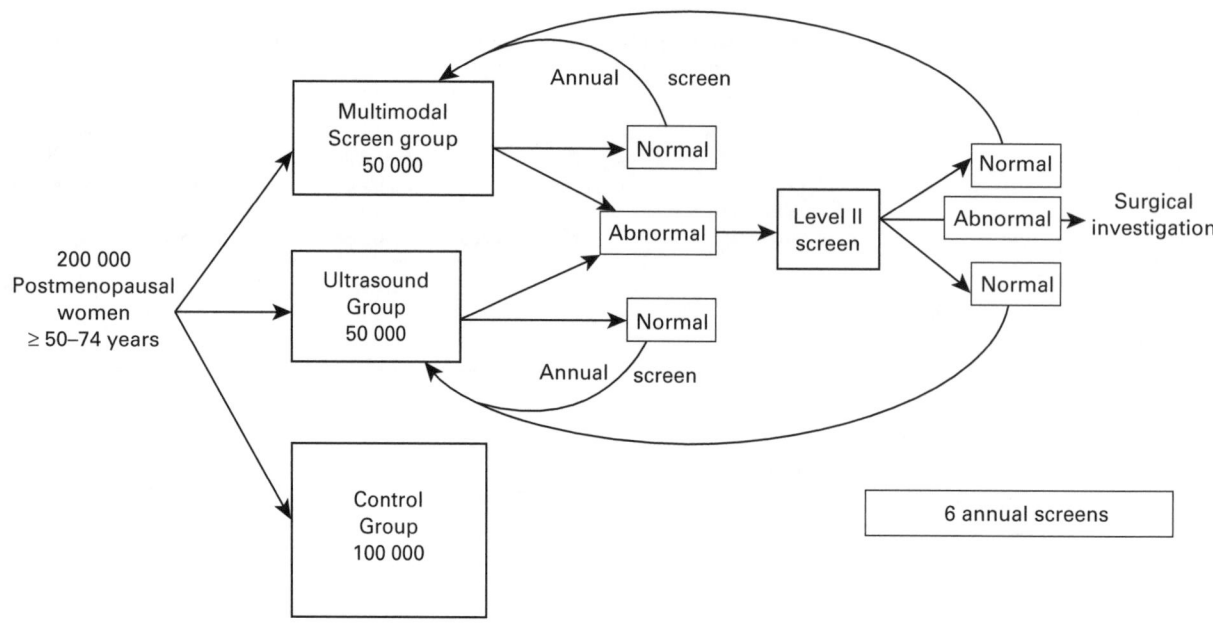

**Figure 16.1** UKCTOCS – trial design. All women followed up for 7 years via the NHS Cancer Registry as well as postal questionnaries

may offer greater sensitivity for early stage disease. An ultrasound-based strategy may have a greater impact on ovarian cancer mortality albeit at a higher price in terms of surgical intervention for false-positive results.[39]

### Current trials in the general population

Randomised controlled trials are now underway in the general population to assess the impact of screening on ovarian cancer mortality. The United Kingdom Collaborative Trial of Ovarian Cancer Screening (UKCTOCS) has started recruiting postmenopausal women from 12 centres in the UK (Figure 16.1): 200 000 women in all will be randomised to either control, screening with ultrasound or multimodal screening. The primary endpoint is impact of screening on ovarian cancer mortality. The study also addresses the issues of target population, compliance, health economics, and physical and psychological morbidity of screening. Results are expected in 10 years (http://www.mds.qmw.ac.uk/gynaeonc/UKCTOCS/).

The Prostate, Lung, Colorectal and Ovarian (PLCO) Cancer Screening Trial has completed enrolling 74 000 women aged 55–74 at 10 screening centres in the USA with balanced randomisation to intervention and control arms. For ovarian cancer, women are screened using both CA125 and transvaginal ultrasound for 3 years and CA125 alone for a further 2 years. Follow up will continue for at least 13 years from randomisation to assess health status and cause of death.[54]

### Trials in a high risk population

In women with strong evidence of a hereditary predisposition, screening is recommended, although there is no conclusive evidence available that screening has an impact on ovarian cancer mortality. As a result a randomised controlled trial of screening in this population is no longer feasible or ethical. Screening is problematic in this population as it includes premenopausal women who have a higher incidence of false-positive CA125 elevations and ultrasound abnormalities. In addition, recent reports suggest that multifocal peritoneal serous papillary carcinoma may be a phenotypic variant of familial ovarian cancer and may be difficult to detect using current screening tests.[55]

In order to develop an optimal screening strategy in the high risk population, a multicentre National Familial Ovarian Cancer Screening Study (UK-FOCSS) involving 5000 "high risk" women is being set up in the UK. This is a prospective study using a standard screening protocol based on annual CA125 measurement and transvaginal ultrasound. The trial design includes collecting and storing serial serum samples for retrospective analysis of CA125 and other markers. The intention is to derive a Familial Risk of Ovarian Cancer Index (FROC), similar to the ROC in use in the general population, which will incorporate in addition to the serial CA125 profile, data on family history and mutation analysis. A similar trial is underway in the USA under the auspices of the Cancer Genetics Network of the National Cancer Institute with the scope for meta-analysis in the future.

## Conclusion

Many aspects of ovarian cancer screening are still poorly understood, including whether or not there are precursor lesions, the rate of disease progression, and to what extent transvaginal ultrasonography and CA125 detect different cancers. Large randomised trials are now underway in the general population to provide definitive data on impact of screening on mortality and address morbidity, health economics, and psychosocial issues. High risk women who request screening should be counselled about the current lack of evidence of its efficacy and encouraged to participate in research trials.

## References

1   Office for National Statistics. *Cancer Statistics: Registrations. Series MB1* 1997;**24**.

2   Werness BA, Eltabbakh GH. Familial ovarian cancer and early ovarian cancer: biologic, pathologic, and clinical features. *Int J Gynecol Pathol* 2001;**20**:48–63.

3   Le T, Krepart GV, Lotocki RJ, Heywood MS. Clinically apparent early stage invasive epithelial ovarian carcinoma: should all be treated similarly? *Gynecol Oncol* 1999;**74**:252–4.

4   Ahmed FY, Wiltshaw E, A'Hern RP *et al*. Natural history and prognosis of untreated stage I epithelial ovarian carcinoma. *J Clin Oncol* 1996;**14**:2968–75.

5   McIndoe WA, McLean MR, Jones RW, Mullins PR. The invasive potential of carcinoma *in situ* of the cervix. *Obstet Gynecol* 1984;**64**:451–8.

6   Lu KH, Bell DA, Welch WR, Berkowitz RS, Mok SC. Evidence for the multifocal origin of bilateral and advanced human serous borderline ovarian tumors. *Cancer Res* 1998;**58**:2328–30.

7   Caduff RF, Svoboda-Newman SM, Ferguson AW, Johnson CM, Frank TS. Comparison of mutations of *Ki-RAS* and *p53* immunoreactivity in borderline and malignant epithelial ovarian tumors. *Am J Surg Pathol* 1999;**23**:323–8.

8   Trope C, Kaern J. Management of borderline tumors of the ovary: state of the art. *Semin Oncol* 1998;**25**:372–80.

9   Darai E, Walker-Combrouze F, Mlika-Cabanne N, Feldmann G, Madelenat P, Scoazec JY. Expression of p53 protein in borderline epithelial ovarian tumors: a clinicopathologic study of 39 cases. *Eur J Gynaecol Oncol* 1998;**19**:144–9.

10  Kupryjanczyk J, Bell DA, Dimeo D, Beauchamp R, Thor AD, Yandell DW. *p53* gene analysis of ovarian borderline tumors and stage I carcinomas. *Hum Pathol* 1995;**26**:387–92.

11  Lodhi S, Najam S, Pervez S. DNA ploidy analysis of borderline epithelial ovarian tumours. *J Pak Med Assoc* 2000;**50**(10):349–51.

12  Crayford TJ, Campbell S, Bourne TH, Rawson HJ, Collins WP. Benign ovarian cysts and ovarian cancer: a cohort study with implications for screening. *Lancet* 2000;**355**:1060–3.

13  Hartge P, Hayes R, Reding D *et al*. Complex ovarian cysts in postmenopausal women are not associated with ovarian cancer risk factors: preliminary data from the prostate, lung, colon, and ovarian cancer screening trial. *Am J Obstet Gynecol* 2000;**183**:1232–7.

14  Einhorn N, Sjovall K, Knapp RC *et al*. Prospective evaluation of serum CA125 levels for early detection of ovarian cancer. *Obstet Gynecol* 1992;**80**:14–18.

15  Jacobs I, Stabile I, Bridges J *et al*. Multimodal approach to screening for ovarian cancer. *Lancet* 1998;**1**:268–71.

16  Jacobs I, Davies AP, Bridges J *et al*. Prevalence screening for ovarian cancer in postmenopausal women by CA 125 measurement and ultrasonography. *BMJ* 1993;**306**:1030–4.

17  Jacobs IJ, Skates S, Davies AP *et al*. Risk of diagnosis of ovarian cancer after raised serum CA 125 concentration: a prospective cohort study. *BMJ* 1996;**313**:1355–8.

18  Jacobs IJ, Skates SJ, MacDonald N *et al*. Screening for ovarian cancer: a pilot randomised controlled trial. *Lancet* 1999;**353**:1207–10.

19  Grover SR, Quinn MA. Is there any value in bimanual pelvic examination as a screening test. *Med J Aust* 1995;**162**:408–10.

20  Adonakis GL, Paraskevaidis E, Tsiga S, Seferiadis K, Lolis DE. A combined approach for the early detection of ovarian cancer in asymptomatic women. *Eur J Obstet Gynecol Reprod Biol* 1996;**65**:221–5.

21  Skates SJ, Xu FJ, Yu YH *et al*. Toward an optimal algorithm for ovarian cancer screening with longitudinal tumor markers. *Cancer* 1995;**76**(Suppl.):2004–10.

22  Xu Y, Shen Z, Wiper DW *et al*. Lysophosphatidic acid as a potential biomarker for ovarian and other gynecologic cancers. *JAMA* 1998;**280**:719–23.

23  Granberg S, Wikland M, Jansson I. Macroscopic characterization of ovarian tumors and the relation to the histological diagnosis: criteria to be used for ultrasound evaluation. *Gynecol Oncol* 1989;**35**:139–44.

24  Menon U, Talaat A, Jeyarajah AR *et al*. Ultrasound assessment of ovarian cancer risk in postmenopausal women with CA125 elevation. *Br J Cancer* 1999;**80**(10):1644–7.

25  Menon U, Talaat A, Rosenthal AN *et al*. Performance of ultrasound as a second line test to serum CA125 in ovarian cancer screening. *Br J Obstet Gynaecol* 2000;**107**:165–9.

26  Bailey CL, Ueland FR, Land GL *et al*. The malignant potential of small cystic ovarian tumors in women over 50 years of age. *Gynecol Oncol* 1998;**69**:3–7.

27  Cohen LS, Escobar PF, Scharm C, Glimco B, Fishman DA. Three-dimensional power Doppler ultrasound improves the diagnostic accuracy for ovarian cancer prediction. *Gynecol Oncol* 2001;**82**:40–8.

28  Kurjak A, Kupesic S, Sparac V, Kosuta D. Three-dimensional ultrasonographic and power Doppler characterization of ovarian lesions. *Ultrasound Obstet Gynecol* 2000;**16**:365–71.

29  Mol BW, Boll D, De Kanter M *et al*. Distinguishing the benign and malignant adnexal mass: an external validation of prognostic models. *Gynecol Oncol* 2001;**80**:162–7.

30  Kehoe S, Lowe D, Powell JE, Vincente B. Artificial neural networks and survival prediction in ovarian carcinoma. *Eur J Gynaecol Oncol* 2000;**21**:583–4.

31  Tailor A, Jurkovic D, Bourne TH, Collins WP, Campbell S. Sonographic prediction of malignancy in adnexal masses using an artificial neural network. *Br J Obstet Gynaecol* 1999;**106**:21–30.

32  Clayton RD, Snowden S, Weston MJ, Mogensen O, Eastaugh J, Lane G. Neural networks in the diagnosis of malignant ovarian tumours. *Br J Obstet Gynaecol* 1999;**106**:1078–82.

33  Biagiotti R, Desii C, Vanzi E, Gacci G. Predicting ovarian malignancy: application of artificial neural networks to transvaginal and color Doppler flow US. *Radiology* 1999;**210**:399–403.

34  Levy G, Levine P, Brennan J, Lerner JP, Monteagudo A, Timor-Tritsch IE. Color flow-directed Doppler studies of ovarian masses. Computer analysis. *J Reprod Med* 1998;**43**:865–8.

35  Newey VR. Classical versus artificial neural network analysis. *Ultrasound Obstet Gynecol* 1997;**10**:5–8.

36  Deligdisch L, Einstein AJ, Guera D, Gil J. Ovarian dysplasia in epithelial inclusion cysts. A morphometric approach using neural networks. *Cancer* 1995;**76**:1027–34.

37  Wilding P, Morgan MA, Grygotis AE, Shoffner MA, Rosato EF. Application of backpropagation neural networks to diagnosis of breast and ovarian cancer. *Cancer Lett* 1994;**77**:145–53.

38  Kappen HJ, Neijt JP. Advanced ovarian cancer. Neural network analysis to predict treatment outcome. *Ann Oncol* 1993;**4**(Suppl. 4):31–4.

39  Menon U, Jacobs I. Ovarian cancer screening in the general population. *Ultrasound Obstet Gynecol* 2000;**15**:350–3.

40  van Nagell JR Jr, DePriest PD, Reedy MB *et al.* The efficacy of transvaginal sonographic screening in asymptomatic women at risk for ovarian cancer. *Gynecol Obstet* 2000;**77**:350–6.

41  DePriest PD, Gallion HH, Pavlik EJ, Kryscio RJ, van Nagell JR, Jr. Transvaginal sonography as a screening method for the detection of early ovarian cancer. *Gynecol Oncol* 1997;**65**:408–14.

42  van Nagell JR Jr, Gallion HH, Pavlik EJ, DePriest PD. Ovarian cancer screening. *Cancer* 1995;**76**:(10 Suppl):2086–91.

43  Sato S, Yokoyama Y, Sakamoto T, Futagami M, Saito Y. Usefulness of mass screening for ovarian carcinoma using transvaginal ultrasonography. *Cancer* 2000;**89**:582–8.

44  Hayashi H, Yaginuma Y, Kitamura S *et al.* Bilateral oophorectomy in asymptomatic women over 50 years old selected by ovarian cancer screening. *Gynecol Obstet Invest* 1999;**47**:58–64.

45  Tabor A, Jensen FR, Bock JE, Hogdall CK. Feasibility study of a randomised trial of ovarian cancer screening. *J Med Screen* 1994; **1**:215–19.

46  Campbell S, Bhan V, Royston P, Whitehead ML, Collins WP. Transabdominal ultrasound screening for early ovarian cancer. *BMJ* 1989;**299**:1363–7.

47  Millo R, Facca MC, Alberico S. Sonographic evaluation of ovarian volume in postmenopausal women: a screening test for ovarian cancer? *Clin Exp Obstet Gynecol* 1989;**16**:72–8.

48  Goswamy RK, Campbell S, Whitehead MI. Screening for ovarian cancer. *Clin Obstet Gynaecol* 1983;**10**:621–43.

49  Kurjak A, Kupesic S. Transvaginal color Doppler and pelvic tumor vascularity: lessons learned and future challenges. *Ultrasound Obstet Gynecol* 1995;**6**:145–59.

50  Vuento MH, Pirhonen JP, Makinen JI, Laippala PJ, Gronroos M, Salmi TA. Evaluation of ovarian findings in asymptomatic postmenopausal women with color Doppler ultrasound. *Cancer* 1995;**76**:1214–18.

51  Parkes CA, Smith D, Wald NJ, Bourne TH. Feasibility study of a randomised trial of ovarian cancer screening among the general population. *J Med Screen* 1994;**1**:209–14.

52  Holbert TR. Screening transvaginal ultrasonography of postmenopausal women in a private office setting. *Am J Obstet Gynecol* 1994;**170**: 1699–703; discussion 1703–4.

53  Schincaglia P, Brondelli L, Cicognani A, *et al.* A feasibility study of ovarian cancer screening: does fine-needle aspiration improve ultrasound specificity? *Tumori* 1994;**80**:181–7.

54  Gohagan JK, Prorok PC, Hayes RB, Kramer BS. The Prostate, Lung, Colorectal and Ovarian (PLCO) Cancer Screening Trial of the National Cancer Institute: history, organization, and status. *Control Clin Trials* 2000;**21**(Suppl.): 251S–272S.

55  Karlan BY, Baldwin RL., Lopez-Luevanos E *et al.* Peritoneal serous papillary carcinoma, a phenotypic variant of familial ovarian cancer: implications for ovarian cancer screening. *Am J Obstet Gynecol* 1999; **180**:917–28.

# 17 Screening for colorectal cancer

*Wendy Atkin*

## Importance of the disease

The large bowel is the fourth most common site for cancer worldwide after lung, stomach and breast, and the fourth most frequent cited cause of cancer death after lung, stomach and liver cancer. There were an estimated 943 000 new cases diagnosed and 510 000 deaths from the disease in 2000.[1] Highest incidence rates occur in North America, Northern Europe, and Australasia where incidence rates rank second after lung cancer. Lowest rates are found in sub-Saharan Africa and India. There have been marked increases in incidence rates in Asian populations who have adopted a Western lifestyle, including the Chinese of Shanghai and Hong Kong, Singaporeans and Japanese, and in Eastern Europe.[2] In higher risk countries rates are increasing more slowly or in some cases have stabilised. In the US there has been a pronounced decrease in incidence and mortality rates in White men and women beginning in the 1980s, but only very small reductions in Black men and women; some researchers[3,4] have speculated that the increased use of sigmoidoscopy and polypectomy have played an important role, although there is some evidence that the increased consumption of fruit and vegetables, non-steroidal anti-inflammatory drugs, and hormone replacement therapy may also be playing a part. In the UK, incidence rates of colorectal cancer increased during the 1970s and 1980s, but in the 1990s rates have stabilised and then fallen slightly in older men and women[5] (Figures 17.1 and 17.2).

In the US and the UK, the estimated probability at birth of eventually developing colorectal cancer is 6% and the probability of dying from the disease is around 3%. Cancer of the colon is equally frequent in men and women but cancer of the rectum is 20–50% more frequent in men.[1]

## Natural history of the disease and potential value of early detection

Survival rates in the US improved substantially during the 1980s and now exceed 60% (SEER Cancer stats 1973–1999) In the 1980s, survival rates in Britain were 8% lower for colon and 4–6% lower for rectal cancer than the average for Europe (40%).[6] The wide differences in colorectal cancer survival across Europe in the 1980s[6] were found to depend to a large extent on the stage at diagnosis. Five-year survival rates for localised disease are 85–90%, compared with 55–60% for regional disease and only 5–8% for distant disease.[7]

Epidemiological, pathological and molecular genetic studies[8–11] have provided convincing evidence that most colorectal cancers arise in adenomatous polyps and that their complete removal arrests the development of cancer at that site.[12] People with familial adenomatous polyposis (FAP) typically have hundreds or thousands of adenomas and have an almost 100% risk of developing cancer. In sporadic disease, the risk of developing metachronous adenomatous polyps or colorectal cancer increases with the number of adenomas detected initially.[13,14] It is not uncommon to see a focus of malignancy within a large adenoma or to see remnant adenomatous tissue adjacent to a carcinoma, particularly in early cancers. It is a less frequent finding in advanced cancers suggesting that the malignant tissue overgrows the adenomatous element. The chance of finding a focus of malignancy within an adenoma grows with increasing size, and with more advanced histology and dysplasia.[8] Molecular genetic studies[11] have provided further evidence for the concept of the adenoma to carcinoma sequence by demonstrating that the adenoma accumulates genetic abnormalities as it becomes larger, more severely dysplastic and progresses to malignancy.

The average duration of the adenoma–carcinoma sequence can be deduced from the difference in the average age at diagnosis of adenomas and of cancers, which in both FAP and sporadic disease is around 10 years.[8,15] In a retrospective study[16] in which patients with unresected colon polyps larger than 1 cm that were followed radiologically, the cumulative risk of developing cancer was 2·5% at 5 years, 8% at 10 years, and 24% at 25 years. The progression of the disease may be faster for flat or depressed adenomas. These have been reported frequently by Japanese surgeons and endoscopists[17,18] but have also been observed in Western patients.[19,20] The proportion of cancers that develop from flat or depressed adenomas is unknown.

## Appropriate groups to treat and intervals to offer screening

A number of groups have an increased risk of developing colorectal cancer. Those at highest risk are those with either

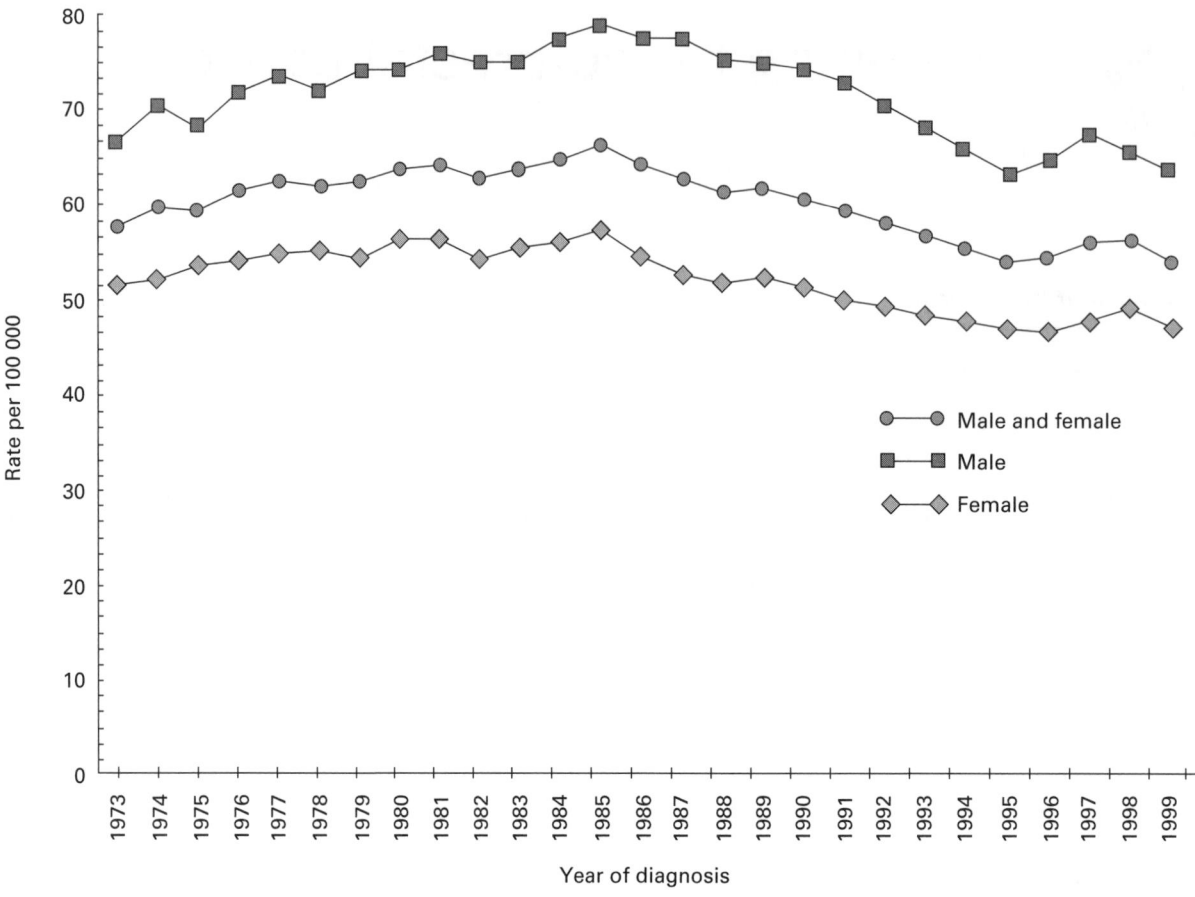

**Figure 17.1**  Age-adjusted rates for colorectal cancer (from *SEER Incidence Age-adjusted Rates, 9 Registries, 1973–1999,* [http://seer.cancer.gov/faststats/html/inc_colorect.html] with permission)

of the dominantly inherited conditions: FAP and hereditary non-polyposis colorectal cancer (HNPCC). Prophylactic colectomy is performed in FAP since the cumulative risk of developing cancer by age 40 approaches 100%. In HNPCC the lifetime risk of colorectal cancer in mutation carriers is 80%[21] and therefore close surveillance is advised. Other groups at moderately increased risk include those with long-standing ulcerative colitis or Crohn's disease,[22] individuals with a personal history of colorectal cancer or large, villous or multiple adenomas,[12] and those with a family history of colorectal cancer. It has been estimated using life-table methods[23,24] that risk is increased two- to three-fold in those with a single affected first-degree relative and five- to six-fold in those with two first-degree relatives.

At least 75% of colorectal cancers develop in people with no known risk factors apart from older age. Colorectal cancer is infrequent below the age of 40 years, but increases rapidly from age 50 with an approximate doubling of incidence with each decade of life. It is probably not worth screening average risk people below age 50 years. The age at which to stop screening is more contentious. The median age of detection of the disease is 69 years in both men and women, so one-half of all cases are diagnosed at age 70 years and above, and 25% of all cases at 80 years and above. However with increasing age, life expectancy decreases, as does the number of life-years saved as a result of screening-initiated treatment of the disease.[25] Most colorectal cancer screening initiatives have focused on the age-group 50–74 years.

The intervals at which to offer screening depend on the target lesion. If the test detects early cancer rather than adenomas, it will need to be offered at least every 2 years, which is thought to be the average lead time for an

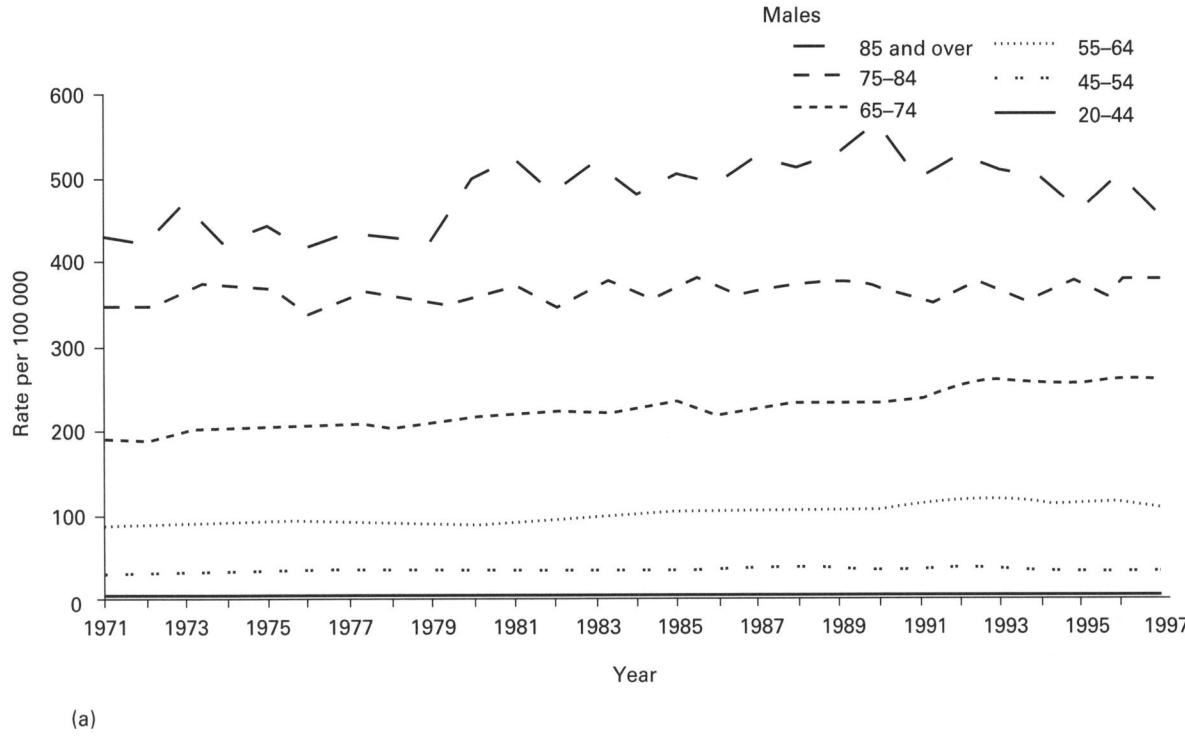

(a)

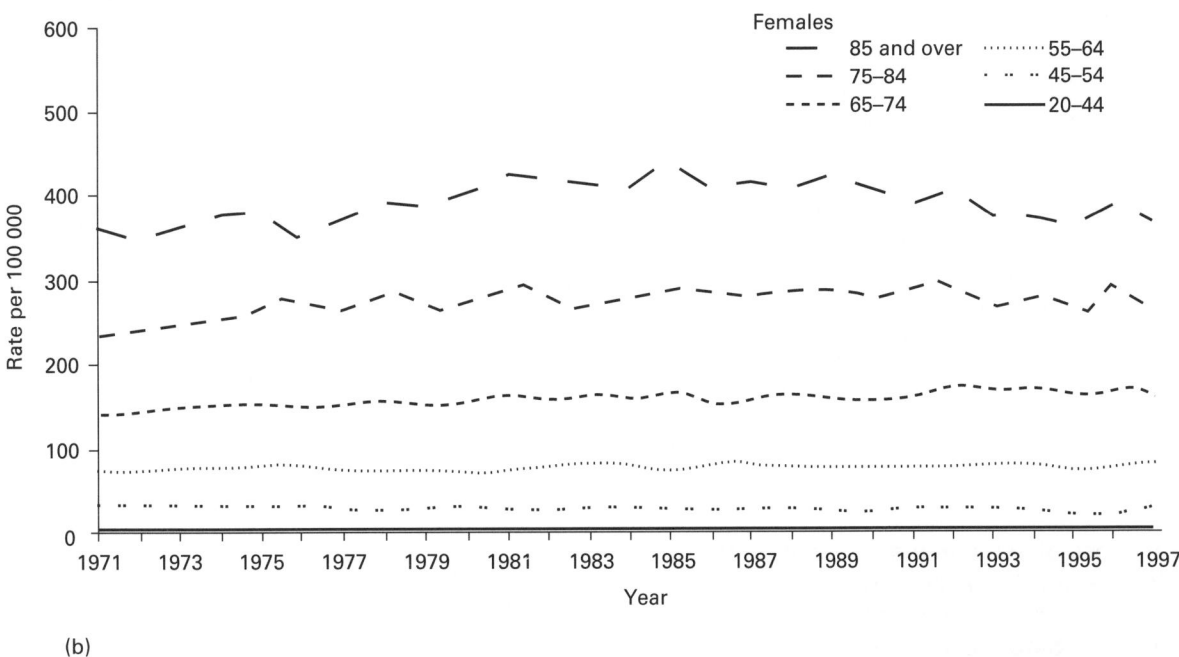

(b)

**Figure 17.2** Age-specific incidence rates for colorectal cancer in males (a) and females (b), England and Wales, 1971–1997 (Taken from *Cancer Trends in England and Wales 1950–1999*,[5] with kind permission from The Stationery Office Limited)

asymptomatic cancer to become symptomatic. If the aim is to detect adenomas, the test can be given much less frequently since adenomas progress slowly to cancer.

## Treatment options following screening

Around 20% of cancers detected during endoscopic screening[26] will be malignant polyps that have only invaded locally and can be removed during endoscopy or by local surgical excision. The others will require open abdominal surgery. At least 50% of colorectal cancers detected at screening will be localised, Dukes' stage A cases,[26,27] and will require no further treatment. This compares with around 10% Dukes' stage A cases amongst patients presenting after symptom onset.[27]

The vast majority of adenomatous polyps are small enough to be removed safely at endoscopy. Only those sufficiently large and sessile to make endoscopic removal impossible or inadvisable will require surgical excision. There are a variety of methods available for endoscopic polypectomy. The specific method will depend on the size and shape of the polyp, but the main aims are to remove the lesion completely without perforating the bowel wall or causing bleeding. It is also desirable to retain all or part of the polyp for histological examination.

Within 3 years of removal of adenomas, around 30–50% of people will have a further neoplasm identified at repeat examination.[13] Some cases are due to truly metachronous neoplasia, while other lesions found at repeat endoscopy are in fact adenomas missed at the first examination.[28,29] However, on the basis of this finding, it is customary to offer colonoscopic surveillance at 3-yearly intervals to all patients following adenoma detection.[30] Because adenomas are very common and colonoscopy is costly and not without risk, it is gradually becoming accepted that people with adenomas should be stratified according to their risk of developing an advanced adenoma or cancer at follow up.[12,31,32] This risk is increased if adenomas are multiple, large, or have villous histology, in contrast to single, small, tubular adenomas where risk is low.[12,33,34] Long-term follow up data from the National Polyp Study[35] suggest subsequent surveillance intervals can be extended to 6 years in this low risk group and, in the context of a screening programme, it may be appropriate to offer no surveillance at all.[36]

## Effectiveness of screening options in terms of incidence/mortality reduction

### Faecal occult blood test (FOBT)

Haemoccult II is the most extensively examined method for colorectal cancer screening. It is a qualitative guaiac-based test designed to detect an elevated level of blood in stool assumed to have been shed from a bleeding neoplasm. The haematin component of haemoglobin in the faecal blood catalyses the oxidation of guaiac in the presence of hydrogen peroxide to produce a blue colour. The test sensitivity is around 30–50% for colorectal cancers but ≤ 20% for adenomas[37] (Table 17.1). It has high specificity of around 98%.[27,38] In practice, this translates to about one case of cancer and three to four adenomas for every 10 positive cases.

The test requires collection of two samples from each of three consecutive stools, which are smeared onto cards and mailed to a laboratory for processing. Colonoscopy is recommended if any of the six cards are positive, since up to 50% will be found to have a cancer or large adenoma (≥ 1 cm). False-positive results may be caused by components of the diet, including vegetables and some fruits, red meat, aspirin, or horseradish; dietary restriction is sometimes advised before and during testing but, when requested, tends to reduce compliance rates.[39,40]

FOBT has been shown, in three large randomised trials (in Minnesota, USA[41,42]; Odense, Denmark[38,43]; and Notthingham, UK[27]) to reduce mortality from CRC by up to 20% if offered biennially, and possibly up to 33% if offered every year. In the US study,[44] CRC incidence rates were reduced by 20% and 17% in the annually and biennially screened groups, respectively, but only 18 years after inception of screening. No incidence reduction has been observed in either of the two European studies,[43] both of which have offered the test at 2-yearly intervals. However, the cohorts have been followed for only 13 years so far and at that stage no effect on incidence was discernable in the US data. In the US trial,[41] the majority of the cards were rehydrated to increase sensitivity by adding a drop of water to the test cards during processing to induce haemolysis. This practice led to an increase in the positivity rates from 2% to 10%. As a result the cumulative colonoscopy rate at 13 years was almost 40% in the annual and 29% in the biennially screened groups (compared with only 4% in the Danish study[43]). It has been suggested that the reduction in incidence rates observed in the US study may be at least in part a consequence of the incidental detection of adenomas in the excess colonoscopies.[45]

Haemoccult is a relatively insensitive test. In a case–control study,[46] only 36% of the FOBTs performed within a year of diagnosis of fatal colorectal cancer yielded positive results. This represents the maximum efficacy of the test even if 100% compliance rates are achieved. Immunochemical tests for haemoglobin or other blood components show greater sensitivity for both CRC and adenomas, but at the expense of lower specificity. Immunochemical tests are used routinely in Japan[47] but there is only limited experience elsewhere.[48,49]

**Table 17.1** Prevalence of adenomas and adenocarcinomas in average risk persons undergoing screening by flexible sigmoidoscopy, faecal occult blood testing or colonoscopy

| First author | Year | Screen | No. of subjects | Adenomas No. | Adenomas % | Adenomas = 1 cm No. | Adenomas = 1 cm % | Cancers No. | Cancers % | Mean age (years) | % Male | Type of test |
|---|---|---|---|---|---|---|---|---|---|---|---|---|
| *Flexible sigmoidoscopy* | | | | | | | | | | | | |
| Meyer[119] | 1980 | | 122 | 9 | 7.4 | | 92 | 1 | 0.8 | 56.6 | 79 | |
| Winnan[120] | 1980 | | 342 | 34 | 9.9 | | | | | 53 | 86 | |
| Spencer[121] | 1983 | | 508 | 55 | 10.8 | | | | | 60 | 45 | |
| Rosevelt[122] | 1984 | | 825 | 57 | 6.9 | | | 3 | 0.4 | 59 | 71F? | |
| McCallum[123] | 1984 | | 1015 | 78 | 7.7 | | | | | 20–89 | 76 | |
| Ujszaszy[124] | 1985 | | 3863 | 305 | 7.9 | 171 | 4.4 | 11 | 0.3 | | | |
| Warden[125] | 1986 | | 632 | 49 | 7.8 | | | | | 60 | | |
| Rozen[126] | 1987 | | 1176 | 38 | 3.2 | | | 4 | 0.3 | 52 | 42 | |
| Neale[127] | 1987 | | 718 | 18 | 2.5 | | | | | 40 | | |
| Yao[128] | 1988 | | 365 | 37 | 10.1 | | | 3 | 0.8 | 63 | 45 | |
| Schertz[129] | 1989 | | 1236 | 137 | 11.1 | | | 15 | 1.2 | | 61 | |
| Shida[130] | 1989 | | 1573 | 134 | 8.5 | 28 | 1.8 | 3 | 0.2 | | 81 | |
| Rex[131] used colonoscope | 1990 | | 500 | 60 | 12.0 | | | 1 | 0.2 | 55 | 93 | |
| Riff[132] | 1990 | | 329 | 26 | 7.9 | 13 | 4.0 | 0 | | 63 | | |
| Cauffman[133] | 1992 | | 1000 | 53 | 5.3 | | | 1 | 0.1 | 61 | 47 | |
| Foley[89] | 1992 | | 900 | 165 | 18.3 | 41 | 4.6 | 8 | 0.1 | 53 | 61 | |
| Wherry[87] | 1994 | | 4005 | 217 | 5.4 | | | 11 | 0.3 | 55 | 66 | |
| Cannon-Albright[134] | 1994 | | 406 | 48 | 11.8 | | | 0 | | 52 | 51 | |
| Olynyk[91] | 1996 | | 342 | 56 | 16.3 | 19 | 5.6 | | | 55–59 | | |
| Verne[90] | 1998 | | 1116 | 76 | 6.8 | | | 4 | 0.4 | | 51 | |
| Paillot[135] | 1999 | | 450 | 22 | 4.9 | 9 | 2.0 | 0 | | | 40 | |
| Collett[136] | 2000 | | 2605 | 352 | 13.5 | 51 | 2.0 | 10 | 0.4 | 55–64 | 59 | |
| Lieberman[63] | 2000 | | 3121 | 554 | 17.7 | 128 | 4.1 | | | 63 | 97 | |
| Imperiale[137] | 2000 | | 1994 | 229 | 11.5 | 26 | 1.3 | | | 60 | 59 | |
| Hoff[138] | 2002 | | 8840 | 141 | 1.6 | | | | | 55–64 | | |
| *Faecal occult blood testing* | | | | | | | | | | | | |
| Kewenter[139] | 1994 | P and R | 41338 | 419 | 1.0 | 238 | 0.6 | 81 | 0.2 | 60–64 | | H II-U |
| Hardcastle[27] | 1996 | P | 44838 | 357 | 0.8 | 311 | 0.7 | 104 | 0.2 | 40–74 | | H II-U |
| | | R (3–6 times) | 88158 | 353 | 0.4 | 271 | 0.3 | 132 | 0.1 | | | |
| Kronborg[38] | 1996 | P | 20672 | | | 68 | 0.3 | 37 | 0.2 | 45–75 | | H II |
| | | R 1 | 18781 | | | 61 | 0.3 | 13 | 0.1 | | | Biennial-U |
| | | R 2 | 17279 | | | 41 | 0.2 | 24 | 0.1 | | | |

*(Continued)*

**Table 17.1** (Continued)

| First author | Year | Screen | No. of subjects | Adenomas | | Adenomas ≥1 cm | | Cancers | | Mean age (years) | % Male | Type of test |
|---|---|---|---|---|---|---|---|---|---|---|---|---|
| | | | | No. | % | No. | % | No. | % | | | |
| | | R 3 | 15 845 | | | 44 | 0.3 | 21 | 0.1 | | | |
| | | R 4 | 14 203 | | | 56 | 0.4 | 25 | 0.2 | | | |
| Lieberman[107] | 2001 | P | 2 885 | 116 | 4.0 | 25 | 0.9 | 12 | 0.4 | 63 | | H II–R |
| Nakama[140] | 2001 | P | 17 432 | | | | | 39 | 0.2 | >40 | | I |
| *Colonoscopy* | | | | | | | | | | | | |
| Lieberman[63] | 2000 | P | 3121 | 1141 | 36.5 | 264 | 8.5 | 30 | 1.0 | 62.9 | | |
| Imperiale[137] | 2000 | P | 1994 | 354 | 17.8 | | | 12 | 0.6 | 59.8 | | |

Abbreviations: H II–U, unhydrated Haemoccult test; H II–R, rehydrated Haemoccult test; I, immunochemical test; P, prevalence; R, rescreening

The feasibility and acceptability of FOBT is now being examined in demonstration pilot projects in Australia (http://www.health.gov.au/pubhlth/strateg/cancer/bowel/index.htm) and in the UK.[50] The UK pilot includes two populations (one in Scotland, one in England) each with around 200 000 people in the age-range 50–69 years. A guaiac test, similar to Haemoccult, is being offered on a single occasion. The results of this 2-year study are due in 2003, after which a decision will be made on whether to offer this form of screening in a programme within the National Health Service.

## Flexible sigmoidoscopy

The 60 cm flexible sigmoidoscope routinely examines the sigmoid colon and rectum where two-thirds of colorectal cancers and adenomas are located. It is usually performed in an endoscopy unit without sedation or analgesia. A single phosphate enema, self-administered around 1 hour before the patient leaves home for the test, is required to clear the lower bowel.[51] The technique is sensitive for the detection of both adenomas and colorectal cancers within its reach.

The detection rates of distal adenomas and cancers at screening flexible sigmoidoscopy in different studies are shown in Table 17.1. Prevalence rates of distal adenomas increase with age during the sixth decade of life but level off after the age of 60 years.[52] Distal adenoma prevalence rates in men are approximately double those in women.[26]

Evidence from case–control and cohort studies indicates that screening by sigmoidoscopy reduces incidence and mortality rates of distal CRC[53–56] by around 60%. In the absence of evidence from a randomised trial, several countries have been unwilling to introduce endoscopic screening. Three trials are currently in progress (in UK,[36] Italy,[57] and US[58]) to address this issue. A 5-year interval is recommended by several professional organisations in the USA,[59,60] although the protection afforded by a single flexible sigmoidoscopy may last for up to 10 years[61] or even longer depending on the age at which it is undertaken.[52] The UK and Italian trials are examining the efficacy of a single flexible sigmoidoscopy screen at around age 60 years and the US trial is examining the efficacy of 5-yearly screening.

In the UK and Italian trials, small polyps are removed during sigmoidoscopy, a practice which has been shown to be safe.[26] Colonoscopy is restricted only to those people who are found to have adenomas with features associated with increased risks of synchronous or metachronous cancer. These features include ≥ 3 adenomas, size ≥ 1 cm, villous histology, severe dysplasia, or malignancy. On these criteria only 5% of people screened will require colonoscopy, compared with 24% if all people found to have any polyps are referred.

The three randomised trials have all reached their recruitment targets but several more years of follow up will be required to determine the effects on incidence and mortality. In the meantime, a population experiment has been ongoing in Northern California where the Health Maintenance Organization, Kaiser Permanente, has been offering such screening at 10-yearly intervals to its members aged over 50 years for the past decade.[62] Uptake rates of 70% have been reported. Colorectal cancer incidence rates have fallen steadily in California and the decrease in left-sided tumours is about twice that of right-sided tumours (24·3% v 11·6%).[3]

## Colonoscopy screening

A limitation of flexible sigmoidoscopy screening is that it does not examine the proximal colon where 40% of adenomas and cancers occur. The finding of an adenoma is associated with an increased likelihood of having adenomas in the proximal colon, so colonoscopy in people with distal neoplasia should enable detection of some proximal neoplasia. A recent study[63] suggested that around 70% of advanced colorectal neoplasia will be detected with this strategy. However, around 50% of proximal neoplasia will occur in the absence of a distal marker and some experts in the US[64,65] have advocated colonoscopy screening to avoid missing these lesions.

Existing data suggest that there is only a moderate additional reduction in incidence and mortality rates with colonoscopy compared with flexible sigmoidoscopy. In a case–control study by Muller and Sonnenberg,[55,66] odds ratios for the development of colon cancer were 0·47 (0·37–0·58) following colonoscopy compared with 0·56 (0·46–0·67) following flexible sigmoidoscopy; odds ratios for colorectal cancer death were respectively 0·24 (0·17–0·35) and 0·38 (0·29–0·49). Kavanagh et al.[67] examined prospectively the risk of CRC in 24 000 people, 3000 of whom had undergone endoscopic screening 8 years previously, 18% by colonoscopy and the remainder by flexible sigmoidoscopy. There was an 80% reduction in stage C and D cancers of the distal large bowel among the screened group, but no reduction in either early or late stage proximal cancer. Data from the National Polyp Study[68] suggest that there is a 75% reduction in colorectal cancer incidence rates following colonoscopic polypectomy. However, these rates might be due solely to an effect on distal cancer. Winawer and Zauber[69] have suggested that a randomised trial is required to examine the efficacy of colonoscopy and a pilot study is in progress.

For the motivated individual, whole colon screening by colonoscopy may give the greatest reassurance, but it may not be suitable for mass population screening because of the personal commitment and the considerable provider resources required. Bowel preparation for colonoscopy requires participants to take a laxative and consume a liquid-only diet on the day before screening. The procedure can be painful so it is usual to give sedation and analgesia. As a result colonoscopy screening requires of the patient at least 36 hours of commitment and time off work compared with only a couple of hours for flexible sigmoidoscopy. Complication rates are also higher (see below). Flexible sigmoidoscopy can be performed competently by nurses,[70,71] while colonoscopy requires the skills of an experienced endoscopist; therefore offering colonoscopy at 10 yearly intervals in the USA presents manpower problems that have yet to be resolved. It is not seen as a viable screening tool in many other countries.

## Imaging techniques

In the precolonoscopy era, barium enema was the only way to examine areas of the bowel proximal to the distal sigmoid colon, apart from surgery. The advent of double contrast barium enema improved the ability to detect smaller lesions such as polyps, but there has been a long debate on the relative merits of barium enema and colonoscopy.[72,73] Proponents have stressed the relative safety of barium enema; critics have stressed the relative insensitivity compared with colonoscopy. In a study of 2193 consecutive colorectal cancers from 21 Indiana hospitals,[74] colonoscopy correctly identified 95% of cancers and barium enema only 83%. Barium enema has been shown[75] to be relatively insensitive for the detection of polyps compared with colonoscopy, detecting only 21%, 42% and 46% respectively of polyps $\leq 5$ mm, 6–10 mm or $> 10$ mm in size.

Computed tomography (CT) and magnetic resonance (MR) colography or colonography are new techniques for imaging the bowel, which may in the future find application in screening for colorectal cancer and polyps. Virtual colonoscopy (CT colography), first described by Vining in 1994,[76] applied complex image rendering techniques to a spiral CT pneumocolon to create 3D graphical images of the colon that simulate a colonoscopy. These techniques require satisfactory bowel cleansing and temporary paralysis of the colon using a muscle relaxant. The technology, both software and hardware, is advancing at a rapid rate and the performance characteristics are improving. For example, it has been reported[77,78] that oral contrast, consumed on the day before screening, may obviate the need for bowel preparation by differentiating faeces from polyps. The techniques appear to have high sensitivity for colorectal cancers and large polyps, but are less sensitive for flat lesions and for smaller polyps.[79] A major limitation at present is the time required to interpret the output (around 15–20 minutes), although computer algorithms are under

development[80] to automatically detect and label suspicious regions, alerting the radiologist to the presence of a polyp. If accuracy improves, if costs can be kept low and if the need for bowel preparation can be eliminated, there may be a role for these methods in screening average risk people.

## DNA-based stool tests

Stool tests have the advantage that they are non-invasive and, despite the universal distaste for handling faecal material, are potentially more convenient for the participant since collection can be performed at home. The past decade has seen enormous advances in the ability to detect the tiny amounts of DNA present in stool which are derived from cells shed from adenomas and cancers. Compared with tissue and blood, extraction of DNA from stool presents special problems as human DNA is often degraded and food digestion products and bacterial contaminants inhibit the polymerase chain reaction. The quantity and quality of the DNA extracted from stools is generally increased in the presence of colorectal neoplasia, probably because there is less efficient degradation by apoptosis of cells shed by tumours compared with fully differentiated cells. However, several recent studies have reported that it is now possible, although still technically difficult, to extract epithelial DNA from 100% of stool samples including those with no neoplasia. Mutations in several genes have been examined including *k-ras*, *APC*, *p53* and *BAT26*.[81–84]

Using a panel of DNA markers, three research groups[81–83] have reported high sensitivity for colorectal cancers and large adenomas. Data so far suggest that, with the exception of *k-ras*, these markers are highly specific and therefore represent a significant improvement over FOBT. However a large NCI study is in progress to examine the sensitivity and specificity of these markers in 10 000 average risk men and women aged over 50 years, all of whom will be examined by colonoscopy as a gold standard for comparison. Whether these stool-based DNA tests will replace or supplement existing methods of screening has yet to be determined. It has been suggested[85] that *BAT26* might be a useful test for the detection of proximal cancers in combination with flexible sigmoidoscopy screening.

## Acceptability of screening methods

In the Nottingham trial of FOBT,[27] 60% of participants completed at least one screening test and 38% completed all the screening tests they were offered (between 3 and 6). These results are similar to experience in Burgundy (France)[86] where during the first five successive rounds of screening, 69% completed at least one round and 37%

completed all five rounds. In the Danish trial,[43] 67% completed the first test. In this study only compliers with the first test were invited for subsequent tests and compliance among this group was 93% at each test. Experience in Nottingham and in France suggests that higher compliance rates are achieved when non-compliers are invited at subsequent rounds.

Reported compliance rates with flexible sigmoidoscopy screening are highly variable. In a US Army screening initiative,[87] attendance was 95%, although flexible sigmoidoscopy screening appeared to be a requirement for overseas posting.[87] An attendance rate of 81% was achieved in Norway,[88] 38% in Ireland[89] and, in the UK,[90] 49% complied with an invitation to undergo flexible sigmoidoscopy screening by their own GP.[90] Lower rates were observed in studies from Australia (12%)[91] and Italy (29%).[92] These rates are still higher than the 6% compliance in a study[93] inviting physicians, dentists and their spouses to undergo screening colonoscopy.

In a survey undertaken in 1999 among Americans aged over 50 years,[94] 40% reported ever having FOBT and 44% ever having a sigmoidoscopy. Compliance with the recommended US screening strategy was 21% for FOBT (having a test within previous year) and 34% for sigmoidoscopy (within previous 5 years); 44% had had either sigmoidoscopy or FOBT during the recommended period.

## Side effects associated with treatment

The main complications of screening are associated with colonoscopy, flexible sigmoidoscopy and surgery. Generally flexible sigmoidoscopy is a much lower risk procedure than colonoscopy, particularly the perforation rate. In the UK flexible sigmoidoscopy screening trial,[26] there was only one perforation in 40 000 despite the removal of more than 19 000 polyps during the procedure. A similar low perforation rate was reported in a 10-year study from the Mayo Clinic[95] (two perforations in 49 500 flexible sigmoidoscopy), and in a screening programme in northern California[103] (two perforations in 109 000 examinations, some of which included polypectomy). In contrast, there is a higher risk of perforation at colonoscopy. In the UK Flexible Sigmoidoscopy trial there were four perforations in 2377 examinations (1:600), all following polypectomy. This perforation rate is similar to that reported in the Nottingham FOBT trial (five in 1474 [1:300] colonoscopies),[97] and in a series from the Mayo Clinic (20 in 10 486 [1:500] colonoscopies).[95] However, in a screening colonoscopy study in average risk men, there were no perforations reported in over 3000 examinations.[63]

Haemorrhage, the next most important complication, is most likely to occur following polypectomy. Waye *et al.*[98]

using data from several prospective studies, estimated the rate to be 1 in 81 if polypectomy had been performed and one in 1352 if it had not. In the UK flexible sigmoidoscopy trial there were only 12 cases in 40 000 (1:3300) flexible sigmoidoscopy examinations (eight following 19 000 [1:2400] polypectomies) and nine cases in 2377 (1:260) colonoscopies (all following polypectomy). Risk of bleeding following polypectomy is minimised by discontinuing anticoagulant drugs several days beforehand.

Endoscopic procedures can induce transient bacteraemia, but prophylactic antibiotics are only needed for patients who are immunosuppressed or who have an implanted mechanical heart valve. Inadequately disinfected endoscopic equipment poses a potential risk of transmission of infection and cases of hepatitis acquired through endoscopy have been reported.[99,100]

Cardiac effects secondary to the use of laxatives or sedatives have been reported in up to 15% of people undergoing colonoscopy.[101] In the FOBT trials the reduction in colorectal cancer mortality observed was of the same order as the increase in mortality from ischaemic heart disease.[102] In a small randomised study of flexible sigmoidoscopy screening in Norway,[103] a 5% increased cardiac mortality was observed in the group undergoing screening. However, in the series from northern California, myocardial infarction was no more frequent at one day, one week or one month following flexible sigmoidoscopy than the remainder of the 52-week period.[96]

Another source of morbidity and mortality is associated with the surgical treatment of early cancers and adenomas too large to be removed endoscopically. Data are scarce but the mortality from elective colorectal surgery varies between 1% and 7%.

## Costs of screening and subsequent work-up

The most commonly used FOBT test (Haemoccult) itself costs less than £1. However, testing needs to be offered at 1- or 2-yearly intervals and it is recommended that test positives are examined by colonoscopy. Positivity rates with the unrehydrated FOBT are around 2% at the initial screen and 1–1·5% thereafter.[27,38] Positivity rates with the rehydrated test vary between 4% and 10%[41] and it has been estimated that cumulative colonoscopy rates over a lifetime of screening make such testing prohibitively expensive.[104]

The costs of colonoscopy, flexible sigmoidoscopy, and polypectomy vary enormously, not only between countries but also between different providers within the same country (Whynes, personal communication). In some countries, flexible sigmoidoscopy costs nearly as much as colonoscopy; clearly, therefore, colonoscopy, which examines the colon more extensively, would be more cost-effective. In other settings, such as in the UK NHS and in managed care, flexible sigmoidoscopy is three to five times less costly than colonoscopy. Accurately costing these procedures is obviously essential in modelling the cost-effectiveness of different screening regimens.

The predicted lifetime costs for localised, regional and disseminated cancer have been estimated to be of the order of $22 000, $44 000, and $58 000 (costs estimated from Group Health Cooperative, Seattle, Washington). However, a recent study[105] suggests that the lifetime costs of early cancers may be greater than late cancers because of the long follow up for early cases and high mortality in late cases.

## Cost effectiveness of different screening strategies

Many different CRC screening strategies have been proposed in the US based on FOBT, sigmoidoscopy, and colonoscopy,[60,106,107] for example, FOBT (unrehydrated or rehydrated) at annual or 2-yearly intervals, sigmoidoscopy at 3-yearly, 5-yearly or 10-yearly intervals or just once at around age 55–60, and colonoscopy at 10-yearly intervals or just once at age 60 or 65 years. In estimating cost-effectiveness, most studies[104,108,109] have used a state-transition Markov model, which simulates the evolution from normal epithelium to adenomatous polyp to malignancy under various assumptions.

There is general agreement that the cost-effectiveness of all strategies for CRC screening (except those using rehydrated FOBT) compare favourably with those for other cancers, such as Pap smear testing for cervical cancer and mammography for early breast cancer detection. The net costs of unrehydrated FOBT are higher than expected since the test is not associated with a decrease in incidence rates,[43] and thereby the costs of treating the disease. By contrast, endoscopic screening, by detecting the disease in the premalignant phase, reduces incidence and avoids the costs of future cancer treatment. Several studies[52,104,110] have shown that the net costs of flexible sigmoidoscopy screening are close to zero and become cost-saving, under some assumptions. Similar claims have been made for a single colonoscopy.[111]

Increasing the interval or reducing the number of screening examinations profoundly reduces costs.[112] Decreasing the age at which screening is first offered increases the number of life-years saved but at much greater cost. Eddy[113] showed that delaying the start of screening from age 40 to 50 reduces costs of FOBT by a factor of two and this became the basis for the US recommendations.[106] Similarly, a single colonoscopy at age 60 saves more lives but is more cost-effective when offered after age 70, when it becomes cost-saving.[111]

There is some controversy about the threshold at which to offer baseline colonoscopy following detection of an adenoma at sigmoidoscopy in order to look for synchronous proximal neoplasia. The risk of advanced neoplasia or colorectal cancer is increased in the presence of multiple or advanced distal adenomas.[12,114] Offering colonoscopy only for high risk rather than for any adenoma potentially increases the feasibility of the screening regimen when resources are limited, by reducing from 12% to 5% the proportion of people referred for colonoscopy.[26] This strategy will inevitably miss some advanced proximal adenomas. However, only around 25% of proximal cancers occur in the presence of a distal marker,[115,116] so sigmoidoscopy is inevitably an ineffective method of detecting proximal neoplasia whatever threshold is used.

The factor that most profoundly affects the costs of all screening regimens is the nearly universal practice of offering 3-yearly surveillance colonoscopy following detection of any adenoma (for discussion see Ransohoff[117]). Depending on the frequency of screening and the proportion of people entering into surveillance, this component can account for up to one-half of the costs of screening programmes.[109,112,118]

## Conclusions

It has now been proven that early detection of colorectal cancer by screening can reduce mortality from the disease. Evidence from case–control studies is highly suggestive that removal of adenomas reduces colorectal cancer incidence rates. The USA is the only country that has advocated endoscopic screening for the purpose of detecting the disease in the premalignant phase, and is the only country in which incidence rates are falling. There are many methods now available for screening for colorectal cancer and adequate evidence of benefit. The precise choice of screening regimen within a particular healthcare setting will depend on issues of acceptability, safety, feasibility and cost-effectiveness. Whatever method of screening is chosen, it will be necessary to perform colonoscopy to a high standard. It is therefore essential that training and quality assurance programmes are in place before screening is implemented.

## References

1  Parkin D, Bray F, Devesa S. Cancer burden in the year 2000. The global picture. *Eur J Cancer* 2001;**37**:4–66.

2  Coleman M, Esteve J, Damiecki P, Arslan A, Renard H. *Trends in cancer incidence and mortality*. Lyon: International Agency for Research on Cancer; 1993.

3  Inciardi J, Lee J, Stijnen T. Incidence trends for colorectal cancer in California: Implications for current screening practices. *Am J Med* 2000;**109**:277–81.

4  Rabeneck L, El-Serag H, Sandler R. Incidence and survival of colorectal cancer in the US:1989–1997. Gastroenterology 2001;**120** (Suppl. 1):A65.

5 Quinn M, Babb P, Brock A, Kirby E, Jones J. *Cancer Trends in England and Wales, 1950–1999*. London: The Stationery Office, 2001.

6 Gatta G, Capocaccia R, Sant M *et al.* Understanding variations in survival for colorectal cancer in Europe: a EUROCARE high resolution study. *Gut* 2000;**47**:533–8.

7 Wingo P, Ries L, Parker S Jr CH. Long-term cancer patient survival in the United States. *Cancer Epidemiol Biomarker Prev* 1998;**7**:269–70.

8 Muto T, Bussey H, Morson B. The evolution of cancer of the colon and rectum. *Cancer* 1975;**36**:2251–70.

9 Morson B, Bussey H, Day D, Hill M. Adenomas of large bowel. *Cancer Surv* 1983:451–77.

10 Jass J. Do all colorectal cancers arise in pre-existing adenomas? *World J Surg* 1989;**74**:45–51.

11 Vogelstein B, Fearon E, Hamilton S *et al.* Genetic alterations during colorectal-tumor development. *N Engl J Med* 1988;**319**:525–32.

12 Atkin W, Morson B, Cuzick J. Long-term risk of colorectal cancer after excision of rectosigmoid adenomas. *N Engl J Med* 1992;**326**:658–62.

13 Winawer S, Zauber A, O'Brien M *et al.* Randomized comparison of surveillance intervals after colonoscopic removal of newly diagnosed adenomatous polyps. *N Engl J Med* 1993;**328**:901–6.

14 Morson B, Williams C, Fruhmorgen P *et al.* Colorectal adenomas: risk of cancer and results of follow-up. *Gastroenterol Int* 1990;**3**:57–62.

15 Winawer S, Zauber A, Diaz B. The National Polyp Study: temporal sequence of evolving colorectal cancer from normal mucosa. *Gastrointest Endosc* 1987;**33**:167.

16 Stryker S, Wolff B, Culp C *et al.* Natural history of untreated colonic polyps. *Gastroenterology* 1987;**93**:1009–13.

17 Muto T, Kamiya J, Sawada T *et al.* Small "flat adenoma" of the large bowel with special reference to its clinicopathologic features. *Dis Colon Rectum* 1985:847–51.

18 Suzuki Y, Honma T, Yoshida H *et al.* Prospective follow-up-study of flat-elevated colorectal adenomas by magnifying colonoscopy. *Gastrointest Endosc* 1997;**45**:377.

19 Hart A, Kudo S, Mackay E, Mayberry J, Atkin W. Flat adenomas exist in asymptomatic people – important implications for colorectal-cancer screening programs. *Gut* 1998;**43**:229–31.

20 Rembacken B, Fujii T, Cairns A *et al.* Flat and depressed colonic neoplasms: a prospective study of 1000 colonoscopies in the UK. *Lancet* 2000;**355**:1211–14.

21 Dunlop M, Farrington S, Carothers A *et al.* Cancer risk associated with germline DNA mismatch repair gene-mutations. *Hum Mol Genet* 1997;**6**:105–10.

22 Itzkowitz S. Inflammatory bowel-disease and cancer. *Gastroenterol Clin N Am* 1997;**26**:129.

23 Lovett E. Family studies in cancer of the colon and rectum. *Br J Surg* 1976;**63**:533–7.

24 John DS, McDermott F, Hopper J *et al.* Cancer risk in relatives of patients with common colorectal cancer. *Ann Intern Med* 1993;**118**:785–90.

25 Law M, Morris J, Wald N. The importance of age in screening for cancer. *J Med Screen* 1999;**6**:16–20.

26 Atkin. UK Flexible Sigmoidoscopy Screening Trial Investigators. Single flexible sigmoidoscopy screening to prevent colorectal cancer; baseline findings of a UK multicentre randomised trial. *Lancet* 2002;**359**:1291–300.

27 Hardcastle J, Chamberlain J, Robinson M *et al.* Randomised controlled trial of faecal-occult-blood screening for colorectal cancer. *Lancet* 1996;**348**:1472–7.

28 Hixson L, Fennerty M, Sampliner R *et al.* Prospective blinded trial of the colonoscopic miss-rate of large colorectal polyps. *Gastrointest Endosc* 1991;**37**:125–7.

29 Rex D, Cutler C, Lemmel G *et al.* Colonoscopic miss rates and adenomas determined by back-to-back colonoscopies. *Gastroenterology* 1997;**112**:24–8.

30 Winawer S, St-John D, Bond J *et al.* Guidelines for the prevention of colorectal cancer: update based on new data. World Health Organization collaborating center for the prevention of colorectal cancer. *Z-Gastroenterol* 1995;**33**:574–6.

31 Grossman S, Milos M, Tekawa I, Jewell N. Colonoscopic screening of persons with suspected risk factors for colon cancer: II. Past history of colorectal neoplasms. *Gastroenterology* 1989;**96**:299–306.

32 Noshirwani C, VanStolk U, Rybicki L, Beck G. Adenoma size and number are predictive of adenoma recurrence: implications for surveillance colonoscopy. *Gastrointest Endosc* 2000;**51**:433–7.

33 Spencer R, Melton L, Ready R, Ilstrup D. Treatment of small colorectal polyps: a population-based study of the risk of subsequent carcinoma. *Mayo Clin Proc* 1984;**59**:305–10.

34 Lotfi A, Spencer R, Ilstrup D, Melton L. Colorectal polyps and the risk of subsequent carcinoma. *Mayo Clin Proc* 1986;**61**:337–43.

35 Zauber A, Winawer S, Bond J *et al.* Long term National Polyp Study (NPS) data on post-polypectomy surveillance. *Endoscopy* 1999;**31**: E13 (abstract).

36 Atkin W, Edwards R, Wardle J *et al.* Design of a multicentre randomised trial to evaluate flexible sigmoidoscopy in colorectal cancer screening. *J Med Screen* 2001;**8**:137–44.

37 Ahlquist D, Wieand H, Moertal C *et al.* Accuracy of fecal occult blood screening for colorectal neoplasia: a prospective study using Hemoccult and Hemoquant. *JAMA* 1993;**269**:1262–7.

38 Kronborg O, Fenger C, Olsen J, Jorgensen O, Sondergaard O. Randomised study of screening for colorectal cancer with faecal-occult-blood test. *Lancet* 1996;**348**:1467–71.

39 Thomas W, Pye G, Hardcastle J, Chamberlain J, Charnley R. Role of dietary restriction in Haemoccult screening for colorectal cancer. *Br J Surg* 1989;**76**:976–8.

40 Rozen P, Knaani J, Samuel Z. Eliminating the need for dietary restrictions when using a sensitive guaiac fecal occult blood test. *Dig Dis Sci* 1999;**44**:756–60.

41 Mandel J, Bond J, Church T *et al.* Reducing mortality from colorectal cancer by screening for fecal occult blood. *N Engl J Med* 1993;**328**:1365–71.

42 Mandel J, Church T, Ederer F, Bond J. Colorectal cancer mortality: Effectiveness of biennial screening for fecal occult blood. *J Natl Cancer Inst* 1999;**91**:434–7.

43 Jorgensen O, Kronborg O, Fenger C. A randomised study of screening for colorectal cancer using faecal occult blood testing: results ater 13 years and seven biennial screening rounds. *Gut* 2002;**50**:29–32.

44 Mandel J, Church T, Bond J *et al.* The effect of fecal occult blood screening on the incidence of colorectal cancer. *N Engl J Med* 2000;**343**:1603–7.

45 Lang C, Ransohoff D. What can we conclude from the randomized controlled trials of fecal occult blood test screening? *Eur J Gastroenterol Hepatol* 1998;**10**:199–204.

46 Selby J, Friedman G, Quesenberry C, Weiss N. Effect of fecal occult blood testing on mortality from colorectal cancer. A case–control study. *Ann Intern Med* 1993;**118**:1–6.

47 Saito H. Screening for colorectal-cancer by immunochemical fecal occult blood testing. *Jpn J Cancer Res* 1996;**87**:1011–24.

48 Rozen P, Knaani J, Samuel Z. Comparative screening with a sensitive guaiac and specific immunochemical occult blood test in an endoscopic study. *Cancer* 2000;**89**:46–51.

49 Castiglione G, Zappa M, Grazzini G *et al.* Screening for colorectal cancer by faecal occult blood test: comparison of immunochemical tests. *J Med Screen* 2000;**7**:35–7.

50 Steele R, Parker R, Patnick J *et al.* A demonstration pilot trial for colorectal cancer screening in the United Kingdom: a new concept in the introduction of healthcare strategies. *J Med Screen* 2001;**8**: 197–203.

51 Atkin W, Hart A, Edwards R *et al.* Single-blind, randomised trial of the efficacy and acceptability of oral Picolax vs self-administered phosphate enema in bowel preparation for flexible sigmoidoscopy screening. *BMJ* 2000;**320**:1504–9 discussion 9.

52 Atkin W, Cuzick J, Northover J, Whynes D. Prevention of colorectal cancer by once-only sigmoidoscopy. *Lancet* 1993;**341**:736–40.

53 Selby J, Friedman G, Jr CO, Weiss N. A case–control study of screening sigmoidoscopy and mortality from colorectal cancer. *N Engl J Med* 1992;**326**:653–7.

54 Newcomb P, Norfleet R, Storer B, Surawicz S, Marcus P. Screening sigmoidoscopy and colorectal cancer mortality. *J Natl Cancer Inst* 1992;**84**:1572–5.

55 Muller A, Sonnenberg A. Prevention of colorectal cancer by flexible endoscopy and polypectomy. A case–controlled study of 32,702 veterans. *Ann Intern Med* 1995;**123**:904–10.

56 Gilbertsen V, Nelms J. The prevention of invasive cancer of the rectum. *Cancer* 1978;**41**:1137–9.

57 Segnan N, Sciallero S, Bonelli L *et al.* Multicentre randomised controlled trial of "once only" flexible sigmoidoscopy screening in Italy-score. *Endoscopy* 1999;**31**(Suppl. 1):E9.

58 Prorok P, Andriole G, Bresalier R *et al.* Design of the Prostate, Lung, Colorectal and Ovarian (PLCO) Cancer Screening Trial. *Control Clin Trials* 2000;**21**(Suppl. 6):273S–309S.

59 Winawer S, Fletcher R, Miller L *et al.* Colorectal-cancer screening – clinical guidelines and rationale. *Gastroenterology* 1997;**112**:594–642.

60 Smith R, vonEschenbach A, Wender R *et al.* American Cancer Society guidelines for the early detection of cancer: Update of early detection guidelines for prostate, colorectal and endometrial cancers. *Cancer J Clin* 2001;**51**:38–75.

61 Selby J, Friedman G. Sigmoidoscopy and mortality from colorectal cancer: the Kaiser-Permanente multiphasic evaluation study. *J Clin Epidemiol* 1988;**41**:427–34.

62 Levin T, Palitz A. Flexible sigmoidoscopy; an important screening option for average-risk individuals. *Gastrointest Endosc Clin N Am* 2002;**12**:23–40.

63 Lieberman D, Weiss D, Bond J *et al.* Use of colonoscopy to screen asymptomatic adults for colorectal cancer. *N Engl J Med* 2000; **343**:162–8.

64 Neugut A, Forde K. Screening colonoscopy: has the time come? *Am J Gastroenterol* 1988;**83**:295–7.

65 Rex K, Johnson A, Lieberman A, Burt R, Sonnenberg A. Colorectal cancer prevention 2000: screening recommendations of the American College of Gastroenterology. *Am J Gastroenterol* 2000;**95**:868–77.

66 Muller A, Sonneberg A. Protection of colorectal cancer by endoscopy against death from colorectal cancer: A case–controlled study among veterans. *Arch Intern Med* 1995;**155**:1741–8.

67 Kavanagh A, Giovannucci E, Fuchs C, Colditz G. Screening endoscopy and risk of colorectal cancer in United States men. *Cancer Causes Control* 1998;**9**:455–62.

68 Winawer S, Zauber A, O'Brien M *et al.* Prevention of colorectal cancer by colonoscopic polypectomy. *N Engl J Med* 1993;**329**: 1977–81.

69 Winawer S, Zauber A. Colonoscopic polypectomy and the incidence of colorectal cancer. *Gut* 2001;**48**:753–6.

70 Maule W. Screening for colorectal cancer by nurse endoscopists. *N Engl J Med* 1994;**330**:183–7.

71 Schoenfeld P, Cash B, Kita J *et al.* Effectiveness and patient satisfaction with screening flexible sigmoidoscopy performed by registered nurses. *Gastrointest Endosc* 1999;**49**:158–62.

72 Thoeni R, Petras A. Detection of rectal and rectosigmoid lesions by double-contrast barium enema examination and sigmoidoscopy. *Radiology* 1982;**142**:59–62.

73 Kewenter J, Brevinge H, Engaras B, Haglind E. The value of flexible sigmoidoscopy and double-contrast barium enema in the diagnosis of neoplasms in the rectum and colon in subjects with a positive hemoccult: results of 1831 rectosigmoidoscopies and double-contrast barium enemas. *Endoscopy* 1995;**27**:159–63.

74 Rex D, Rahmani E, Haseman J *et al.* Relative sensitivity of colonoscopy and barium enema for detection of colorectal cancer in clinical practice. *Gastroenterology* 1997;**112**:17–23.

75 Winawer S, Stewart E, Zauber A *et al.* A comparison of colonoscopy and double-contrast barium enema for surveillance after polypectomy. *N Engl J Med* 2000;**342**:1766–72.

76 Vining D, Gelfand D, Bechtold R *et al.* Technical feasibility of colon imaging with helical CT and virtual reality. *Am J Roentgenol* 1994;**162**(Suppl.):104.

77 Callstrom M, Johnson C, Reed J *et al.* CT colonography of the unprepped colon: an early feasibility study of "virtual preparation". *Gastroenterology* 2000;**118**:A257.

78 Lauenstein T, Goehde S, Ruehm S, Holtmann G, Debatin J. MR colonography with barium-based fecal tagging: Initial clinical experience. *Radiology* 2002;**223**:248–54.

79 Fenlon H. Virtual colonoscopy. *Br J Surg* 2002;**89**:1–3.

80 Summers R, Johnson C, Pusunik L *et al.* Automated polyp detection at CT colonography: Feasibility assessment in a human population. *Radiology* 2001;**219**:51–9.

81 Ahlquist D, Clin M, Rochester M, Harrington J, Shuber A. Detection of altered DNA in stool: feasibility for colorectal neoplasia screening. *Gastroenterology* 1999;**116**:A661.

82 Rengucci C, Maiolo P, Saragoni L *et al.* Multiple detection of genetic alterations in tumors and stool. *Clin Cancer Res* 2001;**7**:590–3.

83 Dong S, Traverso G, Johnson C *et al.* Detecting colorectal cancer in stool with the use of multiple genetic targets. *J Natl Cancer Inst* 2001;**93**:858–65.

84 Traverso G, Shuber A, Levin B *et al.* Detection of APC mutations in fecal DNA from patients with colorectal tumors. *N Engl J Med* 2002;**346**:311–20.

85 Traverso G, Shuber A, Olsson L *et al.* Detection of proximal colorectal cancers through analysis of faecal DNA. *Lancet* 2002;**359**:403–4.

86 Tazi M, Faivre J, Dassonville F *et al.* Participation in fecal occult blood screening for colorectal cancer in a well defined French population: results of five screening rounds from 1988 to 1996. *J Med Screen* 1997;**4**:147–51.

87 Wherry D, Thomas W. The yield of flexible fiberoptic sigmoidoscopy in the detection of asymptomatic colorectal neoplasia. *Surg Endosc* 1994;**8**:393–5.

88 Hoff G, Sauar J, Vatn M *et al.* Polypectomy of adenomas in the prevention of colorectal-cancer – 10 years follow-up of the telemark polyp study.1. a prospective, controlled population study. *Scand J Gastroenterol* 1996;**31**:1006–10.

89 Foley D, Dunne P, Dervan P *et al.* Left-sided colonoscopy and haemoccult screening for colorectal neoplasia. *Euro J Gastroenterol Hepatol* 1992;**4**:925–36.

90 Verne J, Aubrey R, Love S, Talbot I, Northover J. Population based randomised study of uptake and yield of screening by flexible sigmoidoscopy compared with screening by faecal occult blood testing. *BMJ* 1998;**317**:182–5.

91 Olynyk J, Aquilia S, Fletcher D, Dickinson J. Flexible sigmoidoscopy screening for colorectal-cancer in average-risk subjects – a community-based pilot project. *Med J Aust* 1996;**165**:74–6.

92 Senore C, Segnan N, Rossini F *et al.* Screening for colorectal cancer by once only sigmoidoscopy: a feasibility study in Turin, Italy. *J Med Screen* 1996;**3**:72–8.

93 Rex D, Lehman G, Hawes R, Ulbright T, Smith J. Screening colonoscopy in asymptomatic average-risk persons with negative fecal occult blood tests. *Gastroenterology* 1991;**100**:64–7.

94 CDC. Trends in screening for colorectal cancer – United States, 1997 and 1999. *Morbid Mortal Wkly Rep* 2001;**50**:162–6.

95 Anderson M, Pasha T, Leighton J. Endoscopic perforation of the colon: lessons from a 10-year study. *Am J Gastroenterol* 2000;**95**: 3418–22.

96 Robinson M, Hardcastle J, Moss S *et al.* The risks of screening: data from the Nottingham randomised controlled trial of faecal occult blood screening for colorectal cancer. *Gut* 1999;**45**:588–92.

97 Waye J, Kahn O, Auerbach M. Complications of colonoscopy and flexible sigmoidoscopy. *Gastrointest Endosc Clin N Am* 1996;**6**:343–77.

98 Bronowicki J, Venard V, Botte C *et al.* Patient-to-patient transmission of hepatitis-C virus during colonoscopy. *N Engl J Med* 1997;**337**:237–40.

99 Karsenti D, Metman E, Viguier J *et al.* Transmission of hepatitis C virus by colonoscopy: study of 97 "presumed" risk patients. *Gastroenterol Clin Biol* 1999;**23**:985–6.

100 Eckardt V, Kanzler G, Schmitt T, Eckardt A, Bernhard G. Complications and adverse effects of colonoscopy with selective sedation. *Gastrointest Endosc* 1999;**49**:560–5.

101 Ahlquist D. Fecal occult blood testing for colorectal-cancer – can we afford to do this? *Gastroenterol Clin N Am* 1997;**26**:41–55.

102 Thiis-Evensen E, Hoff G, Sauar J *et al.* Population-based surveillance by colonoscopy: Effect on the incidence of colorectal cancer. Telemark Polyp Study I. *Scand J Gastroenterol* 1999;**34**:414–20.

103 Levin T, Conell C, Shapiro J *et al.* Complications of screening sigmoidoscopy. *Gastroenterology* 2001;**120**(Suppl. 1):A65.

104 Frazier A, Colditz G, Fuchs C, Kuntz K. Cost-effectiveness of screening for colorectal cancer in the general population. *JAMA* 2000;**284**:1954–61.

105 Ramsey S, Berry K, Etzioni R. Lifetime cancer-attributable cost of care for long term survivors of colorectal cancer. *Am J Gastroenterol* 2002;**97**:440–5.

106 Levin B, Murphy G. Revision of American Cancer Society recommendations for the early detection of colorectal cancer. *CA-A Cancer J Clin* 1992;**42**:296–9.

107 Lieberman D, Weiss D, Group VACS. One-time screening for colorectal cancer with combined fecal occult-blood testing and examination of the distal colon. *N Engl J Med* 2001;**345**:555–60.

108 Eddy D, Nugent F, Eddy J *et al.* Screening for colorectal cancer in a high-risk population. Results of a mathematical model. *Gastroenterology* 1987;**92**:682–92.

109 Wagner J, Herdman R, Wadhwa S. Cost effectiveness of colorectal cancer screening in the elderly. *Ann Intern Med* 1991;**115**:807–17.

110 Loeve F, Brown M, Boer R *et al.* Endoscopic colorectal cancer screening: a cost-saving analysis. *J Natl Cancer Inst* 2000;**92**: 557–63.

111 Sonnenberg A, Delco F. Cost-effectiveness of a single colonsocopy in screening for colorectal cancer. *Arch Intern Med* 2002;**162**:163–8.

112 Marshall J, Fay D, Lance P. Potential costs of flexible sigmoidoscopy-based colorectal cancer screening. *Gastroenterology* 1996;**111**: 1411–17.

113 Eddy D. Screening for colorectal cancer. *Ann Intern Med* 1990;**113**:373–84.

114 Zarchy T, Ershoff D. Do characteristics of adenomas on flexible sigmoidoscopy predict advanced lesions on baseline colonoscopy? *Gastroenterology* 1994;**106**:1501–4.

115 Lemmel G, Haseman J, Rex D, Rahmani E. Neoplasia distal to the splenic flexure in patients with proximal colon-cancer. *Gastrointest Endosc* 1996;**44**:109–11.

116 Dinning J, Hixson L, Clark L. Prevalence of distal colonic neoplasia associated with proximal colon cancers. *Arch Intern Med* 1994;**154**:853–6.

117 Ransohoff D. Economic impact of surveillance. *Gastrointest Endosc* 1999;**49**:S67–71.

118 Ransohoff D, Lang C, Kuo H. Colonoscopic surveillance after polypectomy: considerations of cost effectiveness. *Ann Intern Med* 1991;**114**:177–82.

119 Meyer C, McBride W, Goldblatt R *et al.* Clinical experience with flexible sigmoidoscopy in asymptomatic and symptomatic patients. *Yale J Biol Med* 1980;**53**:345–52.

120 Winnan G, Berci G, Panesh J *et al.* Superiority of the flexible sigmoidoscope in routine proctosigmoidoscopy. *N Engl J Med* 1980;**302**:1011–12.

121 Spencer R, Wolff B, Ready R. Comparison of the rigid sigmoidoscope and the flexible sigmoidoscope in conjunction with colon X-ray for detection of lesions of the colon and rectum. *Dis Colon Rectum* 1983;**26**:653–5.

122 Rosevelt J, Frankl H. Colorectal cancer screening by nurse practitioner using 60-cm flexible fiberoptic sigmoidoscope. *Dig Dis Sci* 1984;**29**:161–3.

123 McCallum R, Meyer C, Marignani P, Cane E, Contino C. Flexible sigmoidoscopy: diagnostic yield in 1015 patients. *Am J Gastroenterol* 1984;**79**:433–7.

124 Ujszaszy L, Pronay G, Nagy G *et al.* Screening for colorectal cancer in a Hungarian County. *Endoscopy* 1985;**17**:109–12.

125 Warden M, Petrelli N, Herrera L, Mittelman A. The role of colonoscopy and flexible sigmoidoscopy in screening for colorectal carcinoma. *Dis Colon Rectum* 1986;**30**:52–4.

126 Rozen P, Ron E, Fireman Z *et al.* The relative value of fecal occult blood tests and flexible sigmoidoscopy in screening for large bowel neoplasia. *Cancer* 1987;**60**:2553–8.

127 Neale A, Demers R, Budev H, Scott R. Physician accuracy in diagnosing colorectal polyps. *Dis Colon Rectum* 1987;**30**:247–50.

128 Yao Y. Colorectal cancer detection with the 60 cm flexible sigmoidoscope in a solo general internist's office. *J Am Geriatr Soc* 1988;**36**:914–18.

129 Schertz R, Baskin W, Frakes J. Flexible fiberoptic sigmoidoscopy training for primary care physicians: results of a 5-year experience. *Gastrointest Endosc* 1989;**35**:316–20.

130 Shida H, Yamamoto T. Fiberoptic sigmoidoscopy as the first screening procedure for colorectal neoplasms in an symptomatic population. *Dis Colon Rectum* 1989;**32**:404–8.

131 Rex D, Lehman G, Hawes R, O'Connor K, Smith J. Performing screening flexible sigmoidoscopy using colonoscopes: experience in 500 subjects. *Gastrointest Endosc* 1990;**36**:486–8.

132 Riff E, Dehaan K, Garewal G. The role of sigmoidoscopy for asymptomatic patients. Results of three annual screening sigmoidoscopies, polypectomy, and subsequent surveillance colonoscopy in a primary-care setting. *Cleve Clin J Med* 1990;**57**: 131–6.

133 Cauffman JG, Hara J, Rasgon I, Clark V. Flexible sigmoidoscopy in asymptomatic patients with negative fecal occult blood tests. *J Fam Pract* 1992;**34**:281–5.

134 Cannon-Albright L, Bishop T, Samowitz W *et al.* Colonic polyps in an unselected population: prevalence, characteristics, and associations. *Am J Gastroenterol* 1994;**89**:827–31.

135 Paillot B, Czernichow P, Michel P *et al.* Incidence of rectosigmoid adenomatous polyps in subjects without prior colorectal adenoma or cancer: a prospective cohort study. *Gut* 1999;**44**:372–6.

136 Collett J, Olynyk J, Platell C. Flexible sigmoidoscopy screening for colorectal cancer in average-risk people: update of a community-based project. *Med J Aust* 2000;**173**:463–66.

137 Imperiale T, Ransohoff D. Screening for colorectal cancer. *N Engl J Med* 2000;**343**:1653.

138 Hoff G, Bretthauer M, Grotmol T *et al.* Differences in detection rates of colorectal polyps and adenomas among endoscopists in population-based flexible sigmoidoscopy screening. *Digestive Diseases Week*, Conference held in San Francisco 2002:A870.

139 Kewenter J, Brevinge H, Engeras B, Haglind E, Ahren C. Results of screening, rescreening, and follow-up in a prospective randomised study for detection of colorectal cancer by fecal occult blood testing. *Scand J Gastroenterol* 1994;**29**:468–73.

140 Nakama H, Zhang B, Fukazawa K, Zhang X. Comparisons of cancer detection rate and costs for one cancer detected among different age-cohorts in immunochemical occult blood screening. *J Cancer Res Clin Oncol* 2001;**127**:439–43.

# 18 Screening for lung cancer

*John K Gohagan, Pamela M Marcus, Richard M Fagerstrom, William C Black, Barnett S Kramer, Paul F Pinsky, Philip C Prorok*

## How important is lung cancer in public health terms?

Internationally, lung cancer statistics are bleak.[1] Annually, more than a million new cases of lung cancer are diagnosed worldwide and more than 900 000 people die of the disease. Five-year survival following diagnosis is dismal – 14% in the USA and even lower in Europe. Most lung cancers are diagnosed as locally advanced or metastatic disease, with only 22% of cases presenting at an early, and potentially curable, stage. Lung cancer is the leading cancer killer in the USA for both men and women. For males, the USA ranks fifth in World Health Organization age-adjusted standard population mortality statistics behind Hungary, Poland, the Netherlands and Italy. Canada, the UK and most of Europe rank closely below the USA. For females, the USA ranks first, with Denmark, Canada and the UK next in order.

Cigarette smoking is the principal cause of lung cancer. In the USA, where this point has been emphasised for nearly 40 years, cigarette packages by law warn of the risks of smoking, smoking cessation programmes are pervasive, former smokers nearly equal in number current smokers (roughly 46 million) and huge settlements have been awarded in litigation against tobacco companies. Despite these measures, lung cancer persists as the leading cause of cancer-related mortality in the USA, with an increasing fraction of new lung cancers diagnosed in former smokers.

In October 2000, the National Cancer Institute (NCI) of the USA convened its Lung Cancer Progress Review Group (PRG). The PRG was charged with identifying areas of high priority in lung cancer research. The PRG's members – clinicians, scientists, industry representatives and consumer advocates – reviewed the current lung cancer problem and identified research strategies in prevention, early detection, and treatment that have the greatest potential to reduce disease burden. The PRG report began with this troubling picture of lung cancer in the US today[2]:

> Lung cancer is the leading cause of cancer death for both men and women in the USA, killing more people than breast, prostate, colon, and pancreas cancers combined: Fully 85 percent of patients who develop lung cancer die from it. We are still largely ignorant of the molecular events underlying

the development of lung cancer and the mechanisms of resistance to drug and radiation therapy; no agent has been found useful in the prevention of lung cancer; and the benefits of lung cancer screening and early detection are mired in controversy. With half of all lung cancers in the USA now diagnosed in former smokers, it is a sobering reality that tobacco control will ameliorate but not, in the foreseeable future, eliminate the problem of lung cancer.

The PRG characterised the lung cancer problem as "enormous" in scope and noted that:

- "Chemotherapy, surgery, and radiation therapy have had a modest effect on patient outcomes."
- "Molecular events underlying the development of lung cancer are largely unknown."
- "Patients with the earliest surgical stage (T1N0) have disseminated disease between 15 and 30 percent of the time."

## How much is known about the natural history of the disease and the potential of early intervention?

In addition to emphasising the need for smoking cessation initiatives and genetic and aetiologic research, the PRG stressed the importance of research concerning early detection, stating that new imaging:

> approaches (and in particular the application of spiral CT) have the potential to identify small and early lesions that have not been readily accessible in clinical practice through more conventional detection methods ... spiral CT screening offers a unique opportunity to study early carcinogenesis, and potentially to reduce lung cancer mortality. However, the clinical and biological significance of these small and early lesions is not well understood.

Although the search for an efficacious lung cancer screening modality dates back more than 50 years, no screening modality has been shown in randomised controlled trials (RCTs) to reduce lung cancer mortality. Three influential RCTs, constituting the NCI's Early Lung Cancer Detection Project, were conducted in the 1970s and 1980s. Two of them, Johns Hopkins[3] and Memorial Sloan–Kettering,[4] showed no reduction in lung cancer mortality with a regimen of annual chest *x* ray and sputum cytology every 4 months versus annual chest *x* ray alone, indicating that sputum cytology in addition to chest *x* ray was not useful. The third trial, the Mayo Lung Project (MLP), showed no reduction in lung cancer mortality with chest *x* ray and sputum cytology every 4 months versus usual care (with participants in the usual care arm receiving only a recommendation at study entry to receive the two tests annually).[5] As no benefit of sputum cytology was observed in the Johns Hopkins and Memorial Sloan–Kettering trials, the results of the MLP were interpreted to indicate that screening chest *x* ray does not reduce lung cancer mortality.

When the Early Lung Cancer Detection Project was conceived, opinions regarding the usefulness of lung cancer screening were varied. Some institutions, including the Mayo Clinic, recommended annual screening for lung cancer using chest *x* ray and sputum cytology. However, Robert Fontana, a Mayo Clinic physician and Principal Investigator for the MLP, stated that "… when the three NCI-sponsored trials were in the formative stages, it was generally accepted that yearly chest radiography had no appreciable effect on lung cancer mortality".[6] Nevertheless, the trials were carried out. In response to screening enthusiasts, the US National Institutes of Health (NIH) held a consensus development conference on screening for lung cancer while the three trials were still several years away from reporting results. This conference, chaired by Howard Anderson of the Mayo Clinic and John Bailar of the NCI, issued a cautionary report regarding lung cancer screening, in which it was stated that[7]:

> Until the value of screening for lung cancer by these methods has been demonstrated, mass screening programs should be limited to well-designed, controlled clinical trials, with provision for analysis of results and for further diagnostic workup and treatment when indicated. While some screening programs for lung cancer have been initiated among workers in certain industries, caution is strongly recommended in starting any new ones. Screened workers cannot be assured of an overall benefit on the basis of existing data.

A fourth RCT, conducted in Czechoslovakia, provided further evidence that screening with chest *x* ray did not reduce lung cancer mortality (19 lung cancer deaths among 3172 in the screened arm and 13 among 3174 in the control arm).[8] As in the MLP, more lung cancers were diagnosed in the screened arm (108 *v* 82), more screen-detected cancers were resectable (25% *v* 16%), and survival after diagnosis was substantially longer in the screened arm. However, mortality was not reduced in the screened arm. As in the MLP, a larger trial would have been necessary to detect a small reduction in mortality. This trial compared semiannual screening by posteroanterior chest photofluorogram and sputum cytology to 3-year annual

screening and to no screening in a high risk population of men aged 40–64 years.

Over the past 20 years, the findings of NCI's Early Lung Cancer Detection Project and the Czechoslovakian trial have played a central role in shaping policy decisions concerning lung cancer screening. The results of the three US trials convinced the majority of the medical community that screening with either chest *x* ray or state-of-the-art sputum cytology was not effective at reducing lung cancer mortality, and the Czechoslovakian trial added international credence to this conclusion. In 1980, the American Cancer Society revised its previous lung cancer screening recommendations, stating that early detection of lung cancer was not recommended.[9] The national research focus shifted to smoking prevention, with the realisation that cigarette smoking was the primary cause of lung cancer.

The principal investigators of the Memorial Sloan–Kettering trial disagreed with the conclusions of the Early Lung Cancer Detection Project. Maintaining that it was wrong to conclude from these trials that early detection by chest *x* ray or sputum cytology did not lower the probability of death from lung cancer, Melamed and Flehinger wrote[10]:

> A realistic assessment of the current status of lung cancer in the USA, however, permits us only to reaffirm the present importance of identifying lung cancer while the patient is still asymptomatic, and to re-state our view that a decision to advise against efforts to detect lung cancer early is equivalent to a decision not to treat for cure. The weight of evidence continues to support the prudent medical practitioner who recommends regular screening of asymptomatic persons at high risk for lung cancer.

## What are the possible treatment options following screening?

When a lung tumour is limited to the hemithorax and can be completely excised, surgery is the preferred treatment. Screening, as evidenced in the MLP, identifies more early stage (Stage I and II) tumours that can be resected. Disseminated disease, as evidenced by involved lymph nodes, for which chemotherapy is standard treatment, offers much poorer survival prognosis.

## How effective are screening/treatment options in terms of mortality and morbidity?

*Post-hoc* mathematical modelling of the progression kinetics of lung cancer using the Memorial Sloan–Kettering trial data hypothesised that there could be a small mortality reduction attendant to *x* ray screening of less than 20%.[11] Unfortunately, the MLP had inadequate statistical power to identify such a small but clinically important effect. The NCI is currently revisiting this question of effectiveness of lung cancer screening in the Prostate, Lung, Colorectal, and Ovarian (PLCO) Cancer Screening Trial.[12] In the PLCO Trial, the intervention arm is offered an initial and three subsequent annual chest $x$ rays (participants who have never smoked receive only two annual chest $x$ rays) while the control arm receives usual care. This trial has 90% statistical power to detect a 20% reduction in lung cancer mortality. PLCO randomisation concluded at almost 155 000 participants on July 2, 2001; lung cancer screening will conclude in July 2004.

Although lacking the statistical power to identify a small but important reduction in lung cancer mortality, data from the MLP have provided important insights on other issues concerning lung cancer screening. More lung cancers were detected in the screened arm (206 $v$ 160 in the usual care group) and a greater percentage were completely resectable (46% $v$ 32% in the usual care arm). Nevertheless, the cumulative numbers of late stage, unresectable lung cancers in the two groups were almost identical year by year and at no point in the trial was lung cancer mortality significantly lower for the intervention arm.[6] In fact, mortality was a little higher (although not significantly different) in the screened arm (3·2/1000 person-years $v$ 3·0/1000 person-years) at the end of the trial. Strauss *et al.* have interpreted this constellation of findings as indication of a screening benefit and evidence of study flaws, including group incomparability.[13] Others recognise a pattern that strongly suggests overdiagnosis, that is, the diagnosis of cancers that would never have been diagnosed in the absence of screening.[14]

### Extended follow up and reanalysis of the Mayo Lung Project

Marcus and Prorok[15] investigated the possibility that the negative results of the MLP were due to an imbalance of lung cancer risk and prognostic factors across study arms. Using proportional hazards models, the authors examined whether age at entry, history of cigarette smoking, exposure to non-tobacco lung carcinogens and previous pulmonary illnesses confounded the relationship of screening and lung cancer mortality; they also examined whether this relationship was modified by those factors. Neither adjustment for, nor stratification by, these factors altered the original findings of the MLP. To address the possibility that longer follow up of the MLP participants might reveal a mortality reduction, Marcus and colleagues, using a National Death Index Plus search, conducted an additional 14 years of lung cancer mortality follow up for the MLP participants.[16] The result remained the same: lung cancer

mortality was slightly higher for the intervention arm (4·4 deaths per 1000 person-years versus 3·9 per 1000 person-years in the usual care arm; $P$ value = 0·08). These two analyses addressed the major criticisms levelled at the MLP and reinforced the original finding of no reduction in lung cancer mortality with an intense regimen of screening.

All evidence argues against recommending screening for lung cancer by chest $x$ ray or sputum cytology.

### Low dose spiral computed tomography as a lung cancer screening modality

Low dose helical computed tomography (helical CT or spiral CT), an advance in CT technology introduced during the 1990s, has been observed to be more sensitive than chest $x$ ray for identifying lesions in the lung. Low dose spiral CT offers rapid image acquisition at radiation doses substantially below standard high resolution CT making it a candidate for lung cancer screening.[17] The potential for mass screening using spiral CT in Japan was investigated in 1996.[18] Of 5483 smokers and non-smokers between the ages of 40 and 74 years screened in a mobile unit, 279 received work-ups for suspicious findings, 29 underwent surgery, and 23 cancers were diagnosed on the first screen. Some patients received one repeat screen over a 2-year period, and of the 60 cancers detected throughout the period 40 (two-thirds) were not seen on retrospective interpretation of chest radiographs.

The most publicised results regarding the use of low dose spiral CT as a lung cancer screening modality were reported by the NCI-supported Early Lung Cancer Action Project (ELCAP).[19] ELCAP recruited 1000 volunteers at elevated risk of lung cancer (at least 10 pack-years of smoking) and screened them with both chest $x$ ray and low dose spiral CT. In this group, the baseline (prevalence) spiral CT screen detected all non-calcified nodules visible on chest $x$ ray and also identified other lesions: spiral CT detected non-calcified nodules in 233 participants (malignant disease confirmed in 27), while chest $x$ ray detected non-calcified nodules in only 68 participants (malignant disease confirmed in seven). Additionally, four cancers not characterised as nodules were detected by spiral CT. The findings of ELCAP suggest that spiral CT is more sensitive than chest $x$ ray. ELCAP reported finding an additional seven cancers (six non-small cell and one small cell) in this population on repeat screens.[20] Thirty positive screens of the 1184 annual repeat screens resulted in six non-small cell cancers (five of Stage IA) and one small cell cancer. In two instances, the patient died of other causes before diagnostic work-up, the nodules spontaneously resolved in 12, nodules were not enlarging in eight, and eight underwent biopsy for possible cancer. But, because the ELCAP incorporates no equivalent control group for comparison, it lacks the ability to determine the impact of spiral CT screening on mortality or to directly compare harms against possible benefits of screening.

The NCI is also funding a project at the Mayo Clinic in which men and women over 50 years of age with a smoking history of at least 20 pack-years are being screened with spiral CT and sputum cytology.[21] This study in 1 year enrolled 1520 individuals, almost two-thirds of whom were current smokers and the rest former smokers. Indeterminate nodules were found in 775 subjects and 13 lung cancers were diagnosed (12 identified on CT). As with ELCAP, no comparison arm exists in the study for the purpose of assessing the impact of screening on mortality.

There is widespread appreciation that an RCT is needed to determine the mortality reducing efficacy and risks of spiral CT screening for lung cancer. Since early 2000, NCI has sponsored several workshops at which the need for an RCT with ample statistical power to detect a modest reduction in lung cancer mortality was debated and endorsed.[21] The need for an RCT has been argued in the peer-reviewed literature by independent radiologists as well.[14,22]

To assess the feasibility of conducting an RCT of spiral CT for lung cancer screening, the Lung Screening Study (LSS), a 12-month special study within the PLCO Trial, was undertaken in September 2000. The goals were to determine the ability to randomise high risk candidates around the nation to spiral CT versus chest x ray, determine background use of spiral CT, measure cross-over contamination between screening arms, and assess downstream follow up burden. The accrual goal was to randomise 3000 non-PLCO participants aged 55–74 years over a 2-month period at six PLCO screening centres. Randomised individuals received either a single spiral CT or chest x ray screen. Screening was completed on January 31, 2001. Medical record abstracting of diagnostic follow up to positive screens was completed by the end of May 2001. Interest was twice as great as projected, and recruitment mailings had to be discontinued ahead of schedule: 3373 eligible participants were randomised. Previous use of SCT by interested participants was very low at all centres (< 3%). Compliance with screening examinations exceeded 95%. Cross-over contamination from the chest x ray to spiral CT was less than 2%. Positivity rates for SCT and chest x ray were consistent with ELCAP. Investigators plan to publish the data from this feasibility project in 2003.

## New initiatives to evaluate spiral CT

Publication of the ELCAP findings sparked intense international interest in spiral CT for lung cancer screening. Several European countries and the USA are developing

RCT designs to assess the effect of spiral CT screening on mortality. The trial designs under consideration vary by country, as shown in Table 18.1 and the following text. Designs comparing spiral CT to chest x ray reflect the possibility that chest x ray may have a small, but as yet unknown impact on lung cancer mortality. If chest x ray is found in the PLCO Trial to have no effect, these designs will be equivalent to the spiral CT versus usual care design (apart from harms incurred by screening chest x ray and medical management). Randomised controlled trials to evaluate spiral CT for lung cancer screening are under consideration in Denmark, France, Germany, Italy, the Netherlands, Norway and the UK. Israel has begun an RCT, and in the USA, the National Lung Screening Trial, a large RCT, began randomising in the fall of 2002. Table 18.1 summarises the status and designs under consideration. Additional design detail is provided in the subsequent text.

*Denmark (proposed)*: 4000 men and women aged 50–65 years with a smoking history of at least 20 pack-years will be randomised to spiral CT versus usual care. Participants must be current smokers, be able to climb two flights of stairs in 30 seconds with no pausing (measuring fitness for surgery) and have a forced expiratory volume of 1000 ml in one second; they must not have a history of any malignancy (excluding basal cell carcinoma) or other disease that would preclude surgery for lung cancer. Recruitment will be completed in 1 year. Screening will consist of an initial plus five repeat annual screens. Participants in both arms will be invited annually for spirometry, smoking cessation counselling, and quality of life assessment. Participants will be recruited by mail from Copenhagen, Frederiksberg and Copenhagen County. The first interim analysis is expected to be done at the end of the fourth study year.

*France (feasibility phase)*: 40 000 men women aged 50–75 years with a smoking history of at least 15 cigarettes for more than 20 years will be randomised to annual multislice spiral CT. Participants can be current or former smokers, must be able to climb two flights of stairs without significant breathlessness; they must not have current signs or prior history of cancer. Recruitment will be conducted as quickly as possible. Screening will consist of an initial and five repeat screens, and participants will be followed for 10 years. Participants in both arms will receive smoking cessation counselling. Participants will be recruited through 10 000 general practices. Grouped sequential design methods will be employed from the beginning of the study. A pilot phase with enrolled subjects (1000 at the time of writing) is currently underway and is expected to take 2 years.

*Germany (proposed)*: Upto 10 000 men and women aged 50–69 years with at least a 40-year history of smoking will be randomised to spiral CT versus chest x ray. These are intended to contribute to a proposed European collaboration of evaluation of spiral CT screening for lung cancer.

Table 18.1  New randomised controlled trials initiatives

| Country (status) | Smoking history (pack-years) | Size (I/C)* | Randomised by | Calculated effect (%)/power (%) | Screens | Intervention |
|---|---|---|---|---|---|---|
| Denmark (P;m) | 20 | 2000/2000 | Individual | NA | T0 & annual × 5 | SCT v UC |
| France (F;$m) | 15 Cigarettes a day for more than 20 years | 20 000/20 000 | Individual | 20/90 | T0 & annual × 5 | SCT v CXR |
| Germany (P;m) | 40 years | 5000/5000 | Individual | NA | T0 & annual × 4 | SCT v CXR |
| Italy (P;m) | 20 | 6000/6000 | Individual | 35/80 | T0 & annual × 3 | SCT v UC |
| Israel (A;$;m) | 20 | 2500/2500 | Individual | NA | T0 & annual × 5 | SCT v UC |
| Netherlands (A;$m) | 20 Cigarettes a day for 20 years | 8000/16 000 | Individual | 20/90 | ? | SCT v UC |
| Norway (P;m) | 20 | 12 000/12 000 | Individual | ?/80 | T0 & annual × 5 | SCT v UC |
| UK (P;f) | Smokers? | 1000/1000 | Individual | NA | T0 & annual × 1 | SCT v UC |
| UK (P;m) | | 25 000/25 000 | Individual | NA | T0 & annual × 5 | SCT v UC |
| USA (A;$;m) | 30 | 25 000/25 000 | Individual | 20/90 | T0 & annual × 2 | SCT v CXR |

Abbreviations: Status: A, active; P, proposed; $, funded; f, feasibility project; m, mortality endpoint trial; T0, baseline screen; SCT, spiral CT; CXR, chest x ray; UC, usual care
*Size (Intervention/Control) is actual only for the active projects; all else represents approximate planning projections.

Participants can be current or former smokers (if younger than 60 years, former smokers must have quit within the last 5 years), must have a life expectancy of 10 years and be able to undergo chest surgery; they must not have serious illnesses or a history of lung cancer. Recruitment will be completed in 2 years. Screening will consist of an initial and four repeat screens. Participants in both arms will be asked to donate blood for future research. Participants will be recruited via media advertising or direct mail to 2 screening centres in Germany.

*Italy (proposed)*: 12 000 men and women aged 55–69 years with a smoking history of at least 20 pack-years will be randomised to spiral CT versus usual care. Participants can be current or former smokers (former smokers must have quit within the last 10 years), and must be able to undergo curative surgery for lung cancer; they must not have been diagnosed with cancer (except for basal cell carcinoma). Recruitment will be completed in 1 year. Screening will consist of an initial and three repeat screens. Participants in both arms will receive smoking cessation counselling. Participants will be recruited via general practices. The first interim analysis is expected to occur in the sixth study year.

*Israel (active)*: 5000 men and women aged 45–75 years with a smoking history of at least 20 pack-years will be randomised to spiral CT, spirometry and sputum cytology versus usual care. Participants can be current or former smokers (former smokers must have quit within the last 5 years); they must not have active cancer (except skin), a severe heart condition, or a life expectancy of less than 7 years. It is unknown when recruitment will be completed. Screening will consist of an initial screen and five repeat screens. It is unknown whether participants receive other tests or partake in other activities. Participants will be recruited by media and advertising in general practitioner's offices. The date of the first interim analysis is unknown. About 1000 participants were randomised and screened as of June 2001.

*Netherlands (funded, start date May 2003)*: 24 000 men and women aged 50–75 years with an average smoking history of at least 20 cigarettes a day for at least 20 years will be randomised (ratio of 1:2) to CT versus usual care. Participants can be current or former smokers (former smokers must have quit within 5 years), and must have a functional capacity that corresponds with at least 4 metabolic equivalent levels (ACC/AHA) and/or the ability to climb at least 36 steps. Participants must not have a prior history of breast cancer, melanoma, or hypernephroma, and must be willing to undergo curative therapy if lung cancer is detected. Recruitment will be completed in 1 year. The exact screening regimen is unknown. Participants in the

screened arm will donate blood for future research. Participants will be recruited by mail questionnaires using population registries in Rotterdam, Utrecht, Groningen, Haarlem and Leuven (Belgium).

*Norway (proposed)*: 24 000 men and women aged 60–69 years with a smoking history of at least 20 pack-years will be randomised to spiral CT versus usual care. Participants can be current or former smokers (former smokers must have quit within 5 years). Recruitment will be completed in about 1 year. Screening will consist of spiral CT and sputum analysis at the initial visit and annual spiral CT in the subsequent 5 years. Participants in the screened arm will receive spirometry, receive counselling on diet if blood lipids are high, and will donate blood for future research. Participants will be recruited from an established cohort of high risk individuals. The date of the first interim analysis is unknown.

*UK (proposed)*: 2000 men and women aged 60 years will be randomised to spiral CT versus usual care as part of a feasibility project of a larger trial (40 000–60 000). Participants must be current smokers; they must not have any serious illness that would render the person unlikely to benefit from screening. Recruitment to the feasibility project will be completed in 1 year. Screening will consist of one initial screen and one repeat screen. Participants in both arms will be offered a smoking cessation programme. Participants will be recruited through the MRC General Practice Framework.

*USA (active)*: The National Lung Screening Trial (NLST) was developed in part based on the results of the LSS feasibility study. The design calls for 50 000 participants to be randomised to either spiral CT or chest *x* ray. Screening consists of three annual screens (one initial and two repeat). The inclusion criteria are similar to those in the LSS trial (for example, 30 pack-years of smoking, age 55–74, current smoker or former smoker who quit within the last 15 years). Randomisation began in the fall of 2002. The first interim analysis is planned to occur in 2005, and NLST is expected to be completed by 2009.

## How acceptable are screening methods?

Chest *x* ray is a standard clinical procedure and is widely considered to confer low radiation risk (7–12 mrem, compared to annual ambient exposures of about 500 mrem in the USA). The production of sputum for cytologic analysis requires substantial uncomfortable effort from subjects. Spiral CT is a quick and painless screening procedure requiring a 25-second breath hold, which most heavy smokers can achieve when coached effectively.

## What are the costs of screening and subsequent work-up?

Spiral CT screening can cost anywhere from $350 to two or three times that amount in private practice settings. Chest *x* ray may cost about a third as much. Sputum cytology, not a typical procedure, may fall somewhere in the middle. The costs of screening are only the beginning. Follow up procedures to differentially diagnose and treat screen-detected cancers can generate tens of thousands of dollars in charges.

## What is the cost-effectiveness of screening?

Cato *et al.*[23] and Okamoto[24] have attempted to evaluate the potential cost-effectiveness of screening for lung cancer in the USA and Japan, respectively. Each concluded that screening was potentially cost-effective; however, since the true effectiveness of spiral CT or chest *x* ray screening in reducing lung cancer mortality is not known, these analyses relied on postulated benefits of screening. Currently, plans for cost-effectiveness analyses in both PLCO and NLST are being developed. Such analyses will try to estimate the costs associated with a screening programme and weigh these against the beneficial effects of screening, if any. Costs of a screening programme include the costs of the screen, as well as the costs of diagnostic follow up and the costs of treating overdiagnosed cases.

## Unresolved issues

Many issues are yet to be addressed regarding spiral CT screening. Will the high sensitivity of spiral CT result in substantial overdiagnosis, overtreatment and unacceptable harm, or will it be possible to refine the diagnostic process so as to achieve acceptable specificity? ELCAP is applying imaging-based algorithms to determine if lesions detected on spiral CT are growing. Those that appear to be static are considered safe to follow by periodic rescreens. Those that appear to be growing are considered potentially malignant and in need of immediate treatment. It is unclear if this approach will be adequate to minimise harms without diminishing potential efficacy. Uncertainty among experts regarding how to manage the assessment of lesions less than 3 mm in diameter and so called ground-glass opacities was a topic of extensive discussion at the 5th International Conference on Screening for Lung Cancer, October 26–28.[25] Investigators proposing RCTs to evaluate spiral CT are also planning to address screening risks, reliability of image interpretation, optimising the sensitivity/specificity relationship and cost-effectiveness.

In the mean time, advocates of spiral CT screening for lung cancer are active. In the USA newspapers and television advertisements impute benefits to screening. Laypersons and medical professionals are advocating screening, in the belief that screening, if not of proven benefit, is at least not harmful and should be available to all. Waiting to learn if screening is more beneficial than harmful is often considered unacceptable, while doing trials to "further characterise and quantify the risks involved" is acceptable, but should not impede the widespread application of spiral CT screening, some argue.[26]

Recently resurrected enthusiasm for lung cancer screening is based upon intuition and logic rather than carefully controlled trials assessing health outcomes – both good and bad. The history of medicine, for example national neuroblastoma screening in Japan[27,28] tells us that enthusiastic embracement of medical technology – even when well-intended – can lead to unintended harm. In the case of lung cancer screening in particular, trials using chest *x* ray and sputum cytology documented that early calls for widespread implementation were misplaced. The consequences of misplaced enthusiasm can cause harm as well as benefit. It is important to get the answer right. Meticulous application of the scientific method in rigorously designed and conducted trials will not fail us.

## References

1 van Klaveren RJ, Habbema JDF, Pedersen JF, de Koning HJ, Oudkerk M, Hoogsteden HC. Lung cancer screening by low-dose spiral computed tomography. *Eur Respir J* 2001;**18**:857–866.

2 The Report of the Lung Cancer Progress Review Group, 2001 is available on line at http://osp.nci.nih.gov/prg_assess/prg/lungprg/lung_rpt.htm

3 Frost JK, Ball WCJ, Levin ML *et al.* Early lung cancer detection: results of the initial (prevalence) radiologic and cytologic screening in the Johns Hopkins study. *Am Rev Respir Dis* 1984;**130**:549–54.

4 Flehinger BJ, Melamed MR, Zaman MB, Heelan, RT, Perchick, WB, Martini, N. Early lung cancer detection: results of the initial (prevalence) radiologic and cytologic screening in the Memorial Sloan-Kettering study. *Am Rev Respir Dis* 1984;**130**:555–60.

5 Fontana RS, Sanderson DR, Woolner LB, Taylor WF, Miller WE, Muhn JR. Lung cancer screening: the Mayo program. *J Occup Med* 1986;**28**:746–50.

6 Fontana RS, Sanderson DR, Woolner LB *et al.* Screening for lung cancer: a critique of the Mayo Lung Project. *Cancer* 1991;**67**:1155–64.

7 Gordon RS. Lung cancer mortality appears unaffected by roentgenographic and sputum screening in asymptomatic persons. *JAMA* 1979;**241**:1582.

8 Kubik A, Polak J. Lung cancer detection results of a randomized prospective study in Czechoslovakia. *Cancer* 1986;**57**:2427–37.

9 American Cancer Society Report on the cancer-related health check-up: cancer of the lung. *Cancer J Clin* 1980;**30**:199–207.

10 Melamed MR, Flehinger, BJ. Letter to the Editor. *Ann Intern Med* 1989;**111**:764–5.

11 Flehinger BJ, Kimmel M. The natural history of lung cancer in a periodically screened population. *Biometrics* 1987;**43**:127–44.

12 Gohagan JK, Levin DL, Prorok PC, Sullivan, DA, eds. The Prostate, Lung, Colorectal and Ovarian (PLCO) cancer screening trial. *Contro Clin Trials* 2000;**21**(Suppl.):249S–406S.

13  Strauss GM, Gleason RE, Shugarbaker DJ. Screening for lung cancer: another look; a different view. *Chest* 1997;754–68.

14  Black WC. Overdiagnosis: An unrecognized cause of confusion and harm in cancer screening. *J Natl Cancer Inst* 2000;**92**:1280.

15  Marcus PM, Prorok PC. Reanalysis of the Mayo Project data: the impact of confounding and effect modification. *J Cancer Screen* 1999;**6**:47–49.

16  Marcus PM, Bergstralh EJ, Fagerstrom RM *et al.* Lung cancer mortality in the Mayo Lung Project: impact of extended follow-up. *J Natl Cancer Inst* 2000;**92**:1308–16.

17  Naidich DP, Marshall CH, Gribbin C, Arams RS, McCauley DI. Low-dose CT of the lungs: preliminary observations. *Radiology* 1990;**175**:729–31.

18  Sone S, Takashima S, Li F *et al.* Mass screening for lung cancer with mobile spiral computed tomography scanner. *Lancet* 1998;**351**:1242–5.

19  Henschke CI, McCauley DI, Yankelevitz DF *et al.* Early Lung Cancer Action Project: overall design and findings from baseline screening. *Lancet* 1999;**354**:99–105.

20  Henschke CI, Naidich DP, Yankelevitz DF *et al.* Early Lung Cancer Action Project: Initial findings on repeat screening. *Cancer* 2001;**92**:153–9.

21  Division of Cancer Prevention, National Cancer Institute. Proceedings of the Spiral CT Screening for Lung Cancer Workshop, Internal Document, October 26, 1999.

22  Patz EF Jr, Rossi S, Harpole DH, Herndon JE, Goodman PC. Correlation of tumor size and survival in patients with stage 1A non-small cell lung cancer. *Chest* 2000;**117**:1568–71.

23  Cato JJ, Klittich WS, Strauss G. Could chest x-ray screening for lung cancer be cost effective? *Cancer* 2000;**89**:2502–5.

24  Okamoto N. Cost-effectiveness of lung cancer screening in Japan. *Cancer* 2000;**89**:2489–93.

25  5th International Conference on Screening for Lung Cancer, October 26–28, 2001, Weill Medical College of Cornell University, New York.

26  Parles K. Low-dose spiral CT screening. Letter to the Editor. *Chest* 2001;**120**:1042–3.

27  Yamamoto K, Hanada R, Kikuchi A *et al.* Spontaneous regression of localized neuroblastoma detected by mass screening. *J Clin Oncol* 1998;**16**:1265–9.

28  Bessho F. Effect of mass screening on age-specific incidence of neuroblastoma. *Int J Cancer* 1996;**67**:520–2.

# 19 Screening for stomach cancer

*David Forman, Simon Everett, Paul Moayyedi*

Despite declining incidence rates in most developed countries, stomach cancer remains a major public health problem in much of the world especially in parts of South-East Asia, South America and Eastern Europe (Table 19.1). Rates in these high risk areas may be four- or five-fold greater than those in low risk countries such as the USA and Sweden. Males usually have approximately double the rates of females (Table 19.1).

Gastric cancer is the fourteenth most frequent cause of mortality[1] and, after lung cancer, the second most frequent cause of cancer mortality globally – the cause of an estimated 628 000 deaths each year.[2] Projections indicate that the number of new cases is likely to increase in high risk countries due to a combination of population growth and changes in the population age structure.[3] Prognosis is extremely poor with 5-year survival rarely exceeding 25%. In most countries, mortality rates are close to incidence rates (Table 19.1), indicative of the poor survival.

An effective screening modality for stomach cancer could give rise to substantive benefits in terms of a reduction in premature death and a wide range of morbidities associated with both the disease itself and treatments of limited efficacy. Until the early 1990s, the only country where population-based screening for stomach cancer has been seriously considered is Japan, which in the 1960s and 1970s had the highest incidence and mortality rates in the world. The chosen modality for screening in Japan has been barium contrast radiology, usually followed by endoscopy, with the objective of detecting early gastric cancers (EGC), confined to the mucosa or submucosa. These early cancers are then amenable to surgical resection, sometimes using minimally invasive endoscopic techniques. Mass screening for stomach cancer in people over 40 years was introduced in Japan as public health policy in 1983 and approximately 4 million participate annually.[4,5] Although this policy has been subject to some evaluation, there have been no randomised controlled trials conducted in Japan (or anywhere else) of such a screening procedure and, partly for this reason, it has never been adopted elsewhere. After a consideration of the natural history of gastric cancer, the second section of this chapter will consider, therefore, the evidence that exists regarding the efficacy of radiological screening.

**Table 19.1** Age-standardised (world) gastric cancer incidence and mortality rates per 100 000, estimated for the year 2000 in selected countries by sex

| Country | Incidence | | Mortality | |
|---|---|---|---|---|
| | Male | Female | Male | Female |
| Japan | 69·2 | 28·6 | 31·2 | 13·8 |
| Russian Federation | 42·9 | 18·0 | 35·6 | 15·2 |
| Chile | 38·7 | 15·3 | 30·1 | 12·7 |
| China | 36·1 | 17·5 | 27·0 | 13·0 |
| Colombia | 33·2 | 20·5 | 26·4 | 16·4 |
| Portugal | 30·1 | 15·0 | 22·2 | 10·9 |
| Poland | 23·0 | 8·7 | 19·2 | 7·3 |
| Italy | 19·9 | 10·3 | 14·6 | 7·6 |
| Kenya | 12·5 | 9·7 | 10·8 | 8·3 |
| UK | 12·4 | 5·5 | 10·1 | 4·8 |
| Australia | 9·6 | 5·0 | 6·1 | 3·0 |
| Sweden | 8·8 | 4·7 | 7·4 | 4·0 |
| USA | 7·6 | 3·6 | 4·5 | 2·3 |

Source: GLOBOCAN 2000 (International Agency for Cancer Research)

In recent years, a completely different screening strategy has been proposed building on the now established association between the gastric bacterium, *Helicobacter pylori*, and gastric cancer.[6] The objective here is one of primary prevention by testing for, and then eradicating through antibiotic treatment, one of the major causes of stomach cancer. To date, this has not been used as a public health measure in any population but a number of randomised controlled trials evaluating the intervention are now in progress.[7] Thus the third section of the chapter will consider evidence relating to the risks and benefits of such a strategy.

Finally there are a number of clinical conditions that are known to increase the risk of a subsequent diagnosis of stomach cancer and the question arises of whether patients with these conditions should undergo routine surveillance in order to diagnose any cancer at an early stage. The fourth section will thus consider available evidence on the benefits of such surveillance.

## Natural history, precursor lesions and causes of gastric cancer

Gastric cancer is often divided according to the Lauren histological classification into two subtypes: diffuse and intestinal.[8] Both of these appear to develop in a background of chronic gastritis although, whereas the intestinal type is believed to occur through a stepwise series of changes that follow on from this, diffuse cancer may develop in the absence of these changes. These steps were first described by Correa in 1975,[9] although the role of *Helicobacter pylori* infection as a causal factor in this pathway was not appreciated until some 16 years later. In Correa's model, normal gastric mucosa progresses through stages of chronic gastritis, gastric atrophy, and intestinal metaplasia to dysplasia and cancer. The precise order and mechanism for these changes is uncertain, and indeed it is possible that certain events, especially intestinal metaplasia, may be markers of premalignant change rather than being premalignant themselves. The role of *H. pylori* in causing chronic gastritis and accelerating gastric atrophy is, however, now well established. Thus, in an 11-year prospective endoscopic study, the prevalence of atrophy and intestinal metaplasia increased annually by 1·8% and 0·9% respectively in *H. pylori* infected patients, changes that were not seen in uninfected patients.[10] It is postulated that once chronic atrophic gastritis has developed, a series of genotoxic changes may occur in the gastric microenvironment that include elevation of gastric pH, reduction of the concentration of gastric juice, ascorbic acid, and promotion of bacterial proliferation, which may

contribute to increased mucosal oxidative stress and formation of non-dietary carcinogens, such as *N*-nitroso compounds, in gastric juice.[11–13] These processes may increase the chance of mutations developing in gastric epithelial cells, leading to intestinal metaplasia, dysplasia and cancer.

Usually, the chronic inflammatory response associated with *H. pylori* infection involves both antrum and corpus but is most commonly antral predominant. Patients with such pathology are more prone to the development of duodenal ulcer disease. In other patients the gastritis is corpus-predominant and it is these patients who are more likely to develop gastric ulcers, corpus atrophy, intestinal metaplasia, and are at increased risk of gastric cancer.[14] At present the factors that determine which patients will develop corpus- or antral-predominant gastritis are not clear. Strain factors such as the *cagA* and *vacA* genes are associated with increased intensity of inflammatory activity but are not responsible for determining the pattern of disease.[15] What may be of more importance are host factors and the level of basal acid secretion. *H. pylori* flourishes on non-acid secreting epithelium. Usually this is the antrum but in people with low basal acid output *H. pylori* will grow in the corpus leading to corpus inflammation, glandular destruction, and atrophy.[16] Recent studies have demonstrated that polymorphisms of the interleukin-1 gene cluster enhance production of interleukin-1$\beta$ and are associated with hypochlorhydria and gastric cancer. These polymorphisms may thus determine basal acid output, the pattern of *H. pylori* infection and subsequent cancer risk.[17]

Numerous other factors may also play a role in the aetiology of gastric cancer. These include male sex, smoking, family history, dietary factors, previous gastric surgery, and history of pernicious anaemia. Dietary factors have been investigated at length and associations with a decreased risk for gastric cancer include a high level of consumption of fresh fruit, citrus fruit, raw vegetables, wholemeal bread, bran cereals and garlic. Ascorbic acid, $\alpha$-tocopherol, beta-carotene, and selenium have all been identified as protective factors, possibly owing to antioxidant activity. Factors associated with an increased risk for gastric cancer include pickled and fermented vegetables (possibly due to high nitrate levels), beans and other dry legumes (including fava beans), salted or smoked fish, and possibly fresh meats. Nitrite intake is positively associated with gastric cancer risk in some studies and dietary protein intake has also been identified as a risk factor, possibly owing to the presence of secondary and tertiary amines for gastric nitrosation. A high intake of salt is consistently associated with gastric cancer, as is a lack of refrigeration facilities, presumably from the need to pickle and salt food for preservation.[18]

**Table 19.2  Mass screening in Shimane prefecture per annum***

| Parameter | Statistics |
|---|---|
| Total population | 687 895 |
| Target population | 265 884 (38·7%) |
| Participant population | 24 701 (9·3%) |
| Patients with abnormality in barium meal study | 5192 |
| Patients with cancer | 47 |
| Cost of barium meal screening | US$45 |
| Cost of endoscopy | US$127 |

*Data are the mean annual figures between 1979 to 1997 in Shimane prefecture, Japan.[19]

## The Japanese experience with radiological screening

Screening for stomach cancer in Japan has been organised predominantly through municipalities or workplace organisations. Initially a barium meal investigation is performed. If radiological abnormalities are seen endoscopy is performed and the area of abnormality reassessed. The number of gastric cancers detected in these screening programmes is increasing but, within screened populations, screen detection only accounts for less than half of all cases (around 35%), the remainder being diagnosed after investigation of symptoms.[19] Approximately 9–14% of the target Japanese population is screened annually.[19–22] An example of the uptake and costs of screening in a rural region of Japan is illustrated in Table 19.2.

Gastric cancer is detected in approximately 0·2% of initial examinations and approximately half of these diagnoses are of early gastric cancer (EGC).[20,23,24] Barium radiography suffers from a low positive predictive value (between 0·8% and 2·3%), primarily due to the low absolute incidence of gastric cancer.[19,20,25] Although difficult to determine accurately, the sensitivity has been estimated at between 70% and 90%. This figure may be increasing with more refinements to the screening process.[25–27] As the use of privately funded health check-ups increases, endoscopy (which may detect smaller, less advanced cancers) is being used more frequently as the initial screening test.[19]

The detection rate of curable disease has increased gradually in Japan over the past two decades coincident with the introduction of screening. EGC now accounts for around 40% of all newly diagnosed gastric cancers in Japan[28] and more than 50% in referral centres.[29–31] This compares with approximately 10% in Europe.[30] Concomitantly, average tumour size has decreased allowing greater use of endoscopic therapy – 24% of early cancers

were resected by endoscopic mucosal resection in the National Cancer Centre in Tokyo between 1988–1990.[29] Because cancers detected in mass screening programmes comprise a higher proportion of EGC, they exhibit smaller size, less invasion, increased curative resection rate and improved 5-year survival compared to cancers detected by other means, usually after onset of symptoms (Table 19.3).[19,32–34]

Mass population screening using contrast $x$ ray examination has been reported in other areas of high gastric cancer incidence, Venezuela, Chile and Russia[35,36] but, with the exception of results from Venezuela,[37] the impact of these programmes has largely gone unreported.

## Comparative survival studies

Four studies have been published in which gastric cancer survival rates have been compared between patients identified through screening and those identified through other means. These studies are summarised in Table 19.3. All of these studies were retrospective analyses of the outcome of gastric cancer detected in specific institutions. All cancers detected over a given period were included and divided into those detected by screening and those detected by symptoms through the outpatient clinic. As can be seen in Table 19.3, screened cases have a substantially higher rate of EGC detection compared with unscreened cases together with greatly improved 5-year survival (the studies show between a 14% and 37% survival difference, respectively). Such comparisons are very susceptible to lead time bias, although Kampschoer *et al.* claim that the 10 years follow up time available in their study mitigates against such bias.[33] In addition, Kubota *et al.*[19] found that 5-year survival of advanced cancer was better in screened than unscreened patients (61% compared with 29%) making overdiagnosis bias less likely, although this comparison is based on small numbers in the screened group (45 cases). However, these observations do not exclude other forms of bias. In the Kubota *et al.* study,[19] for example, there were more intestinal than diffuse cancers in screened patients (81% intestinal in screened $v$ 65% in unscreened). Since aetiology and prognosis of these two types of cancer may differ, length bias may be present. Likewise, the presence of a higher male:female ratio in the screened group implies selection bias (76% males in the screening group compared with 62% in the non-screening group).

The difficulties in interpreting studies of case fatality or survival data are perhaps illustrated by two cohorts of patients followed over two consecutive 10-year periods between 1971 and 1990.[38] The authors assume that screening rates increased over this period and, presumably

**Table 19.3 Gastric cancer screening in Japan – survival studies**

| Authors | Year | Subjects with gastric cancer* | % with EGC[†] | EGCs limited to mucosa (%) | Size (mean diameter) | Curative resection rate (%) | % Five-year survival | Comments |
|---|---|---|---|---|---|---|---|---|
| Kaibara et al.[34] | 1981 | 184 screened<br>989 other means | 43<br>24 | 44<br>47 | | 79<br>71 | 71<br>55 | |
| Kampschoer et al.[33] | 1989 | 274 screened<br>1859 other means | N/A | | | 91<br>67 | 80 (10 years 79%)<br>56 (10 years 55%) | 10-year follow up reported to reduce effect of lead time bias |
| Hanazaki et al.[32] | 1997 | 189 screened<br>517 other means | 75<br>48 | | | | 86<br>61 | |
| Kubota et al.[19] | 2000 | 196 screened<br>612 other means | 77<br>29 | 57<br>49 | 3·4 cm<br>6·6 cm | 96<br>74 | 81<br>44 | Survival also better in screened patients with advanced cancer – may reduce effect of over diagnosis bias. Different histological types and gender ratios in the two groups |

*Patients with gastric cancer detected either in screening programme or by other means, usually as a result of symptoms in a clinic setting.
[†]The proportion of all gastric cancers that were early gastric cancers.
[‡]5 years and 10 years – 5-year and 10-year survival respectively for all cancers detected.

as a consequence, the proportion of EGC increased from 30% to 48% in the two periods. The 5-year survival rate for EGC was more than 90%, resulting in an improvement in mean 5-year survival for all patients from 54% to 68%. However, the number of advanced cancers stayed the same (183 and 178) and the 5-year survival for advanced cancers did not improve over the study period (44%). Thus, the improvement in 5-year survival may simply reflect registration of greater numbers of EGCs, whilst the number of deaths may not have changed overall.[39] It is evident, therefore, that improvements in survival rates do not necessarily result in an absolute reduction in cancer deaths, underlining the potential for bias in any uncontrolled observational study.[39]

## Cohort studies

Gastric cancer mortality data from cohort studies are also conflicting. The only two such published studies are summarised in Table 19.4. In a large study by Hisamichi *et al.*[24] the cancer mortality rate was significantly lower in screened than unscreened patients over an 18-year follow up period. On the other hand, Inaba *et al.* followed 24 134 subjects and found that screening did not reduce gastric cancer mortality, although the follow up period of 40 months was much shorter.[21] Again, these studies were not randomised and, consequently, are open to selection bias. This may become apparent as different diet, smoking behaviour, parental history of gastric cancer and health beliefs between frequently screened and unscreened individuals.[22,40] In the study of Inaba *et al.*,[21] numerous dietary differences were noted between screened and unscreened patients (higher intakes of beta-carotene, vitamin C, and salt among the screened population), which may affect the risk of gastric cancer developing. Lower all-cause mortality in screened subjects also suggests health-seeking behaviour in these patients and overestimation of the effect of screening on gastric cancer mortality.

## Case–control studies

In case–control studies patients with gastric cancer are matched to disease-free controls and the screening histories compared. All those that have analysed gastric cancer are summarised in Table 19.5. Three have shown that individuals who have died from gastric cancer are about half as likely to have previously had a screening examination and one has shown a similar effect of screening on the diagnosis of advanced cancer.[5,27,41,42] A fifth Venezuelan case–control study, the only one from outside Japan, showed no survival benefit from screening.[37] These studies attempt to control for bias by matching cases and controls – usually by age, sex and address. However, as discussed previously, differences

can be subtle and are usually insufficiently controlled for in this study design.

## Incidence to mortality ratios

Mortality from gastric cancer has been falling worldwide since the 1950s. The rate of decline is similar in most countries, including Japan, and is estimated at about 20% every 5 years.[43] The explanation for this change is uncertain but may relate to dietary factors or changes in *Helicobacter pylori* infection rates. In comparison with other countries, however, the decline in mortality in Japan has been significantly greater than the decline in incidence and this has resulted in a different incidence to mortality ratio (Tables 19.1 and 19.6).[44] This has led some to suggest that detection of early forms of gastric cancer may account, at least in part, for this fall in mortality.[27]

However, an alternative interpretation is that incidence rates are higher in Japan due to the detection and registration of more benign disease that may not have affected the lifespan of the patient had it not been detected. EGC may take many months or years to become advanced. In a study of the natural history of 56 early cancers, half took longer than 44 months to progress beyond the submucosa.[45] This lengthy latent period means that a minority of individuals diagnosed with early gastric cancer may not be affected by it if left undetected. This effect will be greatest where EGC is most common. Furthermore, criteria for diagnosing gastric cancer differ between the West and Japan. Western pathologists require invasion of the lamina propria whereas Japanese pathologists may base the diagnosis on nuclear and glandular changes. As a consequence, Japanese pathologists are more likely to diagnose a gastric lesion as cancer than their Western colleagues, who may label the same lesion as dysplastic.[46] Thus, differences in mortality and incidence rates between different countries are difficult to interpret, cannot be taken as strong evidence of a benefit of screening and may even imply overdiagnosis of cancer.[43,44,47]

## Screening and treatment for *Helicobacter pylori*

Radiological and/or endoscopic diagnosis of early gastric cancer is invasive and likely to be too expensive to consider in Western societies. An alternative screening strategy could involve removing a major environmental carcinogen before the development of malignancy. Such primary prevention would be likely to have a greater impact on gastric cancer mortality than screening for early disease. Although potential primary prevention strategies exist around dietary modifications (such as encouraging low salt, high vitamin C diets), the problems associated with dietary modification

**Table 19.4** Gastric cancer screening in Japan – cohort studies

| Authors | Year | Subjects | Age | Follow up | Relative risk (95% CI) of death from gastric cancer | Relative risk (95% CI) of deaths due to other causes | Comments |
|---|---|---|---|---|---|---|---|
| Hisamichi and Sugawara[24] | 1984 | 4325 screened 2683 unscreened | 40–69 years | 18 years | Gastric cancer mortality rate ($\times 0^{-5}$) Males screened: 61·9 unscreened: 137·2 RR: 0·45 (P <0·005) Females screened: 28·1 unscreened: 53·8 RR: 0·52 (P <0·01) | | Gastric cancer incidence rate also lower (non-significantly) in screened patients. Study details not clearly described |
| Inaba et al.[21] | 1999 | 14 992 unscreened 9142 screened in previous year | >41 years | 40 months | Males: 0·72 (0·31–1·66) Females: 1·46 (0·43–4·90) | Males 0·83 (0·67–1·01) Females 0·77 (0·60–1·01) | Data adjusted for smoking, age, previous peptic ulcer and diet (carotene, vitamin C and salt) |

**Table 19.5  Gastric cancer screening – case–control studies**

| Authors | Year | Subjects | Matching | Odds ratio (95% CI) of death or advanced cancer in screened to unscreened patients | Comments |
|---|---|---|---|---|---|
| Oshima et al[41] | 1986 | 90 gastric cancer deaths, 261 controls | Age (5 years), sex and same location | Death from gastric cancer Males: 0·60 (0·34–1·05)* Females: 0·38 (0·19–0·79) | Calculated for ever screened previously, excluding previous 12 months |
| Fukao et al, after Hisamichi[27] | 1987 | 218 advanced gastric cancer 218 controls | | Diagnosis of advanced cancer Overall: 0·4–0·7 | Odds ratio lower with shorter interval between screenings. (Data taken from Hisamichi, 1989[27]) |
| Pisani et al[37] | 1994 | 241 cases 2410 controls | Age (3 years), sex and same location | Death from gastric cancer Overall: 1·26 (0·83–1·91) Males: 1·52 (0·94–2·47) Females: 0·77 (0·33–1·78) | Study performed in Venezuela Calculated for ever screened previously, excluding previous 6 months |
| Fukao et al[5] | 1995 | 198 gastric cancer deaths 577 controls | Age (3 years), sex and same location | Death from gastric cancer Overall: 0·41 (0·28–0·61) Males: 0·32 (0·19–0·53) Females: 0·63 (0·34–1·16) | Calculated for screening history in previous 5 years |
| Abe et al[42] | 1995 | 800 gastric cancer deaths 2400 controls | Age (3 years), sex and same location | Death from gastric cancer Males: 0·42 (0·28–0·61) Females: 0·48 (0·28–0·82) | Calculated for ever screened previously |

*90% confidence intervals.

**Table 19.6** Worldwide incidence to mortality ratios*

| Population | Incidence: Mortality ratio | |
| --- | --- | --- |
| | Male | Female |
| Japan | 2·1 | 1·9 |
| Norway | 1·2 | 1·3 |
| Poland | 0·8 | 0·9 |
| UK | 1·5 | 1·5 |
| USA | | |
| Black | 1·6 | 1·5 |
| White | 1·8 | 1·5 |
| Iberian peninsula | 0·8 | 0·7 |

*Data age-adjusted to world standard population from Correa *et al.*, 1994.[44]

make, at least in theory, an option of *H. pylori* screening and treatment more achievable.[48]

**The evidence base**

*H. pylori* is a spiral-shaped Gram-negative bacterium that primarily colonises the human stomach. It is one of the most common bacterial infections in the world – possibly as much as half the world's population being infected but with prevalence in developing countries reaching higher levels.[49] Infection is usually acquired in childhood and, once established in the stomach, the host immune response is rarely effective in eradicating the organism. Thus infection and its sequelae are usually lifelong.

The evidence that *H. pylori* infection is a major cause of distal gastric cancer has several strands. The malignancy most commonly arises within a histopathological background of chronic gastritis, which progresses to gastric atrophy, intestinal metaplasia, dysplasia and finally adenocarcinoma.[50,51] Although this pathological sequence was widely accepted before the discovery of *H. pylori* infection, there has since been substantive evidence to demonstrate that infection is the main cause of chronic gastritis and is strongly associated with gastric atrophy and intestinal metaplasia.[52] Several observational studies and randomised controlled trials[53,54] have demonstrated that *H. pylori* eradication reverses chronic gastritis.

The evidence, largely from non-randomised observational studies, that treatment will lead to regression of more advanced histological phenotypes, is difficult to interpret mainly because of insufficient sample size, short length of follow up and problems with endpoint definition. The best evidence has been from a randomised, placebo-controlled trial that assessed the effects of anti-*H. pylori* therapy, vitamin C and beta-carotene with a factorial design[55]: 976 Colombian subjects were randomised and 631 completed

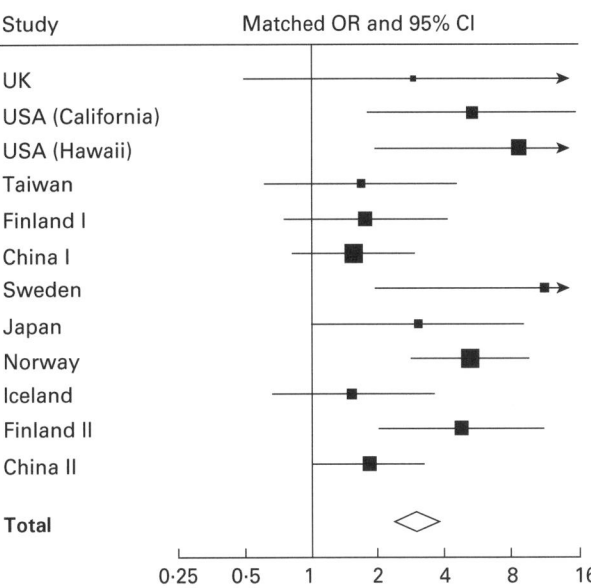

**Figure 19.1**  Pooled analysis of nested case–control studies of the association between *H. pylori* infection and gastric cancer. The diamond (◇) shows odds ratio for all studies combined[59]

follow up for a mean of 6 years. All interventions were associated with a statistically significant regression of intestinal metaplasia and atrophy with no added benefit in combining interventions. In particular, *H. pylori* eradication therapy was associated with a relative risk (RR) of 4·8 (95% CI 1·6–14·2) for regression of atrophy and an RR of 3·1 (95% CI 1·0 to 9·3) for regression of intestinal metaplasia.[55] Another randomised study in China,[54] with only 1 year of follow up, showed a smaller effect on intestinal metaplasia and none on atrophy. Further such randomised studies are in progress in other regions of China, Mexico, Italy and in a European collaborative study.[7]

The evidence derived from epidemiology of gastric cancer *per se* (rather than precancerous lesions) has, to date, largely been from observational studies. A large number of retrospective serological studies have been reported[56] although these have considerable design problems as severe atrophy in the years preceding cancer diagnosis may lead to loss of infection and false negative antibody status.[57,58] The most persuasive epidemiological evidence is summarised in a pooled reanalysis of 12 nested case–control studies from prospective studies (see Figure 19.1). The risk of developing distal gastric cancer showed a statistically significant three-fold increase in *H. pylori* seropositive cases compared with seronegative individuals. This risk increased to almost six-fold if the infection was present at least 10 years before the development of neoplasia.[59]

Two recent prospective cohort studies from Japan have also shown an association between *H. pylori* infection and

**Table 19.7** Systematic review of the accuracy of serology in detecting *Helicobacter pylori* infection[79]

| Country | Kit | Gold standard | Sensitivity (%) | Specificity (%) | Positive LR | Negative LR |
|---------|-----|---------------|-----------------|-----------------|-------------|-------------|
| UK | Premier (Meridian Diagnostics) | Urease, histology | 99 | 99 | 99 | 0·01 |
| USA | | Urease, histology | 74 | 89 | 7 | 0·29 |
| USA | HM-CAP EIA | $^{13}$C-UBT | 98 | 96 | 25 | 0·02 |
| USA | Pyloristat (BioWhittaker) | $^{13}$C-UBT | 99 | 90 | 10 | 0·01 |
| USA | GAP (Bio Rad) | $^{13}$C-UBT | 99 | 26 | 1 | 0·04 |
| France | Pyloristat (BioWhittaker) | Culture, urease | 91 | 86 | 7 | 0·1 |
| USA | Hp Chek | Histology, urease | 88 | 85 | 6 | 0·14 |
| USA | Flexsure HP (SmithKline) | $^{13}$C-UBT | 96 | 95 | 19 | 0·04 |
| France | Pyloriset (Orion Diagnostica) | Culture, urease | 91 | 87 | 7 | 0·1 |

Abbreviations: LR, likelihood ratio; $^{13}$C-UBT, $^{13}$C-urea breath test

cancer consistent with the results of the nested case–control studies.[60,61] In one of these studies, Uemura *et al.*[60] observed the development of gastric cancer in 36 gastroenterology patients over 7 years among 1246 with ongoing *H. pylori* infection compared with no cancers in 280 patients without infection or in 253 who received eradication therapy. In an earlier non-randomised study, the same authors showed that *H. pylori* eradication prevents the recurrence of neoplasia in patients having endoscopic mucosal resection for early gastric cancer.[62]

Randomised controlled trials looking at the effect of *H. pylori* screening and treatment on gastric cancer incidence and mortality are in progress in China and the UK.[7] Difficulties in recruitment have led to the abandonment of randomisation designs in other such studies in Japan and Germany.[63] It will be several years hence before the two ongoing trials report their cancer results.

Alongside the above evidence, geographical correlation studies also lent support to the association,[64,65] although it has been frequently noted that some populations, mainly in developing countries, have extremely high levels of infection prevalence but relatively low gastric cancer rates.[66,67] It is, however, invariably the case that, within populations, both *H. pylori* infection prevalence and gastric cancer incidence are strongly associated with indicators of social deprivation.[68,69] Although not frequently studied, secular trends in *H. pylori* infection prevalence have also declined in common with gastric cancer incidence.[70]

Apart from the epidemiological evidence there are now animal model systems, notably the Mongolian gerbil, in which a direct relationship between *H. pylori* infection and gastric cancer has been observed.[71,72] Many mechanisms have been advanced regarding the process of carcinogenesis within the human stomach subsequent to *H. pylori* infection.[73] In general, it is thought that it is the persistent inflammation of the ongoing infection and accompanying host response that renders the gastric epithelial cells susceptible to carcinogenic challenge.

The foregoing presents evidence supportive of a causal association. The absence of clear results from randomised intervention studies does mean, however, that there is no direct evidence to demonstrate that screening and treatment of *H. pylori* infection would reduce the subsequent risk of cancer. It is not possible currently to assess, for example, whether intervening against *H. pylori* in middle-aged people would be efficacious or whether the process of cancer development may have already advanced too far. Results from the Colombian intervention study of precancerous lesions[53] and the Japanese observational studies[60,61] are encouraging but cannot be readily extrapolated to infer evidence of cancer prevention. With the current evidence base, it is impossible to estimate the likely magnitude of risk reduction following screening or the extent of any adverse effects (see below).

## Evidence relating to the screening test

There are a variety of non-invasive tests for *H. pylori*.[74] Urea breath tests are the most accurate with > 95% sensitivity and specificity but are expensive and have reduced accuracy in subjects taking antibiotics or proton pump inhibitors.[75] Faecal antigen tests may be as accurate as urea breath tests[76] but again the cost of mass screening of populations with this test becomes prohibitive.[77]

Serology has been widely used in epidemiological studies and is probably the most suitable screening test. There are two meta-analyses[78,79] on serology accuracy and tests usually have > 85% sensitivity and specificity (Table 19·7). Testing is relatively inexpensive and medication does not interfere with the accuracy of the test.[80] Near patient serology tests have been developed[81] but the accuracy of these kits varies widely in different communities.[82] Detecting antibodies to *H. pylori* antigens in the saliva is another non-invasive method of diagnosing the infection but, again, the accuracy of this method is inconsistent across different populations.[83]

The accuracy of serology is acceptable for a reasonably wide prevalence of *H. pylori* infection.[84] The positive predictive value of a test, however, becomes poor once the prevalence falls below 25%[74] and, if the proportion of the population infected with *H. pylori* is low, it may be preferable to use a faecal antigen test or urea breath test. Alternatively cut-off values could be altered or a battery of different serology tests could be used to improve accuracy. The negative predictive value of serology is not ideal once the prevalence of *H. pylori* infection rises above 75%[74] and in these situations it may be more appropriate to simply treat the whole population with antibiotics as most will harbour the organism.[85]

The sensitivity and specificity of serology varies in different populations. The reason for this is uncertain but may relate to different strains of *H. pylori* or genetic differences in the population causing diverse immune responses. The kit that is most accurate for the population being screened should be used and the appropriate cut-off should be locally validated.[86]

Treatment for *H. pylori* infection is not 100% effective and it has been suggested that subjects should be tested after treatment to ensure success. Serology is not an accurate test to determine successful *H. pylori* eradication, as the antibody response may be detectable for many years. Urea breath tests or faecal antigen tests are accurate in this situation but economic analyses suggest that follow up testing is unlikely to be cost-effective.[87]

## Evidence relating to treatment

There is a massive amount of evidence available regarding *H. pylori* treatment regimens, much of which has been reviewed elsewhere.[88] *H. pylori* is susceptible to most antibiotics *in vitro* but these are rarely effective in eradicating the organism when used alone.[89] Clinical experience has indicated that the most consistent results are seen when a proton pump inhibitor is combined with two antibiotics: clarithromycin and either amoxicillin or metronidazole for 1 week. Both these "triple-therapy" regimens would be suitable as they achieve 85–95% success rate in eradicating the organism in hospital patients.[90] These eradication rates are seen in motivated patients attending secondary care for cure of their dyspepsia. The regimens may be less efficacious when used in a community screening programme. Indeed in the one trial that evaluated this, the eradication rate was 74% in all evaluable subjects, although it remained at 85% in those that complied with medication.[91]

The advantage of the proton pump inhibitor, clarithromycin, and metronidazole triple therapy is that less acid suppression is needed and a lower dose of clarithromycin is required.[92] The overall cost of the regimen is therefore less, although metronidazole has the disadvantage that it requires abstention from alcohol while the patient is taking the drug. This regimen is also less effective in areas with a high background resistance to this class of drug, although the impact of this is relatively modest.[93] The proton pump inhibitor–amoxycillin–clarithromycin combination is more expensive and is not suitable for the 10% of the population that claims to be allergic to penicillin. It is, therefore, not ideal for a therapy used as a part of a community screening programme.

A combination of a proton pump inhibitor with clarithromycin and metronidazole may be the most suitable treatment in the developed world but clarithromycin is too expensive for many developing countries. A combination of proton pump inhibitor, amoxicillin and metronidazole could be considered in these areas, although this regimen is less efficacious particularly for imidazole-resistant strains of bacteria.[94] The "classical" triple therapy of bismuth salts, tetracycline and metronidazole is another inexpensive alternative for developing nations but the efficacy of this regimen is also compromised in 5–nitroimidazole-resistant strains, and subjects have to take up to 15 tablets a day, which is likely to lead to poor compliance.[95]

## Who should be screened?

*H. pylori* infects over half the world's population and yet only 1% or 2% of these develop gastric cancer. The risk of developing gastric cancer appears to depend on factors associated with the host and the organism.

Relatives of gastric cancer patients infected with *H. pylori* are significantly more likely to have hypochlorhydria and gastric atrophy than their spouses or age-, sex- and social

class-matched controls.[96] Differences in host genetic factors, such as polymorphisms in the interleukin-1β gene,[17] may play a role in determining which infected individuals develop cancer, but at present there are no definitive genetic factors that can be targeted to reduce the number of subjects being offered screening.

Different *H. pylori* strains have varying abilities to cause disease and investigators have identified several genes that make the organism more pathogenic. The majority of these markers require upper gastrointestinal endoscopy and therefore cannot be applied to populations. Antibodies to the cytotoxic associated gene A (cagA) protein, however, can be detected serologically and this could have a potential for community screening. CagA-positive strains of *H. pylori* are more pathogenic than negative strains and have been shown to have a stronger association with gastric cancer.[97] However, subjects harbouring cagA negative strains may still be at greater risk of developing gastric adenocarcinoma compared to those not infected with *H. pylori*.[98] Until a more specific serological marker becomes available, screening and treating all *H. pylori*-infected subjects is likely to have the greatest impact in preventing gastric cancer mortality.[99]

## Additional benefits and potential adverse effects

Community *H. pylori* screening and treatment may reduce mortality from distal gastric cancer. The programme will also reduce the burden of complicated and uncomplicated peptic ulcer disease in the population.[100] A systematic review suggests there may also be a benefit in reducing non-ulcer dyspepsia.[101] There is therefore the possibility of large benefits to the population in terms of more life years and less dyspepsia.

The decline in prevalence of *H pylori* has been mirrored by a rise in gastro-oesophageal reflux disease (GORD). Some case–control and cohort studies have reported a negative association between *H. pylori* infection and GORD, although other results have been conflicting.[102] Confounding factors or bias may explain these results, as two randomised controlled trials have shown that *H. pylori* eradication therapy has no influence on GORD.[103,104]

Two case–control studies have suggested that *H. pylori* infection may protect against gastric cardia cancer and oesophageal adenocarcinoma[105,106] although this finding has not been confirmed by other studies[107] or in a pooled analysis.[59] A small protective effect of *H. pylori* infection on oesophageal or cardia adenocarcinoma cannot be excluded from these data but the effect, if any, is likely to be small and outweighed by the harm the infection causes.

*H. pylori* screening and treatment will lead to an increase in antibiotic exposure to the community, although the impact is likely to be small compared with overall antibiotic prescribing.[108] Nevertheless, this may increase the resistance of other organisms to the antimicrobials used in the regimen. Community-acquired pneumonia, for example, could theoretically be more difficult to treat if a macrolide is used in a an *H. pylori* screening and treatment programme. The magnitude of this effect is difficult to quantify but should be evaluated in randomised controlled trials evaluating the efficacy of this strategy.

All screening programmes will cause anxiety in some individuals.[109] *H. pylori* screening and treatment is unlikely to have any major psychological effects on the population, however, as anxiety scores in over 3000 subjects did not deteriorate after they had been enrolled into this programme, compared with baseline levels.[110] A few individuals are likely to become anxious after being told that they have a potentially carcinogenic infection even after they are given *H. pylori* eradication therapy.

## Economic evidence

Five health economic models have suggested that *H. pylori* screening and treatment is cost-effective.[87,111–114] All have used conservative assumptions and concluded that the programme is cost-effective even at gastric cancer incidences considerably lower than those currently seen in the UK. Two[111,113] of these models have also emphasised that *H. pylori* screening and treatment is unlikely to be cost-effective in subjects less than 40 years of age because the time taken to develop gastric cancer is too long. Four[87,111–113] of these models assumed that *H. pylori* screening and treatment would not have any impact on dyspepsia in the community. A large randomised controlled trial in 2329 subjects showed that *H. pylori* eradication causes a 5% reduction in dyspepsia in the community,[114,115] although interestingly the effect seemed to be limited to men. Economic data were collected during the trial, and men receiving *H. pylori* eradication therapy incurred health service dyspepsia costs reduced by £13·50 per year compared with those receiving placebo.[114] Modelling these data suggested *H. pylori* screening and treatment could actually save money over the lifetime of those being screened and, at even very conservative assumptions, the programme would cost less than £15 000 per life year saved.[114]

These results suggest *H. pylori* screening and treatment is likely to be cost-effective, although all these models assume *H. pylori* eradication will have some impact in reducing the incidence of gastric cancer and this needs confirmation from a randomised controlled trial.

Another advantage of *H. pylori* screening is that it is a one-off procedure, as three cohort studies suggest reinfection rates in adults in developed countries is less than 0·5% per year.[116,117] There is therefore no need to reduce the screening interval. There may also be a pressure to reduce screening age and this will make the programme less cost-effective.[111]

## Surveillance of high risk groups

### Postgastrectomy

The risk of developing gastric cancer following partial gastrectomy for benign ulcer disease is increased. Estimates vary, but overall risk appears to be doubled compared to non-operated controls. This increased risk is not evident (and perhaps even decreased) until 15–20 years after surgery, but rises thereafter.[118] A number of reports have demonstrated higher than expected incidence of gastric cancer in patients surveyed after partial gastrectomy.[119] Such surveys have also demonstrated that a small number of gastric cancers can be detected at an early, resectable stage.[120–123]

However, this group of patients present particular problems, namely their relatively advanced age and the morbidity and mortality of completion gastrectomy.[119] Only a limited number of comparative studies have been performed to assess the effect of surveillance on cancer survival or mortality. In a study by Offerhaus *et al.* the risk of death from gastric cancer did not differ between 962 postgastrectomy patients invited to attend a surveillance programme compared to 633 who were not.[124] A Swedish study compared 354 postgastrectomy patients who accepted surveillance with 484 who declined or were not offered surveillance.[125] After 17 years higher numbers of EGC had been detected in the study group (17 *v* 2) but there were similar numbers of gastric cancer deaths in each group (12 *v* 14).

### Pernicious anaemia

The incidence of gastric cancer in pernicious anaemia is approximately trebled compared to the expected population rate, leading to suggestions that endoscopic surveillance may be beneficial.[126] Reports of such surveillance programmes have demonstrated that gastric cancer can be found in approximately 1–3% of examinees, and that the majority of these are EGCs.[127–130] Surveillance may also detect carcinoid tumours and dysplasia, though the long-term clinical significance and management of these conditions is debatable. However, these reports also include patients diagnosed with EGC who may have been investigated because of symptoms or iron-deficient anaemia. No data comparing survival or mortality in screened and unscreened patients are available, making interpretation of these case series difficult.

## Other high risk categories

It is well established that many gastric cancers develop on a background of chronic gastritis, atrophic gastritis, and intestinal metaplasia. Thus, atrophic gastritis and intestinal metaplasia have been considered by some to be premalignant changes warranting surveillance. A study of annual endoscopies in patients with type III intestinal metaplasia (considered to be the subtype at greatest risk of gastric cancer) compared with historical controls suggested that this approach could increase the detection of EGC.[131] In a more recent study, 166 patients with mixed "high risk" lesions, namely polyps, gastric ulcers, atrophy, intestinal metaplasia, and dysplasia had annual surveillance. Gastric cancer in these patients was detected at an earlier stage and they had better 5-year survival (50% *v* 10%) than patients investigated for dyspepsia.[132] However, neither of these studies had appropriate control groups and overall mortality data are lacking making it difficult to draw firm conclusions.

## Conclusions

The Japanese case–control studies and cohort studies are suggestive of beneficial effect of gastric cancer screening in high risk populations. This is supported by the observational studies. However, these data are significantly open to bias and may profoundly overestimate the beneficial effect.[133] Furthermore, these data are not transferable to other countries in which treatment for gastric cancer may not be as effective. The only way to establish the true margin of benefit, and hence cost-effectiveness, of screening would be within a randomised controlled trial. This is unlikely to happen now in Japan but should be performed if similar screening modalities were to be contemplated in other populations. Likewise, the detection of EGC in high risk groups, such as patients with pernicious anaemia, partial gastrectomy, atrophic gastritis, or intestinal metaplasia, is not proof of benefit and more formal comparison of screened to unscreened patients is required before surveillance can be recommended (category III evidence).

A pooled analysis of prospective nested case control studies has shown that *H. pylori* infection is an important risk factor for the future development of distal gastric cancer. There is also good randomised controlled trial evidence that proton pump inhibitor triple therapy successfully eradicates *H. pylori* and this resolves chronic gastritis, thought to be important in the subsequent development of neoplasia. There is some randomised controlled trial evidence that *H. pylori* eradication may cause regression of gastric atrophy and intestinal metaplasia but, as yet, there are no randomised controlled trial data on the effect of eradication on gastric cancer mortality. The

trials currently in progress[7] are unlikely to provide a definitive answer to the question of whether mortality can be reduced within a reasonable time frame. Whether further appropriately powered trials can be both resourced and successfully initiated is currently debatable. Without an evidence base from such trials, however, it is unlikely that *H. pylori* screening programmes will be implemented on a population basis. It could be argued that an opportunity to accelerate the decline of a fatal cancer would thereby have been lost.

## References

1 Murray CJ, Lopez AD. Global mortality, disability, and the contribution of risk factors: Global Burden of Disease Study. *Lancet* 1997;**349**:1436–42.
2 Pisani P, Parkin DM, Bray F, Ferlay J. Estimates of the worldwide mortality from 25 cancers in 1990. *Int J Cancer* 1999;**83**:18–29.
3 Forman D. Should we go further and screen and treat? *Eur J Gastroenterol Hepatol* 1999;**11**(Suppl. 2):S69–S71.
4 Kawai K. Screening for gastric cancer in Japan. *Clin Gastroenterol* 1978;**7**:605–22.
5 Fukao A, Tsubono Y, Tsuji I, Hisamichi S, Sugahara N, Takano A. The evaluation of screening for gastric cancer in Miyagi Prefecture, Japan: a population-based case-control study. *Int J Cancer* 1995;**60**:45–8.
6 IARC. *Monographs on the evaluation of carcinogenic risks to humans. No. 61.* Lyon, France: IARC, 1994.
7 Forman D. Lessons from ongoing intervention studies. In: Hunt RH, Tytgat GNH, eds. *Helicobacter pylori: Basic Mechanisms to Clinical Care.* Dordrecht: Kluwer, 1998.
8 Lauren P. The two histological main types of gastric carcinoma: diffuse and so-called intestinal-type carcinoma. *Acta Pathol Microbiol Scand* 1965;**64**:31–49.
9 Correa P, Haenszel W, Cuello C, Tannenbaum S, Archer M. A model for gastric cancer epidemiology. *Lancet* 1975;**2**:58–9.
10 Kuipers EJ, Uyterlinde AM, Pena AS *et al.* Long term sequelae of *Helicobacter pylori* gastritis. *Lancet* 1995;**345**:1525–8.
11 Sobala GM, Schorah CJ, Sanderson M *et al.* Ascorbic acid in the human stomach. *Gastroenterology* 1989;**97**:357–63.
12 Davies GR, Simmonds NJ, Stevens TRJ *et al. Helicobacter pylori* stimulates antral mucosal reactive oxygen metabolite production *in vivo. Gut* 1994;179–85.
13 Xu G, Reed P. N-Nitroso compounds in fresh gastric juice and their relation to intragastric pH and nitrite employing an improved analytical method. *Carcinogenesis* 1993;**14**:2547–51.
14 Hansson L, Nyren O, Hsing A *et al.* The risk of stomach cancer in patients with gastric or duodenal ulcer disease. *N Engl J Med* 1996;**335**(4):242–9.
15 Warburton VJ, Everett SM, Mapstone NP, Axon ATR, Hawkey P, Dixon MF. Clinical and histological associations of cagA and vacA genotypes in *Helicobacter pylori* gastritis. *J Clin Pathol* 1998;**51**: 55–61.
16 Lee A, Dixon MF, Danon SJ *et al.* Local acid production and *Helicobacter pylori*: a unifying hypothesis of gastroduodenal disease. *Eur J Gastroenterol Hepatol* 1995;**7**:461–5.
17 El-Omar E, Carrington M, Chow W *et al.* Interleukin-1 polymorphisms associated with increased risk of gastric cancer. *Nature* 2000;**404**: 398–402.
18 Palli D. Dietary factors. *Eur J Gastroenterol Hepatol* 1994;**6**:1076–82.
19 Kubota H, Kotoh T, Masunaga R *et al.* Impact of screening survey of gastric cancer on clinicopathological features and survival: Retrospective study at a single institution. *Surgery* 2000;**128**:41–7.
20 Hisamichi S, Sugawara N, Fukao A. Effectiveness of gastric mass screening in Japan. *Cancer Detect Prevent* 1988;**11**:323–9.
21 Inaba S, Hirayama H, Nagata C *et al.* Evaluation of a screening program on reduction of gastric cancer mortality in Japan: preliminary results from a cohort study. *Prevent Med* 1999;**29**:102–6.

22  Fukao A, Hisamichi, S, Komatsu S *et al.* Comparison of characteristics between frequent participants and non-participants in screening program for stomach cancer. *Tohuku J Exp Med* 1992;**166**:459–69.

23  Shiratori Y, Nakagawa S, Kikuchi A *et al.* Significance of a gastric mass screening survey. *Am J Gastroenterol* 1985;**80**:831–4.

24  Hisamichi S, Sugawara N. Mass screening for gastric cancer by X-ray examination. *Jap J Clin Oncol* 1984;**14**:211–23.

25  Murakami R, Tsukuma H, Ubakata T *et al.* Estimation of validity of mass screening program for gastric cancer in Osaka, Japan. *Cancer* 1990;**65**:1255–60.

26  Yoshida Y, Yamaguchi Y, Tebayashi A, Arisue T, Tamura K, Ichikawa H. Precision in the first stage of the gastric carcinoma mass survey. *Int J Cancer* 1983;**31**:201–6.

27  Hisamichi S. Screening for gastric cancer. *Wld J Surg* 1989;**13**:31–7.

28  Shimizu S, Tada M, Kawai K. Early gastric cancer: its surveillance and natural course. *Endoscopy* 1995;**27**:27–31.

29  Nishi M, Ishihara S, Nakajima T, Ohta K, Ohyama S, Ohta H. Chronological changes of characteristics of early gastric cancer and therapy: Experience in the Cancer Institute Hospital of Tokyo, 1950–1994. *J Cancer Res Clin Oncol* 1995;**121**:535–41.

30  Everett SM, Axon ATR. Early gastric cancer in Europe. *Gut* 1997;**41**:142–50.

31  Maehara Y, Kakeji Y, Oda S, Takahashi I, Akazawa K, Sugimachi K. Time trends of surgical treatment and the prognosis for Japanese patients with gastric cancer. *Br J Cancer* 2000;**83**:986–91.

32  Hanazaki K, Sodeyama H, Wakabayashi M *et al.* Surgical treatment of gastric cancer detected by mass screening. *Hepato-gastroenterology* 1997;**44**:1126–32.

33  Kampschoer GHM, Fujii A, Masuda Y. Gastric cancer detected by mass survey. Comparison between mass survey and out patient detection. *Scan J Gastroenterol* 1989;**24**:813–17.

34  Kaibara N, Kawaguchi H, Nishidoi H *et al.* Significance of mass survey for gastric cancer from the standpoint of surgery. *Am J Surg* 1981;**142**:543–5.

35  Portnoi LM, Kazantseva IA, Isakov VA, Nefedova VI, Gaganov LE. Gastric cancer screening in selected population of Moscow region: retrospective evaluation. *Eur Radiol* 1999;**9**:701–5.

36  Llorens P. Gastric cancer mass survey in Chile. *Semin Surg Oncol* 1991;**7**:339–343.

37  Pisani P, Oliver WE, Parkin DM, Alvarez N, Vivas J. Case-control study of gastric cancer screening in Venezuela. *Br J Cancer* 1994;**69**:1102–5.

38  Ikeda Y, Haraguchi Y, Mori M *et al.* Gastric cancer in a general hospital in Japan. *Semin Surg Oncol* 1994;**10**:150–5.

39  Sasako M, Mann G. Early detection of gastric adenocarcinoma: the key to reduce mortality or an illusion. *Jap J Clin Oncol* 1998;**28**:585–7.

40  Tsubono Y, Fukao A, Hisamichi S, Sugawara N, Hosakawa T. Health belief model and attendance at screenings for gastric cancer in a population of Miyagi, Japan. *Jap J Publ Health* 1993;**40**:255–64.

41  Oshima A, Hirata N, Ubakata T, Umeda K, Fujimoto I. Evaluation of a mass screening program for stomach cancer with a case-control study design. *Int J Cancer* 1986;**38**:829–33.

42  Abe Y, Mitsushima T, Nagatani K, Ikuma H, Minamihara Y. Epidemiological evaluation of the protective effect for dying of stomach cancer by screening programme for stomach cancer with applying a method of case-control study – a study of a efficient screening programme for stomach cancer. *Jap J Gastroenterol* 1995;**92**:836–45.

43  Coleman MP, Esteve J, Damiecki P, Arslan A, Renard H. *Trends in cancer incidence and mortality: IARC Scientific Publications No 121.* Lyon, France: International Agency for Research on Cancer, **19**:193–206 1993.

44  Correa P, Chen VW. Gastric cancer. *Correa & Chen Cancer Surveys* 1994;**19**:55–76.

45  Tsukuma H, Oshima A, Narahara H, Morii T. Natural history of early gastric cancer: a non-concurrent, long term, follow up study. *Gut* 2000;**47**:618–21.

46  Schlemper RJ, Itabashi M, Katobashi M *et al.* Differences in diagnostic criteria for gastric carcinoma between Japanese and Western pathologists. *Lancet* 1997;**349**:1725–9.

47  Everett SM, Axon ATR. Early gastric cancer: disease or pseudodisease? *Lancet* 1998;**351**:1350–2.

48  Hwang H, Dwyer J, Russell RM. Diet, *Helicobacter pylori* infection, food preservation and gastric cancer risk: are there new roles for preventative factors? *Nutr Rev* 1994;**52**:75–83.

49  Xia HH, Talley NJ. Natural acquisition and spontaneous elimination of *Helicobacter pylori* infection: clinical implications. *Am J Gastroenterol* 1997;**92**:1780–7.

50  Correa P. Chronic gastritis as a cancer precursor. *Scan J Gastroenterol* 1984;**104**(Suppl. 1):131–6.

51  You WC, Li JY, Blot WJ *et al.* Evolution of precancerous lesions in a rural Chinese population at high risk of gastric cancer. *Int J Cancer* 1999;**83**:615–19.

52  Dixon MF. Histological responses to *Helicobacter pylori* infection: gastritis, atrophy and preneoplasia. *Baillières Clin Gastroenterol* 1995;**9**:467–86.

53  Schenk BE, Kuipers EJ, Nelis GF *et al.* Effect of *Helicobacter pylori* eradication on chronic gastritis during omeprazole therapy. *Gut* 2000;**46**:615–21.

54  Sung JJ, Lin SR, Ching JY *et al.* Atrophy and intestinal metaplasia one year after cure of *H. pylori* infection: a prospective, randomized study. *Gastroenterology* 2000;**119**:7–14.

55  Correa P, Fontham ET, Bravo JC *et al.* Chemoprevention of gastric dysplasia: randomized trial of antioxidant supplements and anti-*Helicobacter pylori* therapy. *J Natl Cancer Inst* 2000;**92**:1881–8.

56  Huang JQ, Sridhar S, Chen Y, Hunt RH. Meta-analysis of the relationship between *Helicobacter pylori* seropositivity and gastric cancer. *Gastroenterology* 1998;**14**:1169–79.

57  Forman D. The prevalence of *Helicobacter pylori* infection in gastric cancer. *Alim Pharmacol Therap* 1995;**9**(Suppl 2): 71–6.

58  Plummer M, Vivas J, Fauchere JL *et al. Helicobacter pylori* and stomach cancer: a case-control study in Venezuela. *Cancer Epidemiol Biomarker Prevent* 2000;**9**:961–5.

59  Helicobacter and Cancer Collaborative Group. Gastric cancer and *Helicobacter pylori*: a combined analysis of 12 case control studies nested within prospective cohorts. *Gut* 2001;**49**:347–53.

60  Uemura N, Okamoto S, Yamamoto S *et al. Helicobacter pylori* infection and the development of gastric cancer. *N Engl J Med* 2001;**345**:784–9.

61  Yamagata H, Kiyohara Y, Aoyagi K *et al.* Impact of *Helicobacter pylori* infection on gastric cancer incidence in a general Japanese population: the Hisayama study. *Arch Intern Med* 2000;**160**:1962–8.

62  Uemura N, Mukai T, Okamoto S *et al.* Effect of *Helicobacter pylori* eradication on subsequent development of cancer after endoscopic resection of early gastric cancer. *Cancer Epidemiol Biomarker Prevent* 1997;**6**:639–42.

63  Miehlke S, Kirsch C, Dragosics B *et al. Helicobacter pylori* and gastric cancer: current status of the Austrain Czech German gastric cancer prevention trial (PRISMA Study). *Wld J Gastroenterol* 2001;**7**:243–7.

64  Eurogast study group. An international association between *Helicobacter pylori* infection and gastric cancer. *Lancet* 1993;**341**:1359–62.

65  Forman D, Sitas F, Newell DG *et al.* Geographic association of *Helicobacter pylori* antibody prevalence and gastric cancer mortality in rural China. *Int J Cancer* 1990;**46**:608–11.

66  Holcombe C. *Helicobacter pylori*: the African enigma. *Gut* 1992;**33**:429–31.

67  Segal I, Ally R, Mitchell H. *Helicobacter pylori* – an African perspective. *Q J Med* 2001;**44**:561–5.

68  Brown LM. *Helicobacter pylori*: epidemiology and routes of transmission. *Epidemiol Rev* 2000;**22**:283–97.

69  Moayyedi P, Axon ATR, Feltbower R *et al.* Relation of adult lifestyle and socio-economic factors to the prevalence of *Helicobacter pylori* infection. *Int J Epidemiol* 2002;**31**:624–31.

70  Banatvala N, Mayo K, Megraud F, Jennings R, Deeks JJ, Feldman RA. The cohort effect and *Helicobacter pylori*. *J Infect Dis* 1993;**68**:219–21.

71  Hirayama F, Takagi S, Iwao E *et al.* Development of poorly differentiated adenocarcinoma and carcinoid due to long-term *Helicobacter pylori* colonization in Mongolian gerbils. *J Gastroenterol* 1999;**34**:450–4.

72  Fujioka T, Honda S, Tokieda M. *Helicobacter pylori* infection and gastric carcinoma in animal models. *J Gastroenterol Hepatol* 2000;**15**(Suppl):D55–9.

73  Goldstone AR, Quirke P, Dixon MF. *Helicobacter pylori* infection and gastric cancer. *J Patho* 1996;**179**:129–37.

74  Axon ATR, Moayyedi P, Sahay P. Whom, how and when to test for *H pylori* infection. In: Hunt RH, Tytgat GNJ, eds. *Helicobacter pylori: Basic mechanisms to clinical cure.* Dordrecht: Kluwer Academic Publishers, 1996.

75  Atherton JC, Spiller RC. The urea breath test for *Helicobacter pylori.* *Gut* 1994;**35**:723–5.

76  Vaira D, Malfertheiner P, Megraud F *et al.* Diagnosis of *Helicobacter pylori* infection with a new non-invasive antigen-based assay. HpSA European study group. *Lancet* 1999;**354**:30–3.

77  Vakil N. Review article: the cost of diagnosing *Helicobacter pylori* infection. *Alimen Pharmacol Therap* 2001;**15**(Suppl.1):10–15.

78  Loy CT, Irwig LM, Katelaris PH, Talley NJ. Do commercial serology kits for *Helicobacter pylori* infection differ in accuracy? *Am J Gastroenterol* 1996;**91**:1138–44.

79  Roberts AP, Childs S, Rubin G, de Wit NJ. Tests for *Helicobacter pylori* infection: a critical appraisal from primary care. *Fam Pract* 2000;**17**(Suppl.2):S12–S20.

80  Wilcox MH, Dent TH, Hunter JO *et al.* Accuracy of serology for the diagnosis of *Helicobacter pylori* infection – a comparison of eight kits. *J Clin Pathol* 1996;**49**:373–6.

81  Moayyedi P, Carter AM, Catto A, Heppell RM, Grant PJ, Axon ATR. Validation of a rapid whole blood tests for the diagnosis of *Helicobacter pylori* infection. *BMJ* 1997;**314**:119.

82  Stone MA,Mayberry JF, Wicks AC *et al.* Near patient testing for *Helicobacter pylori*: a detailed evaluation of the Cortecs Helisal Rapid Blood test. *Eur J Gastroenterol Hepatol* 1997;**9**:257–60.

83  Moayyedi P, Tompkins DS, Axon AT. Salivary antibodies to *Helicobacter pylori*: screening dyspeptic patients before endoscopy. [Letter] *Lancet* 1994;**344**:1016–17.

84  Moayyedi P, Axon ATR. The usefulness of likelihood ratios in the diagnosis of dyspepsia and gastro-esophageal reflux disease. *Am J Gastroenterol* 1999;**94**:3122–5.

85  Danesh J. *Helicobacter pylori* infection and gastric cancer: systematic review of the epidemiological studies. *Alimen Pharmacol Therap* 1999;**13**:851–6.

86  Cutler AF, Havstad S, Ma CK, Blaser MJ, Perez-Perez GI, Schubert TT. Accuracy of invasive and noninvasive tests to diagnose *Helicobacter pylori* infection. *Gastroenterology* 1995;**109**:136–41.

87  Fendrick AM, Chernew ME, Hirth RA, Bloom BS, Bandekar RR, Scheiman JM. Clinical and economic effects of population-based *Helicobacter pylori* screening to prevent gastric cancer. *Arch Intern Med* 1999;**159**:142–8.

88  Delaney B, Moayyedi P, Forman D. *Helicobacter pylori* infection. *Clinical Evidence* 2002;**7**:414–28.

89  Moayyedi P, Axon ATR. *Helicobacter pylori* eradication: drug regimens. In: Scarpignato C, Bianchi Porro G, eds. *Clinical Pharmacology and Therapy of Helicobacter pylori Infection.* Basel: Karger, 1999.

90  Unge P. What other regimens are under investigation to treat *Helicobacter pylori* infection? *Gastroenterology* 1997;**113**: S131–S148.

91  Moayyedi P, Feltbower R, Crocombe W *et al.* The effectiveness of omeprazole, clarithromycin and tinidazole in eradicating *Helicobacter pylori* in a community screen and treat program. *Alimen Pharmacol Ther* 2000;**14**:719–728.

92  Moayyedi P, Murphy B. *Helicobacter pylori*: a clinical update. *J Appl Microbiol* 2001;1–8.

93  Lind T, Megraud F, Unge P *et al.* The MACH2 Study: Role of omeprazole in eradication of *Helicobacter pylori* with 1-week triple therapies. *Gastroenterology* 1999;**116**:248–53.

94  Bell GD, Bate CM, Axon AT *et al.* Addition of metronidazole to omeprazole/amoxycillin dual therapy increases the rate of *Helicobacter pylori* eradication: a double-blind, randomized trial. *Alimen Pharmacol Therap* 1995;**9**:513–20.

95  Penston, J.G. Review article: *Helicobacter pylori* eradication – understandable caution but no excuse for inertia. *Alimen Pharmacol Therap* 1994;**8**:369–89.

96  El-Omar EM, Oien K, Murray LS *et al.* Increased prevalence of precancerous changes in relatives of gastric cancer patients: critical role of *H. pylori. Gastroenterology* 2000;**118**:22–30.

97  Parsonnet J, Friedman GD, Orentreich N, Vogelman H. Risk for gastric cancer in people with CagA positive or CagA negative *Helicobacter pylori* infection. *Gut* 1997;**40**:297–301.

98  Kikuchi S, Crabtree JE, Forman D, Kurosawa M. Association between infections with CagA-positive or -negative strains of *Helicobacter pylori* and risk for gastric cancer in young adults. Research Group on Prevention of Gastric Carcinoma Among Young Adults. *Am J Gastroenterol* 1999;**94**:3455–9.

99  Harris RA, Owens DK, Witherell H, Parsonnet J. *Helicobacter pylori* and gastric cancer: what are the benefits of screening only for the CagA phenotype of *H. pylori?. Helicobacter* 1999;**4**:69–76.

100  Laine LA. *Helicobacter pylori* and complicated ulcer disease. *Am J Med* 1996;**100**:52S–57S.

101  Moayyedi P, Soo S, Deeks J *et al.* Systematic review and economic evaluation of *Helicobacter pylori* eradication treatment for non-ulcer dyspepsia. *BMJ* 2000;**321**:659–64.

102  Labenz J, Malfertheiner P. *Helicobacter pylori* in gastro-oesophageal reflux disease: causal agent, independent or protective factor? *Gut* 1997;**41**:277–80.

103  Schwizer W, Thumshirn M, Dent J *et al. Helicobacter pylori* and symptomatic relapse of gastro-oesophageal reflux disease: a randomised controlled trial. *Lancet* 2001;**357**:1738–42.

104  Moayyedi P, Bardhan KD, Young L, Dixon MF, Brown L, Axon ATR. The effect if *Helicobacter pylori* eradication on reflux symptoms in gastro-esophageal reflux disease in patients: a randomised controlled trial. *Gastroenterology* 2001;**121**:1120–6.

105  Chow W-H, Blaser MJ, Blot WJ *et al.* An inverse relation between cagA⁺ strains of *Helicobacter pylori* infection and risk of esophageal and gastric cardia adenocarcinoma. *Cancer Res* 1998;**58**:588–90.

106  Hansen S, Melby K, Aase S *et al. Helicobacter pylori* infection and risk of cardia and non-cardia gastric cancer: a nested case-control study. *Scand J Gastroenterol* 1999;**34**:353–60.

107  Limburg PJ, Qiao YL, Mark SD *et al. Helicobacter pylori* seropositivity and subsite-specific gastric cancer risks in Linxian, China. *J Natl Cancer Inst* 2001;**93**:226–33.

108  Moayyedi P, Axon AT. Is there a rationale for eradication of *Helicobacter pylori?* Cost-benefit: the case for. *Br Med Bull* 1998;**54**:243–50.

109  Stewart-Brown, S, Farmer A. Screening could seriously damage your health. *BMJ* 1997;**314**:533–4.

110  Moayyedi P, Feltbower R, Brown J *et al.* Effect of population screening and treatment for *Helicobacter pylori* on dyspepsia and quality of life in the community: a randomised controlled trial. Leeds HELP Study Group. *Lancet* 2000;**355**:1665–9.

111  Parsonnet J, Harris RA, Hack HM, Owens DK. Modelling cost-effectiveness of *Helicobacter pylori* screening to prevent gastric cancer: a mandate for clinical trials. *Lancet* 1996;**348**:150–4.

112  Rupnow MF, Owens DK, Shachter R, Parsonnet J. *Helicobacter pylori* vaccine development and use: a cost-effectiveness analysis using the Institute of Medicine Methodology. *Helicobacter* 1999; **4**:272–80.

113  Sonnenberg A, Inadomi JM. Review article: Medical decision models of *Helicobacter pylori* therapy to prevent gastric cancer. *Alimen Pharmacol Therap* 1998;**12**(Suppl.1):111–21.

114  Mason J, Feltbower R, Crocombe W *et al.* The effect of population *H pylori* screening and treatment on dyspepsia in the community: an economic analysis of a randomised controlled trial. *Alimen Pharmacol Therap* 2002;**16**:559–68.

115  Moayyedi P, Axon ATR. Population screening and treatment of *Helicobacter pylori. Gastroenterology* 2000;**19**:1796–7.

116  Kuipers EJ, Pena AS, van Kamp G *et al.* Seroconversion for *Helicobacter pylori. Lancet* 1993;**342**:328–31.

117  Parsonnet J, Blaser MJ, Perez-Perez GI, Hargrett-Bean N, Tauxe RV. Symptoms and risk factors of *Helicobacter pylori* infection in a cohort of epidemiologists. *Gastroenterology* 1992;**102**:41–6.

118  Toftgaard C. Gastric cancer after peptic ulcer surgery. *Ann Surg* 1989;**210**:159–64.

119  Logan RFA, Langman MJS. Screening for gastric cancer after gastric surgery. *Lancet* 1983;**2**:667–70.

120  Schuman BM, Waldbaum JR, Hiltz SW. Carcinoma of the gastric remnant in a US population. *Gastrointest Endosc* 1984;**30**:71–3.

121 Schrumpf E, Serck-Hanssen A, Stadaas J, Aune S, Myren J, Osnes M. Mucosal changes in the gastric stump 20–25 years after partial gastrectomy. *Lancet* 1977;**2**:467–9.

122 Greene FL. Early detection of gastric remnant carcinoma. The role of gastroscopic screening. *Arch Surg* 1987;**122**:300–3.

123 Greene FL. Management of gastric remnant carcinoma based on the results of a 15–year endoscopic screening program. *Ann Surg* **223**:701–8.

124 Offerhaus GJA, Tersmette AC, Giardiello FM, Huibregtse K, Vandenbroucke JP, Tytgat GNJ. Evaluation of endoscopy for early detection of gastric-stump cancer. *Lancet* 1992;**340**:33–5.

125 Stael von Holstein C, Eriksson B, Huldt B, Hammar E. Endoscopic screening during 17 years for gastric stump carcinoma. A prospective clinical trial. *Scan J Gastroenterol* 1991;**26**:1020–6.

126 Brinton L, Gridley G, Hrubec Z, Hoover R, Fraumeni Jr JF. Cancer risk following pernicious anaemia. *Br J Cancer* 1989;**59**:810–13.

127 Stockbrugger RW, Menon GG, Beilby JOW, Mason RR, Cotton PB. Gastroscopic screening in 80 patients with pernicious anaemia. *Gut* 1983;**24**:1141–7.

128 Armbrechtr U, Stockbrugger RW, Rode J, Menon GG, Cotton PB. Development of gastric dysplasia in pernicious anaemia: a clinical and endoscopic follow up study of 80 patients. *Gut* 1990;**31**:1105–9.

129 Sjoblom SM, Sipponen P, Jarvinen H. Gastroscopic follow up of pernicious anaemia patients. *Gut* 1993;**34**:28–32.

130 Borch K. Epidemiologic, clinicopathologic, and economic aspects of gastroscopic screening of patients with pernicious anaemia. *Scan J Gastroenterol* 1986;**21**:21–30.

131 Rokkas T, Filipe MI, Sladen GE. Detection of an increased incidence of early gastric cancer in patients with intestinal metaplasia type III who are closely followed up. *Gut* 1991;**32**:1110–13.

132 Whiting JL, Sigurdsson A, Rowlands DC, Hallissey MT, Fielding JWL. The long term results of endoscopic surveillance of premalignant gastric lesions. *Gut* 2002;**50**:378–81.

133 Eccles M, Clapp Z, Grimshaw J *et al.* North of England evidence based guidelines development project: methods of guideline development. *BMJ* 1996;**312**:760.

# 20 Screening for melanoma

*Veronique Bataille*

## How important is melanoma in public health terms?

Melanoma has become an important public health issue over the past 20 years because of rising incidence in Caucasian populations (Figure 20.1).[1] It is estimated that over the past 50 years the incidence has risen steadily by around 6% every year leading to a 10-fold increase in incidence since the late 1950s.[2] Current estimates for new cases per year for the year 2000 are 6000 in the UK and 48 000 cases in the USA. However, most recent figures have shown that in parts of USA, Canada, Australia and the UK, the incidence rates have reached a plateau or decreased.[3,4] This downturn in incidence has now been observed over the past 10 years and followed a peak in incidence for the 1930s to 1940s in many Caucasian populations.[5,6] The cause for this decrease in melanoma incidence is not clear, although it has been postulated that changes in sun-seeking behaviour may be responsible, but this has not been formally studied. The lag time between exposure and melanoma is quite long, so possible changes in behaviour are unlikely to have caused a significant impact on melanoma incidence. In terms of world burden, the contribution of melanoma to the cancer epidemic varies according to latitude, ethnic origin and socioeconomic factors, as well the relative contribution of other cancers in respective countries. Estimates in 1990 have shown that melanoma accounts for 1·3% of all cancers and 0·6% of all cancer deaths worldwide. This tumour is more common in younger age groups compared with other cancers and is the most common tumour in age group 25–29 in the USA,[7] so melanoma has a disproportionate impact on young adults.

The most important rise in incidence has been observed for early melanomas. This has led to some debate as to whether the recent melanoma epidemic is genuine or may just reflect a combination of better registration, increase in excision of very early lesions and changes in diagnostic criteria. However, the rise in melanoma has also been observed for thick melanoma tumours with a parallel increase in mortality, which could not be explained by changing diagnostic criteria and excisions.[8,9] Melanoma registration may have improved all over the world, but studies have estimated that melanoma registries

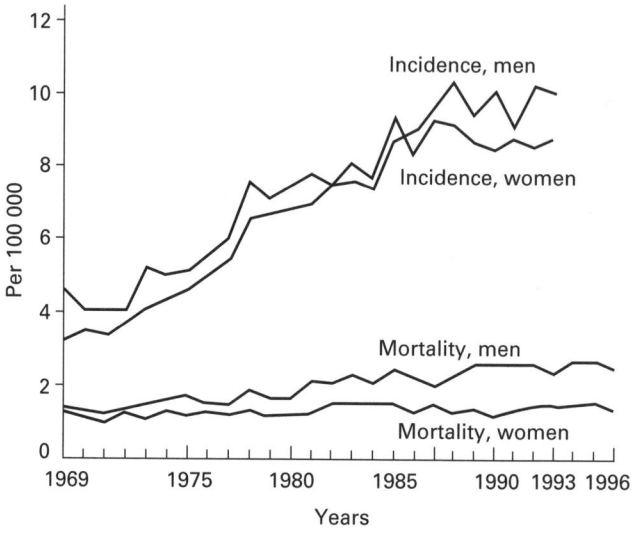

**Figure 20.1** Age-standardised melanoma incidence (1969–1993) and mortality (1969–1996) rates in Canada. Rates are age-standardised to the 1991 Canadian population adjusted for net census undercoverage. (**Data sources**: National Cancer incidence Reporting System, Canadian Cancer Registry, Vital Statistics Data Base)

underestimate the true incidence by as much as 43%.[10,11] In our case–control study of melanoma of the North East Thames region of the UK, the underreporting of melanoma for the period 1990–1994 was 25% (unpublished data). The changes in histological criteria may have had a small impact on very early lesions where the rate of excision has significantly increased. These early lesions are unlikely, however, to have a significant impact on mortality (albeit a possible reverse effect with overall improved mortality). The true biological behaviour of early melanoma is not known and cannot be studied prospectively for obvious ethical reasons. From anecdotal clinical evidence it is possible that some of these early melanomas may never progress or remain static for many years. In our UK studies based on patients with the atypical mole syndrome phenotype, removal of melanocytic lesions for research purposes can reveal melanoma *in situ*, which were totally unsuspected clinically and were completely static clinically (unpublished data).

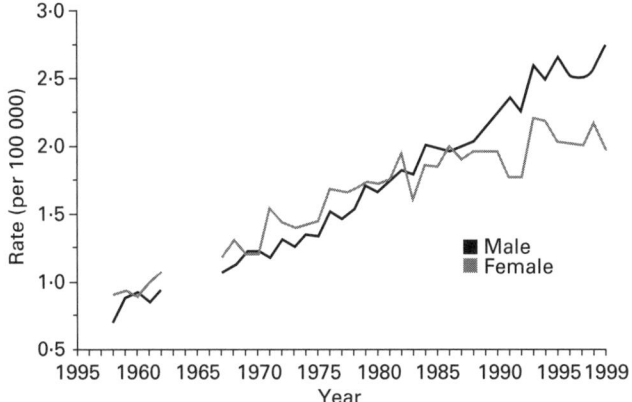

**Figure 20.2** Mortality rates for melanoma in the UK, 1955–1999; all ages. (Source: WHO Cancer Mortality data base)

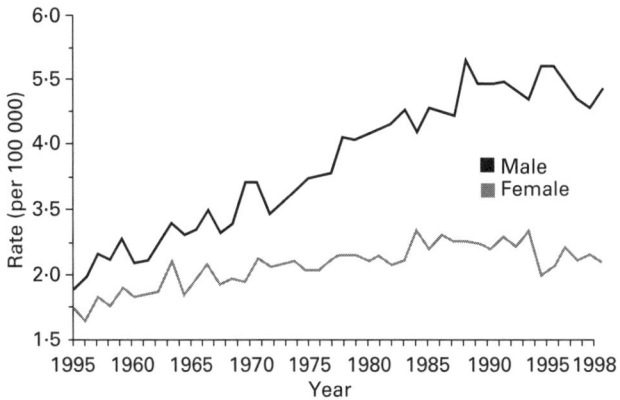

**Figure 20.3** Melanoma mortality rates in Australia, 1955–1998; all ages. (Source: WHO Cancer Mortality database)

After a significant increase in mortality following the sharp rise in incidence over the past several decades, melanoma mortality has been stable and, in some countries, has also shown a decrease over the past 10–20 years, especially in women (Figures 20.1–20.3). This decrease or stability in mortality rates occurred well before the more recent downturn in incidence. Stabilised mortality rates have been observed from the 1980s or even earlier in Australia, some parts of the USA, Sweden, Holland, as well as Scotland (in females only).[12] This decrease in mortality is mostly observed in younger age groups. In older generations, however, mortality rates continue to increase especially in males. Melanoma affects young age groups with a significant number of years of life lost per death.[13] In parallel with incidence rates, a birth cohort effect is observed for mortality with peaks in birth cohorts born between 1920s and 1940s, with declining mortality for birth cohorts born after 1950.[14] These cohort effects can be observed at different times in men and women and the reasons for this gender difference is unclear. It may be due to different sun-seeking behaviour in males and females in identical cohorts. Period effects have also been implicated to explain changes in melanoma mortality over time. Cohort and period effects are important to investigate as they may shed more light on the role of sun exposure and other potential environmental risk factors. Women and patients of higher socioeconomic status have a survival advantage.[15] It is possible that this may, in part, be explained by increased skin awareness in women and higher socioeconomic grouping. However, even after adjusting for tumour thickness, the improved survival in women and higher socioeconomic groups persists, which suggests that factors other than early detection, possibly diet, may be involved.[15]

## How much is known about the natural history of the disease and the potential value of intervention?

Melanoma is a tumour that should be very amenable to prevention and screening. It is one of the cancers for which a significant environmental risk factor, namely sun exposure, has been identified, and behavioural intervention may, in principle, be helpful in its primary prevention. It is also easily accessible and visible to the naked eye, so increased melanoma awareness and early detection are important for its secondary prevention.

## What is the role of primary prevention in melanoma?

Primary prevention of melanoma focuses on informing the public about the deleterious effects of sunlight and attempting to alter behaviour in the sun. The relationship between sun exposure and melanoma has long been established with latitude studies, migration studies and case–control studies. The highest incidence of melanoma is to be found in Queensland, Australia, where high levels of ultraviolet exposure are combined with a susceptible Celtic population, originating mostly from the UK. The incidence in Queensland is around 50 per 100 000 per year compared with 10 per 100 000 per year in Europe. Melanoma is the fourth most common tumour in Australia (including non-melanoma skin cancers) compared with the UK, where it is the 18th most common tumour.[16] Melanoma is equally common in women and men with only small variations in the male/female ratio across the world.[3] In non-Caucasian populations, melanoma is rare and affects different body sites such as palms and soles, which highlights the importance of racial risk factors for this tumour.[17]

The inverse relationship between latitude and melanoma incidence was one of the first pieces of epidemiological evidence linking melanoma to ultraviolet exposure. This gradient is reversed in Europe where the increase in sun exposure in Southern European countries is associated with lower melanoma incidence because of darker skin phenotypes, which are protective.[18] The relationship between melanoma and sun exposure is complex, as cumulative exposure to the sun appears to be protective.[19] Furthermore, whilst sunburns have been shown to be a risk factor for melanoma, the magnitude of the risk is small, with odds ratios in the order of 2. Once adjusted for fair skin phenotypes, the association between sunburns and melanoma often disappear, so this link appears to reflect a specific host susceptibility to ultraviolet light. Many case–control studies have attempted to quantify the number of hours exposed to the sun and it is evident that the relationship between sun and melanoma is not dose-dependent, as exposure can be protective especially in good tanners. The most detrimental exposure appears to be short bursts of intense ultraviolet light exposure especially in childhood.[20] Melanoma body sites also indicate that the relationship with sun exposure is not dose-dependent. Melanoma is more common on intermittently sun-exposed areas especially in young age groups.[21] The association between melanoma and high socioeconomic status has long been known and this may be explained, in part, by increased intermittent and short bursts of sun exposure in "white collar" workers compared with more chronic patterns of sun exposure in manual workers.[22,23]

Behavioural intervention attempting to change population exposure to ultraviolet light via media campaigns first started in Australia and some parts of the USA where the melanoma burden has long been particularly heavy. Whilst media campaigns appear to have significant effects on knowledge, they do not appear to affect behaviour, especially in younger age groups. In Europe, where ultraviolet radiation is much reduced, sun awareness campaigns have also been difficult, as changing sun-seeking behaviour in countries where sunlight exposure is limited is not easy. Successful public health campaigns in Australia cannot necessarily be duplicated in Europe, where the patterns of exposure differ greatly.[24] Even subjects who have close contacts with melanoma patients with greater knowledge about risk factors do not appear to change their behaviour, and other studies have shown that knowledge and behaviour do not correlate.[25,26] Exposure to sunlight provides a feeling of wellbeing and is associated with relaxing and sporting activities. Furthermore, suntan is still regarded as fashionable in most Caucasian populations so reducing exposure is difficult.[27] In terms of reducing sun exposure, shade and clothing are mostly recommended with the addition of sunscreens on parts of the body not protected by clothing. Children should be particularly protected as increased sun exposure before the age of 20 increases melanoma risk more significantly than exposure in adulthood.[20]

Sunscreens have long been promoted for skin cancer prevention but their efficacy in reducing melanoma is unclear.[28] Moreover, recent studies have shown that the use of sunscreens can be associated with an increased risk of melanoma, and this risk is likely to be explained by the suppression of sunburns, which lead to longer exposure to UVR mainly within the UVA range.[29–31] Higher SPF sunscreens also increase mean cumulative sun exposure of young subjects in Europe, which may have a significant impact on doses of UVR a person may be exposed to over a lifetime.[32] Sunscreen use has also been associated with greater number of naevi in children and adolescents, which shows that they may also have significant effects on precursor lesions; long-term follow up studies are needed.[33]

For artificial ultraviolet radiation, the association with melanoma is more controversial as several studies have shown no association between sunbeds and melanoma, whilst others have shown a weak but elevated risk.[34–36] The design of these studies is critical as exposure to natural sunlight acts as a major confounder. Phototherapy for the treatment of psoriasis has also been linked to melanoma but the risk appears to be small, and psoriasis patients receive UVB and PUVA (psoralen + UVA).[37] Gathering data on lifetime exposure to natural and artificial sunlight is a difficult task and case–control designs may not be sensitive enough to detect a true association. New study designs looking at gene–environment interactions may be able to detect significant effects of UVR in genetically susceptible individuals.

It is clear that reducing the occurrence of sunburns is important for skin cancers and skin ageing; it is not known, however, to what extent sun exposure should be reduced and whether this reduction will have an effect on melanoma incidence. More recently, publications have pointed towards the potential protective role of ultraviolet radiation for osteoporosis and solid cancers.[38,39] The incidence of ovarian and colon cancer is also influenced by a latitude gradient with an inverse relationship as observed in melanoma, and it is postulated that this decrease in solid tumours with decreasing latitude may be explained by the anticancer effects of vitamin D following UVR exposure.[40,41] Vitamin D metabolism may play a role in melanoma as it is known to influence the proliferation of a wide variety of cells.[42,43] A recent study showed a negative association between mortality caused by breast, colon, ovarian, and prostate cancer and residential exposure to sunlight.[44] Vitamin D receptor polymorphisms have also shown to be protective in melanoma and more work is needed to investigate the effects of sun avoidance, especially in European countries where UV exposure is only relevant for a few months of the year.[45]

Many questions remained to be answered regarding the association between melanoma and sunlight, such as which part of the UVR spectrum is most detrimental, what doses of UVR exposure are considered excessive in terms of melanoma risk, and what cellular damage caused by UVR is directly implicated in melanoma. Furthermore, the interactions between UVR and melanoma will vary greatly between populations as complex gene–environment interactions are likely depending on skin type and ethnicity. Investigating these complex gene–environment interactions will become possible when the genetic basis for melanoma is better understood. The ultimate goal will be to identify individuals at greatest risk with targeted behavioural intervention.

No significant dietary risk factors have ever been reported for melanoma. However, recent studies have shown a possible protective effect of lipid-lowering drugs in melanoma whilst other have shown a deleterious effect of polyunsaturated fat in women only.[46] In terms of chemoprevention, vitamin A derivatives are potential agents to be explored further. Oral retinoids have already been used successfully for a few human cancers, such as the prevention of head and neck squamous cell cancers, and have also been used in the prevention of non-melanoma skin cancers in patients with xeroderma pigmentosum and Gorlin syndrome.[47] Whilst the role of oral retinoids in melanoma prevention in population at high risk has never been formally studied, topical vitamin A (tretinoin) has been used topically on atypical melanocytic lesions in genetically susceptible individuals. Retinoids were shown to cause significant differentiation and involution of atypical melanocytic lesions in several patients.[48,49] The current limitation for the use of oral retinoids are long-term side effects and teratogenicity, but new formulations may be better tolerated. Although diet, smoking, occupational exposure to chemicals and infections have been investigated in melanoma, none of these potential risk factors has been shown to have a significant role in this tumour. Some studies have suggested links between melanoma and some industrial exposure as well as a protective effect of previous infections; these studies need to take into account many confounding factors, such as economical status and sun-exposure patterns in these populations.

Immunodeficient patients following renal transplantation may have a 100-fold increase in risk of cutanoeus squamous cell carcinomas, but the risk of melanoma after 5 years follow up is much smaller with a 1·6-fold increase after 5 years follow up.[50] Immunosuppression has also been linked to excess of naevi in both adults and children.[51,52] Excess of naevi has also been reported in HIV patients, cardiac transplants as well as children receiving chemotherapy.[53] It may be that longer follow up periods of transplanted patients will reveal a greater risk of melanoma. There is no doubt that immune response is important in melanoma like many other cancers, but levels of immunodeficiency affecting a small group of individuals (mainly transplant patients) are unlikely to be relevant for melanoma prevention in the normal population.

## Host factors and melanoma

Over the past 20 years, epidemiological evidence has shown that host factors (high naevus counts and a fair skin phenotype) are the most powerful predictors of risk for melanoma, and discovering which genes are involved in skin pigmentation and naevus expression will help in understanding melanoma susceptibility. In UK Whites, more than 100 common naevi and the presence of two to three atypical naevi give odds ratios between 5 and 10, whilst fair skin (skin types 1 and 2) is associated with a three-fold increase in melanoma risk (Table 20.1). In the UK, the presence of 100 or more naevi accounts for 22% of melanomas below the age of 40. As naevi numbers decrease significantly with age, only 12% of melanomas are attributable to high numbers of naevi above the age of 40. For all ages, skin type 1 accounts for 9% of all melanomas in the UK.[54]

Apart from the clear genetic basis of skin colour, which is strongly related to melanona risk, melanoma has a genetic basis and does cluster in some families, as many other tumours do, but to what extent genetic factors are implicated in population-based sporadic melanomas is less clear. In melanoma families, progress has been made with the discovery of two melanoma genes: *CDKN2A* or *p16* on chromosome 9 and *CDK4* on chromosome 12. *p16* acts as a true tumour suppressor gene and has a crucial role in cell cycle regulation and senescence.[55] This cyclin-dependent kinase inhibitor may account for up to 25% of familial melanoma whilst *CDK4* mutations on chromosome 12 (which binds to *p16*) have only been found in a few rare families. The *p16* gene has also been linked to multiple melanoma primaries with or without family history of the disease. However, the prevalence of *p16* mutations even in these highly susceptible individuals was low.[56] It is likely that a number of other genes play a role in melanoma and, like other cancers, it is suspected that melanoma has in most cases a complex mode of inheritance. Segregation analyses in Australia based on a large number of melanoma kindreds are in keeping with genetic heterogeneity in melanoma with the rejection of a single major gene or a pure environmental transmission.[57]

**Table 20.1** Odds ratios and attributable proportions for melanoma in the UK in relation to phenotypic features

| | Prevalence in cases (%) | OR (95% CI) | Attributable proportion (%) (95%CI) |
|---|---|---|---|
| *>OR=100 naevi* | | | |
| aged less than 40 years | 28 | 4·4 (2·1–9·0) | 22 (8–64) |
| aged more than 40 years | 15 | 4·5 (2·1–9·4) | 12 (5–32) |
| *2 or more atypical naevi* | | | |
| aged less than 40 years | 26 | 9·2 (3·6–22·4) | 23 (12–43) |
| aged more than 40 years | 14 | 10·8 (3·8–30·9) | 13 (4–42) |
| *Skin type 1* (always burn, never tan) | 12 | 3·2 (1·8–5·7) | 9 (4–21) |

Melanoma families often express a cutaneous phenotype known as the atypical mole syndrome (AMS) (Figures 20.4 and 20.5), which may be regarded mainly as a marker of risk rather than a true precursor phenotype. The rate of malignant transformation of atypical naevi in these high risk patients is thought to be very low, although prospective studies examining the rate of transformation of such lesions have not been carried out, and retrospective data from familial melanoma clinics would be difficult to compare between countries, as clinicians differ in terms of threshold for removal of atypical naevi. It is recommended now that atypical naevi be removed only if the clinical features suggest an early melanoma, whilst in the past many atypical naevi in high risk patients were removed randomly. The presence of the AMS phenotype may increase melanoma a risk by 10–20-fold.[54] It can also be found in other non-melanoma family cancer syndromes, such as familial breast or colon cancer, but the association between the AMS and these non-melanoma (and non-pancreatic) family cancer syndromes needs to be studied further as these may occur by chance. Mutations in the *p16* gene, which appear to be quite specific to melanoma families (as well as pancreatic families), are likely to be implicated in the expression of naevi as well.[58] In UK studies on melanoma families, *p16* mutation carrier status correlates to mean naevus number.[59] It is estimated that up to 60% of the naevus phenotype may be attributed to genetic factors but it appears that the mode of inheritance is complex.[60–62] However, the relationship between *p16* status and naevus number is poorly understood as French melanoma family studies have shown that *p16* status was not correlated to naevus counts.[61] A UK study has also highlighted the complex relationship between excess of naevi, melanoma risk and *p16* status.[63] Screening for *p16* mutations in clinical practice is not recommended at this stage because of its poor predictive value in terms of lifetime risk of melanoma and the fact that knowledge of the mutation status would not change follow up strategies.[55]

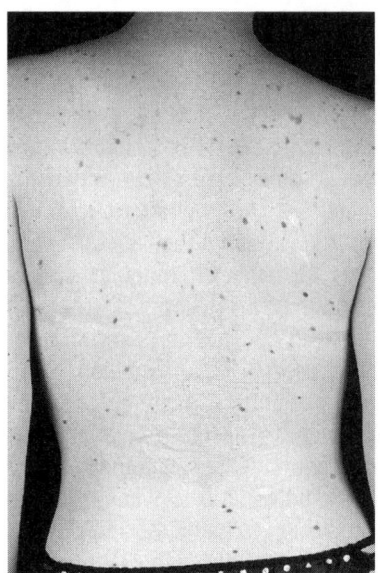

**Figure 20.4** Atypical mole syndrome

Melanoma susceptibility has also been described in the context of various family cancer syndromes. It can be found in families with an excess of breast, throat and gastrointestinal cancers especially pancreatic cancers.[58,64–66] Melanoma can also occur in rarer family cancer syndromes such as retinoblastoma, Li–Fraumeni, and neurofibromatosis type I,[67,68] as well families prone to ocular melanoma, non-Hodgkin lymphoma and nervous system tumours.[69–72] This overall susceptibility to cancer is important to detect by taking a thorough family history in patients with melanoma or the atypical mole syndrome in order to offer genetic counselling and appropriate cancer screening whenever possible. However, care should be taken not to raise anxiety

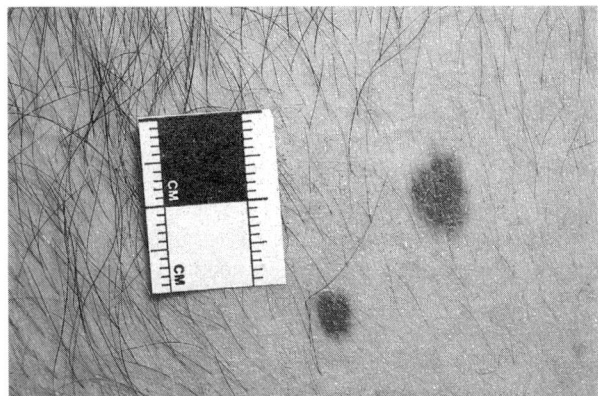

**Figure 20.5**   Close up of atypical naevi

and that genetic counselling in susceptible families is helpful. More studies are needed, however, to determine if the risk of solid tumours other than pancreatic cancer is significantly increased in these susceptible families. The potential link between melanoma and other cancers is important to study as these studies may unravel genetic pathways that melanoma may share with other common cancers.

Many other genes have also been investigated in melanoma including *PTEN*, DNA repair genes, and *MC1R* (melanocortin 1 receptor). However, large studies are needed to establish how useful these genes may be to predict genetically susceptible patients.[73–75] There is no evidence that melanoma patients, including patients with a genetic susceptibility to the disease, have significant defects in DNA repair following UVR exposure, but this has only been assessed on lymphocytes and in a few patients in epidermal cells *in vivo*.[76,77] New techniques using high liquid chromatography can now detect more accurately UV-induced DNA lesions so that milder DNA repair-deficient phenotypes associated with melanoma may come to light in the future. UV-specific DNA mutations in some melanoma tumours, *p16* upregulation in UV-irradiated skin, and the large increase in melanoma in patients with xeroderma pigmentosum suggests that UV damage and repair are likely to have a role in melanoma, and more work is needed in this area.[55,78,79]

Another important risk factor for melanoma is fair skin type with a propensity to sunburn. Individuals with red/blond hair, blue eyes and freckles are most at risk. Polymorphisms in the *MC1R* gene have been linked to a fair hair/skin phenotype with or without freckles. However, the presence of a large number of *MC1R* variants and the complex associations between *MC1R* and skin and hair colour has not helped to detect the real associations between melanoma risk and *MC1R* polymorphisms. It is likely that this association may, in part, reflect the link between melanoma and fair skin phenotypes, but new

*MC1R* variants have now been strongly associated with melanoma irrespective of skin type.[80,81]

With the advances in molecular biology techniques and statistical analyses in the field of genetic epidemiology, new strategies, such as genome wide search, candidate gene approaches, DNA microarrays, and functional assays, are currently being used to discover new melanoma genes. New studies are currently investigating the relative contribution of genes and environment on the expression of naevi. The advantage of studies based on naevi is that this phenotype is a common and continuous trait that is easier to study in large population-based samples, whilst melanoma is relatively rare, and large studies are difficult to set up. Although it is not clear whether naevus genes may be directly relevant for melanoma, the fact that naevi are very powerful predictors of risk suggest that these genes will be relevant. Linkage and association studies are likely to shed some light on new or existing genes that have an important role in melanoma. When new melanoma genes are discovered, epistatic (gene–gene) and gene–environmental interactions will be investigated in more detail. This will require the collaboration of cell biologists, epidemiologists, geneticists, and statisticians.[82] At this stage, however, mutation screening in melanoma remains mainly in the research domain in the UK as its usefulness in screening and follow up strategies remain to be discovered.

## What is the role of secondary prevention in melanoma?

Melanoma is unique in that its detection is amenable to the naked eye. Melanocytic lesions show an array of changes that point towards malignant transformation. The sensitivity and specificity of each clinical feature does vary, and melanoma checklists have been designed in the USA and the UK to help medical practitioners as well as patients.[83] For most tumours, worrying early clinical features such as changes in pigmentation, size and shape allow for these tumours to be picked up early when the chances of survival are high. The important characteristics are asymmetry, irregular pigmentation and borders, and size over 5 mm. Breslow thickness remains to date the most important factor to determine survival. Lesions less than 1 mm in Breslow thickness have a 95% 5-year survival compared with 40% for tumours of 2 mm or more. It is therefore expected that with the implementation of measures to diagnose melanoma earlier, mortality can be significantly reduced. However, there are no randomised studies in the literature formally addressing the role of secondary prevention in the reduction of melanoma mortality.

It is thought that opportunistic screening when patients are consulting general practitioners may be the ideal set up to implement secondary prevention. However, melanoma detection by general practitioners can be poor, as most practitioners will often have never seen a melanoma previously and will have acquired very limited experience in recognising pigmented skin lesions during their medical training. Skin examinations are rarely performed in primary health care and general practitioners, who may feel relatively untrained for the diagnosis of atypical pigmented lesions, will often refer to dermatologists.[84] For detection of potential melanoma in the primary sector or in the workplace, it has been recommended that routine medical checkups include a full skin examination. It has also been proposed that the physical examination of patients during admission for a wide variety of clinical disorders should always include a skin examination, and that medical students should be routinely asked to perform skin examinations as part of their general training. Improved training of physicians is very important in the implementation of secondary prevention as access to dermatologists may be limited, especially in the UK. The diagnosis of pigmented lesions is not always easy and, even within a dermatology department, diagnostic accuracy increases with number of melanomas seen annually and years of dermatology experience. It is recognised that dermatology departments remain the appropriate first point of referral for suspected melanomas once the lesion has been screened by a general practitioner, as dermatologists have the necessary experience to diagnose suspicious lesions.[85]

Whilst primary health workers may be important in diagnosing early melanomas, studies show that in fact up to 60% of all melanomas are self-diagnosed with 15% and 11% diagnosed by the physician and spouse respectively.[86] Women are more melanoma aware and are more likely to self-refer early, which explains, in part, the better survival observed in women.[86] It has been shown that older males are most likely to delay medical advice and are less likely to perform self-examination and this often leads to increase in mortality.[87] Self-examination and public health campaigns raising melanoma awareness are therefore very important in secondary prevention. Patients who self-refer have often detected changes in a lesion but reluctance to seek medical advice and/or lack of skin cancer awareness are the main reasons why melanoma diagnosis may be delayed. In Germany, up to 25% of melanoma patients waited more than 1 year to see a medical practitioner after first seeing changes in their pigmented lesion.[88] Public health campaigns for the primary prevention of melanoma have also been instrumental for secondary prevention in raising melanoma awareness and teaching the public about early changes to watch for in a mole. The need to teach about the most significant signs (major signs) to watch for in a pigmented lesion, such as size and change in shape and/or pigmentation, is important, as the public may believe that bleeding and crusting are the only signs to watch for (minor signs).[89] By the time a melanoma reaches the stage of bleeding and crusting the lesion is usually well advanced and should have been picked up much earlier. Benign melanocytic lesions may also bleed and crust after trauma.

The other avenue in implementing secondary prevention in melanoma is offering access to fast track pigmented lesion clinics. However, retrospective studies have shown that whilst the number of melanomas diagnosed in the pigmented lesion clinic may increase over time, mean tumour thickness did not vary over time, so patients do not appear to be presenting earlier because of the service offered.[90,91] Delays in melanoma diagnosis can also occur if general practitioners do not refer appropriately and carry on sending many suspected melanomas to other routine clinics.[92] Public health campaigns can also be very disruptive for these clinics with a sudden surge in attendance, which affects the care of existing patients and leads to extra costs incurred for biopsy of non-malignant pigmented lesions as well as non-melanoma skin cancers, which will have no impact on mortality.[90,93,94] The general public also finds it difficult to identify if they are in a high risk group or not and self-identification for screening does not seem to target groups most at risk.[95] Although these clinics may be helpful in terms of relieving anxiety (especially after public health campaigns) and raising melanoma awareness, there is no evidence that such services have had an impact on tumour thickness and mortality.[95,96]

Telemedicine is a rapidly expanding area and its use is particularly suited for the diagnosis of skin lesions. This has been piloted in the UK and many other countries and appears to be a fast and safe way to diagnose worrying pigmented lesion.[97,98,99] A recent UK study has shown a sensitivity of 81% and specificity of 73%, which are encouraging figures for the use of telemedicine in the diagnosis of suspicious pigmented lesions.[98] More research is needed in this area to investigate the cost-effectiveness but, more importantly, the safety of teledermatology for the diagnosis of suspicious pigmented lesions.

## Who should be selected for screening and at what interval should screening be offered?

Epidemiological evidence has shown that host factors are the most important elements in determining the risk for melanoma. However, it is not clear which subgroups of the population should be screened for melanoma. This, in part, reflects the fact that melanoma is not a common cancer and that phenotypic risk factors associated with melanoma are common in the general population. Patients with AMS and a family history of melanoma or multiple cancers have a significant risk of developing a melanoma and should be followed up on a 6-monthly or yearly basis.[100] The use of whole body photographs or computer software with an adapted camera is useful to monitor atypical naevi or lesions that may develop *de novo*. AMS patients with a previous history of melanoma should be followed for life, as the risk of a second (or multiple) primary is high.[101] Follow up of patients with a previous melanoma primary show that the second primary is significantly thinner than the first and that patient education is important in recognising the early signs of the disease.[102] Multiple primaries are especially common in patients with AMS, especially in those with a positive family history of melanoma and, although recent US data recommend that all melanoma patients be followed up for life because of the risk of second primary, this only affected 3% of melanomas and may not be warranted, especially as melanoma-aware patients are likely to self-diagnose anyway and re-present to the dermatologist if necessary.[102] Most second primary tumours are also most likely to occur within the first 2 years after the first primary, so the current 5-year follow up recommended for melanoma patients would be adequate.

For individuals with AMS without a family history, the need for screening is less clear as the AMS phenotype is common in Caucasian populations, affecting 2% in the UK and 6% in Australia, so the cost of lifelong regular screening is unlikely to be justified.[54,103] Other risk factors for melanoma are excessive sun exposure in childhood, fair skin type with red or blond hair, freckles, age 50 or over, and male gender. These risk factors taken individually are not sufficient to warrant screening for melanoma, but studies have investigated scoring systems based on combined risk factors to target subjects most at risk of the disease.[104] Future advances in the field of melanoma genetics may reveal important genetic markers, which may become useful in screening genetically susceptible individuals.

## What are the possible treatment options following screening?

Most melanomas are treated with surgery alone, and lesions picked up early with minimal invasion have an excellent prognosis: 70% of melanoma patients will survive their disease with this form of treatment only. The width of excision is at least 1 cm for most invasive melanomas but thickness of the tumour and body site will also determine how wide lesions need to be excised with maximum width of 2–3 cm.[105] Very wide and deep excisions with large skin grafts are no longer recommended as they do not appear to improve survival and cause significant morbidity.

Only 20–30% of tumours will be in the high risk group in terms of recurrence and metastases. It is estimated that 90% of the costs of melanona treatment is attributable to these 20% poor prognosis tumours.[106] The rate of growth of melanoma lesions is not known and anecdotal clinical evidence suggests that in some instances melanoma growth can be slow. However, it is logical to conclude that, if removal is done as early as possible, mortality will be reduced. The levelling off and reduction in mortality observed in many parts of the world especially in females may be, in part, attributed to earlier detection.

## Treatment of more advanced tumours

For adjuvant therapy, the effects on mortality are very disappointing. Melanoma is relatively chemo- and radioresistant, and no chemotherapy (single or combined) or radiotherapy regimens has ever been associated with a significant survival advantage.[107] Most treatments are therefore palliative. Interferon alfa has given some hope for the treatment of advanced tumours with increased disease-free survival and borderline significant increase in long-term survival.[108–110] However, more recent studies have shown that this immunomodulating agent has not yet been associated with a significant longer survival.[111] It has not been easy to reach firm conclusions about the effects of interferon alfa on long-term survival and quality of life, as these studies have used different study protocols in terms of inclusion criteria and different dose regimens ranging from long-term low doses to very high doses. Furthermore, some studies did not reach the number needed to conclude on the effects of interferon alfa on long-term survival and, in some cases, disease-free survival. The high dose regimens cause significant side effects with toxicity often necessitating dose reductions.[108] Morbidity can be significant with interferon alfa treatment and trials are attempting to use smaller but effective doses to reduce toxicity. Studies using published data on interferon alfa in melanoma have estimated (using simulated data from a low dose interferon alfa trial) that the cost per life-year gained was €14 400 after 5 years and €1716 over a lifetime.[112] These costs compare favourably with costs of therapy inside and outside the oncological field. Simulated data from the ECOG trial 1684 estimated the cost per life-year gained to be US $32 6000 after 7 years.[113] However, in the later study, the toxicity of high dose interferon did affect quality of life significantly. More studies should be reaching maturity soon and should provide additional data, which may clarify the position of interferon alfa in terms of cost-effectiveness and beneficial effects on survival in melanoma.

The use of prophylactic lymph node resection is no longer recommended as it has no effect on long-term survival and has significant morbidity. New developments in the field of melanoma staging are also important with the use of sentinel biopsies with or without tyrosinase PCR and these techniques may be helpful in determining which patients need therapeutic lymph node dissection at the earliest stages of node invasion.[114] However, advances in melanoma staging will only be fully appreciated in clinical practice when effective therapies can be offered. For extranodal metastatic disease, treatments differ widely depending on the site and extent of the disease spread, and treatment is palliative.[115]

The guidelines for melanoma treatment in the UK have been published in part by the UK Melanoma Study Group.[116] Current melanoma trials in the UK registered with the National Cancer Registry Network can be found on the National Cancer Research Network website (http://www.ncrn.org.uk). The future for melanoma therapy is likely to be in the development of targeted therapy with vaccines.[117,118] Whilst many different types of vaccines are currently tested in melanoma, results are awaited to confirm their effectiveness and most are only available in the trial setting.

## What side effects are associated with treatment and how common and severe are they?

Current surgical procedures for the removal of melanoma have very low morbidity as the wide and deep excisions with skin grafts are no longer performed. Lymph node dissection can cause long-term lymphoedema, but prophylactic lymph node dissection is no longer recommended so this side effect is less commonly encountered.

Atypical naevi are likely to be removed when subjects undergo screening and the morbidity associated with excision of naevi is not negligible, especially if several lesions are removed. It is important to keep a high threshold for biopsy of pigmented skin lesions and removal should only be warranted if early melanoma is suspected. The removal of many atypical naevi as a primary prevention is not recommended, as this has not been proven to reduce risk and is not cosmetically acceptable.

Adjuvant treatment can cause significant morbidity. Interferon alfa can cause a wide variety of side effects with high dose regimens associated with frequent myelosuppression and/or hepatoxicity.[108,110] The most common side effects are 'flu-like symptoms, fatigue, anorexia, depression, as well as other neuropsychiatric reactions.[119] Other chemotherapy, and immunochemotherapy treatments have, like many cancer treatments, various side effects, but these treatments are usually reserved for patients with very advanced disease who may require control of their disease.

## How effective are the screening/treatment options in terms of mortality and morbidity reduction?

### Screening in the normal population

The question of how effective are population-based detection campaigns for melanoma remains unanswered. Even in Australia where this tumour is a significant burden in terms of public health, the Australian Cancer Society does not recommend population screening.[120] In the USA, the American Academy of Dermatology and American Cancer Society recommend population screening.[121] Since 1985, the American Association of Dermatology has been sponsoring open-access screening clinics with 1 million individuals screened but the impact of these clinics on melanoma mortality in the USA is not yet known. The International Union against Cancer does not recommend screening and the controversy surrounding the need for screening lies in the lack of data to prove its efficacy.[122] Population-based screening initiatives are very expensive and may cause undue anxiety. A population-based screening in the Netherlands has shown that only 0·3% of all lesions screened were histologically confirmed melanomas,[123] and the need to select individuals who are most at risk of the disease for screening is evident.[104] However, this can only be achieved with health campaigns educating the public about risk factors for melanoma.

### Screening of high risk individuals

In patients with AMS who are followed up on a 6-monthly or yearly basis, excision of atypical naevi may be warranted if lesions change over time or if lesions have worrying clinical features suggesting early melanoma. The excision of unstable atypical naevi in high risk groups should, in theory, reduce the risk of melanoma. However, there is no firm evidence in the published literature that the excision of lesions in these high risk patients does decrease melanoma risk. The risk of melanoma is substantially increased in AMS patients (10–50-fold), and clinical evidence clearly demonstrates that atypical naevi do progress to melanoma in these high risk patients, so it is expected that follow up and excisions of unstable lesions is likely to improve mortality. The presence of multiple atypical lesions with a positive family history of the disease can also cause a lot of anxiety and patients welcome regular follow up to the dermatologist. Dermatologists can also give advice about what changes to look for in a mole as well as providing education about reducing sun exposure. Melanoma tumours tend to be thinner in these high risk patients, but this is more to do with self-awareness than close follow up as AMS patients often self-diagnose their lesions.[101] These patients should be followed up by clinicians who are familiar with atypical pigmented lesions as lack of experience may lead to the removal of too many atypical lesions with cosmetic and psychological morbidity. Although the presence of the AMS phenotype is a good indicator of melanoma risk within susceptible families, genetic susceptibility to melanoma can arise in patients without the AMS, so selecting patients who may warrant long-term follow up is not always easy.[63] Genetic markers may be available in the future that may better predict melanoma risk within these families. Studies are needed to assess the role of life long follow up in these high risk groups but there are obvious difficulties in setting up randomised follow up studies for patients with AMS in terms of choosing an adequate control group with obvious ethical issues. Recognising high risk groups is important for general practitioners. A UK study has shown that the recognition of the AMS can be achieved by non-specialist healthcare professionals across Europe by using a scoring system for this phenotype.[124]

Other studies have attempted to use questionnaires to target individuals at risk. A study based in primary care, using a MacKie risk group for melanoma, showed that 4·3% of individuals were in the very high risk group and 4·4% were in the second highest risk group after self-assessment. This assessment reached an agreement of 0·67 (kappa values), 0·60 and 0·43 for freckles moles, and atypical naevi, respectively, when compared with scoring from the general practitioner.[104] It may therefore be possible to use questionnaires for targeted secondary prevention of melanoma, but the cost of such questionnaires compared with media campaigns needs to be evaluated. Furthermore, it is not clear whether general practitioners or dermatologists should be involved in the screening once the target groups are identified. With the shortage of dermatologists in the UK, the burden of melanoma screening on dermatology services is an important issue.

## What are the costs of screening and subsequent work-up?

It is difficult to assess the cost of melanoma screening as this could involve general practitioners or dermatologists, may be opportunistic or campaign-driven, and may involve the general population or only targeted groups. Secondary prevention campaigns do lead to a significant increase in workload for general practitioners, dermatologists and pathologists. Population screening after public health campaigns yields very few melanomas and the poor cost-effectiveness of such programmes is a critical issue.[104,125,126] Furthermore, worrying melanocytic lesions being shown via the media may also raise a lot of anxiety with difficulties in obtaining a fast dermatology referral

especially in the UK. Fast access pigmented lesions clinics have been useful in screening large number of patients but their efficacy in reducing melanoma mortality remains to be seen. It is becoming evident that population screening in Europe is unlikely to be warranted in view of the low prevalence of the disease but studies should investigate ways of targeting high risk individuals. The cost of melanoma screening in countries like the USA and Australia will only be fully evaluated when randomised studies are set up to examine its efficacy in a given population, and costs may still vary significantly between countries.

## What is the cost-effectiveness of screening?

There is no published randomised study evaluating the cost-effectiveness of secondary prevention in melanoma and, even in Australia where melanoma is a significant public health issue, this question has not been formally addressed and remains unanswered. The cost-effectiveness of melanoma screening is, however, an issue that has been addressed in many publications. Some studies have estimated the cost of melanoma screening in the USA and Australia using simulated data. The need for population screening for melanoma remains a controversial issue. In the USA, simulated data suggest that the cost-effectiveness for one-off population screening by a dermatologist at a cost of US $30 per person was US $29 170 per year of life saved (YLS) and this expenditure appeared reasonable compared with other established cancer screenings for cervical and breast tumours.[126] Studies assessing opportunistic screening by primary heathcare workers are needed but will be costly and difficult to set up. The cost-effectiveness of such a public health approach mainly depends on the prevalence of the disease, the sensitivity and specificity of the screening, the compliance of the population screened, and the cost of the screen. It is estimated that for the US data the prevalence of melanoma in the targeted group at a mean age of 50 years should remain above 0·0009 to justify a one-off screening in the normal population.[126] However, these data are based on currently available data on population screening and not randomised studies, so screened individuals are often self-selected and do not represent the normal population. Even in Australia where melanoma is twice as common than in the USA, simulated data show that the cost of screening is still substantial. The cost per year of life saved for screening every 5 years in men over the age of 50 would be Aust. $6853 compared with Aust. $11 102 in women.[127] Increasing the screening to 2-yearly raised the cost significantly. Whilst the cost of melanoma screening may appear high in these studies, it compares favourably with screening costs for breast and cervical cancer screening in the respective countries. However, studies are needed to assess the cost-effectiveness, specificity and sensitivity of screening in the primary care sector, as well as its take-up rate, as it is unlikely that any screening programme will rely solely on dermatologists. The cost-effectiveness of such initiatives can ultimately be judged in the light of the total health budget and the cost-effectiveness of other public health programmes.

## Conclusions

Melanoma is now a relatively common tumour especially in young age groups. It is readily amenable to primary and secondary prevention, although more work is needed to quantify the effects of sun avoidance and the safety of sunscreens in its primary prevention as well as the cost-effectiveness of various screening strategies for secondary prevention. Better training of physicians and health workers, public awareness as well as advances in the field of teledermatology may help in reducing mortality rates. The field of melanoma genetics is shedding light on the pathogenesis of this tumour with cell cycle regulatory genes having an important role in some familial form of the disease. Epidemiological studies over the past 30 years have all pointed towards the importance of host factors for this tumour. Whilst sun exposure is also important, it is becoming more apparent that genes must determine how people respond to mutagenic agents, namely, sun exposure. Discovering genes that determine melanoma susceptibility will help in understanding the complex interactions between genes and the environment in the causation of melanoma, but will also be helpful for the design of behavioural intervention and screening strategies for the prevention of melanoma.

## References

1  Gaudette LA, Gao RN. Changing trends in melanoma incidence and mortality. *Health Rep* 1998;**10**:29–41.

2  Weinstock MA. Issues in the epidemiology of melanoma. *Hematol Oncol Clin N Am* 1998;**12**:681–8.

3  Parkin M, Pisani P, Ferlay J. Estimates of the worldwide incidence of 25 major cancers in 1990. *Int J Cancer* 1999;**80**:827–41.

4  Ries LA, Miller BA, Hankey BF, Kosary CL, Harris A, Edwards BK, eds. *SEER Cancer Statistics Review, 1973–1991*. NIH Pub. No (NIH 94–2789). Bethesda, MD: National Cancer Institute, 1994.

5  Bulliard JL, Cox B, Semenciw R. Trends by anatomic sites in the incidence of cutaneous malignant melanoma in Canada, 1969–1993. *Cancer Causes Control* 1999;407–16.

6  MacKie RM. Incidence of risk factors and prevention of melanoma. *Eur J Cancer* 1999;**34**:S3–S6.

7  Gloster HM, Brodland DG. The epidemiology of skin cancer. *Dermatol Surg* 1996;**22**:217–26.

8  Jemal A, Devesa SS, Hartge P, Tucker MA. Recent trends in cutaneous melanoma incidence amongst whites in the United States. *J Natl Cancer Inst* 2001;**93**:678–83.

9  Marrett LD, Nguyen HL, Armstrong BK. Trends in the incidence of cutaneous malignant melanoma in New South Wales. *Int J Cancer* 2001;**92**:457–62.

10  Brochez L, Verhaege E, Bleyen L, Myny K, De Backer G, Naeyaert JM. Under-registration of melanoma in Belgium: an analysis. *Melanoma Res* 1888;**9**:413–18.

11  Brochez L, Naeyaert JM. Understanding the trends in melanoma incidence and mortality: where do we stand? *Eur J Dermatol* 2001;**10**:71–5.

12  Severi G, Giles GG, Robertson C, Boyle P, Autier P. Mortality from cutaneous melanoma: evidence for contrasting trends between populations. *Br J Cancer* 2000;**82**:1887–91.

13  Osterlind A. Epidemiology of malignant melanoma in Europe. *Acta Oncologica* 1992;**31**:903–8.

14  Jemal A, Devessa SS, Fears TR, Hartge P. Cancer surveillance series: changing patterns of cutaneous malignant melanoma mortality rates among whites in the United States. *J Natl Cancer Inst* 2000;**92**:811–18.

15  MacKie RM, Hole DJ. Incidence and thickness of primary tumours and survival of patients with cutaneous melanoma in relation to socio-economical status. *BMJ* 1996;**312**:1125–8.

16  Armstrong BK, Kricker A. Cutaneous melanoma. *Cancer Surv* 1994;**19**:219–40.

17  Weinstock MA. Epidemiology of melanoma. *Cancer Treat Res* 1993;**49**:29–56.

18  Black RJ, Bray F, Ferlay J, Parkin DM. Cancer incidence and mortality in the European Union: cancer registry data and estimates of national incidence for 1990. *Eur J Cancer* 1999;**135**:1534–6.

19  Elwood JA, Johnson J. Melanoma and sun exposure. An overview of published studies. *Int J Cancer* 1997;**73**:198–203.

20  Whiteman DC, Whiteman AC and Green AC. Childhood sun exposure as a risk factor for melanoma: a systematic review of epidemiologic studies. *Cancer Causes Control* 2001;**12**:69–82.

21  Bulliard JL. Site specific risk of cutaneous malignant melanoma and pattern of sun exposure in New Zealand. *Int J Cancer* 2000;**85**:627–632.

22  Pion IA, Rigel DS, Garfinkel L, Silverman MK, Kopf AW. Occupation and the risk of malignant melanoma. *Cancer* 1995;**75**:637–44.

23  Harrison RA, Haque AU, Roseman JM, Soong SJ. Socio-economic characteristics and melanoma incidence. *Ann Epidemiol* 1998;**8**:327–33.

24  Mellia J, Pendry L, Eiser JR, Harland C, Moss S. Evaluation of primary prevention for skin cancer: a review from a UK perspective. *Br J Dermatol* 2000;**143**;701–8.

25  Jackson A, Wilkinson C, Hood K, Pill R. Does experience predict knowledge and behavior with respect to cutaneous melanoma, moles and sun exposure? Possible outcome measures. *Behav Med* 2000;**26**:74–9.

26  Monfrecola G, Fabbrocini G, Posteraro G, Pini D. What do young people think about the dangers of sunbathing, skin cancer and sunbeds? A questionnaire survey among Italians. *Photodermatol Photoimmunol Photomed* 2000;**16**:15–18.

27  Brandberg Y, Ullen H, Sjoberg L, Holm LE. Sunbathing and sunbed use related to self image in a randomized sample of Swedish students. *Eur J Cancer* 1998;**7**:321–9.

28  Weinstock MA. Do sunscreens increase or decrease melanoma risk: an epidemiological evaluation. *J Invest Dermatol Symp Proc* 1999;**4**:97–100.

29  Westerdahl J, Ingvar C, Masback A, Olsson H. Sunscreen use and malignant melanoma. *Int J Cancer* 2000;**87**:145–50.

30  Vainio H, Bianchini F. Cancer-preventive effects of sunscreens are uncertain. *Scand J Work Environ Health* 2000;**26**:529–31.

31  Autier P, Dore JF, Reis AC *et al.* Suscreen use and intentional exposure to ultraviolet A and B radiation: a double blind randomized trial using personal dosimeters. *Br J Cancer* 2000;**83**:1243–8.

32  Autier P, Dore JF, Negrier S *et al.* Sunscreen use and duration of sun exposure: a double-blind randomized trial. *J Natl Cancer Inst* 1999;**4**:1304–9.

33  Azizi E, Iscovich J, Pavlotsky F *et al.* Use of sunscreen is linked with elevated naevi counts in Israeli school children and adolescents. *Melanoma Res* 2000;**10**:491–8.

34  Westerdahl J, Ingvar C, Masback A, Jonsson N, Olsson H. Risk of cutaneous melanoma in relation to use of sunbeds: further evidence for UV-A carcinogenicity. *Br J Cancer* 2000;**82**:1593–9.

35  Swerdlow AJ, Weinstock MA. Do tanning lamps cause melanoma? An epidemiologic assessment. *J Am Acad Dermatol* 1998;**38**:89–98.

36  Autier P, Dore JF, Lejeune F *et al.* Cutaneous malignant melanoma and exposure to sunlamps or sunbeds. An EORTC multi case-control study in Belgium, France, Germany. EORTC Melanoma Cooperative Group. *Int J Cancer* 1994;**15**:809–13.

37  Stern RS, Nichols KT, Vakeva LH. Malignant melanoma in patients treated for psoriasis with methoxsalen (psoralen) and ultraviolet radiation (PUVA). *N Engl J Med* 1997;**85**:1041–5.

38  Ness AR, Frankel SJ, Gunnell DJ, Smith GD. Are we really dying for a tan? *BMJ* 1999;**319**:114–16.

39  Norton BE, Morris HA. Osteoporosis and vitamin D. *J Cell Biochem* 1992;**49**:19–25.

40  Lefkowitz ES, Graland CF. Sunlight, vitamin D and ovarian cancer mortality rates in US women. *Int J Epidemiol* 1994;**23**:1133–6.

41  Garland CF, Garland FC. Do sunlight and vitamin D reduce the likelihood of colon cancer. *Int J Epidemiol* 1980;**9**:227–31.

42  Bikle DD, NG D, Oda Y, Xie Z. Calcium and vitamin D-regulated keratinocyte differentiation. *Mol Cell Endocrinol* 2001;**25**:161–71.

43  Hansen CM, Binderup L, Hamberg KJ, Carlberg C. Vitamin D and cancer. Effects of 1,25(OH)2D3 and its analogs on growth control and tumorigenesis. *Front Biosci* 2001;**6**:D920, D848.

44  Freedman DM, Dosemeci M, McGlynn K. Sunlight and mortality from breast, ovarian, and non-melanoma skin cancer: a composite death certificate based case–control study. *Occup Environ Med* 2002;**59**:257–62.

45  Hutchinson PE, Osborne JE, Lear JT *et al.* Vitamin D receptor polymorphisms are associated with altered prognosis in patients with malignant melanoma. *Clin Cancer Res* 2000;**6**:498–504.

46  Veirerod MB, Thelle DS, Laake P. Diet and risk of cutaneous melanoma: a prospective study of 50,757 Norwegian men and women. *Int J Cancer* 1997;**71**:600–4.

47  Niles RM. Recent advances in the use of vitamin A (retinoids) in the prevention and treatment of cancer. *Nutrition* 2000;**16**:1084–9.

48  Boxer CM, Bataille V, Newton Bishop JA, Hamby AM, Williams G. Topical tretinoin on atypical naevi. Potential for melanoma chemoprevention. *J Invest Dermatol* 1997;**109**:461.

49  Stam-Posthuma JJ, Vink J, le Cessie S *et al.* Effect of topical tretinoin under occlusion on atypical naevi. *Melanoma Res* 1998; **8**:539–48.

50  Lindelof B, Sigurgeirsson B, Gabel H, Stern RS. Incidence of skin cancer in 5356 patients following organ transplantation. *Br J Dermatol* 2000;**143**:513–19.

51  Szepietowski J, Wasik F, Szepietowski T *et al.* Excess benign melanocytic naevi in renal transplant recipients. *Dermatology* 1997;**194**:17–19.

52  Smith CH, McGregor JM, Barker JN *et al.* Excess melanocytic nevi in children with renal allografts. *J Am Acad Dermatol* 1993;**28**:51–5.

53  Grob JJ, Bastuji-Garin, Vaillant L *et al.* Excess of naevi related to immunodeficiency: a study of HIV-infected patients and renal transplant recipients. *J Invest Dermatol* 1996;**107**:694–7.

54  Bataille V, Bishop JA, Sasieni P *et al.* Risk of cutaneous melanoma in relation to the numbers, types and sites of naevi: a case–control study. *Br J Cancer* 1996;**73**:1605–11.

55  Greene MH. The genetics of hereditary melanoma and nevi. 1998 update. *Cancer* 2000;**86**:2464–77.

56  Hashemi j, Platz A, Ueno T, Stiener U, Ringborg U, Hansson J. CDKN2A germline mutations in individuals with multiple cutaneous melanomas. *Cancer Res* 2000;**60**:6864–7.

57  Aitken JF, Bailey-Wilson J, Green AC, Maclennan R, Martin NG. Segregation analysis of cutaneous melanoma in Queensland. *Genet Epidemiol* 1998;**15**:391–401.

58  Lynch HT, Brand RE, Hogg D *et al.* Phenotypic variation in eight extended CDKN2A germline mutation familial atypical mole melanoma-pancreatic- prone families: the familial atypical mole melanoma-pancreatic carcinoma syndrome. *Cancer* 2002;**94**:84–96.

59  Wachsmuth R, Harland M, Newton Bishop JA. The atypical mole syndrome phenotype is a poor predictor of predisposition in melanoma families. *N Engl J Med* 1998;**6**:2061–7.

60  Bataille V, Snieder H, MacGregor AJ, Sasieni P, Spector TD. Genetics of risk factors for melanoma. An adult twin study of naevi and freckles. *J Natl Cancer Inst* 2000;**92**:457–63.

61  Briollais L, Chompret A, Guilloud-Bataille M, Bressac-de-Paillerets B, Avril MF, Demenais F. Patterns of familial aggregation of three melanoma risk factors: great number of naevi, light phototype and high degree of sun exposure. *Int J Epidemiol* 2000;**29**:408–15.

62  Zhu G, Duffy DL, Eldridge A *et al.* A major quantitative trait locus for mole density is linked to the familial melanoma gene CDKN2: a maximum likelihood combined linkage and association in twins and their sibs. *Am J Hum Genet* 1999;**65**:483–92.

63  Bishop JA, Wachsmuth RC, Harland M *et al.* Genotype/phenotype and penetrance studies in melanoma families with germline CDKN2A mutations. *J Invest Dermatol* 2000;**114**:28–33.

64  Bergman W, Watson P, de Jong J, Lynch HT, Fusaro RM. Systemic cancer and the FAMMM syndrome. *Br J Cancer* 1990;**61**:932–36.

65  Lynch HT, Fusaro RM. Pancreatic cancer and the familial atypical mole multiple mole melanoma (FAMMM) syndrome. *Pancreas* 1991;**6**:127–31.

66  Anderson H, Bladstrom A, Olsson H, Moller TR. Familial breast and ovarian cancer: a Swedish population-based register study. *Am J Epidemiol* 2000;**152**:1154–63.

67  Bataille V, Hiles R, Bishop JA. Retinoblastoma, melanoma and the atypical mole syndrome. *Br J Dermatol* 1995;**132**:134–8.

68  Zoller ME, Rembeck B, Oden A, Samuelsson M, Angervall L. Malignant melanoma and benign tumours with neurofibromatosis type 1 in a defined Swedish population. *Cancer* 1997;**79**:2125–31.

69  Bataille V, Pinney E, Hungerford JL, Cuzick J, Bishop DT, Newton JA. Five cases of co-existent primary ocular and cutaneous melanoma. *Arch Dermatol* 1993;**129**:198–201.

70  Brennan P, Coates M, Armstrong B, Colin D, Bofetta P. Second primary following non-Hodgkin's lymphoma in New South Wales Australia. *Br J Cancer* 2000;**82**:1344–47.

71  Bahuau M, Vidaud D, Jenkins RB *et al.* Germline deletion involving INK4 locus in familial proneness to melanoma and nervous system tumors. *Cancer Res* 1998;**1**:2298–303.

72  Azizi E, Friedman J, Pavlotsky F *et al.* Familial cutaneous malignant melanoma and tumours of the nervous system. An hereditary cancer syndrome. *Cancer* 1995;**1**:1571–8.

73  Winsey SL, Haldar NA, Marsh HP *et al.* A variant within the DNA repair gene XRCC3 is associated with the development of melanoma skin cancer. *Cancer Res* 2000;**15**:5612–16.

74  Rowan A, Bataille V, MacKie R *et al.* Somatic mutations in the Peutz-Jeghers (LKP1/STKII) gene in sporadic malignant melanomas. *J Invest Dermatol* 1999;**112**:509–11.

75  Zhou XP, Gimm O, Hampel H, Nieman T, Walker MJ, Eng C. Epigenetic PTEN silencing in malignant melanoma without PTEN mutation. *Am J Pathol* 2000;**157**:1123–8.

76  Xu G, Snellman E, Bykov VJ, Jansen CT, Hemminki K. Cutaneous melanoma in patients have normal repair-kinetics of ultraviolet-induced DNA repair in skin *in situ*. *J Invest Dermatol* 2000;**114**:628–31.

77  Bataille V, Sasieni P, Nykov V, Cuzick J, Hemminki K. Epidermal cell DNA damage and repair *in vivo* in skin cancer cases and controls. *Br J Dermatol* 2001;**145**(Suppl. 59):133.

78  Cleaver JE. Common pathways for ultraviolet skin carcinogenesis in the repair and replication defective groups of xeroderma pigmentosum. *J Dermatol Sci* 2000;**23**:1–11.

79  Pavey S, Conroy S, Russel T, Gabrielli B. Ultraviolet radiation induces p16/CDKN2A expression in human skin. *Cancer Res* 1999;**1**:4185–9.

80  Itchii-Jones F, Lear JT, Heagerty AH *et al.* Susceptibility to melanoma; influence of skin type and polymorphism in the melanocyte stimulating hormone receptor gene. *J Invest Dermatol* 1998;**111**:218–21.

81  Palmer JS, Duffy DL, Box NF *et al.* Melanocortin-1 receptor polymorphisms and risk of melanoma: is the association explained solely by pigmentation phenotype? *Am J Hum Genet* 2000;**66**:176–86.

82  Berwick M. Gene–environment interaction in melanoma. Forum (Genoa);2000;**10**:191–200.

83  McGovern TW, Litaker MS. Clinical predictors of malignant pigmented lesions. A comparison of the Glasgow seven-point checklist and the American Cancer Society's ABCDs of pigmented lesions. *J Dermatol Surg* 1992;**18**:22–6.

84  Weinstock MA, Martin RA, Risicia PM *et al.* Thorough skin examination for the early detection of melanoma. *Am J Prev Med* 1999;**17**:169–75.

85  Morton CA, MacKie RM. Clinical accuracy of the diagnosis of cutaneous melanoma. *Br J Dermatol* 1998;**138**:283–7.

86  Brady MS, Oliveria SA, Christos PJ *et al.* Patterns of detection in patients with cutaneous melanoma. *Cancer* 2000;**15**:342–7.

87  Oliviera SA, Christos PJ, Halpern AC, Fine JA, Barnhill RL, Berwick M. Evaluation of factors associated with self skin examination. *Cancer Epidemiol Biomarkers Prev* 1999;**8**:971–8.

88  Blum A, Brand CU, Ellwanger U *et al.* Awareness and early detection of cutaneous melanoma; an analysis of factors related to delay in treatment. *Br J Dermatol* 1999;**141**:783–7.

89  Jackson A, Wilkinson C, Pill R. Moles and melanomas – who's at risk, who knows, and who cares? A strategy to inform those at high risk. *Br J Gen Pract* 1999;**49**:199–203.

90  Bataille V, Sasieni P, Curley RK, Cook MG, Marsden RA. Melanoma yield, number of biopsies and missed melanomas in a British teaching hospital pigmented lesion clinic: a 9 year retrospective study. *Br J Dermatol* 1999;**140**:243–8.

91  Duff CG, Melson D, Rigby HS, Kenealy JM, Townsend PL. A 6 year retrospective analysis of the diagnosis of malignant melanoma in a pigmented lesion clinic: even the experts miss malignant melanomas but not often. *Br J Plast Surg* 2001;**54**:317–21.

92  Osborne JE, Bourke JF, Holder J, Colloby P, Graham-Brown RA. The effect of the introduction of a pigmented lesion clinic on the interval between referral by family practitioner and attendance at hospital. *Br J Dermatol* 1998;**138**:418–21.

93  Graham-Brown RA, Osborne JE London SP *et al.* The initial effect on workload and outcome of a public education campaign on early diagnosis and treatment of malignant melanoma in Leicestershire. *Br J Dermatol* 1990;**122**:53–9.

94  Mallet RB, Fallowfield ME, Cook MG *et al.* Are pigmented lesion clinics worthwhile? *Br J Dermatol* 1993;**129**:689–93.

95  Melia J, Moss S, Coleman D *et al.* The relation between mortality and early detection in the Cancer Research Campaign Mole Watcher Study. *Br J Cancer* 2001;**85**:803–7.

96  Eiser JR, Pendry L, Greaves CJ *et al.* Is targeted early detection of melanoma feasible? Self-assessments of risk and attitudes to screening. *J Med Screen* 2000;**7**:199–202.

97  Piccolo D, Smolle J, Wolf IH *et al.* Face to face diagnosis versus telediagnosis of pigmented skin tumours: a teledermoscopic study. *Arch Dermatol* 1999;**135**:1467–71.

98  Joliffe VM, Harris DW, Morris R, Wallacet P, Whittaker SJ. Can we used video images to triage pigmented lesions? *Br J Dermatol* 2001;**145**:904–10.

99  Provost N, Kopf AW, Rabinovitz HS *et al.* Comparison of conventional photographs and telephonically transmitted compressed digitized images of melanomas and dysplastic naevi. *Dermatology* 1998;**196**:299–304.

100  Bataille V. Genetics of familial and sporadic melanoma. *Clin Exp Dermatol* 2000;**25**:464–70.

101  Marghoob AA, Slade J, Kopf AW *et al.* Risk of developing multiple primary cutaneous melanomas in patients with the classic atypical mole syndrome: a case–control study. *Br J Dermatol* 1996;**135**:704–11.

102  Di Fronzo LA, Wanek LA, Morton DL. Ealier diagnosis of second primary melanoma confirms the benefits of patient education and routine post-operative follow up. *Cancer* 2001;**91**:1520–4.

103  Bataille V, Grulich A, Sasieni P *et al.* The association between naevi and melanoma in populations with different sun exposure: a joint case–control study of melanoma in the UK and Australia. *Br J Cancer* 1998;**77**:505–10.

104  Jackson A, Wilkinson C, Ranger M, Pill R, August P. Can primary prevention or selective screening for melanoma be more precisely targeted through general practice? A prospective study to validate a self administered risk score. *BMJ* 1998;**316**:34–8.

105  Kaufmann R. Surgical management of primary melanoma. *Clin Exp Dermatol* 2000;**25**:476–81.

106  Tsao H, Rogers GS, Sober AJ. An estimate of the annual direct cost of treating melanoma. *J Am Acad Dermatol* 1998;**38**:669–80.

107  Whittaker S. Adjuvant therapy in melanoma. *Clin Exp Dermatol* 2000;**25**:497–502.

108  Kirkwood JM, Strawdeman MH, Ernstoff MS *et al.* Interferon alfa-2b adjuvant therapy of high risk resected malignant melanoma. The Eastern Cooperative Oncology Group trial EST 1684. *J Clin Oncol* 1996;**14**:7–17.

109  Pehamberger H, Soyer HP, Steiner A *et al.* Adjuvant interferon alfa-2a treatment in resected primary stage II cutaneous melanoma. Australian Malignant Melanoma Cooperative Group. *J Clin Oncol* 1998;**16**:1425–9.

110  Grob JJ, Dreno B, de la Slamoniere P *et al.* Randomised trial of interferon alpha-2a as adjuvant therapy in resected primary melanoma thicker than 1·5 mm without clinically detectable node metastases. French Cooperative Group on Melanoma. *Lancet* 1998;**351**:1905–10.

111  Philip PA, Flaherty LE. Biochemotherapy for melanoma. *Curr Oncol Rep* 2000;**2**:314–21.

112  Lafuma A, Dreno B, Delaunay M *et al.* Economic analysis of adjuvant therapy with interferon alpha-2a in stage II malignant melanoma. *Eur J Cancer* 2001;**37**:369–75.

113  Hillner BE. Cost-effectiveness assessment of interferon alfa-2b as adjuvant therapy of high risk resected cutaneous melanoma. *Eur J Cancer* 1998;**34**(Suppl. 3):S18–S21.

114  Russell-Jones R, Acland K. Sentinel node biopsy in the management of malignant melanoma. *Clin Exp Dermatol* 2001;**26**:463–8.

115  Becker JC, Kampgen E, Brocker E. Classical chemotherapy for metastatic melanoma. *Clin Exp Dermatol* 2000;**25**:503–8.

116  Roberts DL, Anstey AV, Barlow RJ *et al.* UK guidelines for the management of cutaneous melanoma. *Br J Dermatol* 2002;**146**:7–17.

117  Thompson LW, Brinckerhoff L, Slingluff CL Jr. Vaccination for melanoma. *Curr Oncol Rep* 2000;**2**:292–9.

118  Brown CK, Kirkwood JM. Targeted therapy for melanoma. *Curr Oncol Rep* 2001;**3**:344–52.

119  Weiss K. Safety profile of interferon-alpha therapy. *Semin Oncol* 1998;**25**(Suppl. 1):9–13.

120  Australian Cancer Society. *National cancer prevention policy, 1993.* Sydney: Australian Cancer Society, 1993.

121  Koh HK, Caruso A, Gage I *et al.* Evaluation of melanoma/skin cancer screening in Massachusetts. Preliminary results. *Cancer* 1990;**65**:375–9.

122  International Union Against Cancer. *Melanoma control manual.* Geneva: UICC, 1992.

123  De Rooij MJ, Rampen FH, Schouten LJ, Neumann HA. Skin cancer screening focusing on melanoma yields more selective attendance. *Arch Dermatol* 1995;**131**:422–5.

124  Bishop JA, Bradburn M, Bergamn W *et al.* Teaching non-specialist health care professionals how to identify the atypical mole syndrome phenotype: a multinational study. *Br J Dermatol* 2000;**142**:331–7.

125  De Rooij MJ, Rampen FH, Schouten LJ, Neumann HA. Volunteer melanoma screening. Follow up, compliance and outcome. *Dermatol Surg* 1997;**23**:197–201.

126  Freedberg KA, Geller AC, Miller DR, Lew RA, Koh HK. Screening for malignant melanoma: A cost-effectiveness analysis. *J Am Acad Dermatol* 1999;**41**:738–45.

127  Girgis A, Clarke P, Burton RC, Sanson-Fisher RW. Screening for melanoma by primary health physicians: a cost effectiveness analysis. *J Med Screen* 1996;**3**:47–53.

# Section IV

## Treating tumours of the respiratory system

*Xavier Bonfill, Editor*

# Levels of evidence and grades of recommendation used in *Evidence-based Oncology*

Levels of evidence and grades of recommendation appear within the text in the clinical chapters, for example, **Evidence Level Ia** and **Grade A**.

---

**Levels of evidence**

---

Ia   Meta-analysis of randomised controlled trials (RCTs)
Ib   At least 1 RCT
IIa  At least 1 non-randomised study
IIb  At least 1 other well designed quasi-experimental study
III  Non-experimental, descriptive studies
IV   Expert committee reports or opinions/experience of respected authorities

**Grades of recommendations**

---

A   At least one RCT as part of body of literature of overall good quality and consistency addressing recommendation **Evidence levels Ia, Ib**
B   No RCT but well conducted clinical studies available **Evidence levels IIa, IIb, III**
C   Expert committee reports or opinions/experience of respected authorities in the absence of directly applicable good quality clinical studies **Evidence level IV**

---

From *Clinical Oncology* (2001)**13**:S212
Source of data: MEDLINE, *Proceedings of the American Society of Medical Oncology* (ASCO).

# 21 Lung cancer

*Xavier Bonfill*

## Introduction

Lung cancer is the term used to refer to tumours arising from the respiratory epithelium in the bronchi, bronchioles and alveoli. Four major cell types account for about 88% of all lung cancers: adenocarcinomas, squamous cell carcinomas, large cell carcinomas and small cell carcinomas. Small cell carcinomas represent about 20–25% of cases and the remainder are non-small cell varieties, of which adenocarcinoma is now the most common, having for unknown reasons, recently replaced squamous cell carcinoma as the most frequent histological subtype for all races and sexes combined.[1]

In the year 2000, there were nearly 200 000 lung cancer cases in the 15 member states of the European Union and over one million people around the world died from the disease.[2] Lung cancer is now the leading cause of cancer death for both men and women in the United States,[3] and in England and Wales, where a quarter of all deaths are due to cancer, one in three of these deaths in men and one in 6·5 in women, are due to lung cancer.[4]

The most important single risk factor for lung cancer is smoking, accounting for about 90% of cases[4], but reasons why many heavy smokers do not develop the disease and for the occurrence of the disease in non-smokers are unexplained.[3] Occupational exposure to carcinogens, especially asbestos, increases the risks and there is growing evidence of the contribution of genetic factors.[5]

Over 55% of patients with lung cancer have distant metastases at diagnosis, while about 25% have regional node involvement and only about 15% have localised disease.[1] Although advances in chemotherapy, surgery and radiotherapy have led to a steady increase in survival from 8% in the 1960s to 14% in the 1990s, outlook for the vast majority of people with the disease remains grim.[1] There is clear evidence of a dose–response relationship between smoking and lung cancer,[5] but there nevertheless remain many uncertainties about the aetiology and natural history of the disease. As multidisciplinary research efforts begin to elucidate the complex molecular and cellular processes underlying the disease, there is hope that new treatment approaches may offer an improvement on conventional therapeutic interventions.[4]

Prevention of the disease through implementation of tobacco control policies must continue to be an essential mainstay of lung cancer reduction strategies, but the development and rigorous evaluation of treatment interventions also remains fundamental. As the Lung Cancer Progress Review Group Report of the US National Cancer Institute points out, "It is a sobering reality that tobacco control will ameliorate but not, in the foreseeable future, eliminate the problem of lung cancer".[3]

The International System for Staging Lung Cancer[6] which uses the TNM subsets (T, primary tumour; N, regional lymph nodes; M, distant metastasis) has been adopted by the American Joint Committee on Cancer and the Union Internationale Contre le Cancer, and TNM subsets are grouped into stages (I–IV) for use in both patient management and clinical research.[7]

## References

1 Fauci AS, Braunwald E, Isselbacher KJ *et al.,* eds. *Harrison's Principles of Internal Medicine, 14th edn.* New York: McGraw-Hill, 1998.
2 *Cancer incidence, mortality and prevalence worldwide.* GLOBOCAN 2000. International Agency for Research on Cancer [http://www-dep.iarc.fr].
3 *National Cancer Institute. Report of the Lung Cancer Progress Review Group.* August 2001 [http://prg.nci.nih.gov/lung/finalreport.html].
4 Sethi T. Science, medicine, and the future: Lung cancer. *BMJ* 1997;**314**:652–5.
5 Ginsberg RJ, Vokes EE, Raben A. Non-small cell lung cancer. In: Devita VT Jr, Hellman S, Rosenberg SA. *Cancer. Principles and practice of oncology, 5th edn.* Philadelphia: Lippincott-Raven, 1997.
6 Mountain CF. Revisions in the International System for Staging Lung Cancer. *Chest* 1997;**111**:1710–17.
7 Ries LAG, Eisner MP, Kosary CL eds. *SEER Cancer Statistics Review, 1973–1999.* Bethesda, MD: National Cancer Institute [http://seer.cancer.gov/csr/1973_1999/,2001].

# Non-small cell lung cancer

*Alan Neville, Elinor Thompson*

Non-small cell lung cancer (NSCLC) represents the largest group of lung cancers and includes several histological subtypes of which the most common are adenocarcinoma (40% of all lung cancers), squamous cell carcinoma (30%) and large cell carcinoma (15%).[1] The incidence of NSCLC in men in the United States reached a peak during the 1980s of over 87 cases per 100 000, but is now decreasing. In contrast, although the incidence in women is much lower, it continued to increase until recently and, whereas in 1973 the rate was about one-quarter that of the male level, by 1998 it had risen to over 44 cases per 100 000.[2]

Between 5% and 15% of cases are diagnosed on routine chest *x* ray examination, but the majority of cases present with symptoms and signs related either to the site of growth of the primary tumour, or to the effects of regional spread in the thorax or metastatic spread. About one-third of patients with NSCLC have no evidence of mediastinal node involvement at diagnosis and are therefore suitable for potentially curative surgical intervention, and a further third have stage IV disease.[3] Five-year survival varies from 67% for surgically-pathologically staged T1N0M0 tumours to only 1% for stage IV disease (any T, any N, M1).[4]

Levels of evidence and grades of recommendation for the questions below are given in Table 21.1.

## Does adjuvant or neoadjuvant chemotherapy improve survival in potentially operable patients (stages I, II and resectable stage III)?

### Background

While surgery remains the preferred treatment modality for potential cure for patients with non-small cell lung cancer, only about 50% of all patients will have localised disease at the time of initial presentation and less than one-third are candidates for thoracotomy.[1] Accurate intraoperative staging is required since the most important factors that determine prognosis in patients with early stage disease are the size of the primary tumour and the presence or absence of metastases to local lymph nodes.[4] While patients with pathological stage I disease enjoy survival rates in excess of 50%, for those with N2 disease, thoracic recurrence rates approach 20% and there is a significant risk of distant metastasis.[5] Since the majority of patients with resected disease subsequently suffer systemic recurrence, improvements in survival have been sought through the administration of pre- and postoperative chemotherapy (with or without radiation).

### Answer to question

Meta-analysis of a number of studies of postoperative chemotherapy reveals considerable diversity of results, the direction of the treatment effect dependent on the type of chemotherapy employed. While cisplatin-containing regimens appear to increase survival by about 3% at 2 years, trials using the alkylating agents revealed a 15% increase in the relative risk of death, equivalent to a survival reduction of 4% at 2 years from chemotherapy.

There is evidence from four small randomised controlled trials that for patients with technically resectable stage IIIA disease, the use of preoperative cisplatin-based chemotherapy and postoperative radiotherapy results in superior survival compared with surgery plus postoperative radiotherapy. It is unknown what the benefit of preoperative chemotherapy would be in the absence of postoperative radiotherapy.

### Review of evidence

#### Adjuvant chemotherapy

A systematic review and meta-analysis of individual patient data from 14 trials (4357 patients, 2574 deaths) was identified in which patients underwent surgery with or without adjuvant postoperative chemotherapy. There was considerable heterogeneity across the trials (statistical heterogeneity; $P = 0.02$), although no evidence of heterogeneity within each of the two categories of long-term alkylating drug regimens and cisplatin-based treatments.[6]

Long-term alkylating agents are clearly harmful and trial results favour surgery alone; the combined hazard ratio is 1·15 ($P = 0.005$) in favour of surgery alone. This represents a 15% increase in the relative risk of death from the use of these drugs, reducing survival at 5 years from 50% to 45%.

For postoperative cisplatin-containing regimens, the overall hazard ratio is 0·87 ($P = 0.08$), improving 5-year survival from 50% to 55%, but the 95% confidence limits for absolute difference in survival cross unity, and thus the results are not conclusive of benefit.

This same systematic review also addressed seven randomised trials (807 patients and 619 deaths) in which adjuvant chemotherapy was added to surgery plus postoperative radiotherapy. Six of these studies used a cisplatin-based regimen. While the overall hazard ratio of 0·98 ($P = 0.76$) is marginally in favour of chemotherapy, the 95% confidence intervals again cross unity.

#### Neoadjuvant chemotherapy

Preoperative or neoadjuvant chemotherapy for patients with resectable stage III disease has been addressed in a systematic review.[7] In four trials identified, two small RCTs (60 patients in each with technically resectable stage IIIA disease) were fully reported.[8,9] A pooled analysis of these

**Table 21.1 Non-small cell lung cancer – summary of recommendations**

| Treatment strategy | Recommendation | Level of evidence/ grade of recommendation |
|---|---|---|
| Postoperative adjuvant chemotherapy | Not recommended as survival benefit even with cisplatin regimens is small and toxicity of treatment is significant | **Evidence level Ia, Grade A** |
| Preoperative (neoadjuvant) chemotherapy in stage IIIA disease | Limited evidence that preoperative cisplatin-based chemotherapy should be offered to stage IIIA patients if postoperative radiation is also given | **Evidence level Ia, Grade A** |
| Postoperative radiotherapy (without chemotherapy) | Use of conventional radiotherapy techniques is likely to be ineffective or harmful in patients with completely resected stage I and II disease | **Evidence level Ia, Grade A** |
| Radiotherapy for cure in medically inoperable stage I patients | Given lack of definitive evidence from randomised trials, treatment with radiotherapy should occur in the context of a clinical trial | **Evidence level IIa, Grade B** |
| Combined modality therapy for unresectable stage III disease | Patients > 70 years of age should be offered combined modality therapy as improved survival has been demonstrated. Treatment appears too toxic in those patients < 70 | **Evidence level Ia, Grade A** |
| Hyperfractionation *v* conventional fractionation | Insufficient evidence to recommend altered fractionation radiotherapy | **Evidence level Ia/b, Grade B** |
| Chemotherapy to improve survival and quality of life in stage IV disease patients | Modest improvement in survival and quality of life demonstrated in patients with ECOG performance status 2 or better only | **Evidence level Ia, Grade A** |
| Benefit of second-line chemotherapy | Only docetaxel has demonstrated benefit in survival and quality of life in previously treated patients | **Evidence level Ib, Grade A** |
| Most appropriate palliative radiotherapy for locally advanced symptomatic NSCLC | No recommendation possible based on current evidence for any particular radiotherapy regimen – dose, schedule, fractionation or brachytherapy | **Evidence level III, Grade C** |

two trials found that preoperative chemotherapy versus no chemotherapy significantly improved 2-year survival (OR 0·18; 95% CI 0·06–0·51; $P = 0.001$). In both of these studies, some patients also received postoperative radiation. The trials are small because interim analysis demonstrated significant survival differences between the two groups. Both of these studies have been criticised because patients were staged clinically, not pathologically; the trials included stage T3N0 patients and were not balanced for prognostic factors such as *k-Ras* mutations.[7]

Two further studies have been reported in preliminary form.[10,11] In one, patients (IIIA disease) received preoperative chemotherapy plus surgery plus postoperative chemotherapy or surgery plus postoperative radiation. Interim analysis (27 patients total) showed a median survival advantage for preoperative chemotherapy (28·7 months *v* 15·6 months;

$P = 0.095$). In the other study, the Cancer and Leukemia Group B (CALGB) randomised patients to chemotherapy plus surgery with postoperative chemotherapy and radiation treatment versus radiotherapy followed by surgery and postoperative radiotherapy. This trial closed early owing to poor accrual (47 patients total) and median follow up time was not reported. Median survival was 19 months for those receiving chemotherapy and 23 months for those who did not receive chemotherapy ($P = 0.64$).[11]

## Conclusions

### Implications for practice

Given the toxicity of many of the regimens used in the reported adjuvant studies and the inconclusive and limited survival benefit from adjuvant treatment, postoperative chemotherapy cannot be recommended currently for patients with resected NSCLC. For patients with technically resectable stage IIIA, the evidence from small trials suggests that preoperative cisplatin-based chemotherapy should be offered if the patients also receive postoperative radiotherapy. The implications for treatment are complicated by the fact that stage IIIA disease in some trials includes T3N0, for which surgery alone is usually indicated, as well as T1–3N2. Many surgeons regard the presence of N2 disease as a contraindication to surgery. Thus the recommendations for preoperative chemotherapy and postoperative radiotherapy apply only to those patients with N2 disease for whom surgery is planned.

### Implications for research

Patients with resected NSCLC should be considered for incorporation into new trials of less toxic agents with improved activity against lung cancer in the postoperative setting.

## Does postoperative radiotherapy improve survival in successfully operated patients (with or without mediastinal spread)?

### Background

Surgical excision for early stage non-small cell lung cancer (NSCLC) offers the best chance of cure from the disease. Of the total number of patients presenting with NSCLC, about one-third have no evidence of mediastinal node involvement and are suitable for surgery.[1] But 5-year survival in patients with disease resected with curative intent remains disappointing, ranging from 38% for T3N0 disease to 67% for T1N0 disease[12] and an overall average 5-year survival of about 40%.[13] The effects of adjuvant postoperative radiotherapy (PORT) in improving local disease control and enhancing survival have been investigated in a number of trials, but results have been conflicting as none has had sufficient statistical power to detect a modest survival advantage.[14] A meta-analysis published in 1998 and updated in 2000 found that PORT was detrimental to survival in patients with resected stage I and II disease, although there was no clear evidence of detriment in stage III disease.[13,14] In spite of the conclusions of this study, the debate over the use of adjuvant radiotherapy has continued, partly because of concerns about the use of obsolete techniques in some of the trials included in the meta-analysis, partly because of controversies over the dose and partly because of the unresolved issue of the effect of PORT in stage III N2 disease.[15–17] There have been huge technological advances in radiotherapy in the past 10 years including the introduction of three-dimensional conformal radiotherapy, intensity modulated radiotherapy and more frequent fractionation schedules, the effects of which have yet to be fully evaluated.[18]

### Answer to question

Use of conventional radiotherapy techniques in patients with completely resected stage I and stage II disease is likely to be ineffective or harmful. The benefits versus risks of more modern techniques and fractionation schedules remain unclear, as are the effects of PORT in patients with stage III N2 disease.

### Review of evidence

A systematic review and meta-analysis of individual data on 2128 patients from nine randomised controlled trials[13] (updated January 2000) found that postoperative radiotherapy had a significant adverse effect on survival (HR 1·21; 95% CI 1·08–1·34; $P = 0·001$). This equates to a reduction in overall 2-year survival of 7%, from 55% to 48% at 2 years. The survival curves begin to separate at about 4 months after treatment and remain apart for the following 5 years for which reliable data is available. There were also significant differences in favour of surgery alone, for local and distant recurrence-free survival and for overall recurrence-free survival. Subgroup analysis showed some evidence that patients with stage I disease fared worse with postoperative radiotherapy than those with stage II disease, and there was no clear evidence that the treatment was detrimental for patients with stage III N2 disease. There was no differential effect of treatment with respect to age, sex or histology. There was a 24% reduction in local recurrence among patients who received postoperative radiotherapy compared with those having only surgery, and the authors suggested that this may have been because of the higher death rate in the radiotherapy group, in that these patients died before the tumour recurred.

The possible cause for the reduction in survival in patients who received postoperative radiotherapy is unclear as, although the cause of death was reported in eight of the nine trials, the accuracy of this recording was questioned by the trialists themselves.[14] The fact that the survival difference emerges at about 4 months, increasing over the next few months after which it remains much the same, has led to the suggestion that it was most likely due to radiation-induced pneumonitis.[19]

Patients in the nine trials included in the PORT meta-analysis all had completely resected tumours. A common meta-analysis stage scale was used to overcome differences in the classification systems used in the different trials and, although no patient's tumour was more advanced than stage IIIA, there was variation between trials in the proportion of patients in each stage, and WHO performance status was only available from three trials. The trials in the meta-analysis included data from 1966 to the mid 1990s, a range of radiation doses and schedules were used, and a varying proportion of patients were treated with cobalt-60 (Co60) and linear accelerator (LINAC) machines: one trial used only Co60, two trials used only LINAC, and the remainder used both machines. Treatment with Co60 is no longer considered acceptable and a subanalysis of data from patients treated only with LINAC machines would be interesting. Doses delivered varied from 30 Gy to 60 Gy, number of fractions from 10 to 30, and size of fractions from 1·8 Gy to 3 Gy per day, but there was no evidence that any one dose or schedule was more detrimental than any other.

We found one randomised controlled trial published subsequent to this meta-analysis.[20] This trial, conducted from 1989 to 1997, included 104 patients with stage I disease only, all of whom received CT planned treatment with a linear accelerator. Dose delivered was 50·4 Gy, in fractions of 1·8 Gy per day over 5·5 weeks (28 fractions). In contrast to the PORT findings, this trial found a positive trend for overall survival in favour of the group treated with postoperative radiotherapy, 67% versus 58% (HR 2·4; 95% CI 1·01–5·2; *P*= 0·046). In common with the PORT results, this trial also showed a reduction in local recurrence in the group treated with radiotherapy versus surgery alone (2% *v* 23% respectively). Among patients who received postoperative radiotherapy, six suffered grade 1 acute toxicity and there were 19 cases of postradiation lung fibrosis, with radiological evidence in 18, but no significant impairment of respiratory function. The randomisation procedure and allocation concealment in this trial appeared adequate and analysis was by "intention to treat".

## Conclusions

### Implications for clinical practice

Routine use of postoperative radiotherapy using conventional radiotherapy techniques is not recommended. Evidence from a meta-analysis of individual patient data from nine trials showed that the administration of postoperative radiotherapy after complete resection of stage I and stage II NSCLC has a detrimental effect on survival, although it reduces local recurrence. There was no clear evidence of an adverse effect on survival in patients with more advanced, stage III N2 disease. A recent randomised trial, not included in the meta-analysis showed a positive survival trend in favour of postoperative radiotherapy for patients with stage I disease. Since the effects of more modern radiotherapy techniques and schedules (3D conformal radiotherapy and novel fractionation schedules) as adjuvant therapy remain unclear – these treatments should not occur outside of clinical trials.

### Implications for research

In view of the heterogeneity in the treatment doses, schedules and machines used in the trials included in the PORT meta-analysis, and the conflicting findings from a recently published, non-included RCT, an updated analysis of the pooled data, together with subgroup analysis of those

treated only with a linear accelerator may be relevant. The effects of more modern radiotherapy techniques (3D conformal radiotherapy) and fractionation schedules, such as continuous hyperfractionated accelerated radiotherapy (CHART), in patients with completely resected stage I-IIIA disease, warrant investigation in carefully designed clinical trials. It is important that future trials record accurate data on cause of death in order to distinguish treatment-related deaths from deaths due to lung cancer.[14] It is also essential that precise data on locoregional and distant spread and on the surgical interventions undertaken is recorded.[21,22]

## Can radiotherapy cure patients with stage I disease who are medically inoperable?

### Background

About two-thirds of patients diagnosed with non-small cell lung cancer will be referred for radiotherapy of whom between 10% and 15% will have stage I or II disease classified as medically inoperable.[1] The definition of medically inoperable refers to patients whose lung cancer is technically resectable but whose medical condition makes surgery inadvisable. Patients who refuse surgery are also often considered in this group.[23]

Although current evidence does not support lung cancer screening,[24] recent developments in the development of sputum-based cellular diagnostics[25] and imaging technology[26] are bringing the prospect of an effective screening test ever closer. If these new diagnostic techniques increase the proportion of curable cases diagnosed with early stage disease, the need for evidence-based policy for the management of medically inoperable patients will become urgent.[27] A recent retrospective review of over 20 000 lung cancer patients diagnosed over a 10-year period found that nearly 4% had clinical stage I disease that had been treated non-surgically.[28]

There have been no randomised comparisons of surgery versus radiotherapy in the treatment of early stage lung cancer since the early 1960s,[29] and comparisons between observational series are thwarted by problems in comparing like with like,[30] as survival for the same disease stage may differ depending on whether staging is clinical or pathological (surgical).[31] According to the revised International System for Staging Lung Cancer, 5-year survival in pathologically staged patients with stage IA and IB tumours was 67% and 57% respectively, whereas in those that were clinically staged, respective survivals were 61% and 38%.[4] In contrast, without any treatment, outlook for early stage disease is very poor.[32]

### Answer to question

There is insufficient evidence from randomised trials to assess whether radiotherapy is curative in patients with stage I disease who are medically inoperable.

## Review of evidence

We found no randomised controlled trials that compared immediate radical radiotherapy with best supportive care in patients with stage I non-small cell lung cancer who are medically inoperable. We found one systematic review, which included one randomised controlled study and 26 non-randomised retrospective studies.[30] This review concluded that survival seemed to be better in patients who received radiotherapy compared with those who did not, and that the optimal radiation dose and treatment technique are unknown.

The one randomised study included in the review compared two radiotherapy schedules in 563 patients with pathologically proven, inoperable NSCLC: CHART with 54 Gy in 36 fractions over 12 days versus conventionally fractionated radiotherapy 60 Gy in 30 fractions over 6 weeks.[33] The trial included patients with stage I-IIIB NSCLC and found that in the group as a whole there was an overall improvement in survival of 9% from 20% to 29% ($P=0.008$) with CHART compared with conventional radiotherapy. A subgroup analysis published subsequently to the main report[34] gave details of the effects of the two treatments in patients with stage I-IIA disease. In this subgroup of 169 patients, of whom the majority (163) had stage I disease, 2-year survival was improved in the group receiving CHART as compared with those who received conventional radiotherapy ($37 \pm 5\%$ *v* $24 \pm 5\%$). There was also a smaller improvement in 4-year survival with CHART ($18 \pm 4\%$ *v* $12 \pm 4\%$ for CHART and conventional radiotherapy respectively). The reduction in relative risk of death for patients with stage I-IIA disease was 25% compared with 22% for the whole group.[34] Data on treatment morbidity in patients with stage I disease were not reported separately in this trial. All patients (stages I-IIIB) were defined as being inoperable, but data on the reasons for inoperability (such as whether those with early stage disease included some who were inoperable for medical reasons or because they refused surgery) were not reported. The study authors themselves comment that, with respect to early stage disease, definitive statements regarding the comparability of radiotherapy with other treatment modalities are inadvisable on the basis of these data alone.[34]

In the 26 retrospective studies included in the systematic review, 2-year survival following radiotherapy in patients with stage I/II disease varied between 22% and 72% and 5-year survival varied from 0 to 42%.[30] There was large variation between the studies with respect to patient characteristics (age, performance status, weight loss, comorbidity, proportion being inoperable for medical reasons compared with proportion refusing surgery) and with respect to the dose (range 15–90 Gy) and fractionation schedule of radiotherapy given. None of the 26 retrospective studies nor the randomised controlled study reported data on quality of life.

We found one randomised controlled trial that compared accelerated radiotherapy (60 Gy, 10 fractions, 3 weeks) with standard fraction radiotherapy (60 Gy, 5 fractions, 5 weeks) with or without concurrent chemotherapy in a $2 \times 2$ factorial design.[35] Although this trial included patients with stage I disease, because of the four-arm design, patient numbers in each of the arms were relatively small. Only 19 patients were included in the two radiotherapy-only arms altogether, and no subanalysis of survival by this stage was reported. Another randomised controlled study compared external irradiation plus endobronchial brachytherapy with external irradiation only, in patients with inoperable non-small cell lung cancer.[36] This study also included stage I patients who were prescribed a radical fractionation schedule with or without added brachytherapy, but only nine patients with this stage disease were randomised.

More recent observational studies have shown promising results with radiotherapy, including a 3-year overall survival of 86% in a series of 29 patients with stage I disease, who were medically operable but refused surgery and who were treated with stereotactic radiotherapy.[37]

## Conclusions

### Implications for practice

There is no definitive evidence from randomised trials to determine the risks and benefits of radical radiotherapy in the treatment of medically inoperable stage I non-small cell lung cancer. Results from retrospective reviews indicate that survival may be better with radiotherapy than with no immediate treatment. Optimal doses and fractionation schedules, such as the possible benefits of CHART versus dose escalation in either CHART or conventionally fractionated regimens, are unclear. Radiotherapy of medically inoperable stage I disease should therefore ideally occur within the context of a clinical trial.

### Implications for research

With the development of diagnostic techniques leading to an increasing likelihood of earlier diagnosis of non-small cell lung cancer, there is an urgent need for the development of evidence-based policy for the management of inoperable early disease. The question should be addressed in specifically designed randomised trials, which should stratify data according to patient characteristics, including reasons for inoperability as well as treatment dose and fractionation schedule received. Larger studies of the effects of stereotactic radiotherapy in medically inoperable early stage disease are needed to ascertain whether randomised comparisons with surgery in stage I disease are appropriate.

Some of the retrospective trials that included patients with stage I disease reported relatively high proportions of patients with stage I disease who had declined surgery. Among non-randomised studies included in the Cochrane review, the proportion of patients who were classified as inoperable because they refused surgery varied between 1·4%[38] and 40·8%,[39] and in a more recent observational study this was as high as 58%.[37] Qualitative research is necessary to understand the reasons why substantial proportions of patients with early stage disease refuse surgery when it is currently accepted as the most effective curative intervention. This research could inform both patient education programmes and the development of effective treatment options that are more closely tailored to patient choice.

## In unresectable stage III disease, is the combination of chemotherapy with radiotherapy more effective than radiotherapy alone?

### Background

Most patients with locally advanced unresectable stage IIIB (and some patients with bulky unresected IIIA disease) have disseminated disease at the time of death.[6] The definition of locally advanced disease also includes those patients with a malignant pleural effusion, but now excludes those with T3N0 disease (now staged as IIB) because of their more favourable prognosis compared with those with mediastinal lymph node involvement. Controversy continues regarding which patients with stage IIIA disease should be offered surgery at some point in their management. The inevitable development of metastatic disease in those who present with initially localised disease has led to a number of trials combining chemotherapy with thoracic radiotherapy in a variety of treatment sequences.

### Answer to question

While the observed benefits of chemotherapy in addition to thoracic radiotherapy are modest, systematic reviews have shown improved survival in chemotherapy-treated patients. There is considerably less evidence on the effects of combined treatment on quality of life and the treatment may be too toxic for those older than 70.

### Review of evidence

A systematic review and meta-analysis (22 trials, 3033 patients, and 2814 deaths) and two additional studies were identified, which compared thoracic radiotherapy with or without the addition of chemotherapy for patients with unresectable stage III disease.[6,40,41]

While the overall results from the meta-analysis of 22 studies show a significant benefit for the addition of chemotherapy (HR 0·90; $P = 0·006$), which equates to a 10% reduction in the risk of death, the 11 trials using cisplatin-based chemotherapy provide the strongest evidence (HR 0·87; $P = 0·005$), or a 13% reduction in the risk of death.[6] This is equivalent to an absolute benefit of 4% at 2 years (95% CI 1·0–7·0).

Two additional RCTs not included in the meta-analysis were identified. The first (458 patients) compared 2 months of cisplatin and vinblastine followed by standard radiotherapy, versus either standard or hyperfractionated radiotherapy alone. This study found that combined therapy significantly improved 5-year survival compared with either hyperfractionated therapy (8% $v$ 6%; $P = 0·04$) or with standard radiotherapy alone (8% $v$ 5%; $P = 0·04$).[40]

The second RCT (446 patients) compared radical radiotherapy with or without the addition of up to four cycles of mitomycin, ifosfamide, and cisplatin. In this study, there was no significant difference in survival (11·7 months for combined $v$ 9·7 months for radiotherapy alone).[41] Neither study formally addressed quality of life.

There are some concerns in using combined modality therapy in the elderly. In a quality-adjusted survival analysis of Radiation Therapy Oncology Group (RTOG) studies, patients over the age of 70 had a mean survival of 10·8 months with combined modality therapy versus 13·1 months for radiotherapy alone.[42]

### Conclusions

#### *Implications for practice*

Cisplatin-based chemotherapy should be offered in conjunction with thoracic radiotherapy to patients with locally advanced NSCLC. The optimal dose and fractionation of radiation, and its sequencing with chemotherapy have yet to be established. The analysis of the RTOG studies suggests that caution be exercised in offering combined modality therapy to those older than 70 years of age.

#### *Implications for research*

Future research needs to address the use of newer, less toxic radiosensitising drugs such as gemcitabine in combination with radiotherapy. In addition, the issue of sequential versus concurrent, combined modality treatment requires further study.

## Is hyperfractionated radiation therapy for unresectable stage III non-small cell lung cancer more effective than conventional fractionation?

### Background

Altered fractionation radiation is a type of radiotherapy designed to either increase control of the primary tumour and decrease the toxicity to normal tissues, thereby improving the therapeutic ratio, or to permit greater convenience for patients without compromising primary tumour control and normal tissue effects. Hyperfractionated radiotherapy is defined as the use of two or more fractions daily of smaller than conventional fraction size.[43] This results in an increased total nominal tumour dose compared with standard radiation. The rationale for hyperfractionation is to exploit the enhanced repair capacity of dose-limiting, late-reacting, normal tissues compared with more rapidly proliferating tumours.

Accelerated radiation therapy adds two or more fractions of standard fraction size daily to the same conventional total dose as standard radiotherapy, shortening the overall treatment time, thereby reducing repopulation of cancer cells in rapidly proliferating tumours. Combining hyperfractionation and acceleration in treatment such as CHART is designed to reduce both normal tissue toxicity and the risk of repopulation.

### Answer to question

There is currently insufficient data of high quality to recommend non-accelerated hyperfractionated radiotherapy over standard radiotherapy to patients with stage III disease. There is evidence from one RCT demonstrating that CHART improves survival over standard radiotherapy for patients with unresectable stage III disease.

### Review of evidence

#### Hyperfractionation

We found one systematic review (search date 1999, three RCTs, 442 people) comparing standard hyperfractionation (not CHART) versus conventional radiotherapy.[43] It found no significant difference in 2-year survival (OR 0·67; 95% CI 0·42–1·07; $P = 0·09$).

#### CHART

We found no systematic review or RCTs exclusively in people with stage III NSCLC. One RCT (563 people with non-small cell lung cancer; 61% with stage IIIA or IIIB; 39% with stage I or stage II) compared CHART versus conventional radiotherapy.[33] It found that CHART

significantly improved 2-year survival compared with conventional radiotherapy (Absolute Risk [AR] 29% $v$ 20% with conventional radiotherapy; HR 0·78; 95% CI 0·65–0·94; $P = 0·008$) and improved local tumour control (HR for local control 0·79; 95% CI 0·63–0·98; $P = 0·03$). Despite short-term increases in pain on swallowing and heartburn in the CHART-treated patients, there were no significant differences in long-term morbidity between conventional and altered fractionation schedules.[33,44]

### Conclusions

#### Implications for practice

From those trials designed to improve therapeutic ratios in patients with locally advanced unresectable stage III NSCLC, there is insufficient evidence to recommend standard hyperfractionation over standard radiotherapy. There is evidence from one RCT of a survival benefit with CHART compared with conventional therapy. The potential cost implications of making this the standard care need to be assessed carefully against the potential clinical benefits in different patient groups.

#### Implications for research

Further research preferably in the form of randomised comparisons is required to determine whether CHART is equivalent or superior to standard radiotherapy plus chemotherapy.

## How important is chemotherapy in improving survival and quality of life in patients with advanced disease (stage IV)?

### Background

The majority of patients with NSCLC will die of their disease and thus most treatment is delivered with palliation rather than cure in mind. Attitudes to the treatment of advanced NSCLC have changed over the past 5–10 years, a move from chemotherapeutic nihilism to a recognition of the modest survival and quality-of-life improvements possible with modern drug regimens and appropriate patient selection. Multivariate analyses of factors that predict outcome can guide patient selection. The presence of extrathoracic disease, brain metastasis, and weight loss are associated with a poor prognosis, although patient age and tumour histology do not affect outcome.[45] Clinical trials of chemotherapy have generally excluded patients with an Eastern Cooperative Oncology performance (ECOG) score worse than 2, since patients with even moderately impaired performance status do less well on chemotherapy.

Increasingly, studies of palliative chemotherapy for patients with stage IV NSCLC are evaluating quality of life and economic factors as well as survival as endpoints.

## Answer to question

Chemotherapy (both single agent and combined) can improve survival and quality of life in patients with advanced NSCLC, but the results of a meta-analysis of drugs used over the past 20 years provide no evidence that one particular regimen is better than another. Chemotherapy should be offered only to patients with an ECOG performance status score of 2 or better.

There is limited evidence from one RCT that second-line treatment with docetaxel 75 mg m$^{-2}$ offers a modest survival benefit over best supportive care in patients with good performance status. Effects on quality of life are unclear.

## Review of evidence

### First-line chemotherapy

*Chemotherapy versus best supportive care:* We found four systematic reviews[6,46–48] that addressed survival in people with stage IV non-small cell lung cancer. The most recent review (11 RCTs, 1190 people with advanced disease) compared supportive care versus supportive care plus chemotherapy.[6] It found that, in older trials (from the 1970s), long-term alkylating agents did not significantly improve survival (death with supportive care plus chemotherapy v supportive alone; HR 1·26; 95% CI 0·96–1·66; P= 0·095). However, cisplatin-containing regimens significantly reduced the risk of death at 1 year (HR 0·73 for death with combined treatment v supportive care alone; P< 0·0001), and increased median survival (5·5 v 4 months). It is not possible to deduce from these studies to what extent the observed effects are due to the cisplatin or to all the other drugs in the combinations studied. We found four RCTs that compared single agent chemotherapy versus best supportive care and assessed effects on quality of life.[49–52] Chemotherapeutic agents used were vinorelbine (191 people aged over 70),[49] gemcitabine (300 people),[50] docetaxel (207 people)[51] and paclitaxel (157 people).[52] Overall, the trials consistently found that chemotherapy improved quality of life compared with best supportive care.

*Single agent versus combined chemotherapy:* We found one systematic review (25 RCTs, 5156 people)[53] and four subsequent RCTs.[54–57] The review found that, overall, platinum analogue or vinorelbine-containing combination chemotherapy did not significantly improve 1-year survival compared with platinum analogue or vinorelbine alone (RR 1·10; 95% CI 0·94–1·43).[53] The first subsequent RCT (120 people with advanced disease aged 70 over) found that gemcitabine plus vinorelbine improved survival compared

with vinorelbine alone (at 14 months median follow up, median survival 29 weeks with combined treatment v 18 weeks; P< 0·01).[54] The second RCT (522 chemotherapy-naive people) found that gemcitabine plus cisplatin versus cisplatin alone significantly improved survival (median survival 9·1 months with combination treatment v 7·6 months; P= 0·004).[55] The third RCT (415 people) found a similar result for cisplatin plus vinorelbine versus cisplatin alone (median survival 8 months with combination v 6 months; P= 0·002).[56] The fourth RCT found no significant difference for median survival between cisplatin plus etoposide versus gemcitabine (median survival 6·6 months with gemcitabine v 7·6 months with cisplatin plus etoposide).[57] Some studies have reported improvement in lung cancer symptoms with chemotherapy but over 50% of advanced lung cancer patients treated with chemotherapy reported alopecia, and gastrointestinal and haematological toxicity.[58] One non-systematic review found greater toxicity in patients with Eastern Cooperative Oncology Group performance status 3 or 4.[59]

### Second-line chemotherapy

*Chemotherapy versus best supportive care:* We found two systematic reviews. One[60] (search date not stated) identified 34 single agent and 24 multidrug studies but only two RCTs, only one of which compared chemotherapy with best supportive care, and the other (updated February 2002)[61] also found only one RCT that compared second-line chemotherapy with best supportive care. In this international, multicentre trial,[62] 204 patients with previously treated, locally advanced or metastatic NSCLC received either docetaxel or best supportive care. Patients in the docetaxel arm initially received 100 mg m$^{-2}$ every 21 days but this dose was lowered to 75 mg m$^{-2}$ every 21 days after interim safety monitoring showed a significantly higher toxic death rate in this group. Best supportive care (BSC) included antibiotics, analgesics, transfusions and palliative radiotherapy. There was a modest but significant survival advantage in good performance patients treated with docetaxel 75 mg m$^{-2}$ compared with BSC (median survival 7·5 months v 4·6 months; P= 0·01; and 1-year survival rates 37% v 12%; P= 0·003). Grade 3 or 4 neutropenia was the commonest haematological side effect, occurring in 86% and 67% of the high and lower docetaxel groups respectively. All QOL parameters were reported to have favoured docetaxel, and the use of tumour-related medications was significantly less in this group but detailed data have yet to be published. Intention-to-treat analysis was conducted in this study but the randomisation process and allocation concealment were not described and there were some minor discrepancies in the data within the published report.

*Chemotherapy versus chemotherapy:* Another RCT compared regimens of docetaxel 100 mg m$^{-2}$ (D100) with a regimen of docetaxel 75 mg m$^{-2}$ (D75) and with a control regimen of either vinorelbine or ifosfamide (V/I) in 373 patients with locally advanced or metastatic NSCLC who had relapsed after treatment with one or more platinum-based regimens.[63] Objective partial response favoured docetaxel: 10·8% for D100, 6·7% for D75 versus 0·8% for V/I ($P = 0·001$ and $P = 0·036$ for each dose respectively $v$ V/I), as did the overall time to progression ($P = 0·046$). There was a significant difference in 1-year survival between the D75 group and the V/I (control) group (32% $v$ 19%; $P = 0·025$), although there was no difference in overall survival between any of the three groups. A further survival analysis, censored to account for those in the control group who had chemotherapy after the study ended, also found no significant difference in overall survival, but 1-year survival was better for both docetaxel groups compared with the control ($P < 0·01$). There were non-significant trends for a better response in patient's with good performance status and in those who were platinum-resistant rather than platinum-refractory. Grade 4 neutropenia was significantly greater in patients who received docetaxel compared with the V/I regimen (77% for D100, 54% for D75 $v$ 31% for V/I). Discontinuation of treatment because of treatment-related adverse events occurred in 12·8% of patients on D100, 7·2% of patients on D75, and 4·1% in the V/I group. Preliminary quality-of-life data[64] showed a clinical benefit with docetaxel treatment. The randomisation process and allocation concealment in this study were not reported.

## Conclusions

### Implications for practice

People with Eastern Cooperative Oncology Group performance status 3 or 4 have usually been excluded from RCTs of lung cancer chemotherapy. Newer agents such as vinorelbine, gemcitabine, irinotecan, paclitaxel, and docetaxel produce objective responses in more than 20% of people with advanced lung cancer, and are being studied prospectively alone or in combination with cisplatin or carboplatin in RCTs.[65] Carboplatin has comparable activity to, but a better toxicity profile than, cisplatin in patients with stage IV non-small cell lung cancer.[65]

Only docetaxel has been evaluated for use as second-line therapy in randomised trials. One trial found a modest survival benefit with docetaxel 75 mg m$^{-2}$ compared with best supportive care, and the other found an improvement in 1-year survival with docetaxel compared with vinorelbine/ ifosfamide but no significant difference in overall survival. High levels of toxicity were found with docetaxel 100 mg m$^{-2}$ To our knowledge detailed quality-of-life data are still to be published from both trials.

### Implications for research

Even with the introduction of new chemotherapeutic agents, currently available single and multiagent regimens appear to have reached a plateau in terms of response rate and survival benefit over best supportive care. An alternative strategy is to explore the potential of biological agents, particularly anti-angiogenesis factors and retroviral-vector transport of *p53* tumour-suppressor genes into lung tumours. Clinical trials using these agents have begun and, if successful, will be likely to change the direction of research in the systemic therapy of advanced lung cancer.

Future randomised trials need to clarify the optimal second-line (and subsequent) chemotherapy regimens in relation to the type and dose of the first-line regimen, as well as individual patient and tumour characteristics. Response to previous platinum-containing agents needs to be carefully documented with clear definitions of "sensitive" and "refractory" to treatment, as well as time intervals between the last chemotherapy course, disease progression and initiation of subsequent chemotherapy regimens. Trials of other chemotherapeutic agents as second-line therapy should consider using docetaxel 75 mg m$^{-2}$ as the standard comparator regimen. Measuring quality of life in people with lung cancer remains a serious challenge, yet this is an extremely important endpoint in clinical trials of chemotherapy in poor performance status patients.

## What is the most appropriate regimen of palliative radiotherapy for locally advanced and symptomatic NSCLC?

### Background

The currently accepted, evidence-based treatment for selected patients with locally advanced, unresectable lung cancer (stage III) is combined chemotherapy and radical radiotherapy.[66] There is nevertheless a group of patients for whom this treatment has failed or for whom chemotherapy is contraindicated. Although the emphasis of treatment in such patients is symptom palliation rather than cure, the optimal interventions for maximising quality of life are unresolved. Studies have shown that much of radiation oncologists' time is spent giving palliative radiotherapy to patients with advanced disease but, since dose regimens and schedules have developed empirically and have not been subject to rigorous evaluation, there is considerable variation in practice.[67]

### Answer to the question

The question of whether palliative radiotherapy offers a significant benefit in terms of survival, symptom control or quality of life compared with best supportive care has not been adequately assessed in randomised controlled trials. Evidence from studies comparing different radiotherapy regimes suggests that, compared with lower dose, hypofractionated schedules, higher doses cause greater toxicity, with no advantage in symptom control, although there may be a modest survival advantage in good performance status patients. The optimal palliative radiotherapy regimen remains to be determined.

## Review of evidence

### *External beam radiotherapy*

We found only one RCT that compared palliative radiotherapy with best supportive care for the treatment of advanced non-small cell lung cancer.[68] This trial was small and preliminary published results relating to only the first 86 patients (80% of the sample) found no significant differences between patients treated with radiotherapy (40 Gy in two courses of 20 Gy over 5 days split by a 2-week interval) and the control group.

A systematic review (updated June 2001)[67] has addressed the questions as to which regimens of palliative radiotherapy are the most effective in achieving control of thoracic symptoms with the least toxicity, and whether there is an association between higher doses and increased survival. The review identified 10 RCTs (nine published, one unpublished) that compared at least one RT regimen with another.

A quantitative meta-analysis was inappropriate because of the wide range of regimens given in the studies (from 10 Gy in a single fraction to 60 Gy in 30 fractions over 6 weeks), variations in patient characteristics (age, performance status, histological confirmation of NSCLC), and different outcome assessment methods.

Symptoms were assessed by different methods in the 10 RCTs and no study used differential measures to determine the degree of relief obtained by radiotherapy. Only five of the 10 studies included both patient- and clinician-assessed symptoms using standardised instruments, while three studies relied on clinician assessment only, one study used a patient questionnaire, and the remaining study did not assess symptoms.

All the RCTs found a consistent improvement in symptoms following radiotherapy which persisted for some time after treatment but, since none of these studies included a control group who received no treatment or best supportive care, it was not possible to determine the extent of placebo effect.

*Survival:* Only two of the trials included in the systematic review showed any difference in survival between higher and lower dose treatment groups. One of these,[69] the only trial that had sufficient statistical power to detect a 5%

improvement at 1 or 2 years, found that a modest survival benefit (36% v 31% at 1 year; HR 0·82; 95% CI 0·69–0·99) was obtained with a higher dose of RT (39 Gy in 13 fractions over 2·5 weeks; N = 254) compared with a lower dose (17 Gy in 2 fractions over 8 days; N = 255) in good performance status patients. Median survival was 9 months in the 13-fraction group compared with 7 months in the two-fraction group, and at 2 years the survival rates were 12% and 9% in these groups, respectively. Another smaller study[70] supported these findings in that a large survival advantage (48% v 28% at 1 year, 18% v 6% at 2 years, median survival 12 v 8·3 months) was found in patients (N = 79) who received a higher dose (50 Gy in 25 fractions over 5 weeks) compared with those (N = 81) who received a lower dose (40 Gy in 10-fraction split course with 4-week gap). In this study, which did not report confidence intervals, patients seemed to be of generally better performance status, some were asymptomatic, and only 43% were aged over 60.

*Toxicity:* The occurrence of more acute side effects in patients who received higher equivalent doses of RT was a consistent finding in the studies included in the systematic review. Radiation oesophagitis was the best documented (four studies) but there was also evidence of more tiredness and anorexia with a higher dose regime.[69] The risks of radiation myelopathy in patients undergoing palliative radiotherapy calculated from an analysis of the pooled data from the three MRC RCTs were reported separately.[71] Five cases of radiation myelopathy were reported amongst 1048 patients treated, three amongst patients who received 17 Gy in two fractions, and two cases in patients who received 39 Gy in 13 fractions.

The systematic review found no evidence that giving higher doses (or higher biological effective doses) results in better thoracic symptom control. In contrast there was strong evidence of greater toxicity, particularly radiation oesophagitis with higher dose regimens. The reviewers therefore recommended the use of short, hypofractionated regimens in the majority of patients, with particular care to avoid high doses to the spinal cord.

### *Brachytherapy*

We found no randomised trial that compared brachytherapy with best supportive care. We found two randomised trials that assessed the effectiveness of brachytherapy (intraluminal radiotherapy) in relation to external radiotherapy. One RCT compared endobronchial brachytherapy (EBT) with external beam radiotherapy (XRT).[72] In this study 99 patients (79 men, 20 women; mean age 68) with histologically confirmed, inoperable NSCLC received either a single exposure of EBT, 15 Gy, 1 cm from an iridium source in the bronchus or eight exposures of XRT, 30 Gy over 10–12 days. There were improvements in symptoms with both treatments. There was more acute morbidity in the XRT group compared with the EBT group, but at 8 weeks there was significantly greater patient-assessed symptom palliation in the XRT group compared with the EBT group, with differences being significant for chest pain, anorexia, tiredness and nausea. With the exception of tiredness, this difference was no longer significant at 16 weeks. There was a trend for greater palliation in clinician assessed symptoms following XRT but this was not significant. Duration of palliation was greater following XRT than EBT and there was a modest but significant survival gain in those treated initially with XRT (median survival 287 *v* 250 days). Interestingly this study found a significant disagreement between doctors' and patients' assessments of symptoms, with doctors consistently underestimating the severity of breathlessness, anorexia, tiredness and nausea.

The other recent trial[36] assessed the effectiveness of brachytherapy combined with external irradiation, with external irradiation alone. This study, which ended prematurely because of poor accrual, analysed data on 95 patients randomised to receive either XRT alone or a combination of XRT and EBT. There was no difference in dyspnoea response (primary outcome) between the two groups, although in the group receiving both treatments there was a significantly higher rate of radiological re-expansion of the collapsed lung as well as significant improvements in the inspiratory vital capacity compared with the group receiving XRT only. There was a temporary beneficial effect of the combined therapy on mean dyspnoea scores which disappeared after 3 months and did not translate into an improvement in global quality of life or functioning. The beneficial effect of the treatment combination appeared to be restricted to patients whose tumour was obstructing the main bronchus. There was no significant survival difference between the two groups.

## Conclusions

### *Implications for practice*

It is not possible to draw firm conclusions for practice based on current evidence. A systematic review of randomised comparisons of different doses and fractionation schedules of radiotherapy was hampered by clinical heterogeneity between studies which made meta-analysis impossible. While the qualitative review found no evidence that higher doses gave greater palliation, there was evidence that they gave more acute toxicity. There was evidence from two trials, that a higher dose regimen gave a modest but significant survival benefit compared with a lower dose regimen. In view of this evidence, short-course, low dose palliative therapy should be given ideally within the context of clinical trials that are organised to ensure homogeneity in

both patient characteristics and treatment interventions. In patients with good performance status and non-metastatic disease there may be a case for giving higher dose radiotherapy to gain a modest survival benefit at the cost of greater toxicity. There is currently no evidence from randomised trials that supports the use of palliative brachytherapy either alone or in combination with external radiotherapy unless there is obstruction of the main bronchus.

### *Implications for research*

The need for a larger randomised trial comparing palliative external radiotherapy with best supportive care using updated radiotherapy techniques should be considered. If a randomised trial is deemed unethical or there are accrual problems, comparative individual patient data by disease stage and performance status are required from trials using homogeneous treatment interventions and standardised methods of assessing outcomes. Since the emphasis of palliative radiotherapy in patients with advanced disease for whom other treatment options have failed or are inappropriate, is symptom control, the use of standardised instruments for assessing symptoms and quality of life is essential.

## References

1 Ginsberg RJ, Vokes EE, Raben A. Non-small cell lung cancer. In: Devita VT Jr, Hellman S, Rosenberg SA. *Cancer. Principles and practice of oncology, 5th edn*. Philadelphia: Lippincott-Raven, 1997.
2 Ries LAG, Eisner MP, Kosary CL *et al.*, eds. *SEER Cancer Statistics Review, 1973–1999*, Bethesda, MD: National Cancer Institute [http://seer.cancer.gov/csr/1973_1999/,2001].
3 Fauci AS, Braunwald E, Isselbacher KJ *et al.*, eds. *Harrison's Principles of Internal Medicine, 14th edn*. New York: McGraw-Hill, 1998.
4 Mountain CF. Revisions in the International System for Staging Lung Cancer. *Chest* 1997;**111**:1710–17.
5 Feld R, Rubinstein LV, Weisenberger TH, Lung Cancer Study Group. Sites of recurrence in resected stage I non-small cell lung cancer: a guide for future studies. *J Clin Oncol* 1984;**2**:1352–9.
6 Non-small Cell Lung Cancer Collaborative Group. Chemotherapy for non-small cell lung cancer (Cochrane Review). In: *Cochrane Library*, Issue 2. Oxford: Update Software, 2002.
7 Goss G, Paszat L, Newman T *et al.* Use of preoperative chemotherapy with or without post-operative radiotherapy in technically resectable stage IIIA non-small cell lung cancer. *Cancer Prev Control* 1998;**2**:32–9.
8 Rosell R, Gomez-Codina J, Camps C *et al.* A randomised trial comparing preoperative chemotherapy plus surgery alone in patients with non-small cell lung cancer. *N Engl J Med* 1994;**330**:153–8.
9 Roth JA, Atkinson EN, Fossella F *et al.* Long-term follow-up of patients enrolled in a randomised trial comparing perioperative chemotherapy and surgery with surgery alone in resectable stage IIIA non-small cell lung cancer. *Lung Cancer* 1998;**21**:1–6.
10 Pass HI, Pogrebniak HW, Steinberg SM *et al.* Randomised trial of neoadjuvant therapy for lung cancer: interim analysis. *Ann Thoracic Surg* 1992;**53**:992–8.
11 Elias AD, Hendon J, Kumer P *et al.* A phase III comparison of "best local-regional therapy" with or without chemotherapy for stage IIIA

T1-T3N2 non-small cell lung cancer. *Proc Am Soc Clin Oncol* 1997;**16**:A1611.

12  Pisters KM. The role of chemotherapy in early-stage (stage I and II) resectable non-small cell lung cancer. *Semin Radiat Oncol* 2000;**10**:274–9.

13  PORT Meta-analysis Trialists Group. Postoperative radiotherapy for non-small cell lung cancer (Cochrane Review). In: *Cochrane Library*, Issue 2. Oxford: Update Software, 2002.

14  PORT Meta-analysis Trialists Group. Post-operative radiotherapy in non-small cell lung cancer: systematic review and meta-analysis of individual patient data from nine randomised controlled trials. *Lancet* 1998;**352**:257–63.

15  Machtay M, Lee JH, Shrager JB, Kaiser LR, Glatstein E. Risk of death from intercurrent disease is not excessively increased by modern postoperative radiotherapy for high-risk resected non-small cell lung carcinoma. *J Clin Oncol* 2001;**19**:3912–17.

16  Bonner JA, Tincher SA, Fiveash JB. Balancing the possible effectiveness of postoperative radiotherapy for non-small cell lung cancer against the possible detriment of radiation-induced toxicity. *J Clin Oncol* 2001;**19**:3905–7.

17  Vallières E. Adjuvant radiation therapy after complete resection of non-small-cell lung cancer. *J Clin Oncol* 2002;**20**:1427–9.

18  Symonds RP. Recent advances in radiotherapy. *BMJ* 2001;**323**: 1107–10.

19  Munro AJ. What now for postoperative radiotherapy for lung cancer? *Lancet* 1998;**352**:250–1.

20  Trodella L, Granone P, Valente S *et al.* Adjuvant radiotherapy in non-small cell lung cancer with pathological stage 1: definitive results of a phase III randomized trial. *Radiat Oncol* 2002;**62**:11–19.

21  Touboul E, Deniaud-Alexandre E, Pereira R, Deluen F. Postoperative radiotherapy after complete resection of stage II (N1) non-small cell lung cancer: reasons for not proposing it. *Rev Pneumonol Clin* 2000;**56**:287–92.

22  Machtay M. Postoperative radiotherapy in non-small-cell lung cancer. *Lancet* 1998;**352**:1385–6.

23  Dosoretz DE, Katin MJ, Blitzer PH *et al.* Medically inoperable lung carcinoma: the role of radiation therapy. *Semin Radiat Oncol* 1996;**6**:98–104.

24  Manser RL, Irving LB, Stone C, Byrnes G, Abramson M, Campbell D. Screening for lung cancer. (Cochrane Review). In: Cochrane Library, Issue 2. Oxford: Update Software, 2002.

25  Mulshine JL, De Luca LM, Dedrick RL, Tockman MS, Webster R, Placke ME. Considerations in developing successful, population-based molecular screening and prevention of lung cancer. *Cancer* 2000;**89**(Suppl.):2465–7.

26  Ellis SM, Husband JE, Armstrong P, Hansell DM. Computed tomography screening for lung cancer: back to basics. *Clin Radiol* 2001;**56**:691–9.

27  McGarry RC, Song G, des Rosiers P, Timmerman R. Observation-only management of early stage, medically inoperable lung cancer(*): poor outcome. *Chest* 2001;**121**:1155–8.

28  Motohiro A, Ueda H, Komatsu H, Yanai N, Mori T. Prognosis of non-surgically treated, clinical stage I lung cancer patients in Japan. *Lung Cancer* 2002;**36**:65–9.

29  Morrison R, Deeley TJ, Cleland WP. The treatment of carcinoma of the bronchus: a clinical trial to compare surgery and supervoltage radiotherapy. *Lancet* 1963;**i**:683–4.

30  Rowell NP, Williams CP. Radical radiotherapy for stage I/II non-small cell lung cancer in patients not sufficiently fit for of declining surgery (medically inoperable) (Cochrane Review). In: *Cochrane Library*, Issue 2. Oxford: Update Software, 2002.

31  Zierhut D, Bettscheider K, Schubert K, van Kampen M, Wannenmacher M. Radiation therapy for stage I and II non-small cell lung cancer (NSCLC): *Lung Cancer* 2001;**34**:S39–S43.

32  Vrdoljak E, Miše K, Sapunar D, Rozga A, Marušicm M. Survival analysis of untreated patients with non-small-cell lung cancer. *Chest* 1994;**106**:1797–800.

33  Saunders M, Dische S, Barrett A, Harvey A, Griffiths G, Parmar M, (on behalf of the CHART steering committee). Continuous, hyperfractionated, accelerated radiotherapy (CHART) versus conventional radiotherapy in non-small-cell lung cancer: mature data

from the randomised multicentre trial. *Radiother Oncol* 1999;**52**: 137–48.

34  Bentzen SM, Saunders MI, Dische S, Parmar MK. Updated data for CHART in NSCLC: further analyses. *Radiother Oncol* 2000;**55**:86–7.

35  Ball D, Bishop J, Smith J *et al.* A randomised phase III study of accelerated or standard fraction radiotherapy with or without concurrent carboplatin in inoperable non-small cell lung cancer: final report of an Australian multi-centre trial. *Radiother Oncol* 1999; **52**:129–36.

36  Langendijk H, de Jong J, Tjwa M *et al.* External irradiation versus external irradiation plus endobronchial brachytherapy in inoperable non-small cell lung cancer: a prospective randomized study. *Radiother Oncol* 2001;**58**:257–68.

37  Uematsu M, Shioda A, Suda A *et al.* Computed tomography-guided frameless stereotactic radiotherapy for stage I non-small-cell lung cancer: a 5 year experience. *Int J Radiat Oncol Biol Phys* 2001;**51**: 666–7.

38  Sibley GS, Jamieson TA, Marks LB, Anscher MS, Prosnitz LR. Radiotherapy alone for medically inoperable stage I non-small cell lung cancer: the Duke experience. *Int J Radiat Oncol Biol Phys* 1998;**40**: 149–54.

39  Jeremic B, Shibamoto Y, Acimovic L, Milisavljevic S. Hyperfractionated radiotherapy alone for clinical stage I non-small cell lung cancer. *Int J Radiat Oncol Biol Phys* 1997;**38**:521–5.

40  Sause W, Kolesar P, Taylor S *et al.* Final results of a phase III trial in regionally advanced unresectable non-small cell lung cancer: Radiation Therapy Oncology Group, Eastern Cooperative Oncology Group and Southwest Oncology Group. *Chest* 2000;**117**:358–64.

41  Cullen MH, Billingham CM, Woodroofe AD *et al.* Mitomycin, Ifosfamide and Cisplatin in unresectable non-small cell lung cancer: effects on survival and quality of life. *J Clin Oncol* 1999;**17**:3188–94.

42  Mousas B, Scott C, Sause W *et al.* The benefit of treatment intensification is age and histology dependent in patients with locally advanced non-small cell lung cancer (NSCLC): a quality adjusted survival analysis of Radiation Therapy Oncology Group (RTOC) chemoradiation studies. *Int J Radiat Oncol Biol Phys* 1999;**45**: 1143–9.

43  Yu E, Lochrin C, Dixon P *et al.* Altered fractionation of radical radiation therapy in the management of unresectable non-small cell lung cancer. *Curr Oncol* 2000;**7**:98–109.

44  Bailey AJ, Parmar MKB, Stephens RJ. Patient-reported short-term and long-term physical and psychological symptoms: results of the continuous hyperfractionated accelerated radiotherapy (CHART) randomised trial in non-small cell lung cancer. *J Clin Oncol* 1998;**16**:3082–93.

45  Albain KS, Crowley JJ, LeBlanc M, Livingston RB. Survival determinants in extensive-stage non-small cell lung cancer: the Southwest Oncology Group experience. *J Clin Oncol* 1991;**9**:1618–26.

46  Gilli R, Oxman AD, Julian JA. Chemotherapy for advanced non-small cell lung cancer: How much benefit is enough? *J Clin Oncol* 1993;**11**:1866–72.

47  Souquet PJ, Chauvin F, Boissel JP *et al.* Polychemotherapy in advanced non small cell lung cancer: a meta-analysis. *Lancet* 1993;**342**:19–21.

48  Marino P, Pampaliona S, Preatoni A *et al.* Chemotherapy versus supportive care in advanced non-small cell lung cancer: results of a meta-analysis of the literature. *Chest* 1994;**106**:861–5.

49  Elderly Lung Cancer Vinorelbine Study Group. Effects of vinorelbine on quality of life and survival of elderly patients with non-small cell lung cancer. *J Natl Cancer Inst* 1999;**91**:66–72.

50  Anderson H, Hopwood P, Stephens RJ *et al.* Gemcitabine plus best supportive care (BSC) versus BSC in inoperable non-small cell lung cancer in a randomised trial with quality of life as the primary outcome. *Br J Cancer* 2000;**83**:447–53.

51  Roszkowski K, Pluzanska A, Krzakowski M *et al.* A multicenter, randomised phase III study of docetaxel plus best supportive care versus best supportive care in chemo-naive patients with metastatic or non-resectable localised non-small cell lung cancer (NSCLC). *Lung Cancer* 2000;**27**:145–57.

52  Ranson M, Davidson N, Nicolson M *et al.* Randomised trial of paclitaxel plus supportive care versus supportive care for patients with

advanced non-small cell lung cancer. *J Natl Cancer Inst* 2000;**92**:1074–80.

53   Lilenbaum RC, Langenberg P, Dickersin K. Single agent versus combination chemotherapy in patients with advanced non-small cell lung cancer: A meta-analysis of response, toxicity and survival. *Cancer* 1998;**82**:116–26.

54   Frasci G, Lorusso V, Panza N *et al.* Gemcitabine plus vinorelbine versus vinorelbine alone in elderly patients with advanced non-small cell lung cancer. *J Clin Oncol* 2000;**18**:2529–36.

55   Sandler AB, Nemunaitis J, Denham C *et al.* Phase III trial of gemcitabine plus cisplatin versus cisplatin alone in patients with locally advanced or metastatic non-small cell lung cancer. *J Clin Oncol* 2000;**18**:122–30.

56   Wozniak AG, Crowley JJ, Balcerzak SP *et al.* Randomised trial comparing cisplatin with cisplatin plus vinorelbine in the treatment of advanced non-small cell lung cancer: a Southwest Oncology Group study. *J Clin Oncol* 1998;**16**:2459–65.

57   Bokkel-Huinink WW, Bergman B, Chemaissani A *et al.* Single-agent gemcitabine: an active and better tolerated alternative to standard cisplatin-based chemotherapy in locally advanced or metastatic non-small cell lung cancer. *Lung Cancer* 1999;**26**:85–94.

58   Le Chevalier T, Brisgand D, Douillard J-Y *et al.* Randomized study of vinorelbine and cisplatin versus vindesine and cisplatin versus vinorelbine alone in advanced non-small cell lung cancer: results of a European multicenter trial including 612 people. *J Clin Oncol* 1994;**12**:360–7.

59   Bunn PA Jr, Kelly K. New chemotherapeutic agents prolong survival and improve quality of life in non-small cell lung cancer: a review of literature and future directions. *Clin Cancer Res* 1998;**4**:1087–100.

60   Huisman C, Smit EF, Postmus PE. Second-line chemotherapy in relapsing or refractory non-small cell lung cancer: A review. *J Clin Oncol* 2000;**18**:3722–30.

61   Bonfill X, Serra C, Sacristán M, Nogué M, Losa F, Montesinos J. Second-line chemotherapy for non-small cell lung cancer (Cochrane Review). In: *Cochrane Library*, Issue 2. Oxford: Update Software, 2002.

62   Shepherd FA, Dancey J, Ramlan R. Prospective randomised trial of docetaxel versus best supportive care in patients with non-small cell lung cancer previously treated with platinum-based chemotherapy. *J Clin Oncol* 2000;**18**:2095–103.

63   Fossella FV, DeVore R, Kerr RN. Randomized phase III trial of docetaxel versus vinorelbine or ifosfamide in patients with advanced non-small cell lung cancer previously treated with platinum-containing regimens. *J Clin Oncol* 2000;**18**:2354–62.

64   Miller VA, Fossella FV, DeVore R *et al.* Docetaxel benefits lung cancer symptoms and quality of life in a randomized phase III trial of non-small cell lung cancer patients previously treated with platinum-based therapy. *Proc Am Soc Clin Oncol* 1999;**18**:491a (Abs. 1895).

65   Bunn PA Jr. Review of therapeutic trials of carboplatin in lung cancer. *Semin Oncol* 1989;**16**:27–33.

66   Neville A. Lung cancer. In: Barton S, ed. *Clinical Evidence*, Issue 6. London: BMJ Publishing Group, 2001.

67   Macbeth F, Toy E, Coles B, Melville A, Eastwood A. Palliative radiotherapy regimens for non-small cell lung cancer (Cochrane review). In: *Cochrane Library*, Issue 2. Update Software, 2002.

68   Expósito J, Linares A, Cano C, del Moral R, Martínez M, Hernández V. Papel de la radioterapia en el cáncer de pulmón no microcítico avanzado. Primeros resultados de un ensayo randomizado. [Role of radiotherapy in advanced non-small cell lung cancer. First results from a randomised trial]. *Oncología* 1994;**17**:399–405.

69   MRC Lung Cancer Working Party, Macbeth F, Bolger JJ, Hopwood P *et al.* Randomised trial of palliative two-fraction versus more intensive 13-fraction radiotherapy for patients with in-operable non-small cell lung cancer and good performance status. *Clin Oncol* 1996;**8**:167–75.

70   Reinfuss M, Glinski B, Kowalska T *et al.* Radiotherapie du cancer bronchique non a petites cellules de stade III, inopérable, asymptomatique. Resultats definitifs d'un essai prospectif randomisé (240 patients) [Radiotherapy in stage III, irresectable, asymptomatic, non-small cell lung cancer. Final results of a prospective randomised study of 240 patients]. *Cancer Radiotherapie* 1999;**3**:475–9.

71   MRC lung cancer working party, Macbeth F, Wheldon TE, Girling DJ *et al.* Radiation myelopathy: estimates of risk in 1048 patients in three randomised trials of palliative radiotherapy for non-small cell lung cancer. *Clin Oncol* 1996;**8**:176–81.

72   Stout R, Barber P, Burt P *et al.* Clinical and quality of life outcomes in the first United Kingdom randomized trial of endobronchial brachytherapy (intraluminal radiotherapy) vs. external beam radiotherapy in the palliative treatment of inoperable non-small cell lung cancer. *Radiother Oncol* 2000;**56**:323–7.

# Small cell lung cancer (SCLC)

*Alan Neville*

## Background

Small cell lung cancer (SCLC) accounts for 20–25% of all lung cancers.[1] About 70% patient present with a perihilar mass and a similar proportion will be found to have Extensive Stage Disease at diagnosis (defined by the Veteran's Administration Lung Cancer Student Group Criteria).[2] Less than 15% of patients present with a peripheral nodule.[3] Less than 10% of patients show a mixture of SCLC with another histologic component of NSCLC.[4] Compared to NSCLC, SCLC exhibits neuroendocrine properties, *C-myc* oncogene amplification, *BCL-2* expression (75–95%), *p53* gene inactivation (75–100%) and *Retinoblastoma* gene inactivation (~ 90%).[5] These molecular disturbances are associated with a type of lung cancer which metastasises readily, yet exhibits greater sensitivity to chemotherapy than NSCLC. Systemic chemotherapy is the mainstay of treatment for all patients with SCLC, yet even with chemotherapy, plus thoracic irradiation and the selective use of radiation, the median survival of even limited stage disease patients is only 18–24 months with a 2-year survival of 20%.[1]

## What is the role of surgery in the management of SCLC?

## Background

Since SCLC is a widely metasising tumour with dissemination to lymph nodes and or distant metastatic sites in more than 90% of patients at the time of initial presentation, it is clear that any local treatment modality alone, such as surgery or radiation will constitute inadequate therapy. Despite the fact that SCLC is a highly chemosensitive tumour, the 2-year survival rate is 20% or less in most series and, for patients with limited stage disease, the most common site of treatment failure is the area of the primary tumour and its hilar or mediastinal draining lymph nodes.

Although thoracic irradiation has been shown to improve control at the primary disease site and increase patient survival, local failure rates remain at 25–30% even after radiation. This high local failure, even after combined radiation and chemotherapy, has led some investigators to postulate that control of the main site of bulk disease in the chest by surgery, followed by systemic chemotherapy to eradicate distant micrometastases might result in an increased long-term survival.

Investigators have also considered the issue of the treatment of combined modality treatment for patients who have both small cell and non-small cell histologies, which occurs in about 5–10% of cases of what appears at first to be SCLC. For patients with localised mixed histology tumours, a combination of chemotherapy to treat the small cell histology and surgery to remove the left chemosensitive small cell histology constitutes rational therapy. Despite the rationale for offering surgery to a select group of patients with SCLC, either before or after chemotherapy, there is only one RCT which has addressed whether the addition of surgery to combination chemotherapy and radiation treatment can prolong survival for patients with limited stage SCLC.

## Answer to the question

There are no randomised controlled trials supporting the use of surgery for patients with small cell lung cancer. A number of phase II trials have shown that selected patients are curable with a combined modality approach with chemotherapy and surgery. The patients who appear to benefit from this combined modality approach are those with very early stage disease (that is, T1–2 N0). Since fewer than 10% of patients with SCLC are found with this very early stage of disease, randomised controlled trials will probably never be feasible to answer the question of the value of surgery in small cell lung cancer.

## Evidence

We found a single RCT reported by the Lung Cancer Study Group in 1994. Limited disease stage SCLC patients[6] were given induction chemotherapy using cyclophosphamide, doxorubicin, vincristine and etoposide in the early phase of the trial, and cyclophosphamide, doxorubicin and vincristine in the later phase of the study. Patients received five cycles of chemotherapy and were then restaged to assess the possibility of thoracotomy and pulmonary resection. Eligible patients were subsequently randomised to undergo surgical resection by radiation treatment to the chest as well as prophylactic cranial radiation or to radiation treatment alone. Following chemotherapy, 144 patients (42%) of those enrolled originally were randomised, but of the 68 randomised to surgery, six did not undergo thoracotomy. A complete pathological response was found in 18% of patients who underwent surgery. Interestingly, 11% of patients who underwent resection were found to have non-small cell pathology, that is, mixed tumours. Of note, clinical and surgical TNM stages after chemotherapy were the same in only 20 patients and postchemotherapy clinical staging was found to be quite inaccurate. Median survival of those randomised to surgery was 15·4 months versus 18·6 months for those who received radiation to the chest (*P* = 0·78 log-rank). Fourteen patients were deemed medically inoperable. There are no other RCTs of either surgery followed by chemotherapy or chemotherapy followed by surgery.

## Conclusions

With one relatively small RCT to consider, it is difficult to draw definitive conclusions about the role of surgery in limited stage SCLC. Given that 10% of patients in the Lung Cancer Study Group protocol did not receive the treatment that they had been randomised to, which compounded the risk of a Type II error, the fact that patients did not receive the current standard cisplatin and etoposide chemotherapy, and that most patients had either T3 or N2 tumours, the results of this one RCT cannot answer the question as to whether patients with T1–2 N0 disease, particularly those with a peripheral nodule, should undergo surgery followed by chemotherapy. Retrospective analyses and phase II studies, but not RCTs, have suggested that patients with T1–2, N0 small cell tumours are potentially curable, with a combination of chemotherapy and surgery, the sequencing of which appears to be immaterial.[3]

## What is the benefit of adding irradiation to chemotherapy in limited stage SCLC?

### Background

Recognition that even with multiagent chemotherapy including cisplatin and etoposide, disease recurrences most commonly occurred at the sites of initial bulk disease, a number of RCTs have investigated the combination of chest irradiation and chemotherapy for patients with limited stage SCLC. The two modalities of treatment have been delivered concurrently, sequentially or in alternating manner. Most trials have used concurrent chemotherapy and irradiation, with the rationale of shortening overall treatment time, increasing treatment intensity, and taking advantage of the synergy observed when radiation-sensitising chemotherapy drugs are used with radiation. These advantages are offset to some extent by increased toxicity from concurrent administration of the two modalities, particularly oesophagitis, pneumonitis and myelosuppression.

Two meta-analyses have demonstrated a significant survival advantage for adding thoracic irradiation to chemotherapy for limited stage SCLC. However, most of the trials reviewed in the two meta-analyses used cyclophosphomide or doxorubicin-based chemotherapy and not the current standard of cisplatin and etoposide;

discussions of the toxicity of combined modality therapy are thus difficult to interpret and, furthermore, no firm conclusions can be made from the meta-analyses regarding the optimal timing and sequencing of chemotherapy and irradiation.

## Answer to the question

The addition of local chest irradiation to standard cisplatin-based chemotherapy improves both local and control and overall survival in patients with limited stage SCLC. Furthermore, both local disease control and progression-free survival are probably improved when higher doses of irradiation are given, but the optimal dose has yet to be established. There is conflicting evidence as to whether the irradiation should be administered early or late in the course of treatment, although evidence supports the administration of concurrent rather than sequential treatments with the two modalities.

Based on currently available published data, there is insufficient evidence to offer hyperfractionated irradiation to patients with limited disease SCLC.

## Evidence

We found two systematic reviews of adding thoracic irradiation to chemotherapy in people with limited stage small cell lung cancer. The first review (search date 1992; 13 RCTs; 2573 people; range 52–426 people) found that 3-year survival was significantly higher with radiation plus chemotherapy versus chemotherapy alone (15% *v* 10%; *P* = 0·001).[7] The second review (search date not stated; 11 pooled data from nine of the RCTs; 1521 people) found that local control was achieved in 50% with radiation versus 25% with chemotherapy alone (ARR 25%; 95% CI 17–34).[8]

### Timing of radiation

We found one systematic review (search date 1999; four RCTs; 927 people), which added early versus late thoracic radiotherapy to chemotherapy,[9] and two additional RCTs.[10,11] The first of these RCTs compared initial with delayed accelerated hyperfractionated irradiation.[10] Chemotherapy consisted of cisplatin and etoposide. Patients (107 randomised) received either early (1–4 weeks) or late (weeks 6–9) twice daily radiation (1·5 Gy per dose to total dose of 54 Gy). Five-year survival rates were 30% versus 15% (*P* = 0·027), early versus late.

A second RCT, reported twice in abstract and once in a non-systematic review article[11] randomised 228 eligible patients receiving four cycles of cisplatin and etoposide to concurrent (started day 2 of chemotherapy cycle 1) or sequential (after cycle 4 completed). Two-year survival rate was 55·3% in the concurrent group versus 25·4% in the sequential group (significance not given).

### Dose

We found one RCT (333 people) comparing standard dose radiotherapy (25 Gy over 2 weeks) versus high dose radiotherapy (37·5 Gy over 3 weeks).[12] It found no significant difference in overall survival between the groups.

### Fractionation

We found two RCTs.[13,14] One RCT found that hyperfractionation (twice daily treatment) versus conventional fractionation significantly improved 5-year survival (26% with hyperfractionation versus 16% with conventional fractionation; $P = 0·04$).[13] The second RCT found no significant difference in 3-year survival (34% with 50·4 Gy in 29 fractions daily $v$ 29% with 48 Gy in 32 fractions twice daily; $P = 0·46$).[14]

### Harms

The risk of treatment-related death was more than twice as high in people given thoracic irradiation compared with those receiving chemotherapy alone (29/884 [3·3%] $v$ 12/841 [1·4%]; OR 2·54; 95% CI 1·90–3·18).[8] The incidence of oesophagitis was also higher in those treated with twice daily irradiation.[13]

## Conclusions

The results of the published meta-analysis have demonstrated both survival benefit and improved local control for combined thoracic irradiation with combination cisplatin and etoposide for patients with limited disease SCLC. Combined modality therapy should therefore be the standard of care. While it is clear from the meta-analyses that treatment toxicity is increased significantly when concurrent combined modality therapy is used, the studies analysed did not use cisplatin-based chemotherapy, the current standard. It is likely, however, that the addition of concurrent irradiation to cisplatin-based chemotherapy does increase overall toxicity.

## What is the best chemotherapy treatment for patients with SCLC?

## Background

Despite the marked sensitivity of SCLC to chemotherapy, 2- and 5-year survival rates are low owing to the frequent occurrence of chemoresistance after induction of primary chemotherapy. For patients with limited stage disease, 2-year survival rates of up to 20% are being achieved using chemotherapy plus thoracic irradiation and prophylactic cranial radiation. For patients with extensive stage disease, who are the majority with SCLC, median survival with combination chemotherapy remains at 7–9 months, with few survivors at 2 years. Twenty years of clinical trials have improved the situation for these patients by only about 2 months. Two approaches have been taken to improve the survival of patients with SCLC:

- to increase the dose intensity of currently available chemotherapeutic regiments
- to introduce new agents.

Although optimal drug combinations and schedules for the treatment of SCLC remain to be defined, there are two published meta-analyses examining the use of cisplatin compared with other regimens, but no systematic reviews or meta-analyses of dose intensification. One recently published RCT compares the standard cisplatin and etoposide combination versus cisplatin plus irinotecan in patients with extensive stage SCLC.

## Evidence

The first meta-analysis examining the evidence for using cisplatin in the treatment of SCLC was published in 2000 (search date 1999).[15] Nineteen RCTs involving previously untreated and histologically or cytologically proven SCLC patients were included in the analysis. RCTs examined compared a cisplatin-containing regimen versus a regimen without this alkylating agent. A total of 4054 eligible patients were randomised between a cisplatin-containing regimen (1814 patients) and a regimen without cisplatin (2240 patients). This meta-analysis showed that patients receiving a cisplatin-containing regimen had a lower risk of death at 6 months with an OR of 0·74 (95% CI 0·59–0·94; $P = 0·006$). The OR of being a responder in a cisplatin-containing regimen was 1·35 (95% CI 1·18–1·55; $P < 0·0001$). Using the DerSimonian and Laird method of estimating effect size, the authors concluded there was no increased risk of toxic death in those receiving cisplatin-containing regimens versus those who received chemotherapy without cisplatin (probability of toxic death in cisplatin group 0·031 $v$ non-cisplatin 0·027; $P = 0·23$).

There are no systematic reviews or meta-analyses of dose-intensive therapy for SCLC. A number of different approaches towards SCLC chemotherapy dose intensification have been published. These include increasing the dose of conventional chemotherapy drugs, increasing of dose intensity of chemotherapy drugs with haematopoietic stem cell support, reduction of the chemotherapy cycle duration, or lastly, the addition of other chemotherapy drugs to the standard cisplatin and etoposide combination. Interpretation of these studies is confounded by the admixture of both limited and extensive stage disease patients in some of the studies while others restricted eligibility to one or other of the stages of the disease. In addition, RCTs such as a recent comparison of a four-drug combination versus cisplatin and etoposide employed a schedule of cisplatin and etoposide in 4-week cycle which is non-standard. Median survival in the experimental group was 10·5 months versus 9·3 months ($P=0\cdot0067$ log-rank). For this 5-week prolongation of median survival, 67% of the patients in the four-drug treatment arm of the study required antibiotic infusions for febrile neutropenia, and there was a 9% treatment-related mortality.[16]

Studies in which high dose chemotherapy with autologous bone marrow support was provided have omitted concurrent thoracic irradiation in limited disease stage patients. One RCT of 403 patients randomised between a 3-week cycle of doxorubicin, cyclophosphamide, and etoposide versus a 2-week cycle supported with granulocyte colony-stimulating factor demonstrated that, although overall survival was longer in the dose intense group (HR 0·8; 95% CI 0·65–0·99; $P=0\cdot04$), the metastasis-free survival in the limited disease stage subgroup, of which there were 152 patients in each arm, was similar in the two groups (HR 0·95; 95% CI 0·75–1·21; $P=0\cdot67$). In addition, median survival of limited disease patients randomised to the dose intense treatment arm, was only 14–15 months, considerably less than the 18 months expected from standard treatment with chemotherapy and thoracic irradiation.[17]

We found one RCT comparing cisplatin and one of the newer chemotherapeutic agents, irinotecan, versus the standard cisplatin and etoposide combination in the treatment of extensive stage SCLC: 154 patients (77 in each arm) were randomised. Median survival was 12·8 months in the irinotecan group (95% CI 11·7–15·2 months) and 9·4 months in the etoposide group (95% CI, 8·1–10·8 months log-rank test). At 2 years, survival in the irinotecan plus cisplatin group was 19·5% (95% CI 10·6–28·3, significance not stated) and in the etoposide plus cisplatin group, 5·2% (95% CI 0·2–10·2). One of the flaws of this study was that full information concerning treatment after disease progression was not available although no patient was lost to follow up and the estimates of overall survival were thought to be reliable.[18]

## Conclusions

While there has been enthusiasm for increasing the intensity of chemotherapy treatment of SCLC, given its initial chemosensitivity, there is currently no evidence to suggest that such intensive treatment as the addition of extra drugs to the standard cisplatin and etoposide

combination or increasing the absolute dose with bone marrow support is likely to lead to increased survival. There has been a plateau in survival from recent studies of the systemic treatment of SCLC. A number of additional chemotherapeutic agents such as the taxanes and topoisomerase inhibitors have shown some early promise in phase II studies but randomised controlled trials will be required to assess whether the addition of these new drugs or substitution of these new drugs for one of the existing standard agents will further improve the outcome for SCLC patients. Lack of significant progress in extending the survival of patients with SCLC has led investigators to turn to the evaluation of alternative treatment strategies including the use of biological agents. A number of studies including those using matrix metalloproteinase inhibitors are currently under evaluation, but these trials are not yet mature and survival results are not available.

## What is the role of single agent oral etoposide in the treatment of extensive stage SCLC patients?

### Background

Patients with extensive stage SCLC have a poor prognosis with only 5–10% of patients surviving 2 years. The primary aim of chemotherapy for these patients is to palliate symptoms. Enthusiasm for the use of oral etoposide, particularly in poor prognosis or elderly patients, was based on a number of earlier findings. Firstly, it was shown that the antitumour cytotoxicity of etoposide is greatest after lengthy exposure to low plasma concentrations and that this is best achieved by oral administration of the drug.[19] This benefit is mitigated, however, by the variability between and within patient biovariability of oral etoposide.[20]

In previously untreated patients, uncontrolled phase II studies reported responses in up to 70% of patients and survival comparable to that seen with the use of multiagent intravenous chemotherapy in patients with extensive stage disease. An assumption was made that oral etoposide would be preferable to intravenous chemotherapy with respect to side effects, even if there were no survival benefit from its use.

Oral etoposide is obviously easier to administer than combination intravenous chemotherapy.

### Answer to the question

We found three RCTs comparing the use of oral etoposide with intravenous chemotherapy in patients with SCLC. Survival was uniformly inferior in patients receiving oral etoposide as a single agent and, while acute nausea and vomiting were less when oral etoposide was administered, all other aspects of symptom control and quality of life were either the same or worse in the oral etoposide group.

## Evidence

There are no meta-analyses or systematic reviews of the use of oral etoposide versus combination chemotherapy in patients with extensive stage SCLC. Three RCTs have been published. Two RCTs from the United Kingdom, the Medical Research Council Lung Cancer Working Party Trial and the London Lung Cancer Group Trial, terminated early on the recommendation of their data monitoring committees based on a significant difference in survival. In the first study, 339 patients were randomly allocated to four cycles of 50 mg of oral etoposide twice daily for 10 days (171 patients) or an intravenous regimen of etoposide and vincristine, or cyclophosphamide, doxorubicin and vincristine (168 patients). Survival was inferior in the oral etoposide group (HR 1·35; 95% CI 1·03–1·79; $P = 0·03$). Median survival was 130 days in the oral etoposide group and 183 days in the control group (significance not stated). Haematological toxicity, particularly anaemia was 29% in the oral etoposide group and 21% in the intravenous chemotherapy group (significance not stated). There was no increase in the prevalence of fever or bronchopneumonia in the oral etoposide group.[21]

The second UK trial employed an etoposide regimen of 100 mg twice daily for 5 days, compared with intravenous chemotherapy consisting of alternating cycles of cisplatin plus etoposide, followed by cyclophosphamide, doxorubicin, and vincristine.[22] Each group received six cycles of chemotherapy every 3 weeks. Survival at 1 year in the oral etoposide group was 9·8% versus 19·3% for intravenous chemotherapy (95% CI 0·3–18·7; $P < 0·05$) The median survivals were 5·9 months with intravenous chemotherapy and 4·8 months with oral etoposide (significance not stated). With the use of the Rotterdam symptom checklist and a daily diary card, quality of life was assessed in these patients. On overall quality of life on the Rotterdam checklist, oral etoposide produced inferior results compared with intravenous chemotherapy ($P < 0·01$), but the oral treatment was comparable in effects on psychological wellbeing and physical symptoms. On the daily diary card, oral etoposide proved worse than intravenous chemotherapy when appetite, pain, sleep, mood and general wellbeing were assessed (sleep $P < 0·02$; other symptoms $P < 0·01$). Oral etoposide treatment was preferable to intravenous chemotherapy only in regards to acute nausea ($P < 0·01$).

The third RCT from Denmark randomised 65 patients to carboplatin intravenously and high dose oral etoposide (240 mg m$^{-2}$) given orally on days 1–3 versus oral etoposide 50 mg per day from day 1 to 14 of a 4-week cycle.[23] The rate of progression was three times higher in the group receiving oral etoposide ($P = 0·006$, Fisher's exact test, 2-sided value). Median overall survival in the intravenous chemotherapy group was 211 days (95% CI 1·38–2·58) and 155 days in the oral etoposide group (95% CI 1·13–2·02; $P = 0·095$). Quality of life was not assessed in this third study.

## Conclusions

Despite the early promise from phase II studies showing that patients with SCLC do in fact respond to oral etoposide, evidence from three RCTs show that there is no benefit either in terms of survival or quality of life in poor performance status patients. Given the simplicity of administration of oral etoposide, however, the development of oral preparations of some of the newer chemotherapeutic drugs such as topotecan may allow the development of effective and well-tolerated oral combination drug regimens for elderly or poor performance patients with SCLC.

## What is the role of prophylactic cranial irradiation in the treatment of SCLC?

### Background

CNS involvement commonly complicates the course of SCLC. Brain metastases are present at the time of initial diagnosis in about 10% patients.[24] However, autopsy studies demonstrate an incidence of 65%, suggesting that brain metastases are a common cause of treatment failure in those who have achieved a complete response to prior chemoirradiation.[24] RCTs published since 1980 have established the efficacy of prophylactic cranial irradiation (PCI) in reducing the cumulative incidence of brain metastases, but the survival benefit has remained controversial. Optimal dose, fractionation and timing of the radiation have not been established and there are still unresolved issues about possible long-term neurological toxicity of the treatment.

### Answer to the question

Evidence from a number of RCTs shows that PCI reduces the frequency of brain metastases and increases disease-free survival in SCLC patients with both limited and extensive stage disease who have achieved a complete remission with initial chemotherapy or chemotherapy plus irradiation. RCTs in which patients have been followed for up to 2 years suggests that PCI does not produce significant cognitive dysfunction.

## Evidence

We found one systematic review (search date not stated, seven RCTs, 987 people) of cranial irradiation for people with SCLC in complete remission.[25] The review used individual participant data from included RCTs. Of the people studied, 12% in the irradiation group and 17% in the control group had extensive stage disease at presentation. Meta-analysis found that cranial irradiation significantly improved survival (RR of death at 3 years 0·84; 95% CI 0·73–0·97, corresponding to a 5·4% increase in survival) and increased disease-free survival (RR of recurrence or death at 3 years 0·76; 95% CI 0·65–0·86). Subgroup analysis identified survival benefit only for men and not for women, but the difference in survival between the two subgroups was not significant ($P = 0·07$). The cumulative incidence of brain metastases was decreased (RR 0·46; 95% CI 0·38–0·57). Larger doses of radiation led to a greater decrease in brain metastases ($P = 0·02$), but did not influence survival significantly ($P = 0·89$).

One of the RCTs was a three arm trial carried out from 1987 to 1995 in which 314 patients with SCLC were randomised to one of two PCI protocols (36 Gy over 18 fractions or 24 Gy in 12 fractions) or observation.[26] To improve accrual the PCI arms were condensed to one PCI arm of clinician's choice of PCI protocol, versus observation. In this trial, the number of brain metastases developing in those given the lower radiation dose was not significantly different from the control group (HR 0·71; 95% CI 0·36–1·43, no $P$ value given), while there was a clear difference using the higher dose (HR 0·16; 95% CI 0·07–0·36;

$P = 0·0007$). This suggests a dose–response effect. This trial also showed a trend for survival advantage for PCI-treated patients (HR 0·86; 95% CI 0·66–1·12; $P = 0·25$ log-rank).

None of the trials cited in the meta-analysis addressed the optimum timing of PCI in relation to induction chemotherapy and thoracic irradiation. All patients received PCI after completion of their initial treatment and assessment of complete response. A non-systematic review of 40 trials of PCI, which included trials in which patients received PCI before achieving a complete response, and 11 RCTs, of which two were included in the previously described meta-analysis, concluded that the same dose of PCI has a greater effect if given early (that is, within 60 days of starting chemotherapy).[27] This means that some patients would be receiving chemotherapy and PCI either concurrently, the toxicity of which is undetermined. Despite the opposing theoretical arguments for giving PCI before or after the patient achieves a complete response (CR), the International Association for the Study of Lung Cancer concluded that optimal timing of PCI remains unknown.[28]

Two RCTs have examined cognitive function as outcomes for PCI therapy. In one RCT, neurologists made five assessments of SCLC patients in CR randomised to PCI or observation initially pre-PCI, and then at four periods over 48 months. Two-year cumulative incidence of neuropsychological changes was the same in both groups, and CT scans of the brain performed at the same intervals as the neurological examinations were not significantly different in the number of abnormalities (PCI 27% $v$ observation 21%; RR 1·48; $P = 0·60$ log-rank).[29]

**Table 21.2  Summary of recommendations for small cell lung cancer**

| Treatment strategy | Recommendation | Level of evidence/grade of recommendation |
|---|---|---|
| Surgical resection | Reasonable for patients with T1–2 N0 tumours | **Evidence level IIa, Grade B** |
| Addition of irradiation to chemotherapy in limited stage disease | Local control and survival both improved with combined modality treatment. Conflicting evidence on timing and dose of irradiation | **Evidence level Ia, Grade A** |
| Best chemotherapy treatment | Cisplatin and etoposide remain standard, Increasing drug dose or the number of drugs has not increased patient survival | **Evidence level Ia, Grade A** |
| Single agent oral etoposide for extensive stage SCLC patients | Compared to combination chemotherapy, oral etoposide offers no survival benefit or improved quality of life | **Evidence level Ib, Grade A** |
| Prophylactic cranial irradiation | PCI reduces frequency of brain metastasis and increases disease-free survival in SCLC patients with either limited or extensive stage disease | **Evidence level Ia, Grade A** |

In a second RCT a subgroup of 136 patients (84 received PCI, 52 observation) out of a total of 314 patients underwent cognitive assessment. No statistical comparison was made, but the authors reported no difference between PCI and the observation group in "sustained deterioration" of cognitive function.[26]

## Conclusions

SCLC patients with either limited or extensive stage disease should be offered PCI if they have achieved CR from initial chemoradiation therapy. The evidence from meta-analysis demonstrates that PCI reduces brain metastases and can increase overall survival (Table 22.2). Future research needs to address optimal dose and timing of PCI. Since patient follow up is relatively short in many studies, the potential longer term cognitive toxicity and quality-of-life issues in PCI-treated patients remain to be addressed.

## References

1 Carney, DN. Lung cancer – Time to move on from chemotherapy. *N Engl J Med* 2002;**346**:126–7.
2 Green RA, Humphrey E, Close H *et al.* Alkylating agents in bronchogenic carcinoma. *Am J Med* 1969;**46**:516–25.
3 Shepherd FA. Surgical management of small cell lung cancer. In: Pass HI, Mitchell JB, Johnson DH *et al.*, eds. *Lung Cancer, Principles and Practice, 2nd edn.* Philadelphia, PA: Lippincott Williams and Wilkins, 2002.
4 Travis WD, Linder J and Mackay B. Classification, histology, cytology and electron microscopy. In: Pass HI, Mitchell JB, Johnson DH *et al.* eds. *Lung Cancer, Principles and Practice, 2nd edn.* Philadelphia, PA: Lippincott Williams and Wilkins, 2002.
5 Wistuba II, Gazdar AF, Minne JD. Molecular genetics of small cell lung carcinoma. *Semin Oncol* 2001;**28**(Suppl. 4):3–13.
6 Lad T, Plantadori S, Thomas P *et al.* A prospective randomized trial to determine the benefit of surgical resection of residual disease following response of small cell lung cancer to combination chemotherapy. *Chest* 1994;**106**(Suppl.):3205–3235.
7 Pignon JP, Arriagada R, Ihde DC *et al.* A meta-analysis of thoracic radiotherapy for small-cell lung cancer. *N Engl J Med* 1992;**327**:1618–24.
8 Warde P, Payne D. Does thoracic irradiation improve survival and local control in limited-stage small cell carcinoma of the lung? A meta-analysis. *J Clin Oncol* 1992;**10**:890–5.
9 Okawara G, Gagliardi A, Evans WK *et al.* The role of thoracic radiotherapy as an adjunct to standard chemotherapy in limited-stage small-cell lung cancer. *Curr Oncol* 2000;**7**:162–72.
10 Jeremic B, Shibamoto Y, Acimovic L *et al.* Initial versus delayed accelerated hyperfractionated radiation therapy and concurrent chemotherapy in limited small-cell lung cancer. A randomized study. *J Clin Oncol* 1997;**15**:893–900.
11 Tsukada H, Yokoyama A, Goto K *et al.* Concurrent versus sequential radiotherapy for small cell lung cancer. *Semin Oncol* 2001;**28**(Suppl. 4):23–6.
12 Coy P, Hodson I, Payne DG *et al.* The effect of dose of thoracic irradiation on recurrence in patients with limited stage small cell lung cancer. Initial results of a Canadian Multicentre Randomized Trial. *Int J Radiat Oncol Biol Phys* 1988;**14**:219–26.
13 Turrisi AT, Kim K, Blum R *et al.* Twice-daily compared with once-daily thoracic radiotherapy in limited small-cell lung cancer treated concurrently with cisplatin and etoposide. *N Engl J Med* 1999;**340**:265–71.
14 Bonner JA, Sloan JA, Shanahan TG *et al.* Phase III comparison of twice-daily split-course irradiation versus once-daily irradiation for patients with limited stage small-cell lung carcinoma. *J Clin Oncol* 1999;**17**:2681–91.
15 Pujol JL, Carestia, Davies, JP. Is there a case for cisplatin in the treatment of small cell lung cancer? A meta-analysis of randomized trials of a cisplatin-containing regimen versus a regimen without this alkylating agent. *Br J Cancer* 2000;**83**:8–15.
16 Pujol JL, Davies JP, Riviere A *et al.* Etoposide plus cisplatin with or without the combination of 4-epidoxombicin plus cyclophosphamide in treatment of extensive small-cell lung cancer: a French Federation of Cancer Institutes Multicentre Phase III randomized study. *J Natl Cancer Inst* 2001;**93**:300–8.
17 Thatcher N, Girling DJ, Hopwood P *et al.* Improving survival without reducing quality of life in small cell lung cancer patients by increasing the dose-intensity of chemotherapy with granulocyte colony-stimulating factor support: Results of a British Medical Research Council Multicentre Randomized Trial. *J Clin Oncol* 2000;**18**:395–404.
18 Noda K, Nishikawa Y, Kawahara M *et al.* Irinotecan plus cisplatin compared with etoposide plus cisplatin for extensive small cell lung cancer. *N Engl J Med* 2002;**346**:85–91.
19 Payne DG. The role of radiation oncology in small cell lung cancer. *Crit Rev Oncol Hematol* 1994;**16**:113–27.
20 DeJong RS, Mulder NH, Dijksterhuis D *et al.* Review of current clinical experience with prolonged (oral) etoposide in cancer treatment. *Anticancer Res* 1995;**15**:2319–330.
21 Medical Council of Canada Working Party. Comparison of oral etoposide and standard intravenous multidrug chemotherapy for small cell lung cancer: A stopped multicentred randomized trial. *Lancet* 1996;**348**:563–6.
22 Souhami RL, Spiro SG, Rudd RM *et al.* Five day oral etoposide treatment for advanced small cell lung cancer: randomized comparison with intravenous chemotherapy. *J Natl Cancer Inst* 1997;**89**:577–80.
23 Pfifer P, Rytter C, Madsen EL *et al.* RE: Five-day oral etoposide treatment for advanced small-cell lung cancer: randomized comparison with intravenous chemotherapy. *J Natl Cancer Inst* 1997;**89**:1892.
24 Stakel RA. Diagnosis, staging and prognostic factors of small cell lung cancer. *Curr Opin Oncol* 1991;**3**:306–11.
25 Auperin A, Arriagada R, Pignon JP *et al.* Prophylactic cranial irradiation for people with small-cell lung cancer in complete remission. *N Engl J Med* 1999;**341**:476–84.
26 Gregor A, Cull A, Stephens RJ *et al.* Prophylactic cranial irradiation is indicated following complete response to induction therapy in small cell lung cancer. Results of a multicentre randomized trial. *Eur J Cancer* 1997;**33**:1752–8.
27 Suwinski R, Lee SP, Withers HR. Dose-response relationship for prophylactic cranial irradiation in small cell lung cancer. *Int J Radiat Biol Phys* 1998;**40**:797–806.
28 Ihde D, Souhami B, Comis R *et al.* Consensus report: Small cell lung cancer. *Lung Cancer* 1997;**17**(Suppl. 1):519.
29 Arriaga R, LeChevalier T, Borie F *et al.* Prophylactic cranial irradiation for patients with small-cell lung cancer in complete remission. *J Natl Cancer Inst* 1995;**87**:183–190.

# 22 Malignant pleural mesothelioma

*Ferran Ariza, Miquel Mateu, Ramón Rami-Porta, Mireia Serra*

Malignant pleural mesothelioma is a fatal neoplasm arising from the mesothelial cells of the pleura. It is a relatively rare disease, with about 2800 new cases seen in the USA every year[1] and an annual incidence of up to 10–15/100 000 in older males in most Western European countries.[2] The incidence of mesothelioma is increasing and a peak is expected in many developed countries within the next two decades owing to the long latency period between exposure to asbestos and the development of clinical symptoms.[3] The association between exposure to asbestos and mesothelioma was first reported by Wagner *et al.* in 1960[4] and subsequently confirmed by other authors.[5–15] Today, asbestos exposure is commonly accepted as the main aetiological factor, although non-asbestos-related malignant mesothelioma has been reported and discussed.[16–17]

Three pathological types of mesothelioma have been described: sarcomatous, epithelial and mixed. Different prognostic scoring staging systems have been proposed (Butchart, IMIG TNM, EORTC, CALGB) but there is no general consensus as to the most appropriate.[18] The prognosis for malignant pleural mesothelioma is generally poor with a median survival for untreated patients of 6 to 18 months from the time of diagnosis.[19] The disease spreads asymptomatically along the pleura and clinical presentation is often late in the natural history, with invasion of the chest wall, lung substance and mediastinal structures.[20] The tumour may also metastasise, but patients usually die from local complications. Poorer prognosis has been associated with sarcomatous cell type, low haemoglobin, high white blood cell count, poor performance status. and male sex.[18]

Levels of evidence and grades of recommendation are given in Table 22.1.

## What are the effects of chemotherapy for malignant pleural mesothelioma?

### Background

Several reviews have concluded that no single agent or combined chemotherapy modality has been shown to be effective in improving survival rates for mesothelioma. One review[21] reported that some chemotherapy agents have marginal activity, but selection of young patients with good prognosis for the more intensive treatments may have resulted in erroneous conclusions about effectiveness. Furthermore, occasional prolonged survival of untreated patients has been described in many reports and may have biased the interpretation of results. Another review[19] found that, although responses to single agent chemotherapy have been reported, impact on survival rates has not been clearly proven. Diagnosis of the disease at an early stage seems to be the most important factor for the success of the treatment. Another review[22] noted that, although numerous agents have been tested, few have shown any clear benefit. Because of the low prevalence of this disease, most trials have been small and have had insufficient power to detect statistical significance.

## Review of evidence

### Single agent chemotherapy

We found no systematic reviews. One small RCT compared doxorubicin (N = 15) versus cyclophosphamide (N = 16) in 32 patients with malignant pleural mesothelioma.[23] Reporting of results and statistical analysis was limited. No partial or complete remissions were seen in any patient. One trial compared the platinum analogues JM8 and JM9 in 16 patients with pleural malignant mesothelioma.[24] No differences in either response rates or emetogenesis were seen. However, JM8 was better tolerated and could therefore be given in an outpatient situation in significantly more cases (62·5% for JM8 *v* 12·5% for JM9; $\chi^2 = 10·3$; df = 1, $P < 0·005$).

### Combined chemotherapy in malignant mesothelioma

We found no systematic reviews, but identified two small RCTs that compared combined chemotherapy regimens. Neither found statistically significant differences in response rates, relapse-free survival or overall survival.

One RCT compared cisplatin plus mitomycin (C + M; N = 35) versus cisplatin plus doxorubicin (C + D; N = 35) in 70 patients with pleural (N = 66) and peritoneal (N = 4) mesotheliomas.[25] Some patients had undergone prior surgery and/or radiotherapy. No significant differences were found in the overall response rates (26% for C + M; 95% CI 12%–43% *v* 14% for C + D; 95% CI 5%–30%), time to treatment failure (3·6 months for C + M *v* 4·8 months for C + D; log-rank $P = 0·59$), and overall survival (median survival of 7·7 months for C + M *v* 8·8 months for C + D;

**Table 22.1  Mesothelioma – levels of evidence/grades of recommendation**

| Question | Answer | Levels of evidence | Grade of recommendations | Comments |
|---|---|---|---|---|
| Does chemotherapy improve survival in patients with malignant pleural mesothelioma? | Unknown | | | Neither systematic reviews nor well-designed RCTs comparing single and multimodality chemotherapy regimens, either as a single or adjuvant treatment were found |
| Is chemotherapy useful as a palliative treatment in patients with malignant pleural mesothelioma? | Unknown | | | Neither systematic reviews nor RCTs comparing chemotherapy to best supportive care were found |
| Does radiotherapy improve survival in patients with malignant pleural mesothelioma? | Unknown | | | Neither systematic reviews nor well-designed RCTs comparing standard and fractionated radiotherapy schemes, either as a single or adjuvant treatment were found |
| Is radiotherapy useful as a palliative treatment in patients with malignant pleural mesothelioma? | Unknown | | | Neither systematic reviews nor RCTs comparing radiotherapy to best supportive care were found |
| Is radiotherapy useful in preventing malignant mesothelioma seeding after diagnostic pleural invasive procedures? | Yes | Evidence level Ib | Grade A/B | Only one small RCT |
| Can radical surgery improve survival in malignant pleural mesothelioma? | Unknown | | | Neither systematic reviews nor RCTs comparing radical surgery to best supportive care were found |
| Is any surgical intervention more effective than any other in achieving symptom palliation in mesothelioma? | Unknown | | | Neither systematic reviews nor RCTs comparing surgical interventions were found. Evidence from two observational studies favours pleuroscopy and pleurodesis with talc or partial pleurectomy to control pleural effusion |

log-rank $P = 0.75$). Overall tolerance of treatments was considered good. For combined grades 3 (severe) and 4 (life-threatening) toxicity, C + D patients were found to have more leucopenia (46% *v* 17%, $P = 0.01$) and alopecia (49% *v* 3%; $P = 0.001$) and C + M patients were found to have more thrombocytopenia (43% *v* 17%; $P = 0.02$).

The other RCT compared cyclophosphamide, imidazole carboxamide and adriamycin (CIA, N = 40) versus cyclophosphamide and adriamycin (CA, N = 36) in 76 patients with advanced stage malignant pleural (N = 53) and peritoneal (N = 23) mesotheliomas.[26] Some patients had undergone prior chemotherapy, surgery or radiotherapy. Differences in overall survival (median survival of 25 weeks for CIA *v* 30 weeks for CA), response rates (13% for CIA *v* 11% for CA) and relapse-free survival (9 weeks for CIA *v* 14 weeks for CA) were not found to be statistically significant. Patients in the CIA group had higher grade 3 or greater leucopenia rates than patients in the CA group (46% *v* 38%) (statistical significance not indicated). Eighty five per cent of CIA patients and 67% of CA patients had non-haematological toxicities (nausea, vomiting, stomatitis and/or diarrhoea) (statistical significance not indicated).

### *Neoadjuvant and adjuvant chemotherapy*

We found no systematic reviews nor RCTs that assessed neoadjuvant or adjuvant chemotherapy. In both RCTs described above (combined chemotherapy) patients having prior surgery, radiotherapy, chemotherapy, or no prior therapy were all mixed within the same treatment group so the role of adjuvant chemotherapy could not be determined separately.

One small, non-randomised trial[27] compared surgery plus intrapleural chemotherapy (with or without additional systemic chemotherapy), surgery plus radiotherapy, and surgery alone. Patients receiving intrapleural chemotherapy had lower survival rates, shorter median time to progression and a had shorter survival time than those who did not. Differences in overall survival and time to progression for patients who did and did not receive standard chemotherapy (intrapleural plus systemic) were not statistically significant (see section below on Neoadjuvant or adjuvant radiotherapy).

One non-randomised trial compared radiotherapy (N = 31) with radiotherapy plus doxorubicin and cyclophosphamide (N = 16) in 47 patients.[28] Comparisons between both groups were not considered possible since only patients with better prognosis factors after radiotherapy were offered chemotherapy.

### *Palliative chemotherapy*

We found no systematic reviews or RCTs comparing chemotherapy with best supportive care.

## Conclusions

### *Implications for clinical practice*

There is no strong evidence supporting the use of chemotherapy in malignant mesothelioma.

### *Implications for research*

Large, well-designed randomised controlled trials are needed to define the possible role of chemotherapy for

mesothelioma. RCTs comparing chemotherapy versus best supportive care alone should be carried out and the role of single agent chemotherapy versus combined chemotherapy regimens should be clarified. The effects of neoadjuvant and adjuvant chemotherapy should also be studied.

## What are the effects of radiotherapy for malignant pleural mesothelioma?

### Background

Several reviews have concluded that radiotherapy does not improve survival rates in mesothelioma but whether it is useful or not as a palliative treatment remains unclear. Two reviews[29,30] have concluded that radiotherapy is not curative but is useful for symptom palliation. Combinations of therapies have been tried but most studies have been uncontrolled and the results are impossible to interpret because of selection bias. Another review suggested that palliative radiotherapy is problematic since differences between tumour cytotoxicity and pulmonary tolerance are small and radiation pneumonitis may significantly impair quality of life.[31] Other authors have commented that, although radiotherapy does not offer worthwhile prolonged disease control when used in isolation, it has an important role as part of multimodality therapy.[32] Many reviews have concluded that radiotherapy is useful for prophylaxis against needle-track metastases.[21,33,34]

### Review of evidence

### *Neoadjuvant or adjuvant radiotherapy*

We found no systematic reviews or RCTs. One small, non-randomised trial[27] compared surgery plus intrapleural chemotherapy with (N = 7) or without (N = 6) additional systemic chemotherapy, N = 13), surgery plus radiotherapy (N = 4) and surgery alone (N = 3).

*Survival and time to progression:* Patients receiving intrapleural chemotherapy had lower survival rates than those who did not (median of 9 months *v* 21 months; *P* = 0·04). Median time to progression was longer for patients not receiving intrapleural chemotherapy (12 months *v* 6 months; *P* = 0·01). Patients receiving postoperative radiotherapy lived longer (38 months) than those undergoing surgery alone (13 months) and those having surgery plus intrapleural chemotherapy (9 months); both overall survival and time to progression were significantly longer (*P* = 0·05 and *P* = 0·04, respectively) in patients receiving postoperative radiotherapy than in the other groups combined. Differences in overall survival and time to progression for the patients who did and did not receive standard chemotherapy (intrapleural plus systemic) were not statistically significant (16 *v* 9 months and 7 *v* 5 months, respectively).

*Toxicity and palliation:* Data on toxicity and palliation were reported, but no comparisons between groups or tests of statistical significance were shown.

One non-randomised trial compared outcomes in patients with malignant pleural mesothelioma, who received either no treatment (N = 64), surgery alone (N = 28), chemotherapy (N = 12, prior surgery in 8) or radiotherapy (N = 12, prior surgery in 8).[35] No significant differences in survival were found between treatment groups or between treated and untreated patients (median survival of 20, 19, 18 and 18 months for surgery alone, chemotherapy, radiotherapy and untreated patients, respectively). Data on toxicity and palliation were reported for each group, but no comparisons between groups or tests of statistical significance were shown.

One non-randomised trial compared six different radiotherapy schedules of altered fractionation in a combined modality programme (surgery, chemotherapy and radiotherapy) in 57 patients.[36] The schemes were:

- hemithorax irradiation I (N = 8), consisting of conventional fractionation (20 Gy given in 10 fractions of 2 Gy) with prior CYVADIC chemotherapy (cyclophosphamide, vincristine, doxorubicin, dacarbazine);
- hemithorax irradiation II (N = 17), consisting of split-course (Gy given in 25 fractions of 2·2 Gy) plus a 15 Gy boost (given in six fractions of 2·5 Gy) with prior CYVADIC chemotherapy given to five patients with stage III disease;
- hemithorax irradiation III (N = 6), consisting of hyperfractionation (70 Gy given in 56 fractions of 1·25 Gy) with prior mitoxantrone chemotherapy;
- hemithorax irradiation IV (N = 11), consisting of hyperfractionation and hypofractionation (35 Gy given in 28 fractions of 1·25 Gy followed by 36 Gy given in 9 fractions of 4 Gy) with prior 4-epirubicin chemotherapy;
- hemithorax irradiation V (N = 5), consisting of hypofractionation (38·5 Gy given in 11 fractions of 3·5 Gy) with prior etoposide chemotherapy;
- hemithorax irradiation VI (N = 10), consisting of conventional fractionation and hypofractionation (20 Gy given in 10 fractions of 2 Gy followed by 30 Gy given in 10 fractions of 3 Gy) with prior amonafide chemotherapy.

All patients underwent thoracotomy prior to the above treatment; 16 patients had biopsy only, one had pleuropneumonectomy and the rest underwent parietal pleurectomy or partial resection of the tumour. No significant differences in survival were seen between the treatment groups.

### Palliative radiotherapy

We found no systematic reviews or randomised controlled trials comparing radiotherapy versus best supportive care only.

### Radiotherapy for preventing malignant seeding after invasive diagnosis procedures

One small trial randomised 40 patients to either receive (N = 20) or not receive (N = 20) local radiotherapy after invasive diagnostic procedures.[37] None of the patients receiving local radiotherapy developed subcutaneous nodules at the entry site of thoracoscopy trocars, chest tubes and/or cytology or biopsy needles, while eight in the control group did (0% *v* 40%; *P* < 0·001). Tolerance of local radiotherapy was reported to be excellent.

## Conclusions
### Implications for clinical practice

There is no strong evidence supporting the use of radiotherapy in malignant mesothelioma. There is weak evidence from one small RCT, which lacked statistical power, that local radiotherapy may be effective in preventing malignant seeding after diagnostic invasive procedures.

### Implications for research

Large, well-designed randomised controlled trials are needed to define the possible role of radiotherapy for mesothelioma. RCTs comparing radiotherapy versus best supportive care should be carried out. The role of neoadjuvant and adjuvant radiotherapy should be further studied.

## Can radical surgery improve survival in malignant pleural mesothelioma?

### Background

Surgical treatment of malignant pleural mesothelioma ranges from extrapleural pneumonectomy to pleural decortication with maximal excision of tumour tissue.[35,39] This surgery is very aggressive with a perioperative mortality from 3% to 15%. Furthermore, the term "radical surgery" is inexact, as it is very difficult to achieve complete excision of the tumour because it infiltrates through the muscles, diaphragm, mediastinal soft tissue, and mediastinal organs.

### Review of evidence

We found no systematic review or randomised controlled trial comparing radical surgery with best supportive care, and we found only two non-randomised, prospective clinical trials. One trial[39] compared extrapleural pneumonectomy with palliative treatment in 83 patients, and the second, which was terminated prematurely[35] and included only 12 patients, compared pleurectomy plus intrapleural and systemic chemotherapy with palliative treatment. No significant differences were found between extrapleural pneumonectomy, pleurectomy, and palliative care, for either median overall survival, which was 10 months, or 2-year survival, which was 20% in all groups in both trials. The disease-free interval was longer in the surgical group, but this had no influence in survival.

We selected four descriptive studies, with more than 75 cases in each, in whom the surgical intervention depended on the patient's clinical status and disease extension[35] and which together gave a combined total of 620 patients with malignant pleural mesothelioma. In these studies survival was compared following pleurectomy, extrapleural pneumonectomy, and best supportive care, and, wherever possible, surgery was combined with chemotherapy,[40–42] radiotherapy,[41,42] or brachytherapy.[40] There were no significant differences in mean survival, which ranged from 20 months[35] to 5 months,[40] or in 1-year (82%), 2-year (30%), or 4-year (10%) survival[35] Five-year survival was reported in only one study (9·1%).[42]

We found one randomised controlled trial that compared survival in 63 patients with malignant pleural mesothelioma who received maximum debulking surgery (pleurectomy or pneumonectomy) with postoperative immunotherapy, with or without intraoperative photodynamic therapy (PDT).[43] Type of resection and numbers of immunochemotherapy cycles delivered were comparable in the two groups. Debulking to 5 mm was not possible in 15 patients. Median survival in the 48 patients who received their assigned treatment was 14 months, with no significant differences between the PDT and no PDT groups in median survival, median progression-free time, or sites of first recurrence.

## Conclusions

### *Implications for clinical practice*

Radical surgical treatment consisting of extrapleural pneumonectomy for diffuse malignant pleural mesothelioma is not recommended. Evidence from two non-randomised clinical trials and four selected descriptive studies showed no evidence that surgery increases survival. There is currently no curative surgical treatment for this uncommon tumour.

## Is any surgical intervention more effective than any other in achieving symptom palliation in mesothelioma?

### Background

The aim of palliative surgery for mesothelioma is to improve symptoms of thoracic pain and dyspnoea. To relieve pain, pleurectomy to reduce tumour size may be undertaken. Where there is dyspnoea in the presence of pleural effusion, a pleuroscopy is indicated, firstly to obtain a pathological diagnosis, but also to drain the effusion and to perform a pleurodesis with irritative substances (talc, tetracyclines, chemotherapeutic agents).

### Review of evidence

We identified two non-randomised clinical trials that compared palliative surgical treatment consisting of pleural decortication, with chemotherapy, radiotherapy, or no treatment.[35,39] No differences were found in either study in 2-year survival (20% *v* 18·5%), but decortication controlled pleural effusion better than the other treatment modalities. In other descriptive studies we found that palliative treatment consisting of partial pleurectomy,[41] and pleurodesis with talc poudrage[44] to control a pleural effusion or growing tumour, improved respiratory symptoms such as dyspnoea, but not pain.[42]

### Conclusions

#### *Implications for clinical practice*

Where a mesothelioma is associated with a pleural effusion, pleuroscopy and pleurodesis with talc or partial pleurectomy can allow accurate anatomopathological diagnosis, and control an effusion and palliate dyspnoea.

#### *Implications for research*

The role and effectiveness of surgery as part of a multimodality treatment approach should be investigated.

It has been suggested[35] that there may be a case for screening people exposed to asbestos and the feasibility of this should be investigated.

### References

1  Price B. Analysis of current trends in United States mesothelioma incidence. *Am J Epidemiol* 1997;**145**:211–18.
2  La Vecchia C, Decarli A, Peto J, Levi F, Tomei F, Negri E. An age, period and cohort analysis of pleural cancer mortality in Europe. *Eur J Cancer Prev* 2000;**9**:179–84.

3    Briton M. The epidemiology of mesothelioma. *Semin Oncol* 2002;**29**:18–25.

4    Wagner JC, Sleggs EA, Marchand P. Diffuse pleural mesothelioma and asbestos in the North Western Cape Province. *Br J Ind Med* 1960;**17**:260–71.

5    Fowler PBS, Sloper JC, Warner EC. Exposure to asbestos and mesothelioma of the pleura. *BMJ* 1964;**2**:211–13.

6    Selikoff IJ, Churg J, Hammond EC. The occurrence of asbestosis among insulation workers in the United States. *Ann NY Acad Sci* 1965;**132**:139–55.

7    Nurminen M. The epidemiologic relationship between pleural mesothelioma and asbestos exposure. *Scand J Work Environ Health* 1975;**1**:128–37.

8    Kucuksu N, Thomas W, Ezdinli EZ. Chemotherapy of malignant diffuse mesothelioma. *Cancer* 1976;**37**:1265–74.

9    Newhouse ML, Thompson H. Mesothelioma of pleura and peritoneum following exposure to asbestos in the London area. 1965. *Br J Ind Med.* 1993;**50**:769–78.

10   Gennaro V, Ceppi M, Boffetta P, Fontana V, Perrotta A. Pleural mesothelioma and asbestos exposure among Italian oil refinery workers. *Scand J Work Environ Health* 1994;**20**:213–15.

11   Kishimoto T. [Relationship between asbestos exposure and malignant pleural mesothelioma: occurrence near the old Japanese naval shipyard]. *Nihon Kyobu Shikkan Gakkai Zasshi* 1994;**32**(Suppl.):250–6. [in Japanese]

12   Sakellariou K, Malamou-Mitsi V, Haritou A *et al.* Malignant pleural mesothelioma from nonoccupational asbestos exposure in Metsovo (north-west Greece): slow end of an epidemic?. *Eur Respir J* 1996;**9**:1206–10.

13   Schneider J, Straif K, Woitowitz HJ. Pleural mesothelioma and household asbestos exposure. *Rev Environ Health* 1996;**11**:65–70.

14   Metintas M, Ozdemir N, Hillerdal G *et al.* Environmental asbestos exposure and malignant pleural mesothelioma. *Respir Med* 1999;**93**:349–55.

15   Iwatsubo Y, Pairon JC, Boutin C. Pleural mesothelioma: dose-response relation at low levels of asbestos exposure in a French population-based case-control study. *Am J Epidemiol* 1998;**148**:133–42.

16   Peterson JT Jr, Greenberg SD, Buffler PA. Non-asbestos-related malignant mesothelioma. A review. *Cancer* 1984;**54**:951–60.

17   Gun RT. Mesothelioma: is asbestos exposure the only cause? *Med J Aust* 1995;**162**:429–31.

18   Steele JP, Rudd RM. Malignant mesothelioma: predictors of prognosis and clinical trials. *Thorax* 2000;**55**:725–6.

19   Ryan CW, Herndon J, Vogelzang NJ. A review of chemotherapy trials for malignant mesothelioma. *Chest* 1998;**113**(Suppl. 6):66S–73S.

20   Aisner J. Current approach to malignant mesothelioma of the pleura. *Chest* 1995;**107**(Suppl.):332S–344S.

21   Boutin C, Schlesser M, Frenay C, Astoul P. Malignant pleural mesothelioma. *Eur Resp J* 1988;**12**:972–81.

22   Falkson G, Alberts AS, Falkson HC. Malignant pleural mesothelioma treatment: the current state of the art. *Cancer Treat Rev* 1988;**15**:231–42.

23   Sorensen PG, Bach F, Bork E, Hansen HH. Randomized trial of doxorubicin versus cyclophosphamide in diffuse malignant pleural mesothelioma. *Cancer Treat Rep* 1985;**69**:1431–2.

24   Cantwell BM, Franks CR, Harris AL. A phase II study of the platinum analogues JM8 and JM9 in malignant pleural mesothelioma. *Cancer Chemother Pharmacol* 1986;**18**:286–8.

25   Chahinian AP, Antman K, Goutsou M *et al.* Randomized phase II trial of cisplatin with mitomycin or doxorubicin for malignant mesothelioma by the Cancer and Leukemia Group B. *J Clin Oncol* 1993;**11**:1559–65.

26   Samson MK, Wasser LP, Borden EC *et al.* Randomized comparison of cyclophosphamide, imidazole carboxamide, and adriamycin versus cyclophosphamide and adriamycin in patients with advanced stage malignant mesothelioma: a Sarcoma Intergroup Study. *J Clin Oncol* 1987;**5**:86–91.

27   Sauter ER, Langer C, Coia LR, Goldberg M, Keller SM. Optimal management of malignant mesothelioma after subtotal pleurectomy: revisiting the role of intrapleural chemotherapy and postoperative radiation. *J Surg Oncol* 1995;**60**:100–5.

28   Linden CJ, Mercke C, Albrechtsson U, Johansson L, Ewers SB. Effect of hemithorax irradiation alone or combined with doxorubicin and cyclophosphamide in 47 pleural mesotheliomas: a nonrandomized phase II study. *Eur Respir J* 1996;**9**:2565–72.

29   Sterman DH, Kaiser LR, Albelda SM. Advances in the treatment of malignant pleural mesothelioma. *Chest* 1999;**116**:504–20.

30   Lee YC, Light RW, Musk AW. Management of malignant pleural mesothelioma: a critical review. *Curr Opin Pulm Med* 2000;**6**:267–74.

31   Antman KH. Natural history and epidemiology of malignant mesothelioma. *Chest* 1993;**103**(Suppl. 4):373S–376S.

32   Butchart EG. Contemporary management of malignant pleural mesothelioma. *Oncologist* 1999;**4**:488–500.

33   Gross-Goupil M, Ruffie P. Malignant pleural mesothelioma. *Bull Cancer* 1999;(Suppl. 3):43–54.

34   Astoul P. Pleural mesothelioma. *Cuur Opin Pulm Med* 1999;**5**:259–68.

35   Law MR, Gregor A, Hodson ME, Bloom HJ, Turner-Warwick M. Malignant mesothelioma of the pleura: a study of 52 treated and 64 untreated patients. *Thorax* 1984;**39**:255–9.

36   Holsti LR, Pyrhonen S, Kajanti M *et al.* Altered fractionation of hemithorax irradiation for pleural mesothelioma and failure patterns after treatment. *Acta Oncol* 1997;**36**:397–405.

37   Boutin C, Rey F, Viallat JR. Prevention of malignant seeding after invasive diagnostic procedures in patients with pleural mesothelioma. A randomized trial of local radiotherapy. *Chest* 1995;**108**:754–8.

38   Rusch VW, Piantadosi S, Holmes E. The role of extrapleural pneumonectomy in malignant pleural mesothelioma. A lung cancer study group trial. *J Thorac Cardiovasc Surg* 1991;**102**:1–9.

39   Rusch VW. Trials in malignant mesothelioma. LCSG 851 and 882. *Chest* 1994;**106**:359S–362S.

40   Calavrezos A, Koschel G, Hüsselmann H, Taylessani A, Heilmann HP, Fabel H. Malignant mesothelioma of the pleura. *Klin Wochenschr* 1988;**66**:607–13.

41   McCormack P, Nagasaki F, Hilaris BS, Martini N. Surgical treatment of pleural mesothelioma. *J Thorac Cardiovasc Surg* 1982;**84**:834–42.

42   Takagi K, Tsuchiya R, Watanabe Y. Surgical approach to pleural diffuse mesothelioma in Japan. *Lung Cancer* 2001;**31**:57–65.

43   Pass HI, Temeck BK, Kranda K *et al.* Phase III randomised trial of surgery with or without intraoperative photodynamic therapy and postoperative immunochemotherapy for malignant pleural mesothelioma. *Ann Surg Oncol* 1997;**4**:628–33.

44   Cantó A, Guijarro R, Arnau A, Galbis J, Martorell M, Garcia Aguado R. Videothoracoscopy in the diagnosis and treatment of malignant pleural mesothelioma with associated pleural effusions. *Thorac Cardiovasc Surg* 1997;**45**:16–19.

# Section V

## Treating tumours of the gastrointestinal tract

*Peter Simmonds, Editor*

# Levels of evidence and grades of recommendation used in *Evidence-based Oncology*

Levels of evidence and grades of recommendation appear within the text in the clinical chapters, for example, **Evidence level Ia** and **Grade A**.

---

**Levels of evidence**

---

Ia   Meta-analysis of randomised controlled trials (RCTs)
Ib   At least 1 RCT
IIa  At least 1 non-randomised study
IIb  At least 1 other well designed quasi-experimental study
III  Non-experimental, descriptive studies
IV   Expert committee reports or opinions/experience of respected authorities

**Grades of recommendations**

---

A   At least one RCT as part of body of literature of overall good quality and consistency addressing recommendation **Evidence levels Ia, Ib**
B   No RCT but well conducted clinical studies available **Evidence levels IIa, IIb, III**
C   Expert committee reports or opinions/experience of respected authorities in the absence of directly applicable good quality clinical studies **Evidence level IV**

From *Clinical Oncology* (2001)**13**:S212
Source of data: MEDLINE, *Proceedings of the American Society of Medical Oncology* (ASCO).

# 23 Cancer of the oesophagus

*Ian Chau, David Cunningham*

The worldwide incidence of oesophageal cancer is increasing with a marked rise in the incidence of adenocarcinoma.[1] It is estimated that over 400 000 new cases of oesophageal cancer were diagnosed in 2000 worldwide accounting for 340 000 deaths.[2] In the USA, 13 000 new cases of oesophageal cancer with 12 600 deaths were estimated to have occurred in 2002.[3] Long-term outcome for these patients are poor ranging from 6% in England and Wales, 8% in Europe, to 13·7% in the USA.[4,5] In patients with localised cancer, surgery is often considered the standard treatment, but results are unsatisfactory. Multimodality treatment using chemotherapy and radiotherapy have been used to improve on the results achieved by surgery and can provide cure in selected patients without surgical intervention. In patients with locally advanced and metastatic disease, surgical resection is generally not recommended and chemo(radio)therapy is the preferred treatment. Mechanical measures including dilatation and stenting complement antineoplastic treatment in the management of malignant dysphagia.

## Epidemiology

The increase in the incidence of adenocarcinoma of oesophagus, particularly in the lower oesophagus and oesophagogastric junction, has attracted most attention. The cumulative rates (that is, lifetime cancer rates) for adenocarcinoma of oesophagus vary widely between genders, between countries, between different ethnicity within the same country, and within the same ethnicity residing in different countries.[6] The highest rate occurred in the Scottish men with a cumulative rate of 0·6% compared to 0·27% in US White men and 0% in Korea, Thailand and Estonia. There are also substantial differences in the cumulative rates of oesophageal squamous cell carcinoma (SCC) by ethnicity and gender.[6]

The mechanism for this increase in adenocarcinoma of oesophagus is still not fully understood. However, the widespread nature of gastro-oesophageal reflux disease (GORD) in the general population (symptoms of GORD occur monthly in 50% of US adults and weekly in almost 20%) and the development of Barrett's oesophagus from long-term GORD may play a role.[7] Barrett's oesophagus is a change in the lining of the oesophagus from its usual squamous epithelium to columnar epithelium. It appears to be a common precursor lesion to adenocarcinoma of the oesophagus. The risk of cancer among individuals with Barrett's oesophagus is unclear. Studies examining this risk reported 40–125 times increase in relative risk to that of the general population. However, given the low baseline incidence of adenocarcinoma of oesophagus, the absolute risk is approximately 0·5% per patient-year (that is, the risk of any given patient with Barrett's oesophagus developing cancer in a year is approximately 1 in 200) in recent large longitudinal studies and meta-analysis.[7,8]

The degree of dysplasia in Barrett's oesophagus has been found to be the most predictive factor for subsequent progression to adenocarcinoma. Those with high grade dysplasia have an excess risk of 25% for the development of cancer. Pharmacological therapies such as proton pump inhibitors neither avert progression to adenocarcinoma of the oesophagus in those with Barrett's oesophagus nor cause substantial regression in the amount of metaplastic tissue present. They have not been proven to decrease the cancer risk associated with the condition and currently have no role in chemoprevention. No prospective randomised data are available to show that endoscopic surveillance of individuals with Barrett's oesophagus would prolong survival. However, the American College of Gastroenterologists recommends surveillance endoscopy in patients with Barrett's oesophagus with decreasing interval in patients with severe dysplasia.[9]

## Staging investigations

Accurate staging of oesophageal cancer is essential as this will identify individuals most likely to benefit from aggressive therapy. Staging remains the most accurate method for predicting overall prognosis. The options available for initial staging include computer tomography (CT), endoscopic ultrasound (EUS), positron emission tomography (PET), and minimal invasive surgical staging using thoracoscopy and laparoscopy. With the advent of multimodality therapy using radiotherapy, chemotherapy and surgery, it becomes more important to evaluate the accuracy of these imaging techniques as it may influence the decision on initial management, and whether surgery is necessary after chemotherapy and radiotherapy.

## Endoscopic ultrasound

EUS combines the diagnostic access of endoscopy with the versatility of ultrasonography and has been in use since the early 1980s. The oesophagus is shown on EUS as five concentric rings of alternating echogenicities. The TNM staging system is used by EUS. Tumour involvement is diagnosed as a hypoechoic disruption of the layers. T1 tumours penetrate to the third EUS (submucosa) layer of the oesophageal wall, T2 tumours penetrate to the fourth EUS (muscularis propria) layer of the oesophageal wall, T3 tumours extend through the fourth EUS layer (invading adventitia) and T4 tumours extend into adjacent structures (for example, aorta, trachea and pericardium). When staging for lymph node involvement, EUS not only assesses the size of lymph node, but can give additional information such as lymph node shape, border characteristics and central echogenecity.

A systematic review assessed the staging performance of EUS in oesophageal cancer.[10] In 13 studies identified, the sensitivity for EUS in assessing T-staging was between 71·4% and 100% and specificity was 66·7–100%. Sensitivity of lymph node staging of gastro-oesophageal carcinoma was found to be between 59·5–97·2% and specificity was 40·0–100%. In the studies that compared EUS with CT, the latter imaging modality was found to have a sensitivity range of 40–80% and a specificity range of 14·3–97% for tumour staging and a sensitivity of 40·0–79·3% and specificity of 25·0–66·7% for lymph node staging. It appears that CT has a wide range of sensitivity and specificity for staging owing to the limited number of studies that compared EUS with CT. EUS is a highly accurate tool in pretreatment locoregional staging for oesophageal cancer, and complements CT scan findings to provide more accurate staging. Impassable stenosis represents a challenge for EUS and reduces its accuracy. Miniprobes capable of traversing very tight stenoses are available, but their accuracy has not yet been fully evaluated.

After neoadjuvant therapy, the accuracy of EUS to assess tumour using TNM classification is considerably lower, to about 40–50%.[11] Difficulties in assessing post-treatment tumour response are attributed to the problems in resolving fibrosis, inflammation with residual tumours. Other studies have attempted to correlate tumour response and survival with other parameters on EUS.[12,13] Reduction in tumour cross-sectional area has been shown to correlate with pathological response and improved survival.[12]

## Positron emission tomography

PET represents an advance over CT scanning in the screening for distant metastases. However, PET is usually unable to resolve metastatic deposits of less than 1 cm and it lacks anatomical definition. It has greater accuracy in detecting distant lymph node metastasis compared to locoregional lymph node metastasis. It also does not allow accurate differentiation in T-staging of the local tumours. The primary advantage of PET imaging is its improved diagnostic value for distant metastatic sites, which may substantially affect patient management decisions.[14–18] Complementary information from CT and EUS especially with regard to locoregional nodal staging would enhance the accuracy of the overall clinical staging of oesophageal cancer and allow more informed management decisions to be made. PET has been shown to differentiate responding and non-responding adenocarcinoma or SCC after cisplatin-based polychemotherapy,[19] or chemoradiation (CRT) with 5-FU infusion.[20]

## Treatment of localised oesophageal cancer

### Surgery

In patients who are found to have localised carcinoma of the oesophagus after optimal staging work-up, the intention of management is to cure. Surgery has been considered as the treatment of choice. However, despite curative resection, the 5-year survival rate remains no more than 20%. Radiotherapy has been used as single modality for the curative management of patients with oesophageal cancer, but there is a lack of well-designed randomised controlled trials to determine which treatment approach is superior. In order to improve the unsatisfactory outcome achieved by surgery alone, several strategies have been pursued: preoperative chemotherapy, preoperative radiotherapy, preoperative CRT and definitive CRT without surgery (Figure 23.1).

### Preoperative chemotherapy

Preoperative chemotherapy has been used in an attempt to reduce the size of the primary tumour and eliminate micrometastatic disease with the aim of improving disease-free and overall survival. A Cochrane systematic review addressed this issue.[21] Seven randomised trials were identified including 1653 patients. Out of these patients, 1267 were derived from two studies – the US Intergroup study,[22] and the United Kingdom (UK) Medical Research Council (MRC) OEO2 study.[23] All trials evaluated patients with SCC except for the US Intergroup and MRC trial, which also included adenocarcinoma. All studies used cisplatin-based chemotherapy. In addition, two studies also continued chemotherapy in the postoperative period. Pooling data together, there was no difference in survival at 1 year but a significant decrease in mortality at 2 years (OR 0·80; 95% CI 0·65–0·99).

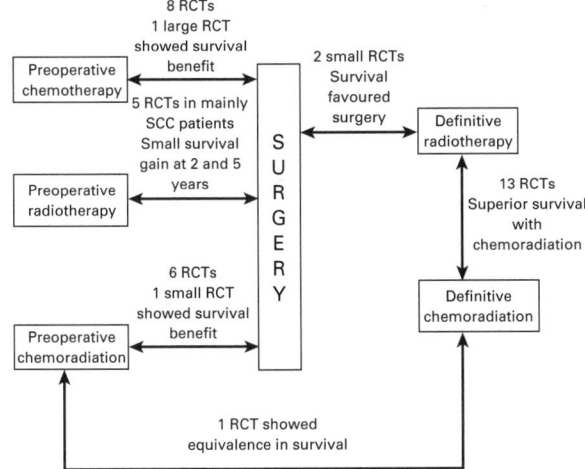

**Figure 23.1** Treatment strategies for localised oesophageal cancer. RCT, randomised controlled trial; SCC, squamous cell carcinoma

The recently published MRC OEO2 study is the largest study evaluating the role of preoperative chemotherapy in oesophageal cancer[23]: 802 previously untreated patients were randomly assigned to two cycles of 3-weekly cisplatin (80 mg m$^{-2}$) and fluorouracil (1000 mg m$^{-2}$) daily for 4 days followed by surgical resection or surgery alone. Overall survival was better in the preoperative chemotherapy arm (Hazard Ratio [HR] 0·79; 95% CI 0·67–0·93; $P = 0·004$) compared to surgery. Two-year survival rates were 43% in preoperative chemotherapy arm and 34% in the surgery arm. The second largest study was conducted in the US where 440 eligible patients were randomly allocated to preoperative three cycles of cisplatin (100 mg m$^{-2}$) and fluorouracil (1000 mg m$^{-2}$) daily for 5 days every 4 weeks followed by surgical resection or surgery alone.[22] Postoperative chemotherapy with a reduced dose of cisplatin was advocated in patients with disease that was stable or responsive to treatment. No difference in survival was found between the two arms (HR 1·07; 95% CI 0·87–1·32). Two-year survival rates were 35% in preoperative chemotherapy arm and 37% in surgery alone arm.

The conflicting results between the MRC and the Intergroup studies could not be accounted for by differing baseline characteristics of the study populations. Although both cisplatin and fluorouracil were used in the chemotherapy arm, different doses and number of cycles were given. The toxic effects from the larger individual and total doses of chemotherapy given in the Intergroup study may potentially diminish the survival benefit. In the MRC study, individual clinicians could choose to give preoperative RT to patients randomised to either arm, but this was well balanced with 9% of patients in each arm receiving preoperative radiotherapy. The treatment effects were similar for SCC and adenocarcinoma in both the MRC and the Intergroup studies. Table 23.1 shows the comparison between the MRC OEO2 and US Intergroup studies.

Another meta-analysis has recently been published assessing the role of preoperative chemotherapy.[24] In this meta-analysis, 11 randomised controlled trials were included involving 1976 patients, which also included two trials excluded from the Cochrane systematic review because they had not provided survival data. However, this new meta-analysis derived survival data from graphically presented survival curves, which may be subject to interpretation errors. In addition a further trial published since the Cochrane systematic review was included.[25] Pooling data together, this new meta-analysis found no benefit in the use of chemotherapy with odds ratios of 1·00 (95% CI 0·76–1·30; $P = 0·98$) for 1-year survival, 0·88 (95% CI 0·62–1·24; $P = 0·45$) for 2-year survival and 0·77 (95% CI 0·37–1·59; $P = 0·48$) for 3-year survival. This meta-analysis also found that patients treated with surgery alone were more likely to have an oesophageal resection, but those treated with chemotherapy and surgery were more likely to have a complete (R0) resection. A clinical response to chemotherapy was observed in 31% of patients and 5% had complete pathological responses (pCR). Chemotherapy did not affect locoregional or distant cancer recurrence. Table 23.2 shows a summary of meta-analyses conducted to evaluate treatment strategies for localised carcinoma of the oesophagus.

**Table 23.1    Comparison between Medical Research Council (MRC) OEO2 and United States Intergroup studies**

| Parameter | MRC[23] | | US Intergroup[22] | |
| --- | --- | --- | --- | --- |
| | Surgery | Chemotherapy + surgery | Surgery | Chemotherapy + surgery |
| No. of patients | 402 | 400 | 227 | 213 |
| Median survival | 13·3 months | 16·8 months | 16·1 months | 14·9 months |
| 2-year survival | 34% | 43% | 37% | 35% |

**Table 23.2** Meta-analyses of treatment strategies for localised carcinoma of the oesophagus

| Reference | No. of studies included | No. of patients included | Risk ratio in survival (95% confidence interval) | | | Comments |
|-----------|------------------------|--------------------------|---------------|---------------|---------------|----------|
| | | | 1-year | 2-year | 3-year | |
| *Preoperative chemotherapy v surgery alone* | | | | | | |
| Malthaner et al,[21] | 7 | 1653 | 1·03 (0·78, 1·36) | 0·80 (0·65, 0·99) | 0·85 (0·61, 1·19) | 2-year survival benefit in favour of preoperative chemotherapy |
| Urschel et al,[21] | 11 | 1976 | 1·00 (0·76, 1·30) | 0·88 (0·62, 1·24) | 0·77 (0·37, 1·59) | No benefit seen with preoperative chemotherapy in this meta-analysis, but may have methodological limitations |
| *Preoperative radiotherapy v surgery alone* | | | | | | |
| Arnott et al,[26] | 5 | 1147 | | 0·89 (0·78, 1·01) | | Overall risk ratio given. Borderline significant survival advantage in favour of preoperative radiotherapy |
| *Chemoradiation v radiotherapy alone* | | | | | | |
| Wong et al,[27] | 8 | 769 | 0·61 (0·44, 0·84) | 0·53 (0·32, 0·88) | 0·28 (0·02, 4·12) | Studies for concomitant chemoradiation showed a survival advantage for chemoradiation |
| Wong et al,[5] | 5 | 453 | 0·69 (0·35, 1·38) | 1·08 (0·61, 1·89) | 1·21 (0·09, 17·08) | Studies for sequential chemoradiation did not show a survival advantage for chemoradiation. Pooling concomitant and sequential chemoradiation studies supported the use of chemoradiation over radiotherapy alone. Results of 3-year survival have wide confidence interval due to small number of studies reporting 3-year survival |

The data from the two largest trials evaluating preoperative chemotherapy are conflicting. The MRC study showed a 2-year survival advantage and has led to the adoption of preoperative chemotherapy as standard treatment in the UK and some other European countries. However, in North America, clinical practice has been greatly influenced by the negative results from the Intergroup study, and thus patients are not routinely offered chemotherapy before surgery Evidence level Ia, Grade A.

## Preoperative radiotherapy

It is recognised that locoregional recurrences are frequent even after potentially curative resection. Preoperative radiotherapy may provide better local control, thereby improving survival. A systematic review was published pooling results from five randomised studies involving 1147 patients.[26] Most patients (89%) had SCC. The overall HR was 0·89 ($P = 0·06$) improving 2-year survival from 30% to 34% and 5-year survival from 15% to 18% with the use of preoperative radiotherapy. Same degree of benefit was evident in different patient subgroups by gender, age and tumour location with preoperative RT. As the absolute gain in survival was small and the majority of patients included in these studies had SCC, which nowadays is often treated with definitive CRT, preoperative RT is not recommended as standard Evidence level Ia, Grade A.

## Chemoradiation (CRT)

Combined chemotherapy and radiotherapy with or without surgery have been pursued for an additive or synergistic effect over radiotherapy alone. This may occur from intensifying the effect on local disease, as well as reducing subsequent failures from occult distant disease. This strategy may also increase the resection rate. A large number of uncontrolled studies have been published testing the role of preoperative CRT. In a total of 2704 patients from 46 non-randomised trials, a median survival ranging from 8 to 37 months and 3-year survival from 8% to 55% were seen; 24% of patients treated by preoperative CRT achieved pCR.[28]

Six randomised trials comparing preoperative CRT followed by surgery with surgery alone in resectable oesophageal cancer have been published.[29–34] Three used concomitant CRT whereas the other three gave CRT in sequential fashion. Four studies recruited patients with SCC only, one recruited adenocarcinoma only, and one with both histologies. Only one trial showed a statistically significant improvement in overall survival in favour of preoperative CRT.[34] This study included 113 patients with adenocarcinoma, and the surgery alone arm performed worse than expected with a median survival of 11 months only. Notably there were nearly three times more patients with pathological

stage III in the surgery alone arm compared with those that received preoperative CRT. This study was closed before planned accrual because of a survival advantage in CRT arm during interim analysis. Recently the largest randomised trial conducted in Australasia was reported.[35] In this study, 256 patients were randomised to receive one cycle of preoperative cisplatin (80 mg m$^{-2}$) and fluorouracil (800 mg m$^{-2}$ per day) for 4 days followed by radiotherapy (35 Gy in 15 fractions) or surgery alone; 61% of patients had adenocarcinoma. No differences in median survival was detected between the two arms (CRT 21 months $v$ surgery 18 months; $P = 0·32$). Pathological CR was achieved in 15·2% of patients. Treatment-related mortality occurred in 4·6% of patients with no differences between the two arms. Preoperative CRT therefore remains investigational and is not recommended as standard practice Evidence level Ib, Grade A.

Combined CRT has also been compared with RT alone in localised oesophageal cancer. In a recent systematic review, 13 randomised studies were included.[27] Eight studies used concomitant CRT with a total of 769 patients whereas five used sequential CRT involving a total of 453 patients. Six studies contained SCC exclusively whereas the remaining seven studies included both histology. The majority of patients included suffered from locally advanced disease.

Pooling data from studies using concomitant CRT showed a benefit in favour of CRT over RT at 1 year (OR 0·61; 95% CI 0·44–0·84; $P = 0·003$) and at 2 years (OR 0·53; 95% CI 0·32–0·88; $P < 0·009$). Follow up in these studies was short, and long-term survival rates cannot be ascertained with accuracy. One study showed a significant survival advantage whereas the others showed no significant benefit with the concomitant CRT approach over RT alone.[36] Pooling data from studies using sequential CRT did not show significant survival benefit.

However, pooling data from both sequential and concomitant approach supported the use of combined CRT over RT alone. The mortality rates for RT alone were 67% at 1 year with an absolute risk reduction of 9% with CRT and 86% at 2 years with an absolute risk reduction of 10% with CRT. The overall rate of local failure was significantly lowered by 15% (95% CI 4–26%) with combined modality, and this could serve as a surrogate measure of improvement in quality of life in this group of patients Evidence level Ia, Grade A.

### Preoperative CRT versus definitive CRT alone

In a recently reported randomised study in France, 455 patients with locally advanced but resectable carcinoma of oesophagus were treated with two cycles of 3-weekly fluorouracil (800 mg m$^{-2}$ per day) days 1–5 and cisplatin (75 mg m$^{-2}$ on day 2 or 15 mg m$^{-2}$/day on days 1–5) followed by RT (20 Gy protracted or 15 Gy split course)[37];

259 patients with at least partial response were randomised between surgery or an additional three cycles of fluorouracil/cisplatin given with the same treatment schedule. Similar median survival (CRT + surgery 17·7 months *v* definitive CRT 19·3 months) and 2-year survival (CRT + surgery 34% *v* definitive CRT 40%; *P* = 0·56) were seen between the two arms. However, treatment-related mortality was much higher in the CRT + surgery arm compared with definitive CRT (9% *v* 1%, respectively).

Definitive CRT may therefore represent an alternative strategy to avoid major surgery. However, in this French study, only patients with responding disease were randomised; therefore an adequately powered, carefully stratified, multicentre comparison of preoperative CRT with definitive CRT is required to define whether surgery could be omitted for all patients **Evidence level Ib, Grade A**.

### Toxicity of CRT

Acute toxicity is increased with CRT during preoperative treatment. However, postoperative morbidity and mortality were comparable with surgery alone. Compared with preoperative RT, CRT increased the risk of grade 3–4 acute toxicities by 17% with no increase in late toxicities.[11]

## Postoperative adjuvant therapy

Adjuvant therapy has been shown to be beneficial in several solid tumours. However, oesophagectomy is associated with considerable perioperative morbidity compared to, for example, breast surgery. Therefore postoperative treatment is less well tolerated and has not been evaluated as extensively as preoperative treatment.

Adjuvant RT has been tested in three randomised studies. No improvement in survival was demonstrated by the use of adjuvant RT, although there was a reduction in the incidence of local recurrence. This approach is also associated with a significant risk of toxicity. Indeed, two of the studies showed a disadvantage in survival (attributable to treatment-related deaths) with postoperative RT and this approach is generally not recommended. However, in patients with residual disease after surgery and for whom the risk of local recurrence and its associated morbidity is high, the use of postoperative RT may convey local control benefit[11] **Evidence level Ib, Grade A**.

Adjuvant chemotherapy was evaluated in two studies in which only patients with SCC were included. Cisplatin-based chemotherapy was used in both studies.[38,39] In the first study, conducted by the Japan Clinical Oncology Group, 205 patients were randomised to receive two cycles of cisplatin (70 mg m$^{-2}$) and vindesine (3 mg m$^{-2}$) postoperatively or surgery alone. Five-year survival rates were similar between the two arms (48·1% in the surgery plus chemotherapy arm *v* 44·9% in the surgery alone group).[38] However, 5-year survival rates of both groups appear to be superior to those seen in other contemporary trials.

In a second study, 120 patients were randomised to receive cisplatin (100 mg m$^{-2}$) and fluorouracil (1000 mg m$^{-2}$/day) for 5 days for a total of 6–8 months[39]; 58 patients with micro- and macroscopic residual disease were included. No differences in survival outcome were seen with postoperative chemotherapy and this approach is therefore not recommended as routine practice **Evidence level Ib, Grade A**.

Adjuvant CRT has been tested in a US Intergroup study in which 556 patients with resected adenocarcinoma of the stomach or oesophagogastric junction were randomly assigned to surgery plus adjuvant CRT or surgery alone.[40] In this study, approximately 20% of patients had oesophagogastric tumours. Chemotherapy (fluorouracil 425 mg m$^{-2}$ per day and leucovorin 20 mg m$^{-2}$ per day for 5 days) was started on day 1 and was followed by CRT 28 days after the start of the first cycle of chemotherapy. CRT consisted of 45 Gy of radiation in 25 fractions with a reduced dose of fluorouracil and leucovorin on the first 4 and last 3 days of radiotherapy. Two further cycles of chemotherapy were given 1 month after the completion of radiotherapy. Three-year survival rates were 50% in the CRT group and 41% in the surgery-only group (HR 1·35; 95% CI 1·09–1·66; *P* = 0·005). Three-year relapse-free survival was also significant better in the adjuvant CRT group (CRT arm 48%; surgery alone arm 31%; *P* < 0·001). However, although extensive (D2) nodal resection was recommended in this study, only 10% of patients underwent a D2 dissection, 36% had a D1 dissection, and 54% had a D0 lymphadenectomy (that is, a resection in which not all of the N1 nodes were removed). In addition, 54% of patients had grade 3/4 haematological toxicity and 33% had grade 3/4 gastrointestinal toxicity with CRT. Only 64% of patients undergoing adjuvant CRT completed the protocol treatment.

In North America, postoperative CRT is now regarded as standard treatment in patients with resected carcinoma of stomach and oesophagogastric junction. This practice has not been widely adopted in Europe because it is thought that the radiation therapy may merely compensate for the less radical lymphadenectomy performed in the US Intergroup study compared with the standard surgical approach in Europe **Evidence level Ib, Grade A**. A large UK MRC study has just finished recruitment in which 503 patients with resectable carcinoma of the lower third of oesophagus and stomach were randomly allocated to chemotherapy before and after surgery or surgery alone. Those patients randomised to perioperative chemotherapy

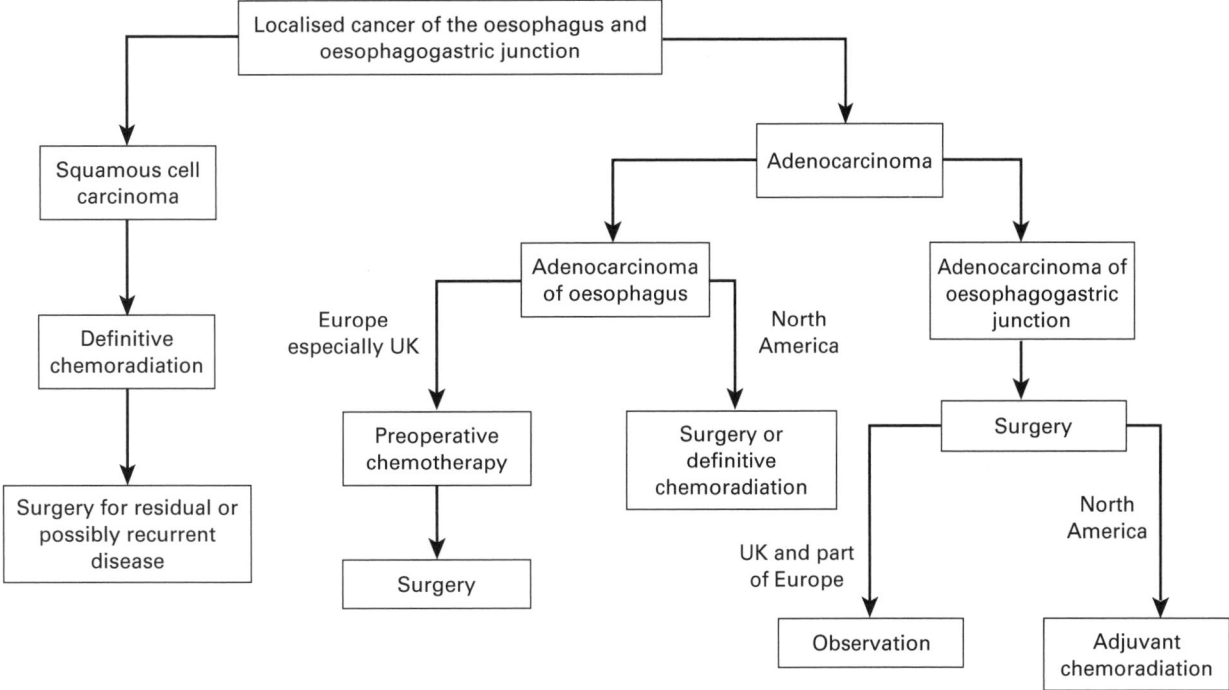

**Figure 23.2**  Treatment paradigm for localised oesophageal cancer

arm received epirubicin (50 mg m$^{-2}$), cisplatin (60 mg m$^{-2}$) and protracted venous infusion of fluorouracil (200 mg m$^{-2}$/day) repeated every 3 weeks (ECF regimen) for three cycles before and three cycles after surgery. The results of this study would shed more light on the role of pre- and postoperative treatment in patients with resected carcinoma of oesophagus.

## Clinical practice and future research

With data emerging from both uncontrolled single arm and randomised controlled studies, the current paradigm for the treatment of localised oesophageal cancer varies between North America and Europe including the UK (Figure 23.2). A recent US Pattern of Care study analysed 400 patients with oesophageal cancer who had received radiation as a component of their care; 62% of patients had SCC; 300 patients received CRT and of these, 54% received definitive CRT without surgery, 13·25% received CRT preoperatively and 7·75% received CRT postoperatively[41]; 100 patients received RT alone and of these, 20·25% received definitive RT without surgery, 1·25% received RT preoperatively, and 3·5% received RT postoperatively. Definitive CRT without surgery was the most frequently used regimen for patients with both SCC and adenocarcinoma and for all stages of disease. Consistent with data from randomised trials, patients who received definitive CRT had a better 2-year survival compared with RT as a single modality (39% *v* 20·6%; *P* = 0·027). Two-year locoregional failure was also significantly less with definitive CRT as compared with definitive RT alone (30% *v* 57·9%; *P* = 0·0031). Patients who received preoperative CRT had a higher survival rate (63% *v* 39% at 2 years) and a lower rate of locoregional failure (22% *v* 30% at 2 years) than those who received definitive CRT, but these differences were not significant (*P* = 0·11 and *P* = 0·52 respectively).

Patients who underwent preoperative treatment and achieved pCR had a significantly better survival than those who did not achieve pCR. In addition, locoregional and distant disease recurrences were also reduced in patients who had pCR.[28] Current strategies to increase pCR rates include integrating taxanes, camptothecins new platinum compounds, oral fluoropyrimidines and other new anticancer therapies. However, whether these new agents will improve survival remains to be seen.

## Palliative chemotherapy

In patients with metastatic disease, palliative chemotherapy is given with the intention of prolonging

**Table 23.3** Response rate of ECF and MCF according to anatomical sites and histology in a large randomised study[47]

|  | No. of responders in ECF arm (%) | No. of responders in MCF arm (%) | P |
|---|---|---|---|
| *Anatomical sites* |  |  |  |
| Oesophagus (N = 181) | 36 (39·6%) | 46 (51·1%) | 0·119 |
| Oesophagogastric junction (N = 121) | 34 (57·6%) | 27 (43·6%) | 0·122 |
| Stomach (N = 235) | 45 (37·2%) | 45 (39·5%) | 0·719 |
| *Histology* |  |  |  |
| Squamous cell carcinoma (N = 58) | 7 (36·8%) | 9 (47·4%) | 0·63 |
| Adenocarcinoma (N = 461) | 107 (45·3%) | 97 (43·1%) | 0·511 |

Abbreviations: ECF, epirubicin, cisplatin and protracted venous infusion of fluorouracil; MCF, mitomycin C, cisplatin and protracted venous infusion of fluorouracil

survival, relieving symptoms and improving quality of life. Results from randomised studies comparing the use of chemotherapy with best supportive care in patients with advanced disease are inconclusive. In one study, 39% of patients included had complete resection of primary tumours but had lymph node involvement rather than advanced disease.[42] In the other two studies, the chemotherapy regimens used would not be regarded as standard.[43,44]

Several studies have compared different chemotherapy regimens in patients with advanced or metastatic oesophageal cancer. Epirubicin, cisplatin and protracted infusion of fluorouracil (ECF) has been tested in two large randomised studies against FAMTX (fluorouracil, doxorubicin and methotrexate),[45,46] and MCF (mitomycin C, cisplatin and fluorouracil).[47] In the first study of 274 patients with adenocarcinoma of oesophagus and stomach, ECF resulted in a superior response rate (46% *v* 21%; *P* = 0·00003), median (8·7 months *v* 6·1 months; *P* = 0·0005) and 2-year survival (14% *v* 5%; *P* = 0·03) compared with FAMTX.[45,46] Following this study, ECF was tested against MCF in the largest randomised study in advanced oesophagogastric cancer involving 580 patients with adenocarcinoma, SCC, or undifferentiated carcinoma. Median survival was similar between the two treatment arms (ECF 9·4 months *v* MCF 8·7 months), but better global quality of life score was achieved with ECF.[47] An overall response rate of 42·4%,[48] was seen with ECF in this study with no differences between various anatomical locations or histology (Table 23.3) **Evidence level Ib, Grade A** .

## Clinical practice and future research

The combination of cisplatin and infused fluorouracil with or without another chemotherapeutic agent has been used most commonly in previously untreated patients with metastatic oesophageal cancer. ECF, tested in two large randomised studies, remains one of the reference regimens for this disease. No chemotherapy regimens are considered as standard in second-line setting. However, survival remains poor for these patients and new drugs are being evaluated, although no randomised phase III data on survival are available. Taxanes such as paclitaxel and docetaxel are active single agents in oesophageal cancer with response rates of 15–30%. Combinations of paclitaxel and cisplatin with or without fluorouracil have been tested in several phase II studies. Three-drug regimen of paclitaxel, cisplatin and 5-FU resulted in considerable haematological and gastrointestinal toxicities.[48] This prompted studies to investigate cisplatin and paclitaxel without 5-FU incorporating haemopoietic growth factor support. Although gastrointestinal toxicity was less severe without fluorouracil, paclitaxel and cisplatin still resulted in significant myelosuppression with 11% treatment-related deaths.[49]

Irinotecan, a semisynthetic derivative of the natural alkaloid camptothecin which interacts with topoisomerase-I, has been evaluated as part of the combination therapy with cisplatin in oesophageal cancer.[50,51] The results of these studies have demonstrated irinotecan as an active agent with response rates of 58%. In a randomised phase II study, irinotecan combined with 5-FU suggested a better survival compared with irinotecan/cisplatin.[52] Irinotecan/infused 5-FU/leucovorin has also been shown to have response rate of 20% in second-line setting in patients who were refractory to cisplatin/fluorouracil treatment.[53]

Oxaliplatin, a third generation platinum compound, is being tested in a randomised phase III study with a $2 \times 2$ factorial design where oxaliplatin is used in place of cisplatin in the ECF regimen. Capecitabine, an oral fluoropyrimidine, is also being tested in the same study in place of 5-FU in the ECF regimen. Preliminary results showed antitumour activity with both oxaliplatin and capecitabine in oesophagogastric cancer.[54]

Molecular targeted therapy has shown activity in several solid tumours and it is being investigated in oesophageal cancer. Epidermal growth factor receptor (EGFR) signalling pathway influences cell differentiation, proliferation, migration, angiogenesis, and apoptosis.[55] Cetuximab is a monoclonal antibody directed against EGFR and appears to have synergistic effect with chemotherapy and radiotherapy. Studies evaluating the combination of cetuximab and chemo(radio)therapy in carcinoma of oesophagus are currently recruiting. Studies have also commenced evaluating oral EGFR tyrosine kinase inhibitors including ZD1839 and OSI 774 in oesophageal cancer. Marimastat, a matrix metalloproteinase inhibitor, has been tested in a randomised study in inoperable gastric adenocarcinoma and a trend towards survival advantage was seen in the marimastat group. Subset analysis revealed patients who received prior chemotherapy had better survival in the marimastat group.[56] Epidemiological studies have also suggested use of non-steroidal anti-inflammatory drugs (NSAID) may reduce incidence of oesophageal cancer,[57–59] presumably through inhibition of cyclooxygenase (COX) 2, an enzyme inducible by cytokines, growth factors, and oncogenes, and thereby contributes to the synthesis of prostaglandins in inflamed and neoplastic tissues. Studies are being planned to investigate the use of NSAID or COX 2 inhibitors in patients with Barrett's oesophagus.

## Conclusion

For patients with localised oesophageal cancer, the current treatment paradigm is to give definitive CRT for patients with squamous cell carcinoma and reserve surgical salvage for those with residual disease after definitive CRT. However, for adenocarcinoma of oesophagus, preoperative chemotherapy is becoming the standard treatment in the UK and parts of Europe, whereas patients in North America receive surgery alone or definitive CRT without surgery. For those patients with adenocarcinoma of oesophagogastric junction, surgery alone is the current standard treatment in the UK, whereas postoperative adjuvant CRT would be strongly considered in North American patients.

Cisplatin and fluorouracil-based chemotherapy regimens are used most widely in those with advanced or metastatic disease. New drugs such as taxanes, irinotecan, oxaliplatin, and oral fluoropyrimidines are being tested in ongoing phase III studies to assess their impact on survival. Inhibitions of molecular targets, such as EGFR, matrix metalloproteinases, COX and angiogenic factors, may further improve survival after an understanding of their optimal integration with currently available cytotoxic drugs in the treatment of oesophageal cancer.

## References

1  Blot WJ, McLaughlin JK. The changing epidemiology of esophageal cancer. *Semin Oncol* 1999;**26**:2–8.
2  Ferlay J, Bray F, Pisani P *et al.* GLOBOCAN 2000-Cancer Incidence, Mortality and Prevalence Worldwide, Version 1.0. *IARC CancerBase* No. 5. Lyon: IARC Press, 2001.
3  *Cancer Facts & Figures 2002.* American Cancer Society, 2002.
4  SEER Cancer Statistic Review, 1973–1998. Bethesda, MD: National Cancer Institute, 2001.
5  Office for National Statistics. *Cancer Survival Trends in England & Wales 1971–1995.* Office for National Statistics, 1999.
6  Corley DA, Buffler PA. Oesophageal and gastric cardia adenocarcinomas: analysis of regional variation using the Cancer Incidence in Five Continents database. *Int J Epidemiol* 2001;**30**: 1415–25.
7  Shaheen N, Ransohoff DF. Gastroesophageal reflux, Barrett esophagus, and esophageal cancer: scientific review. *JAMA* 2002;**287**:1972–81.
8  Shaheen NJ, Crosby MA, Bozymski EM, Sandler RS. Is there publication bias in the reporting of cancer risk in Barrett's esophagus? *Gastroenterology* 2000;**119**:333–8.
9  Sampliner RE. Practice guidelines on the diagnosis, surveillance, and therapy of Barrett's esophagus. The Practice Parameters Committee of the American College of Gastroenterology. *Am J Gastroenterol* 1998;**93**:1028–32.
10  Kelly S, Harris KM, Berry E *et al.* A systematic review of the staging performance of endoscopic ultrasound in gastro-oesophageal carcinoma. *Gut* 2001;**49**:534–9.
11  Wong R, Malthaner R. Esophageal cancer: a systematic review. *Curr Probl Cancer* 2000;**24**:297–373.
12  Chak A, Canto MI, Cooper GS *et al.* Endosonographic assessment of multimodality therapy predicts survival of esophageal carcinoma patients. *Cancer* 2000;**88**:1788–95.
13  Hirata N, Kawamoto K, Ueyama T *et al.* Using endosonography to assess the effects of neoadjuvant therapy in patients with advanced esophageal cancer. *Am J Roentgenol* 1997;**169**:485–91.
14  Kato H, Kuwano H, Nakajima M *et al.* Comparison between positron emission tomography and computed tomography in the use of the assessment of esophageal carcinoma. *Cancer* 2002;**94**:921–8.
15  Lerut T, Flamen P, Ectors N *et al.* Histopathologic validation of lymph node staging with FDG-PET scan in cancer of the esophagus and gastroesophageal junction: A prospective study based on primary surgery with extensive lymphadenectomy. *Ann Surg* 2000;**232**: 743–52.
16  Flamen P, Lerut A, Van Cutsem E *et al.* The utility of positron emission tomography for the diagnosis and staging of recurrent esophageal cancer. *J Thorac Cardiovasc Surg* 2000;**120**:1085–92.
17  Meltzer CC, Luketich JD, Friedman D *et al.* Whole-body FDG positron emission tomographic imaging for staging esophageal cancer comparison with computed tomography. *Clin Nucl Med* 2000;**25**:882–7.

18 Rice TW. Clinical staging of esophageal carcinoma. CT, EUS, and PET. *Chest Surg Clin N Am* 2000;**10**:471–85.

19 Weber WA, Ott K, Becker K *et al.* Prediction of response to preoperative chemotherapy in adenocarcinomas of the esophagogastric junction by metabolic imaging. *J Clin Oncol* 2001;**19**:3058–65.

20 Brucher BL, Weber W, Bauer M *et al.* Neoadjuvant therapy of esophageal squamous cell carcinoma: response evaluation by positron emission tomography. *Ann Surg* 2001;**233**:300–9.

21 Malthaner R, Fenlon D. Preoperative chemotherapy for resectable thoracic esophageal cancer. *Cochrane Database Syst Rev* 2001;**1**: CD001556.

22 Kelsen DP, Ginsberg R, Pajak TF *et al.* Chemotherapy followed by surgery compared with surgery alone for localized esophageal cancer. *N Engl J Med* 1998;**339**:1979–84.

23 Medical Research Council Oesophageal Cancer Working Group Surgical resection with or without preoperative chemotherapy in oesophageal cancer: a randomised controlled trial. *Lancet* 2002;**359**:1727–33.

24 Urschel JD, Vasan H, Blewett CJ. A meta-analysis of randomized controlled trials that compared neoadjuvant chemotherapy and surgery to surgery alone for resectable esophageal cancer. *Am J Surg* 2002;**183**:274–9.

25 Ancona E, Ruol A, Santi S *et al.* Only pathologic complete response to neoadjuvant chemotherapy improves significantly the long term survival of patients with resectable esophageal squamous cell carcinoma: final report of a randomized, controlled trial of preoperative chemotherapy versus surgery alone. *Cancer* 2001;**91**:2165–74.

26 Arnott SJ, Duncan W, Gignoux M *et al.* Preoperative radiotherapy for esophageal carcinoma. *Cochrane Database Syst Rev* 2000;CD001799.

27 Wong R, Malthaner R. Combined chemotherapy and radiotherapy (without surgery) compared with radiotherapy alone in localized carcinoma of the esophagus. *Cochrane Database Syst Rev* 2001;**1**.

28 Geh JI. The use of chemoradiotherapy in oesophageal cancer. *Eur J Cancer* 2002;**38**:300–13.

29 Apinop C, Puttisak P, Preecha N. A prospective study of combined therapy in esophageal cancer. *Hepatogastroenterology* 1994;**41**:391–3.

30 Bosset JF, Gignoux M, Triboulet JP *et al.* Chemoradiotherapy followed by surgery compared with surgery alone in squamous-cell cancer of the esophagus. *N Engl J Med* 1997;**337**:161–7.

31 Le Prise E, Etienne PL, Meunier B *et al.* A randomized study of chemotherapy, radiation therapy, and surgery versus surgery for localized squamous cell carcinoma of the esophagus. *Cancer* 1994;**73**:1779–84.

32 Nygaard K, Hagen S, Hansen HS *et al.* Pre-operative radiotherapy prolongs survival in operable esophageal carcinoma: randomized, multicenter study of pre-operative radiotherapy and chemotherapy. The second Scandinavian trial in esophageal cancer. *World J Surg* 1992;**16**:1104–9.

33 Urba SG, Orringer MB, Turrisi A *et al.* Randomized trial of preoperative chemoradiation versus surgery alone in patients with locoregional esophageal carcinoma. *J Clin Oncol* 2001;**19**:305–13.

34 Walsh TN, Noonan N, Hollywood D *et al.* A comparison of multimodal therapy and surgery for esophageal adenocarcinoma. *N Engl J Med* 1996;**335**:462–7.

35 Burmeister BH, Smithers BM, Fitzgerald L *et al.* A randomized phase III trial of preoperative chemoradiation followed by surgery (CR-S) versus surgery alone (S) for localized resectable cancer of the esophagus. *Proc Am Soc Clin Oncol* 2002;**21**:130A.

36 Cooper JS, Guo MD, Herskovic A *et al.* Chemoradiotherapy of locally advanced esophageal cancer: long-term follow-up of a prospective randomized trial (RTOG 85–01). Radiation Therapy Oncology Group. *JAMA* 1999;**281**:1623–7.

37 Bedenne L, Michel P, Bouche O *et al.* Randomized phase III trial in locally advanced esophageal cancer: radiochemotherapy followed by surgery versus radiochemotherapy alone (FFCD 9102). *Proc Am Soc Clin Oncol* 2002;**21**:130A.

38 Ando N, Iizuka T, Kakegawa T *et al.* A randomized trial of surgery with and without chemotherapy for localized squamous carcinoma of the thoracic esophagus: the Japan Clinical Oncology Group Study. *J Thorac Cardiovasc Surg* 1997;**114**:205–9.

39 Pouliquen X, Levard H, Hay JM *et al.* 5-Fluorouracil and cisplatin therapy after palliative surgical resection of squamous cell carcinoma of the esophagus. A multicenter randomized trial. French Associations for Surgical Research. *Ann Surg* 1996;**223**:127–33.

40 Macdonald JS, Smalley SR, Benedetti J *et al.* Chemoradiotherapy after surgery compared with surgery alone for adenocarcinoma of the stomach or gastroesophageal junction. *N Engl J Med* 2001;**345**: 725–30.

41 Coia LR, Minsky BD, Berkey BA *et al.* Outcome of patients receiving radiation for cancer of the esophagus: results of the 1992–1994 Patterns of Care Study. *J Clin Oncol* 2000;**18**:455–62.

42 Levard H, Pouliquen X, Hay JM *et al.* 5-Fluorouracil and cisplatin as palliative treatment of advanced oesophageal squamous cell carcinoma. A multicentre randomised controlled trial. The French Associations for Surgical Research. *Eur J Surg* 1998;**164**:849–57.

43 Mannell A, Becker PJ, Melissas J, Diamantes T. Intubation v. dilatation plus bleomycin in the treatment of advanced oesophageal cancer. The results of a prospective randomized trial. *S Afr J Surg* 1986;**24**:15–19.

44 Schmid EU, Alberts AS, Greeff F *et al.* The value of radiotherapy or chemotherapy after intubation for advanced esophageal carcinoma – a prospective randomized trial. *Radiother Oncol* 1993;**28**:27–30.

45 Waters JS, Norman A, Cunningham D *et al.* Long-term survival after epirubicin, cisplatin and fluorouracil for gastric cancer: results of a randomized trial. *Br J Cancer* 1999;**80**:269–72.

46 Webb A, Cunningham D, Scarffe JH *et al.* Randomized trial comparing epirubicin, cisplatin, and fluorouracil versus fluorouracil, doxorubicin, and methotrexate in advanced esophagogastric cancer. *J Clin Oncol* 1997;**15**:261–7.

47 Ross P, Nicolson M, Cunningham D *et al.* Prospective randomized trial comparing mitomycin, cisplatin, and protracted venous-infusion fluorouracil (PVI 5-FU) with epirubicin, cisplatin, and PVI 5-FU in advanced esophagogastric cancer. *J Clin Oncol* 2002;**20**:1996–2004.

48 Ilson DH, Ajani J, Bhalla K *et al.* Phase II trial of paclitaxel, fluorouracil, and cisplatin in patients with advanced carcinoma of the esophagus. *J Clin Oncol* 1998;**16**:1826–34.

49 Ilson DH, Forastiere A, Arquette M *et al.* A phase II trial of paclitaxel and cisplatin in patients with advanced carcinoma of the esophagus. *Cancer J* 2000;**6**:316–23.

50 Ajani JA, Baker J, Pisters PW *et al.* CPT-11 plus cisplatin in patients with advanced, untreated gastric or gastroesophageal junction carcinoma: results of a phase II study. *Cancer* 2002;**94**:641–6.

51 Ilson DH, Saltz L, Enzinger P *et al.* Phase II trial of weekly irinotecan plus cisplatin in advanced esophageal cancer. *J Clin Oncol* 1999;**17**:3270–5.

52 Pozzo C, Bugat R, Peschel C *et al.* Irinotecan in combination with CDDP or 5-FU and folinic acid is active in patients with advanced gastric or gastro-oesophageal junction adenocarcinoma: final results of a randomised phase II study. *Proc Am Soc Clin Oncol* 2002;**20**:134A.

53 Assersohn L, Rigg A, Cunningham D *et al.* A phase II trial of irinotecan and 5-fluorouracil (5FU) and folinic acid (FA) in patients with oesophago-gastric carcinoma who had progressed or relapsed within 3 months of 5FU-based chemotherapy. *Proc Am Soc Clin Oncol* 2002;**21**:157A.

54 Tebbutt N, Norman A, Cunningham D *et al.* Randomised, multicentre phase III study comparing capecitabine with fluorouracil and oxaliplatin with cisplatin in patients with advanced oesophago-gastric cancer interim analysis. *Proc Am Soc Clin Oncol* 2002;**21**:131A.

55 Ciardiello F, Tortora G. A novel approach in the treatment of cancer: targeting the epidermal growth factor receptor. *Clin Cancer Res* 2001;**7**:2958–70.

56 Bramhall SR, Hallissey MT, Whiting J *et al.* Marimastat as maintenance therapy for patients with advanced gastric cancer: a randomised trial. *Br J Cancer* 2002;**86**:1864–70.

57 Morgan G, Vainio H. Barrett's oesophagus, oesophageal cancer and colon cancer: an explanation of the association and cancer chemopreventive potential of non-steroidal anti-inflammatory drugs. *Eur J Cancer Prev* 1998;**7**:195–9.

58 Farrow DC, Vaughan TL, Hansten PD *et al.* Use of aspirin and other nonsteroidal anti-inflammatory drugs and risk of esophageal and gastric cancer. *Cancer Epidemiol Biomarkers Prev* 1998;**7**:97–102.

59 Sharp L, Chilvers CE, Cheng KK *et al.* Risk factors for squamous cell carcinoma of the oesophagus in women: a case-control study. *Br J Cancer* 2001;**85**:1667–70.

# 24 Gastric carcinoma

*Alexandria Phan, Jaffer Ajani*

## Background

### Epidemiology

Gastric cancer is more common than oesophageal cancer is in Western countries. An estimated 21 600 new cases of gastric carcinoma and 12 400 deaths as a result of the disease were expected in the USA in 2002. However, worldwide, gastric cancer is the second most common neoplasm, representing approximately 10% of new cancer cases and accounting for more than 12% of all cancer deaths. The incidence and mortality rates of this disease have been declining in most countries. Men are more frequently afflicted by gastric cancer than women at a ratio of approximately 2:1. Also, the incidence of gastric cancer increases with age with most cases occurring between the ages of 65 and 74 years. Gastric cancer is most prevalent in Asian countries with almost 40% of newly diagnosed cases found in China. However, when adjusted for age, the highest occurrence rate of new gastric cancer cases is in Japan. In addition, from 1992 to 1997, only 21% of patients having gastric cancer presented with localised disease, and in all patients as a whole, the 5-year survival rate is 20% or less.[1,2]

### Aetiology and risk factors

Diet and environment have been implicated in the development of gastric cancer. Specifically, a diet low in vegetables and fruits and high in salts and nitrates has been associated with an increased risk of gastric carcinoma.[3] Occupational exposure to carcinogens in coal mining and processing of nickel, rubber and timber has also been reported to increase the risk of gastric cancer.[4–7] Studies have also reported an association between gastric adenocarcinoma and intestinal metaplasia.[8] In yet another study, intestinal metaplasia was found in 94% of resected gastric cancers, suggesting that it is a premalignant condition.[9] Furthermore, both prior gastric resection of benign disease and pernicious anaemia have been anecdotally reported to be associated with an increased risk of gastric malignancies, and *Helicobacter pylori* infection is a contributing factor in gastric carcinogenesis. The genetic abnormalities associated with gastric cancer have not been fully elucidated, although a number of abnormalities have been described, particularly those of the *p53* and *APC* genes.

## Clinical manifestations

Most gastric cancers are at an advanced stage when diagnosed. Presenting signs and symptoms are often non-specific and typically include pain, early satiety, weight loss, vomiting, and anorexia; haematemesis is the presenting manifestation in 10–20% of patients. Peritoneal implants, abdominal mass, ascites, hepatomegaly and nodal involvement are among the other possible physical findings.

## Screening and diagnosis

Routine screening of gastric cancer is generally not performed in Western countries. However, routine mass screening for gastric cancers is performed in Japan. Methods of screening include endoscopy and barium *x* ray. Once a diagnosis is obtained, the staging work-up may include CT scans and endoscopic ultrasound. Laprascopic staging is also used commonly.

## Pathology

Adenocarcinoma is the predominant form of gastric cancer, accounting for approximately 95% of all cases. Histologically, adenocarcinomas are classified as intestinal or diffuse; the mixed type occurs rarely. Intestinal-type cancer is characterised by cohesive cells that form gland-like structures and is often preceded by intestinal metaplasia. Diffuse-type cancer is composed of infiltrating cells that infrequently form masses or ulcers. Other histologic types, including squamous cell carcinomas, lymphomas, small cell carcinomas, carcinoid tumours, leiomyosarcomas and gastrointestinal soft tissue sarcomas are infrequent.

## Staging and prognosis

Currently, the most frequently used staging system for gastric cancers is the TNM system (Box 24.1). The Japanese staging system relies on anatomic distribution but the American Joint Committee on Cancer (AJCC) system relies on the number of involved nodes. Traditional prognostic factors for gastric cancer include the depth of tumour penetration and number of involved nodes. It had been suggested that aneuploidy and diffuse-type adenocarcinoma have a poorer outcome. Finally, the prognostic significance

**Box 24.1 TNM staging system for gastric cancer**

**Primary tumour (T)**

| | |
|---|---|
| Tx | Primary tumour cannot be assessed |
| T0 | No evidence of primary tumour |
| Tis | Carcinoma *in situ*: intraepithelial tumour with invasion of the lamina propria |
| T1 | Tumour invades lamina propria or submucosa |
| T2 | Tumour invades mucularis propria or subserosa |
| T3 | Tumour penetrates serosa (visceral involvement) without invasion of adjacent structures |
| T4 | Tumour invades adjacent structures |

**Regional lymph nodes (N)**

| | |
|---|---|
| Nx | Regional node(s) cannot be assessed |
| N0 | No regional lymph node metastasis |
| N1 | Metastasis in 1–6 regional lymph nodes |
| N2 | Metastasis in 7–15 regional lymph nodes |
| N3 | Metastasis in > 15 regional lymph nodes |

**Distant metastases (M)**

| | |
|---|---|
| Mx | Distant metastasis cannot be assessed |
| M0 | No distant metastases |
| M1 | Distant metastases |

| AJCC Stage grouping | | | | 5-year survival rate (%) |
|---|---|---|---|---|
| Stage 0 (*in situ*) | Tis | N0 | M0 | >90 |
| Stage IA | T1 | N0 | M0 | 60–80 |
| Stage IB | T1 | N1 | M0 | |
| | T2 | N0 | M0 | 50–60 |
| Stage II | T2 | N2 | M0 | |
| | T2 | N1 | M0 | |
| | T3 | N0 | M0 | 30–40 |
| Stage IIIA | T2 | N2 | M0 | |
| | T3 | N2 | M0 | |
| | T4 | N0 | M0 | 20 |
| Stage IIIB | T3 | N2 | M0 | 10 |
| Stage IV | T4 | N1–2 | M0 | |
| | Any T | N3 | M0 | |
| | Any T | Any N | M1 | <5 |

**Box 24.2 Treatment according to stage of gastric cancer**

| Stage | Standard treatment option |
|---|---|
| 0 | Surgery |
| IA | Surgery |
| IB | Surgery ± chemoradiation |
| II | Surgery ± chemoradiation |
| IIIA | Surgery ± chemoradiation |
| IIIB | Palliative chemotherapy, radiotherapy ± surgery, neoadjuvant chemoradiation |
| IV | Palliative chemotherapy, radiotherapy ± surgery, neoadjuvant chemoradiation |

treatment of gastric cancer depends on the disease stage at the time of diagnosis (Box 24.2).

## Locoregional disease – surgery

The current treatment recommendation for patients having locoregional gastric cancer is surgical resection. The objectives of this treatment are to confirm resectability, completely remove the cancer, provide pathologic staging, and re-establish gastrointestinal continuity. Laparoscopy has emerged as an excellent tool for evaluating the extent of disease prior to surgery. Subtotal gastrectomy, when possible, is preferred over total gastrectomy, as it leads to comparable survival but lower morbidity. The recommended margin of resection is 5 cm of normal gastric tissue. The extent of gastric resection depends on the location and size of the primary tumour.

The extent of lymph node dissection at the time of gastrectomy continues to be controversial. D1 lymphadenectomy involves only the removal of perigastric lymph nodes, while D2 lymphadenectomy involves the removal of lymph nodes along the coeliac, left gastric, splenic and hepatic arteries. Retrospective data have shown that extended lymphadenectomy (D2 dissection or greater) is associated with more precise staging, improved locoregional control and enhanced survival in comparison with historical controls. The more extensive lymph node resection is safe and does not increase morbidity.[10] However, it also has been shown that resection of the higher echelon of lymph nodes should be done only by experienced surgeons in large centres. In addition, prospective Western studies comparing D1 and D2 lymphadenectomy have demonstrated higher postoperative morbidity and mortality without a significant improvement of long-term survival.[11–13] **Evidence level Ib** For the purpose of proper N-staging, the recent AJCC classification requires removal and examination of at least 15 lymph nodes.

Patients with T3-T4 tumours are at the highest risk for locoregional recurrence after potentially curative surgery

of various oncogenes and tumour suppressor genes is currently under investigation.

## Treatment

The only potentially curative treatment modality for localised gastric cancer is surgery; however, overall 5-year survival rate often does not exceed 40%. Patients having unresectable localised gastric cancers but no evidence of metastatic disease can be expected to survive 5–6 months. Palliative measures for advanced gastric cancer can include surgery, radiotherapy and chemoradiotherapy; palliative resection or bypass is often not recommended. Also, the

regardless of their nodal and metastatic status. Even patients having node-negative disease (T3N0) have a gastric cancer-related mortality rate of about 50% within 5 years. However, mortality is significantly worse in patients having positive nodes.

## Locoregional disease – preoperative therapy

Because surgical resection is the only curative treatment modality, several clinical trials have been carried out to attempt to improve the success of gastric cancer treatment. Prompted by the promising results and acceptable toxicity of preoperative chemoradiation in other parts of the gastrointestinal tract, such as the oesophagus and rectum, there is growing enthusiasm for this modality in gastric cancer. Preoperative therapy used for this disease has included radiotherapy, chemotherapy, and chemoradiotherapy. In addition, Safran *et al.*[14] reported preliminary data on preoperative chemoradiotherapy using paclitaxel (Taxol) in patients having T2-T4 N0-N3 adenocarcinoma. They found an overall response rate of 63% with acceptable toxicity.

## Locoregional disease – adjuvant therapy

The 5-year survival rate after "curative resection" for gastric cancer is only 30–40%. Treatment failure in these cases stems from a combination of local or regional recurrence and distant metastasis. This has stimulated interest in adjuvant and postoperative therapy in the hope of improving treatment results.

Postoperative chemotherapy for gastric carcinoma is largely ineffective. Numerous prospective, randomised trials have been conducted in the United States and Europe, producing conflicting results. For example, Hermans *et al.*,[15] in a meta-analysis of 123 trials, 11 of which could be analysed for crude mortality odds, showed no improvement in survival after adjuvant chemotherapy. However, at the 1998 American Society of Clinical Oncology (ASCO) meeting, Earle *et al.*[16] presented a reanalysis of the literature. Twelve trials met the criteria for inclusion in this meta-analysis. They found a small survival benefit in the group that received adjuvant chemotherapy. Currently, postoperative adjuvant chemotherapy is not recommended. **Evidence level Ia**

The study, INT-0116, was designed to evaluate postoperative adjuvant chemoradiation in these patients. A total of 556 patients having adenocarcinoma of the gastro-oesophageal junction were randomised to either receive postoperative chemoradiation or undergo observation after curative resection. The chemoradiotherapy regimen consisted of one cycle of 5-FU (425 mg m$^{-2}$)/leucovorin (LV) (20 mg m$^{-2}$) given daily for five cycles followed by 4500 cGy of radiation (180 cGy per day) given with 5-FU/LV (40 mg m$^{-2}$ and 20 mg m$^{-2}$) on days 1 through 4 and the last 3 days of irradiation. One month after the completion of

irradiation, two cycles of daily 5-FU/LV (425 and 20 mg m$^{-2}$, respectively) were given five times daily at monthly intervals. At a median follow up of 3·3 years, the 3-year disease-free survival rate was 49% in the treatment group and 32% in the observation group, while the 3-year overall survival rate was 52% in the treatment group and 41% in the observation group. These differences were statistically significant. The median survival duration was also improved from 27 to 42 months in the two arms of the study. As a result of this large trial, postoperative chemoradiation is now considered a standard of care for R0 resected high risk locally advanced adenocarcinoma of the stomach and gastroesophageal junction.[17] **Evidence level Ib**

## Metastatic disease – chemotherapy

Standard treatments for advanced or metastatic gastric cancer have not been well established. The most commonly administered chemotherapy agents with objective response rates in gastric cancer include mitomycin C, doxorubicin, 5-FU and cisplatin. Monotherapy with these agents results in 15–20% response rates and responses with combination chemotherapy regimens increase to 30–60%. Despite the higher responses and toxicity, no clinical or survival benefit for any combination regimens over those of 5-FU alone have been observed.[18] In this study of 252 patients randomised to either 5-FU alone, or 5-FU/doxorubicin/cisplatin, or 5-FU/doxorubicin/methyl-CCNU with triazinate, no survival advantage over the 5-FU alone arm was observed. Various combinations of chemotherapy have been evaluated in phase II clinical trials performed with variable response rates. However, prospective phase III trials failed to demonstrate a superior regimen. Newer agents including the Japanese TS-1, taxanes, and other topoisomerase inhibitors used in combination chemotheraputic regimens have produced promising results. Patients with advanced or metastatic gastric cancer should be encouraged to enrol in clinical trials.

## Discussion

The major advance in the treatment of locoregional gastric carcinoma has been the new standard of adjuvant chemoradiotherapy following a curative resection. Laparoscopy is more or less established as a staging procedure prior to surgery. Staging with endoscopic ultrasonography has improved. New strategies will include the use of preoperative approaches and incorporation of new agents. Similar to carcinoma of the oesophagus, the use of molecular markers to predict response and survival is needed. Preoperative chemoradiotherapy needs to be further investigated in this disease.

**Table 24.1  Selected results of postoperative/adjuvant chemoradiation for gastric cancer**

| Study | No. of patients | Treatment | Survival (%)*(months) |
|---|---|---|---|
| GITSG | 71 | Methyl CCNU + 5-FU | 50 (56) |
| | 71 | No adjuvant | 31 (33) |
| ECOG | 91 | Methyl CCNU + 5-FU | 57 (33) |
| | 89 | No adjuvant | 57 (37) |
| VASOG | 66 | Methyl CCNU + 5-FU | 39 (25·2) |
| | 68 | No adjuvant | 38 (25·2) |
| Estape | 33 | Mitomycin C | 76 (No reached) |
| | 37 | No adjuvant | 30 (12) |
| Allum | 141 | Mitomycin C + 5-FU | 28 (16) |
| | 140 | Mitomycin C + 5-FU + CMFV | 10 (16) |
| | 130 | No adjuvant | 18 (15) |
| Nakajima | 81 | Mitomycin C + 5-FU + AraC | 68 (>60) |
| | 83 | Mitomycin C + UFT + AraC | 63 (>60) |
| | 79 | No adjuvant | 51 (>60) |
| MacDonald | 83 | 5-FU + adriamycin + mitomycin C | 32 |
| | 93 | No adjuvant | 28 |
| Coombes | 133 | 5-FU + adriamycin + mitomycin C | 46 (36) |
| | 130 | No adjuvant | 18 (15) |
| Krook | 61 | 5-FU + adriamycin | 32 (36) |
| | 64 | No adjuvant | 33 (34) |
| Nakajima | 288 | Mitomycin C + 5-FU + UFT | 86 (>60) |
| | 285 | No adjuvant | 83 (>60) |
| Neri | 48 | 5-FU + leucovorin + epirubicin | 20 (20·4) |
| | 55 | No adjuvant | 25 (13·9) |
| Hallissey | 138 | 5-FU + adriamycin + mitomycin C | 19 (17·3) |
| | 153 | RT | 12 (12·9) |
| | 145 | No adjuvant | 20 (14·7) |
| Tsavaris | 42 | 5-FU + epirubicin + mitomycin | 64 |
| | 42 | No adjuvant | 81 |

Abbreviations: 5-FU, fluorouracil; CCNU, lomustine; AraC, cytarabine; CMFV, cyclophosphamide, methotrexate, 5-FU and vincristine; UFT, tetrahydrofuranyl derivative of 5-FU; RT, radiotherapy; MS, median survival; DFS, disease-free survival
*Survival (%, months MS, months DFS whenever data is available) at 5 years.

# References

1  Devesa SS, Fraumeni JF Jr, The rising incidence of gastric cardia cancer. *J Natl Cancer Inst* 1999;**91**:747–9.

2  Terry MB, Gaudet MM, Gammon MD. The epidemiology of gastric cancer. *Semin Radiat Oncol* 2002;**12**:111–27.

3  Neugut AI, Hayek M, Howe G. Epidemiology of gastric cancer. *Semin Oncol* 1996;**23**:281–91.

4  Gonzalez CA, Sanz M, Marcos G *et al.* Occupation and gastric cancer in Spain. *Scand J Work Environ Health* 1991;**17**:240–7.

5  Kneller RW, Gao YT, McLaughlin JK *et al.* Occupational risk factors for gastric cancer in Shanghai, China. *Am J Ind Med* 1990;**18**:69–78.

6  Parent ME, Siemiatycki J, Fritschi L. Occupational exposures and gastric cancer. *Epidemiology* 1998;**9**:48–55.

7  Tsuda T, Mino Y, Babazono A, Shigemi J, Otsu T, Yamamoto E. A case-control study of the relationships among silica exposure, gastric cancer, and esophageal cancer. *Am J Ind Med* 2001;**39**:52–7.

8  Sugimura T, Matsukura N, Sato S. Intestinal metaplasia of the stomach as a precancerous stage. *IARC Sci Publ* 1982;**39**:515–30.

9  Lei DN, Yu JY. Types of mucosal metaplasia in relation to the histogenesis of gastric carcinoma. *Arch Pathol Lab Med* 1984;**108**:220–4.

10  Brennan MF, Karpeh MS Jr. Surgery for gastric cancer: the American view. *Semin Oncol* 1996;**23**:352–9.

11  Bonenkamp JJ, Hermans J, Sasako M, van de Velde CJ. Extended lymph-node dissection for gastric cancer. Dutch Gastric Cancer Group. *N Engl J Med* 1999;**340**:908–14.

12  Cuschieri A, Lezoche E, Morino M *et al.* EAES multicentre prospective randomized trial comparing two-stage vs single-stage management of patients with gallstone disease and ductal calculi. *Surg Endosc* 1999;**13**:952–7.

13  Cuschieri A, Weeden S, Fielding J *et al.* Patient survival after D1 and D2 resections for gastric cancer: long-term results of the MRC randomized surgical trial. Surgical Co-operative Group. *Br J Cancer* 1999;**79**:1522–30.

14  Safran H, Akerman P, Cioffi W *et al.* Paclitaxel and concurrent radiation therapy for locally advanced adenocarcinomas of the pancreas, stomach, and gastroesophageal junction. *Semin Radiat Oncol* 1999;**9**:53–7.

15  Hermans J, Bonenkamp JJ, Boon MC *et al.* Adjuvant therapy after curative resection for gastric cancer: meta-analysis of randomized trials. *J Clin Oncol* 1993;**11**:1441–7.

16  Earle CC, Maroun JA. Adjuvant chemotherapy after curative resection for gastric cancer in non-Asian patients: revisiting a meta-analysis of randomised trials. *Eur J Cancer* 1999;**35**:1059–64.

17  Macdonald JS, Smalley SR, Benedetti J *et al.* Chemoradiotherapy after surgery compared with surgery alone for adenocarcinoma of the stomach or gastroesophageal junction. *N Engl J Med* 2001;**345**:725–30.

18  Cullinan SA, Moertel CG, Wieand HS *et al.* Controlled evaluation of three drug combination regimens versus fluorouracil alone for the therapy of advanced gastric cancer. North Central Cancer Treatment Group. *J Clin Oncol* 1994;**12**:412–16.

# 25 Pancreatic cancer

*Paula Ghaneh, Conor Magee, John P Neoptolemos*

## Introduction: incidence and mortality

Pancreatic ductal adenocarcinoma remains one of the most difficult cancers to treat. It is the commonest cancer affecting the exocrine pancreas and is one of the major causes of cancer death. There are approximately 28 000 deaths per year in the USA **Evidence level III**[1] and 40 000 per year in Europe **Evidence level III**.[2] The incidence and mortality ratios are roughly equivalent, indeed the latest estimated figures from the IARC for the year 2000 demonstrate that there will be 217 000 new cases and 213 000 deaths from pancreatic cancer worldwide **Evidence level III**.[2] The majority of patients present with advanced disease resulting in a rather low resection rate especially outside of regional specialist units.[3] Those patients who undergo pancreatic resection demonstrate a median survival of 10–18 months and a 5-year survival rate of 17–24% **Evidence level III**.[3–6] The late presentation is responsible in part for the poor overall median survival of 3–5 months and poor long-term survival rate of 0·4–5·0% **Evidence level III**.[3–6] Nevertheless, there have been major improvements in operative mortality and morbidity in the past decade through the development of specialist regional centres[3] and encouraging evidence of improved long-term survival with the use of adjuvant chemotherapy as shown in the ESPAC-1 trial **Evidence level Ib**.[7] The evidence base around specialist units has grown substantially and now clearly shows that this has resulted in: a reduced postoperative mortality that is a continuous effect, with no threshold, unaffected by case mix and only a possible single surgeon effect; reduced postoperative morbidity; reduced postoperative length of stay and cost; an increased resection rate; and probable increased long-term survival.[3] In parallel with these clinical advances, recent remarkable progress has been made in understanding the key molecular events in pancreatic cancer. It is hoped that this knowledge will provide the basis for novel and effective diagnostic and therapeutic approaches in the near future.

## Background

### Aetiology

The principle risk factors are smoking, chronic pancreatitis, hereditary pancreatitis and an inherited predisposition for pancreatic cancer *per se* or part of certain familial cancer syndromes. The main risk factor is cigarette smoking and accounts for around 25–30% of cases **Evidence levels IIb, III**.[8–10]

The risk from chronic pancreatitis is of the order of 5–15-fold **Evidence level III**[10,11] and hereditary pancreatitis is associated with a 50- to 70-fold risk and a cumulative lifetime risk to the age of 75 years of 40% **Evidence level III**.[12,13] The mode of parental transmission of the disease does not affect the risk of developing pancreatic cancer **Evidence level III**[13,14] as was once believed **Evidence level III**.[12]

Pancreatic cancer may also occur in three other situations in which there is an inherited predisposition.

- There appears to be an inherited component to pancreatic cancer in up to 10% of patients with pancreatic cancer in the absence of familial pancreatic cancer and other cancer syndromes **Evidence levels IIb, III**.[15,16]
- There is an increased incidence of pancreatic cancer in individuals from families with familial pancreatic cancer in which the disease appears to be transmitted in an autosomal dominant manner with impaired penetrance. Two recent studies have shown that around 17–19% of these families may have disease-causing *BRCA2* mutations in both Jewish and non-Jewish populations **Evidence level III**.[17,18] Also a susceptibility locus on chromosome 4q32–34 has been identified in one large kindred with familial pancreatic cancer **Evidence level III**.[19]
- An increased risk of pancreatic cancer may occur as part of another cancer syndrome including familial atypical multiple mole melanoma (FAMMM), hereditary non-polyposis colorectal carcinoma (HNPCC), familial breast–ovarian cancer syndromes, familial adenomatous polyposis (FAP) and most notably Peutz–Jeghers syndrome (PJS), but probably not Li–Fraumeni syndrome.[20]

Germline mutations involving the *BRCA1* and *2* genes are associated with breast and breast/ovarian cancer families, somatic mutations of which have been found in sporadic pancreatic cancer **Evidence level III**.[21] Germline mutations of *p16* are found in FAMMM and these correlate with an excessive incidence of pancreatic cancer **Evidence level III**.[22]

## Recommendations

- Continued health education to avoid tobacco consumption should lower the risk of developing pancreatic cancer Grade B.
- Continued health education to avoid excess alcohol consumption should lower the risk of developing chronic pancreatitis Grade B.
- All patients with an increased inherited risk of pancreatic cancer should be referred to a specialist centre offering specialist clinical advice and genetic counselling and, where appropriate, genetic testing such as for *BRCA2* mutations Grade B.

## Molecular pathogenesis

As with other cancers, the pathogenesis of pancreatic cancer involves an accumulation of genetic and molecular changes that result in a malignant phenotype with invasive potential. Studies in sporadic pancreatic cancer have revealed activation of key oncogenes such as *K-ras* Evidence level III [23] and inactivation of important tumour suppressor genes such as *p53*, *p16* and *SMAD4* in a large proportion of cases Evidence level III. [24-26] These changes promote uncontrolled cell growth and failure of programmed cell death and abnormalities in growth factors and growth factor receptors also contribute to the malignant phenotype. [27] Disruption of the normal regulation of the extracellular matrix involving the matrix metalloproteinases (MMPs) and tissue inhibitors of matrix metalloproteinases (TIMPs), and increase in the expression of angiogenic factors such as vascular endothelial growth factor (VEGF) and platelet derived endothelial cell growth factor (PDECGF) also contribute to the invasive potential of tumour cells. [27] *K-ras* mutation subtype has been shown to be significantly related to survival Evidence level III [28] but inactivation of tumour suppressor genes *p16*, *p53* and *p21I*, and expression of apoptotic genes *bax* and *bcl-2* have not been found to be of any prognostic significance Evidence level III. [29] Expression of wild-type *p53*, however, may predict responsiveness to chemotherapy Evidence level III. [30] It is hoped that these molecular markers may have a clinically useful prognostic role in patient management in the future – the molecular understanding for pancreatic cancer is the basis for emerging gene therapy trials. [31]

## Recommendations

- Further investigation of the pathogenesis of pancreatic cancer is essential to identify new therapeutic targets and also novel diagnostic and prognostic markers Grade B.

## Screening

Based on the prevalence of undiagnosed pancreatic cancer and the sensitivity and specificity of potential screening techniques, primary screening for pancreatic cancer unfortunately is not applicable to the general population at the present time. [20] The molecular analysis of key genes involved in pancreatic cancer however may be of importance for secondary screening of high risk groups, notably chronic pancreatitis, hereditary pancreatitis, Peutz–Jeghers syndrome and familial pancreatic cancer. [20]

There are various serum and surface proteins such as CA19·9, CA494, CA50, CA242, TPA, Dupan2, Spa-1, Muc1 and cytokeratins 7,8,18,19 that have been found to be elevated or overexpressed in pancreatic cancer. The most commonly used marker in everyday practice, CA19·9, has a sensitivity of 70–90% and specificity of 90% Evidence level III. [32] False positives frequently occur in benign obstructive jaundice and chronic pancreatitis even in the absence of bile duct obstruction and ascites. These markers have a very poor sensitivity for early lesions and their sensitivity and specificity, given the prevalence of pancreatic cancer in the general population, renders current tumour markers unsuitable for screening. Nevertheless, they have a role in diagnosis in general practice prompting referral to a specialist centre. Investigational secondary screening programmes for pancreatic cancer are in place for familial pancreatic cancer, certain familial cancer syndromes and hereditary pancreatitis Evidence level III. [20,33]

A key recommendation of the Consensus Guidelines developed by the International Association of Pancreatology is that patients with an inherited predisposition to pancreatic cancer should be referred to specialist centres capable of providing expert clinical assessment of pancreatic diseases, genetic counselling and advice on secondary screening Evidence level IV. [34]

The European Registry of Hereditary Pancreatitis and Familial Pancreatic Cancer (EUROPAC) has been established to identify families with hereditary pancreatitis and familial pancreatic cancer and develop strategies for early detection of pancreatic ductal adenocarcinoma in such high risk groups (The Study Co-ordinator, EUROPAC, Department of Clinical Genetics, Alder Hey Children's Hospital, Eaton Road, Liverpool, L12 2AP, UK; Email: europac@liv.ac.uk; website: http://www.liv.ac.uk/surgery/ europac.html). [20]

## Recommendations

- Primary screening for pancreatic cancer in the general population is not feasible at present Grade B.
- Secondary screening for pancreatic cancer in high risk cases should only be part of an investigational programme Grade B.

## How is the diagnosis made?

Pancreatic cancer classically presents with painless jaundice, weight loss, and back pain (70–90%). The initial

**Table 25.1** Imaging techniques in pancreatic cancer

| Reference | Technique | No. | Sensitivity (%) | Specificity | Accuracy | Resected (%) |
|-----------|-----------|-----|-----------------|-------------|----------|--------------|
| 36 | Laparoscopy | 38 | 35 | 100 | 60 | 40 |
|    | Lap US |   | 88 | 92 | 89 |   |
| 39 | Spiral CT | 55 | 64 | 88 | – | – |
|    | Lap US |   | 77 | 96 | – |   |
| 40 | Spiral CT | 21 | 63 | 100 | 86 | 62 |
|    | EUS |   | 75 | 77 | 76 |   |
| 35 | CT | 88 | 80 | 72 | 76 | 48 |
| 37 | MRCP | 37 | 83–8 | 96·6 | – | – |
|    | ERCP |   | 70–3 | 94·3 | – |   |
| 41 | EUS | 95 | 78 | 93 | 85 | – |
|    | ERCP |   | 81 | 88 | 84 |   |
| 38 | Spiral CT | 35 | 53 | – | – | – |
|    | EUS |   | 93 | – | – |   |
|    | FDG-PET |   | 87 | – | – |   |

Abbreviations: ERCP, endoscopic retrograde cholangiopancreatography; EUS, endoscopic ultrasound scan; FDG-PET, fluorodeoxyglucose positron emission tomography; Lap US, laparoscopic ultrasound; MRCP, magnetic resonance cholangiopancreatography

symptoms, however, may be non-specific thus delaying diagnosis. Patients may also present with late onset diabetes mellitus without obesity, acute or chronic pancreatitis, acute cholangitis, duodenal obstruction, or deep venous thrombosis. Signs may include jaundice, hepatomegaly, palpable gallbladder, an abdominal mass and ascites. Initial investigations include blood tests for anaemia, clotting profile, liver function tests and serum CA19·9. At present there is no single ideal diagnostic modality for pancreatic cancer. Advances in technology have meant that the sensitivity for detecting smaller lesions is improving and also identification of extrapancreatic spread of disease.

### Non-invasive imaging techniques

Transabdominal ultrasound is usually the initial investigation and can detect most tumours over 2 cm in size, dilatation of the biliary and main pancreatic ducts and possible extrapancreatic spread, notably liver metastases. Diagnostic accuracy reaches 75% with this method (Table 25.1) **Evidence levels IIa, III**.[35–41] Contrast-enhanced CE-CT scan is the single most useful imaging procedure and can achieve diagnostic rates of 97% for pancreatic cancer[40] (Figure 25.1a–c) **Evidence level IIb**. The accuracy for predicting unresectable lesions is 90% but the accuracy of predicting resectable **Evidence level IIb** lesions is much less at 80–85%. False negatives prior to laparotomy are mainly due to small hepatic metastases under 1 cm and small peritoneal deposits. Spiral CE-CT has almost 100% accuracy in predicting unresectable disease, and allows 3D reconstruction of anatomy **Evidence level IIb**.[40] The detection rates for pancreatic cancer are similar to CE-CT.

Magnetic resonance imaging (MRI) allows for similar results to spiral CE-CT but may be less easy to interpret than CE-CT but is useful for patients who cannot receive intravenous contrast. Positron emission tomography (PET) can differentiate inflammatory conditions from tumours and the accuracy continues to improve; presently the sensitivity is only 71–87% with specificity of around 64–80%. The latest MRI machines with large magnets can give magnetic resonance cholangiopancreatography (MRCP) images perhaps as good as endoscopic cholangiopancreatography (ERCP) **Evidence level IIb**.[37]

### Invasive imaging techniques

ERCP can be used to visualise the biliary tree and pancreatic duct. Stents can be placed to relieve obstruction and biopsies, or brush cytology can be carried out for diagnosis. Positive cytology from sampling during ERCP was found in 87 (59·6%) of 147 patients with pancreatic cancer **Evidence level III**.[42] Percutaneous transhepatic cholangiography (PTC) may be used to visualise the biliary tree and relieve jaundice in patients who cannot undergo ERCP because of difficult anatomy or previous surgery. Endoscopic ultrasound (EUS) is increasingly being used (Figure 25.2a, b) and demonstrates a sensitivity of 95% and specificity of 80% with a positive predictive value of 95% and negative predictive value of 80% for malignant masses **Evidence levels IIa, IIb**.[38,41] EUS can be combined with fine needle aspiration (FNA) to obtain biopsy with a sensitivity of 86–96%. The sensitivity, specificity, positive predictive value and negative predictive value of EUS-guided pancreatic FNA diagnosis in 47 patients with

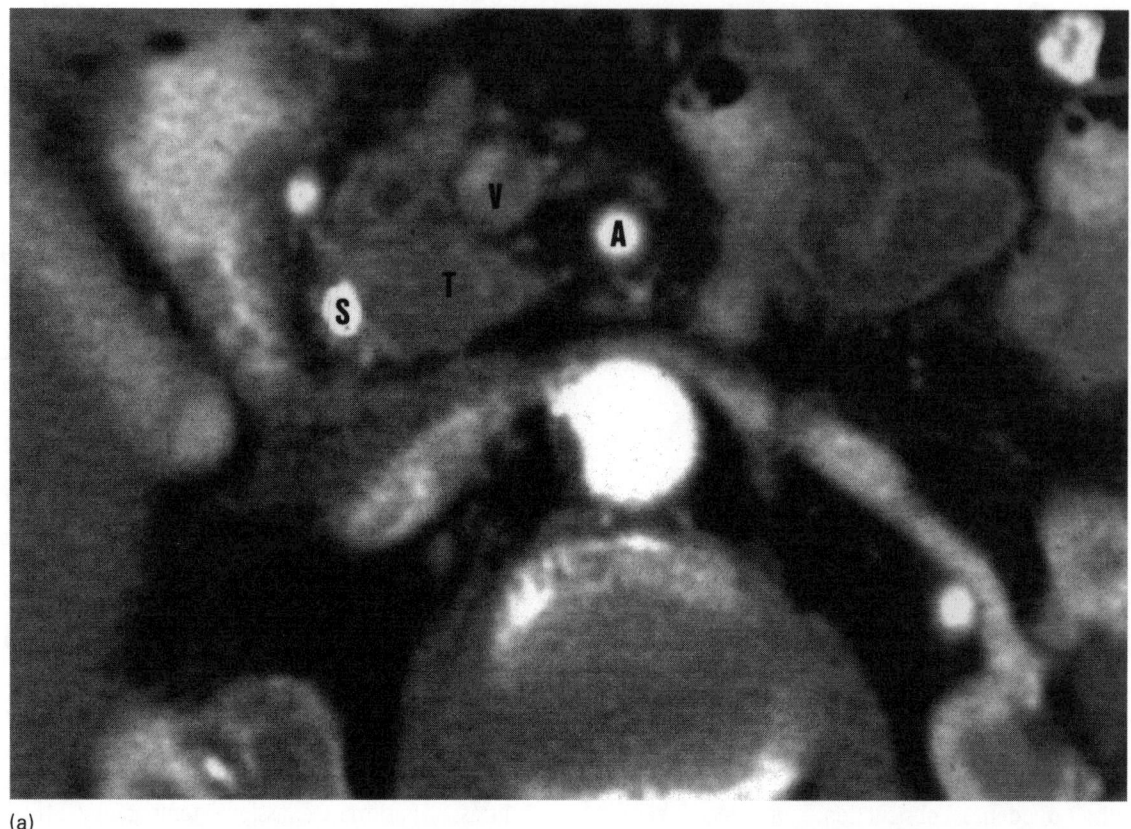

(a)

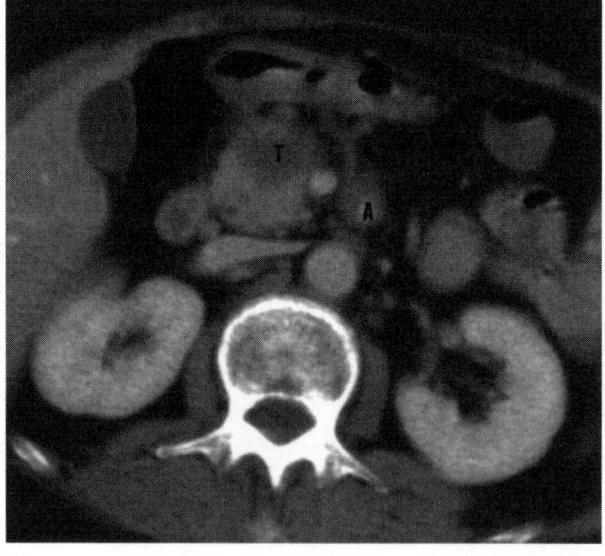

(b)

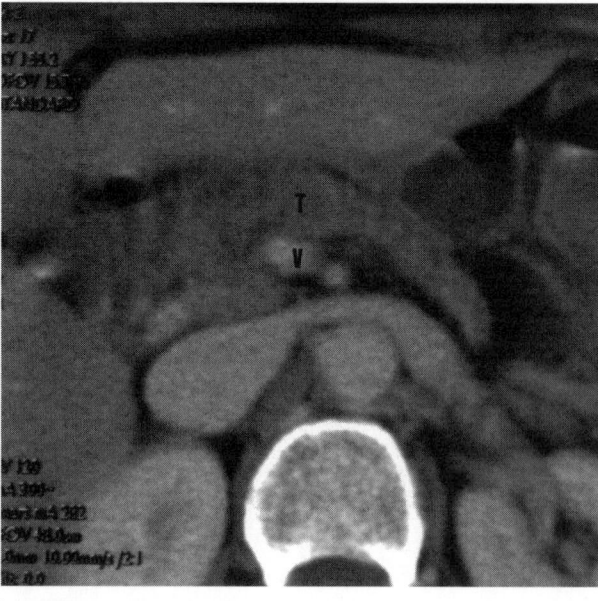

(c)

**Figure 25.1**  (a) Contrast-enhanced spiral CT scan of the pancreas. Arterial phase showing a 2 cm tumour in the uncinate process (T) and a stent is present (S). This was a resectable tumour. (b) Contrast-enhanced spiral CT scan (portal venous phase) of a small pancreatic tumour (T). There is encasement of the superior mesenteric artery (A). This tumour was unresectable (c) Contrast-enhanced spiral CT scan (portal venous phase) showing a pancreatic tumour (T) in contact with the superior mesenteric vein (V). This tumour required a resection of a segment of the portal vein. V, superior mesenteric vein; A, superior mesenteric artery.

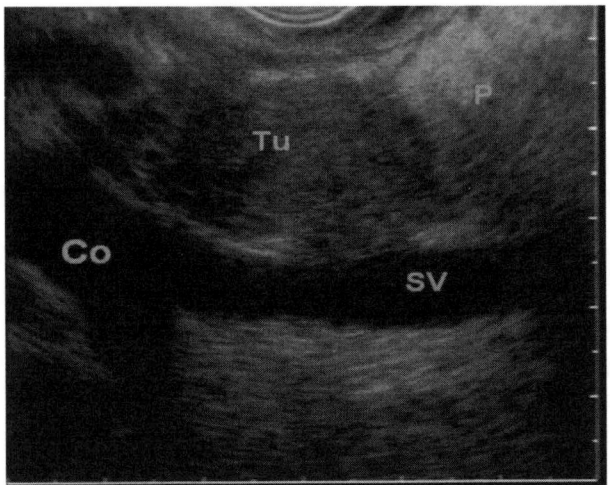

(a)

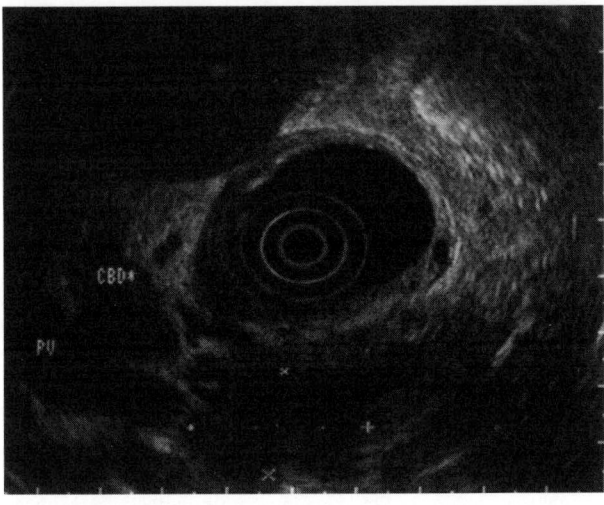

(b)

**Figure 25.2** (a) Endoscopic ultrasound scan demonstrating a 5 cm tumour (Tu) in the head of the pancreas that is close to the superior mesenteric vein (SV). This tumour was resectable. (b) Endoscopic ultrasound scan demonstrating a tumour (arrow) invading the portal vein (PV) and obstructing the common bile duct (CBD). This tumour was not resectable. P, pancreas; Co, confluence of the superior mesenteric vein, splenic vein and hepatic portal vein

malignancy was 64%, 100%, 100%, and 16% respectively **Evidence level III**.[43] The drawbacks of EUS are that it is less effective for assessing nodal involvement and cannot adequately assess distant disease such as liver metastases.

Laparoscopy allows direct exploration in patients with equivocal imaging findings and biopsies may be taken under direct vision. Combined with spiral CT, it increases resectability rates to 91% reducing unnecessary laparotomies. Washout for peritoneal cytology may also be performed.

Peritoneal cytology has been shown to be positive in 58% of patients who may have unresectable tumours or have a limited postoperative survival. Laparoscopic ultrasound (LUS) enables intraoperative scanning of the liver and pancreas to be performed and predicts resectability in over 90%. Percutaneous FNA biopsy may be used to obtain a diagnosis in patients who are deemed inoperable on imaging. The sensitivity, specificity and accuracy of percutaneous FNA biopsy in the diagnosis of 270 patients with pancreatic carcinoma was 69%, 100%, and 75% respectively **Evidence level III**.[44] Fears that percutaneous FNA would result in higher frequencies of positive peritoneal cytology and reduced survival following resection are not supported by current series **Evidence level IIa**.[45,46] Our policy is to avoid percutaneous FNA unless the disease is unresectable.

Most centres use a combination of CE-spiral CT with EUS or ERCP or MRCP, and also routine or selective use of laparoscopy combined with LUS. Vascular involvement of the superior mesenteric vessels is of major importance when resectability is being assessed, and current imaging protocols are aimed at improving this factor. Although laparoscopy plus LUS results in an alteration in clinical decision making in 10–20% of cases, it has been suggested that this is superfluous given the equivalent outcome between surgical and endoscopic bypass procedures. Presently we perform this routinely in order to avoid open surgery if at all possible, and for logistical reasons to optimise operating theatre and postoperative critical care unit usage.

### Recommendations

- Clinical symptoms and signs suggestive of pancreatic cancer (painless jaundice, weight loss, back pain, late onset diabetes mellitus without obesity, unexplained acute or chronic pancreatitis or acute cholangitis, duodenal obstruction, or deep venous thrombosis) should be assessed using transabdominal ultrasound **Grade B**.

- The use of contrast-enhanced helical CT is the gold standard for non-invasive staging of pancreatic cancer **Grade B**.

- Selective use of other modalities such as MRCP, ERCP, and PET may contribute further information but should not be used exclusively **Grade B**.

- Endosonography and/or laparoscopy with laparoscopic ultrasound may be appropriate in selective cases **Grade B**.

- Attempts should be made during the course of investigative endoscopic procedures to obtain a tissue diagnosis **Grade B**.

- Tissue diagnosis should be sought in all cases deemed unresectable **Grade C**.

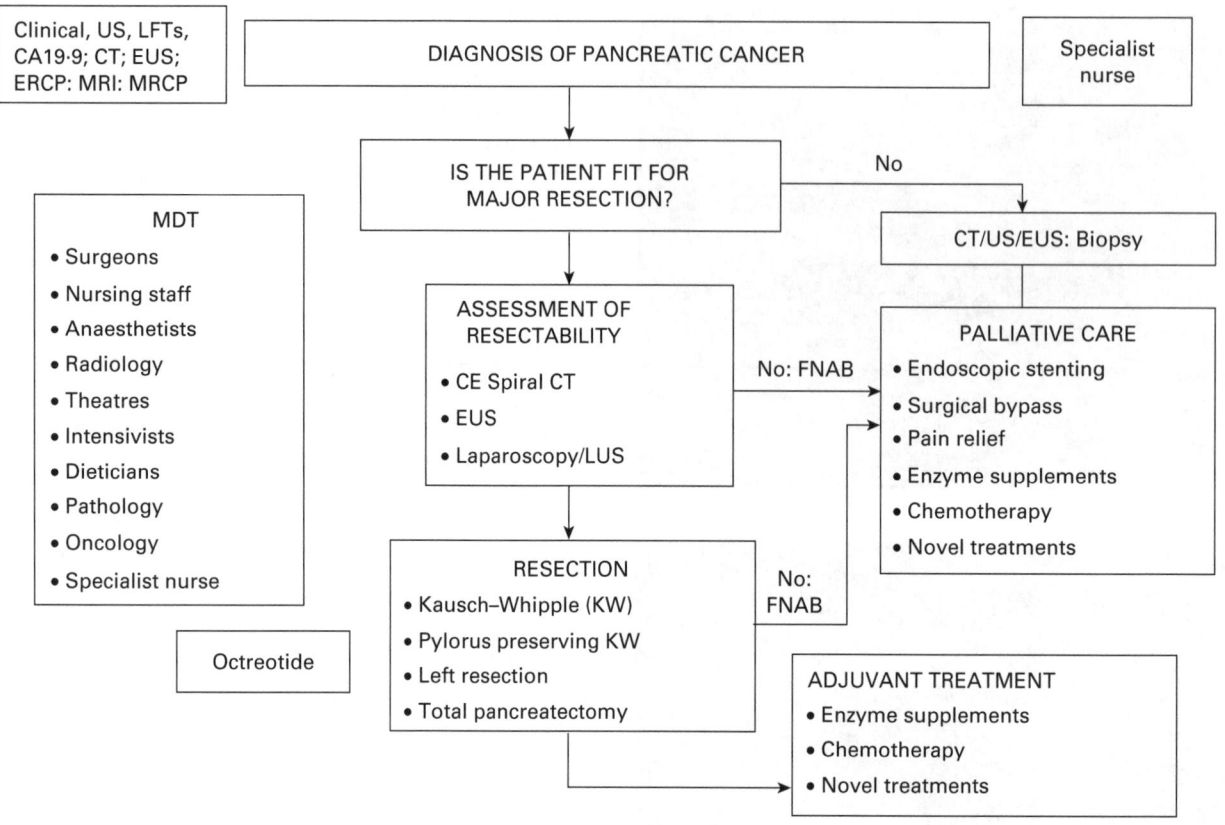

**Figure 25.3** Algorithm for the management of patients with pancreatic cancer.
US, transabdominal ultrasound scan; CT, computed tomography; EUS, endoluminal ultrasound; ERCP, endoscopic retrograde cholangiopancreatography; MRI, magnetic resonance imaging; MRCP, magnetic resonance cholangiopancreatography; MDT, multidisciplinary team; FNAB, fine needle aspiration biopsy

- Transperitoneal techniques of tissue biopsy have poor sensitivity and should be avoided in cases where resection is possible **Grade C**.

## Treatment

The management of a patient with suspected pancreatic cancer requires the immediate input of a pancreas cancer specialist nurse and the involvement of the regional pancreas tumour multidisciplinary team (Figure 25.3).

### What are the options for non-resectable pancreatic cancer?

Symptom control and quality of life are extremely important in the palliation of patients with pancreatic cancer. Intractable pain is a major problem for these patients and often necessitates the use of high dose opiate analgesia. Alternative approaches include intraoperative neurolytic coeliac plexus block, which has demonstrated benefit in randomised trials **Evidence level Ib**.[47] Percutaneous CT-guided neurolytic coeliac plexus block

shows reasonable results in patients with cancers in the head of the pancreas but not in those with cancers in the body and tail of the pancreas **Evidence level IIb**.[48] The overall success rate (78%) of coeliac plexus block using endoluminal ultrasound is similar (74%) to that using CT **Evidence level IIb**.[48] There have been encouraging results from the use of bilateral or unilateral thoracoscopic splanchnicectomy **Evidence level III**.[49] Weight loss can be a marked feature of pancreatic cancer that to a large extent, at least initially, is due to pancreatic exocrine insufficiency from obstruction of the main pancreatic duct and subsequent fibrosis of the distal gland. Pancreatic exocrine insufficiency may also contribute to abdominal pain and bloating. When pancreatic enzyme supplements are given to patients with advanced pancreatic cancer they enjoy a better quality of life and improved symptom score **Evidence level Ib**.[50]

### *Endoscopic palliation*

The majority of patients will present with advanced disease that is not amenable to curative resection. The major

**Table 25.2    Results of combination chemotherapy regimens in advanced pancreatic cancer**

| Reference | Period | No. of patients | Regimen | Median survival (months) | P value |
|-----------|--------|-----------------|---------|--------------------------|---------|
| 60* | – | 21 | 5-FU + MT + VC + CY + MMC | 11 | |
| | | 19 | Untreated control | 2·1 | 0·00006 |
| 61* | 1973–77 | 65 | 5-FU + CCNU | 3 | |
| | | 87 | Untreated control | 3·9 | 0·17 |
| 62* | 1989–91 | 23 | 5-FU + AM+MMC | 8·1 | |
| | | 20 | Untreated control | 3·2 | 0·002 |
| 63* | 1991–95 | 47 | 5-FU + FA + /-ET | 6 | |
| | | 43 | Best supportive care | 2·5 | 0·01 |

Abbreviations: 5-FU, 5-fluorouracil; A, doxorubicin; AM, adriamycin; CCNU, carmustine; CY, cyclophosphamide; ET, etoposide; FA, folinic acid; MMC, mitomycin C; MT, methotrexate; P, cisplatin; VC, vincristine
*Randomised controlled trial.

symptom requiring intervention is obstructive jaundice. Biliary stenting using ERCP is the preferred option with the combined PTC-endoscopy approach, used only if the former is technically not possible. Recurrent jaundice is a relatively common complication of stenting because of stent occlusion or migration, and approximately 20% of stented patients develop gastric outlet obstruction requiring further intervention. Self-expanding metal stents have greatly reduced the risk of acute cholangitis and obstruction **Evidence level Ib**.[51,52] Metal stents are, however, very expensive compared with plastic ones, and evidence supports the use of metal stents for patients with a good prognosis (locally advanced primary tumour 3 cm) and plastic ones for those patients with metastases and tumours over 3 cm in diameter **Evidence level Ib**.[53] The life of a plastic stent is approximately 3 months. Expandable metal stents may also be deployed endoscopically for duodenal obstruction with an immediate success rate of 67–87% with complications in up to 25%, including perforation, fistula and bleeding. Recurrent obstruction occurs in up to 23% due to stent migration or fracture **Evidence level III**.[54]

### Surgical palliation

Surgical bypass can be used to relieve jaundice and duodenal obstruction preferably with the use of a Roux-en-Y loop choledochojejunostomy and gastrojejunostomy. In trials comparing endoscopic stenting and surgical bypass procedures, acute cholangitis and bile leaks are more common in bypass procedures. There is a case for surgery, however, to reduce the number of rehospitalisations to treat recurrent jaundice. In a series of 56 patients using a single loop biliary and gastric bypass, only four needed subsequent biliary stenting (of which two were permanent) and no reoperations were required before death **Evidence level III**.[55] Prophylactic gastrojejunostomy has been evaluated in a randomised trial and found to decrease the incidence of late gastric outlet obstruction **Evidence level Ib**.[56]

### Chemotherapy

Pancreatic ductal adenocarcinoma is highly resistant to conventional methods of cytotoxic and radiotherapy treatment. There are few chemotherapeutic agents that have been shown to have reproducible response rates of more than 15%; 5-fluorouracil (5-FU) is an inhibitor of thymidylate synthetase that is essential for synthesis of DNA nucleotides and has been the most widely used in advanced pancreatic cancer giving a median survival of around 5–6 months.[57] A large randomised trial of 5-FU alone, versus 5-FU + methotrexate + vincristine + cyclophosphamide + mitomyc in C or 5-FU + doxorubicin + cisplatin found greater toxicity in the combination regimens with no difference in survival compared to 5-FU alone **Evidence level Ib**.[58] Capecitabine (Xeloda) is a novel oral, fluoropyrimidine carbamate that is sequentially converted to 5-FU by three enzymes located in the liver and in tumours including pancreatic cancer. In a phase II trial, 10 (24%) of 42 patients experienced a clinically beneficial response with an overall response rate of ·95 **Evidence level IIb**.[59] There have been four randomised trials comparing chemotherapy with a no-treatment control arm, three of which demonstrated a survival benefit in patients who received active treatment (Table 25.2) **Evidence level Ib**.[60–63]

Overall these studies suggest a role for chemotherapy but the survival time is limited, and recently there has been some emphasis on clinical benefit response. In a randomised study comparing 5-FU with the nucleoside analogue gemcitabine, median survival times were 4·4 months and 5·7 months, a 1-year survival rate of 2% versus 18%, and a clinical benefit response of 5% versus 24% respectively **Evidence level III**.[64] Newer trials are now comparing various combinations of gemcitabine with other agents including the Cancer Research UK GEM-CAP trial comparing gemcitabine alone or with capecitabine. There are now many other combinations being tested in clinical trials as doublet or triplet therapy including the incorporation of novel agents (Table 25.3).

**Table 25.3**  Novel therapeutic approaches to pancreatic cancer currently undergoing clinical trials

| Therapeutic approach | Mode of action |
|---|---|
| *Cytotoxics* | |
| Nucleoside analogues | **Gemcitabine (Gemzar)** is an S-phase nucleoside (deoxycytidine) analogue (diflourodeoxycytidine) that is phosphorylated stepwise by deoxycytidine kinase (also stimulated by gemcitabine) to diflourodeoxycytidine triphosphate incorporated into nascent DNA to inhibit DNA synthesis. This enables the insertion of a further base pair before DNA polymerase is inhibited (masked termination) making DNA repair more difficult. Gemcitabine also inhibits ribonucleotide reductase reducing the pool of dNTPs and inhibits deoxycytidine monophosphate deaminase involved in its degradation. The fixed dose rate regimen may be better; being used in numerous trials of doublet and triplet therapies and as a radiosensitiser. **Troxacitabine (Troxatyl)** is a dioxolane nucleoside analogue of cytidine that is incorporated into DNA during replication inhibiting DNA polymerase and DNA synthesis. Unlike other cytidine analogues, troxacitabine is not degraded by cytidine deaminases. Undergoing phase II/III trials |
| Antimetabolites | **Raltitrexed (Tomudex)** is a second generation thymidylate synthetase inhibitor with more potency than 5-FU. **Permetrexed (Alimta, LY231514)** is a new generation antifolate with inhibitory activity against multiple enzymes involved in pyrimidine and purine metabolism, including thymidylate synthase, glycinamide ribonucleotide formyltransferase and dihydrofolate reductase that causes concentration- and time-dependent apoptosis. Systemic toxicity is reduced by coadministration of folic acid and vitamin B12, and dexamethasone prevents an associated skin rash. **Capecitabine (Xeloda)** is an oral, tumour-selective fluoropyrimidine carbamate that is sequentially converted to 5-FU by three enzymes located in the liver and in tumours. The final step is the conversion of 5′ deoxy-5-fluorouridine to 5-FU by thymidine phosphorylase in tumours. It circumvents dihydropyrimidine dehydrogenase catabolism and its activity mimics that of continuously infused 5-FU. These are being used in numerous doublet and triplet therapies phase II/III trials. **ZD9331** is a novel oral non-polyglutamated antifolate thymidylate synthase inhibitor. This enzyme is crucial for DNA synthesis and catalyses the reductive methylation of dUMP to form thymidylate, which is subsequently converted to dTTP; currently undergoing phase II trials |
| Topoisomerase-I inhibitors | DNA topoisomerases reduce the tortional stress on DNA induced by replication and transcription by forming short-lived breaks (nicking) in the strand of DNA followed by a religation step. Topoisomerase-I inhibitors (irinotecan [CPT-11, Camptosar], camptothecin, topotecan, rubitecan and DX-8951f) act to slow this step and also prevent release of the topoisomerase from the DNA. The net result of these two processes is an increase in double-stranded breaks that induces apoptosis. Phase III trials are in progress |
| Taxanes | The microtubular complex is essential for maintaining cellular architecture, transport and motility and polarity during cell division. The taxanes (paclitaxel, docetaxel [taxotere]) are semisynthetic compounds produced by the endophytic fungus, *Taxomyces andreannae*, found on the inner surface of the bark of the Pacific or European Yew tree. Taxanes are microtubule inhibitors that bind to tubulin, but they have a different mode of action to the vinca alkaloids (another class of antimicrotubule agents). Taxanes bind to β-tubulin and promote microtubule assembly and prevent depolymerisation. The net result is the formation of stable non-functional complexes and disruption of other microtubule functions, also causing cell cycle arrest (G2 and M phases) by inhibiting function of the mitotic spindle. Cell cycle arrest at these points renders the cell sensitive to radiation. Taxanes may also induce production of TNF-α and inhibit angiogenesis |
| Platinum analogues | These form adducts with DNA inhibiting transcription and replication causing cell death. Oxaliplatin is a third-generation platinum analogue (a diaminocyclohexane platinum derivative) that may have activity in tumours resistant to cisplatin or carboplatin and have an additive/synergistic activity in doublet or triplet therapy. Phase II/III trials are in progress |

(Continued)

**Table 25.3** *(Continued)*

| Therapeutic approach | Mode of action |
| --- | --- |
| Acylfulvenes | These are chemically modified toxins produced by the mushroom *Omphalotus illudens* and called acylfulvenes. Hydroxymethylacylfulvene (HMAF or irofulven) forms adducts with proteins, DNA and RNA, inducing single-strand DNA breaks, S-phase arrest and caspase-dependent apoptosis. Phase III trial is in progress |
| Proteasome inhibitors | The 26S proteasome is a key part of the system that degrades regulatory proteins that govern cell trafficking, transcription factor activation, cell cycle regulation and apoptosis. PS-341 is a reversible and specific inhibitor of the proteasome in early clinical development |
| Cyclo-oxygenase-2 inhibitors | Specific cyclo-oxygenase-2 (COX-2) inhibitors have been found to reduce proliferation, inhibit angiogenesis and promote apoptosis. First generation COX-2 inhibitors include celecoxib and rofecoxib, and second-generation agents include parecoxib, valdecoxib and etoricoxib. A number of these are undergoing early clinical trials |
| Polyamine analogues | Polyamines (putrescine, spermine and spermidine) are ubiquitous organic cations that are essential for growth and differentiation. Depletion by polyamine analogues (diethylnorspermine, DENSPM) leads to disruption of chromatin and cell structure resulting in apoptosis |
| Histone deacytylator inhibition | CI-994 (N-acetyl dinaline, PD 123654) is a novel oral agent active in a broad variety of human tumour xenografts causing inhibition of both histone deacetylation and the G1 to S transition phase of the cell cycle. Phase II studies are in progress |
| *Biologicals* | |
| Matrix metalloproteinase inhibitors (MMPs) | MMPs are a large family of cell surface and secreted zinc-containing enzymes that are differentially overexpressed in pancreatic cancer and are essential for cell invasion, angiogenesis and metastasis. The MMP inhibitor marimastat was shown not to be superior to gemcitabine in advanced pancreatic cancer and the results of an adjuvant trial are awaited. More selective MMP inhibitors are being developed |
| Farnesyl transferase inhibitors | Around 80–90% of pancreas tumours have mutant *K-ras* inducing a continuous intracellular growth signal. For its action *K-ras* must be anchored to the cell surface by farnesyl groups involving farnesyl transferase. Farnesyl transferase inhibitors (R115777, Zarnestra) block the farnesylation of newly synthesised *K-ras*, which therefore becomes functionally inactive. Phase III trials are in progress |
| Anti-Erb-B2 antibodies | Erb-B2 is a mutated cell surface receptor (part of the epidermal growth factor receptor family) that functions as an oncogene and is overexpressed in 20–30% of pancreas tumours. Herceptin (Trastuzumab) is an antibody to Erb-B2 that blocks extracellular mitogenic signalling and has been found to be very effective in patients with breast cancer who overexpress Erb-B2. Trials in pancreatic cancer are in progress |
| Anti-EGFR antibodies | Epidermal growth factor receptor (EGFR) is a growth factor that is overexpressed in most pancreatic cancers whose ligands include EGF and TGFα. Erbitux (IMC-C225) is an EGFR monoclonal antibody that blocks intracellular mitogenic signals inhibiting tumour growth and also angiogenesis. Other antibodies include ABX-EGF and EMD7200. Phase I/II clinical trials are in progress |
| Tyrosine kinase inhibitors | These agents (ZD1839, OSI-774 [Tarceva], PKI 166 and CI-1033) inhibit the active intracellular domain (tyrosine kinase) of the EGF receptor leading to cell death and inhibition of angiogenesis. Phase III trials are in progress |
| Anti-CEA antibodies | Carcinoembryonic antigen (CEA) is highly expressed in pancreatic tumours. Greatly improved humanised monoclonal antibodies directed against CEA that may be tagged with toxic agents are now undergoing phase I/II trials |

*(Continued)*

**Table 25.3** (Continued)

| Therapeutic approach | Mode of action |
|---|---|
| Anti-angiogenic agents | Angiogenic factors such as vasoendothelial growth factor (VEGF) and their receptors are vital for the growth of tumours and the establishment and development of metastases. Anti-angiogenic agents (TNP-470; thalidomide) are being evaluated in phase III trials |
| Gene-directed enzyme prodrug therapy (GDEPT) | GDEPT introduces an enzyme gene (mammalian or non-mammalian) into a tumour cell that is expressed converting a non-toxic drug into a toxic cancer-killing agent. One such system is the ifosfamide-CYP2B1 combination. The non-toxic oxazaphosphorine, ifosfamide, is converted into 4-hydroxyifosfamide by hepatic cytochrome P450 enzymes (including the 2B1 isoform, CYP2B1). In turn 4-hydoxy-ifosfamide decays to phosphoramide mustard, which alkylates DNA, and acrolein, which alkylates proteins. This principle, although not GDEPT itself, is currently under clinical development. Microcapsules containing an established cell line overexpressing the CYP2B1 gene are injected into pancreatic tumours followed by systemic administration of ifosfamide |
| Replication-selective oncolytic viruses | Adenoviral infection of mammalian cells leads to cell death due to lysis following viral replication. Around 50–70% pancreatic cancers lack wild-type *tp53* tumour suppresser gene function. Onyx-015 is an E1B-55 *kDa* gene-deleted adenovirus that replicates selectively in cells lacking functional *p53* either because of *tp53* gene mutations or because they carry a *p14ARF* gene mutation (the protein of which interacts with *p53*). A phase I trial using intratumour injection of the virus showed rather than localised antitumour activity only |
| Ras peptide immunotherapy | Mutant K-ras peptide may be used to stimulate host immune response that may destroy tumour cells. Autologous antigen presenting cells may also be transduced with synthetic K-ras peptides, identical to those found in the patient and reintroduced into the patient; phase III trials are in progress |
| Gastrin vaccination | The hormone gastrin is a potent growth factor for pancreas tumour cells. The G17DT therapeutic vaccine (formerly Gastrimmune) consists of the amino terminal portion of gastrin linked to a diphtheria toxoid that *in vivo* generates antibodies blocking gastrin interaction with the CCK-2 receptor. Both passive and active immunisation are effective. Two pivotal phase III trials are in progress: in the USA, G17DT is used in combination with gemcitabine versus gemcitabine alone, and in Europe the comparison is between G17DT alone and gemcitabine alone |
| HCG vaccination | Human chorionic gonadotrophin (HCG) promotes tumour growth, angiogenesis and metastases. Avicine is a therapeutic cancer vaccine developed from HCG peptides. A multicentre phase II clinical trial of Avicine has shown similar survival to gemcitabine with an even better effect for the combination |
| GM-CSF vaccination | Granulocyte macrophage-colony stimulating factor (GM-CSF) is a cytokine involved in the recruitment and differentiation of antigen presenting cells optimising the tumour immune response. The GAX(R) vaccine (called) is generated by transduction of tumour cells derived from each individual patient with a retroviral vector carrying the GM-CSF gene, lethally irradiated and reintroduced into the patient. A phase II trial is evaluating the adjuvant use of GVAX(R) in combination with radiation and chemotherapy |
| Heat shock protein–peptide vaccination | Heat shock proteins (HSPs) act as intracellular chaperones maintaining a wide range of proteins in the correct conformation and acting as shuttle vectors. Purification of HSP-peptide complexes from tumour cells pulls out peptides from which tumour-specific vaccines can be generated. Autologous HSP-peptide complexes (HSPPC-96) are being prepared from patients with pancreatic cancer and used to stimulate an immune response. A phase I study is in progress |
| Virulizin | This is an immune response modifier (derived from bovine bile) that stimulates the production of TNFα from tumour cells promoting apoptosis and also leads to tumour recruitment of macrophages. A phase III trial is in progress |
| 13-*cis*-retinoic acid (Accutane) | This retinal promotes cellular differentiation and growth arrest. A phase II pilot trial of 13-*cis*-retinoic acid and interferon alfa yielded a survival time of almost 8 months |

## Chemoradiotherapy

Radiotherapy has been widely used for the treatment of pancreatic cancer. The main drawback is the limit on the dosage owing to the close proximity of adjacent radiosensitive organs. External beam radiotherapy is routinely used with 5-FU as a radiosensitising agent (chemoradiotherapy), although gemcitabine is now being evaluated as an alternative radiosensitiser. There have been many non-randomised and randomised studies but none has compared EBRT with an untreated control group. The results of these studies can show median survival times of 7–15 months, but these were in highly selected groups of patients **Evidence level III**.[65–67] Good local disease control rates are observed but the extent to which this translates into improved survival times cannot be determined. Attempts to increase the dose of radiation without increasing the toxic side effects include the use of intraoperative radiotherapy (IORT) and hyperfractionation protocols. IORT alone does not produce superior survival times than EBRT and has been used to boost EBRT **Evidence level III**.[68,69] Newer techniques such as conformal radiotherapy are now being used but these studies almost invariably employ follow-on chemotherapy once the chemoradiotherapy has been completed. Thus the survival effect from the combination therapy compared with chemoradiotherapy alone or chemotherapy alone has never been clearly established.

## Combination therapy

The rationale for combination chemoradiation and follow-on chemotherapy is to produce good local control and systemic destruction of disease. The Gastrointestinal Tumour Study Group (GITSG) undertook the pivotal study, which randomised three groups of patients with advanced pancreatic cancer to either 60 Gy EBRT (with radiosensitising 5-FU) with or without follow-on 5-FU versus 40 Gy EBRT with radiosensitising 5-FU and follow-on 5-FU **Evidence level Ib**.[70] The median survival times per group were 40, 23, and 42 weeks respectively indicating that high dose chemoradiotherapy alone was actually inferior to combination therapy.

The Eastern Cooperative Oncology Group (ECOG) randomly allocated 91 patients to receive either bolus 5-FU once weekly, or to 40 Gy chemoradiotherapy with bolus 5-FU, followed by weekly maintenance 5-FU. The median survival times were 8·2 and 8·3 months respectively, with significantly more toxicity experienced by patients treated in the combined modality arm **Evidence level IIb**.[71] These findings were subsequently contradicted by a much smaller GITSG study of only 43 patients in which they were randomly allocated to streptozocin, mitomycin C, and 5-FU triplet chemotherapy (SMF) versus chemoradiotherapy (with concomitant 5-FU) followed by maintenance SMF.

The median survival rate for the combined-modality arm was significantly better than the SMF only group (32 weeks versus 42 weeks respectively) **Evidence level IIb**.[72]

A more recent study used hyperfractionated, accelerated radiotherapy and simultaneous application of 5-FU and folinic acid with follow-on chemotherapy according to response, every 4 weeks. The total tumour dose of 44·8 Gy was applied in two daily fractions of 1·6 Gy, resulting in 10 fractions per week to achieve a median survival time of 12·7 months **Evidence level III**.[73] The absence of phase III trials to test the benefits of newer forms of chemoradiotherapy either alone or in combination in advanced pancreatic cancer prevents an accurate estimate of any treatment benefit.

Although these and more recent studies suggest a reasonable survival time with chemoradiotherapy and maintenance chemotherapy, the results are not convincingly better than chemotherapy alone. Temporary pain relief, however, is typically reported in as many as 40–80% of patients given chemoradiation in phase II studies **Evidence levels Ib, III**.[74,75]

## Regional chemotherapy

Regional therapy is used to deliver high doses of the cytotoxic to the tumour bed whilst reducing harmful systemic side effects. A variety of regimens have been used with and without radiotherapy in small retrospective groups of patients **Evidence level III**.[76] There have been very encouraging results in response rates but in highly selected groups of patients. This approach requires experienced operators and facilities. An important outcome of this approach has been the downstaging of certain tumours. These patients have been able to undergo resection following regional therapy. Regional therapy offers good local control and reduction in hepatic disease, but there is still disease progression from peritoneal deposits and distant disease.

## Novel therapy

The greater understanding of the molecular events involved in pancreatic carcinogenesis has prompted the development of new treatments. These are currently being assessed in preclinical and early clinical trials (Table 25.3). There are several immunotherapeutic strategies under assessment including vaccination of patient-specific mutant *K-ras* peptide **Evidence level III**[77] and heat shock protein tumour peptide complexes from the patient. *Ex vivo* approaches include transducing tumour cells with immune genes such as *GM-CSF* or pulsing dendritic cells prior to reinjection. Gene therapy approaches have used introduction of tumour suppressor genes into pancreatic cancer, gene-directed enzyme pro-drug therapy (GDEPT) **Evidence level III**[78] and the use of the ONYX 015 virus, which only lyses cells with an abnormal *p53* pathway **Evidence level III**.[79] Whilst a GDEPT-like approach produced some tumour responses[78] the ONYX 015 did not.[79] Anti-angiogenic agents may reduce tumour circulation but this has not produced good results yet. MMPs are important in the balance of the extracellular matrix and have a role in angiogenesis, and a range of MMP inhibitors have been developed. Marimastat, an oral MMP inhibitor **Evidence level III**,[80] has been shown to have a dose–response effect but at the highest dose was not superior to gemcitabine **Evidence level Ib**.[81]

### Recommendations

- Neurolytic coeliac plexus block should be considered as part of palliative care in pancreatic cancer **Grade A**.
- Chemoradiation should be considered for severe pain **Grade B**.
- Pancreatic enzyme supplements should be used to maintain weight and increase quality of life **Grade A**.
- Endoscopic biliary stenting should be used in malignant biliary obstruction **Grade A**.
- Metal stents should be used in patients with defined parameters (locally advanced tumour < 3 cm diameter), plastic stents should be used otherwise **Grade A**.
- Prophylactic gastrojejunostomy may prevent late gastric outlet obstruction **Grade A**.
- Duodenal obstruction and gastric outlet obstruction should be treated surgically **Grade C**.
- Chemotherapy may benefit patients with advanced pancreatic cancer **Grade A**.
- Where possible, patients with advanced pancreatic cancer should be offered treatment with novel therapeutics as part of a randomised, controlled, clinical trial **Grade C**.

### How should we approach resectable pancreatic cancer?

All surgically fit patients with potentially resectable disease should proceed to surgical exploration in a regional centre. There is no clear evidence that preoperative endoscopic stenting is either of benefit or harmful in terms of surgical outcome **Evidence levels Ia, III**,[82–87] but it may facilitate logistical planning of staging and treatment. Metal stents must be avoided in patients who have tumours that may be resectable because of the tissue reaction they invoke **Evidence level IV**.

The majority of pancreatic cancers affect the head of the pancreas and are removed by pancreaticoduodenectomy. It was first successfully performed by Walter Kausch in Berlin in 1909[88] and later popularised by Allan O Whipple in 1935.[89] The procedure removes head, neck and uncinate process of the pancreas, the duodenum, the distal stomach, and the gallbladder, a small part of the proximal jejunum and the biliary tree distal to the junction of the choledochus

and cystic duct, all performed *en bloc* to include the locoregional lymph nodes. The standard method of reconstruction includes a pancreaticojejunostomy, a hepaticojejunostomy, and a gastrojejunostomy. This has been refined to a pylorus-preserving Whipple resection where a duodenojejunostomy is performed. There are various methods of reconstruction involving the pancreatic anastomosis. Our unit favours the duct-to-mucosa pancreaticojejunostomy **Evidence level Ib**[90] with the use of an externally draining pancreatic stent that may reduce postoperative complications **Evidence level III**.[91]

Pancreaticoduodenectomy is now a routine procedure in larger surgical units dealing with pancreatic cancer. A consensus statement on standard operative technique and pathological reporting has been published to enable more accurate interpretation of results from different centres **Evidence level IV**.[92] Reports from specialised centres indicate that the procedure can now be performed with a significantly decreased mortality rate of 5% or less **Evidence level IIa**.[93] Surgical technique varies but the best results are achieved using meticulous surgery by practised surgeons. The low mortality rates are associated with the units having a high throughput of patients rather than a particular surgeon being a factor.[3] Surgery-related postoperative morbidity has also decreased in recent years, but it still ranges from 20% to 54% **Evidence level III**.[94] The main complications are fistula, delayed gastric emptying, pulmonary problems, bleeding and intra-abdominal abscess. The reoperation rate is 4–9% with high reoperative mortality rates of 23–67% **Evidence level III**.[94] The use of somatostatin analogue octreotide in the immediate postoperative period has been shown to reduce the incidence of postoperative complications in four multicentre placebo-controlled randomised trials **Evidence level Ib**,[95–98] but not in two single-centre open-labelled trials **Evidence level Ib**.[99,100] The use of postoperative somatostatin analogues is now part of the surgical approach of many pancreatic centres including our own.

Resection rates in the UK have been low in the past (2·6%) **Evidence level III**[6] but recent data have shown little in the way of an increase (4%) **Evidence level II**.[101] In comparison, resection rates in regional units are much higher, around 40%,[3] but even so they are associated with a much lower postoperative mortality rate than in non-specialist, lower-volume units **Evidence level III**.[3,102] In an attempt to improve the survival following standard resections, more extensive radical surgery involving a radical lymph node dissection and retroperitoneal tissue clearance along with a pancreaticoduodenectomy has been proposed by a number of Japanese groups and others **Evidence level III**.[103–105] Clearly, with more lymph nodes harvested, this permits more accurate staging but the retrospective nature of these studies precludes any firm conclusion. The interpretation of these results is also difficult because of differences between the UICC and Japanese Pancreas Society (JPS) staging systems owing to the phenomenon of "stage migration". This is best demonstrated in the study of Satake *et al.* **Evidence level IIa**[106] who analysed a large cohort of patients with the two systems. There was a better survival for each stage (stages I–IV) with the JPS system when compared with the UICC system, yet the overall 5-year survival (11%) was obviously the same since exactly the same patients were used.

There has been only one randomised trial that has addressed the question of radical or conventional lymphatic resection **Evidence level IIa**.[107] This was a multicentre, randomised trial that compared the standard pancreatic-oduodenectomy with and without a more extensive lymph node dissection. There was no significant difference in survival between the two groups although *post hoc* analysis suggested better survival in patients with nodal involvement. In the light of these findings the ultimate benefit of extended lymphadenectomy still requires further evaluation. At the present time the accepted approach is to use either the classic Kausch–Whipple procedure or the pylorus preserving pancreaticoduodenectomy, both of which produce similar long-term survival **Evidence level IIb**.[108]

## Recurrence

The lack of survival benefit associated with radical resection may be due in part to the pattern of recurrence following surgery. The majority of patients will go on to develop disease recurrence, which is usually at the resection site, the peritoneum and the liver **Evidence level III**.[109–114] The majority of tumour recurrences have been shown to occur within 2 years of surgery **Evidence level III**.[112,114] Liver metastases frequently develop early following resection, indicating the presence of micrometastases at the time of surgery. Local recurrences by contrast tend to appear at a later stage. Although some authors have advocated extended resection and lymph node dissection as a means of reducing locoregional failure, extended resection has been associated with a local recurrence of up to 80% **Evidence level III**.[115] The reasons as to why there is recurrence following an apparently successful resection include residual retroperitoneal disease and an aggressive invasive phenotype, as shown by a very high frequency of perineural, lymphatic and vascular invasion. These local and distant patterns of recurrence highlight a need for therapy that is effective both locoregionally and systemically. The best predictors of outcome following surgery also reflect the causes of disease relapse. The most powerful independent predictors are grade and the diameter of the primary tumour and lymph node status) **Evidence level Ib**.[7]

## Should we use adjuvant therapy

Even with optimum surgical intervention, the survival data for patients with pancreatic cancer are poor, the pattern of disease progression and recurrence are clear indications for the use of additional treatment modalities. Until recently the evidence for the use of adjuvant therapy was relatively poor but this has now greatly improved.

### Neoadjuvant therapy

The use of preoperative therapy has the potential advantages of downstaging the tumour to increase resectability rates and avoiding long delays in instituting therapy after surgery, which occur with adjuvant treatment, but randomised trials are lacking. Most regimens are a form of chemoradiotherapy (Table 25.4),[116–123] producing resection rates as high as 60% and negative resection margin rates in the order of 90% instead of 80% **Evidence level Ib**.[7] Following neoadjuvant treatment patients are restaged (up to 6 months later) and those who have developed metastases (perhaps up to 50%) will not go on to surgery; a prognostically favourable subgroup is thereby selected. Moreover, it may be impossible to distinguish between the prognostically favourable group of patients with intrapancreatic bile duct cancer from those with pancreatic ductal adenocarcinoma because of the effects of the neoadjuvant treatment on histology of the primary tumour. Most studies report median survival rates between 16 and 19 months (Table 25.4).[116–123] One study reported a remarkable median survival rate of 32 months but it is likely that that this is due to the aforementioned biases within a superselect group given the equally remarkable median survival rate of 21 months in the unresected group **Evidence level IIb**.[123] The largest comparative study found that neither the survival nor the pattern of disease recurrence was significantly different between neoadjuvant and adjuvant therapy **Evidence level IIb**.[119] At the present time neoadjuvant therapy cannot be recommended as a treatment option unless part of a clinical trial.

### Adjuvant therapy

There have been surprisingly few randomised studies and only recently have these included large numbers of patients (Table 25.5).[7,124–132] Bakkevold *et al.*[126] from Norway, randomised 61 patients to receive six courses of chemotherapy (FAM regimen) or no chemotherapy. Median survival was significantly better in the FAM group (23 months) versus the no chemotherapy group (11 months). Unfortunately this benefit did not extend to 5-year survival, which was 4% and 8% for each group, respectively. There was considerable toxicity with this regimen: only 24 out of 30 patients started therapy and only 13 managed to

**Table 25.4** Neoadjuvant therapy for pancreatic cancer

| Reference | Year | No. of patients | Regimen | Resection rate Nos (%) | Positive resection margin (Nos) | Median survival (months) | Actuarial survival (%) 3-year | Actuarial survival (%) 5-year |
|---|---|---|---|---|---|---|---|---|
| 116 | 1994 | 23 | EBRT | 17/23 (74) | – | – | – | 22 |
| 117 | 1994 | 27 | EBRT+5-FU+MMC | 13/27 (48) | 0/13 | 16 | 43 | – |
| 118 | 1996 | 39 | EBRT+5-FU+IORT | 39/39 (100) | 7/39 | 19 | – | 19 (4 years) |
| 119 | 1997 | 41 | EBRT+5-FU | 41/91 (51) | 5/41 | 19·2 | – | – |
| 120 | 1998 | 53 | EBRT+5-FU+MMC | 24/53 (45) | – | 15·7 | – | – |
| 121 | 1999 | 25 | 5-FU+EBRT+MMC+CPP | 5/25 (20) | – | – | – | – |
| 122 | 2000 | 14 | 5-FU+EBRT+CPP | 9/14 (64) | – | – | – | – |
| 123 | 2000 | 68 | EBRT+5-FU+STREP+CPP | 20/68 (29) | – | 32 | 32 | – |
| | | | | 48 NR (71) | – | 21 | 13 | – |

Abbreviations: 5-FU, 5-fluorouracil; CDDP, cisplatinum; CPP, cisplatin; DPD, dipyridamole; EBRT, external beam radiotherapy; FA, folinic acid; IORT, intraoperative radiotherapy; MMC, mitomycin C; NR, not resectable; STP, streptozocin

**Table 25.5** Results of adjuvant therapy in patients who have undergone resection for pancreatic cancer

| Reference | Year | No. of patients | Radiotherapy (Gy) | Chemotherapy | Median survival (months) | Actuarial survival (%) | | | |
|---|---|---|---|---|---|---|---|---|---|
| | | | | | | 1-year | 2-year | 3-year | 5-year |
| 124* | 1985 | 21 | EBRT 40 | 5-FU | 20 | 67 | 42 | 24 | 18 |
| | | 22 | – | – | 11 | 50 | 15 | 7 | 8 |
| 125 | 1987 | 30 | EBRT 40 | 5-FU | 18 | – | 46 | – | – |
| 126* | 1993 | 30 | – | 5-FU/DOX/MMC | 23 | 70 | – | 70 | 4 |
| | | 31 | – | – | 11 | 45 | – | 30 | 8 |
| 104 | 1996 | 56 | EBRT 45 | 5-FU | 20 | – | 35 | – | – |
| 128 | 1997 | 53 | – | – | 13·5 | – | 30 | – | – |
| | | 99 | EBRT 40–45 | 5-FU | 21 | – | 44 | – | – |
| | | 21 | EBRT 50–57 | 5-FU+FA | 17·5 | – | 22 | – | – |
| 129 | 1998 | 35 | EBRT 40 | 5-FU | 13 | 56 | 38 | 29 | 15 |
| 130 | 1999 | 23 | EBRT | 5-FU+FA | 15·9 | – | – | – | – |
| 131 | 1999 | 30 | EBRT | 5-FU | 26 | – | – | – | – |
| | | 8 | EBRT | | 5·5 | – | – | – | – |
| 132* | 1999 | 54 | – | – | 12·6 | – | – | – | 10 |
| | | 60 | EBRT 40 | – | 17·1 | – | – | – | 20 |
| 75 | 2000 | 10 | EBRT | 5-FU+FA+CPP | 17 | – | – | – | – |
| 7* | 2001 | 238 238 | – | 5-FU+FA | 20 | – | – | – | – |
| | | | – | – | 14 | – | – | – | – |
| 7* | 2001 | 235 235 | EBRT 40 | – | 15·5 | – | – | – | – |
| | | | – | – | 16·1 | – | – | – | – |

Abbreviations: 5-FU, 5-fluorouracil; CPP, cisplatin; EBRT, external bean radiotherapy; FA, folinic acid.
*Randomised controlled trial.

complete all six cycles of FAM. The GITSG trial in the 1970s explored the combination of chemoradiotherapy and follow-on chemotherapy in patients who had undergone pancreaticoduodenectomy and had microscopically negative resection margins (R0) **Evidence level Ib**.[124] A total of 43 patients were randomised to receive either 40 Gy (with radiosensitising 5-FU) and then weekly 5-FU or surgery alone. The median survival was 20 months in the treated group and 11 months in the surgery-only group, and the 2-year survival rates were 42% and 15%, respectively,[124] which translated into 5-year survival rates of 18% and 8%, respectively **Evidence level Ib**.[125]

The European Organisation for Research and Treatment of Cancer (EORTC) organised a multicentre trial (largely with units in Holland, Belgium, and northern France) comparing adjuvant chemoradiotherapy (40 Gy and concomitant infusional 5-FU but no follow-on chemotherapy) with surgery alone in patients with various tumours of the head of the pancreas, including bile duct and ampullary cancers **Evidence level Ib**.[132] Only 114 of the 218 patients actually had pancreatic ductal adenocarcinoma. There was no significant difference in median survival (17·1 months with treatment and 12·6 months with observation) and 5-year survival (20% and 10%), nor was there any significant difference in the survival of those patients with the other types of cancer. This study was, however, underpowered and therefore it was difficult to draw a meaningful conclusion.

The experience of UK Pancreatic Cancer Trials Group (UKPACA)[129] was instrumental in the design of the ESPAC-1 trial **Evidence level Ib**,[7] which commenced in 1994. This pivotal multicentre randomised trial compared the effects of adjuvant chemoradiotherapy (40 Gy with radiosensitising 5-FU) versus no chemoradiotherapy and chemotherapy (5-FU plus folinic acid for 6 months) versus no chemotherapy using a 2 × 2 factorial design. Patients randomised to both groups first received the chemoradiotherapy followed by the chemotherapy, and patients randomised to control on both counts had active follow up and best supportive care. A total of 591 patients were randomised of which 541 had pancreatic ductal adenocarcinoma. The key findings were that chemoradiotherapy had no survival benefit (chemoradiation median survival 15·5 months *v* no chemoradiation 16·2 months), chemotherapy probably had a survival benefit (chemotherapy median survival 19·7 months *v* no chemotherapy median survival 14 months), and there was a significant improvement in quality of life after surgery, irrespective of the use of or type of adjuvant therapy. Twenty per cent of patients had a microscopically positive (R1) resection margin and these too had a prolonged survival with chemotherapy (but not with chemoradiation) and also had an improvement in quality of life **Evidence level Ib**.[133]

Unexpectedly the combination of chemoradiotherapy with chemotherapy in the ESPAC-1 trial reduced the survival effect of chemotherapy, creating uncertainty as to the true benefit of adjuvant chemotherapy. Whilst there was no doubt as to the lack of value in the use of adjuvant chemoradiotherapy, the surgery-only group had exceptionally good survival compared with other studies, which questions the effect of adjuvant chemotherapy **Evidence level Ib**.[7] The ESPAC-3 trial is currently under way and is randomising patients who have undergone pancreatic resection to one of three arms: 5-FU + folinic acid, gemcitabine alone, or observation. A total of 990 patients will be recruited over the next few years from countries in Europe as well as Australia and Canada. Thus ESPAC-3 will establish the true benefit of adjuvant chemotherapy and indicate the type of chemotherapy that should form the basis for future combinations.

### Recommendations

- Surgical resection should be confined to specialist centres, to increase resection rates and decrease hospital morbidity and mortality **Grade B**.
- Endoscopic biliary drainage prior to surgery does not influence surgery **Grade B**.
- Pancreaticoduodenectomy with or without pylorus preservation is the most appropriate procedure **Grade B**.
- Extended resections *de necessitaire* are acceptable, although extended resection *de principe* does not improve survival **Grade B**.
- Neoadjuvant therapies should only be administered as part of a clinical trial **Grade B**.
- Adjuvant chemoradiation has not been shown to improve survival in the absence of maintenance chemotherapy **Grade A**.
- Adjuvant 5-FU based chemotherapy may prolong life and improve quality of life, but needs to be more clearly defined through further clinical trials and cannot be recommended as standard treatment **Grade A**.

### Organisation and delivery of pancreatic cancer services

The provision of pancreatic cancer services in the UK is undergoing profound changes driven by a desire to use evidence-based findings to improve patient outcome. Many studies have shown the benefit of pancreatic surgery being undertaken by appropriately trained surgeons in specialised centres **Evidence level IIa**.[93,134]

The NHS Executive Evidence *Improving outcomes in upper gastrointestinal cancers*[135,136] was published in 2001 and recommended the establishment of designated cancer units and cancer centres. In the context of pancreatic cancer, the cancer units were anticipated to be based in hospitals with sufficient diagnostic and therapeutic facilities to allow likely diagnoses to be made and assessment of patients' ability to undertake interventional, possibly curative, treatments. In addition, cancer units will be expected to provide adequate palliative care treatment. The cancer centre is expected to be supraregional serving a population of 2–4 million and offering services equal to that of cancer units but with specialist facilities to allow precise staging of pancreatic disease, pancreatic surgery (including intensive care, dietician, physiotherapy support), further palliative procedures requiring combined radiological/endoscopic/surgical input, additional histopathology services, and the ability to act as a nexus for national and international trials. It is to be expected that such a centre should provide facilities for basic research into pancreatic cancer.

At present such reorganisation of the NHS has only just begun; it may be that there exist "islands of excellence" where single-handed surgeons offer safe, effective pancreatic surgery in smaller district general hospitals. It is acceptable and pragmatic to allow this situation to occur in the interim until cancer centres are fully established.

### Recommendations

- All pancreatic cancer surgery should be carried out by appropriately trained and experienced surgeons **Grade B**.
- Cancer centres for pancreatic cancer should be established **Grade C**.

## Conclusions

Pancreatic cancer still remains a formidable disease to diagnose and treat. Surgical approaches have become more standardised and are safer, with much improvement in both morbidity and mortality in specialised centres. Diagnosis has improved, using conventional imaging methods and appropriate treatment decisions can be made because of these improvements. Palliative treatment is improving, including the use of endoscopic stent placement, effective pain relief and pancreatic enzyme supplementation. Chemotherapy regimens can prolong survival in patients with advanced disease without sacrificing their quality of life. At the present time, only pancreatic resection can improve survival significantly. A further survival benefit may be achievable using adjuvant chemotherapy but not radiochemotherapy. The molecular mechanisms, which are responsible for pancreatic cancer, may represent hope for the future with respect to earlier diagnosis and targeted treatments, using novel genetic and biological approaches.

No surgeon should be undertaking pancreatic cancer surgery unless 30 or more resections per year are being performed[134] and within a regional pancreas tumour centre.[135,136]

In the past there has been a nihilistic approach to patients with pancreatic cancer, but we are now entering a very encouraging phase in the diagnosis and treatment of pancreatic cancer. The information and resources now available can result in a reasoned approach to the treatment of patients with pancreatic cancer to ensure the best outcome with an optimum quality of life.

## References

1 Greenlee RT, Hill-Harmon MB, Murray T, Thun M. Cancer statistics, 2001. *CA Cancer J Clin* 2001;**51**:15–36.
2 Parkin DM, Bray FI, Devesa SS. Cancer burden in the year 2000. The global picture. *Eur J Cancer* 2001;**37**(Suppl.8):4–66.
3 Andren-Sandberg A, Neoptolemos J. Resection for pancreatic cancer in the new millenium. *Pancreatology* 2002;**2**:431–9.
4 Sener SF, Fremgen A, Menck HR, Winchester DP. Pancreatic cancer: a report of treatment and survival trends for 100,313 patients diagnosed from 1985–1995, using the National Cancer Database. *J Am Coll Surg* 1999;**189**:1–7.
5 Sohn TA, Yeo CJ, Cameron JL *et al.* Resected adenocarcinoma of the pancreas-616 patients: results, outcomes, and prognostic indicators. *J Gastrointest Surg* 2000;**4**:567–79.
6 Bramhall SR, Allum WH, Jones AG, Allwood A, Cummins C, Neoptolemos JP. Treatment and survival in 13,560 patients with pancreatic cancer, and incidence of the disease, in the West Midlands: an epidemiological study. *Br J Surg* 1995;**82**:111–15.
7 Neoptolemos JP, Dunn JA, Stocken DD *et al.* Adjuvant chemoradiotherapy and chemotherapy in resectable pancreatic cancer: a randomised controlled trial. *Lancet* 2001;**358**:1576–85.
8 Coughlin SS, Calle EE, Patel AV, Thun MJ. Predictors of pancreatic cancer mortality among a large cohort of United States adults. *Cancer Causes Control* 2000;**110**:915–23.
9 Harnack LJ, Anderson KE, Zheng W, Folsom AR, Sellers TA, Kushi LH. Smoking, alcohol, coffee, and tea intake and incidence of cancer of the exocrine pancreas: the Iowa Women's Health Study. *Cancer Epidemiol Biomarkers Prev* 1997;**62**:1081–6.
10 Talamini G, Bassi C, Falconi M *et al.* Alcohol and smoking as risk factors in chronic pancreatitis and pancreatic cancer. *Dig Dis Sci* 1999;**44**:1303–11.
11 Lowenfels AB, Maisonneuve P, Cavallini G *et al.* Pancreatitis and the risk of pancreatic cancer. International Pancreatitis Study Group. *N Engl J Med* 1993;**328**:1433–7.
12 Lowenfels AB, Maisonneuve P, DiMagno EP *et al.* Hereditary pancreatitis and the risk of pancreatic cancer. International Hereditary Pancreatitis Study Group. *J Natl Cancer Inst* 1997;**89**:442–6.
13 Howes N, Wong T, Greenhalf W *et al.* Pancreatic cancer risk in Hereditary Pancreatitis in Europe. *Digestion* 2000;**61**:300.
14 Lerch MM, Ellis I, Whitcomb DC *et al.* Maternal inheritance pattern of hereditary pancreatitis in patients with pancreatic carcinoma. *J Natl Cancer Inst* 1999;**91**:723–4.
15 Tersmette AC, Petersen GM, Offerhaus GJ *et al.* Increased risk of incident pancreatic cancer among first-degree relatives of patients with familial pancreatic cancer. *Clin Cancer Res* 2001;**7**:738–44.
16 Silverman DT, Schiffman M, Everhart J *et al.* Diabetes mellitus, other medical conditions and familial history of cancer as risk factors for pancreatic cancer. *Br J Cancer* 1999;**80**:1830–7.
17 Murphy KM, Brune KA, Griffin C *et al.* Evaluation of candidate genes MAP2K4, MADH4, ACVR1B, and BRCA2 in familial pancreatic cancer: deleterious BRCA2 mutations in 17%. *Cancer Res* 2002;**62**:3789–93.

18 Hahn SA, Greenhalf W, Ellis I *et al.* BRCA2 germ line mutations in familial pancreatic carcinoma. *J Natl Cancer Inst* 2003;**95**(3):214–21.

19 Eberle MA, Pfutzer R, Pogue-Geile KL *et al.* A new susceptibility locus for autosomal dominant pancreatic cancer maps to chromosome 4q32–34. *Am J Hum Genet* 2002;**70**:1044–8.

20 Wong T, Howes N, Threadgold J *et al.* Molecular diagnosis of early pancreatic ductal adenocarcinoma in high-risk patients. *Pancreatology* 2001;**1**:486–509.

21 Lal G, Liu G, Schmocker B *et al.* Inherited predisposition to pancreatic adenocarcinoma: role of family history and germ-line p16, BRCA1, and BRCA2 mutations. *Cancer Res* 2000;**60**:409–16.

22 Lynch HT, Brand RE, Hogg D *et al.* Phenotypic variation in eight extended CDKN2A germline mutation familial atypical multiple mole melanoma-pancreatic carcinoma-prone families: the familial atypical mole melanoma-pancreatic carcinoma syndrome. *Cancer* 2002;**94**: 84–96.

23 Klimstra DS, Longnecker DS. K-ras mutations in pancreatic ductal proliferative lesions. *Am J Pathol* 1994;**145**:1547–50.

24 Dergham ST, Dugan MC, Kucway R *et al.* Prevalence and clinical significance of combined K-ras mutation and p53 aberration in pancreatic adenocarcinoma. *Int J Pancreatol* 1997;**21**:127–43.

25 Rozenblum E, Schutte M, Goggins M *et al.* Tumor-suppressive pathways in pancreatic carcinoma. *Cancer Res* 1997;**57**:1731–4.

26 Hahn SA, Schutte M, Hoque AT *et al.* DPC4, a candidate tumor suppressor gene at human chromosome 18q21·1. *Science* 1996;**271**: 350–3.

27 Magee CJ, Greenhalf W, Howes N, Ghaneh P, Neoptolemos JP. Molecular pathogenesis of pancreatic ductal adenocarcinoma and clinical implications. *Surg Oncol* 2001;**10**:1–23.

28 Kawesha A, Ghaneh P, Andren-Sandberg A *et al.* K-ras oncogene subtype mutations are associated with survival but not expression of p53, p16(INK4A), p21(WAF-1, cyclin D1, erbB-2 and erbB-3 in resected pancreatic ductal adenocarcinoma. *Int J Cancer* 2000;**89**: 469–74.

29 Ghaneh P, Kawesha A, Evans JD, Neoptolemos JP. Molecular prognostic markers in pancreatic cancer. *J Hepatobiliary Pancreat Surg* 2002;**9**:1–11.

30 Nio Y, Dong M, Uegaki K *et al.* Comparative significance of p53 and WAF/1-p21 expression on the efficacy of adjuvant chemotherapy for resectable invasive ductal carcinoma of the pancreas. *Pancreas* 1999;**18**:117–26.

31 Magee CJ, Ghaneh P, Hartley M, Sutton R, Neoptolemos JP. The role of adjuvant therapy for pancreatic cancer. *Expert Opin Investig Drugs* 2002;**11**:87–107.

32 Tanaka N, Okada S, Ueno H, Okusaka T, Ikeda M. The usefulness of serial changes in serum CA19–9 levels in the diagnosis of pancreatic cancer. *Pancreas* 2000;**20**:378–81.

33 Brentnall TA, Bronner MP, Byrd DR, Haggitt RC, Kimmey MB. Early diagnosis and treatment of pancreatic dysplasia in patients with a family history of pancreatic cancer. *Ann Intern Med* 1999;**131**:247–55.

34 Ulrich C, Diseases amotTISoH. Pancreatic Cancer in hereditary pancreatitis- Consensus guidelines for prevention, screening and treatment. *Pancreatology* 2001;**1**:412–441.

35 McCarthy MJ, Evans J, Sagar G, Neoptolemos JP. Prediction of resectability of pancreatic malignancy by computed tomography. *Br J Surg* 1998;**85**:320–5.

36 John TG, Greig JD, Carter DC, Garden OJ. Carcinoma of the pancreatic head and periampullary region. Tumor staging with laparoscopy and laparoscopic ultrasonography. *Ann Surg* 1995;**221**: 156–64.

37 Adamek HE, Albert J, Breer H, Weitz M, Schilling D, Riemann JF. Pancreatic cancer detection with magnetic resonance cholangiopancreatography and endoscopic retrograde cholangiopancreatography: a prospective controlled study. *Lancet* 2000;**356**:190–3.

38 Mertz HR, Sechopoulos P, Delbeke D, Leach SD. EUS, PET, and CT scanning for evaluation of pancreatic adenocarcinoma. *Gastrointest Endosc* 2000;**52**:367–71.

39 Van Delden OM, Phoa SS. Comparison of laparoscopic US and contrast-enhanced spiral CT in the staging of potentially resectable tumours of the pancreatic head region. *Radiology* 1997;**205**:SS619.

40 Howard TJ, Chin AC, Streib EW, Kopecky KK, Wiebke EA. Value of helical computed tomography, angiography, and endoscopic ultrasound in determining resectability of periampullary carcinoma. *Am J Surg* 1997;**174**:237–41.

41 Glasbrenner B, Schwarz M, Pauls S, Preclik G, Beger HG, Adler G. Prospective comparison of endoscopic ultrasound and endoscopic retrograde cholangiopancreatography in the preoperative assessment of masses in the pancreatic head. *Dig Surg* 2000;**17**:468–74.

42 Stewart CJ, Mills PR, Carter R *et al.* Brush cytology in the assessment of pancreatico-biliary strictures: a review of 406 cases. *J Clin Pathol* 2001;**54**:449–55.

43 Bhutani MS, Hawes RH, Baron PL *et al.* Endoscopic ultrasound guided fine needle aspiration of malignant pancreatic lesions. *Endoscopy* 1997;**29**:854–8.

44 Linder S, Blasjo M, Sundelin P, von Rosen A. Aspects of percutaneous fine-needle aspiration biopsy in the diagnosis of pancreatic carcinoma. *Am J Surg* 1997;**174**:303–6.

45 Leach SD, Rose JA, Lowy AM *et al.* Significance of peritoneal cytology in patients with potentially resectable adenocarcinoma of the pancreatic head. *Surgery* 1995;**118**:472–8.

46 Merchant NB, Conlon KC, Saigo P, Dougherty E, Brennan MF. Positive peritoneal cytology predicts unresectability of pancreatic adenocarcinoma. *J Am Coll Surg* 1999;**188**:421–6.

47 Polati E, Finco G, Gottin L, Bassi C, Pederzoli P, Ischia S. Prospective randomized double-blind trial of neurolytic coeliac plexus block in patients with pancreatic cancer. *Br J Surg* 1998;**85**:199–201.

48 Rykowski JJ, Hilgier M. Efficacy of neurolytic celiac plexus block in varying locations of pancreatic cancer: influence on pain relief. *Anesthesiology* 2000;**92**:347–54.

49 Leksowski K. Thoracoscopic splanchnicectomy for control of intractable pain due to advanced pancreatic cancer. *Surg Endosc* 2001;**15**:129–31.

50 Bruno MJ, Haverkort EB, Tijssen GP, Tytgat GN, van Leeuwen DJ. Placebo controlled trial of enteric coated pancreatin microsphere treatment in patients with unresectable cancer of the pancreatic head region. *Gut* 1998;**42**:92–6.

51 Davids PH, Groen AK, Rauws EA, Tytgat GN, Huibregtse K. Randomised trial of self-expanding metal stents versus polyethylene stents for distal malignant biliary obstruction. *Lancet* 1992;**340**:1488–92.

52 Knyrim K, Wagner HJ, Pausch J, Vakil N. A prospective, randomized, controlled trial of metal stents for malignant obstruction of the common bile duct. *Endoscopy* 1993;**25**:207–12.

53 Prat F, Chapat O, Ducot B *et al.* Predictive factors for survival of patients with inoperable malignant distal biliary strictures: a practical management guideline. *Gut* 1998;**42**:76–80.

54 Park KB, Do YS, Kang WK *et al.* Malignant obstruction of gastric outlet and duodenum: palliation with flexible covered metallic stents. *Radiology* 2001;**219**:679–83.

55 Isla AM, Worthington T, Kakkar AK, Williamson RC. A continuing role for surgical bypass in the palliative treatment of pancreatic carcinoma. *Dig Surg* 2000;**17**:143–6.

56 Lillemoe KD, Cameron JL, Hardacre JM *et al.* Is prophylactic gastrojejunostomy indicated for unresectable periampullary cancer? A prospective randomized trial. *Ann Surg* 1999;**230**:322–30.

57 Haycox A, Lombard M, Neoptolemos J, Walley T. Review article: current treatment and optimal patient management in pancreatic cancer. *Aliment Pharmacol Ther* 1998;**120**:949–64.

58 Cullinan S, Moertel CG, Wieand HS *et al.* A phase III trial on the therapy of advanced pancreatic carcinoma. Evaluations of the Mallinson regimen and combined 5-fluorouracil, doxorubicin, and cisplatin. *Cancer* 1990;**65**:2207–12.

59 Cartwright TH, Cohn A, Varkey JA *et al.* Phase II study of oral capecitabine in patients with advanced or metastatic pancreatic cancer. *J Clin Oncol* 2002;**20**:160–4.

60 Mallinson CN, Rake MO, Cocking JB *et al.* Chemotherapy in pancreatic cancer: results of a controlled, prospective, randomised, multicentre trial. *BMJ* 1980;**281**:1589–91.

61 Frey C, Twomey P, Keehn R, Elliott D, Higgins G. Randomized study of 5-FU and CCNU in pancreatic cancer: report of the Veterans Administration Surgical Adjuvant Cancer Chemotherapy Study Group. *Cancer* 1981;**47**:27–31.

62  Palmer KR, Kerr M, Knowles G, Cull A, Carter DC, Leonard RC. Chemotherapy prolongs survival in inoperable pancreatic carcinoma. *Br J Surg* 1994;**81**:882–5.

63  Glimelius B, Hoffman K, Sjoden PO *et al.* Chemotherapy improves survival and quality of life in advanced pancreatic and biliary cancer. *Ann Oncol* 1996;**7**:593–600.

64  Burris HA, 3rd, Moore MJ, Andersen J, Green MR, Rothenberg ML, Modiano MR *et al.* Improvements in survival and clinical benefit with gemcitabine as first-line therapy for patients with advanced pancreas cancer: a randomized trial. *J Clin Oncol* 1997;**15**:2403–13.

65  Gunderson LL, Nagorney DM, Martenson JA, Donohue JH, Garton GR, Nelson H, *et al.* External beam plus intraoperative irradiation for gastrointestinal cancers. *Wld J Surg* 1995;**19**:191–7.

66  Komaki R, Wadler S, Peters T *et al.* High-dose local irradiation plus prophylactic hepatic irradiation and chemotherapy for inoperable adenocarcinoma of the pancreas. A preliminary report of a multi-institutional trial (Radiation Therapy Oncology Group Protocol 8801. *Cancer* 1992;**69**:2807–12.

67  Tisdale BA, Paris KJ, Lindberg RD, Jose B, Spanos WJ, Jr. Radiation therapy for pancreatic cancer: a retrospective study of the University of Louisville experience. *South Med J* 1995;**88**:741–4.

68  Gunderson LL, Martin JK, Kvols LK *et al.* Intraoperative and external beam irradiation +/− 5-FU for locally advanced pancreatic cancer. *Int J Radiat Oncol Biol Phys* 1987;**13**:319–29.

69  Garton GR, Gunderson LL, Nagorney DM *et al.* High-dose preoperative external beam and intraoperative irradiation for locally advanced pancreatic cancer. *Int J Radiat Oncol Biol Phys* 1993;**27**:1153–7.

70  Moertel CG, Frytak S, Hahn RG *et al.* Therapy of locally unresectable pancreatic carcinoma: a randomized comparison of high dose (6000 rads) radiation alone, moderate dose radiation (4000 rads + 5-fluorouracil), and high dose radiation + 5-fluorouracil: The Gastrointestinal Tumor Study Group. *Cancer* 1981;**48**:1705–10.

71  Klaassen DJ, MacIntyre JM, Catton GE, Engstrom PF, Moertel CG. Treatment of locally unresectable cancer of the stomach and pancreas: a randomized comparison of 5-fluorouracil alone with radiation plus concurrent and maintenance 5-fluorouracil – an Eastern Cooperative Oncology Group study. *J Clin Oncol* 1985;**3**:373–8.

72  GITSG. Treatment of locally unresectable carcinoma of the pancreas: comparison of combined modality therapy (chemotherapy plus radiotherapy) to chemotherapy alone. Gastrointestinal Tumor Study Group. *J Natl Cancer Inst* 1988;**80**:751–5.

73  Prott FJ, Schonekaes K, Preusser P *et al.* Combined modality treatment with accelerated radiotherapy and chemotherapy in patients with locally advanced inoperable carcinoma of the pancreas: results of a feasibility study. *Br J Cancer* 1997;**75**:597–601.

74  Shinchi H, Takao S, Noma H *et al.* Length and quality of survival after external-beam radiotherapy with concurrent continuous 5-fluorouracil infusion for locally unresectable pancreatic cancer. *Int J Radiat Oncol Biol Phys* 2002;**53**:146–50.

75  Andre T, Balosso J, Louvet C *et al.* Combined radiotherapy and chemotherapy (cisplatin and 5-fluorouracil) as palliative treatment for localized unresectable or adjuvant treatment for resected pancreatic adenocarcinoma: results of a feasibility study. *Int J Radiat Oncol Biol Phys* 2000;**46**:903–11.

76  Muchmore JH, Preslan JE, George WJ. Regional chemotherapy for inoperable pancreatic carcinoma. *Cancer* 1996;**78**(Suppl.):664–73.

77  Gjertsen MK, Bakka A, Breivik J *et al.* Vaccination with mutant ras peptides and induction of T-cell responsiveness in pancreatic carcinoma patients carrying the corresponding RAS mutation. *Lancet* 1995;**346**:1399–400.

78  Mulvihill S, Warren R, Venook A *et al.* Safety and feasibility of injection with an E1B-55 kDa gene-deleted, replication-selective adenovirus (ONYX-015) into primary carcinomas of the pancreas: a phase I trial. *Gene Ther* 2001;**8**:308–15.

79  Lohr M, Hoffmeyer A, Kroger J *et al.* Microencapsulated cell-mediated treatment of inoperable pancreatic carcinoma. *Lancet* 2001;**357**:1591–2.

80  Evans JD, Stark A, Johnson CD *et al.* A phase II trial of marimastat in advanced pancreatic cancer. *Br J Cancer* 2001;**85**:1865–70.

81  Bramhall SR, Rosemurgy A, Brown PD, Bowry C, Buckels JA. Marimastat as first-line therapy for patients with unresectable pancreatic cancer: a randomized trial. *J Clin Oncol* 2001;**19**:3447–55.

82  Povoski SP, Karpeh MS, Jr, Conlon KC, Blumgart LH, Brennan MF. Preoperative biliary drainage: impact on intraoperative bile cultures and infectious morbidity and mortality after pancreaticoduodenectomy. *J Gastrointest Surg* 1999;**3**:496–505.

83  Martignoni ME, Wagner M, Krahenbuhl L, Redaelli CA, Friess H, Buchler MW. Effect of preoperative biliary drainage on surgical outcome after pancreatoduodenectomy. *Am J Surg* 2001;**181**:52–9 discussion 87.

84  Sewnath ME, Karsten TM, Prins MH, Rauws EJ, Obertop H, Gouma DJ. A meta-analysis on the efficacy of preoperative biliary drainage for tumors causing obstructive jaundice. *Ann Surg* 2002;**236**:17–27.

85  Sewnath ME, Birjmohun RS, Rauws EA, Huibregtse K, Obertop H, Gouma DJ. The effect of preoperative biliary drainage on postoperative complications after pancreaticoduodenectomy. *J Am Coll Surg* 2001;**192**:726–34.

86  Pisters PW, Hudec WA, Hess KR *et al.* Effect of preoperative biliary decompression on pancreaticoduodenectomy- associated morbidity in 300 consecutive patients. *Ann Surg* 2001;**234**:47–55.

87  Marcus SG, Dobryansky M, Shamamian P *et al.* Endoscopic biliary drainage before pancreaticoduodenectomy for periampullary malignancies. *J Clin Gastroenterol* 1998;**26**:125–9.

88  Kausch W. Carcinom der papilla duodeni und seine radikale entfernung. *Beitr Klin Chir* 1912;7839–486.

89  Whipple AO, Parsons WB, Mullens CR. Treatment of carcinoma of the ampulla of vater. *Ann Surg* 1935;**102**:763–9.

90  Yeo CJ, Cameron JL, Maher MM *et al.* A prospective randomized trial of pancreaticogastrostomy versus pancreaticojejunostomy after pancreaticoduodenectomy. *Ann Surg* 1995;**222**:580–92.

91  Roder JD, Stein HJ, Bottcher KA, Busch R, Heidecke CD, Siewert JR. Stented versus nonstented pancreaticojejunostomy after pancreato-duodenectomy: a prospective study. *Ann Surg* 1999;**229**:41–8.

92  Pedrazzoli S, Beger HG, Obertop H *et al.* A surgical and pathological based classification of resective treatment of pancreatic cancer. Summary of an international workshop on surgical procedures in pancreatic cancer. *Dig Surg* 1999;**16**:337–45.

93  Birkmeyer JD, Siewers AE, Finlayson EV *et al.* Hospital volume and surgical mortality in the United States. *N Engl J Med* 2002;**346**:1128–37.

94  Halloran CM, Ghaneh P, Bosonnet L, Hartley M, Sutton R, Neoptolemos JP. Complications of pancreatic cancer resection. *Dig Surg* 2002;**19**:138–46.

95  Buchler M, Friess H, Klempa I *et al.* Role of octreotide in the prevention of postoperative complications following pancreatic resection. *Am J Surg* 1992;**163**:125–31.

96  Pederzoli P, Bassi C, Falconi M, Camboni MG. Efficacy of octreotide in the prevention of complications of elective pancreatic surgery. Italian Study Group. *Br J Surg* 1994;**81**:265–9.

97  Montorsi M, Zago M, Mosca F *et al.* Efficacy of octreotide in the prevention of pancreatic fistula after elective pancreatic resections: a prospective, controlled, randomized clinical trial. *Surgery* 1995;**117**:26–31.

98  Friess H, Beger HG, Sulkowski U *et al.* Randomized controlled multicentre study of the prevention of complications by octreotide in patients undergoing surgery for chronic pancreatitis. *Br J Surg* 1995;**82**:1270–3.

99  Lowy AM, Lee JE, Pisters PW *et al.* Prospective, randomized trial of octreotide to prevent pancreatic fistula after pancreaticoduodenectomy for malignant disease. *Ann Surg* 1997;**226**:632–41.

100  Yeo CJ, Cameron JL, Lillemoe KD *et al.* Does prophylactic octreotide decrease the rates of pancreatic fistula and other complications after pancreaticoduodenectomy? Results of a prospective randomized placebo-controlled trial. *Ann Surg* 2000;**232**:419–29.

101  NYCRIS. *Key sites study.* 2000. Northern and Yorkshire Cancer Registry and Information Service.

102  Neoptolemos JP, Russell RC, Bramhall S, Theis B. Low mortality following resection for pancreatic and periampullary tumours in 1026 patients: UK survey of specialist pancreatic units. UK Pancreatic Cancer Group. *Br J Surg* 1997;**84**:1370–6.

103  Ishikawa O, Ohhigashi H, Sasaki Y *et al.* Practical usefulness of lymphatic and connective tissue clearance for the carcinoma of the pancreas head. *Ann Surg* 1988;**208**:215–20.

104 Nagakawa T, Nagamori M, Futakami F *et al.* Results of extensive surgery for pancreatic carcinoma. *Cancer* 1996;**77**:640–5.

105 Ohigashi H, Ishikawa O, Tamura S *et al.* Pancreatic invasion as the prognostic indicator of duodenal adenocarcinoma treated by pancreatoduodenectomy plus extended lymphadenectomy. *Surgery* 1998;**124**:510–5.

106 Satake K, Nishiwaki H, Yokomatsu H *et al.* Surgical curability and prognosis for standard versus extended resection for T1 carcinoma of the pancreas. *Surg Gynecol Obstet* 1992;**175**:259–65.

107 Pedrazzoli S, DiCarlo V, Dionigi R *et al.* Standard versus extended lymphadenectomy associated with pancreatoduodenectomy in the surgical treatment of adenocarcinoma of the head of the pancreas: a multicenter, prospective, randomized study. Lymphadenectomy Study Group. *Ann Surg* 1998;**228**:508–17.

108 Di Carlo V, Zerbi A, Balzano G, Corso V. Pylorus preserving pancreaticoduodenectomy versus conventional Whipple operation. *Wld J Surg* 1999;**23**:920–5.

109 Whittington R, Bryer MP, Haller DG, Solin LJ, Rosato EF. Adjuvant therapy of resected adenocarcinoma of the pancreas. *Int J Radiat Oncol Biol Phys* 1991;**21**:1137–43.

110 Westerdahl J, Andren-Sandberg A, Ihse I. Recurrence of exocrine pancreatic cancer – local or hepatic? *Hepatogastroenterology* 1993;**40**:384–7.

111 Zerbi A, Fossati V, Parolini D *et al.* Intraoperative radiation therapy adjuvant to resection in the treatment of pancreatic cancer. *Cancer* 1994;**73**:2930–5.

112 Griffin JF, Smalley SR, Jewell W *et al.* Patterns of failure after curative resection of pancreatic carcinoma. *Cancer* 1990;**66**:56–61.

113 Sperti C, Pasquali C, Piccoli A, Pedrazzoli S. Recurrence after resection for ductal adenocarcinoma of the pancreas. *Wld J Surg* 1997;**21**:195–200.

114 Amikura K, Kobari M, Matsuno S. The time of occurrence of liver metastasis in carcinoma of the pancreas. *Int J Pancreatol* 1995;**17**:139–46.

115 Kayahara M, Nagakawa T, Ueno K, Ohta T, Takeda T, Miyazaki I. An evaluation of radical resection for pancreatic cancer based on the mode of recurrence as determined by autopsy and diagnostic imaging. *Cancer* 1993;**72**:2118–23.

116 Ishikawa O, Ohigashi H, Imaoka S *et al.* Is the long-term survival rate improved by preoperative irradiation prior to Whipple's procedure for adenocarcinoma of the pancreatic head? *Arch Surg* 1994;**129**:1075–80.

117 Coia L, Hoffman J, Scher R *et al.* Preoperative chemoradiation for adenocarcinoma of the pancreas and duodenum. *Int J Radiat Oncol Biol Phys* 1994;**30**:161–7.

118 Staley CA, Lee JE, Cleary KR *et al.* Preoperative chemoradiation, pancreaticoduodenectomy, and intraoperative radiation therapy for adenocarcinoma of the pancreatic head. *Am J Surg* 1996;**171**:118–25.

119 Spitz FR, Abbruzzese JL, Lee JE *et al.* Preoperative and postoperative chemoradiation strategies in patients treated with pancreatico-duodenectomy for adenocarcinoma of the pancreas. *J Clin Oncol* 1997;**15**:928–37.

120 Hoffman JP, Lipsitz S, Pisansky T, Weese JL, Solin L, Benson AB, 3rd. Phase II trial of preoperative radiation therapy and chemotherapy for patients with localized, resectable adenocarcinoma of the pancreas: an Eastern Cooperative Oncology Group Study. *J Clin Oncol* 1998;**16**:317–23.

121 White R, Lee C, Anscher M *et al.* Preoperative chemoradiation for patients with locally advanced adenocarcinoma of the pancreas. *Ann Surg Oncol* 1999;**6**:38–45.

122 Wanebo HJ, Glicksman AS, Vezeridis MP *et al.* Preoperative chemotherapy, radiotherapy, and surgical resection of locally advanced pancreatic cancer. *Arch Surg* 2000;**135**:81–8.

123 Snady H, Bruckner H, Cooperman A, Paradiso J, Kiefer L. Survival advantage of combined chemoradiotherapy compared with resection as the initial treatment of patients with regional pancreatic carcinoma. An outcomes trial. *Cancer* 2000;**89**:314–27.

124 Kalser MH, Ellenberg SS. Pancreatic cancer. Adjuvant combined radiation and chemotherapy following curative resection. *Arch Surg* 1985;**120**:899–903.

125 Douglass HO, Jr. Further evidence of effective adjuvant combined radiation and chemotherapy following curative resection of pancreatic cancer. Gastrointestinal Tumor Study Group. *Cancer* 1987;**59**:2006–10.

126 Bakkevold KE, Arnesjo B, Dahl O, Kambestad B. Adjuvant combination chemotherapy (AMF) following radical resection of carcinoma of the pancreas and papilla of Vater – results of a controlled, prospective, randomised multicentre study. *Eur J Cancer* 1993;**5**:698–703.

127 Conlon KC, Klimstra DS, Brennan MF. Long-term survival after curative resection for pancreatic ductal adenocarcinoma. Clinicopathologic analysis of 5-year survivors. *Ann Surg* 1996;**223**:273–9.

128 Yeo CJ, Abrams RA, Grochow LB *et al.* Pancreaticoduodenectomy for pancreatic adenocarcinoma: postoperative adjuvant chemoradiation improves survival. A prospective, single-institution experience. *Ann Surg* 1997;**225**:621–36.

129 Neoptolemos JP, Group MotUPC. Adjuvant radiotherapy and follow-on chemotherapy in patients with pancreatic cancer: Results of the UK Pancreatic Cancer study (UKPACA-1). *GI Cancer* 1998;**2**:235–45.

130 Abrams RA, Grochow LB, Chakravarthy A *et al.* Intensified adjuvant therapy for pancreatic and periampullary adenocarcinoma: survival results and observations regarding patterns of failure, radiotherapy dose and CA19–9 levels. *Int J Radiat Oncol Biol Phys* 1999;**44**:1039–46.

131 Paulino AC. Resected pancreatic cancer treated with adjuvant radiotherapy with or without 5-fluorouracil: treatment results and patterns of failure. *Am J Clin Oncol* 1999;**22**:489–94.

132 Klinkenbijl JH, Jeekel J, Sahmoud T *et al.* Adjuvant radiotherapy and 5-fluorouracil after curative resection of cancer of the pancreas and periampullary region: phase III trial of the EORTC gastrointestinal tract cancer cooperative group. *Ann Surg* 1999;**230**:776–82; discussion 782–4.

133 Neoptolemos JP, Moffitt DD, Dunn JA *et al.* The influence of resection margins on survival for patients with pancreatic cancer treated by adjuvant chemoradiation and/or chemotherapy within the ESPAC-1 randomized controlled trial. *Ann Surg* 2001;**238**:758–68.

134 Birkmeyer JD, Warshaw AL, Finlayson SR, Grove MR, Tosteson AN. Relationship between hospital volume and late survival after pancreaticoduodenectomy. *Surgery* 1999;**126**:178–83.

135 NHS Executive. *Guidance on commissioning cancer services. Improving outcomes in upper gastrointestinal cancers. The Evidence.* London: Department of Health, 2001.

136 NHS Executive. *Guidance on commissioning cancer services. Improving outcomes in upper gastrointestinal cancers. The Manual.* London: Department of Health, 2001.

# 26 Hepatobiliary cancers

*Philip J Johnson*

This chapter seeks to define the optimal management of patients with primary hepatobiliary cancers. The most common of these, hepatocellular carcinoma (HCC), serves as the focus of the review; cholangiocarcinoma, a less frequent clinical problem is dealt with briefly at the end of the chapter.

## Background

Progress in the acquisition of evidence-based therapies for hepatobiliary cancers has been slow and disappointing. A recent attempt to undertake a meta-analysis of non-surgical methods of treatment led the authors to conclude that it was probably an impossible task, so poor was the quality of the available data.[1] An understanding of the reasons why the treatment of such a common tumour as HCC, evokes so little consensus among practitioners and has been so poorly studied in terms of clinical trials, gives important insights into the major management problems.

- The disease is most common in populations where the infrastructure to undertake prospective randomised clinical trials is least developed. This geographical problem is compounded by the widely held perception that tumours of different aetiologies have different natural histories and different response rates to therapeutic regimens. Thus, for example, it is widely perceived (though with little data to support the contention) that the prognosis of the disease in Japan, where most cases will be related to hepatitis C virus (HCV) infection will be different from that in China where most cases are hepatitis B virus (HBV) related. The results of the clinical trials may not "travel".

- Most patients with HCC have two diseases: chronic liver disease (usually at the stage of cirrhosis) of some type, usually virus- or alcohol-related and HCC. These two diseases have independent natural histories. Thus, in HCC patients with advanced cirrhosis, the potential to improve survival, even if the tumour could be completely eradicated, may be limited. This may be one reason why several therapeutic studies have convincingly demonstrated tumour necrosis, and yet such "responses" have seldom translated into survival advantage.

- There is increasing evidence that large tumours of the liver, primary or secondary, may not change in size even if there is very significant tumour cell kill. This limits the credibility that can be attached to phase II studies in which response rates are calculated on the basis of conventional tumour size-related criteria.

On the basis of current evidence it would be ethical to enter most HCC patients into randomised controlled trials (RCTs) that have a control arm of "best supportive therapy". Indeed a number of such studies have recently emanated from Europe, and are the most valuable source of data available. However, in many areas of the world the fact that several current treatments are clearly effective in destroying tumour tissue, even without a demonstrable survival advantage, has inhibited physicians in recruiting patients, and patients consenting, to enter RCTs with a "no active treatment" arm.

## Is there a role for surgical resection and orthotopic liver transplantation?

It is widely held that surgical resection is the definitive treatment for HCC, and the only one that offers the hope of cure or, at least, long-term survival. This treatment has not been subjected to an RCT, but in nearly all series, the survival curve flattens out at around 25–40%. Generally agreed figures for survival would be 75% at 1 year, 50% at 5 years, and 33% at 10 years with an operative mortality of 5–15%, the higher figure being applicable to those with more advanced cirrhosis (reviewed in reference no.2). The morbidity would be a combination of disease recurrence (usually intrahepatic) and early postoperative hepatic decompensation.[3–5]

In interpreting the evidence the sceptical reader would note that the performance status of patients undergoing surgery is much better than that of an HCC patient group as a whole. Even in the absence of any treatment, early studies showed that survival of up to 3 years was not uncommon in patients with a small HCC, and a more recent European study described a group of patients who, in the absence of any treatment, had 1-, 2-, and 3-year survival figures of 87%, 65% and 50% respectively.[6] This group was characterised as having "early tumours" – asymptomatic and without

267

vascular invasion – not too different from the group of patients who constitute the surgical resection experience. They also noted that figures for mortality and survival are a function of the clinical status of the patients who undergo surgical resection and thus the figures in any series can be readily manipulated by patient selection. Nonetheless it is a reasonable assumption that some HCC patients are indeed cured of their cancer by resection and this does not appear to occur with other forms of treatment.

However, most patients (80%) have unresectable disease at presentation because of poor liver function (about 75% will have underlying chronic liver disease), bilobar disease, comorbid diseases, major blood vessel involvement, or extra hepatic metastases. The overall resectability rate for HCC is thus only 10–25%.[2,7,8] If the disease is unresectable, the prognosis is poor with an overall median survival of only a few months or years. Even amongst those who undergo surgical resection, there is a recurrence rate of up to 83% at 5 years.[3-5] If the reason for non-resectability is poor underlying liver function, then liver transplantation is the best approach.[9] Mazzafero *et al.* reported an actuarial survival rate of 75%, and an 83% disease-free survival rate at 4 years[10] after liver transplantation. This group of patients were required to have tumours smaller than 5 cm in diameter and less than three in number. If the patient has an even smaller tumour, or the tumour is detected unexpectedly at the time of liver transplantation for end-stage liver disease, the results are even better.

Thus a reasonable conclusion, based on the available evidence, is that all patients with HCC should be assessed to determine if their disease is resectable. It is important that this opinion should be gained from a centre with experience in liver surgery. If the disease is not resectable on the grounds of underlying liver insufficiency, then orthotopic liver transplantation should be considered where this is an available option. The question of transplantation for patients who have tumours, which could be resected by conventional surgery, remains controversial depending among other things, on the availability of donors.[7,8]

### Measures to decrease postoperative recurrence

A recently reported prospective randomised trial suggests that administration of a single dose of intrahepatic arterial lipiodol I[131] (1850 MBq), after complete resection, significantly decreased the rate of recurrence (from 59% to 28·5%), and increased the overall survival rate.[11]

### Are locoregional treatments useful?

Strictly speaking surgical resection and liver transplantation should be regarded as a form of "locoregional" treatment.

However, in clinical practice "locoregional treatment" is usually taken to comprise those approaches that seek to directly destroy the tumour tissue by some means other than surgical removal. The broad consensus is that these treatments are less "radical" than surgical resection and are applied with the primary intention of palliation rather than cure. This line is beginning to blur in the case of techniques such as percutaneous ethanol injection.

There are four broad approaches to locoregional treatment, and multiple themes based on each of these. It has been well documented that the wide variety of possible treatments reflects the fact than none is very effective or obviously better than the others. None of these has been shown in a prospective RCT to be better than no treatment; neither has one been shown to be better than the other. The various approaches are classified below and examples of each are described briefly.

The first approach is based on the observation that primary liver tumours derive the bulk of their blood supply from the hepatic artery, whereas the remaining liver is predominantly supplied by the portal vein. This offers some degree of selectivity or tumour "targeting":

- arterial embolisation
- intra-arterial chemotherapy
- use of lipiodol to target intra-arterial chemotherapy (transarterial chemoembolisation – TACE)
- selective internal radiation.

The second approach involves the direct intratumoural injection of some noxious agents such as:

- alcohol
- acetic acid
- hot water.

The third seeks to destroy tumour tissue by more "physical" means:

- focused ultrasound ablation
- radiofrequency ablation
- cryoablation.

The distinction between the latter two approaches is not clear-cut.

### Hepatic artery embolisation

This is achieved by injecting various embolic materials, under fluoroscopic control, at the time of diagnostic hepatic arteriography into the tumour feeding vessels and has largely replaced surgical ligation of the hepatic artery. Effective embolisation is often associated with fever, pain and vomiting for up to 5 days after which it subsides spontaneously. Although more than half the patients show clear evidence of tumour regression, clinical experience and a recent prospective randomised controlled trial suggest that there is no improvement in overall survival.[12,13] The procedure can be repeated on several occasions. It may be particularly effective in pain relief. The presence of Child's grade C cirrhosis is a relative contraindication.

## Intra-arterial combination chemotherapy

Direct infusion of cytotoxic agents into the hepatic artery may allow an increase in drug exposure (the time/concentration interval) of the tumour up to 400-fold (depending on the properties of the drug employed) so that dose limiting toxicity may become "regional", that is, hepatic and not systemic.[14] There is little doubt that the response rates are significantly higher than for the same treatment administered systemically.[15] However, enthusiasm is tempered by the high toxicity and the suspicion that much of the apparent benefit is related to the fact that patients with better performance status are selected for this approach.

## Use of lipiodol to target intra-arterial chemotherapy

When lipiodol, an oily contrast medium, is injected into the hepatic artery at the time of arteriography, subsequent CT scanning shows that it is cleared from normal hepatic tissues but accumulates in malignant tumours.[16] Lipiodol has therefore been used as a vehicle for targeting cytotoxic drugs. In so-called "trans-arterial chemoembolisation" (TACE), an attempt is made to enhance the effect of arterial embolisation, as described above, by the addition of chemotherapy. Typically, 60 mg of doxorubicin is mixed with 15 ml of lipiodol and injected into the tumour-feeding arteries. This is followed by embolisation with 0·5–1 mm of gelatin cubes. Side effects and complications are mainly related to the embolisation and have been described above. The procedure has, until recently, been widely regarded as standard treatment for inoperable disease. Although there is tumour regression in over 50% of cases, recent prospective randomised trials have again confirmed the efficacy of the procedure in terms of achieving high response rates, but have failed to document any improvement in survival.[17,18]

Nonetheless, TACE remains widely practised. Proponents remain unconvinced by the clinical trials,[17,18] identifying within them several problems. The large number of participating centres, each only contributing a small number of patients, the variation in operator technique and the varying degrees of embolisation achieved, were all concerns.

## Selective internal radiation (SIR) with yttrium-90 microspheres

Yttrium-90, a pure beta emitter, has a mean penetration in tissue of about 2·5 mm. It can be incorporated into glass or ceramic beads (microspheres) that will lodge in tumour vessels after injection into tumour-feeding arteries during hepatic arteriography. With such an approach, tolerance of the liver to the effects of radiation is higher than expected from external radiation, and a therapeutic dose of radiation can be delivered without causing radiation hepatitis. The degree of lung shunting must be determined before administration of the radioisotope because of the risk of radiation pneumonitis. A pretreatment technetium-99m macroaggregated albumin (Tc-MAA) scan with gamma camera scanning to predict the percentage of lung shunting and the relative tumour to non-tumour uptake ratio (T/N ratio) is therefore performed. Those with high lung shunting (> 15%) and poor T/N ratio are not suitable for yttrium-90 microsphere treatment. The majority of patients have a significant tumour response and, in up to 10% of patients treated by this approach, initially unresectable tumours may become resectable and long-term survivors have been described.[19]

## Direct chemical attack

The second locoregional approach, typified by alcohol injection, delivers the therapeutic agent percutaneously, directly into the tumour. Over the past two decades there have been numerous variations on this theme. The account given here outlines some of the more commonly used approaches.

### *Percutaneous alcohol injection (PEI)*

Under real time ultrasonic or CT guidance about 5 ml of sterile 95% ethanol is injected through a 20-cm long, 21- or 22-gauge needle, into the tumour. The procedure is repeated depending on the size of the tumour and extent of necrosis obtained. The advantage of this approach is its simplicity, lack of side effects and cheapness. On the other hand, whilst small tumours (< 2 cm) only require three to four sessions, larger tumours may require up to 20. Many workers have found it difficult to gain a homogeneous distribution of alcohol throughout the lesion. The patient often complains of mild pain and some fever. If the alcohol escapes into the peritoneal cavity, severe pain ensues. This can be avoided by very slow infiltration of the alcohol.

Survival at 1, 3 and 5 years has been reported to be 96%, 72% and 51% for Child's A cirrhosis; 90%, 72% and 48% for Child's B cirrhosis and 94%, 25% and 0% for Child's C cirrhosis, respectively.[20] Although prospective randomised trials have not been undertaken, with the use of historical control groups it appears that, at least over the first 3 years after treatment, results are similar to those obtained by surgical resection.[21–23] Other injection agents, such as acetic acid, are currently being assessed.[24]

### *Thermal ablation*

Local heating or cooling of the tumour can be an effective means of destroying local disease. The first approach, *cryotherapy*, involves freezing the tumour using a probe inserted directly into the lesion. More recently, radiofrequency (RF) and microwaves have been used to heat tumours up to 70°C. There are several advantages over PEI including shorter treatment time, and the facility to attack a larger tumour more efficiently. However, such benefits have to be balanced against a higher rate of severe complications and the limited number of sites that are suitable for treatment because of nearby critical structures.[25–29]

After three decades of experience with locoregional therapy some broad consensus seems to be emerging. Response rates are consistently higher than those that can be achieved by systemic therapy. There is no doubt that all the locoregional therapies described above are capable of causing extensive and selective tumour destruction; this has led to their widespread adoption. However, where prospective randomised trials have been undertaken, none has yet been proven to be better than any other or, indeed, better than no treatment at all. Several reasons probably combine to account for this state of affairs.

- The "selective" treatment may in fact cause damage to a significant part of the non-tumorous liver.
- In patients whose liver function is already precarious, this may have a major negative impact on survival. The survival of the patients is, in large part, related to their underlying liver function, so that reduction in tumour load may have only a small impact on overall survival.
- The techniques used in locoregional treatment may be very operator-dependent. We cannot be certain that patients treated by different operators are in fact receiving the same treatment. This is of particular importance when patients are entered into multicentre trials.
- We know from surgical resection, itself a form of locoregional treatment, that recurrence, presumably from pre-existing micrometastases, is the rule. Since patients being treated by locoregional therapies will generally have more advanced disease, it is even more likely that they will develop further intrahepatic metastases even if the treatment of the primary lesion is effective.

### Is systemic therapy useful?

HCC is widely considered to be chemotherapy resistant. Response rates for single cytotoxic agent chemotherapy are low and durable remission is rare. The most widely used single cytotoxic agent for HCC has been doxorubicin, an anthracycline. In a review of the overall response rate by Nerenstone *et al.*, from 13 published trials, the typical response rate was about 20% with a median survival of 4 months.[30] Complete remissions have been described but are seldom durable. A prospective trial that randomised 60 patients to receive either doxorubicin or no active treatment reported an increase in survival from a median value of 7 weeks for the control arm to 11 weeks for the doxorubicin arm.[31] However, in systematic reviews of randomised trials of doxorubicin therapy, no significant survival effect was discernable.[32,33] The dose-limiting toxicity of doxorubicin is mainly cardiac and bone marrow suppression. Treatment with doxorubicin is relatively contraindicated in patients with concomitant heart disease and the dosage should be reduced if the liver function is poor (total bilirubin more than two times the upper limit of the reference range). No other systemic therapies have fared significantly better; systemic therapy should be confined to clinical trials.[34]

### Combination chemotherapy

Combination chemotherapy appears to give a higher response rate, though again the duration of remission is usually short. In general, even for well-selected patients, the expected objective response for combination chemotherapy is only around 20–30% and, as such, seems unlikely to have a significant impact on survival.[34]

Nonetheless some encouraging reports have emerged recently. Patt *et al.* used a four-drug systemic intra-arterial combination chemobiotherapy (cisplatin, recombinant interferon alfa-2b, doxorubicin, and 5-fluorouracil [PIAF]) and reported a complete pathological remission in a case of disseminated HCC.[35] A phase II study, using the same drug combination but modified to an outpatient intravenous treatment,[36] involved 50 patients with unresectable HCC and reported an objective response rate of 26% (all partial responses). Although the response rate was not high, nine of the 13 partial responders had their disease rendered resectable. Histopathological examination of the resected specimens confirmed complete pathological remission in four patients. The same group has recently updated their results and reported 15 cases (including the nine cases reported earlier) of unresectable HCC that underwent surgical resection for the residual lesion(s) after partial response to PIAF.[37] There were eight complete pathological remissions out of the 15 cases and in the remainder there was over 95% necrosis.

Thus for systemic chemotherapy we can conclude that single-agent doxorubicin gives a response rate of around 15–20% and, with combination therapy, this figure rises to around 20–35%. HCC is clearly not entirely chemotherapy-resistant, but systemic therapy should still be largely confined to clinical trials.

## Antihormonal therapy

An alternative systemic approach has been endocrine manipulation. Early small studies with anti-oestrogenic and anti-androgenic agents showed some promise.[38] However, recent large-scale prospective controlled studies have refuted any role for anti-androgenic agents or tamoxifen.[39–41] In a recent small prospective controlled study, octreotide led to a significant improvement in survival (13 months in the treated group *v* 4 months in the control group). Although there were no reported "responses", octreotide appears worthy of larger scale studies.[42]

## HCC therapy – conclusions

There is no good evidence that any systemic or hormonal therapy is effective. Similarly, although locoregional treatments are clearly effective in causing tumour necrosis, any benefit in terms of survival remains to be proven. Surgical resection appears to cure a small percentage of patients and, where available, liver transplantation appears highly effective in selected patients. Neither has ever been proven in clinical trials. We should remember the case for benefit is unproven; this is quite different from saying that no effect exists.

Rather than a call for "more clinical trials" or "better drugs", a consensus into the design of clinical trials in HCC is more important. We need to agree on approaches to stratification, staging and control-arm therapies before expending more resources on the actual trials.

## Cholangiocarcinoma

Cholangiocarcinomas are rare tumours of the biliary tract that are best classified according to their anatomical situation – intrahepatic (10%), perihilar (70%), or distal (20%). Intrahepatic cholangiocarcinomas, also known as peripheral cholangiocarcinoma, present and are managed in a similar way to HCC in the non-cirrhotic liver. The only effective treatment is surgical resection and results are similar to those obtained in HCC.[43]

Hilar cholangiocarcinomas, on the other hand, present with jaundice and abdominal pain. The optimal treatment is

again complete surgical resection, and this often involves partial hepatectomy. About 10–20% of cases are candidates for resection and several long-term survivors have now been recorded.[44–47] Adjuvant therapy is of no proven benefit. The high incidence of portal lymph node spread has led to particularly poor results from liver transplantation.[47,48] Where surgical resection proves impossible, either surgical bypass or biliary endoprostheses are options[49] but survival is typically only in terms of a few months. Referral to specialist units for assessment is mandatory if optimal therapy is to be offered.

## References

1 Mathurin P, Rixe O, Carbonell N *et al.* Review article: overview of medical treatments in unresectable hepatocellular carcinoma – an impossible meta-analysis? *Aliment Pharmacol Ther* 1998;**12**:111–26.
2 De Matteo RP, Fong Y, Blumgart LH. Surgical treatment of malignant liver tumours. *Ballière's Clin Gastroenterol* 1999;**13**:557–74.
3 Nagao T, Panis Y, Farges O, Benhamou JP, Fekete F. Intrahepatic recurrence after resection of hepatocellular carcinoma complicating cirrhosis. *Ann Surg*, 1991;**241**:114–17.
4 Nagao T, Inoue S, Yoshimi F *et al.* Postoperative recurrence of hepatocellular carcinoma. *Ann Surg* 1990;**211**:28–33.
5 Nagasue N, Uchida M, Makino Y *et al.* Incidence and factors associated with intrahepatic recurrence following resection of hepatocellular carcinoma. *Gastroenterology* 1993;**105**:488–94.
6 Llovet JM, Bustamante J, Castells A *et al.* Natural history of untreated nonsurgical hepatocellular carcinoma: rationale for the design and evaluation of therapeutic trials. *Hepatology* 1999;**29**:62–7.
7 Llovet JM, Bruix J, Gores GJ. Surgical resection versus transplantation for early hepatocellular carcinoma; clues for the best strategy. *Hepatology* 2000;**31**:1019–21.
8 Llovet JM, Foster J, Bruix J. Intention-to-treat analysis of surgical treatment for early hepatocellular carcinoma: resection versus transplantation. *Hepatology* 1999;**30**:1434–40.
9 Heneghan MA, O'Grady JG. Liver transplantation of malignant liver disease. *Ballière's Clin Gastroenterol* 1999;**13**:575–91.
10 Mazzaferro V, Regalia E, Doci R *et al.* Liver transplantation for the treatment of small hepatocellular carcinoma in patients with cirrhosis. *N Engl J Med* 1996;**334**:693–9.
11 Lau WY, Leung TWT, Ho SKW *et al.* Adjuvant intra-arterial lipiodol-iodine-131-labelled lipiodol for resectable hepatocellular carcinoma – a prospective randomised trial. *Lancet* 1999;**353**:797–801.
12 Bruix J, Castells A, Montanya X *et al.* Phase II study of transarterial embolisation in European patients with hepatocellular carcinoma: need for controlled trials. *Hepatology* 1994;**20**:643–50.
13 Bruix J, Llovet JM, Castells A *et al.* Transarterial embolization versus symptomatic treatment in patients with advanced hepatocellular carcinoma: results of a randomized, controlled trial in a single institution. *Hepatology* 1998;**27**:1578–83.
14 Chen HSG, Gross JF. Intra-arterial infusion of anticancer drugs: theoretic aspects of drug delivery and review of responses. *Cancer Treat Rep* 1980;**64**:31–40.
15 Carr BI, Iwatsuki S, Starzl TE, Selby R, Madariaga J. Regional cancer chemotherapy for advanced stage hepatocellular carcinoma. *J Surg Oncology* 1993;**3**(Suppl.):100–3.
16 Yumoto Y, Jinno K, Tokuyama K *et al.* Hepatocellular carcinoma detected by iodized oil. *Radiology*, 1985;**154**:19–24.
17 Group d'Etude et de Traitement du Carcinome Hepatocellulaire. A comparison of lipiodol chemoembolization and conservative treatment for unresectable hepatocellular carcinoma. *N Engl J Med* 1995;**332**:1256–61.
18 Pelletier G, Ducreux M, Gay F *et al.* Treatment of unresectable hepatocellular carcinoma with lipiodol chemoembolization: a

multicenter randomized trial. Groupe CHC. *J Hepatol* 1998;**29**: 129–34.

19  Lau WY, Ho S, Leung WT *et al.* Selective internal radiation therapy for inoperable hepatocellular carcinoma with intraarterial infusion of yttrium$^{90}$ microspheres. *Int J Rad Oncol Bio Phys* 1998;**40**:583–7.

20  Castells A, Bruix J, Bru C *et al.* Treatment of small hepatocellular carcinoma in cirrhotic patients: a cohort study comparing surgical resection and percutaneous ethanol injections. *Hepatology* 1993;**18**: 1121–6.

21  Llovet JM, Bruix J, Capurro S, Vilano R for the BCLC Group. Longer term survival after ethanol injection for small hepatocellular carcinoma in 100 cirrhotic patients. Relevance of maintained success. *J Hepatol* 1999;**30**:100–4.

22  Kotoh K, Sakai H, Sakamoto S *et al.* The effect of percutaneous ethanol injection therapy on small solitary hepatocellular carcinoma is comparable to that of hepatectomy. *Am J Gastroenterol* 1994;**89**:194–8.

23  Vilana R, Bruix J, Bru C, Ayuso C, Sole M, Rodes J. Tumor size determines the efficacy of percutaneous ethanol injection for the treatment of small hepatocellular carcinoma. *Hepatology* 1992;**16**:353–7.

24  Ohnishi K. Comparison of percutaneous acetic acid injection and percutaneous ethanol injection for small hepatocellular carcinoma. *Hepatogastroenterology* 1998;**3**:1254–8.

25  Crews KA, Kuhn JA, McCarty TM *et al.* Cryosurgical ablation of hepatic tumors. *Am J Surg* 1997;**174**:614–18.

26  De Sanctis JT, Goldberg N, Mueeler PR. Percutaneous treatment of hepatic neoplasms: a review of current techniques. *Cardiovasc Intervent Radiol* 1998;**21**:273–96.

27  Solbiati L. New applications of ultrasonography: interventional ultrasound. *Eur J Radiol* 1998;**27**(Suppl. 2):S200–S206.

28  Rossi S, Buscarini E, Garbagnati F *et al.* Percutaneous treatment of small hepatic tumors by an expandable RF needle electrode. *Am J Roentgen* 1998;**170**:1015–22.

29  Sato M, Watanabe Y, Ueda S *et al.* Microwave coagulation therapy for hepatocellular carcinoma. *Gastroenterology* 1996;**110**:1507–14.

30  Nerenstone SR, Ihde DC, Friedman MA. Clinical trials in primary hepatocellular carcinoma: current status and future directions. *Cancer Treat Rev* 1988;**15**:1–31.

31  Lai CL, Wu PC, Chan GC *et al.* Doxorubicin versus no antitumor therapy in inoperable hepatocellular carcinoma. A prospective randomized trial. *Cancer* 1988;**62**:479–83.

32  Mathurin P, Rixe O, Carbonell N *et al.* Review article: overview of medical treatments in unresectable hepatocellular carcinoma – an impossible meta-analysis? *Aliment Pharmacol Ther* 1998;**12**:111–26.

33  Simonetti RG, Leberati A, Angiolini C *et al.* Treatment of hepatocellular carcinoma: A systematic review of randomized controlled trials. *Ann Oncol* 1997;**8**:117–36.

34  Leung WT, Johnson PJ. Systemic therapy for hepatocellular carcinoma. *Semin Oncol* 2001;**28**:514–29.

35  Patt YZ, Hoque A, Roh M *et al.* Durable clinical and pathologic response of hepatocellular carcinoma to systemic and hepatic arterial administration of platinol, recombinant interferon alpha 2B, doxorubicin, and 5-fluorouracil: a communication. *Am J Clin Oncol* 1999;**22**:209–13.

36  Leung TWT, Patt YZ, Lau WY *et al.* Complete pathological remission is possible with systemic combination chemotherapy for inoperable hepatocellular carcinoma. *Clin Cancer Res* 1999;**5**:1676–81.

37  Lau WY, Leung WT, Lai BS *et al.* Pre-operative systemic chemoimmunotherapy and sequential resection for unresectable hepatocellular carcinoma. *Ann Surg* 2001;**233**:236–41.

38  Chow PKH, Soo KC. Hormonal therapy in hepatocellular carcinoma. The current scientific and clinical evidence. *Asian J Surg* 2000;**23**:56–63.

39  (No authors listed). Tamoxifen in treatment of hepatocellular carcinoma: a randomised controlled trial. CLIP Group. *Lancet* 1998;**352**:17–20.

40  Castells A, Bruix J, Bru C *et al.* Treatment of hepatocellular carcinoma with tamoxifen: a double-blind placebo-controlled trial in 120 patients. *J Gastroenterol* 1995;**109**:917–22.

41  Grimaldi C, Bleiberg H, Gay F *et al.* Evaluation of antiandrogen therapy in unresectable hepatocellular carcinoma: results of a European Organisation for Research and Treatment of Cancer multicentric double-blind trial. *J Clin Oncol*, 1998;**16**:411–17.

42  Kouroumalis E, Skordilis P, Thermos K, Vasilaki A, Moschandrea J, Manousos ON. Treatment of hepatocellular carcinoma with octreotide: a randomised controlled study. *Gut* 1998;**42**:442–7.

43  Casavilla FA, Marsh JW, Iwatsuki S *et al.* Hepatic resection and transplantation for peripheral cholangiocarcinoma. *J Am Coll Surg* 1997;**185**:429–36.

44  Pitt HA, Dooley WC, Yeo CJ *et al.* Malignancies of the biliary tree. *Curr Probl Surg* 1995;**31**:1.

45  Ahrendt SA, Cameron JL, Pitt HA. Current management of patients with perihilar cholangiocarcinoma. In: Cameron JL, ed. *Advances in Surgery, vol 30*. St. Louis: Mosby, 1996.

46  Klempnauer J, Ridder GJ, von Wasielewski R *et al.* Resectional surgery of hilar cholangiocarcinoma: a multivariate analysis of prognostic factors. *J Clin Oncol* 1997;**15**:947–54.

47  Saldinger PF, Blumgart LH. Resection of hilar cholangiocarcinoma – a European and United States experience. *Hepatobil Surg* 2000;**7**: 111–14.

48  Iwatsuki S, Todo S, Marsh JW *et al.* Treatment of hilar cholangiocarcinoma (Klatskin tumors) with hepatic resection or transplantation. *J Am Coll Surg* 1998;**187**:353–64.

49  Jarnagin WR, Burke E, Powers C *et al.* Intrahepatic biliary enteric bypass provides effective palliation in selected patients with malignant obstruction at the hepatic duct confluence. *Am J Surg* 1998;**175**: 453–60.

# 27 The treatment of cancers of the small bowel

*ER Copson, TJ Iveson*

The infrequent occurrence of malignant tumours within the small intestine compared with the large bowel is a well-documented, if poorly understood phenomenon. Despite the fact that the small intestine accounts for three-quarters of the length of the alimentary canal and over 90% of its mucosal surface, small intestinal tumours comprise only 1–5% of gastrointestinal cancers.[1] Protective factors may include rapid cell turnover, an alkaline environment, the relative absence of bacteria and low levels of activating enzymes of precarcinogens.[2] A number of histological subtypes are seen at this site, including adenocarcinomas, lymphomas, sarcomas and neuroendocrine tumours. Distinct geographical differences are seen in the incidences of these tumour types (Table 27.1). Whilst lymphomas predominate in the Far East and Third World, the most common malignant tumour of the small bowel in the Western world is adenocarcinoma and this chapter will therefore focus on this condition. In view of the rarity of all these tumours, all published reports to date are in the form of retrospective series, and no randomised trials of different chemotherapy regimens exist.

## Background

### Adenocarcinomas of the small intestine

Adenocarcinomas represent 28–47% of neoplastic small bowel tumours in British and American series,[4] with an age-adjusted incidence in the United States of 1 per 100 000.[5] Regional variations correlate with prevalence rates for colonic cancers, but not gastric cancer.[6] Peak incidence occurs in the 6th and 7th decades of life and there is a slight male preponderance.[7] Young age is associated with increased incidence of local and distant spread at presentation.[8] The majority of tumours arise in the duodenum (54%) and occur with decreasing frequency in the jejunum (28%) and ileum (18%).[9] Periampullary tumours constitute a special anatomical entity, present earlier, and have a better overall prognosis than duodenal tumours[10]; data pertaining to these tumours have therefore not been included in this chapter.

**Table 27.1 Worldwide variation in small bowel cancers[3]**

| Histological subtype | Proportion of cases |
| --- | --- |
| Adenocarcinoma | 8% (Nigeria) to 56% (Canada) |
| Carcinoid | 2% (Japan) to 45% (Saskatchewan) |
| Sarcoma | 3% (Israel) to 30% (Sweden) |
| Lymphoma | 7% (Sweden) to 68% (Nigeria, Israel) |

### Aetiology and pathology

It has been suggested that an adenoma–carcinoma sequence analogous to that implicated in colonic malignancies occurs within the small intestine.[11] In a study of 12 duodenal adenocarcinomas, Achille *et al.*[12] found that 75% exhibited mutations in either the *K-ras* or *p53* genes. The mutations in *K-ras* were at sites similar to those seen in colorectal neoplasms. Younes *et al.*[13] similarly reported that *K-ras* mutations appear to play a significant role in the pathogenesis of duodenal adenocarcinomas, but are not important in ileal or jejunal tumours. Certain polyposis syndromes such as familial adenomatous polyposis (FAP) are associated with a higher risk of development of small bowel malignancies; the lifetime risk of upper GI cancer is 5–10% in an FAP patient.[14] Small bowel cancer has also been reported in association with Peutz–Jeghers syndrome.[14]

Other conditions linked to an increased frequency of adenocarcinomas of the small intestine include Crohn's disease, ulcerative colitis, cystic fibrosis, peptic ulcer disease, multiple endocrine neoplasia, von Recklinghausen's disease and coeliac disease.[3,16] Alcohol intake, cigarette smoking, dietary factors and cholecystectomy have all also been implicated in the causation of this condition.[2] A greater than eight-fold increase in second malignancies has been reported in association with small bowel tumours.[17]

## Presentation

Adenocarcinomas of the small intestines, as with all small bowel neoplasms, classically present insidiously with non-specific symptoms. Intermittent abdominal pain (42–83%), anaemia (18–75%), bleeding (13–68%), nausea and vomiting (27–34%), and weight loss (23–87%) all invoke a wide range of differential diagnoses.[3] As a result, a significant delay in diagnosis is commonly seen. In an analysis of 77 cases, the average delay to appropriate investigation was 8·2 months, with a further 4-month delay before the definitive diagnosis was made.[18] Obstruction is usually a late feature owing to the liquid contents of the small bowel; it was the presenting problem in 13% of cases in a series of 54 small bowel tumours.[10]

## Diagnosis and staging

Barium contrast studies and upper gastrointestinal endoscopy are usually sufficient for diagnosis of proximal lesions. Diagnosis of tumours located more distally may require enteroclysis or enteroscopy. Ileal cancers associated with Crohn's disease present a particular diagnostic challenge as they frequently mimic inflammatory exacerbations. CT scanning is limited in its value in assessing the primary tumour but is indicated to evaluate for distant metastases. Endoscopic ultrasound or MRI may provide additional information regarding surrounding structures to surgeons contemplating curative resection.[4] Raised serum levels of carcinoembryonic antigen (CEA) in cases of small bowel cancer have been described but there are no reports of its diagnostic potential in this condition.

Tumours of the small bowel are usually classified by the conventional TNM system and American Joint Committee on Cancer staging system[19] (Boxes 27.1 and 27.2). Howe *et al.* found that 2·7% of patients presented with stage 0 disease, 12% with stage I disease, 27% with stage II disease, 26% with stage III disease and 32·3% with stage IV disease.[8] In the same series 50% of tumours were moderately differentiated, 15% were well differentiated, 33·9% were poorly differentiated and 1·5% were anaplastic.

## Prognosis

Modern published series report 5-year survival figures of 17–45%.[1,20] In the largest series published so far, of 4995 cases of small bowel adenocarcinomas, the overall 5-year disease-free survival was 30·5% with a median survival of 17·7 months.[8] Survival was poorer in patients with duodenal tumours and patients aged over 75 years, while poorly differentiated tumours, advanced stage of tumour and the presence of distant metastases were all also adverse prognostic features. Some smaller series have, however,

---

**Box 27.1 Staging of small bowel cancer (TNM classification)[19]**

TX  Primary tumour not evaluated
T0  No pathological evidence of tumour
Tis  *In situ* cancer
T1  Invades lamina propria or submucosa
T2  Invades muscularis propria
T3  Invades < 2 cm beyond serosa or non-peritonealised perimuscular tissue (mesentery or retroperitoneum)
T4  Perforates visceral peritoneum or invades adjacent structure > 2 cm

NX  Nodes not evaluated
N0  No regional nodes
N1  Lymph node metastases

MX  Metastases not evaluated
M0  No metastases
M1  Distant metastases

---

**Box 27.2 Staging of small bowel cancer (AJCC system)[19]**

(American Joint Committee on Cancer, 1993)

Stage 0  TisN0M0
Stage 1  T1 or 2N0M0
Stage 2  T3 or 4N0M0
Stage 3  Any TN1M0
Stage 4  Any T; Any NM1

---

found no association between nodal status or tumour differentiation and outcome.[21–23]

## What is the role of surgery?

Surgical resection of the primary tumour is the mainstay of treatment for small bowel cancer. In the largest published series to date, a review of 4995 patients diagnosed with small bowel tumours between 1985 and 1995, a total of 88·1% underwent surgery.[8] This was described as cancer-directed surgery in 67·6% of cases and non-cancer-directed in 20·4% of patients. A significantly smaller percentage of patients with duodenal tumours (52%) underwent surgery with curative intent than those with ileal or jejunal tumours (90%). Most studies report curative resection rates of 40–65%.[24–26] A number of retrospective series have reported significantly improved survival in patients who have a curative resection, compared with those who do not.[6,20,21,24,26] In their series of 22 patients who underwent resection of a primary small bowel adenocarcinoma, Brucher *et al.*[20] found that a local R0 resection could be achieved in 18 patients, 1 patient had microscopic residual tumour (R1) and 3 patients had a local R2 resection. The median survival time in patients with incompletely resected tumours (3 months) was significantly shorter than in those with completely resected tumours (> 40 months).

As 22–71% of patients with duodenal adenocarcinomas present with positive regional lymph nodes, and a finite 5-year survival rate is reported in this situation, curative resection of duodenal carcinomas should always include a systematic regional lymphadenectomy, regardless of the tumour's location.[27] However, resection of small bowel neoplasms together with their lymphatic drainage is complicated by the anatomy of the superior mesenteric artery and its branches.[8] A truly radical nodal resection is not generally possible as it would disrupt this blood vessel and compromise the vascular supply to the remaining small bowel and it has been postulated that this is one of the reasons for the poor long-term survival of patients with small bowel adenocarcinoma **Evidence level III** .[28]

## Which operation should be performed?

No randomised studies have assessed the various surgical techniques available. Most published articles recommend the segmental resection of jejunal and ileal tumours *en bloc* with draining regional lymph nodes at laporotomy. There has been one report of successful laparoscopic-assisted resection for jejunal carcinoma.[29] No long-term follow up information is yet available.

Distal duodenal tumours are generally also managed by segmental resection, including the mesentery.[7] Whether a pancreaticoduodenectomy or a pancreas-preserving operation is the appropriate procedure for more proximal lesions is currently the subject of debate. No randomised controlled trials have been performed to compare the outcomes of these two procedures. Sohn *et al.*[23] reported a significant improvement in survival for patients undergoing pancreaticoduodenectomy compared with segmental resection in a series of 48 duodenal adenocarcinomas. Poor survival (14% 5-year disease-specific survival) was also described by Maher *et al.*[30] in a series of 11 cases treated by pancreas-sparing surgery. However, the former group of patients had a 25% rate of positive resection margins, whilst the latter series included seven cases of stage III and IV disease. Other published series have all shown no significant differences in survival between patients undergoing pancreaticoduodenectomy or pancreas-sparing surgery,[31–34] and Kaklamonos *et al.* reported comparable retrieval of lymph nodes with both procedures.[35] Similar morbidity and mortality rates (0–13%) have been reported for both types of surgery.[7]

The use of endoscopic resection with a submucosal injection technique has been described in the treatment of early duodenal cancers. In a Japanese series 14 tumours (20 mm or less in diameter) were resected either *en bloc* (12) or in a piecemeal fashion (2).[36] No long-term follow up data have been published **Evidence level III**.

## What is the role of non-curative surgery?

Surgical resection of the primary tumour can still be appropriate in patients with locally advanced disease or distant metastases to palliate symptoms and avoid or relieve bowel obstruction. Laparoscopic procedures may offer benefits over open operations in this group of patients. A retrospective analysis of 13 open gastrojejunostomies for symptomatic duodenal obstruction secondary to biliary malignancies versus nine laparoscopic procedures found no differences in mortality and complication rates, but a significantly shorter hospital stay was required by the laparoscopic group.[37] Endoscopic and fluoroscopic procedures are also now available for duodenal stenting **Evidence level III**.[38]

## Is neoadjuvant treatment recommended?

Data regarding the preoperative treatment of small bowel tumours consist of only one phase II trial of chemoradiation. Yeung *et al.*[39] describe four patients with duodenal adenocarcinomas who received neoadjuvant radiotherapy (1·8 Gy per day to a total dose of 50·4 Gy) with concurrent 5-fluorouracil (1 g m$^{-2}$ per day) on days 2–5 and 29–32, and mitomycin C (10 g m$^{-2}$) on day 2 only. Surgical resection was performed 4–6 weeks after completion of chemoradiation and, at histological review, the four resected duodenal specimens contained no residual tumour. These patients were still alive without recurrence at 12, 23, 35 and 40 months.[40] Therefore there is no evidence of benefit for neoadjuvant therapy at present **Evidence level III** .

## Is adjuvant chemotherapy recommended?

There have been no randomised controlled trials to assess the value of adjuvant chemotherapy after the resection of small bowel tumours and only three retrospective studies describe the use of systemic cytotoxics in this setting. Cunningham *et al.*[26] reported the use of adjuvant chemotherapy in 11 of 29 patients who underwent curative resections of ileal adenocarcinomas. Postoperative chemotherapy was given at the discretion of the supervising physician and no details of the treatment regimes used are described. A median survival of 9·5 months was seen in patients receiving chemotherapy, while those who did receive adjuvant treatment had a median survival of 26 months. However, the number of patients involved was too small to draw any statistical conclusions regarding the value of adjuvant treatment.

The other two reports of adjuvant chemotherapy document one patient each. Gillen et al.[41] treated one patient with 5-fluorouracil and folinic acid following resection of a duodenal adenocarcinoma. This patient developed recurrent disease at 18 months but was still alive at the time of the report. The patient described by Haq et al.[42] died of sepsis 3 weeks after commencing chemotherapy **Evidence level III**.

## Is palliative chemotherapy beneficial?

The use of chemotherapy in the treatment of patients with locally advanced or metastatic disease has also yet to be assessed in a randomised controlled trial. In the National Cancer Data Bank series chemotherapy was administered to 25·8% of 4995 patients with small bowel tumours between 1985–1995.[8] Chemotherapy was given to 35·4% of patients with locoregional disease and to 36·9% of those with distant metastases; 13·5% received chemotherapy after surgery and a further 4·0% were treated with a combination of surgery, chemotherapy, and radiation. For 5·3%, chemotherapy was the sole treatment modality used.

Since 1980, outcome data has been published on a total of 51 patients treated with chemotherapy for locally advanced or metastatic adenocarcinoma of the small intestine (see Table 27.2). These publications mostly consist of very small series or case reports. A variety of chemotherapy regimens have been described, but most have included 5-fluorouracil. In general, combination therapies have appeared to have more effect on survival than single agent regimens.[8] The three largest series to date are those of Jigyasu et al., Crawley et al. and Ouriel et al. Jigyasu et al.[43] reported 21 courses of various chemotherapy regimens in 14 patients with metastatic disease. One partial response and two minor responses were seen whilst nine patients had stable disease. Ouriel et al.[25] treated 12 patients with 5-fluorouracil-based regimens and described a beneficial effect on survival in both patients with metastatic disease (mean survival of 10·7 months compared with 4 months in untreated patients) and patients with locally recurrent tumours (mean survival 11·5 months compared with 7·9 months).

Most recently, Crawley et al.[44] reported the use of protracted venous infusion 5-fluorouracil-based chemotherapy in eight patients with inoperable disease. Overall a response rate of 37·5% was seen and symptomatic benefits were documented. Treatment was generally well tolerated with toxicity mainly limited to grades 0–2 **Evidence Level III**.

## What is the role of radiotherapy?

Tumours of the small bowel are generally considered to be relatively radioresistant[48] and it is well recognised that radiation treatment of the small intestine is limited by the

**Table 27.2  Published series of chemotherapy use in small bowel adenocarcinomas**

| Reference | No. of patients | Stage of disease | Treatment regimen | Overall survival (months) |
|---|---|---|---|---|
| Ouriel et al.[25] | 6 | Metastatic | 5-FU + others | 11·5 |
| | 6 | Recurrent local | 5-FU + others | |
| Jigyasu et al.[43] | 14 | Metastatic | 5-FU, adriamycin, mitomycin C, CCNU, cyclophosphamide | 9·0 |
| Haq et al.[42] | 1 | Metastatic | 5-FU | 1·0 |
| | 1 | Metastatic | 5-FU + doxorubicin | 12·0 |
| Niemic et al.[46] | 1 | Metastatic | 5-FU + doxorubicin + cisplatin | >31 |
| Zuchetti et al.[47] | 2 | Metastatic | 5-FU + doxorubicin + mitomycin | 31·5 |
| Bauer et al.[24] | 10 | Not specified | 5-FU, others | 5·5 |
| Frost et al.[49] | 1 | Locally advanced | 5-FU + radiation | 86·0 |
| Witham et al.[45] | 1 | Metastatic | 5-FU | >30·0 |
| Crawley et al.[44] | 8 | Metastatic + locally advanced | 5-FU + others | 13·0 |

potential for severe gastrointestinal toxicity. To date there have been no randomised controlled trials to assess the value of radiation in the adjuvant or palliative management of this malignancy. In a retrospective series describing 4995 cases of small bowel tumours between 1985 and 1995 from data submitted to the National Cancer Data Base, Howe et al.[8] found that 11·2% of these patients received radiation therapy. This group comprised 8·2% of patients with localised disease, 15·6% of patients with regional disease, and 11·5% of those with distant metastases. Radiotherapy was given more frequently to patients with duodenal tumours (15·4%) than those with jejunal or ileal sites of disease. No details of the radiation regimens used are described. A median survival of 15·9 months was reported for patients who underwent surgery and radiation. Further published information on the use of radiation in small bowel malignancies is minimal, consisting of seven patients treated at four separate centres, with limited survival data.[25,49–51] A patient with jejunal adenocarcinoma who received 5-fluorouracil and radiotherapy did, however, survive for 86 months.[49]

At present therefore, no meaningful conclusions can be formed regarding the use of radiotherapy in small bowel malignancies. It has been suggested that the most appropriate use of radiation might be within an intraoperative setting, using radiation to treat residual microscopic or macroscopic disease while shielding adjacent organs.[52] Clinical trials are required to assess this approach **Evidence level III**.

## Conclusions

Small intestinal adenocarcinomas are rare tumours and literature on their optimal management is sparse. Current information suggests that early surgical resection of locally confined tumours results in the best outcomes. No prospective trials have evaluated the addition of adjuvant chemotherapy, although modest response rates to chemotherapy are seen in more advanced disease. Randomised controlled trials are urgently required to assess the different surgical techniques currently used and to analyse the benefit of adjuvant chemotherapy, as well as to evaluate the response rates of different chemotherapy regimens in advanced disease. Such trials would require multicentre cooperation to achieve adequate patients numbers and the establishment of a national database of small intestine adenocarcinomas might facilitate these developments.

## Neuroendocrine tumours

A number of different neuroendocrine tumours (NET) can arise in the small intestine, including carcinoids, gastrinomas, somatostatinomas, vipomas, schwannomas, and paragangliomas. All these tumours have the potential to produce both local effects such as obstruction of the bowel and systemic symptoms through overproduction of specific bioactive peptides. The majority of NET are well-differentiated, expressing the markers of neuroendocrine differentiation such as Chromogranin A(CgA), and have low proliferative rates as assessed by nuclear Ki-67 expression. Anaplastic NET show histological similarity to small cell lung cancers and behave aggressively with rapid growth and early development of metastases.[53] By far the most common small intestine neuroendocrine tumours are carcinoids but the overall incidence of these is still only 0·28 per 100 000 per year.[54] As a consequence of their rarity, published data on the management of gastrointestinal neuroendocrine neoplasms almost always refer to a heterogeneous collection of varying histologies, dominated by carcinoids. Reports to date have also frequently combined information on small bowel neuroendocrine tumours with those arising in other primary sites, particularly the pancreas. This section will focus on the available evidence for the management of small bowel carcinoids using surgery, chemotherapy and biotherapy techniques.

## Carcinoid tumours

Twenty-nine per cent of all carcinoids occur in the small bowel with 70% of these being sited in the appendix.[55] Like adenocarcinomas, the peak incidence of this condition occurs in the sixth and seventh decade,[56] and clinical manifestations also tend to be vague. These tumours grow slowly and patients have symptoms for a median of 2 years (and up to 20 years) before diagnosis.[57] Lymph node metastases are present in 20–45% of cases at presentation.[55] Features of the carcinoid syndrome, namely intermittent abdominal cramps, diarrhoea, flushing bronchospasm, and cyanosis, are seen in approximately 10% of patients and require the release of peptides such as serotonin, kallikrein, 5-hydroxytryptophan, neurotensin and substance P. The liver is capable of metabolising large quantities of serotonin and accordingly, carcinoid syndrome only occurs when tumour tissue is drained by a blood supply that bypasses the liver, or when metastases occur within the liver itself.[58] The overall 5-year survival for all carcinoid tumours, regardless of primary site has been reported to be 50·4%.[59] However, Modlin et al.[55] found overall survival to be less than 2 years when the carcinoid syndrome is present at diagnosis.

### *What is the role of surgery?*

Surgery remains the only curative procedure for neuroendocrine tumours of the small bowel. In the case of appendiceal carcinoids, approximately 36% of them are discovered as incidental findings following surgery for "classical" appendicitis. Providing the tumour is < 1 cm (70–90% of cases) a simple appendicectomy is accepted as a curative procedure. An increased risk of metastases is seen as the size of the tumour increases and surgical intervention should therefore be extended to a right hemicolectomy for all appendiceal carcinoids that are 2 cm or larger.[60] Appendiceal carcinoid tumours less than 2 cm in size but with positive regional lymph nodes should also be managed with a formal right hemicolectomy.[61]

Neuroendocrine tumours sited elsewhere in the small bowel are associated with a high risk of lymph node metastases (ranging from 44% for a < 1 cm tumour to 85% for > 1 cm tumours). They should therefore always be resected *en bloc* with removal of lymph node drainage pathways.[62] Proximal duodenal lesions frequently require pancreaticoduodenectomy.[58]

Midgut carcinoids can frequently cause mechanical small bowel obstruction owing to either direct tumour involvement or fibrosis of the surrounding mesentery. Debulking of either locally advanced or metastatic lesions can therefore also be an important palliative procedure.[63] Partial resections can, however, expose the patient to a risk of bleeding and there is also a theoretical risk of disseminating the tumour into the peritoneum.[60]

Of patients with hepatic metastases, less than 10% are candidates for radical surgical excision. Debulking hepatic metastases may palliate systemic symptoms of carcinoid syndrome but published results are inconsistent. Response rates of approximately 50% have been reported but mean durations of symptom relief vary between 6 and 39 months. Orthoptic liver transplantations have been performed for metastatic carcinoid tumours, but at present the role of this procedure is unclear. The largest published series so far (15 transplantations between 1989 and 1994) is encouraging, however, with a 5-year survival rate of 69% in highly selected patients **Evidence level III**.[64]

### Pharmacological therapies in the management of carcinoid syndrome

Somatostatin is a 14-amino acid peptide with a short half-life (2 minutes) that inhibits the release of various hormones by binding to somatostatin receptors. The observation that somatostatin receptors are found on over 80% of carcinoid tumours led to the development of longer acting somatostatin analogues for use in both the detection and treatment of carcinoid tumours. Octreotide and lanreotide are octapeptides which bind to somatostatin receptor subtypes 2 and 5 and are the most widely tested drugs of this type. Their effects are thought to occur via induction of tyrosine phosphatases by receptor type 2 and the inhibition of calcium flux through receptor 5.[65]

To date data have been published describing the effect of somatostatin analogues in over 1000 patients with carcinoid

syndrome. Standard subcutaneous dosing of octreotide (100–300 micrograms per day divided into two or three doses) results in symptomatic improvement in a median of 60% of patients, with a biochemical response in 70%.[66] Objective tumour shrinkage occurs however in only approximately 5% of patients.[67] High dose octreotide treatment (> 3000 micrograms per day) results in similar symptomatic and biochemical responses, with objective tumour responses increased slightly to 11%.[68] Side effects of octreotide are generally mild but include fat malabsorption and gallstone formation.

Recently, slow-release formulations of both octreotide (somatostatin-LAR) and lanreotide (lanreotide-PR) have become available. Switching patients from regular octreotide to somatostatin-LAR (20–30 mg intramuscularly once per month) was associated with continuing biochemical response in 80% of patients. Similar data have been published for lanreotide-PR 30 mg given intramuscularly every 2 weeks, with a biochemical response rate of 50%. A significant improvement in quality of life was reported during treatment with the longer acting formula.[67]

Interferon alfa was adopted by Oberg *et al.* as a potential treatment for carcinoid tumours in 1982 because of its recognised capacity to stimulate natural killer cell function and control hormone secretion.[65] Data describing this treatment in over 400 patients have now been published, but there have been no randomised trials. Using doses of between 3 and 9 MU of IFNα, three to seven times a week (titrated to maintain a leucocyte count of $3 \cdot 0 \times 10^9$ per litre) has achieved biochemical response rates of 50% with significant tumour reduction in 15%. The median duration of response was 32 months and 35% of patients showed disease stabilisation with no further growth.[67] Side effects of fatigue and 'flu-like symptoms occurred in 15–20% of patients and frequently necessitated dose reductions.

The addition of IFNα may potentiate the effects of somatostatin analogues in patients previously resistant to this treatment. Tiensuu Janson *et al.*[69] reported a biochemical response rate of 77% following the introduction of 5 MU INFα three times a week but no significant tumour reduction was seen **Evidence level IIa**.

### What is the role of radiation therapy?

External irradiation has not been found to be of value in the treatment of gastrointestinal neuroendocrine tumours, with the exception of palliating pain from bone, skin, or brain metastases.[70] However, there is now some evidence to suggest that targeted irradiation may be beneficial to patients with the carcinoid syndrome. Meta-iodobenzylguanidine (MIBG) is structurally similar to noradrenaline and is therefore taken up into the majority of NET cells by the amine precursor uptake mechanism. 131-Iodine labelled MIBG has been extensively used for imaging NET and since

1987 a few centres have also published experience of its therapeutic use. Hoefnagel *et al.*[71] reported the then worldwide results of therapeutic use of [131]I in 52 patients with metastatic carcinoid disease. Symptomatic responses were seen in 65%, although only 15% had evidence of objective tumour shrinkage. Mukherjee *et al.*[72] published a retrospective analysis of [131]I-MIBG treatment of 18 patients with carcinoid syndrome. In their series, 44% achieved symptomatic improvement but a biochemical response was documented in only 17% of cases with tumour shrinkage occurring in only 11%.

More recently, a radiolabelled somatostatin analogue, [90]Y-DOTATOC, has been developed. A phase II trial of its use in 41 patients with neuroendocrine tumours resulted in symptomatic responses in 83% of those with carcinoid syndrome.[73] Objective tumour responses were seen in 24%. Both [90]Y-DOTATOC and 131-MIBG appear to be well tolerated treatments but further trials are required to fully assess these treatments **Evidence level IIb**.

### What is the role of chemotherapy?

Reviewing published literature to assess the efficacy of chemotherapy in the treatment of small bowel carcinoids is complicated by a number of issues. As previously commented, many studies have included other neuroendocrine tumours, or primary carcinoids arising elsewhere. Studies also tend to comprise small numbers of patients and only four randomised controlled trials have been published. In addition, differing criteria of response have been used, varying from symptomatic and biochemical responses to objective assessment of tumour shrinkage by formal imaging.[74] Chemotherapy does appear to be of benefit to patients with pancreatic neuroendocrine tumours. Combinations of streptozocin with 5-fluorouracil or with doxorubicin have achieved partial remissions in 40–60% of patients with advanced disease, with associated median survivals of 2 years (see Table 27.3). Classical midgut carcinoids, however, respond far less well to conventional cytotoxics. Trials of single agents have generally resulted in response rates of less than 20%. Studies of combinations of streptozocin, 5-fluorouracil, cyclophosphamide, and doxorubicin have also resulted in short lived responses in only 15–33% of patients (Table 27.3).

In contrast, a response rate of 67% has been described in anaplastic, poorly differentiated carcinoids treated with cisplatin plus etoposide, a combination commonly used to treat smallcell lung cancers.[79] This regimen has also been associated with a similar response rate in carcinoids of the foregut.

As a consequence of these findings, Oberg recommends that systemic chemotherapy as a first-line treatment approach should be reserved for tumours with a high proliferation index (> 10% Ki67) regardless of the primary site.[67] In all other cases, cytotoxic use should be limited to fit patients with unresectable tumours that have not responded to biotherapy or chemoembolisation[86] **Evidence level IIb**.

### Liver targeted therapies

It is very common for a carcinoid patient's clinical course to be dominated by liver metastates, with tumour mass causing local pain even when symptoms of the carcinoid syndrome are not present. Hepatic metastases from NET are usually hypervascular and this has provided the rationale for hepatic artery occlusion as a potential treatment. Various series of hepatic artery embolisation and hepatic artery ligations have been published. The largest describes gel foam embolisations in 29 patients with metastatic midgut carcinoids.[87] An overall objective response was seen in 52%, with a median duration of 12 months. The 5-year survival rate was 60% but there was a 10% rate of serious complications. There have been no controlled trials to compare this technique with other procedures, and side effects can include pain, haemorrhage, sepsis and hepatic dysfunction.

As it is assumed that embolisation-induced ischaemia sensitises tumour cells to cytotoxic drugs, a number of centres have now gone on to combine chemotherapy with hepatic artery occlusion (Table 27.4). The use of a doxorubicin emulsion as the embolising agent has been associated with a response rate of 95% but of median duration of 8·5 months and with significant adverse effects.[92] Hepatic arterial occlusion followed by doxorubicin plus dacarbazine chemotherapy alternated with fluorouracil plus streptozocin chemotherapy has resulted in an 80% objective regression rate with a median duration of 18 months,[93] and similar results have been confirmed in more recent series.[59] There have however been no randomised trials to compare these techniques with systemic chemotherapy alone and further studies are required to fully evaluate the role of chemoembolisation **Evidence Level III**.

### Conclusions

The large variation in tumour growth seen in patients with carcinoids arising in the small bowel calls for an individual treatment approach for each patient. Surgical resection of the primary tumour in the absence of any disseminated disease remains the only curative approach. Control of hormone-mediated symptoms by somatostatin analogues can considerably enhance quality of life in cases of carcinoid syndrome and the addition of interferon alfa may potentiate the effects of these. Classical well-differentiated midgut carcinoids do not respond well to systemic chemotherapy and such treatment should be kept in reserve for use after failure of biotherapy. Anaplastic

**Table 27.3   Published series of chemotherapy use in neuroendocrine tumours**

| Reference | No. of patients | Histology | Stage | Regimen | Response rate (%) | Time to progression (months) | Overall survival |
|---|---|---|---|---|---|---|---|
| Moertel and Hanley[75] | 118 | Carcinoid, mixed site | Metastatic | Streptozocin + 5-FU<br>Streptozocin + cyclophosphamide | 33<br>26 | | –<br>– |
| Van Hazel et al.[76] | 32 | Carcinoid | Metastatic | Dacarbazine<br>Dactinomycin | 13·3<br>5·8 | 4·2<br>2·3 | 10·9<br>6·5 |
| Engstrom et al.[77] | 172 | Carcinoid | Advanced and metastatic | STZ + 5-FU<br>Doxorubicin | 22<br>21 | 7·2<br>6·0 | 14·8<br>11·1 |
| Moertel et al.[78] | 16 | Carcinoid | Metastatic | Cyclophosphamide + methotrexate | 0 | – | – |
| Moertel et al.[79] | 18<br>27 | Anaplastic Well-differentiated | Metastatic | Etoposide + cisplatin | 67<br>7 | 8mo | 19 |
| Bukowski et al.[80] | 56<br>9 | Carcinoid | Metastatic | FAC-S*<br>FC-S† | 31<br>22 | – | 10·8<br>10·8 |
| Rougier et al.[81] | 24 | Mixed site Carcinoids + NET | Metastatic | 5-FU + doxorubicin + cisplatin | 15 | – | – |
| Di Bartolomeo et al.[82] | 38 | Mixed | Advanced Metastatic | Dacarbazine + epirubicin + 5-FU | 18 | 5 | – |
| Mitry et al.[83] | 41<br>11 | Anaplastic Well-differentiated | Advanced Metastatic | Etoposide + cisplatin | 41·5<br>9·4 | 9·2<br>8·5 | 15<br>– |
| Fjallskog et al.[84] | 36 | Mixed | Metastatic | Cisplatin + etoposide | 50 | 9 | – |
| Bajetta et al.[85] | 72 | Mixed | Advanced and metastatic | 5-FU, dacarbazine + epirubicin | 24·4 | 21 | 38 |

*5-Fluorouracil, doxorubicin, streptozocin + cyclophosphamide.
†5-Fluorouracil, streptozocin + cyclophosphamide.

carcinoids, however, have shown good response rates to cisplatin- and etoposide-containing regimens. Chemoembolisation is a promising technique but randomised trials are required to compare the effects of this invasive procedure with other management strategies and ongoing trials of targeted irradiation should further evaluate the efficacy of this new development.

## Lymphomas

In Europe and the United States, lymphomas represent 15–20% of malignant small bowel tumours. Non-Hodgkin's (NH) lymphomas of the gastrointestinal tract account for 5–20% of all NH lymphomas and the gut is the common extranodal site of disease.[94] The majority of those found in the small intestine are intermediate or high grade B-cell lymphomas. Less frequent forms are mucosa-associated lymphoid tissue lymphomas (MALTomas) and T-cell lymphomas, associated with coeliac disease. Although patients frequently undergo surgery to obtain a diagnosis, the mainstay of treatment is systemic chemotherapy dictated by the histological nature of the lymphoma. The expected 5-year survival of a primary small intestinal lymphoma is currently 25–30%.[3] IPSID (immunoproliferative small intestinal disease) represents a special form of MALTomas prevalent in the Middle East and thought to have an infective aetiology. It is associated with a 70% complete response rate with antibiotic therapy.[95]

**Table 27.4  Published series of chemotherapy use in pancreatic neuroendocrine tumours**

| Reference | No. of patients | Histology | Stage | Regimen | Response rate (months) | Time to progression (months) |
|---|---|---|---|---|---|---|
| Moertel et al.[88] | 84 | Mixed pancreatic NET | Advanced | Streptozocin | 63 | |
| | | | | Streptozocin + 5-FU | 36 | |
| Moertel et al.[89] | 20 | Mixed pancreatic NET | Advanced | Doxorubicin | 20 | |
| Moertel et al.[90] | 105 | Mixed pancreatic NET | Advanced | Streptozocin + doxorubicin | 69 | 20 |
| | | | | Streptozocin + 5-FU | 45 | 6·9 |
| | | | | Clortozocin | 30 | 6·9 |
| Eriksson et al.[92] | 31 | Mixed pancreatic NET | Advanced metastatic | Streptozocin + 5-FU | 54 | 23 |

## Sarcomas

Leiomyosarcomas are the fourth most common small bowel malignancy. The most frequent site of occurrence is the jejunum, followed by the ileum and the duodenum. These tumours often grow to a significant size before producing symptoms. Surgical resection is the only documented effective treatment for leiomyosarcomas of the small intestine, with *en bloc* resection of the neoplasm required together with the adjacent mesentery. There is no evidence for any role of chemotherapy or radiotherapy in the management of this condition.[3] Prognosis is poor with a maximum 5-year survival of 33% reported so far.[96]

## References

1   Zollinger RM, Sternfeld WC, Schreiber H. Primary neoplasms of the small intestine. *Am J Surg* 1986;**151**:654–8.
2   Neugut AI, Jacobsen JS, Suh S *et al.* The epidemiology of cancer of the small bowel. *Cancer Epidemiol Biomarker Prev* 1998;**7**:243–51.
3   Neugut AI, Marvin MR, Rella VA, Chabot JA. An overview of adenocarcinoma of the small intestine. *Oncology* 1997;**11**:529–36.
4   Gill SS, Heuman DM, Mihas AA. Small intestinal neoplasms. *J Clin Gastroenterol* 2001;**33**:267–282.
5   Attanoos R, Williams GT. Epithelial and neuroendocrine tumours of the duodenum. *Semin Diagn Pathol* 1991;**8**:149–62.
6   Miles RM, Crawford D, Duras S. The small bowel tumour problem. *Ann Surg* 1979;**189**:732–8.
7   Hutchins RR, Bani Hani A, Kojodjojo P, Ho R, Snooks SJ. Adenocarcinoma of the small bowel. *Aust NZ J Surg* 2001;**71**:428–37.
8   Howe JR, Karnell LH, Menck MR, Scott-Conner C. Adenocarcinoma of the small bowel. Review of the National Cancer Data Base. *Cancer* 1999;**86**:2693–706.
9   Chow WH, Linet MS, McLaughlin JK *et al.* Risk factors for small intestine cancer. *Cancer Causes Control* 1996;**4**:163–9.
10  Naef M, Buhlmann M, Metzger D, Baer HU. Periampullary carcinomas: A special entity of duodenal tumours. *Swiss Surg* 1999;**5**:11–13.
11  Sellner F. Investigations on the significance of the adenoma-carcinoma sequence in the small bowel. *Cancer* 1990;**66**:702–15.
12  Achille A, Baron A, Zamboni G *et al.* Molecular pathogenesis of sporadic duodenal cancer. *Br J Cancer* 1998;**77**:760–5.
13  Younes N, Fulton N, Tanaka R *et al.* The presence of K-12 ras mutations in duodenal adenocarcinomas and the absence of ras mutaions in other small bowel adenocarcinomas and carcinoid tumours. *Cancer* 1997;**79**:1804–8.
14  Heiskanen I, Kellokumpu I, Jarvinen H. Management of duodenal adenomas in 98 patients with familial adenomatous polyposis. *Endoscopy* 1999;**31**:412–16.
15  Hidalgo L, Villanueva A, Soler T *et al.* Molecular changes in adenocarcinoma of the small intestine associated with Peutz-Yeghers syndrome. *Rev Esp Enferm Dig* 1996;**88**:137–40.
16  Veyrieres M, Baillet P, Hay JM *et al.* Factors influencing long-term survival in 100 cases of small intestine primary adenocarcinoma. *Am J Surg* 1997;**173**:237–9.
17  Ripley D, Weinerman BH. Increased incidence of second malignancies associated with small bowel adenocarcinoma. *Can J Gastroenterol* 1997;**11**:65–8.
18  Maglinte DD, O'Connor K, Bessette J *et al.* The role of the physician in the late diagnosis of primary malignant tumours of the small intestine. *Am J Gastroenterol* 1991;**86**:304–8.
19  American Joint Committee on Cancer. Small intestine. In: Beahrs OH, Henson DE, Hutter RVP, Kennedy BJ, eds. *Handbook for the staging of cancer.* Philadelphia: Lippincott, 1993.
20  Brucher BL, Stein HJ, Roder JD *et al.* New aspects of prognostic factors in adenocarcinomas of the small bowel. *Hepato-gastroenerology* 2001;**48**:727–32.
21  North JH, Pack MS. Malignant tumours of the small intestine: A review of 144 cases. *Am Surg* 2000;**66**:46–51.
22  Rose DM, Hochwald SN, Klimstra DS, Brennan MF. Primary duodenal adenocarcinoma: A ten-year experience with 79 patients. *J Am Coll Surg* 1996;**183**:89–96.
23  Sohn TA, Lillemoe KD, Cameron JL *et al.* Adenocarcinoma of the duodenum: Factors influencing long-term survival. *J Gastrointest Surg* 1998;**2**:79–87.
24  Bauer RL, Palmer ML, Bauer AM *et al.* Adenocarcinoma of the small intestine: 21-year review of diagnosis, treatment and prognosis. *Ann Surg Oncol* 1994;**1**:183–8.
25  Ouriel K, Adams JT. Adenocarcinoma of the small intestine. *Am J Surg* 1984;**147**:66–71.
26  Cunningham JD, Aleali R, Aleali M *et al.* Malignant small bowel neoplasms. *Ann Surg* 1997;**225**:300–6.

27  Lai ECS, Doty JE, Irving C, Tompkins RK. Primary adenocarcinoma of the duodenum: analysis of survival. *Wld J Surg* 1988;**12**:695–701.

28  Wilson JM, Melvin DB, Gray GF, Thorbjarnarson B. Primary malignancies of the small bowel: a report of 96 cases and review of the literature. *Ann Surg* 1974;**180**:175–9.

29  Tanimura S, Higashino M, Fukunaga Y, Osugi H. Laparoscopy-assisted resection for jejunal carcinoma. *Surg Laparosc Endosc Percutan Tech* 2001;**11**:287–8.

30  Maher MM, Yeo CJ, Lillemoe KD *et al.* Pancreaticoduodenectomy for infra-ampullary duodenal pathology. *Am J Surg* 1996;**171**:62–7.

31  Almwark A, Anderson A, Lasson A. Primary carcinoma of the duodenum. *Ann Surg* 1980;**191**:13–18.

32  Delcore R, Thomas JH, Forster J *et al.* Improving respectability and survival in patients with primary duodenal carcinoma. *Am J Surg* 1993;**166**:626–31.

33  Joesting DR, Beart JRW, van Heerden JA *et al.* Improving survival in adenocarcinoma of the duodenum. *Am J Surg* 1981;**141**:228–31.

34  Lillemoe K, Imbembo AL. Malignant neoplasms of the duodenum. *Surg Gynaecol Obstet* 1980;**150**:822–6.

35  Kaklamanos IG, Bathe OF, Franceschi D *et al.* Extent of resection in the management of duodenal adenocarcinoma. *Am J Surg* 2000;**179**:37–41.

36  Hirasawa R, Ilishi H, Tatsuta M, Ishiguro S. Clinicopathologic features and endoscopic resection of duodenal adenocarcinomas and adenomas with the submucosal saline injection technique. *Gastrointest Endosc* 1997;**46**:507–13.

37  Bergamaschi R, Marvik R, Thoresen JE *et al.* Open versus laparoscopic gastrojejunostomy for palliation in advanced pancreatic cancer. *Surg Laparosc Endosc* 1998;**8**:92–6.

38  Soetikno RM, Carr-Locke DL. Expandable metal stents for gastric-outlet, duodenal and small-intestinal obstruction. *Gastro-intest Endosc Clin N Am* 1999;**9**:447–58.

39  Yeung RS, Weese JL, Hoffman JP *et al.* Neoadjuvant chemoradiation in pancreatic and duodenal carcinoma. *Cancer* 1993;**72**:2124–33.

40  Coia L, Hoffman J, Scher R *et al.* Preoperative chemoradiation for adenocarcinoma of the pancreas and duodenum. *Int J Radiat Oncol Biol Phys* 1994;**30**:161–7.

41  Gillen CD, Wilson CA, Walmsley RS *et al.* Occult small bowel adenocarcinoma complicating Crohn's disease: A report of three cases. *Postgrad Med J* 1995;**71**:172–4.

42  Haq MM, Blumenthal BJ, Culotta RJ *et al.* Small bowel adenocarcinoma: A report of three cases and review of literature. *Texas Med* 1985;**81**:51–3.

43  Jigyasu D, Bedikian AY, Stroehlein JR. Chemotherapy for primary adenocarcinoma of the small bowel. *Cancer* 1984;**53**:23–5.

44  Crawley C, Ross P, Nowman A, Hill A, Cunningham D. The Royal Marsden experience of small bowel adenocarcinoma treated with protracted venous infusion 5-flourouracil. *Br J Cancer* 1998;**78**:508–10.

45  Witham M, Harnett PR. Adenocarcinoma of the duodenum with liver metastases. Complete remission and long-term survival with 5-flourouracil chemotherapy – a case report. *Am J Clin Oncol* 1996;**19**:305–6.

46  Niemiec TR, Senekjian EK, Montag AG. Adenocarcinoma of the small intestine presenting as an ovarian mass. *J Reproduct Med* 1989;**43**:917–20.

47  Zuchetti F, Bellantone R, Frontera D *et al.* Adenocarcinoma of the small intestine. *Int Surg* 1991;**76**:230–4.

48  Herbsman H, Wetstein L, Rosen Y. Tumours of the small intestine. *Curr Probl Sur* 1980;**17**:121–8.

49  Frost DB, Mercado PD, Tyrell JS. Small bowel cancer: A 30 year review. *Ann Surg Oncol* 1994;**1**:290–5.

50  Sakker S, Ware CC. Carcinoma of the duodenum: comparison of surgery, radiotherapy and chemotherapy. *Br J Surg* 1973;**60**:867–72.

51  Temple DF, Adenocarcinoma of the small intestine (25 year review-Roswell Park). *J Florida Med Assoc* 1986;**73**:526–8.

52  Abe M, Takahashi M, Yabumoto E *et al.* Clinical experiences with intraoperative radiotherapy of locally advanced cancers. *Cancer* 1980;**45**:40–8.

53  Solcia E, Rindi G, Paolotti D *et al.* Clinicopathological profile as a basis for classification of the endocrine tumours of the gastroenteropancreatic tract. *Ann Oncol* 1999;**10**:S9–S15.

54  Olney JR, Urdenata LF, Al-Jurf AS *et al.* Carcinoid tumours of the gastrointestinal tract. *Am Surg* 1985;**51**:37–41.

55  Modlin Im, Sandor A. An analysis of 8305 cases of carcinoid tumours. *Cancer* 1997;**79**:813–29.

56  Kulke MH, Meyer RJ. Carcinoid tumours. *N Engl J Med* 1999;**340**:858–68.

57  Vinik AI, McCleod MK, Fig LM *et al.* Clinical features, diagnosis and localisation of carcinoid tumours and their management. *Gastroenterol Clin N Am* 1989;**8**:865–9.

58  Moertel CG. Treatment of the carcinoid tumour and the malignant carcinoid syndrome. *J Clin Oncol* 1983;**1**:727–33.

59  Kaltsas G, Mukherjee JJ, Plowman PN, Grossman AB. The role of chemotherapy in the nonsurgical management of malignant neuroendocrine tumours. *Clin Endocrinol* 2001;**55**:575–87.

60  Falconi M, Bettini R, Scarpa A *et al.* Surgical strategy of gastrointestinal neuroendocrine tumours. *Ann Oncol* 2001;**12**:S101–S103.

61  Deans GT, Spence RA. Neoplastic lesions of the appendix. *Br J Surg* 1995;**82**:299–306.

62  Basson MD, Ahlman H, Wangberg B *et al.* Biology and management of the midgut carcinoid. *Am J Surg* 1993;**165**:288–97.

63  Sweeney JF, Rosemurgy AS. Carcinoid tumours of the gut. *Cancer Control* 1997;**4**:18–24.

64  Le Treut YP, Delpero JR, Dousset B *et al.* Results of liver transplantation in the treatment of metastatic neuroendocrine tumours. A 31-case French multicentric report. *Ann Surg* 1997;**225**:355–64.

65  Oberg K. Carcinoid tumours: current concepts in diagnosis and treatment. *Oncologist* 1998;**3**:339–45.

66  Harris A, Redfern JS. Octreotide treatment of carcinoid syndrome: Analysis of published dose titration data. *Aliment Pharmacol Ther* 1995;**9**:387–94.

67  Oberg K. Chemotherapy and biotherapy in the treatment of neuroendocrine tumours. *Ann Oncol* 2001;**12**:S111–S114.

68  Imam H, ErikssonB, Lukinius A *et al.* Induction of apoptosis in neuroendocrine tumours of the digestive system during treatment with somatostatin analogues. *Acta Oncol* 1997;**36**:607–14.

69  Tiensuu Janson E, Ahlström H, Andersson T, *et al.* Octreotide and interferon alfa: a new combination for the treatment of malignant carcinoid tumours. *Eur J Cancer* 1992;**28**:1647A–50A.

70  Keane TS, Rider WP, Harwood HR *et al.* Whole body radiation in the management of the metastatic carcinoid tumour. *Int J Radiat Oncol Biol Phys* 1981;**7**:1519–21.

71  Hoefnagel CA. Metaiodobenzylguanidine and somatostatin in oncology: role in management of neural crest tumours. *Eur J Nucl Med* 1994;**43**:336–43.

72  Mukerjee JJ, Kaltsas GA, Islam N *et al.* Treatment of metastatic carcinoid tumours, phaeochromocytoma, paraganglioma and medullary carcinoma of the thyroid with [131]I-meta-iodobenzylguanidine. *Clin Endocrinol* 2001;**55**:47–60.

73  Waldherr C, Pless M, Maecke HR *et al.* The clinical value of [90]Y-DOTA-D-Phe-Tyr-octreotide ([90]Y-DOTATOC) in the treatment of neuroendocrine tumours: a clinical phase II study. *Ann Oncol* 2001;**12**:941–5.

74  Veenhof CHN. Pancreatic endocrine tumours, immunotherapy and gene therapy: chemotherapy and interferon therapy of endocrine tumours. *Ann Oncol* 1999;**10**(Suppl.4):S185–S187.

75  Moertel CG, Hanley JA. Combination chemotherapy trials in metastatic carcinoid tumours and the malignant carcinoid syndrome. *Cancer Clin Trials* 1979;**2**:327–34.

76  Van Hazel GA, Rubin J, Moertel CG. Treatment of metastatic carcinoid tumour with dactinomycin and dacarbazine. *Cancer Treat Rep* 1983;**67**:583–5.

77  Engstrom PF, Lavin PT, Moertel CG *et al.* Streptozocin plus fluorouracil versus doxorubicin therapy for metastatic carcinoid tumour. *J Clin Oncol* 1984;**2**:1255–9.

78  Moertel CG, O'Connell MJ, Reitemeier RJ, Rubin J. Evaluation of combined cyclophosphamide and methotrexate therapy in the

treatment of metastatic carcinoid tumour and malignant carcinoid syndrome. *Cancer Treat Rep* 1984;**68**:665–7.

79  Moertel CG, Kvols LK, O'Connell MJ, Rubin J. Treatment of neuroendocrine carcinomas with combined etoposide and cisplatin. Evidence of major therapeutic in the anaplastic variants of these neoplasms. *Cancer* 1991;**68**:227–32.

80  Bukowski Rm, Johnson KG, Peterson RF *et al.* A phase II trial of combination chemotherapy in patients with metastatic carcinoid tumours. A Southwest Oncology Group Study. *Cancer* 1987;**60**:2891–5.

81  Rougier P, Oliveira J, Ducreux M *et al.* Metastatic carcinoid and islet cell tumours of the pancreas: phase II trial of the efficacy of combination chemotherapy with 5-fluorouracil, doxorubicin and cisplatin. *Eur J Cancer* 1991;**27**:1380–2.

82  Di Bartolomeo M, Bajetta E, Bochicchio AM *et al.* A phase II trial of dacarbazine, flourouracil and epirubicin patients with neuroendocrine tumours. A study by the Italian Trials in Medical Oncology Group. *Ann Oncol* 1995;**6**:77–9.

83  Mitry E, Baudin E, Ducreux M *et al.* Treatment of poorly differentiated neuroendocrine tumours with etoposide and cisplatin. *Br J Cancer* 1999;**81**:1351–5.

84  Fjallskog ML, Granberg DP, Welin Sl *et al.* Treatment with cisplatin and etoposide in patients with neuroendocrine tumours. *Cancer* 2001;**92**:1101–7.

85  Bajetta E, Ferrari L, Procopio G *et al.* Efficacy of a chemotherapy combination for the treatment of metastatic neuroendocrine tumours. *Ann Oncol* 2002;**13**:614–21.

86  Rougier P, Mitry E. Chemotherapy in the treatment of neuroendocrine malignant tumours. *Digestion* 2000;**62**(Suppl.1):73–8.

87  Eriksson BK, Larsson EG, Skogseid BM *et al.* Liver embolisations of patients with malignant neuroendocrine gastrointestinal tumours. *Cancer* 83;**2**:293–301.

88  Moertel CG, Hanley JA, Johnson LA. Streptozocin alone compared with streptozocin plus fluorouracil in the treatment of advanced islet-cell carcinoma. *N Engl J Med* 1980;**303**:1189–94.

89  Moertel CG, Lavin PT, Hahn RG. Phase II trial of doxorubicin therapy for advanced islet cell carcinoma. *Cancer Treat Rep* 1982;**66**:1567–9.

90  Moertel CG, Lefkopoulo M, Lipsitz *et al.* Streptozocin-doxorubicin, streptozocin-fluorouracil or chlortozocin in the treatment of advanced islet-cell carcinoma. *N Engl J Med* 1992;**326**:519–23.

91  Eriksson B, Oberg K. An update of the medical management of malignant endocrine pancreatic tumours. *Acta Oncol* 1993;**32**:203–8.

92  Clouse ME, Perry L, Stuart K, Stokes KR. Hepatic arterial chemoembolisation for metastatic neuroendocrine tumours. *Digestion* 1994;**55**(Suppl.3):2–97.

93  Moertel CG, Johnson CM, McKusick MA *et al.* The management of patients with advanced carcinoid tumours and islet cell carcinomas. *Ann Intern Med* 1994;**120**:302–9.

94  D'Amore F, Chhristen BE, Brincker H *et al.* Clinicopathological features and prognostic features in extra-nodal non-Hodgkin's lymphomas. *Eur J Cancer* 1991;**27**:1201–8.

95  Salimi M, Spinelli JJ. Chemotherapy of Mediterranean abdominal lymphoma: retrospective comparison of chemotherapy protocol in Iranian patients. *Am J Clin Oncol* 1996;**19**:18–22.

96  Blanchard DK, Budde JM, Hatch III GF *et al.* Tumours of the small intestine. *Wld J Surg* 2000;**24**:421–9.

# 28 The treatment of carcinoma of the colon and rectum

*M Michael, JR Zalcberg*

Colorectal cancer (CRC) accounts for the fourth highest number of cancer cases and the third highest cancer mortality rate in the developed world. When localised to the bowel wall and/or regional lymph nodes, it is highly treatable, often curable. Treatment in this setting is thus aimed towards a reduction in disease recurrence. Advanced CRC, however, is not curable in the majority of cases, with treatment achieving only a modest increase in overall survival (OS). The aim here is therefore to maintain or improve quality of life (QoL) with the reduction of disease-related symptoms (DRS).

In this chapter we will provide an evidence-based overview for the treatment approaches of both localised and advanced CRC, in an attempt to answer common questions faced by clinicians in this discipline (Figure 28.1). The basis of management needs to be both individualised and multidisciplinary. The scope of this chapter, however, will not include a discussion of colorectal tumour biology, its aetiology, including premalignant conditions and familial syndromes, or strategies for its prevention or screening.

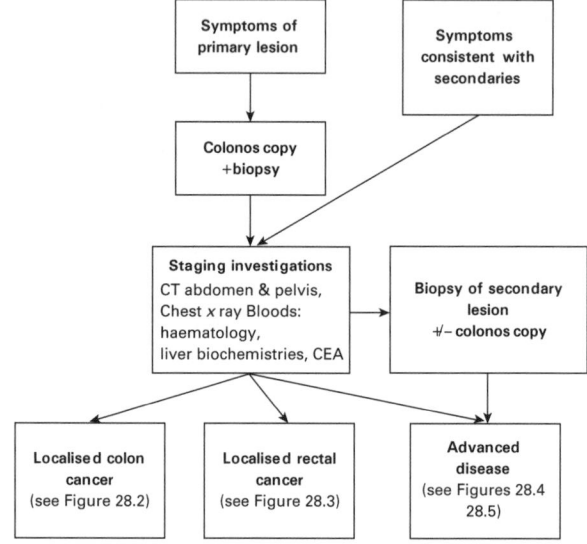

**Figure 28.1** The management schema for newly diagnosed colorectal cancer. CEA, carcinoembryonic antigen; CT, computed tomography; CXR, chest *x* ray

## Background

### Incidence and mortality rates

Worldwide 700 000 new cases of CRC are reported each year accounting for the fourth highest number of cancer cases after prostate, breast and lung in the developed world.[1] Its incidence increases with age from 0·7/100 000 at ages 20–24 to 430/100 000 at 80–85, increasing linearly from the 5th decade of life, with a male preponderance, 1·5 relative to females, at all ages.[1,2] It accounts for the third highest cancer mortality rate, with annual mortality rates about 50% relative to its incidence.[2]

CRC shows a significant geographical variation, varying at least 10-fold from developing to developed countries, and together with migrant studies reflects the importance of environmental effects upon its aetiology.[3,4] Rectal cancer has a similar geographical distribution as colon cancer. However, there is less variation between countries.[5]

### Pathology

Overall for the large bowel, 69% of the cancers arise in the colon and 31% in the rectum.[6] The anatomical localisation of colonic cancers is as follows: caecum (22%), ascending colon (12%), transverse colon (10%), descending colon (7%) and sigmoid colon (35%). Over several decades there has been a distal to proximal shift in the anatomical distribution of CRC.[7] Adenocarcinomas account for 90–95% of colorectal cancers, classified as well to poorly differentiated. Less common variants include mucinous and signet ring cell adenocarcinomas, poorly differentiated cancers with some neuroendocrine features. Rare histological types include squamous cell, adenosquamous, small cell and medullary carcinomas, sarcomas (usually leiomyosarcomas) and carcinoids.

**Table 28.1** The TNM staging classification of colorectal cancer and its comparison to the Aster–Coller Modification of Dukes' and AJCC/UICC staging systems[13,14]

| TNM classification | | AJCC/UICC Stage | TNM into stage groupings | Aster–Coller Modification of Dukes' staging |
|---|---|---|---|---|
| Primary tumour (T) | Tx: Primary tumour cannot be assessed | 0 | Tis, N0, M0 | |
| | T0: No evidence of primary tumour | I | T1, N0, M0 | A |
| | | | T2, N0, M0 | |
| | Tis: Carcinoma *in situ*: intraepithelial or invasion of the lamina propria* | II | T3, N0, M0 | B1 |
| | | | T4, N0, M0 | B2 |
| | T1: Tumour invades submucosa | III | Any T, N1, M0 | C1 |
| | | | Any T, N2, M0 | C2 |
| | T2: Tumour invades muscularis propria | IV | Any T, Any N, M1 | D[§] |
| | T3: Tumour invades through the muscularis propria into the subserosa, or into non-peritonealised pericolic or perirectal tissues[†] | | | |
| | T4: Tumour directly invades other organs or structures, and/or perforates visceral peritoneum[‡] | | | |
| Regional lymph nodes (N)[†] | N0: No regional lymph node metastasis | | | |
| | NX: Regional nodes cannot be assessed | | | |
| | N1: Metastasis in 1 to 3 regional lymph nodes | | | |
| | N2: Metastasis in 4 or more regional lymph nodes | | | |
| Distant metastasis (M) | MX: Distant metastasis cannot be assessed | | | |
| | M0: No distant metastasis | | | |
| | M1: Distant metastasis | | | |

*Tis includes cancer cells confined within the glandular basement membrane (intraepithelial) or lamina propria (intramucosal) with no extension through the muscularis mucosae into the submucosa.
[†]A tumour nodule greater than 3 mm in diameter in the perirectal or pericolic fat without histologic evidence of a residual node in the nodule is classified as regional perirectal or pericolic lymph node metastasis. A tumour nodule 3 cm or less in diameter is classified in the T category as a non-contiguous extension, that is T3.
[‡]Direct invasion in T4 includes invasion of other segments of the colorectum by way of the serosa; for example, invasion of the sigmoid colon by a carcinoma of the caecum.
[§]Added subsequently to the classification.

## Staging classification of cancers of the colon and rectum

The prognosis of CRC is determined by pathological (postresection) and radiological findings indicating the depth of tumour penetration, extent of involved lymph nodes and presence of distant metastases.[8–12] The TNM (Tumour, Node, Metastasis) classification, has been accepted as the preferred staging system rather than the older Dukes' or the Modified Astler-Coller classification.[13,14] However, the TNM system has substantial similarities with these other classifications when grouped into stages, emphasising its prognostic relevance (Table 28.1).

## Clinical staging of colorectal cancer

Following the diagnosis of the primary lesion, or metastatic site, radiological imaging, usually CT scan of the chest, abdomen and pelvis, are performed to assess the anatomical extent of locoregional and distant disease (Figure 28.1). Carcino-embryonic antigen (CEA) is not a recommended screening test for the diagnosis.[15] For rectal primaries, endorectal ultrasound and pelvic MRI provide additional detail on the extent of rectal wall penetration, perirectal lymph node involvement and invasion of adjacent viscera. Positron emission tomography is proving useful in staging, for the detection of otherwise

**Table 28.2** Local failure, disease-free survival (DFS) and overall survival (OS) rates for resected colonic cancer[18-21]

| AJCC/UICC stage | TNM stage | Local failure rates (%) | 5-year DFS rates (%) | 5-year OS rates (%) |
|---|---|---|---|---|
| Stage 0 | Tis, N0, M0 | | | 100 |
| Stage I | T1, N0, M0 | 3 | 90 | >90 |
| | T2, N0, M0 | | | |
| Stage II | T3, N0, M0 | 2 | 75 | 85 |
| | T4, N0, M0 | 33 | 64–70 | 64–75 |
| Stage III | Any T, N1, M0 | 32–40 | 38–60 | 45–60 |
| | Any T, N2, M0 | | | |
| Stage IV | Any T, Any N, M1 | | | 3 |

occult metastases not visualised by structural imaging and for the work-up of patients being considered for curative hepatic metastectomy.[16,17]

## Patterns of spread

Cancers of the colon and rectum can spread either by lymphatics, or haematogenously, via the portal and systemic circulation and via transcoelemic routes.

Spread to lymph nodes is common, increasing with local stage, and is a major adverse prognostic factor, as illustrated in the OS seen for patients with resected Dukes' C versus B disease (Table 28.2). Spread generally follows an orderly progression from the locoregional to retroperitoneal and subsequently to mediastinal and supraclavicular nodes. Atypical or retrograde nodal spread can occur by aberrant lymphatic channels or by lymphatic obstruction.[22,23]

Up to 8–25% of patients present *de novo* with metastases, up to a third of these have metastases limited to the liver.[24-28] The liver similarly represents the commonest site of abdominal relapse following resection of the localised primary ranging from 17–57%.[21,29] The lungs are the next most common site either isolated in 3–9% or combined with other sites in 21–30%.[30-32] An analysis of necropsy data from 1541 patients who had died from CRC found that other sites of metastases included adrenals (31%), bone marrow (27%), brain (11%), skin (15·4%), kidney (13%), pleura (12%), pancreas (9%), abdominal wall, ureter/bladder and gallbladder (4%).[33]

Peritoneal spread by implantation can occur at diagnosis or as a result of surgical manipulation of the primary. During surgical manipulation, implantation of exfoliated cancer cells can occur within abdominal wounds, laparoscopic port sites or into the bowel lumen with deposits in the anastomosis or in the bowel distally.

## Is the categorisation of patients with CRC into prognostic groups of clinical utility?

From various lines of evidence, several prognostic factors have been identified at diagnosis to be predictive of survival. Only recently have there been attempts to consolidate all these factors into predictive models for OS, and hence indicate those patients that should be considered for therapy in the localised or advanced setting.

### Prognostic factors for resectable local disease

#### Patient factors

Patients less than 40 years of age at presentation have tumours that tend to be poorly differentiated and more advanced in stage relative to the elderly. Even stage for stage relative to the elderly, their disease has a more aggressive course with a poorer OS.[34-36] However, a pooled analysis of 3351 patients, from three randomised trials of adjuvant postoperative chemotherapy versus observation, found no significant interaction between age and efficacy in terms of OS and time to recurrence.[37] Most prospective trials and retrospective series have identified females as having better outcome following curative resection.[38-44]

#### Tumour-related factors

The pathological stage is the single most important prognostic factor in terms of disease-free survival (DFS) and OS. The local and distant failure rates for surgically resected colon cancer increase with stage together with a corresponding decrease in OS (Table 28.2).[18-21] Rectal cancers have local recurrence rates ranging from 0% for stage A, to 25–35% in stage B2 and 40% in stage C.[9,19-21,45-48]

**Table 28.3** Categorisation of pathologic prognostic factors (factors linked to outcome) and predictive factors (factors predicting response to therapy) in CRC: College of American Pathologists Consensus Statement 1999[49]

| Categories and their criteria | Factors included into category |
|---|---|
| *Category I*<br>Factors definitely proven to be of prognostic importance based on evidence from multiple statistically robust published trials used in patient management | Pathological (p) T and pN category of TNM staging<br>Blood or lymphatic vessel invasion<br>Residual tumour: positive margins<br>Elevated preoperative CEA |
| *Category IIA*<br>Factors extensively studied and shown to be of prognostic and/or predictive value, sufficient to be included in a pathological report, but remain to be validated by statistically robust studies | Tumour grade<br>Radial margin status (resected specimens with non-peritonealised surfaces)<br>Residual tumour post neoadjuvant therapy |
| *Category IIB*<br>Factors shown to be promising in multiple studies but lacking sufficient data for inclusion into category I or IIA | Histological type<br>Histological features associated with MSI*<br>MSI-*H*† DCC‡ gene allelic loss<br>Tumour border configuration: pushing versus infiltrating |
| *Category III*<br>Factors not sufficiently studied to determine their prognostic value | DNA content. Other molecular markers except those in IIB; perineural invasion; microvessel density; tumour-cell associated proteins or carbohydrates; peritumoural fibrosis and inflammatory response; focal neuroendocrine differentiation; nuclear organising regions; proliferation indices |
| *Level IV*<br>Factors well studied and shown to have no prognostic significance | Tumour size<br>Gross tumour infiltration |

*Histologic features associated with microsatellite instability (MSI): host lymphoid response to tumour, medullary, or mucinous histologic type.
†MSI-*H*: high degree of MSI.
‡DCC: deleted in colon cancer.

The College of American Pathologists have formulated a consensus statement addressing prognostic factors in CRC following a review of all medical literature and their stratification based upon the level of evidence (Table 28.3).[49] Factors in Level I, definitively proven to be of prognostic significance based on evidence from multiple statistically robust published trials and used in management, include: pathological (p)TNM staging, regional lymph node metastases, blood or lymphatic vessel invasion, positive resection margins.[49]

Several investigators have confirmed that obstruction is an independent prognostic factor predictive of poorer survival.[38,50–52] Rectal primaries are associated with a poorer prognosis, reflecting a greater tendency for local recurrence relative to colon primaries.[40,53–55] Within the colon, it appears that right-sided tumours are associated with a better prognosis and benefit from adjuvant chemotherapy.[43,54,56] This may reflect the differing distribution and importance of prognostic markers such as *p53* and microsatellite instability (MSI) in proximal versus distal tumours.[57,58]

## Prognostic factors for advanced disease

A multivariate analysis of 3825 patients with advanced CRC has been performed to identify the clinical determinants of survival with 5-fluorouracil (5-FU)-based regimens.[59] The data was drawn from three phase II and 19 randomised phase III trials, and was separated into a learning and validation set. Twenty-three potential predictors, laboratory, clinical and tumour-related, were assessed and those found to be significant are summarised in

**Table 28.4** Clinical determinants of survival in patients with advanced CRC treated with 5-FU-based regimens: categorisation into risk groups based on a multivariate analysis of 3825 patients[59]

| Risk groups | Variables (laboratory, clinical, tumour)* | Median survival (months) |
|---|---|---|
| Low | ECOG 0/1, only 1 tumour site | 15 |
| Intermediate | ECOG 0/1, > 1 tumour site, ALP < 300 U litre$^{-1}$ | 10·7 |
| | or | |
| | ECOG > 1, only 1 tumour site, WBC count < 10 × 10$^9$ litre$^{-1}$ | |
| High | ECOG 0/1, > 1 tumour site, ALP ≥ 300 U litre$^{-1}$ | 6·1 |
| | or | |
| | ECOG > 1, > 1 tumour site, WBC count > 10 × 10$^9$/litre$^{-1}$ | |

*Abbreviations: ALP, alkaline phosphatase; ECOG, Eastern Cooperative Oncology Group; WBC, white blood cell

**Table 28.5** Clinical factors of independent prognostic importance ($P < 0.05$) for survival in patients with CRC derived from recent trials

| Parameter | Clinical state or therapy* | Reference |
|---|---|---|
| *Patient factors: clinical* | | |
| Performance status | Unresected hepatic metastases | 60, 61 |
| | 5-FU-based regimens | 62–65 |
| | Oxaliplatin-based regimen | 66 |
| | Irinotecan-based regimens | 67, 68 |
| Weight loss | Hepatic metastases | 60, 69 |
| Age | Irinotecan | 70 |
| Asymptomatic state | Hepatic metastases | 71 |
| | 5-FU + LV in advanced disease | 63, 69 |
| *Patient factors: laboratory* | | |
| ↓ Serum albumin | Hepatic metastases | 60 |
| ↑ Lactate dehydrogenase | Oxaliplatin-based regimens | 66 |
| | Irinotecan-based regimens | 68 |
| Haemoglobin > 11 g litre$^{-1}$ | Irinotecan v BSC | 67 |
| ↑ Se alkaline phosphatase | Hepatic metastases | 71 |
| | Oxaliplatin-based regimens | 66 |
| *Tumour-related factors* | | |
| Liver v non-liver metastases | Irinotecan-based regimens | 67, 68 |
| | Oxaliplatin-based regimens | 66 |
| | 5-FU-LV regimens | 65 |
| Extent of liver involvement > 30% | Unresected hepatic metastases | 60, 61 |
| No. of involved organs | Irinotecan-based regimens | 67, 68 |
| | Oxaliplatin-based regimens | 66, 70 |

*BSC, best supportive care.

Table 28.4.[59] Patients were hence subdivided into three risk groups, low to high, based on a combination of these factors, with corresponding median survivals of 15, 10·7 and 6·1 months, respectively.[59] These findings have also been confirmed by other randomised phase III trials and meta-analyses (Table 28.5).

**Table 28.6  Oncogenes assessed for prognostic significance for survival in patients with colorectal cancer**

| Marker and method of evaluation | Clinical state | Prediction of survival | Reference |
|---|---|---|---|
| *p53* | | | |
| IMH | Dukes' B2 and C; D | No prognostic value | 72, 73 |
| | Stages I–III rectal cancer | IPF for DFS | 74 |
| PCR | Dukes' D | No prognostic value | 75 |
| | Dukes' B and C | No prognostic value | 76 |
| PCR, IMH | Dukes' C | Normal *p53*, IPF for survival benefit by chemotherapy | 58 |
| *Ras mutation* | | | |
| PCR | Stages A–D | Negative IPF for survival | 77, 78 |
| *c-myc* | | | |
| PCR | Stages A–D | ↑ Expression with normal *p53* correlated with better survival | 79 |
| *EGFR* | | | |
| IMF | Stages A–D | ↑ Expression negative IPF for survival | 80 |
| *Ras + p53 mutations* | | | |
| PCR | Stages A–D | Poor prognosis | 79 |
| *TGF-β-1* | | | |
| NR | Stages A–D | Poor prognosis for Stage D treated with chemotherapy | 81 |
| *p21* | | | |
| IMH | T1–4, N0–3, M0; NR | IPF for survival | 82, 83 |
| *Chromosomal imbalance* | | | |
| SNP | Dukes' A and B | Allelic imbalance in chromosome 8p and/or, 18q, IPF for survival | 84 |
| *DCC* | | | |
| IMH | Stages II and III | Loss of DCC IPF for reduced survival | 85 |
| *Chromosomal LOH, TGF-β-1 and MSI* | | | |
| PCR | Stage II and III + 5-FU-based chemotherapy | 18q allele + MSI-S and TGF-β-1 mutation + MSI-H IPF for OS and DFS following adjuvant chemotherapy | 41 |

Abbreviations: DCC, deleted in colon cancer; DFS, disease-free survival; EGFR, epidermal growth factor receptor; IMH, immunohistochemistry; IPF, independent prognostic factor; LOH, loss of heterozygosity; MSI, microsatellite instability; MSI-H, -high; MSI-S, -stable; NR, not reported; OS, overall survival; SNP, single nucleotide polymorphism; TGF, transforming growth factor

## Molecular prognostic factors for localised and advanced disease

A significant number of prognostic markers have been examined in an attempt to identify correlations with outcome, but as a whole do not provide a definite argument for their clinical utility (Tables 28.6 and 28.7).[104] **Evidence level III, Grade B**. There is marked heterogeneity of stages and treatment within and between studies as well as of the methodology for marker evaluation. Often single markers are assessed; however, other covariables may be significant in combination. The correlations drawn from one population in the past may not be applicable to patients presenting in 2002, given recent advances in treatment and diagnostic approaches.

Several large studies reflect these problems. A meta-analysis of 28 published articles, involving 4416 patients, has evaluated the importance of *p53* (23 using immunohistochemistry (IMH), eight DNA sequencing).[105] The IMH studies showed that *p53* status correlated

**Table 28.7   Other molecular markers assessed for prognostic significance in patients with colorectal cancer**

| Marker | Method of evaluation | Clinical state or therapy | Prediction of survival | Reference |
|---|---|---|---|---|
| *Cell proliferation* | | | | |
| PCNA | IMH | Stage D | Positive correlation with OS | 86 |
| *Apoptosis markers* | | | | |
| Bcl-2 | IMH | Stages A–D | No association | 87 |
| *Angiogenesis* | | | | |
| VEGF | IMH | Stages A–D | ↑ Expression negative IPF for OS | 88 |
| TP | PCR | Stage D | ↓ Expression correlated with ↑ OS | 89, 90 |
| *Adhesion molecules* | | | | |
| CD-44 and cytokeratin-19 | IMH | Dukes' B and C | ↑ Expression positive IPF for OS and DFS | 91 |
| E-cadherin | IMH | NR | ↓ Expression negative IPF for OS | 92 |
| Beta-catenin | IMH | Localised rectal cancer | No correlation for DFS | 93 |
| *Microsatellite instability* | | | | |
| | PCR | Stages I–IV | MSI-H IPF for survival | 94 |
| | PCR | Stages B2, C | MSI-H and 8p allelic imbalance, IPF for OS and recurrence | 95 |
| | PCR | Stages A–D | IPF for prolonged survival | 96 |
| *Targets of chemotherapy or metabolic enzymes* | | | | |
| TS | PCR | Stage D | ↓ Expression correlated with better survival | 75 |
| | IMH | Stage D | ↓ Expression correlated with poorer survival | 97, 98 |
| | IMH | Stages A–D | ↓ Expression correlated with poorer survival | 99 |
| | IMH | Dukes' B2 and C, | No correlation with OS and DFS | 72 |
| | IMH | Stages B and C | Expression inversely related to survival for surgery alone | 42 |
| TS polymorphism | PCR | Stage C | Double repeat polymorphism 2RR/2RR (↓ TS) correlated with ↑ survival | 100 |
| DPD | PCR | Stage D | Low gene expression correlated with ↑ survival | 75 |
| *General markers* | | | | |
| Sialyl-Le(x) antigen | IMH | Stages II–IV | IPF for OS in stages II and III | 101 |
| CEA | Serum analysis | Stages IV + 5-FU + LV | Negative IPF for survival | 102, 103 |

Abbreviations: CEA, carcinoembryonic antigen; DFS, disease-free survival; DPD, dihydropyrimidine dehydrogenase; IMH, immunohistochemistry; IPF, independent prognostic factor; MSI, micro-satellite instability; MSI-H, -high; NR, not reported; OS, overall survival; PCNA, proliferating cell nuclear antigen; TP, thymidine phosphorylase; TS, thymidylate synthase

significantly in surgically treated patients for DFS but not for OS, and the reverse order was found after DNA sequencing of *p53*. No influence was observed for patients treated by surgery and radiotherapy. The conclusions are limited, as the analysis was not based on individual patient data.[105]

## Are prognostic markers of any use?

In terms of postoperative adjuvant therapy, at present treatment is based on pathological stage, as will be discussed below. For advanced disease, patients in poor prognostic groupings may benefit the most from treatment, in terms of palliative benefit or OS, however they are often excluded from clinical trials. Performance status is by far the most widely reported and consistent factor across several studies of advanced CRC **Evidence level Ia, Grade A**. This is not unexpected as it provides a crude measure of global QoL and disease load. However, performance status also can determine the tolerance and hence aggressiveness of therapy as well as physician bias. At present the use of molecular prognostic markers to guide therapy in patients with CRC is not recommended[106] **Evidence level III, Grade B**.

## The treatment of localised colon cancer

### The importance of surgical technique and the surgeon for the treatment of localised disease

The primary treatment of localised colonic cancer is hemicolectomy with ligation of the major vascular supply and wide regional lymphadenectomy. The aim is to achieve histologically clear resection margins both at the proximal and distal ends and radially. Preoperative chemoradiotherapy may be required prior to *en bloc* resection in cases where the primary invades adjacent viscera (Figure 28.2).

The lymph node dissection allows for staging in addition to prognostic information as discussed above. The surgical technique and the surgeon do have an impact on patient outcome. A retrospective analysis of the INT-0089 trial, which randomised patients with resected stage II and III disease to receive one of four different 5-FU-based adjuvant regimens, found a positive correlation between the number of nodes removed and survival, independent of the number of pathologically involved nodes ($P = 0.0001$ for overall, disease-specific and DFS). Survival rose as more nodes were removed, implying a greater likelihood of identifying true node-negative and -positive cases.[12] Retrospective surgical series have well documented that surgical technique as well as survival rates vary considerably amongst surgeons, based on their level of special interest.[107,108] Laparoscopic techniques are being increasingly used, but until randomised trials are completed they cannot be considered as standard **Evidence level III, Grade B**.

### Adjuvant chemotherapy for stage II and III colon cancer: who and with what?

#### Who to treat?

Patients with Dukes' C and B2 colon cancer after surgical resection alone have a 5-year survival rate of between

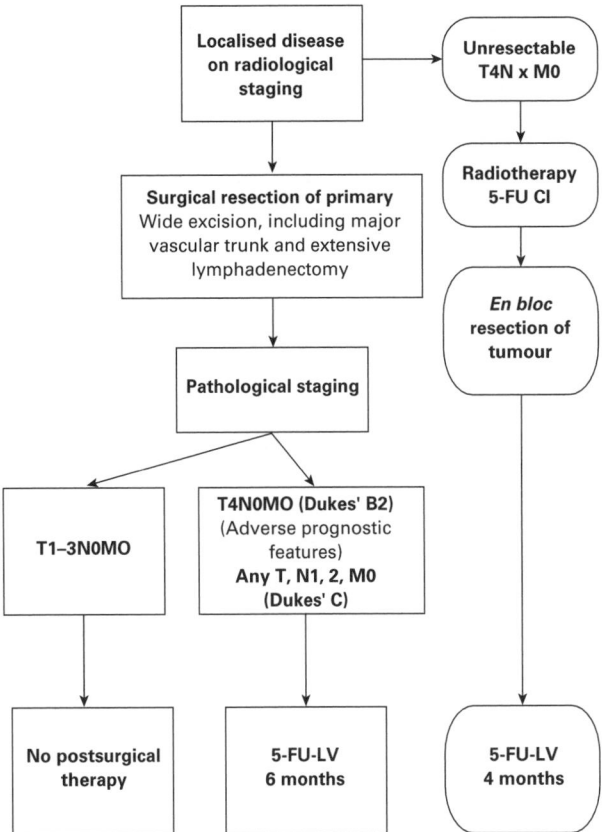

**Figure 28.2** The management of localised colon cancer. CI, continuous infusion; LV, leucovorin; 5-FU, 5-fluorouracil

45–60% and 64–75%, respectively.[19–21] The inability to cure all such patients is a direct consequence of residual occult disease at the time of surgery. Adjuvant chemotherapy is offered to such high risk patients with the aim to decrease relapse and improve OS by attempting to eliminate microscopic residual disease (Figure 28.2).

Two recent meta-analyses have been reported which support the efficacy of adjuvant chemotherapy.[109,110] The largest and most recent from the Colorectal Cancer Collaborative Group analysed 50 trials involving 18 000 patients. The death rate was reduced by 11% ($P = 0.001$) in patients receiving prolonged systemic chemotherapy. The major benefit was seen in patients with Dukes' C disease.[109]

### The optimal regimen for adjuvant chemotherapy?

The major advances in adjuvant chemotherapy for resected CRC were made in the early 1990s, with the biomodulation of 5-FU with either levamisole (Lev) or leucovorin (LV, folinic acid) (Table 28.8). The two recent meta-analyses above had shown that the reduction in

**Table 28.8   Randomised adjuvant chemotherapy trials for resected colon cancer**

| Trial name or organisation and reference | Treatment arms | No. of patients (median follow up in years) | Stage | DFS | OS | Comment |
|---|---|---|---|---|---|---|
| IMPACT[111] | 5-FU-HD LV, every 4 weeks × 6 | 1526 (3) | B, C | 71 | 83 | |
| | Observation | | | 62 ($P < 10^{-4}$) | 78 ($P = 0.03$) | |
| NCCTG[112] | 5-FU-Lev, 12 months | 1296 (6·5) | B, C | 67 | 74 | No benefit in stage B. |
| | Lev (stage C), 12 months | | | 53 | 65 | No benefit for Lev alone |
| | observation | | | 48 | 64 | |
| Intergroup-0089[113] | 5-FU-Lev × 12 months | 3759 | II, III | 56 | 63 | Lev provided no added |
| | 5-FU-Lev-LD LV × 12 months | (5) | | 60 | 67 | benefit to 5-FU-LV |
| | 5-FU-LD LV × 6 cycles, | | | 60 | 66 | |
| | 5-FU-HD LV × 4 cycles | | | 59 | 65 | |
| QUASAR[114] | 5-FU-LD LV ± Lev | 4927 | A–C | 36 | 70·1 | No added |
| | 5-FU-HD LV ± Lev | (3) | | 35·8 | 71·1 | benefit by |
| | Weekly or every 4 weeks | | | | | Lev. HD-LV equivalent to LD-LV |
| NSABP C03[115] | MOF | 1081 | B, C | 63 | 77 | |
| | 5-FU-HD LV | (3) | | 73 ($P = 4 \times 10^{-4}$) | 84 ($P = 0.003$) | |
| NCCTG[116] | 5-FU-LD LV × 6 cycles every 4 weeks | 317 (5) | II, III | 74 | 74 | |
| | Observation | | | 58 ($P < 0.01$) | 63 ($P < 0.02$) | |
| NCCTG-NCIC[117] | 5-FU-LV-Lev, 6 months | 891 (5) | II, III | 63 | 70 | No difference for |
| | 5-FU-LV-Lev, | | | 57 | 63 | 6 *v* 12 months. |
| | 5-FU-Lev, 6 months | | | 58 | 60 | 5-FU-Lev × 6 months |
| | 5-FU-Lev, 12 months | | | 63 | 68 | inferior ($P < 0.01$) |

*(Continued)*

**Table 28.8** *(Continued)*

| Trial name or organisation and reference | Treatment arms | No. of patients (median follow up in years) | Stage | DFS | OS | Comment |
|---|---|---|---|---|---|---|
| NSABP C04[118] | 5-FU-HD LV, weekly | 2151 | II, III | 65 | 74 | No benefit |
| | 5-FU-Lev | (5) | | 60 | 70 | for Lev |
| | 5-FU-HD LV-Lev | | | 64 | 73 | added to 5-FU-LV |

Abbreviations: DFS, disease-free survival; 5-FU, 5-fluorouracil; HD, high dose; LD, low dose; LV, folinic acid, leucovorin; Lev, levamisole; MOF, semustine, vincristine, fluorouracil; OS, overall survival

mortality by modulation of 5-FU by LV or Lev (29%, $P = 0.007$; 22%, $P = 0.01$, respectively) was significantly larger than that for unmodulated 5-FU (6%, $P = 0.11$).[109,110] The NCCTG study has demonstrated the benefit of 5-FU plus Lev relative to observation or Lev alone in reducing tumour recurrence and improving OS in patients with Dukes' C disease.[112] The IMPACT, NSABP C03 and NCCTG trials have all demonstrated the advantage of 5-FU plus LV relative to their respective control arms including observation or the 5-FU-semustine-vincristine (MOF) combination (Table 28.8).[111,115,116]

Since these studies and meta-analyses, several large multicentre randomised trials have been performed to define the optimal 5-FU-based regimen: that is, the combination with high or low dose LV (HDLV, LDLV respectively) and/or Lev in patients with B2 and C colon cancer (Table 28.8). One of the largest was the Intergroup-0089 trial, a four-arm trial involving 3760 patients with high risk stage II/III disease.[113] The other large trial, the QUASAR study, evaluated the role of Lev and dose of LV in stage I–III colorectal cancer.[114] The study enrolled 4927 patients who were randomised to HDLV versus LDLV (175 mg $v$ 25 mg) respectively, and to Lev versus placebo. The patients were allowed to receive, by physician choice, two different 5-FU regimens: 5-FU (370 mg m$^{-2}$) given weekly ($\times$ 30 weeks) versus the same daily dose $\times$ 5 (repeated 4 weekly) for 6 months.[114,119]

These large randomised studies have shown that 5-FU/HDLV is equivalent to 5-FU/LDLV at least as administered in the daily $\times$ 5, 4-weekly regimen. They also show that the weekly regimen of 5-FU-LV is equivalent but less toxic compared with a 4-weekly regimen. However, the addition of Lev provides no additional survival benefit and should no longer be used.[113,114,117–119] The efficacy of adjuvant chemotherapy for 12 months provides no further benefit compared with a 6-month duration.[113,117] **Evidence level Ib, Grade A**.

### Is adjuvant therapy appropriate for patients with Dukes' B colon cancer?

The efficacy of systemic adjuvant chemotherapy for patients with Dukes' B colon cancer has still not been confirmed. A pooled analysis of 1016 patients with B2 colon cancer from the IMPACT trial, in which patients were randomised to 5-FU-LV versus observation, found chemotherapy did not provide a significant advantage in terms of event-free survival (EFS) (82% $v$ 80%, respectively) or OS (76% $v$ 73%, respectively) after a median follow up of 5.75 years.[120] Another analysis evaluated 5-FU-HD or LDLV in 998 patients with Dukes' B colon cancer from five randomised trials: the 5-year EFS for control and 5-FU-LV arms was 74% and 77% ($P = 0.051$) and the 5-year OS was 81% and 83% ($P = 0.036$), respectively.[121] However in contrast, when the results from the NSABP C01–4 trials were also pooled to compare the efficacy of chemotherapy in 1565 patients with Dukes' B relative to Dukes' C disease, regardless of stage, there was a reduction in mortality, DFS and recurrence by chemotherapy: the reduction for Dukes' B was of a similar magnitude to that seen for Dukes' C disease.[122]

The issue is far from clarified: the ideal trial to answer this question in a disease with a 5-year survival rate of 75% will require at least 15 000 patients.[123] Prognostic factors, as described above, may identify those patients with Dukes' B disease that would most benefit from adjuvant chemotherapy. Based on the evidence thus far, it would be correct to propose that patients with Dukes' B disease should be offered observation alone **Evidence level Ib, Grade A**. However, there has been a trend to treat those with Dukes' B2 disease, with other poor prognostic factors including young age, perforation or obstruction (Figure 28.2). The alternatives need to be carefully discussed with the patient.

### Is there a role for alternative approaches of adjuvant chemotherapy?

*Portal vein infusion (PVI) adjuvant chemotherapy:* This is a mechanism to a deliver high concentration of 5-FU to the liver, being the commonest site of relapse, with the advantage of first pass metabolism reducing systemic exposure and hence toxicity. A meta-analysis evaluated data from 10 randomised trials (3999 patients), comparing PVI with surgery alone: at 5 years there was a 4·7% increase in survival ($P = 0·006$) in favour of PVI. However there was no reduction in the number of patients who developed hepatic metastases as the first site of metastasis.[124]

The AXIS trial (which has been reported in abstract form) randomised 3583 patients with resected CRC to PVI 5-FU over 7 days versus no further therapy. PVI provided patients with curative resection an estimated 2.5% reduction in 5-year survival ($P = 0·02$), 4% in those with colon cancer.[125] This has not been confirmed by two other recent randomised trials.[126,127]

*Continuous infusional 5-FU:* Two randomised trials have thus far been completed comparing modulated bolus 5-FU to infusional regimens in patients with Dukes' B and C colon cancer. The first, a SWOG study, randomised patients to bolus 5-FU-LV + Lev versus CI 5-FU + Lev.[128] The second trial randomised patients to CI 5-FU for 12 weeks versus 6 months bolus 5-FU-LV.[129] The infusional regimens provided no advantage over the bolus schedules in terms of OS, but with reduced toxicity as expected.

*Antibody therapy: Mab17-1A:* A monoclonal antibody to a 34-kd glycoprotein on the cell surface of epithelial cells has been evaluated as targeted therapy in patients with resected Dukes' C colon cancer. Despite a positive randomised phase II trial, subsequent large multicentre phase III studies of 17-1A both as monotherapy and in combination with 5-FU-based chemotherapy versus chemotherapy alone have failed to demonstrate consistent efficacy.[7,130–133]

A phase III North American trial randomised 1421 patients with resected stage III disease to 5-FU-based adjuvant therapy with and without Mab17-1A. At 3 years, the trial showed an OS benefit in favour of the experimental arm (81·6% *v* 78·9%, $P = 0·023$), but failed to demonstrate a statistically significant advantage for DFS.[133] Its development program was terminated in 2000.

*New cytotoxic agents:* As will be discussed below there are several new agents apart from 5-FU that have demonstrated activity in advanced CRC and are now being evaluated in the adjuvant setting. The PETACC-1 trial in which patients with Dukes' C colon cancer were randomised to either raltitrexed, a thymidylate synthase inhibitor, or to 5-FU-LV bolus regimen was terminated by excess toxic deaths in the raltitrexed arm.[7] Other agents being assessed include oral 5-FU prodrugs

(capecitabine and UFT), oxaliplatin-5-FU, and irinotecan-5-FU combinations.[134,135]

At present bolus 5-FU-LV regimens remain the gold-standard for adjuvant chemotherapy in patients with resected colon cancer **Evidence level Ia, Grade A**.

## The treatment of locally advanced rectal cancer

### Is total mesorectal excision the new gold standard for rectal cancer surgery?

For rectal cancer, principal surgical approaches comprise anterior resection (AR) or abdominoperineal resection (APR), the choice depending in part on the position of the primary lesion. Local recurrences in surgical series, subject to the technique used and experience of the surgeon, range from 0% for T1 (stage A), to 25–65% for tumours with penetration through the bowel wall or with nodal involvement (T3, 4 or N1; stages B and C).[9,19–21,45–48,136] With modern adjuvant therapy, isolated local recurrences have been reduced to less than 10–15%[137–140] (Table 28.9).

Local recurrence is commonly a result of incomplete circumferential clearance when the tumour extends beyond the muscularis propria.[144] Sharp dissection of the mesorectum (that is, total mesorectal excision, TME) of rectal cancers has been reported to reduce local recurrence rates in comparison to conventional techniques where the mesorectum is left intact. The intial case series of 200 patients who underwent TME, reported a 5-year local and overall recurrence rate of 4% and 18%, respectively, and at 10 years 4% and 19%, respectively.[145] Similar results had been achieved in a randomised Dutch trial with TME alone as its control arm (Table 28.9).[140] Nevertheless, the TME technique has shown a lack of reproducibility in some centres with higher recurrence rates, emphasising the need for rigorous quality control.[146–148] A randomised trial of TME versus conventional surgery has not been performed and is unlikely to be completed, given the increasing acceptance of the former.

Sphincter sparing surgery (SSS), by various techniques, has also been evaluated in order to reduce APR rates and the need for colostomy. Relative to APR, operative mortality rates and recurrence rates are similar for such procedures.[149] Randomised trials are lacking, with outcome hence being a reflection of careful patient selection.

### Adjuvant therapy for rectal cancer

Radiation therapy, from the 1950s, has been the major mode of adjuvant therapy, and shown to reduce locoregional relapse.[150] The current gold standard was postoperative chemoradiotherapy; however, this has been challenged by recent phase III randomised trials (Figure 28.3).

**Table 28.9** Patterns of failure and survival parameters following adjuvant therapies for stages II and III rectal cancer

| Trial name or organisation and reference | Treatment[a] | No. of patients (median follow up in years) | LR only (%) | DFS (%) | OS (%) |
|---|---|---|---|---|---|
| Stockholm II Trial[47] | RT→S[b] | 272 | 13 | 32[e] | |
| | S[b] | 285[c,d] (8·8) | 27 | 47 | |
| Swedish Rectal Cancer Trial[141] | RT→S | 553 | 11 | 58 | |
| | S | 557 (5) | 27 | 48 | |
| Dutch Colorectal Cancer Group[140] | RT→TME | 1861 | 2·4 | 82 | |
| | TME | (2) | 8·2 | 81·8 | |
| O'Connell[142] | S→5-FU(+ Se)→ RT-bolus 5-FU →5-FU(+ Se) | 660 (4) | 47 | 60 60 | |
| | S→5-FU(+Se) →RT-CI 5-FU →5-FU(+ Se) | | 37 | 70 | |
| Intergroup INT-0114[139] | S→5-FU→RT-5-FU→5-FU | 1792 | 6 | 62 | 78[f] |
| | S→5-FU/LV→RT-5-FU/LV →5-FU/LV | (4) | 4 | 68 | 80 |
| | S→5-FU/Lev→RT-5-FU →5-FU/Lev | | 5 | 62 | 79 |
| | S→5-FU/Lev/LV →RT-5-FU/LV →5-FU/Lev/LV | | 4 | 62 | 79 |
| NSABP R-01[143] | S | 184 | 25 | 30 | 43 |
| | S→MOF | 187 | 21 | 42 | 53 |
| | S→RT | 184 (6·3) | 16 | (5) | 41 |
| GITSG[9] | S | 58 | 40 | 36 | |
| | S→RT-5-FU→5-FU-Se | 46 (5) | 33 | 56 | |
| Krook[46] | S | 204 | 25 | | 34 |
| | S→5-FU-Se→RT-5-FU →5-FU-Se | (5) | 13·5 | | 52 |
| GITSG[137] | S→RT-5-FU→5-FU-Se, 12 months | 95 | 11 | 54 | 66 |
| | S→RT-5-FU→5-FU, 6 months | 104 (3) | 15 | 68 | 75 |
| NSABP R-02[138] | S→MOF or 5-FU/LV[h] | 348 | 14 | 50 | 58 |
| | S→MOF or 5-FU/LV[h] →RT-5-FU→ MOF or 5-FU/LV | 346 (8) | 8 | 50 | 58 |

*(Continued)*

**Table 28.9**   (*Continued*)

[a]Abbreviations: CI, continuous infusion; DFS, disease-free survival; 5-FU, 5-fluorouracil; Lev, levamisole; LR, local relapse; LV, leucovorin; MOF; semustine, vincristine, 5-FU; OS, overall survival; RT, radiotherapy; s, surgery; Se, semustine; TME, total mesorectal excision.
[b]Curative surgery if Dukes' A–C.
[c]7% in surgery arm and 11% in combined arm had distant metastases at trial entry.
[d]Results summarised from patients who underwent curative surgical resection.
[e]Cancer-related survival.
[f]Overall survival calculated at 3 years.
[g]Combined chemoradiotherapy arm only.
[h]Females only entered into 5-FU-leucovorin arms based upon results of NSABP R-01.[143]

### Postoperative therapy: does radiation provide any benefit over chemotherapy alone?

The major advantage of postoperative adjuvant therapy is the selection of appropriate patients based on pathological staging. However, it entails irradiation of a hypoxic surgical bed and a potential large radiation field incorporating a significant volume of small bowel. Treatment can also be delayed to allow time for the patient to recover from surgery.

A meta-analysis has evaluated 2157 patients from eight randomised trials comparing the outcomes of surgery followed by postoperative radiotherapy with surgery alone.[151] The radiation schedules assessed had biologically effective doses (BED) in excess of 30 Gy, with total dose/fraction ranging from 25 Gy in five fractions to 45 Gy in 25 fractions. Overall, postoperative radiotherapy resulted in a marginally improved OS of 58·6% versus 57·5% for surgery alone ($P = 0·04$), and a reduction in isolated local recurrence at 5 years (15·3% $v$ 22·9%, respectively, $P = 0·0002$), but no reduction in risk of any recurrence.[151]

Chemotherapy had been added to increase local control rates by radiosensitisation, and to reduce the high distant failure rates. The major randomised trials reported have been summarised in Table 28.9. The NSABP R-02 trial randomised patients to MOF or 5-FU-LV chemotherapy with or without radiotherapy (combined with bolus 5-FU).[138] Radiation therapy was associated with a reduction in locoregional recurrence compared with surgery alone (16% $v$ 25%, respectively, $P = 0·06$) and with chemotherapy alone (8% $v$ 13%, respectively, $P = 0·02$). However, it did not provide a reduction in DFS or OS ($P = 0·90$ and $P = 0·89$, respectively), regardless of the chemotherapy type.[138] The results of this trial have initiated considerable debate over the role of postoperative radiotherapy. It must be noted that specific modes and schedules of radiographic assessment were not mandated, and also the delay from surgery to the commencement of radiotherapy of up to 21 weeks may explain the lack of benefit from radiotherapy. In addition, there was no strict quality control of the surgical technique

apart from an independent review of the hospital surgical reports. Few studies in the above meta-analysis had used chemotherapy, so no comparisons of the effectiveness of radiotherapy in the presence or absence of chemotherapy were possible.

### What is the optimal chemotherapy regimen for postoperative chemoradiotherapy?

Trials have demonstrated that semustine provided no additional benefit over 5-FU alone in combination with radiotherapy, and that 5-FU CI was superior to bolus 5-FU in terms of OS and distant failure (Table 28.9).[137,142] The Intergroup (INT)-0114 trial found at 4 and 7.4 years follow up, that no comparative advantage was seen for either 5-FU, 5-FU/LV, 5-FU/Lev, or 5-FU/LV/Lev combined with radiotherapy with regard to OS, DFS and incidence of distant failure.[44,139] It is not clear if infusional 5-FU is superior to bolus 5-FU-LV in this setting.

### Is the short course intensive preoperative radiotherapy (25 Gy in five fractions) equivalent to preoperative chemoradiotherapy (50–60 Gy, 5-FU-based)?

*Preoperative radiotherapy:* The advantages for preoperative radiotherapy include tumour downstaging to improve resectability; decreased tumour seeding; minimising toxicity to normal tissues by reduction of radiation field size; reducing radiation to small bowel, which is not fixed in the pelvis, and increasing radiosensitivity of the well-oxygenated tumour bed.[152] Overtreating patients with early stage disease is avoided by current staging techniques including CT scan, pelvic MRI, endorectal ultrasound and FDG-PET (as discussed above).

A meta-analysis has been reported using summary data from 14 randomised trials up to 1999 involving 6426 patients, comparing preoperative radiation followed by surgery with surgery alone. The radiation schedule varied between studies from: 5 Gy in 1 fraction to 45 Gy in 25 fractions at five per week, and BED ranging from 7·5 Gy to

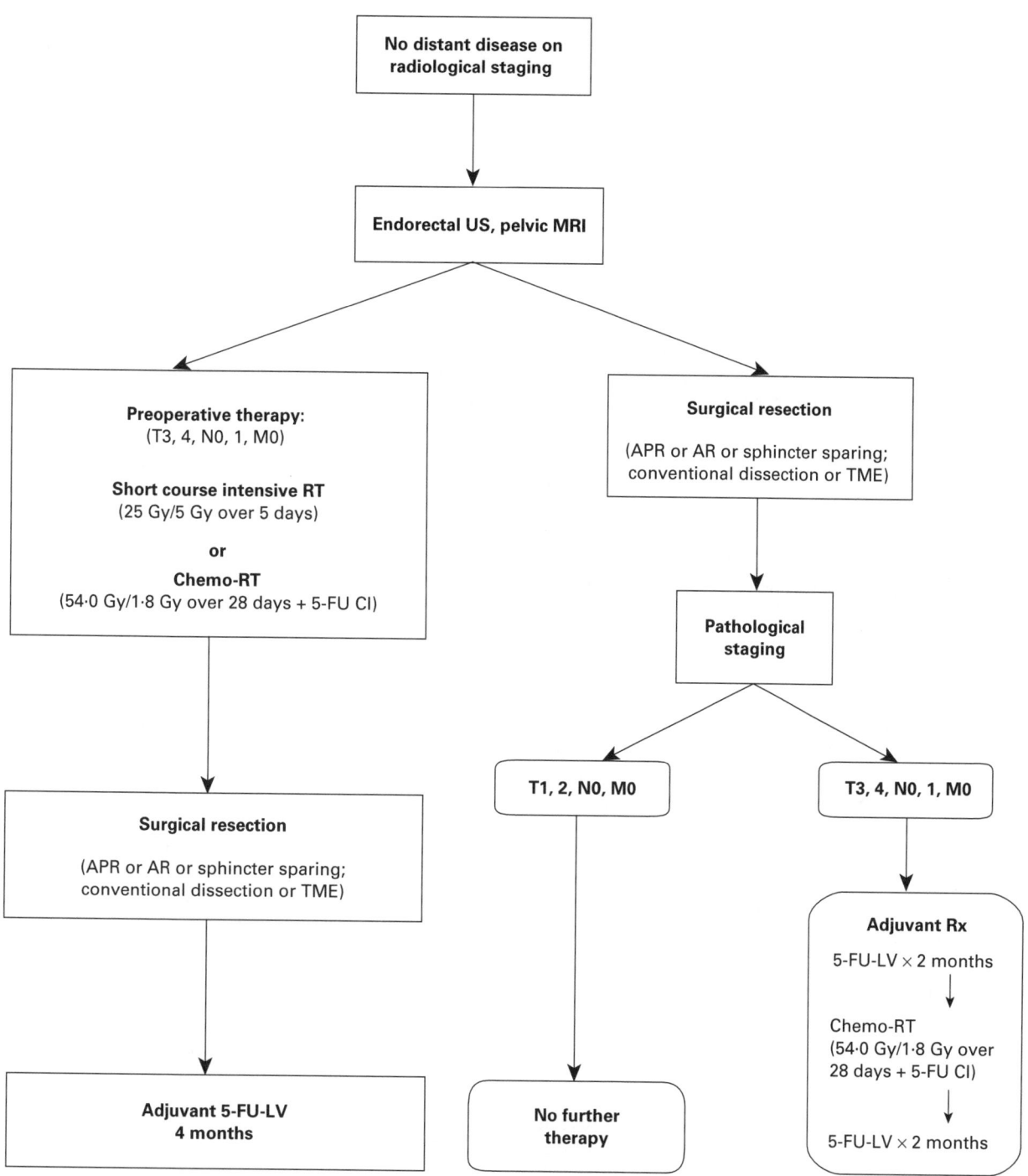

**Figure 28.3** The treatment of localised rectal cancer. (APR, abdominal perineal resection; AR, anterior resection; CI, continuous infusion; 5-FU, 5-fluorouracil; LV, leucovorin; MRI, magnetic resonance imaging; RT, radiotherapy; Rx, treatment; TME, total mesorectal excision; #, fraction.)

53·1 Gy. Radiotherapy plus surgery compared with surgery alone reduced the 5-year mortality rate (OR 0·84; 95% CI 0·72–0·98; P = 0·03); as well as the cancer-related mortality (OR 0·71; P < 0·001) and local recurrence rate (OR 0·49; P < 0·001). There was a trend to improved OS for patients with Dukes' B and C disease.[153] Mortality data according to

Dukes' stage was missing from several trials that may have influenced the analysis. The largest of these trials have been summarised in Table 28.9.[47,141]

A further meta-analysis, on this occasion using individual patient data, analysed 28 randomised trials comparing the outcomes of surgery plus preoperative or postoperative radiotherapy with surgery alone. The reduction in risk of local and overall recurrence by preoperative radiotherapy was confirmed, with the advantage extending out to 10 years.[151] There was a trend towards greater efficacy of preoperative radiotherapy with a BED in excess of 30 Gy. Cancer-related deaths were reduced compared with surgery alone (45% $v$ 50%, $P = 0.0003$), however, deaths from other causes were increased (8% $v$ 4%, $P < 0.0001$).[151] This analysis concluded that short intensive course preoperative radiotherapy appears to be as effective as longer schedules.[151]

The increase in non-cancer deaths was statistically significant in two trials that used anterior-posterior field arrangements with high dose per fraction (5 Gy). This technique tended to irradiate large volumes of normal tissues, hence greater toxicity, compared with multiple field (three or four) approaches.[154,155] The reduced mortality of the latter more modern technique has been confirmed by subsequent series.[141,156,157]

Short-term preoperative radiotherapy has been to shown to provide additional benefit to TME for the reduction of local recurrence. The Dutch Colorectal Cancer Group have reported a multicentre trial, which randomised 1861 patients with resectable rectal cancer either to TME or to preoperative radiotherapy (25 Gy in five fractions) followed by TME 1 week later. The trial was characterised by rigorous quality control for standardisation of the TME techniques, radiation planning and pathological reporting (Table 28.9). The local recurrence rate was 8·2% versus 2·4%, respectively ($P < 0.001$), the benefit was greatest for T2 and T3 tumours ($P = 0.01$ and $P < 0.001$, respectively).[140] The irradiated patients had shown more perineal complications ($P = 0.08$) in cases of APR; however, no difference in postoperative mortality was observed (4·0% $v$ 3·3%).[158]

*Preoperative chemotherapy* There have been several modest sized phase II trials combining conventional fractionated radiation therapy (45–50 Gy) with 5-FU-based chemotherapy in the preoperative setting.[159–162] Pathological response rates range from 15% to 30%, with 3-year survival rates of approximately 90% and local failure rates of less than 5%. SSS was achievable in up to 89% of patients deemed to require an APR at baseline.[159–161] However, its efficacy has not yet been confirmed by randomised phase III trials. The EORTC 22921 trial is randomising patients with T3/4, NX disease to preoperative radiotherapy (45 Gy, 1·8 Gy fractions over

5 weeks) with or without concurrent 5-FU/LV.[163] The issue is also being addressed by an Australasian randomised phase III trial evaluating short course intensive preoperative radiotherapy (25 Gy in five fractions) versus conventional fractionated preoperative chemoradiotherapy (50·4 Gy/1·8 Gy fractions over 5·5 weeks) with CI 5-FU, followed postoperatively by four courses of adjuvant 5-FU/LV as in the Mayo regimen (Ngan S, personal communication; 2001). A similar Polish trial is also planned with the preoperative chemoradiation comprising of 50 Gy over 5·5 weeks with bolus 5-FU/LV.[164]

### Is preoperative chemoradiation superior to postoperative chemoradiation?

Three randomised trials have been developed to assess this question in patients with clinically resectable T3 rectal cancer, using conventional radiation doses and techniques and concurrent 5-FU-based chemotherapy. The NSABP R-03 trial randomised patients to two cycles of chemotherapy followed by 50·4 Gy radiation plus 5-FU-LV in weeks 1 and 5 and subsequent surgery after 8 weeks versus the same regimen postoperatively. The trial was closed by poor accrual as preoperative chemoradiotherapy has become more widely used. An interim analysis of the first 116 patients found no difference in severe acute toxicities. About two-thirds of patients who were deemed to require an APR, underwent SSS.[165] A second US trial, the intergroup INT-0147 study, was also closed early owing to poor accrual.

The only current phase III study is the German CAO/ARO/AI0094 trial randomising patients with T3/4 or N+ disease to either two cycles of 5-FU concurrent with 50·4 Gy radiation followed by surgery 4–6 weeks later, or to two postoperative cycles of 5-FU concurrent with 55·8 Gy; an additional four cycles of 5-FU are given following surgery or radiation respectively. Interim results have been reported for 417 of the planned 800 cohort, with the preoperative treatment being associated with reduced grade 3 or 4 diarrhoea (7% $v$ 14%) and similar rates of perioperative complications compared with postoperative therapy. Final results are eagerly awaited.[166]

### The optimal therapy of localised rectal cancer

Preoperative and postoperative therapy have both proved to be effective, each with its own potential advantages and disadvantages as discussed above **Evidence level Ia, Grade A**. For example, postoperative therapy is associated with more complications, including a greater incidence of late adverse effects especially small bowel obstruction, radiation enteritis as well as sphincteric disturbances relative to the preoperative setting.[167,168]

However, their relative superiority over the other awaits confirmation by the current randomised trials. On the basis of anatomic staging, patients with extensive local disease or nodal involvement may be treated with preoperative therapy **Evidence level Ia, Grade A**. In resected cases, adjuvant therapy may be reserved for those with adverse pathological features (that is, transmural penetration or nodal involvement) **Evidence level Ia, Grade A**. In patients with resected early stage disease at low risk of recurrence or where morbidity of radiotherapy is considered significant, radiation may be deleted and the patient treated with adjuvant chemotherapy alone if indicated (Figure 28.3).[169]

Further advances may be made with the incorporation of new chemotherapy agents, combined with radiotherapy.[170-175] Biological markers predictive of prognosis and response to therapy may in future also assist to optimise patient selection, as discussed below.

## Advanced colorectal cancer

### Introduction

#### Definition

Advanced disease can be defined as either:

- locally recurrent disease that is not amenable to definitive or salvage local therapy owing to its extent or prior therapy, or
- metastatic disease (TxNxM1, stage 4 disease) that is not amenable to potentially curative surgical resection.

#### Epidemiology of advanced colorectal cancer

Approximately 10–25% of patients with CRC will present with distant metastases, depending on the series.[176] A further 25% will develop distant disease at some point in time following definitive local therapy, subject to tumour stage and mode of therapy.

#### Proportion of patients who will die of advanced disease and their life expectancy

Overall, less than 50% of patients with CRC are cured and the remainder will eventually die from their disease. For patients with stage IV disease at diagnosis or at relapse, the 5-year survival is less than 5%.[177] Prognosis of inoperable, advanced CRC depends on a variety of prognostic factors, including performance status and extent of disease as outlined above. Thus survival ranges from 30·7% to 70% at 1 year, subject to the treatment and study.[63,66,178–182] In the subsequent years the survival rate falls precipitously to less than 10% at 3 years and subsequently declines very slowly beyond 5 years.

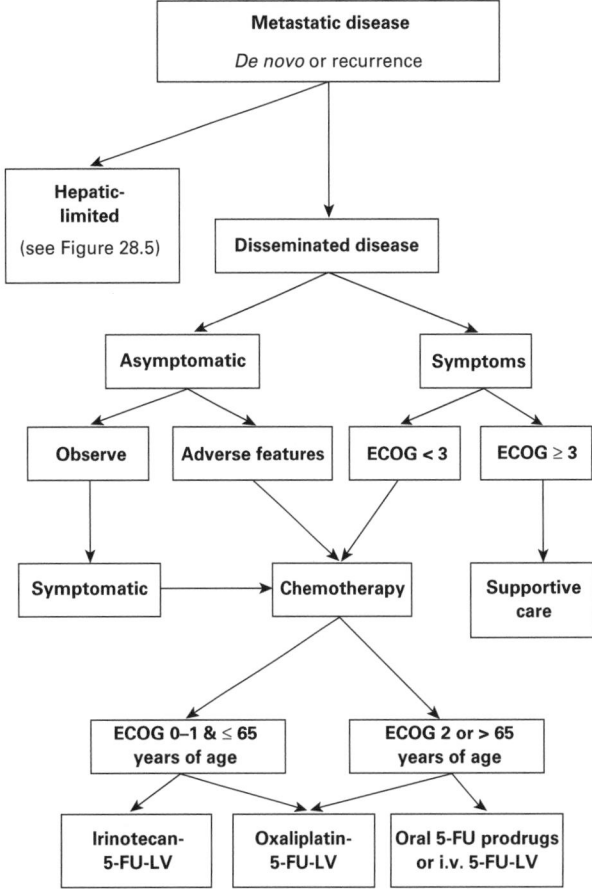

**Figure 28.4** The management of advanced colorectal cancer. 5-FU, 5-fluorouracil; LV, leucovorin

## Treatment options for patients with advanced colorectal cancer

The treatment options for patients with advanced CRC must always be patient-directed. Unless patients have resectable liver metastases, cure cannot be achieved with systemic therapy, although life may be significantly prolonged. In addition another important aim is to improve QoL with a reduction in disease-related symptoms. Gains from treatment must not be offset by significant treatment-related toxicity. The management pathway for these patients is illustrated in Figure 28.4. The treatment approach for patients with metastases limited to the liver will be discussed in the next section.

## Systemic chemotherapy for advanced colorectal cancer

### Does systemic therapy provide advantages over BSC in terms of QoL and survival?

There have been two meta-analyses that have analysed randomised trials of chemotherapy versus BSC in patients

**Table 28.10  Randomised trials comparing chemotherapy to best supportive care in patients with advanced CRC**

| Reference | Clinical setting | Arm | No. of patients | Median survival (months) | Comments |
|---|---|---|---|---|---|
| Scheithauer[184] | No prior therapy | Cisplatin/5-FU/LV<br>BSC | 24<br>12 | 11<br>5<br>($P=0.006$) | No difference in QoL, 2 BSC patients had crossed over |
| NGTATG[179] | Chemo-naive and no symptoms | MTX-5-FU-LV<br>Delayed therapy once Sx | 92<br>90 | 14<br>9<br>($P<0.02$) | 51 had delayed therapy. Median symptom-free period 10 *v* 2 months ($P<0.001$) |
| Hafstrom[185] | Non-resectable liver metastases | HAO-IP 5-FU<br>BSC | 32<br>28 | 17<br>8<br>($P=0.0039$) | |
| Allen-Mersch[186] | Non-resectable liver metastases | HAI 5-FUDR<br>BSC | 51<br>49 | 13·5<br>7·5<br>($P=0.03$) | Maintenance of QoL scores for symptoms, anxiety and depression |
| Rougier[187] | Non-resectable liver metastasis | HAI 5-FUDR<br>BSC or 5-FU/LV | 81<br>82 | 15<br>11<br>($P<0.02$) | 50% in BSC arm treated at a median of 4 months |
| Gerard[188] | Hepatic metastasis | HAL+IP 5-FU<br>HAL | 35<br>32 | 12<br>12 | |
| Ackland[189] | No prior therapy | 5-FU-LV<br>Delayed therapy once Sx | 84<br>84 | 12 months | 68% had delayed therapy. No difference in OS |
| Cunningham[67] | Progression on 5-FU | Irinotecan<br>BSC | 189<br>90 | 9·2<br>6·5<br>($P=0.001$) | QoL parameters improved except diarrhoea |

Abbreviations: BSC, best supportive care; 5-FU, 5-fluorouracil; 5-FUDR, floxuridine; HAI, hepatic artery infusion; HAL, hepatic artery ligation; HAO, hepatic artery occlusion; IP, intraportal; LV, folinic acid, leucovorin; MTX, methotrexate; OS, overall survival; QoL quality of life; Sx, symptoms

with advanced CRC.[178,183] The Colorectal Cancer Collaborative Group used individual patient data from 7 of the 13 considered trials.[178] The second from Canada, used summary data from 7 trials.[183] Both concluded that chemotherapy reduces the risk of death from 20–35% at 1 year, with possible benefit extending to 24 months.[178,183] These meta-analyses, a direct consequence of the trials they evaluated, provide scant information in terms of QoL and toxicity. In the Colorectal Cancer Collaborative Group study, QoL data were available for six of the 13 studies, and in three of these the chemotherapy arms showed superior results for QoL. However, it must be noted that the instruments were not always validated or specific to cancer. Only one study compared toxicity in both arms of the

trial.[178] The majority of these studies have been summarised in Table 28.10.

The results must be placed in the context of patients in the trial setting. The majority of studies documented 80% or more of the patients entered had a performance status of at least ECOG 0–1 or a median Karnofsky performance status (KPS) of 80–100, not necessarily typical of the vast majority of patients who present with inoperable advanced CRC. On the other hand the majority of these studies used older chemotherapy regimens and hence may underestimate the effect compared with modern chemotherapy approach.

As these meta-analyses do not provide any conclusions for the QoL benefits of chemotherapy, we must depend upon data from randomised phase III trials (Table 28.11). The

**Table 28.11  Quality of life (QoL) benefits provided by chemotherapy in patients with advanced CRC**

| Reference | Indication | Treatment arms | QoL instrument | Result |
|---|---|---|---|---|
| Hill[190] | Chemo-naive | CI 5-FU<br>CI 5-FU+αIF | EORTC-QLQ-C30 | Maintenance of QoL with αIF |
| Caudry[191] | Chemo-naive | 5-FU-LV<br>CI-5-FU+Cy+Mito-C | LASA | No difference in QoL |
| NGTATG[179] | Chemo-naive | 5-FU-MTX-LV<br>5-FU | NR | Symptom relief with no adverse effects: 45% MTX arm v 23% |
| Earlam[192] | Chemo-naive | BSC<br><br>5-FU<br>HAI 5-FUDR | RSC, SIP, HAD | QoL impaired by 5-FU v BSC<br>HAI sustained QoL v 5-FU |
| Glimelius[193] | Chemo-naive, asymptomatic | 5-FU-MTX-LV<br>Observation | NR | Maintenance of QoL and ↑symptom-free survival |
| Glimelius[194] | Chemo-naive, symptomatic | 5-FU-MTX-LV<br>5-FU-LV | NR | Improved QoL in parallel with objective + subjective response |
| Sullivan[195] | Chemo-naive | 5-FU<br>5-FU-LV | FLIC | QoL ↑ or stable in 89%, correlated with survival |
| Poon[63] | Chemo-naive | 5-FU<br>5-FU-HD/LD-LV,<br>5-FU-LD/HD-MTX<br>5-FU-CDDP | ECOG PS, DRS | Improved PS, weight and DRS in favour of combinations |
| Cunningham[31] | Chemo-naive | Tomudex<br>5-FU-LV | EORTC-QLQ-C30 | Improved pain and global QoL in both arms |
| de Gramont[66] | Chemo-naive | Ox-5-FU-LV<br>5-FU-LV | EORTC-QLQ-C30 | No difference between arms, QoL decline delayed in Ox arm |
| Saltz[68] | Chemo-naive | Ir-5-FU-LV<br>5-FU-LV<br>Ir | EORTC-QLQ-C30 | No difference between arms |

Abbreviations: αIF, interferon alfa; BSC, best supportive care; CDDP, cisplatin; CI, continuous infusion; Cy, cyclophosphamide; DRS, disease-related symptoms; EORTC-QLQ-C30, European Organisation for Research and Treatment of Cancer Quality of Life Questionnaire-C30; FLIC, Functional Living Index-Cancer; HAD, Hospital Anxiety and Depression scale; HD, high dose; Ir, Irinotecan LASA, linear analogue symptom scales; LD, low dose; LV, leucovorin, folinic acid; Mito-C, mitomycin-C; MTX, methotrexate; NGATG, Nordic Gastrointestinal Tumour Adjuvant Therapy Group; NR, not recorded; Ox, Oxaliplatin: RSC, Rotterdam Symptom Control; SIP, Sickness Impact Profile

instruments used vary considerably from performance status assessment and descriptive measures of DRS to cancer-specific QoL instruments. The majority demonstrate that modern systemic chemotherapy is associated with an improvement in QoL in patients with advanced CRC relative to BSC or to less active regimens. The improvement is associated with a reduction in DRS such as pain and weight loss, and has been correlated to tumour response.[67,194,196]

Any gains in QoL by an enhanced response must not be offset by increased toxicity. A French randomised trial involved 420 patients who were treated with the LVFU2 regimen (a combination of LV plus CI/bolus 5-FU) with and without oxaliplatin. In the oxaliplatin arm patients had a significantly longer progression-free survival (PFS) of 9 versus 6·2 months, and response rate of 50·7% versus 22·3% relative to the control. QoL was not improved statistically, which may be a consequence of a significant increase in 5-FU-related toxicities relative to the control arm. In addition, 18·2% patients overall had grade 3 neurotoxicity, which was reversible in only 74%.[66]

### When is the best time to treat patients who present with advanced CRC?

Symptomatic patients should be offered systemic chemotherapy given the benefits discussed above, but with certain caveats. The treatment of the asymptomatic patient is less straightforward (Figure 28.4). Two trials have randomised asymptomatic patients to immediate therapy or to observation with therapy at the onset of symptoms (Table 28.10).[179,189] Only in one was there a significant increase in OS for immediate therapy (14 versus 9 months, $P < 0·02$). In the control arm, only 50% actually had received therapy, hence complicating the interpretation of the results.[179] Asymptomatic patients should be offered therapy in the following circumstances:

- if the patient is keen to receive treatment;
- if there is disease that has demonstrated a rapid progression within vital structures such as liver or lungs;
- if there is extensive peritoneal disease, with a high risk of viscus obstruction.

### Which regimen is optimal for the individual patient?

The choice of regimen must be individualised, considering the patient, medical comorbidities, end-organ function, geography and compliance.

### 5-Fluorouracil-based regimens and biomodulation: what is the optimal regimen?

5-FU, via several anabolic steps, acts by several mechanisms including inhibition of TS, with the depletion of thymidine nucleotides for DNA synthesis; incorporation into RNA resulting in impaired RNA function; incorporation of FU into DNA, and subsequent damage.[197,198] This agent was introduced into clinical practice over 40 years ago and still remains the cornerstone of treatment of advanced CRC.

### Bolus v CI as a method of administering 5-FU

Two methods have been used to administer 5-FU, either as a bolus injection, over 1–3 minutes or as a CI given over 1 hour to several days or weeks, with different mechanisms of action (that is, RNA dysfunction and TS inhibition,

respectively).[199] The CI regimens achieve a dose intensity up to 3–4 times greater than for bolus, but drug exposure is limited by a linear increase in drug clearance.[200]

Two meta-analyses have been reported from the Meta-analysis Group in Cancer, evaluating both the toxicity and efficacy of CI 5-FU relative to bolus administration.[64,201] Both evaluated individual patient data from 1219 patients entered in seven randomised trials, two of which had biomodulation with LV in both arms. The analyses of efficacy derived from 1103 patients showed an overall tumour response of 22% (CR 3%) for CI versus 14% for the bolus, with an RR of 0·55 (95% CI 0·41–0·75) in favour of 5-FU CI ($P = 0·0002$). The trend for CI was only significant in three of the seven trials: not including the two trials with biomodulation.[64] Continuous infusion 5-FU showed a small significant advantage over bolus for median survival, 12·1 versus 11·3 months (hazard ratio 0·88; 95% CI 0·78–0·99; $P = 0004$). Modulation by LV provided no advantage though the result was based on too few patients (see the next section).[64]

The toxicity meta-analysis showed that CI 5-FU was associated with significantly less neutropenia (31% $v$ 4%, $P < 0·001$) and greater hand–foot syndrome (34% $v$ 13%, $P < 0·001$) relative to bolus; however, there was no statistical difference for other non-haematological toxicities.[201] CI 5-FU requires central venous access devices with potential complications such as thrombosis and line sepsis and the need for expensive ambulatory pumps.

The duration of the 5-FU bolus was not detailed in the meta-analysis. Given the different clinical behaviour of 5-FU when given by rapid injection (< 5 minutes) compared with short-term (> 20 minutes) infusions, the conclusions of the meta-analysis need to be considered with caution. As only two studies in the analysis were biomodulated with LV, the superiority of CI 5-FU over 5-FU combined with LV cannot be inferred (see next section).

### 5-FU biomodulation

The binding of dFUMP to TS is stabilised and dependent on the presence of reduced folates 5,10-CH2-FH4 acid, whose intracellular concentrations can be increased by the LV (5-formyl-5,6,7,8-tetrahydrofolate or folinic acid). The end result is the enhanced formation and stabilisation of the ternary complex with dFUMP and TS (and reduced folinic acid) and hence inhibition of DNA synthesis.

At least 15 randomised phase III trials have been reported comparing 5-FU plus LV to 5-FU alone, using the weekly or daily $\times$ 5 schedule, monthly 5-FU regimens. Ten of such studies, involving 1381 patients, have been evaluated in a meta-analysis.[65] In the 5-FU and LV arms, the overall response rate was 23% versus 11% in the 5-FU alone arm with an OR of 0·45 (95% CI 0·36–0·60; $P < 10^{-7}$).

The response OR were 0·36 (95% CI 0·24–0·55) for the four trials adding weekly LV, and 0·29 (95% CI 0·17–0·49) for the three trials adding monthly LV. There was no survival advantage achieved by biomodulation and the lack of difference persisted when excluding the trials where cross-over had occurred.[65]

A survival advantage has been reported in a phase III randomised trial from the Swiss Group for Clinical Cancer Research, which randomised 306 patients to either FU 400 mg m$^{-2}$/day, days 1–5, every 4 weeks with and without LV 20 mg m$^{-2}$/day, days 1–5. There was a 3-month median PFS advantage ($P = 0·0001$), and median survival of 12·4 months versus 10 months ($P = 0·02$) in favour of the LV arm.[69]

Studies in the past two decades have attempted to define the optimal biomodulated 5-FU regimen in terms of LV dose (HD $v$ LD) and 5-FU schedule (weekly or daily × 5 every month) (Table 28.12). No significant difference has been observed for survival, objective or symptomatic response between the biomodulated weekly versus monthly regimens regardless of LV dose.[28,63,181,202–208] LD-LV biomodulation appears to be as effective as HD-LV with substantially reduced cost and toxicity. The HD-LV weekly regimens were associated with more diarrhoea but less stomatitis and neutropenia than the LD-LV monthly regimens.

### Combined CI-biomodulated 5-FU regimens

A modulated infusional 5-FU regimen, combines the advantages of both approaches in terms of efficacy and toxicity profile and has been a major focus of clinical research. A phase III trial had randomised 448 patients with untreated CRC to receive either monthly bolus 5-FU (425 mg m$^{-2}$) plus LV (20 mg m$^{-2}$) days 1–5, or to a bimonthly regimen of intravenous LV 200 mg m$^{-2}$ over 2 hours, followed by 5-FU bolus 400 mg m$^{-2}$ and 22-hour 5-FU CI 600 mg m$^{-2}$ for 2 consecutive days.[209] The response for the bimonthly regimen was 32·6% versus 14·4% ($P = 0·0004$) and the PFS was 27·65 weeks versus 22 weeks ($P = 0·0012$) in favour of the experimental arm. However, median survival was not statistically different.[209]

A German trial has also compared HD-LV plus high dose 5-FU CI relative to CI alone or modulation with interferon alfa, confirming the superior response rate and time to progression of the combined approach.[210]

### Oral 5-FU prodrugs

Oral fluoropyrimidines have been developed as an alternative to intravenous therapy, by overcoming the first pass effect of intestinal/systemic dihydropyrimidine dehydrogenase (DPD). Oral agents are generally preferred by patients, provided there is no loss of efficacy, hence the interest in this approach. At present five such agents have

entered clinical trials: capecitabine (Xeloda®), UFT (tegafur and uracil) + LV (Orzel®), eniluracil, S-1 and BOF A-2.[211] The first three have been compared with intravenous LV modulated 5-FU regimens in randomised phase III trials (Table 28.13).

Capecitabine is a fluoropyrimidine carbamate that is absorbed unchanged and converted to 5-FU by three enzymatic steps. The terminal step is catalysed by thymidine phosphorylase (TP), which has greater activity in tumour cells relative to normal host tissues. Two randomised trials (non-US and US centres) have been reported comparing it to intravenous bolus 5-FU plus LV (Table 28.13).[212,213] The studies demonstrated superior response rates, but no significant difference in median TTP or OS. From the non-US study, and supported by the other trial, the capecitabine arm demonstrated significantly lower incidence of grade 3–4 stomatitis (1·3% $v$ 13·3%), neutropenia, and neutropenic fever, but more grade 3–4 hand–foot syndrome (16·3% $v$ 0·3%) and hyperbilirubinaemia ($P < 0·001$).[212] A medical resource analysis derived from the first trial found fewer hospital admissions, reduced hospital stays for adverse event treatment, and less need for supportive care drugs, such as antibiotics or haematological growth factors.[218]

The second agent is a combination of oral uracil and tegafur (UFT™). Tegafur is a prodrug metabolised to 5-FU, whose bioavailability is increased by uracil inhibiting DPD. UFT has been combined with oral LV (Orzel) and directly compared with bolus 5-FU-LV in two randomised phase III trials (Table 28.13).[214,215] Both trials have demonstrated equivalence of this combination relative to bolus 5-FU-LV, in terms of response rate, median survival, but with significantly fewer episodes of febrile neutropenia, infection, and grade 3–4 mucositis, and less requirement for supportive medications ($P < 0·001$).[214,215]

Oral 5-FU has also been combined with eniluracil (776C85), a potent inhibitor of DPD.[219] Two phase III trials have compared eniluracil plus oral 5-FU to intravenous 5-FU + LV as in the Mayo regimen (Table 28.13). In both studies, despite equivalent response rates, OS and PFS were inferior; this has led to the agent being withdrawn from further study.[216,217] S-1 represents an oral combination of tegafur together with chloro-2,4-dihydropyridine, an inhibitor of DPD, and potassium oxonate, an inhibitor of orolate phosphoribosyltransferase, which catalyses the conversion of uracil to UMP. In a phase II trial it had demonstrated similar activity to infusional 5-FU and LV: a 35% response rate in 62 patients.[220] Phase III trials have not been reported as yet.

### The optimal 5-FU regimen?

The combined modulated bolus infusional regimens appear superior to bolus 5-FU schedules, although they have

**Table 28.12  Randomised trials evaluating the biomodulation of 5-FU by leucovorin (folinic acid)**

| Reference | No. of patients | Regimen (mg m$^{-2}$) | Overall response rate (%) | Median survival (months) | Toxicity |
|---|---|---|---|---|---|
| Wang[202] | 96 | 5-FU 425, LV 20, days 1–5, q 4 weeks | 10·6 | 15·8 | |
| | | 5-FU 400, LV 20, weekly | 14·3 (NS) | 18·4 (NS) | ↑ G3/4 diarrhoea ($P = 0.029$) |
| Buroker[203] | 372 | 5-FU 425 + LV 20, days 1–5, q 4 weeks | 35 | 9·3 | ↑ Leuckopenia, mucositis |
| | | 5-FU 600 + LV 500, weekly × 6, q 8 weeks | 31 (NS) | 10·7 (NS) | ↑ Diarrhoea |
| Poon[63][†] | 192 | 5-FU 500, D1–5, q 5 weeks | 10 | 7·7 | |
| | | 5-FU 370 + LV 200, days 1–5, q 4 weeks[‡] | 26[§] | 12·2[§] | 30% severe stomatitis[§] |
| | | 5-FU 370 + LV 20, days 1–5, q 4 weeks[‡] | 43[§] | 12·0[§] | 26% severe stomatitis[§] |
| Labianca[204] | 422 | 6S-LV 100 + 5-FU 370, days 1–5, q 4 weeks | 9·3 | 11 | No difference in toxicity profile |
| | | 6S-LV 10 + 5-FU 370, days 1–5, q 4 weeks | 10·7 (NS) | 11 (NS) | |
| Leichmann[181][†] | 528 | 5-FU 500, days 1–5, q 5 weeks | 29 | 14 | Arms 1, 2: 47% grade 3–4 neutropenia and 27% grade 3–4 diarrhoea |
| | | 5-FU 425, LV 20, days 1–5, q 4 weeks | 27 | 14 | |
| | | 5-FU 600, LV 500, weekly × 6, q 8 weeks | 21 | 13 | |
| | | 5-FU CI, 200/d × 28, q 5 weeks | 29 | 15 | |
| | | 5-FU CI, 200 per day × 28, q 5 weeks + LV 20, weekly | 26 | 14 | |
| | | 5-FU 2600, 24 hour CI, weekly | 25 (NS) | 15 (NS) | |
| O'Connell[205] | 208 | 5-FU 500, days 1–5, q 4 weeks | 10 | 8 | Increased stomatitis in LV arms |
| | | 5-FU 500, LV 20, days 1–5, q 4 weeks | 43[§] | 12[§] | |
| | | 5-FU 500, LV 200, days 1–5, q 4 weeks | 26[§] | 12[§] | |
| Ychou[206] | 83 | 5-FU 400, 1-hour CI, LV 20, days 1–5, q 4 weeks | 16·2 | 11·5 | |
| | | 5-FU 500, 1 hour CI, LV 200, days 1–5, q 4 weeks | 8·3 (NS) | 10·8 (NS) | |
| Goldberg[207] | 926 | 5-FU 370, l-LV 100, days 1–5, q 4 weeks[‡] | 28 | 12 | No difference in toxicity profile |
| | | 5-FU 370 i.v., LV 375, p.o[¶], days 1–5, q 4 weeks[‡] | 34 | 12 | |
| | | 5-FU 370, LV 200, days 1–5, q 4 weeks[‡] | 34 | 12 (NS) | |

Abbreviations: 6S, stereoisomer; CI, continuous infusion; i.v., intravenous; LV, leucovorin, or folinic acid; NS, non-significant difference; p.o., per orally

[†]5-Fluorouracil ± LV arms only.

[‡]Chemotherapy repeated at 4 and 8 weeks, then every 5 weeks.

[§]$P < 0.05$ relative to 5-FU alone.

*l*-LV, *L*-stereoisomer of LV.

[¶]Oral *d,l*-LV given 125 mg m$^{-2}$ hourly for 3 hours followed by 5-FU on the fourth hour.

**Table 28.13** Randomised trials comparing oral 5-FU prodrugs to intravenous 5-FU-leucovorin regimens in patients with advanced CRC

| Agent | Reference | Arms | No. of patients | Overall response rate (%) | Overall survival (months) |
|---|---|---|---|---|---|
| Capecitabine | Van Cutsem[212] | Capecitabine* | 301 | 18·9 | 13·2 |
| | | i.v. 5-FU-LV[†] | 301 | 15·0 | 12·1 |
| | Hoff[213] | Capecitabine* | 302 | 25·8 | 12·5 |
| | | i.v. 5-FU-LV[†] | 303 | 11·6 | 13·3 |
| UFT | Pazdur[214] | UFT[‡] + LV | 409 | 12·0 | 12·4 |
| | | i.v. 5-FU-LV[†] | 407 | 15·0 | 13·4 |
| | Carmichael[215] | UFT + LV[‡] | 195 | 11·0 | 12·2 |
| | | i.v. 5-FU-LV[†] | 185 | 9·0 | 11·9 |
| Eniluracil | Levin[216] | Eniluracil + oral 5-FU[§] | 485 | 12·2 | 13·3 |
| | | i.v. 5-FU-LV[†] | 479 | 12·7 | 14·5 |
| | Van Cutsem[217] | Eniluracil + oral 5-FU[§] | 268 | 11·6 | 11·1 |
| | | i.v. 5-FU-LV[†] | 263 | 14·4* | 14·9 |

*1250 mg m$^{-2}$, q 12 hours, for 14 days, q 3 weeks.
[†]5-FU, 425 mg m$^{-2}$ per day + LV, 20 mg m$^{-2}$ per day, days 1–5, q 4 weeks.
[‡]UFT, 330 mg m$^{-2}$ per day + LV, 75–90 mg$^1$ per day for 28 days, q 5 weeks.
[§]Eniluracil, 11·5 mg m$^{-2}$ per day + oral 5-FU, 1·15 mg m$^{-2}$ per day, b.i.d, for 28 days, q 5 weeks.
*Hazard ratio 0·77, 95% CI 0·62–0·95, in favour of control arm.

the requirement for pumps and central venous access devices **Evidence level Ia, Grade A**. Capecitabine and Orzel represent alternatives to the bolus intravenous 5-FU-LV regimens, in selected patients, based on their equivalent (but not superior) efficacy and favourable toxicity profile **Evidence level Ia, Grade A**. Conclusions regarding their equivalence with other 5-FU regimens, such as combined modulated bolus infusional regimens, await further study, and cannot be inferred at this time. Compliance as for all oral medications, and potential risks of continued self-administration by patients despite moderate to severe toxicities are also major concerns with these oral agents.

## Raltitrexed

Raltitrexed is a quinazoline folate analogue, designed as a direct and specific TS inhibitor, unlike the actions of 5-FU described above. It is taken up into cells by the reduced folate membrane carrier system, where it is polyglutamated, leading to prolonged TS inhibition.[221] Four randomised phase III trials involving over 2000 patients have been reported, with inconsistent results in terms of radiological response and survival time parameters relative to bolus and infusional 5-FU regimens.[32,222–224] A phase III trial randomised 905 patients with chemo-naive advanced CRC to either two different infusional 5-FU regimens (Lokich and de Gramont) or to raltitrexed. There was no difference in OS between arms; however, the raltitrexed arm was associated with greater toxicity, including 18 treatment-related deaths, and inferior QoL.[224]

The use of raltitrexed was associated with significantly greater frequency of clinically significant transaminitis. In addition, when compared with the infusional 5-FU regimens, raltitrexed was associated with a worsening of QoL, with 4% treatment-related mortality.[224] However, the use of raltitrexed resulted in a reduction of outpatient hospital visits and costs for supportive drugs for adverse events.[225,226] Its place as single-agent therapy seems unclear, although it may have a role in patients who are intolerant to 5-FU or combination therapy.

## Irinotecan (CPT-11)

CPT-11 is a campothecin analogue that acts by inhibiting topoisomerase-I, an enzyme that breaks and hence relaxes torsionally strained supercoiled DNA to enable replication and transcription.[227] CPT-11 is converted to its most active moiety, SN-38 (7-ethyl-10-hydroxy-campthecin), which stabilises the topoisomerase-I bridged DNA breaks, referred to as "cleavable complexes". Collision of the replication fork with these cleavable complexes results in replication arrest and cell death.[228] Delayed onset diarrhoea and myelosuppression are the major dose-limiting toxicities.[229,230]

Two pivotal randomised phase III trials evaluated the addition of irinotecan to a 5-FU-LV bolus or infusional

**Table 28.14**  Randomised trials of irinotecan and oxaliplatin 5-FU-based regimens in untreated advanced colorectal cancer

| Reference | Treatment | Progression-free survival (months) | Overall survival (months) | Overall response rate (%) |
|---|---|---|---|---|
| Saltz[68] | Irinotecan + 5-FU-LV | 7·0[a] | 14·8[a] | 39[a] |
| | Irinotecan | 4·2 | 12·0 | 18 |
| | 5-FU-LV[b] | 4·3 | 12·6 | 21 |
| Doulliard[180] | Irinotecan + 5-FU-CI + LV[c,d] | 7·2 | 17·4 | 34·8 |
| | 5-FU-LV[e,f] | 6·5 | 14·1 ($P=0.03$) | 21·9 ($P=0.005$) |
| De Gramont[66] | LV5-FU2 | 6·2 | 14·7 | 22·3 |
| | LV5-FU2 + oxaliplatin | 9·0 ($P=0.0003$) | 16·2 ($P=0.12$) | 50·7 ($P=0.0001$) |
| Giacchetti[231] | 5-FU-LV CM[g] | 6·1 | 19·9 | 16 |
| | Oxaliplatin + 5-FU-LV CM[h] | 8·7 ($P<0.05$) | 19·4 | 53 ($P<0.001$) |
| Grothey[232] | 5-FU-LV[b] | 5·6 | | 21·5 |
| | 5-FU 24 hours CI + LV + oxaliplatin[i] | 8·0 ($P=0.0001$) | | 51·4 |
| Tournigand[233] | FOLFIRI[j]→FOLFOX[k] | 8·4 (first line) | | 57·5→21 |
| | FOLFOX→FOLFIRI | 8·9 (first line) | | 56→7 |
| Goldberg[234] | Irinotecan + 5-FU-LV | 6·9 | 14·1 | 29 |
| | FOLFOX | 8·7 | 18·6[l] | 38[l] |
| | Irinotecan + oxaliplatin[m] | 6·7 | 16·5 | 28 |

[a]$P<0.04$, relative to 5-FU-LV.

[b]5-FU, 425 mg m$^{-2}$ per day, bolus + LV 20 mg m$^{-2}$ per day, days 1–5, q 4 weeks.

[c]Irinotecan + DeGramont 5-FU-LV regimen: irinotecan 180 mg m$^{-2}$ + 5-FU 400 mg m$^{-2}$ bolus, 600 mg m$^{-2}$ every 22 hours CI + LV 200 mg m$^{-2}$, days 1 and 2, q 2 weeks.

[d]Irinotecan + AIO 5-FU-LV regimen: irinotecan 80 mg m$^{-2}$ + 5-FU 2300 mg m$^{-2}$ 24-hour CI + LV 500 mg m$^{-2}$, weekly.

[e]DeGramont 5-FU-LV regimen: 5-FU 400 mg m$^{-2}$ bolus, 600 mg m$^{-2}$ every 22 hours CI + LV 200 mg m$^{-2}$, days 1 and 2, q 2 weeks.

[f]AIO 5-FU-LV regimen: 5-FU 2600 mg m$^{-2}$ every 24 hours CI + LV 500 mg m$^{-2}$, weekly.

[g]5-FU-LV CM: LV 300 mg m$^{-2}$ + 5-FU 700 mg m$^{-2}$, chronomodulated days 1–5, q 3weeks.

[h]Oxaliplatin + 5-FU-LV CM: oxaliplatin 125 mg m$^{-2}$, CI 6 hours, day 1 + LV 300 mg m$^{-2}$ + 5-FU 700 mg m$^{-2}$, chronomodulated days 1–5, q 3 weeks.

[i]5-FU 2000 mg m$^{-2}$, 24 hours, CI + LV 500 mg m$^{-2}$ + oxaliplatin 50 mg m$^{-2}$, 2-hour CI, weekly × 4, q 5 weeks.

[j]FOLFIRI: irinotecan, 180 mg m$^{-2}$, day 1 + LV, 200 mg m$^{-2}$, day 1 + 5-FU bolus 400 mg m$^{-2}$, day 1 followed by 5-FU 46-hour CI 2·4–3 g m$^{-2}$, q 2 weeks.

[k]FOLFOX: oxaliplatin 100 mg m$^{-2}$, day 1 + LV, 200 mg m$^{-2}$, day 1 + 5-FU bolus 400 mg m$^{-2}$, day 1 followed by 5-FU 46-hour CI 2·4–3 g m$^{-2}$, q 2 weeks.

[l]$P<0.03$, relative to irinotecan+5-FU-LV.

[m]Irinotecan 200 mg m$^{-2}$ + oxaliplatin 85 mg m$^{-2}$, q 3 weeks.

regimen in chemo-naive patients with advanced CRC.[68,180] The first randomised patients to bolus 5-FU-LV (Mayo regimen) or to irinotecan alone (125 mg m$^{-2}$ per week × 4, every 6 weeks) or to irinotecan plus 5-FU-LV (125 mg m$^{-2}$ per week; 500 mg m$^{-2}$ per week; 20 mg m$^{-2}$ per week × 4, every 6 weeks, respectively) with the endpoints being PFS and OS.[68] Patients entered had a median age of 60, and over 50% had an ECOG performance status of 1 or 2. The results are summarised in Table 28.14, and demonstrate a modest survival benefit relative to the control arms, despite a doubling of response rates. Grade 3 and 4 diarrhoea was seen in the irinotecan-5-FU-LV, irinotecan alone, and the 5-FU-LV arms at a rate of 22·7%, 31% and 13·2% respectively. As expected, the Mayo regime was associated with a greater grade 3/4 neutropenia and mucositis relative to irinotecan-5-FU/LV. There were no significant QoL differences between the arms, and all three arms were associated with a 1% treatment-related death rate.[68]

The use of the bolus irinotecan/5-FU-LV regimen in one trial for advanced CRC (NCCTG N9741) and another in the adjuvant setting (CALBG C89803) had apparently resulted in an excessive number of early deaths compared with the original trial reported above.[235] An independent analysis of these trials found that patients treated with this regimen had a three-fold higher rate of treatment-induced or -exacerbated death than patients treated on the other arms. It was concluded that, with careful monitoring of patients in addition to dose delay or reduction for unresolved toxicities and aggressive supportive therapy, this regimen could be administered safely.[236]

In the second phase III trial, 387 patients were randomised to receive one of two infusional 5-FU-LV regimens with and without irinotecan, with the primary endpoint being response rate. The results are summarised in Table 28.14 and concur with the first trial. Toxicities included a grade 3–4 diarrhoea rate of 44% in the irinotecan arm versus 25·6% in the control ($P = 0·055$) arm, and QoL was not significantly different in the groups.[180]

Two European randomised phase III trials have compared irinotecan to either BSC or an infusional 5-FU regimen in the second-line setting.[67,237] In both trials irinotecan was given at a dose of 350 mg m$^{-2}$ every 3 weeks, or 300 mg m$^{-2}$ if the WHO performance status was 2 or patients were 70 years of age or over. In the first trial the 1-year survival was 36·2% in the irinotecan group versus 13·8% in the supportive care arm, with a median survival of 9·2 versus 6·5 months, respectively ($P = 0·0001$) (Table 28.10). Irinotecan provided significant palliative and QoL benefits: including prolongation of pain-free survival and time to definitive QoL deterioration ($P < 0·002$, $P = 0·003$, respectively) as well as improvement in several EORTC-QLQ-C30 scores.[67] The second study randomised 267 patients to irinotecan or to best infusional 5-FU-based regimen, with the results being similar to the first in terms of survival parameters and palliative benefit.[237] In both trials, patients had failed a prior 5-FU-based regimen. These two trials suggest that irinotecan should be the standard second-line agent in patients who have progressed on a 5-FU-based regimen. However, in view of its toxicity profile and modest improvement in survival, it appears to be a reasonable approach only in those patients with a good performance status.[238]

## Oxaliplatin

Oxaliplatin is a diaminocyclohexane (DACH) carrier ligand-based platinum compound, which, unlike other platinum compounds, has shown efficacy in CRC. It forms intrastrand, and less commonly interstrand, cross-links inhibiting DNA synthesis to a greater degree relative to cisplatin and carboplatin. The increased efficacy is thought to be due to the bulky DACH carrier ligand.[239,240] Preclinical studies had confirmed additive or synergistic effects with 5-FU, which have led to subsequent clinical trials evaluating this combination.[241]

Randomised trials have confirmed its place in both chemo-naive and previously treated patients. Three randomised phase III trials have compared two different first-line 5-FU-LV regimens with the same regimen with the addition of oxaliplatin (Table 28.14). The first trial randomised 420 patients to the LV5-FU2 regimen (LV 200 mg m$^{-2}$, 5-FU 400 mg m$^{-2}$ bolus, 5-FU 600 mg m$^{-2}$ per day, 22-hour CI, days 1 and 2) or to LV5-FU2 with oxaliplatin 85 mg m$^{-2}$ over 2 hours on day 1.[66] The primary endpoint was a prolongation in PFS: as many patients at the time of failure can now be salvaged with active second-line regimens, this endpoint seems a logical choice over OS. The response rate was doubled; however, the improvement in PFS was 2·8 months ($P = 0·0003$).[66] The addition of oxaliplatin to the LV5-FU2 regimen exacerbated the toxicities common to modulated 5-FU and was associated with significant neurotoxicity, as discussed in the section above (*Does systemic therapy provide advantages over BSC in terms of QoL and survival?*).[66] The second trial randomised 200 patients to receive either a chronomodulated 5-FU regimen or the same regimen with the addition of oxaliplatin, and confirmed the results of the first study (Table 28.14).[231] A third trial reported in abstract form only, had randomised 252 patients with untreated advanced CRC to either bolus 5-FU-LV (Mayo regimen) or to weekly high dose 24-hour 5-FU infusion plus oxaliplatin (Table 28.14) and again confirmed a doubling of response rates with comparable toxicity.[232]

The role of oxaliplatin relative to irinotecan as first-line therapy has been further supported from the results of two randomised trials. The first is a French study, published in abstract form, which randomised approximately 220 patients to receive an infusional 5-FU/LV-irinotecan regimen (FOLFIRI) or infusional 5-FU/LV-oxaliplatin regimen (FOLFOX) as first-line therapy, with cross-over at progression. The primary endpoint was time to progression after the second-line therapy (Table 28.14).[233] There was no significant difference between the first-line regimens in terms of response rates (FOLFIRI 57·5% *v* FOLFOX 56%), and in PFS and OS.[233] The second, the Intergroup N9741 trial, randomised patients to one of six chemotherapy arms – the interim results from three arms (oxaliplatin plus infusional 5-FU-LV, irinotecan plus bolus 5-FU-LV and irinotecan plus oxaliplatin) have been published in abstract form.[234] After 795 patients were randomised, the interim analysis had found superior efficacy for the oxaliplatin-5-FU-LV arm in terms of OS, PFS and toxicity, relative to the irinotecan arm, entailing closure of the latter (Table 28.14).[234] However, approximately 60% of patients in each arm had second-line therapy on progression. The superiority of the oxaliplatin-5-FU-LV arm to an irinotecan-infusional 5-FU regimen (that is, FOLFIRI) cannot be implied by these results.

Phase II trials involving 5-FU-refractory patients treated with oxaliplatin combined with 5-FU-LV have produced objective response rates of between 13–45%, PFS ranging from 5 to 10 months and a median OS of 9–17 months.[242–245] The beneficial effect of adding oxaliplatin to the same bolus or infusional 5-FU regimen on which patients had previously progressed, has also been confirmed by several studies.[245,246] A response rate of 21% was observed in patients treated with second-line oxaliplatin-5-FU following progression on an irinotecan-infusional 5-FU regimen.[233]

## Mitomycin-C

Two randomised phase III trials have demonstrated superior activity of mitomycin-C plus CI 5-FU versus CI 5-FU alone or a circadian-timed infusional 5-FU regimen, with overall response rates for the mitomycin-C arms of 54% and 40% respectively.[247,248] The first had demonstrated an advantage in terms of PFS and QOL; however, OS was not significantly increased.[247] Mitomycin-C in combination with infusional 5-FU has also shown response rates of up to 16% in 5-FU-refractory patients.[249] Its role in patients who have progressed on irinotecan or oxaliplatin is undefined as yet.

## New combinations

Combinations of the drugs discussed above are now entering phase I/II trials including the oral 5-FU prodrugs combined with oxaliplatin or with irinotecan, or combinations of irinotecan with oxaliplatin, etc. The newer regimens are also being combined with biological agents such as angiogenesis inhibitors (vascular endothelial growth factor inhibitors), epidermal growth factor receptor antagonists (C225, ZD1839), farnesyl transferase inhibitors, and cyclo-oxygenase-2 inhibitors. The usefulness of this approach must await the results of randomised phase III trials.

## *The selection of chemotherapy regimens in chemo-naive and previously treated patients*

The number of active agents available to patients with advanced CRC has increased over the past decade providing for greater individualisation of therapy. As seen above, most phase III first-line studies have not specified a second-line regimen on progression, hence the correct sequence of regimens remains to be clarified. Based on the currently reported randomised trials, certain recommendations can be made (Figure 28.4). For patients with previously untreated advanced colorectal cancer the options include the following.

- Patients with good performance status (ECOG 0–1) and no confounding medical comorbidities, as represented in the reported phase III trials should be offered an irinotecan- or oxaliplatin-5-FU-containing regimen **Evidence level Ib, Grade A**. It appears that oxaliplatin- infusional 5-FU-LV may be superior to irinotecan-bolus-5-FU-LV but equivalent to the irinotecan-infusional 5-FU-LV regimen. Oxaliplatin also provides the potential advantage of providing a downstaging effect to allow metastectomy (see section below on *What is the role of neoadjuvant chemotherapy prior to surgical resection of hepatic metastases?*).

- Patients with significant medical comorbidities or elderly patients over 65 years of age, or patients with performance status ECOG 2 should be offered a 5-FU regimen, either one of the 5-FU-FA regimens, modulated infusional 5-FU regimens or oral 5-FU prodrugs **Evidence level Ib, Grade A**. The latter would be preferred given the convenience of oral medication, provided patients are compliant and have an understanding of the actions to be taken if significant toxicities develop.

- Raltitrexed alone may be considered for those patients intolerant of 5-FU or who need to travel long distances for treatment, especially if the oral agents are not available or suitable.

The choice of second-line treatment offered to patients is determined by their clinical status, prior treatment given and its tolerance:

- single-agent irinotecan,[67,237] irinotecan plus infusional 5-FU-LV regimen, or oxaliplatin plus infusional 5-FU-LV regimen[233] **Evidence level Ib, Grade A**;
- infusional 5-FU: there are reports indicating response rates of 10–15% in patients with infusional regimens who have failed to respond to bolus 5-FU-LV[250,251] **Evidence level IIa, Grade B**;
- mitomycin-C in combination with infusional 5-FU **Evidence level IIa, Grade B**.

There is no recommended third-line regimen outside of clinical trials, and expert palliative care alone should be considered in all such patients.

## Local therapies for hepatic metastases

## Hepatic resection

Approximately 25% of patients will present with metastatic disease confined to the liver at the time of

**Table 28.15** Results of surgical resection of isolated hepatic metastases from advanced colorectal cancer

| Reference | No. of patients | 5-year survival (%) | Median survival (months) | Operative mortality (%) |
|---|---|---|---|---|
| Scheele[255] | 376 | 39 | 28 | 4 |
| Hughes[256] | 859 | 33 | NR | NR |
| Rosen[257] | 280 | 25 | 34 | 4 |
| Gayowiski[258] | 204 | 32 | NR | 1 |
| Schlag[259] | 122 | 30 | 32 | 4 |
| Fong[260] | 456 | 38 | 46 | 2·8 |
| Adson[261] | 141 | 25 | NR | 4 |

NR, not recorded.

diagnosis and another 25% will develop hepatic secondaries during their disease course. The OS of patients with untreated hepatic metastases ranges from 4–9 months up to 24 months, but with less than 3% overall surviving 5 years.[24,252–255]

Surgical resection of hepatic metastases remains the treatment of choice for patients with disease confined to the liver. The results of the larger case series are summarised in Table 28.15. In the majority, the 5-year survival is in excess of 25–38%, with a median survival of over 30 months.[176,255–261] Mortality rates from surgery are generally less than 5%, a consequence of a better understanding of hepatic anatomy, optimal patient selection, and improved postoperative care.[262]

Patient selection mandates that there should be no disease outside the liver as determined by detailed preoperative staging, including CT or MRI and increasingly FDG-PET. In addition, the extent of hepatic involvement and the relationship of lesions to vascular structures needs to be defined. Series evaluating FDG-PET as a staging modality in such patients have found that this technique had altered management in 11–49% of cases.[16,263,264] Intraoperative staging with laparoscopy, prior to laparotomy, and intraoperative hepatic ultrasound are also essential, the latter demonstrating additional metastatic deposits in 50% of patients (Figure 28.5).[265,266]

Prognostic factors predictive of survival following surgical resection include patient characteristics, stage and histologic grade of the primary tumour, and the characteristics of the liver metastases. The latter appear to be the most important factor determining long-term survival and include the following: the status of resection margins,[255,256,258,260,267–269] four or more tumour deposits,[258,260] tumour size,[260] bilobar distribution, lymph node involvement, and invasion of adjacent organs.[258,260] The presence of adverse prognostic factors does not contraindicate patients from undergoing an attempted curative resection. In one series of 456 patients who underwent hepatic resection, those with multiple metastases (three or more, or bilobar) or short disease-free

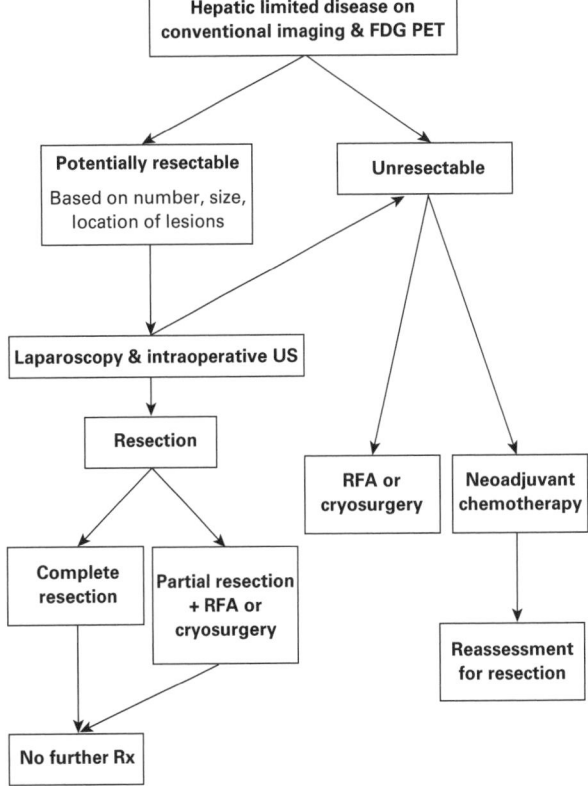

**Figure 28.5** The management of hepatic limited metastatic disease. FDG PET, fluorodeoxyglucose positron emission tomography; RFA, radiofrequency ablation; RT, radiotherapy; Rx, treatment; US, ultrasound

interval had a 5-year survival rate of over 24%, and of those with positive resection margins, 17% were alive at 5 years.[260] The presence of extrahepatic disease is generally regarded as an exclusion for resection, the only exception being patients with isolated pulmonary and limited hepatic metastases that have demonstrated a slow rate of disease progression.[270]

Patients with synchronous primary and hepatic metastases, despite the adverse effect on survival, should be considered for surgery if the lesions are otherwise resectable.[270] In general, the resection is performed as a staged procedure: the primary tumour is resected first, followed by a formal hepatic resection at a latter date, allowing time for occult metastases to declare themselves. Non-randomised studies have shown that such an approach provides similar outcomes compared with a combined resection.[271,272]

The majority of patients (70%) will still die from metastatic disease after hepatic resection. Sites of recurrence include the liver alone (21–41%), extrahepatic site (10–50%, in particular lung alone; 21%), and liver plus extrahepatic site (7–69%).[259,260,273–275] In isolated hepatic recurrence, where feasible, repeat resections have been performed with a 3-year survival rate of 33% in one series.[276]

### Is there a role for adjuvant therapy (hepatic arterial infusional [HAI] and/or systemic therapy) following resection of hepatic metastases?

HAI is based on the premise that hepatic metastases derive most of their blood supply from the hepatic artery rather than the portal vein as for the rest of the hepatic parenchyma. Delivery of chemotherapy via HAI allows for higher concentrations of the cytotoxic to be delivered to the metastasis, relative to systemic delivery. However, efficient hepatic drug extraction and metabolism would reduce the systemic drug exposure and hence systemic toxicity. Most regimens have used the 5-fluoro-2'-deoxyuridine (FUDR), a drug similar to 5-FU in terms of efficacy, but which has greater hepatic extraction.[277]

Three recent randomised phase III trials have evaluated the role of postoperative adjuvant chemotherapy in resected patients (Table 28.16). The first study from the German Cooperative on Liver Metastases, observed that postoperative HAI, with 5-FU/LV, provided no additional benefit to surgery alone in terms of median survival, liver PFS and overall PFS.[278] The second study randomised patients following surgery to systemic chemotherapy (5-FU-based) with or without HAI with FUDR. No significant median survival or PFS difference between the arms were observed. Liver PFS was in favour of the combined therapy at 2 years (90% v 60%, P < 0·01), which was maintained up to 7 years (Table 28.16).[279]

The final study, an Intergroup trial, randomised patients following surgery to observation or to systemic and HAI therapy. The results for liver progression-free and recurrence-free survival are based on 75 patients who actually received the planned therapy, rather than on an intention-to-treat analysis.[280] This has lead to difficulties in the interpretation of the results.[281] Postresection "adjuvant" systemic therapy with 5-FU-LV in two randomised studies has not shown a significant benefit in terms of DFS and OS.[282,283]

The use of postresection HAI ± systemic chemotherapy in the form assessed by these studies cannot be recommended as standard therapy **Evidence level Ib, Grade A**. The staging and treatment of advanced CRC has advanced significantly since the commencement of these trials with introduction of more efficacious agents, as discussed above. The role of neoadjuvant therapy and the identification of active combinations for systemic and HAI treatment will require validation by randomised trials. Surgery alone still represents the standard of care in most centres.

### What is the role of neoadjuvant chemotherapy prior to surgical resection of hepatic metastases?

The usefulness of neoadjuvant chemotherapy to increase the potential for a curative resection has been a more recent concept (Figure 28.5). A retrospective study reported on approximately 150 patients with unresectable hepatic metastases who received chronomodulated oxaliplatin plus 5-FU-LV. The objective response rate was 59%, with 78% of these responders undergoing resection with clear margins. The estimated 5-year survival rate for chemotherapy and surgery was 58%.[284] Phase III trials are awaiting completion, and no conclusions can be drawn in the interim.

### Can hepatic arterial infusional chemotherapy (HAI) for unresectable hepatic metastases be dispensed with?

There have been several randomised trials that have compared HAI with FUDR to systemic FUDR, or to systemic 5-FU, or to no or delayed therapy in patients with unresectable metastatic disease limited to the liver.[186,187,285–289] The Meta-Analysis Group in Cancer has analysed these trials involving 654 patients with the two endpoints of interest being tumour response rate and OS.[290] The objective tumour response was 41% for the HAI arms and 14% for systemic therapy: overall response ratio was 0·25 (95% CI 0·16–0·40; P < 10^{-10}). No survival advantage was observed for individual trials comparing HAI to systemic chemotherapy or to the combination: median survival time of 16 versus 12·2 months (P = 0·14).[290] This interpretation was limited by the absence of individual patient data from one of the larger trials assessed. A further meta-analysis of these trials, with complete individual patient data on this occasion, comparing regional versus systemic chemotherapy, confirmed a 10% survival advantage

**Table 28.16** Results of randomised trials of postoperative adjuvant chemotherapy (HAI, systemic) following resection of hepatic metastases

| Reference | No. of patients (follow up) | Treatment | Median survival (months) | Liver-PFS[a] | PFS (months) |
|---|---|---|---|---|---|
| Lorenz[278] | 226 (70% > 18 months) | Surgery<br>Surgery + HAI[b] | 41<br>35<br>(NS) | 24 months<br>22 months<br>(NS) | 14<br>14<br>(NS) |
| Kemeny[279] | 156 (5 years) | Surgery + systemic[c]<br>Surgery + systemic[d] + HAI[e] | 59<br><br>72<br>(NS) | 60%<br><br>90%[f]<br>($P<0.01$) | 17<br><br>37<br>(NS) |
| Kemeny[280] | 109 (4.25 yrs) | Surgery<br>Surgery + Systemic + HAI[g] | 47<br>34<br>(NS)[h] | 43%[i]<br>67%<br>($P=0.03$)[j] | 25.2%[k]<br>45.7%<br>($P=0.04$)[j] |

[a]Abbreviations: L-PFS, liver-progression free survival; OS, overall survival; NS, non-significant to the 0.05 level; PFS, progression-free survival.
[b]HAI: LV 200 mg m$^{-2}$ bolus + 5-FU 1000 mg m$^{-2}$, CI 24 hours, days 1–5, q 4 weeks × 6 cycles.
[c]5-FU 370 mg m$^{-2}$ + LV 200 mg m$^{-2}$ bolus, days 1–5, q 4 weeks × 6 cycles or 5-FU 1000 mg m$^{-2}$ per day, CI 24 hours, days 1–5, q 4 weeks × 6 cycles (if past exposure to 5-FU/LV).
[d]5-FU 325 mg m$^{-2}$ + LV 200 mg m$^{-2}$, bolus, days 1–5, q 4 weeks × 6 cycles or 5-FU 850 mg m$^{-2}$, CI 24 hours, days 1–5, q 4 weeks × 6 cycles (if past 5-FU/LV).
[e]FUDR 0.25 mg kg$^{-1}$ per day, CI 24 hours, days 1–14, every 21 days × 6 cycles.
[f]At 2 years.
[g]HAI; FUDR, 0.05–0.2mg/kg per day, days 1–14, every 4 weeks × 4 cycles. Systemic chemotherapy, commenced from day 15 of HAI cycle, 5-FU 200 mg m$^{-2}$ per day, CI over 14 days. After HAI, 5-FU 300 mg m$^{-2}$ per day, days 1–14, q 4 weeks × 8 cycles.
[h]Based on intention to treat analysis (109 patients).
[i]Based on 75 assessable patients, not on intention to treat.
[j]4 years.
[k]Recurrence-free survival at 4 years.

at 1 year in favour of FUDR HAI ($P=0.041$), but was not significant at 2 years (6%, $P=0.124$).[291]

Recent trials have included what would be considered standard systemic chemotherapy in their control arms. A multicentre trial from Germany randomised patients to HAI 5-FU/LV versus intravenous 5-FU/LV, or to HAI FUDR, with median survival times of 18.7, 17.6, and 12.7 months, respectively. There was no significant difference on comparison between pairs of treatment arms.[292] Current directions are now focusing on irinotecan and oxaliplatin being given by HAI as well as systemically to improve results. Intra-arterial yttrium-90 microspheres combined with FUDR by HAI has shown intial promising results compared with FUDR alone in a small randomised trial.[293]

HAI requires the operative placement of an infusion device and intra-arterial catheter and is associated with catheter-related complications as well as chemical hepatitis (16–79%), biliary sclerosis (10%), gastritis and gastroduodenal ulceration (8–20%).[187,285–288] At present, HAI for unresectable hepatic metastases cannot be considered as standard of care, and should be used only by experienced oncologists in circumstances that prevent patients receiving chemotherapy with other equally active systemic approaches **Evidence level Ia, Grade A**.

### Is the role of local hepatic ablative therapies defined in the treatment of hepatic metastases?

Cryotherapy and radiofrequency ablation (RFA) have been used to treat unresectable hepatic metastases often as an adjunct or an alternative to surgical resection (Figure 28.5). Cryotherapy requires a formal laparotomy with intra-operative ultrasound guidance, whereas RFA can be performed intraoperatively or via percutaneous probes. Studies to date have been performed in highly selected but differing populations of patients, some in combination with surgical resection.

Tumour control rates with RFA range from 70% to 90% and 3-year survival rates 33%.[294,295] The majority of cryosurgery series are small in number, with reported 1- and 2-year survival rates of over 70% and 50%, respectively, and 5-year DFS rates of 15% to 28%. Cryotherapy is associated with a greater risk of complications relative to RFA, including haemorrhage, biliary fistula, hepatic or subphrenic abscess, and, rarely, hepatic failure.[296–299] In one large series, 136 patients with unresectable hepatic metastases underwent cryotherapy, with a median OS of 30 months: 20 patients underwent re-cryotherapy and 65% had failed outside the liver.[300] Despite their widespread use, cryotherapy and RFA cannot be considered as standard therapeutic approaches in the absence of well designed trials **Evidence level IIa, Grade B**.

External beam radiotherapy has also been used to palliate symptomatic hepatic metastases, with an improvement in pain in 80–90% of cases.[301,302] More recently, stereotactic single and hypofractionated radiation therapy has been given to hepatic malignancies in order to attain a highly localised cytotoxic dose.[303,304] In a recent series, 60 hepatic lesions from 37 patients were treated with an escalated dose from 14 Gy to 26 Gy: 54 of the 55 lesions were locally controlled after 6 weeks with 32 objective responses.[304] Randomised trials are required to clarify the role of this approach.

## Are there markers predictive of response to therapy that may allow for individualisation of treatment?

### Molecular factors that predict for greater efficacy to adjuvant chemotherapy, independent of tumour stage

Identification of molecular changes within cancer cells may provide a far better insight into tumour biology by defining predictors of the natural history of individual tumours as well as the role of chemotherapy. The molecular markers that have been evaluated in regard to the efficacy of adjuvant chemotherapy include *TS*, *p53* and *Ki-ras* (Table 28.17). MSI has also been assessed with conflicting results. A population-based retrospective cohort study of 656 patients with resected Dukes' C disease demonstrated that patients with MSI-high tumours had a marked survival benefit from adjuvant chemotherapy (90% *v* 35%, at 54 months median follow up, $P < 0.0007$) relative to patients who were MSI-stable.[43] However, a pooled molecular analysis of randomised adjuvant chemotherapy trials, demonstrated that patients with MSI-high tumours receiving 5-FU-based therapy had a trend to poorer OS compared with no therapy ($P = 0.07$), implying that such

patients do not benefit from therapy.[308] Thus this area requires further clarification.

## Factors predictive of response in patients with advanced disease

### *Patient-derived factors*

Clinical factors predictive of response from meta-analyses and a number of studies using 5-FU-based regimens and newer agents, such as oxaliplatin and irinotecan, have been summarised in Table 28.18. Discordant identification of predictors of response in trials evaluating similar regimens can occur by variation in patient selection, presence of measurable disease, metastatic sites, biochemical parameters as well as dose intensity and regimen.[312]

Apart from the treatment effect, the identified patient-derived factors predictive for response are inconsistent, in stark contrast to those seen for survival (Table 28.18). Performance status was found to be predictive of response in two meta-analyses, the first evaluating bolus versus CI 5-FU and the second 5-FU modulation by interferon alfa.[64,310] In the phase III trial of infusional 5-FU-LV with and without irinotecan, the independent predictive factors for response by multivariate analysis apart from irinotecan were weight loss ($P = 0.009$) and time from diagnosis to first metastasis ($P = 0.001$).[180]

### *Tumoural factors predictive of response to chemotherapy*

Molecular predictors of response that have been evaluated include *TS DPD*, *TP* and *p53*. Several studies have demonstrated in patients with advanced CRC that an increased expression of *TS* (mRNA, protein levels and enzyme activity) is associated with a reduced response to 5-FU-based therapy.[75,97,99,313,314] Its expression has been correlated to polymorphisms within the enhancer region of the *TS* promoter gene. The 2R/2R polymorphism resulted in a reduced TS content and hence better response to 5-FU-based therapy and OS.[100,315]

The mean *TP* mRNA levels in one clinical study were found to be 2·6 times greater in non-responding tumours compared with responding tumours.[90] *DPD* is the major catabolic enzyme for the fluoropyrimidines that may contribute to drug resistance. Studies in human cancer cell lines and resected tumour samples have demonstrated that its activity and mRNA expression were independent factors related to 5-FU sensitivity.[316–318] Mutations in the *p53* tumour suppressor gene has also been inconsistently correlated with response to therapy.[73,86,98,319]

The utility of multiple markers has also been assessed. One study attempted to correlate the gene expression of *DPD*, *TS* and *TP* to 5-FU response. Colorectal tumours with

**Table 28.17  Molecular markers predictive of response following adjuvant therapy for localised colorectal cancer**

| Marker | Detection | Primary and stage | Treatment modality | Correlation | Reference |
|---|---|---|---|---|---|
| *p53* | IMH, PCR-SSCP | Rectum, LA | Preoperative CT/RT | ↑ Expression/or mutation no correlation | Elsaleh[305] |
| | IMH, PCR-SSCP | CRC, stage III | S $v$ S+5-FU-Lev | CT provided maximal OS benefit if normal *p53*. ($P$=0·041) | Elsaleh[58] |
| Enhancer region polymorphism in TS gene promoter | PCR | Dukes' C, CRC | 5-FU-based | Homozygous (3R/3R), no benefit from CT | Iacopetta[100] |
| | PCR | Rectum, LA | Preoperative 5-FU/RT | Homozygous (3R/3R) ↓ response ($P$=0·036) Trend to ↓ 3-year DFS | Villafranca[306] |
| TS expression | IMH | CRC, Dukes' B and C | S $v$ S+5-FU CT | ↑ Expression correlated with ↑ DFS for CT arm ($P$=0·02) | Edler[42] |
| *Ki-ras* mutation | PCR | CRC, Dukes' C | 5-FU-LV or 5-FU-Lev | Non-Asp mutations IPF for OS benefit from CT | Gnanasampanthan[307] |
| LOH 18q alleles | PCR | Stages II[†] and III | S or S+CT[‡] | No LOH+MS-S, ↑ 5-year DFS+OS following CT ($P$=0.05) | Watanabe[41] |
| MSI | PCR | Stage C | S+CT | IPF for survival following chemotherapy | Elsaleh[43] |
| TGF-β1 | PCR | Stages II[†] and III | S or S+CT[‡] | Type II TGF-β1 receptor mutation and MSI correlated with ↑ 5-year DFS+OS following CT ($P$=0·04) | Watanabe[41] |

Abbreviations: Asp, aspartate; CRC, colorectal; CT, chemotherapy; DFS, disease-free survival; IPF, independent prognostic factor; LA, locally advanced; Lev, Levamisole; LOH, loss of heterozygosity; LV, leucovorin; MSI, microsatellite instability; MS-S, Microsatellite-stable; OS, overall survival; PCR-SSCP, polymerase chain reaction/single strand conformation polymorphism; RT, radiotherapy; S, surgery; TGF, transforming growth factor; TS, thymidylate synthase.
[†]High risk stage II.
[‡]From two randomised trials with the following arms: 5-FU+Lev, Lev alone, 5-FU+LV (low dose or high dose), 5F+LV+Lev.

**Table 28.18  Predictive factors for response in advanced disease**

| Factor | Clinical indication | Treatment | Predictive factors for response | Reference |
|---|---|---|---|---|
| *Patient characteristics* | | | | |
| Extent of prior therapy | 5-FU resistant | Ox + 5-FU-LV | $\geq$ 3 prior regimens, $\downarrow$ response | 309 |
| Weight loss | Chemo-naive | Ir-5-FU-LV *v* 5-FU-LV | Loss $\leq$ 5%, $P = 0.009$ | 180 |
| Time from diagnosis to metastasis | 5-FU resistant | Ir | $\geq$ 9 months, $\uparrow$ ORR, $P = 0.24$ | 70 |
| Performance status | 5-FU resistant | Ox + 5-FU-LV | WHO PS $\geq$ 2, $\downarrow$ ORR | 309 |
| | Chemo-naive | 5-FU CI *v* 5-FU bolus | ECOG 0 *v* 1 *v* 2 +, $P < 0.0001$ | 64 |
| Tumour markers | Chemo-naive | 5-FU-LV-based | Baseline CEA significant predictor | 103 |
| Number of organs involved | 5-FU resistant | Ir | 1 *v* > 1 organ involved, $P = 0.008$ | 70 |
| Synchronous *v* metachronous metastases | Chemo-naive | Ox+5-FU-LV *v* 5-FU-LV | OR = 1.57, $P = 0.031$ | 66 |
| Site of metastases | Chemo-naive | 5-FU-based therapy | $P = 0.0001$ | 202 |
| | Chemo-naive | $\alpha$-IF + 5-FU-LV *v* 5-FU-LV | Liver confined $\uparrow$ ORR, $P < 10^{-4}$ | 310 |
| *Treatment effect* | | | | |
| 5-FU modulation by LV | Chemo-naive | 5-FU-LV *v* 5-FU | 5-FU-LV weekly, $P < 10^{-5}$; 5-FU-LV monthly, $P < 10^{-5}$ | 65 |
| Experimental 5-FU regimen | Chemo-naive | i.v. bolus 5-FU *v* experimental 5-FU* | OR = 0.48, $P < 0.001$ | 311 |
| Irinotecan | Chemo-naive | Ir-5-FU-LV *v* 5-FU-LV | | 68, 180 |
| Oxaliplatin | Chemo-naive | Ox+5-FU-LV *v* 5-FU-LV | OR = 1.84, $P = 0.0001$ | 66 |
| *Treatment toxicity* | | | | |
| Grade 3 or 4 neutropenia or diarrhoea | 5-FU resistant | Ir | OR = 1.66, $P = 0.041$ | 70 |

Abbreviations: Ir, irinotecan; IF, interferon; OR, odds ratio; ORR, overall response rate; Ox, oxaliplatin; LV, leucovorin
*Experimental 5-FU regimens: 5-FU + leucovorin, 5-FU + methotrexate, 5-FU continuous infusion, intra-arterial infusion of floxiuridine.

expression values of all three below their individual non-response cut-off levels had a response rate of 92% to 5-FU.[75] In a series of 50 patients with advanced CRC treated with irinotecan plus 5-FU-LV, concomitant low expression of topoisomerase 1 and TS had a response rate of 28% versus 41% for all other groups.[320]

## Local palliative therapies for the treatment of advanced CRC

Palliative locally directed therapy in patients with advanced CRC, subject to the site, can take the form of external beam radiotherapy with or without concurrent chemotherapy for local disease or metastases, to endoscopic laser, stent insertion, or surgery for symptomatic primary lesions.

## Can locally recurrent colorectal cancer be salvaged with the aim for cure?

In the case of rectal cancer, isolated recurrence ranges from 25–40% following conventional surgery alone, to 13–25% following adjuvant chemoradiotherapy, and to 4–8% for TME, often associated with significant local symptoms and poor QoL.[46,145,147,321] Surgical salvage by local excision of anastomotic recurrence or *en bloc* resection of involved adjacent organs and/or pelvic structures, in highly selected patients can provide a 30–50% 5-year survival rate and a 50% long-term local control rate.[321–325] A series from the MD Anderson Cancer Center reported on 43 patients with locally recurrent rectal cancer involving pelvic viscera, sacrum, or pelvic sidewalls, that were treated with preoperative chemoradiation (25 with additional intraoperative radiotherapy). At surgery, 33 had macroscopic complete resection, 29 had negative microscopic margins and no patient required sacropelvic resection. The 5-year survival rate for the entire group was 37%.[326]

## What is the optimal regimen of radiotherapy for the palliation of recurrent rectal cancer?

Several series have been reported on the palliation of symptomatic recurrent/inoperable rectosigmoid malignancies using varying radiation schedules.[327–333] A few of these have also combined 5-FU with radiotherapy for radiosensitisation.[328,329,334] Symptomatic relief had been achieved in 65–100% for pain, 100% for bleeding and 24% for mass effect.[327–329,331–333] Up to a third of patients achieved symptom control up to 6 months following radiotherapy alone.[331]

Given the nature of the studies it is unclear whether a dose–response relationship exists for the palliation of symptoms and the duration of their control.[327–329] The exact role of chemotherapy either combined with radiotherapy or alone is not clear.

## Intraluminal palliative approaches for symptomatic local disease in patients who are unfit for surgery

Patients with symptomatic local disease who are unfit for surgical resection or colostomy can be palliated with local endoscopic measures such as laser therapy or stent insertion. Several series have reported on the use of endoscopic laser therapy to lesions of the rectum or distal colon for the relief of symptoms such as obstruction, bleeding, mucous discharge and diarrhoea.[335–339] Its usefulness is limited as it is often required to be repeated every 1 to 2 months to maintain symptom control.

Endoscopic stents (plastic, endocoil, or self-expanding metallic) have been used to relieve obstruction and to also prolong the interval between laser therapies. The reported series have been small; however, stenting of obstructive lesions can be accomplished in 64–100% of lesions depending on the series and site, either as a final palliative measure or prior to definitive surgery. In those lesions successfully dilated, long-term luminal patency is maintained in up to 63–100%.[340–344]

## Conclusions

1  The treatment of colorectal cancer needs to be both individualised and multidisciplinary.

2  Staging defines the extent of local disease as well the presence of metastases. FDG-PET is becoming increasingly important in this process.

3  Pathological stage remains the major prognostic factor in terms of outcome. In the adjuvant setting, molecular markers predictive of survival and response remain to be elucidated. For advanced inoperable disease, performance status remains the most important prognostic factor in terms of outcome **Evidence level Ia, Grade A**.

4  For localised colorectal cancer, surgery with wide lymphadenectomy is the primary therapy.

5  Adjuvant therapy for stage III colon cancer comprises of one of several standard 5-FU-LV combinations over 6 months **Evidence level Ia, Grade A**. Infusional regimens appear to be equivalent to bolus regimens **Evidence level Ib, Grade A**. Adjuvant therapy is reasonable for selected patients with Dukes' B disease. However, the data are inconsistent.

6  The treatment of localised rectal cancer is in a state of change. On the basis of anatomic staging, patients with extensive local disease or with nodal involvement may be treated with preoperative therapy (that is, chemoradiotherapy or preoperative radiotherapy followed by TME) **Evidence level Ib, Grade A**. In resected cases, adjuvant chemoradiotherapy may be reserved for those with adverse operative pathological features, including transmural penetration or nodal involvement, at high risk of local recurrence **Evidence level Ib, Grade A**. In patients with resected early stage disease, at low risk of recurrence or where morbidity of radiotherapy is considered significant, radiation may be deleted **Evidence level Ia, Grade A**.

7  *Advanced disease*: systemic chemotherapy provides benefits in terms of improved QoL and prolonged survival relative to best supportive care.

- In patients with previously untreated advanced colorectal cancer the options are based on performance status and medical condition. (a) Patients with good performance status (ECOG 0–1) and few confounding medical comorbidities, should be offered an irinotecan or oxaliplatin-containing regimen **Evidence level Ib, Grade A**. (b) Patients with significant medical comorbidities, elderly patients over 65 years of age, or patients with performance status (ECOG 2), should be offered a 5-FU regimen, either one of the 5-FU-LV regimens: modulated infusional 5-FU regimens or oral 5-FU prodrugs **Evidence level Ib, Grade A**. The latter would be preferred given the convenience of oral medication, provided patients are compliant and have an understanding of the actions to be taken if significant toxicities develop.

(c) Raltitrexed may be considered for those patients intolerant of 5-FU or who need to travel long distances for treatment, especially if the oral agents are not available or suitable.

- In the second-line setting, treatment is determined by the clinical status, choice and tolerance to prior therapy. Options include: (a) single agent irinotecan or in combination with an infusional 5-FU-LV regimen **Evidence level Ib, Grade A**; (b) oxaliplatin plus infusional 5-FU-LV regimen **Evidence level Ib, Grade A**; (c) infusional 5-FU **Evidence level IIa, Grade B**; (d) mitomycin-C in combination with infusional 5-FU **Evidence level IIa, Grade B**.

- There is no recommended third-line regimen and hence patients wanting to receive more chemotherapy should be entered into relevant clinical trials. Palliative care is appropriate at all later stages of illness.

8  At present there are no consistent clinically useful predictors of response to chemotherapy in the adjuvant or advanced setting **Evidence level III, Grade B**.

9  Patients with resectable hepatic-limited metastases should be offered potentially curative surgical resection. The use of postresection HAI with or without systemic chemotherapy cannot be recommended as standard therapy **Evidence level Ib, Grade A**. Neoadjuvant chemotherapy to increase the potential for a curative resection may be potentially useful, but is unproven in randomised trials **Evidence level IIa, Grade B**.

10  HAI cannot be considered standard of care in patients with unresectable hepatic-limited metastases at the present time **Evidence level Ia, Grade A**. Despite their widespread use, cryotherapy and RFA cannot be considered as standard therapeutic approaches in the absence of well-designed trials. RFA is probably the preferred ablative technique because of its non-operative use and lower toxicity.

11  Locally recurrent rectal cancer that is not amenable to surgical salvage can be treated with radiotherapy either alone or with chemotherapy or both. This provides good palliation and in some cases the potential for downstaging to allow resection **Evidence level IIa, Grade B**.

12  Symptomatic primary disease in patients unfit for resection may be palliated by endoscopic laser or stent **Evidence level III, Grade B**.

## References

1  Ries LAG, Eisner MP, Kosary CL *et al.* eds. *SEER Cancer Statistics Review*, 1973–1998, Bethesda MD: National Cancer Institute, 2002.

2  Pisani P, Parkin DM, Bray F, Ferlay J. Estimates of the worldwide mortality from 25 cancers in 1990. *Int J Cancer* 1999;**83**:18–29.

3  Haenszel W, Kurihara M. Studies of Japanese migrants. I. Mortality from cancer and other diseases among Japanese in the United States. *J Natl Cancer Inst* 1968;**40**:43–68.

4  McMichael AJ, McCall MG, Hartshorne JM *et al.* Patterns of gastrointestinal cancer in European migrants to Australia: The role of dietary change. *Int J Cancer* 1980;**25**(Suppl.):431–7.

5  Parkin DM, Pisani P, Ferlay J. Global cancer statistics. *CA Cancer J Clin* 1999;**49**:33–64.

6  Schottenfeld D. Epidemiology. In: Cohen AM, Winawer SJ, eds. *Cancer of the colon, rectum and anus.* New York: McGraw-Hill, 1995.

7  Ragnhammar P, Hafstrom L, Nygren P *et al.* A systematic overview of chemotherapy effects in colorectal cancer. *Acta Oncol* 2001;**40**: 282–308.

8  Gastrointestinal Tumor Study Group. Adjuvant therapy of colon cancer- Results of a prospectively randomized trial. *N Engl J Med* 1984;**310**:737–43.

9  Gastrointestinal Tumor Study Group. Prolongation of the disease free survival in surgically treated rectal cancer. *N Engl J Med* 1985;**312**:1465–72.

10  Wolmark N, Fisher ER, Wieand HS *et al.* The relationship of depth of penetration and tumor size to the number of positive nodes in Dukes C colorectal cancer. *Cancer* 1984;**53**:2707–12.

11  Tepper JE, O'Connell MJ, Niedzwiecki D *et al.* Impact of number of nodes retrieved on outcome in patients with rectal cancer. *J Clin Oncol* 2001;**19**:157–63.

12  Le Voyer TE, Sigurdso ER, Hanlon AL *et al.* Colon cancer survival is associated with increasing number of lymph nodes removed. A secondary analysis of INT-0089. *Proc Am Soc Clin Oncol* 2000;**21**:925(abstr).

13  Colon and rectum. In: American Joint Committee on Cancer. *Manual for staging of cancer, 5th edn.* Philadelphia: JB Lippincott, 1997.

14  Dukes CE. The classification of cancer of the rectum. *J Pathol* 1932;**35**:323–32.

15  Bast RC, Ravdin P, Hayes DF *et al.* 2000 Update of recommendations for the use of tumor markers in breast and colorectal cancer: Clinical practice guidelines of the American Society of Clinical Oncology. *J Clin Oncol* 2001;**19**:1865–78.

16  Ruers TJ, Langenhoff BS, Neeleman N *et al.* Value of positron emission tomography with [F-18]fluorodeoxyglucose in patients with colorectal liver metastases: a prospective study. *J Clin Oncol* 2002;**20**:388–95.

17  Abdel-Nabi H, Doerr RJ, Lamonica DM *et al.* Staging of primary colorectal carcinomas with fluorine-18 fluorodeoxyglucose whole-body PET: correlation with histopathologic and CT findings. *Radiology* 1998;**206**:755–60.

18  Aster VB, Coller FA. The prognostic significance of direct extension of carcinoma of the colon and rectum. *Ann Surg* 1954;**139**:846–51.

19  Fuchs CS, Mayer RJ. Adjuvant chemotherapy for colon and rectal cancer. *Semin Oncol* 1995;**22**:472–87.

20  Minsky BD, Mies C, Rich TA *et al.* Potentially curative surgery of colon cancer: Patterns of failure and survival. *J Clin Oncol* 1988;**6**:106–18.

21  Willet CG, Tepper JE, Cohen AM *et al.* Failure patterns following curative resection of colonic carcinoma. *Ann Surg* 1984;**200**:685–90.

22  Grinell RS. The grading and prognosis of carcinoma of the colon and rectum. *Ann Surg* 1939;**109**:500–3.

23  Grinnell RS. Lymphatic block with atypical and retrograde lymphatic metastasis and spread in carcinoma of the colon and rectum. *Ann Surg* 1966;**163**:272–80.

24  Bengmark S, Hafstrom L. The natural history of primary and secondary malignant tumors of the liver: The prognosis for patients with hepatic metastases from colonic and rectal carcinoma verified by laparotomy. *Cancer* 1969;**23**:198–23.

25  Greenway B. Hepatic metastases from colorectal cancer: Resection or not. *Br J Surgery* 1988;**75**:513–19.

26  Wood CG, Gillis CR, Blumgart LH. A retrospective study the natural history of patients with liver metastases from colorectal cancer. *J Clin Oncol* 1976;**2**:285–8.

27  Taylor B, Langer B, Falk RE *et al.* Role of resection in the management of metastases to the liver. *Can J Surg* 1983;**26**:215–17.

28 Petrelli N, Douglas OH, Herrera L *et al.* The modulation of fluorouracil with leucovorin in metastatic colorectal carcinoma: A randomized phase III trial. *J Clin Oncol* 1989;**7**:1419–26.

29 Gilbert JM. Distribution of metastases at necropsy in colorectal cancer. *Clin Exp Metastasis* 1983;**1**:97–101.

30 Sugarbaker PH, Gianola FJ, Dwyer A *et al.* A simplified plan for follow up of patients with colon and rectal cancer supported by prospective studies of laboratory and radiologic test results. *Surgery* 1987;**102**:79–87.

31 Cunningham D, Zalcberg JR, Rath U *et al.* Tomudex (ZD1694): results of a randomised trial in advanced colorectal cancer demonstrate the efficacy and reduced mucositis and leucopenia. The Tomudex Colorectal Cancer Study Group. *Eur J Cancer* 1995;**31A**:1945–54.

32 Cocconi D, Cunningham D, Van Cutsem E *et al.* Open, randomized, multicenter trial of raltitrexed versus fluorouracil plus high dose leucovorin in patients with advanced colorectal cancer. *J Clin Oncol* 1998;**16**:2943–52.

33 Weiss L, Grundmann E, Torhosrt J *et al.* Haematogenous metastatic patterns in colonic carcinoma: an analysis of 1541 necroscopies. *J Pathol* 1986;**150**:195–203.

34 Behbehani A, Sakwa M, Ehrlichman R *et al.* Colorectal carcinoma in the young. *Aust NZ J Surg* 1985;**55**:149–52.

35 Taylor MC, Pounder D, Ali Ridhaa NH *et al.* Prognostic factors in colorectal carcinoma of young adults. *Can J Surg* 1988;**31**:150–3.

36 Adkins RB, DeLozier JB, McKnight WG *et al.* Carcinoma of the colon in patients 35 years of age and younger. *Am Surg* 1987;**53**:141–5.

37 Sargent DJ, Goldberg RM, Jacobson SD *et al.* A pooled analysis of adjuvant chemotherapy for resected colon cancer in elderly patients. *N Engl J Med* 2001;**345**:1091–7.

38 Chapius PH, Dent OF, Fisher R *et al.* A multivariate analysis of clinical and pathological variables in prognosis after resection of large bowel cancer. *Br J Surg* 1985;**72**:698–702.

39 Isbister WH, Fraser J. Survival following surgical resection for colorectal cancer: A New Zealand national study. *Dis Colon Rectum* 1985;**28**:725–7.

40 Wolters U, Stutzer H, Keller HW, Schroder U, Pichlmaier H. Colorectal cancer- a multivariate analysis of prognostic factors. *Eur J Surg Oncol* 1996;**22**:592–7.

41 Watanabe T, Wu TT, Catalano PJ *et al.* Molecular predictors of survival after adjuvant chemotherapy for colon cancer. *N Engl J Med* 2001;**344**:1196–206.

42 Edler D, Glimelius B, Hallstrom M *et al.* Thymidylate synthase expression in colorectal cancer: A prognostic and predictive marker of benefit from adjuvant fluorouracil-based chemotherapy. *J Clin Oncol* 2002;**20**:1721–28.

43 Elsaleh H, Joseph D, Grieu F, Zeps N, Spry N, Iacopetta B. Evidence for tumour site and gender specific survival benefit from adjuvant chemotherapy in colorectal cancer. *Lancet* 2000;**355**:1745–50.

44 Tepper JE, O'Connel D, Niedzwiecki D *et al.* Adjuvant therapy in rectal cancer: Analysis of stage, sex, and local control – Final report of Intergroup 0114. *J Clin Oncol* 2002;**20**:1744–50.

45 Rich T, Gunderson LL, Lew R *et al.* Patterns of recurrence of rectal cancer after potentially curative surgery. *Cancer* 1983;**52**:1317–29.

46 Krook JE, Moertel CG, Gunderson LL *et al.* Effective surgical adjuvant therapy for high-risk rectal carcinoma. *N Engl J Med* 1991;**324**:709–15.

47 Martling A, Holm T, Johansson H *et al.* The Stockholm II trial on preoperative radiotherapy in rectal carcinoma: long-term follow-up of a population-based study. *Cancer* 2001;**92**:896–902.

48 Fisher B, Fisher ER, Redmond C. A brief overview of findings from NSABP trials of adjuvant therapy. *Recent Results Cancer Res* 1984;**96**:55–65.

49 Compton CC, Fielding LP, Burgart LJ *et al.* Prognostic factors in colorectal cancer. College of American Pathologists Consensus Statement 1999. *Arch Pathol Lab Med* 2000;**124**:979–94.

50 Wolmark N, Wieand HS, Rockette HE *et al.* The prognostic significance of tumour location and bowel obstruction in Dukes B and C colorectal cancer. Findings from the NSABP clinical trials. *Ann Surg* 1983;**198**:743–52.

51 Steinberg SM, Barkin JS, Kaplan RS *et al.* Prognostic indicators of colonic tumours: The Gastrointestinal Tumour Group experience. *Cancer* 1986;**57**:1866–70.

52 Serpell JW, McDermott FT, Katrivessis H *et al.* Obstructing carcinomas of the colon. *Br J Surg* 1989;**76**:965–9.

53 Enblad P, Adami HO, Bergstrom R *et al.* Improved survival of patients with cancers of the colon and rectum? *J Natl Cancer Inst* 1988;**80**:589–91.

54 Eisenberg B, DeCosse JJ, Hartford F *et al.* carcinomas of the colon and rectum: The natural history reviewed in 1704 patients. *Cancer* 1982;**49**:1131–4.

55 Kune GA, Kune S, Field B *et al.* Survival in patients with large-bowel cancer. *Dis Colon Rectum* 1990;**33**:938–46.

56 Laurie JA, Moertel CG, Fleming TR *et al.* Surgical adjuvant therapy of large-bowel carcinoma: an evaluation of levamisole and the combination of levamisole and fluorouracil. The North Central Cancer Treatment Group and the Mayo Clinic. *J Clin Oncol* 1989;**7**:1447–56.

57 Diez M, Medrano M, Muguerza JM *et al.* Influence of tumor localization on the prognostic value of P53 protein in colorectal adenocarcinomas. *Anticancer Res* 2000;**20**:3907–12.

58 Elsaleh H, Powell B, McCaul K *et al.* P53 alteration and microsatellite instability have predictive value for survival benefit from chemotherapy in stage III colorectal carcinoma. *Clin Cancer Res* 2001;**7**:1343–9.

59 Kohne CH, Cunningham D, Di Costanzo F *et al.* Clinical determinants of survival in patients with 5-fluorouracil-based treatment for metastatic colorectal cancer: results of a multivariate analysis of 3825 patients. *Ann Oncol* 2002;**13**:308–317.

60 Kemeny N, Niedzwiecki D, Shurgot B, Oderman P. Prognostic variables in patients with hepatic metastases from colorectal cancer. Importance of medical assessment of liver involvement. *Cancer* 1989;**63**:742–7.

61 Rougier P, Milan C, Lazorthes F *et al.* Prospective study of prognostic factors in patients with unresected hepatic metastases from colorectal cancer. Foundation Francaise de Cancerolologie Digestive. *Br J Surg* 1995;**82**:1397–400.

62 Thirion P, Wolmark N, Haddad E *et al.* Survival impact of chemotherapy in patients with colorectal metastases confined to the liver: A re-analysis of 1458 non-operable patients. *Ann Oncol* 1999;**10**:1317–20.

63 Poon MA, O'Connell MJ, Moertel CG *et al.* Biochemical modulation of fluorouracil: evidence of significant improvement in survival and quality of life in patients with advanced colorectal carcinoma. *J Clin Oncol* 1989;**7**:1407–18.

64 Meta-Analysis Group in Cancer. Efficacy of intravenous continuous infusion of 5-fluorouracil compared with bolus administration in advanced colorectal cancer. *J Clin Oncol* 1998;**16**:301–8.

65 Advanced Colorectal Cancer Meta-Analysis Project. Modulation of fluorouracil by leucovorin in patients with advanced colorectal cancer: evidence in terms of response rate. *J Clin Oncol* 1992;**10**:896–90.

66 de Gramont A, Figer AA, Seymour M *et al.* Leucovorin and fluorouracil with and without oxaliplatin as first line treatment in advanced colorectal cancer. *J Clin Oncol* 2000;**18**:2938–47.

67 Cunningham D, Pyrhonen S, James RD *et al.* Randomised trial of irinotecan plus supportive care versus supportive care alone after fluorouracil failure for patients with metastatic colorectal cancer. *Lancet* 1998;**352**:1413–18.

68 Saltz LB, Cox JV, Blanke C *et al.* Irinotecan plus fluorouracil and leucovorin for metastatic colorectal cancer. Irinotecan Study Group. *N Engl J Med* 2000;**343**:905–14.

69 Borner MM, Castiglione M, Bacchi M *et al.* The impact of adding low dose leucovorin to monthly 5-fluorouracil in advanced colorectal carcinoma: results of a phase III trial. Swiss Group for Clinical Cancer Research (SAKK). *Ann Oncol* 1998;**9**:535–41.

70 Freyer G, Rougier P, Bugat P *et al.* Prognostic factors for tumour response, progression free survival and toxicity in metastatic colorectal cancer patients given irinotecan as second-line chemotherapy after 5-FU failure. CPT-11 F205, F220, F221 and V222 study groups. *Br J Cancer* 2000;**83**:431–7.

71 Earlam, S, Glover C, Fordy C, Burke D, Allen-Mersh TG. Relation between tumor size, quality of life and survival in patients with colorectal liver metastases. *J Clin Oncol* 1996;**14**:171–5.

72 Allegra CJ, Parr AL, Wold LE *et al.* Investigation of the prognostic and predictive value of thymidylate synthase, p53, and Ki-67 in patients with locally advanced colon cancer. *J Clin Oncol* 2002;**20**:1735–43.

73  Brett MC, Pickard M, Green B *et al.* p53 protein overexpression and response to biomodulated 5-fluorouracil chemotherapy in patients with advanced colorectal cancer. *Eur J Surg Oncol* 1996;**22**:182–5.

74  Schwandner O, Schiedeck TH, Bruch HP, Duchrow M, Windhoevel U, Broll R. p53 and Bcl-2 as significant predictors of recurrence and survival in rectal cancer. *Eur J Cancer* 2000;**36**:348–56.

75  Salonga D, Danenberg KD, Johnson M *et al.* Colorectal tumors responding to 5-fluorouracil have low gene expression levels of dihydropyrimidine dehydrogenase, thymidylate synthase, and thymidine phosphorylase. *Clin Cancer Res* 2000;**6**:1322–7.

76  Soong R, Powell B, Elsaleh H *et al.* Prognostic significance of TP53 gene mutation in 995 cases of colorectal carcinoma. Influence of tumour site, stage, adjuvant chemotherapy and type of mutation. *Eur J Cancer* 2000:**36**:2053–60.

77  Elnatan J, Goh HS, Smith DR. C-KI-RAS activation and the biological behaviour of proximal and distal colonic adenocarcinomas. *Eur J Cancer* 1996;**32A**:491–7.

78  Benhattar J, Losi L, Chaubert P, Givel JC, Costa J. Prognostic significance of K-ras mutations in colorectal cancer. *Gastroenterology* 1993;**104**:1044–8.

79  Smith DR, Goh HS. Overexpression of the c-myc proto-oncogene in colorectal carcinoma is associated with a reduced mortality that is abrogated by point mutation of the p53 tumor suppressor gene. *Clin Cancer Res* 1996;**2**:1049–53.

80  Mayer A, Takimoto M, Fritz E, Schellander G, Kofler K, Ludwig H. The prognostic significance of proliferating cell nuclear antigen, epidermal growth factor receptor, and mdr gene expression in colorectal cancer. *Cancer* 1993;**71**:2454–60.

81  Robson H, Anderson E, James RD, Schofield PF. Transforming growth factor beta 1 expression in human colorectal tumours: an independent prognostic marker in a subgroup of poor prognosis patients. *Br J Cancer* 1996;**74**:753–8.

82  Ropponen KM, Kellokoski JK, Lipponen PK *et al.* p21/WAF1 expression in human colorectal carcinoma: association with p53, transcription factor AP-2 and prognosis. *Br J Cancer* 1999;**81**:133–140.

83  Zirbes TK, Baldus SE, Moenig SP *et al.* Prognostic impact of p21/waf1/cip1 in colorectal cancer. *Int J Cancer* 2000;**89**:14–18.

84  Zhou W, Goodman SN, Galizia G *et al.* Counting alleles to predict recurrence of early-stage colorectal cancers. *Lancet* 2002;**359**:219–25.

85  Shibata D, Reale MA, Lavin P *et al.* The DCC protein and prognosis in colorectal cancer. *N Engl J Med* 1996;**335**:1727–32.

86  Paradiso A, Rabinovich M, Vallejo C *et al.* p53 and PCNA expression in advanced colorectal cancer: response to chemotherapy and long-term prognosis. *Int J Cancer* 1996;**69**:437–41.

87  Schneider HJ, Sampson SA, Cunningham D *et al.* Bcl-2 expression and response to chemotherapy in colorectal adenocarcinomas. *Br J Cancer* 1997;**75**:427–31.

88  Amaya H, Tanigawa N, Lu C *et al.* Association of vascular endothelial growth factor expression with tumour angiogenesis, survival and thymidine phosphorylase/platelet-derived endothelial growth factor expression in human colorectal cancer. *Cancer Lett* 1997;**119**:227–35.

89  Ishikawa T, Sekiguchi P, Pukase Y *et al.* Positive correlation between the efficacy of capecitabine and doxifluridine and the ratio of thymidine phosphorylase to dihydropyrimidine dehydrogenase activities in tumors in human cancer xenografts. *Cancer Res* 1998;**58**:685–90.

90  Metzger R, Danenberg K, Leichman CG *et al.* High basal level gene expression of thymidine phosphorylase (platelet-derived endothelial cell growth factor) in colorectal tumors is associated with nonresponse to 5-fluorouracil. *Clin Cancer Res* 1998;**4**:2371–6.

91  Bhatavdekar JM, Patel DD, Chikhlikar PR *et al.* Molecular markers are predictors of recurrence and survival in patients with Dukes B and Dukes C colorectal adenocarcinoma. *Dis Colon Rectum* 2001;**44**:523–33.

92  Kimura T, Tanaka S, Haruma K *et al.* Clinical significance of MUC1 and E-cadherin expression, cellular proliferation, and angiogenesis at the deepest invasive portion of colorectal cancer. *Int J Oncol* 2000;**16**:55–64.

93  Gunther K, Brabletz T, Kraus C *et al.* Predictive value of nuclear beta-catenin expression for the occurrence of distant metastases in rectal cancer. *Dis Colon Rectum* 1998;**41**:1256–61.

94  Gafa R, Maestri I, Matteuzzi M *et al.* Sporadic colorectal adenocarcinomas with high-frequency microsatellite instability. *Cancer* 2000;**89**:2025–37.

95  Halling KC, French AJ, McDonnell SK *et al.* Microsatellite instability and 8p allelic imbalance in stage B2 and C colorectal cancers. *J Natl Cancer Inst* 1999;**91**:1295–303.

96  Gryfe R, Kim H, Hsieh ETK *et al.* Tumor microsatellite instability and clinical outcome in young patients with colorectal cancer. *N Engl J Med* 2000;**342**:69–77.

97  Corsi DC, Ciaprarrone M, Zannoni G *et al.* Predictive value of thymidylate synthase expression in resected metastases of colorectal cancer. *Eur J Cancer* 2002;**38**:527–34.

98  Paradiso A, Simone G, Petroni S *et al.* Thymidylate synthase and p53 primary tumour expression as predictive factors for advanced colorectal cancer patients. *Br J Cancer* 2000;**82**:560–7.

99  Edler D, Kressner U, Ragnhammar P *et al.* Immunohistochemically detected thymidylate synthase in colorectal cancer: an independent prognostic factor of survival. *Clin Cancer Res* 2000;**6**:488–92.

100  Iacopetta B, Grieu F, Joseph D, Elsaleh H. A polymorphism in the enhancer region of the thymidylate synthase promoter influences the survival of colorectal cancer patients treated with 5-fluorouracil. *Br J Cancer* 2001;**85**:827–30.

101  Grabowski P, Mann B, Mansmann U *et al.* Expression of SIALYL-Le(x) antigen defined by MAb AM-3 is an independent prognostic marker in colorectal carcinoma patients. *Int J Cancer* 2000;**88**:281–6.

102  Massacesi C, Norman A, Price T, Hill M, Ross P, Cunningham D. A clinical nomogram for predicting long-term survival in advanced colorectal cancer. *Eur J Cancer* 2000;**36**:2044–52.

103  Fountzilas G, Gossios K, Zisiadis A *et al.* Prognostic variable in patients with advanced colorectal cancer treated with fluorouracil and leucovorin-based chemotherapy. *Med Pediatr Oncol* 1996;**26**:305–17.

104  McLeod HL, Murray GI. Tumour markers of prognosis in colorectal cancer. *Br J Cancer* 1999;**79**:191–203.

105  Petersen S, Thames HD, Nieder C, Petersen C, Baumann M. The results of colorectal cancer treatment by p53 status: treatment-specific reviews. *Dis Colon Rectum* 2001;**44**:322–33.

106  Allegra C. Thymidylate synthase levels: Prognostic, predictive, or both? *J Clin Oncol* 2002;**20**:1711–13.

107  McArdle CS, Hole D. Impact of variability among surgeons on postoperative morbidity and mortality and ultimate survival. *BMJ* 1991;**302**:1501–5.

108  Reinbach DH, McGregor JR, Murray GD, O'Dwyer PJ. Effect of the surgeon's specialty interest on the type of resection performed for colorectal cancer. *Dis Colon Rectum* 1994;**37**:1020–3.

109  Gray R. Adjuvant therapy: how effective, and for which patients? A meta-analysis. *Proc Eur Cancer Conf Org* 1997;**9**:288(abstr).

110  Dube S, Heyen F, Jenicek M. Adjuvant chemotherapy in colorectal carcinoma. *Dis Colon Rectum* 1997;**40**:35–41.

111  International Multicentre Pooled Analysis of Colon Cancer Trials Investigators. Efficacy of adjuvant fluorouracil and folinic acid in colon cancer. *Lancet* 1995;**345**:939–44.

112  Moertel CG, Fleming TR, Macdonald JS *et al.* Fluorouracil plus levamisole as effective adjuvant therapy after resection of stage III colon carcinoma: a final report. *Ann Intern Med* 1995;**122**:321–6.

113  Haller DG, Catalano PJ, Macdonald JS, Mayer RJ. Fluorouracil, leucovorin and levamisole adjuvant therapy for colon cancer: five-year final report of Int-0089. *Proc Am Soc Clin Oncol* 1998;**17**:982(abstr).

114  QUASAR Collaborative Group. Comparison of fluorouracil with additional levamisole, higher-dose folinic acid, or both, as adjuvant chemotherapy for colorectal cancer: a randomized trial. *Lancet* 2000;**355**:1588–96.

115  Wolmark N, Rockette H, Fisher B *et al.* The benefit of leucovorin-modulated fluorouracil as post-operative adjuvant therapy for primary colon cancer: results from National Surgical Adjuvant Breast and Bowel Project protocol C-03. *J Clin Oncol* 1993;**11**:1879–97.

116  O'Connell MJ, Mailliard JA, Kahn MJ *et al.* Controlled trials of fluorouracil low-dose leucovorin given for 6 months as post-operative adjuvant therapy for colon cancer. *J Clin Oncol* 1997;**15**:246–50.

117  O'Connell MJ, Laurie JA, Kahn M *et al.* Prospectively randomized trial of postoperative adjuvant chemotherapy in patients with high-risk colon cancer. *J Clin Oncol* 1998;**16**:295–300.

118  Wolmark N, Rockette H, Mamounas E *et al.* Clinical trial to assess the relative efficacy of fluorouracil and leucovorin, fluorouracil and levamisole, and fluorouracil, leucovorin and levamisole in patients with Dukes' B and C carcinoma of the colon: Results from National Surgical Adjuvant Breast and Bowel Project Protocol C-04. *J Clin Oncol* 1999;**17**:3553–9.

119  Kerr DJ, Gray R, McConkey C *et al.* Adjuvant chemotherapy with 5-fluorouracil, L-folinic acid and levamisole for patients with colorectal cancer: Non-randomised comparison of weekly versus four-weekly schedules – less pain, same gain. *Ann Oncol* 2000;**11**:947–55.

120  International Multicentre Pooled Analysis of B2 Colon Cancer Trials Investigators. Efficacy of adjuvant fluorouracil and folinic acid in B2 colon cancer. *J Clin Oncol* 1999;**17**:1356–63.

121  Erlichman C, Marsoni S, Seitz JF *et al.* Event free and overall survival is increased by FUFA in resected B colon cancer: a pooled analysis of five randomized trials. *Proc Am Soc Clin Oncol* 1997;**17**:991(abstr).

122  Mamounas E, Wieand S, Wolmark N *et al.* Comparative efficacy of adjuvant chemotherapy in patients with Dukes' B versus Dukes' C colon cancer: results from four National Surgical Adjuvant Breast and Bowel Project adjuvant studies (C-01, C-02, C-03, and C-04) *J Clin Oncol* 1999;**17**:1349–55.

123  Harrington DP. The tea leaves of small trials. *J Clin Oncol* 1999;**17**:1336–8.

124  Liver Infusion Meta-analysis Group. Portal vein chemotherapy for colorectal cancer: a meta-analysis of 4000 patients in 10 studies. *J Natl Cancer Inst* 1997;**89**:497–505.

125  James RD *et al.* Intraportal 5–FU and Peri-Operative Radiotherapy (RT) in the Adjuvant Treatment of Colorectal Cancer – 3681 Patients Randomised in the UK Coordinating Committee on Cancer Research (UKCCCR) AXIS Trial. *Proc Am Soc Clin Oncol* 1999;**18**:1013(abstr).

126  Rougier P, Sahmoud T, Nitti D *et al.* Adjuvant portal-vein infusion of fluorouracil and heparin in colorectal cancer: a randomised trial. European Organization for Research and Treatment of Cancer Gastrointestinal Tract Cancer Cooperative Group, the Gruppo Interdisciplinare Valutazione Interventi in Oncologia, and the Japanese Foundation for Cancer Research. *Lancet* 1998;**351**:1677–81.

127  Labianca R, Boffi L, Marsoni S *et al.* A randomized trial of intraportal versus systemic versus intraportal and systemic adjuvant chemotherapy in patients with resected Dukes B and C colon carcinoma. *Proc Am Soc Clin Oncol* 1999;**18**:1014(abstr).

128  Poplin E, Benedetti J, N Estes N *et al.* Phase III randomized trial of bolus 5-FU/leucovorin/levamisole versus 5-FU continuous infusion/levamisole as adjuvant therapy for high risk colon cancer (SWOG 9415/INT-0153). *Proc Am Soc Clin Oncol* 2000;**19**:931(abstr).

129  Saini A, Cunningham D, Norman A *et al.* Multicentre randomized trial of protracted venous infusion 5 FU compared to 5 FU/folinic acid as adjuvant therapy for colorectal cancer. *Proc Am Soc Clin Oncol* 2000;**19**:928(abstr).

130  Riethmuller G, Holz E, Schlimok G *et al.* Monoclonal antibody therapy for resected Dukes' C colorectal cancer: seven-year outcome of a multicenter randomized trial. *J Clin Oncol* 1998;**16**:1788–94.

131  Dencausse Y, Hartung G, Sturm J, Post S, Queisser W, Mannhaim K. Prospective randomised study of adjuvant therapy with edrecolmab (Panorex®) of stage II colon cancer – Interim analysis. *Proc Am Soc Clin Oncol* 2001;**20**:2198(abstr).

132  Schwartzberg LS. Clinical experience with edrecolomab: a monoclonal antibody therapy for colorectal carcinoma. *Crit Rev Oncol Hematol* 2001;**40**:17–24.

133  Fields AL, Keller AM, Schwartzberg L *et al.* Edrecolomab (17–1A antibody) (EDR) in combination with 5-fluorouracil (FU) based chemotherapy in the adjuvant treatment of stage III colon cancer: results of a randomised North American phase III study. *Proc Am Soc Clin Oncol* 2002;**21**:508(abstr).

134  de Gramont A, Boni C, Navarro M *et al.* Oxaliplatin/5–FU/LV in adjuvant colon cancer: safety results of the international randomized MOSAIC trial. *Proc Am Soc Clin Oncol* 2002;**21**:525(abstr).

135  Coppola FS, Arca R, Ferro A *et al.* A phase III randomized trial (COLON-OXALAD) of adjuvant therapy for very high risk colon cancer (CC) patients (pts) with oxaliplatin (OXA) ± bolus 5-fluorouracil (5-FU)/folinic acid (FA): a toxicity report. *Proc Am Soc Clin Oncol* 2002;**21**:656(abstr).

136  Gunderson LL, Sosin H. Areas of failure found at reoperation (second or symptomatic look) following "curative surgery" for adenocarcinoma of the rectum. Clinicopathologic correlation and implications for adjuvant therapy. *Cancer* 1974;**34**:1278–92.

137  Gastrointestinal Tumor Study Group. Radiation therapy and fluorouracil with or without semustine for the treatment of patients with surgical adjuvant adenocarcinoma of the rectum. *J Clin Oncol* 1992;**10**:549–57.

138  Wolmark N, Wieand S, Hyams DM *et al.* Randomized trial of postoperative adjuvant chemotherapy with or without radiotherapy for carcinoma of the rectum: National Surgical Adjuvant Breast and Bowel Project Protocol R-02. *J Natl Cancer Inst* 2000;**92**:388–96.

139  Tepper JE, O'Connell MJ, Petroni GR *et al.* Adjuvant post-operative fluorouracil-modulated chemotherapy combined with pelvic radiation therapy for rectal cancer: Initial results of Intergroup 0114. *J Clin Oncol* 1997;**15**:2030–9.

140  Kapiteijn E, Marijnen CAM, Nagategaal ID *et al.* Preoperative radiotherapy combined with total mesorectal excision for resectable rectal cancer. *N Engl J Med* 2001;**345**:638–46.

141  Swedish Rectal Cancer Trial. Improved survival with pre-operative radiotherapy in rectal cancer. *N Engl J Med* 1997;**336**:980–7.

142  O'Connell MJ, Martenson JA, Wieand HS *et al.* Improving adjuvant therapy for rectal cancer by combining protracted infusion fluorouracil with radiation therapy after curative surgery. *N Engl J Med* 1994;**331**:502–7.

143  Fisher B, Wolmark N, Rockette H *et al.* Postoperative adjuvant chemotherapy or radiation therapy for rectal cancer: results from NSABP protocol R-01. *J Natl Cancer Inst* 1988;**80**:21–9.

144  Quirke P, Durdey P, Dixon MF, Williams NS. Local recurrence of rectal adenocarcinoma due to inadequate surgical resection. Histopathological study of lateral tumour spread and surgical excision. *Lancet* 1986;**1**:996–9.

145  MacFarlane JK, Ryall RD, Heald RJ. Mesorectal excision for rectal cancer. *Lancet* 1993;**341**:457–60.

146  Goldberg S, Klas JV. Total mesorectal excision in the treatment of rectal cancer: a view from the USA. *Semin Surg Oncol* 1998;**15**:87–90.

147  Enker WE. Total mesorectal excision – the new golden standard of surgery for rectal cancer. *Ann Med* 1997;**29**:127–33.

148  Bolognese A, Cardi M, Muttillo IA, Barbarosos A, Bocchetti T, Valabrega S. Total mesorectal excision for surgical treatment of rectal cancer. *J Surg Oncol* 2000;**74**:21–3.

149  Williams NS, Durdey P, Johnston D. The outcome following sphincter-saving resection and abdominoperineal resection for low rectal cancer. *Br J Surg* 1985;**72**:595–8.

150  Stearns MW, Quan SH, Deddish MR. Preoperative roentgen therapy for cancer of the rectum. *Surg Gynecol Obstet* 1959;**111**:507.

151  Colorectal Cancer Collaborative Group: Adjuvant radiotherapy for rectal cancer: a systematic overview of 8507 patients from 22 randomised trials. *Lancet* 2001;**358**:1291–304.

152  Minsky BD. Adjuvant therapy for rectal cancers: Results and controversies. *Oncology* 1998;**12**:1129–39.

153  Camma C, Giunta M, Fiorica F, Pagliaro L, Craxi A, Cottone M. Preoperative radiotherapy for resectable rectal cancer: A meta-analysis. *JAMA* 2000;**284**:1008–15.

154  Stockholm Colorectal Cancer Study Group. Preoperative short-term radiation therapy in operable rectal cancer: a prospective randomised trial. *Cancer* 1990;**66**:49–55.

155  Goldberg PA, Nicholls RJ, Porter NH, Love S, Grimsey JE. Long-term results of a randomized trial of short course low dose adjuvant pre-operative radiotherapy for rectal cancer: reduction in local treatment failure. *Eur J Cancer* 1994;**30**:1602–6.

156  Cedermark B, Johansson H, Rutgrist L Wilking N. The Stockholm I trial of preoperative short-term radiotherapy in operable rectal carcinoma. A prospective randomized trial. Stockholm Colorectal Cancer Study Group. *Cancer* 1995;**75**:2269–75.

157 Stockholm Colorectal Cancer Study Group. Randomized study on pre-operative radiotherapy in rectal carcinoma. *Ann Surg Oncol* 1996;**3**:423–30.

158 Marijnen CA, Kapiteijn E, van De Velde CJ *et al.* Acute side effects and complications after short term preoperative radiotherapy combined with total mesorectal excision in primary rectal cancer: report of a multicenter randomized trial. *J Clin Oncol* 2002;**20**:817–25.

159 Grann A, Feng C, Wong D *et al.* Preop combined modality therapy for uT3 rectal cancer. *Proc Am Soc Clin Oncol* 2000;**19**:967(abstr).

160 Bosset JF, Magnin V, Maignon P *et al.* Preoperative radiochemotherapy in rectal cancer: long term results of a phase II trial. *Int J Radiat Oncol Biol Phys* 2000;**46**:323–7.

161 Chari RS, Tyler D, Ansher M *et al.* Preoperative radiation and chemotherapy in the treatment of adenocarcinoma of the rectum. *Ann Surg* 1995;**221**:778–86.

162 Ngan SY, Burmeister BH, Fisher R *et al.* Early toxicity from preoperative radiotherapy with continuous infusion 5-fluorouracil for resectable adenocarcinoma of the rectum: a Phase II trial for the Trans-Tasman Radiation Oncology Group. *Int J Radiat Oncol Biol Phys* 2001;**50**:883–7.

163 Bosset JF, Pierart M, Glabbeke MV. Preoperative radiochemotherapy versus preoperative radiotherapy with or without post-operative chemotherapy: progress report of the EORTC 22921 rectal trial. *Radiother Oncol* 2000;**56**:S52.

164 Hu KS, Harrison LB. Adjuvant therapy for resectable rectal adenocarcinoma. *Semin Surg Oncol* 2000;**19**:336–49.

165 Hyams DM, Mamounas E, Petrelli N *et al.* A clinical trial to evaluate the worth of preoperative multimodality therapy in patients with operable carcinoma of the rectum: a progress report of National Surgical breast and Bowel Project Protocol R-03. *Dis Colon Rectum* 1997;**40**:131–9.

166 Sauer R, Fietkau R, Martus R *et al.* Adjuvant and neoadjuvant radiochemotherapy for advanced rectal cancer – first results of the German multicentre phase III trial. *Int J Radiat Oncol Biol Phys* 2000;**48**:17(abstr).

167 Ooi BS, Tjandra JJ, Green MD. Morbidities of adjuvant chemotherapy and radiotherapy for resectable rectal cancer: an overview. *Dis Colon Rectum* 1999;**42**:403–18.

168 Marijnen CA, Glimelius B: The role of radiotherapy in rectal cancer. *Eur J Cancer* 2002;**38**:943–52.

169 Haller DG. Defining the optimal therapy for rectal cancer. *J Natl Cancer Inst* 2000;**92**:361–2.

170 Ngan S, Zalcberg J, Kell A *et al.* Phase I study of capecitabine combined with radiotherapy for locally advanced potentially operable rectal cancer. *Proc Am Soc Clin Oncol* 2001;**20**:591(abstr).

171 Hoff PM, Janjan N, Saad ED *et al.* Phase I study of preoperative oral uracil and tegafur plus leucovorin and radiation therapy in rectal cancer. *J Clin Oncol* 2000;**18**:3529–34.

172 Sebag-Montefiore D, Tim M, Stephen F, Glynne-Jones R, Meadows H. A phase I dose escalation study of oxaliplatin when given in combination with 5-fluorouracil, low dose folinic acid and synchronous pre-operative radiotherapy in locally advanced rectal cancer. *Proc Am Soc Clin Oncol* 2001;**20**:585(abstr).

173 Klautken G, Kirchner R, Hopt U, Fietkau R. Continuous infusion of 5-FU and weekly irinotecan with concurrent radiotherapy as neoadjuvant treatment for locally advanced or recurrent rectal cancer. *Proc Am Soc Clin Oncol* 2001;**20**:555(abstr).

174 Valentini V, Morganti AG, Fiorentino G *et al.* Chemoradiation with raltitrexed and concomitant preoperative radiotherapy has potential in the treatment of stage II/III resectable rectal cancer. *Proc Am Soc Clin Oncol* 1999;**18**:987(abstr).

175 Botwood N, James R, Vernon C, Price P. Raltitrexed (Tomudex) and radiotherapy can be combined as postoperative treatment for rectal cancer. *Ann Oncol* 2000;**11**:1023–8.

176 Hughes KS, Rosenstein RB, Songhorabodi S *et al.* Resection of the liver for colorectal carcinoma metastases. A multi-institutional study of long-term survivors. *Dis Colon Rectum* 1988;**31**:1–4.

177 Hermann R. Systemic treatment of advanced colorectal cancer. *Eur J Cancer* 1993;**29A**:583–6.

178 Simmonds PC, Colorectal Cancer Collaborative Group. Palliative chemotherapy for advanced colorectal cancer: systematic review and meta-analysis. *BMJ* 2000;**321**:531–5.

179 Nordic Gastrointestinal Tumor Adjuvant Therapy Group (NGTATG). Expectancy or primary chemotherapy in patients with asymptomatic colorectal cancer: A randomized trial. *J Clin Oncol* 1992;**10**:904–11.

180 Doulliard JY, Cunningham D, Roth AD *et al.* Irinotecan combined with fluorouracil compared with fluorouracil as first line treatment for metastatic colorectal cancer: a multicentre randomised trial. *Lancet* 2000;**355**:1041–7.

181 Leichman CG, Fleming TR, Muggia FM *et al.* Phase II study of fluorouracil and its modulation in advanced colorectal cancer. *J Clin Oncol* 1995;**13**:1303–11.

182 Labianca R, Pancera G, Aitini C *et al.* Folinic acid + 5-fluorouracil versus equidose 5-FU in advanced colorectal cancer. Phase III study of GISCAD (Italian Group for the study of Digestive Tract Cancer). *Ann Oncol* 1991;**2**:673–79.

183 Jonker DJ, Maroun JA, Kocha W. Survival benefit of chemotherapy in metastatic colorectal cancer: meta-analysis of randomized controlled trials. *Br J Cancer* 2000;**82**:1789–94.

184 Scheithauer W, Rosen H, Kornek GV, Sebesta C, Depisch D. Randomised comparison of combination chemotherapy plus supportive care with supportive care alone in patients with metastatic colorectal cancer. *BMJ* 1993;**306**:752–5.

185 Hafstrom L, Engaras B, Holmberg SB *et al.* Treatment of liver metastases from colorectal cancer with hepatic artery occlusion, intraportal 5-fluorouracil infusion, and oral allopurinol. A randomized clinical trial. *Cancer* 1994;**74**:2749–56.

186 Allen-Mersh TG, Earlam S, Fordy C, Abrams K, Houghton J. Quality of life and survival with continuous hepatic-artery floxuridine infusion for colorectal liver metastases. *Lancet* 1994;**344**:1255–60.

187 Rougier P, Laplanche A, Huguier M *et al.* Hepatic arterial infusion of floxuridine in patients with liver metastases from colorectal carcinoma: long-term results of a prospective randomized trial. *J Clin Oncol* 1992;**10**:1112–18.

188 Gerard A, Buyse M, Pector JC *et al.* Hepatic artery ligation with and without portal infusion of 5–FU. A randomized study in patients with unresectable liver metastases from colorectal carcinoma. The E.O.R.T.C. Gastrointestinal Cancer Cooperative Group (G.I. Group). *Eur J Surg Oncol* 1991;**17**:289–94.

189 Ackland, SP Moore M, Jones M *et al.* A meta-analysis of two randomized trials of early chemotherapy in asymptomatic metastatic colorectal cancer. *Proc Am Soc Clin Oncol* 2001;**20**:526(abstr).

190 Hill M, Norman A, Cunningham D *et al.* Impact of protracted venous infusion fluorouracil with or without interferon alfa-2b on tumor response, survival, and quality of life in advanced colorectal cancer. *J Clin Oncol* 1995;**1**:2317–23.

191 Caudry M, Bonnel C, Floquet A *et al.* A randomized study of bolus fluorouracil plus folinic acid versus 21-day fluorouracil infusion alone or in association with cyclophosphamide and mitomycin-C in advanced colorectal carcinoma. *Am J Clin Oncol* 1995;**18**:118–25.

192 Earlam S, Glover C, Davies M, Fordy C, Allen-Mersh TG. Effect of regional and systemic fluorinated pyrimidine chemotherapy on quality of life and in colorectal liver metastasis patients. *J Clin Oncol* 1997;**15**:2022–9.

193 Glimelius B, Graf W, Hoffman K, Pahlman L, Sjoden PO, Wennberg A. General condition of asymptomatic patients with advanced colorectal cancer receiving palliative chemotherapy. A longitudinal study. *Acta Oncol* 1992;**31**:645–51.

194 Glimelius B, Hoffman K, Graf W, Pahlman L, Sjoden PO. Quality of life during chemotherapy in patients with symptomatic advanced colorectal cancer. The Nordic Gastrointestinal Tumor Adjuvant Therapy Group. *Cancer* 1994;**73**:556–62.

195 Sullivan BA, McKinnis R, Laufman LR. Quality of life in patients with metastatic colorectal cancer receiving chemotherapy: a randomized, double-blind trial comparing 5-FU versus 5-FU with leucovorin. *Pharmacotherapy* 1995;**15**:600–7.

196 Glimelius B. Biochemical modulation of 5-Fluorouracil: a randomized comparison of sequential methotrexate, 5-fluorouracil and leucovorin versus sequential 5-fluorouracil and leucovorin in patients with advanced symptomatic colorectal cancer. The Nordic Gastrointestinal Tumor Adjuvant Therapy Group. *Ann Oncol* 1993;**4**:235–40.

197 Grem JL. 5-fluoropyrimidines. In: Chabner BA, Longo DL eds. *Cancer Chemotherapy and Biotherapy: Principles and Practice. 2nd edn.* Philadelphia: Lippincott-Raven 1996.

198 Diasio RB, Harris BE. Clinical pharmacology of 5-fluorouracil. *Clin Pharmacokinet* 1989;**16**:215–37.

199 Sobero AF, Aschele C, Bertino JR. Fluorouracil in colorectal cancer – A tale of two drugs: Implications for biochemical modulation. *J Clin Oncol* 1997;**15**:368–81.

200 Erlichman C, Fine S, Elhakim T. Plasma pharmacokinetics of 5-FU given by continuous infusion with allopurinol. *Cancer Treat Rep* 1986;**70**:903–4.

201 Meta-Analysis Group in Cancer. Toxicity of fluorouracil in patients with advanced colorectal cancer: Effect of administration schedule and prognostic factors. *J Clin Oncol* 1998;**16**:3537–41.

202 Wang WS, Lin JK, Chiuo TJ *et al.* Randomized trial comparing weekly bolus 5-fluorouracil plus leucovorin versus monthly 5-day 5-fluorouracil plus leucovorin in metastatic colorectal cancer. *Hepatogastoenterology* 2000;**47**:1599–603.

203 Buroker TR, O'Connell MJ, Wieand HS *et al.* Randomized comparison of two schedules of fluorouracil and leucovorin in the treatment of advanced colorectal cancer. *J Clin Oncol* 1994;**12**:14–20.

204 Labianca R, Cascinu F, Frontini L *et al.* High- versus low- dose levo-leucovorin as a modulator of 5-fluorouracil in advanced colorectal cancer: a 'GISCAD' phase III study. Italian Group for the Study of Digestive Tract Cancer. *Ann Oncol* 1997;**8**:169–74.

205 O'Connell MJ. A phase III trial of 5-fluorouracil and leucovorin in the treatment of advanced colorectal cancer. A Mayo Clinic/North Central Cancer Treatment Group study. *Cancer* 1989;**63**:1026–30.

206 Ychou M, Fabbro-Peray P, Perney P *et al.* A prospective randomized study comparing high- and low-dose leucovorin combined with same dose 5-fluorouracil in advanced colorectal cancer. *Am J Clin Oncol* 1998;**21**:233–6.

207 Goldberg RM, Hatfiled AK, Kahn M *et al.* Prospectively randomized North Central Cancer Treatment Group trial of intensive-course fluorouracil combined with the l-isomer of intravenous leucovorin, oral leucovorin or intravenous leucovorin for the treatment of advanced colorectal cancer. *J Clin Oncol* 1997;**15**:3320–9.

208 Jager E, Heike M, Bernhard H *et al.* Weekly high dose leucovorin versus low-dose leucovorin combined with fluorouracil in advanced colorectal cancer: results of a randomised trial. Study Group for Palliative Treatment of Metastatic Colorectal Cancer Study Protocol 1. *J Clin Oncol* 1996;**14**:2274–9.

209 de Gramont A, Bosset J-F, Milan C *et al.* Randomized trial comparing monthly low-dose leucovorin and fluorouracil bolus with bimonthly high-dose leucovorin and fluorouracil bolus plus continuous infusion for advanced colorectal cancer. *J Clin Oncol* 1997;**15**:808–15.

210 Kohne CH, Schoffski P, Wilke H *et al.* Effective biomodulation by leucovorin of high-dose infusion fluorouracil given as a weekly 24-hour infusion: results of a randomized trial in patients with advanced colorectal cancer. *J Clin Oncol* 1998;**16**:418–26.

211 Diasio RB. Current status of oral chemotherapy for colorectal cancer. *Oncology* 2001;**15**:(3 Suppl. 5):16–20.

212 Van Cutsem E, Twelves C, Cassidy J *et al.* Oral capecitabine compared with intravenous fluorouracil plus leucovorin in patients with metastatic colorectal cancer: results of a large phase III study. *J Clin Oncol* 2001;**19**:4097–106.

213 Hoff PM, Anasari R, Batist G *et al.* Comparison of oral capecitabine versus intravenous fluorouracil plus leucovorin as first-line treatment in 605 patients with metastatic colorectal cancer: *J Clin Oncol* 2001;**19**:2282–92.

214 Pazdur R, Doulliard J-Y, Skillings JR *et al.* Multicentre phase III trial of 5-fluorouracil or UFT in combination with leucovorin in patients with metastatic colorectal cancer. *Proc Am Soc Clin Oncol* 1999;**19**:1009(abstr).

215 Carmichael J, Popiela T, Radstone S *et al.* Randomized comparative study of ORZEL® (oral uracil/tegafur (UFT™)) plus leucovorin versus parenteral 5-fluorouracil plus LV in patients with metastatic colorectal cancer. *Proc Am Soc Clin Oncol* 1999;**19**:1015(abstr).

216 Levin J, Schilsky R, Burris H *et al.* North American phase III study of oral eniluracil plus oral 5-fluorouracil versus intravenous 5-FU plus leucovorin in the treatment of advanced colorectal cancer. *Proc Am Soc Clin Oncol* 2001;**21**:523(abstr).

217 Van Cutsem E, Sorensen J, Cassidy J *et al.* International phase III study of oral eniluracil plus 5-fluorouracil versus intravenous (IV) 5-FU plus leucovorin (LV) in the treatment of advanced colorectal cancer. *Proc Am Soc Clin Oncol* 2001;**20**:522(abstr).

218 Twelves C, Boyer M, Findlay M et al. Capecitabine (Xeloda) improves medical resource use compared with 5-fluorouracil plus leucovorin in a phase III trial conducted in patients with advanced colorectal cancer. *Eur J Cancer* 2001;**37**:597–604.

219 Baker SD, Peang Khor S, Adjei AA *et al.* Pharmacokinetic, oral bioavailability, and safety study of fluorouracil in patients treated with 776C85, an inactivator of dihydropyrimidine dehydrogenase. *J Clin Oncol* 1996;**14**:3085–96.

220 Ohtsu A, Baba H, Sakata Y *et al.* Phase II study of S-1, a novel oral fluoropyrimidine derivative in patients with metastatic colorectal carcinoma. S-1 Cooperative Colorectal Carcinoma Study Group. *Br J Cancer* 2000;**83**:141–5.

221 Bleiberg H. Colorectal cancer – Is there an alternative to 5-FU? *Eur J Cancer* 1997;**33**:536–41.

222 Cunningham D, Zalcberg JR, Rath U *et al.* Final results of a randomised trial comparing Tomudex® (raltitrexed) with 5-fluorouracil plus leucovorin in advanced colorectal cancer. *Ann Oncol* 1996;**7**:961–5.

223 Pazdur R, Vincent M. Raltitrexed (Tomudex®) versus 5-fluorouracil and leucovorin in patients with advanced colorectal cancer. *Proc Am Soc Clin Oncol* 1997;**16**:801(abstr).

224 Maughan TS, James RD, Kerr DJ *et al.* Comparison of survival, palliation, and quality of life with three chemotherapy regimens in metastatic colorectal cancer: a multicentre randomised trial. *Lancet* 2002;**359**:1555–63.

225 Ross P, Heron J, Cunningham D. Costs of treating advanced colorectal cancer: A retrospective comparison of treatment regimens. *Eur J Cancer* 1996;**32A**(Suppl.):S13–S17.

226 Elliot R. Analysis of drug costs for the management of chemotherapy related side effects in advanced colorectal cancer. *J Oncol Clin Pharmacol* 1996;**2**:186–90.

227 Chen AY, Liu LF. DNA topoisomerases: Essential enzymes and lethal targets. *Ann Rev Pharmacol Toxicol* 1994;**34**:191–218.

228 Hsiang YH, Lihou MG, Liu LF. Arrest of replication forks by drug-stabilized topoisomerase-I-DNA cleavable complexes as a mechanism of cell killing by campothecin. *Cancer Res* 1989;**49**: 5077–82.

229 Bleiberg H, Cvitkovic E. Characterization and clinical management of CPT-11 (Irinotecan)-induced adverse events: The European perspective. *Eur J Cancer* 1996;**32A**:S18–S23.

230 Rothenberg ML. Topoisomerase I inhibitors: Review and update. *Ann Oncol* 1997;**8**:837–55.

231 Giacchetti S, Perpoint B, Zidani R *et al.* Phase III multicenter randomized trial of oxaliplatin added to chronomodulated fluorouracil-leucovorin as first-treatment of metastatic colorectal cancer. *J Clin Oncol* 2000;**18**:136–47.

232 Grothey A, Deschler B, Kroening H *et al.* Bolus 5-fluorouracil/folinic acid (Mayo) versus weekly high dose 24-hr 5-FU infusion/FA and oxaliplatin in advanced colorectal cancer. Results of a phase III trial. *Proc Am Soc Clin Oncol* 2001;**20**:496(abstr).

233 Tournigand C, Louvet C, Quinaux E *et al.* FOLFIRI followed by FOLFOX versus FOLFOX followed by FOLFIRI in metastatic colorectal cancer: Final results of a phase III study. *Proc Am Soc Clin Oncol* 2001;**20**:494(abstr).

234 Goldberg RM, Morton RF, Sargent DJ *et al.* N9741:Oxaliplatin or CPT-11 +5-fluorouracil/leucovorin or oxaliplatin + CPT-11 in advanced colorectal cancer. Initial toxicity and response data from a GI Intergroup study. *Proc Am Soc Clin Oncol* 2002;**21**:511(abstr).

235 Sargent DJ, Niedzwiecki D, O'Connell MJ, Schilsky RL. Recommendation for caution with irinotecan, fluorouracil, and leucovorin for colorectal cancer. *N Engl J Med* 2001;**345**:144–5.

236 Rothenberg ML, Meropol NJ, Poplin EA, Van Cutsem E, Wadler S. Mortality associated with irinotecan plus bolus fluorouracil/leucovorin: Summary findings of an independent panel. *J Clin Oncol* 2001;**19**:3801–7.

237  Rougier P, Van Custem, Bajetta E *et al*. Randomised trial of irinotecan versus fluorouracil by continuous infusion after fluorouracil failure in patients with metastatic colon cancer. *Lancet* 1998;**352**:1407–12.

238  O'Connell MJ. Irinotecan for colorectal cancer: a small step forward. *Lancet* 1998;**352**:1402.

239  Woynarowski JM, Chapman WG, Napier C, Herzig MC, Juniewicz P. Sequence- and region-specificity of oxaliplatin adducts in naked and cellular DNA. *Mol Pharmacol* 1998;**54**:770–7.

240  Raymond E, Faivre S, Woynarowski JM *et al*. Oxaliplatin: mechanisms of action and antineoplastic activity. *Semin Oncol* 1998;**25**(Suppl. 5):4–12.

241  Raymond E, Buquet-Fagot C, Djelloul S *et al*. Antitumor activity of oxaliplatin in combination with 5-fluorouracil and the thymidylate synthase inhibitor AG337 in human colon and breast and ovarian cancers. *Anticancer Drugs* 1997;**8**:876–85.

242  Brienza S, Bensmaine MA, Soulie P *et al*. Oxaliplatin added to 5-FU-based therapy in the treatment of pretreated patients with advanced colorectal carcinoma: results from the European compassionate-use program. *Ann Oncol* 1999;**10**:1311–16.

243  Gerard B, Bleiberg H, Van Daele D *et al*. Oxaliplatin combined to 5-fluorouracil and folinic acid: an effective therapy in patients with advanced colorectal cancer. *Anticancer Drugs* 1998;**9**:301–5.

244  de Gramont A, Vignoud J, Tournigand C *et al*. Oxaliplatin with high-dose leucovorin and 5-fluorouracil 48-hour continuous infusion in pretreated metastatic colorectal cancer. *Eur J Cancer* 1997;**33**:214–19.

245  Andre T, Louvet C, Raymond E. Bimonthly high-dose leucovorin and 5-fluorouracil infusion and oxaliplatin for metastatic colorectal cancer resistant to the same leucovorin and 5-fluorouracil regimen. *Ann Oncol* 1998;**9**:1251–3.

246  Van Cutsem E, Szanto J, Roth A *et al*. Evaluation of the addition of oxaliplatin to the same Mayo or German 5-FU regimen in advanced colorectal cancer. *Proc Am Soc Clin Oncol* 1999;**18**:900(abstr).

247  Ross P, Norman A, Cunningham D *et al*. A prospective randomised trial of protracted venous infusion 5-fluorouracil with or without mitomycin C in advanced colorectal cancer. *Ann Oncol* 1997;**8**:995–1001.

248  Price T, Cunningham D, Hickish T *et al*. Phase III study of chronomodulated vs protracted venous infusional 5-fluorouracil both combined with mitomycin in first line therapy for advanced colorectal carcinoma. *Proc Am Soc Clin Oncol* 1999;**18**:1008(abstr).

249  Chester JD, Dent JT, Wilson G, Ride E, Seymour MT. Protracted infusional 5-fluorouracil with bolus mitomycin-C in 5-FU-resistant colorectal cancer. *Ann Oncol* 2000;**11**:235–7.

250  Mori A, Bertoglio S, Guglielmi A *et al*. Activity of continuous infusion 5-fluorouracil in patients with advanced colorectal cancer clinically resistant to bolus 5-fluorouracil. *Cancer Chemother Pharmacol* 1993;**33**:179–80.

251  Falcone A, Allegrini G, Lencioni M *et al*. Protracted continuous infusion of 5-fluorouracil and low-dose leucovorin in patients with metastatic colorectal cancer resistant to 5-fluorouracil bolus-based chemotherapy: a phase II study. *Cancer Chemother Pharmacol* 1999;**44**:159–63.

252  Begtsson G, Carlsson G, Hafstrom L *et al*. Natural history of patients with untreated liver metastases from colorectal cancer. *Am J Surg* 1981;**141**:586–9.

253  Wagner JS, Adson MA, Van Heerden JA *et al*. The natural history of hepatic metastases from colorectal cancer. *Ann Surg* 1984;**199**:502–7.

254  Goslin R, Steele G Jr, Zamcheck N, Mayer R, MacIntyre J. Factors influencing survival in patients with hepatic metastases from adenocarcinoma of the colon and rectum. *Dis Colon Rectum* 1982;**25**:749–54.

255  Scheele J, Stangl R, Altendorf-Hofmann A *et al*. Indicators of prognosis after hepatic resection for colorectal secondaries. *Surgery* 1991;**110**:13–29.

256  Hughes K, Simon R, Songhorabodi S *et al*. Resection of liver for colorectal carcinoma metastases: A multi-institutional study of indications for resection. Registry of hepatic metastases. *Surgery* 1988;**103**:278–88.

257  Rosen CB, Nagorney DM, Taswell HF *et al*. Perioperative blood transfusion and determination of survival after resection of metastatic colorectal carcinoma. *Ann Surg* 1992;**216**:493–505.

258  Gayowski TJ, Iwatsuki S, Madariaga JR *et al*. Experience in hepatic resection for metastatic colorectal cancer: analysis of clinical and pathologic risk factors. *Surgery* 1994;**116**:703–11.

259  Schlag P, Hohenberger P, Holting T *et al*. Hepatic arterial infusion chemotherapy for liver metastases of colorectal cancer using 5-FU. *Eur J Surg Oncol* 1990;**16**:99–104.

260  Fong Y, Cohen AM, Fortner JG *et al*. Liver resection for colorectal metastases. *J Clin Oncol* 1997;**15**:938–46.

261  Adson MA, van Heerden JA, Adson MH *et al*. Resection of liver metastases from colorectal cancer. *Arch Surg* 1984;**119**:647–51.

262  Busch E, Kemeny MM. Colorectal cancer: Hepatic-directed therapy – Role of surgery, regional chemotherapy and novel modalities. *Semin Oncol* 1995;**22**:494–508.

263  Topal B, Flamen P, Aerts R *et al*. Clinical value of whole-body emission tomography in potentially curable colorectal liver metastases. *Eur J Surg Oncol* 2001;**27**:175–9.

264  Boykin KN, Zibari GB, Lilien DL, McMillan RW, Aultman DF, McDonald JC. The use of FDG-positron emission tomography for the evaluation of colorectal metastases of the liver. *Am Surg* 1999;**65**:1183–5.

265  Machi J, Isomoto H, Yamashita Y *et al*. Intraoperative ultrasonography in screening for liver metastases from colorectal cancer: Comparative accuracy with traditional procedures. *Surgery* 1987;**101**:678–84.

266  Charnley R, Morris D, Dennsion A *et al*. Detection of colorectal liver metastases using intraoperative ultrasonography. *Br J Surg* 1991;**78**:45–8.

267  Seifert JK, Bottger TC, Weigel TF, Gonner U, Junginger T. Prognostic factors following liver resection for hepatic metastases from colorectal cancer. *Hepatogastroenterology* 2000;**47**:239–46.

268  Imamura H, Matsuyama Y, Shimada R *et al*. A study of factors influencing prognosis after resection of hepatic metastases from colorectal and gastric carcinoma. *Am J Gastroenterol* 2001;**96**:3178–84.

269  Sugihara K, Hojo K, Moriya Y *et al*. Patterns of recurrence after hepatic resection for colorectal metastases. *Br J Surg* 1993;**80**:1032–5.

270  Adson MA: Resection of liver metastases- When is it worthwhile. *Wld J Surg* 1987;**11**:511–20.

271  Vogt P, Raab R, Ringe B *et al*. Resection of synchronous liver metastases from colorectal cancer. *Wld J Surg* 1991;**15**:62–7.

272  Lyass S, Zamir G, Matot I, Goitein D, Eid A, Jurin O. Combined colon and hepatic resection for synchronous colorectal liver metastases. *J Surg Oncol* 2001;**78**:17–21.

273  Hughes KS, Simon R, Songhorabodi S *et al*. Resections of the liver for colorectal carcinoma metastases: a multi-institutional study of patterns of recurrence. *Surgery* 1986;**100**:278–84.

274  Doci R, Gennari L, Bignami P *et al*. One hundred patients with hepatic metastases from colorectal cancer treated by resection. Analysis of prognostic determinants. *Br J Surg* 1991;**78**:797–801.

275  van Ooijen B, Wiggers T, Meijer S *et al*. Hepatic resection of colorectal metastases in the Netherlands- A multi-institutional 10-year study. *Cancer* 1992;**70**:28–34.

276  Nordlinger B, Vaillant JC, Guiguet M *et al*. Survival benefit of repeat liver resections for recurrent colorectal metastases. One-hundred and forty-three cases. *J Clin Oncol* 1994;**12**:1491–6.

277  Ensminger WD, Gyves JW. Regional chemotherapy of neoplastic disease. *Pharmacol Ther* 1983:**21**:277–93.

278  Lorenz M, Muller HH, Schramm H *et al*. Randomized trial of surgery versus surgery followed by adjuvant hepatic arterial infusion with 5-fluorouracil and folinic acid for liver metastases of colorectal cancer. *Ann Surg* 1998;**228**:756–62.

279  Kemeny N, Huang Y, Cohen AM *et al*. Hepatic arterial infusion of chemotherapy after resection of hepatic metastases from colorectal cancer. *N Engl J Med* 1999;**341**:2039–48.

280  Kemeny MM, Sudeshna A, Gray B *et al*. Combined modality treatment for resectable metastatic colorectal carcinoma to the liver: Surgical resection of hepatic metastases in combination with

continuous infusion of chemotherapy – An intergroup study. *J Clin Oncol* 2002;**20**:1499–505.

281 Nordlinger B, Rougier P. Liver metastases from colorectal cancer: The turning point. *J Clin Oncol* 2002;**20**:1442–5.

282 Langer B, Bleiberg H, Labianca R *et al.* Fluorouracil plus l-leucovorin versus observation after potentially curative resection of liver or lung metastases from colorectal cancer (CRC): results of the ENG (EORTC/NCIC CTG/GIVIO) randomized trial. *Proc Am Soc Clin Oncol* 2002;**21**:592(abstr).

283 Portier G, Rougier Ph, Milan C *et al.* Adjuvant systemic chemotherapy using 5-fluorouracil and folinic acid after resection of liver metastases from colorectal origin. Results of an intergroup phase III study (trial FFCD/ACHBTH/AURC 9002). *Proc Am Soc Clin Oncol* 2002;**21**:528(abstr).

284 Giacchetti S, Itzhaki M, Gruia G *et al.* Long-term survival of patients with unresectable colorectal cancer liver metastases following infusional chemotherapy with 5-fluorouracil, leucovorin, oxaliplatin and surgery. *Ann Oncol* 1999;**10**:663–9.

285 Hohn DC, Stagg RJ, Friedman MA *et al.* A randomized trial of continuous intravenous versus hepatic intra-arterial floxiuridine in patients with colorectal cancer metastatic to the liver: the Northern California Oncology Group trial. *J Clin Oncol* 1989;**7**:1646–54.

286 Kemeny N, Daly J, Reichman B, Geller N, Botet J, Oderman P. Intrahepatic or systemic infusion of fluorodeoxyuridine in patients with liver metastases from colorectal cancer. A randomized trial. *Ann Intern Med* 1987;**107**:459–65.

287 Chang AE, Schneider PD, Sugarbaker PH *et al.* A prospective randomized trial of regional versus systemic continuous 5-fluorodeoxyuridine chemotherapy in the treatment of colorectal hepatic metastases. *Ann Surg* 1987;**206**:685–93.

288 Martin JK, O'Connell MJ, Wieand HS *et al.* Intra-arterial floxuridine v systemic fluorouracil for hepatic metastases from colorectal cancer. A randomized trial. *Arch Surg* 1990;**125**:1022–7.

289 Kemeny MM, Goldberg D, Beatty JD *et al.* Results of a prospective randomized trial of continuous regional chemotherapy and hepatic resection as treatment of hepatic metastases from colorectal cancer. *Cancer* 1986;**57**:492–8.

290 Meta-analysis Group in Cancer. Reappraisal of hepatic arterial infusion in the treatment of nonresectable liver metastases from colorectal cancer. *J Natl Cancer Inst* 1996;**88**:252–8.

291 Harmantas A, Rotstein L, Langer B. Regional versus systemic chemotherapy in the treatment of colorectal carcinoma metastatic to the liver. *Cancer* 1996;**78**:1639–45.

292 Lorenz M, Muller HH. Randomized, multicenter trial of fluorouracil plus leucovorin administered either via hepatic arterial or intravenous infusion versus fluorodeoxyuridine administered via hepatic arterial infusion in patients with nonresectable liver metastases from colorectal carcinoma. *J Clin Oncol* 2000;**18**:243–54.

293 Van Hazel G, Gray BN, Anderson J. Randomised phase III trial of SIR-spheres® plus chemotherapy versus chemotherapy alone in patients with colorectal hepatic metastases. *Proc Am Soc Clin Oncol* 1999;**18**:1026(abstr).

294 De Baere T, Elias D, Dromain C *et al.* Radiofrequency ablation of 100 hepatic metastases with a mean follow up of more than 1 year. *Am J Roentgenol* 2000;**175**:1619–25.

295 Solbiati L, Ierace T, Tonolini M, Osti V, Cova L. Radiofrequency thermal ablation of hepatic metastases. *Eur J Ultrasound* 2001; **13**:149–58.

296 Neeleman N, Wobbes T, Jager GJ, Ruers TJ. Cryosurgery as treatment modality for colorectal liver metastases. *Hepatogastroenterology* 2001;**48**:325–9.

297 Morris DL, Ross WB. Australian experience of cryoablation of liver tumors: metastases. *Surg Oncol Clin N Am* 1996;**5**:391–7.

298 Ravikumar TS, Kane R, Cady B, Jenkins R, Clouse M, Steele G Jr. A 5-year study of cryosurgery in the treatment of liver tumors. *Arch Surg* 1991;**126**:1520–3.

299 Ravikumar TS. Interstitial therapies for liver tumors. *Surg Oncol Clin N Am* 1996;**5**:365–77.

300 Weaver ML, Ashton JG, Zemel R. Treatment of colorectal metastases by cryotherapy. *Semin Surg Oncol* 1998;**14**:163–70.

301 Sherman DM, Weichselbaum R, Order SE *et al.* Palliation of hepatic metastasis. *Cancer* 1978;**41**:2013–17.

302 Leibel SA, Pajak TF, Massullo V *et al.* A comparison of misonidazole sensitized radiation therapy to radiation therapy alone for the palliation of hepatic metastases: Results of Radiation Therapy Oncology Group randomized prospective trial. *Int J Rad Oncol Biol Phys* 1987;**13**:1057–64.

303 Sato M, Uematsu M, Yamamoto F *et al.* Feasibility of frameless stereotactic high-dose radiation therapy for primary or metastatic liver cancer. *J Radiosurg* 1998;**1**:233–8.

304 Herfarth KK, Debus J, Lohr F *et al.* Stereotactic single-dose radiation therapy of liver tumours: results of a phase I/II trial. *J Clin Oncol* 2001;**19**:164–70.

305 Elsaleh H, Robbins P, Joseph D *et al.* Can p53 alterations be used to predict tumour response to pre-operative chemo-radiotherapy in locally advanced rectal cancer? *Radiother Oncol* 2000;**56**:239–44.

306 Villafranca E, Okruzhnov Y, Dominguez MA *et al.* Polymorphisms of the repeated sequences in the enhancer region of the thymidylate synthase gene promoter may predict downstaging after preoperative chemoradiation in rectal cancer. *J Clin Oncol* 2001;**19**:1779–86.

307 Gnanasampanthan G, Elsaleh H, McCaul K, Iacopetta B. Ki-ras mutation type and the survival benefit from adjuvant chemotherapy in Dukes' C colorectal cancer. *J Pathol* 2001;**195**:543–8.

308 Ribic CM, Sargent DJ, Moore MJ *et al.* Tumor microsatellite instability and the benefit of 5-FU based chemotherapy in stage II & III colon cancer: a pooled molecular reanalysis of randomized chemotherapy trials. *Proc Am Soc Clin Oncol* 2002;**21**:509(abstr).

309 Bensmaine MA, Marty M, de Gramont A *et al.* Factors predicting efficacy of oxaliplatin in combination with 5-fluorouracil (5-FU) +/– folinic acid in a compassionate-use cohort of 481 5-FU-resistant advanced colorectal cancer patients. *Br J Cancer* 2001;**85**:509–17.

310 Meta-Analysis Group in Cancer. Alpha-interferon does not increase the efficacy of 5-fluorouracil in advanced colorectal cancer. *Br J Cancer* 2001;**84**:611–20.

311 Buyse M, Thirion P, Carlson RW, Burzykowski T, Molenberghs G, Piedbois P. Relation between tumour response to first-line chemotherapy and survival in advanced colorectal cancer: a meta-analysis. Meta-Analysis Group in Cancer. *Lancet* 2000;**356**:373–8.

312 Labianca R, Pancera G, Luporini G. Factors influencing response rates for advanced colorectal cancer chemotherapy. *Ann Oncol* 1996;**7**:901–6.

313 Leichman CG, Lenz HJ, Leichman L *et al.* Quantitation of intratumoral thymidylate synthase expression predicts for disseminated colorectal cancer response and resistance to protracted infusion fluorouracil and weekly leucovorin. *J Clin Oncol* 1997: **15**:3223–9.

314 Yamachika T, Nakanishi H, Inada K *et al.* A new prognostic factor for colorectal carcinoma, thymidylate synthase, and its therapeutic significance. *Cancer* 1998;**82**:70–7.

315 Pullarkat ST, Ghaderi V, Ingles SA *et al.* Human thymidylate synthase gene polymorphism determines response to 5-FU chemotherapy. *Proc Am Soc Clin Oncol* 2000;**19**:942(abstr).

316 Nita ME, Tominaga O, Nagawa H *et al.* Dihydropyrimidine dehydrogenase but not thymidylate synthase expression is associated with resistance to 5-fluorouracil in colorectal cancer. *Hepato-gastroenterology* 1998;**45**:2117–22.

317 Beck A, Etienne MC, Cheradame S *et al.* A role for dihydropyrimidine dehydrogenase and thymidylate synthetase in tumour sensitivity to fluorouracil. *Eur J Cancer* 1994;**30A**:1517–22.

318 Ichikawa W, Uetake H, Yamada H *et al.* Expression of dihydropyrimidine dehydrogenase in primary lesion predicts the anti-tumour effect in 5-fluorouracil based chemotherapy for gastrointestinal tract cancer. *Proc Am Soc Clin Oncol* 2000;**19**:1114(abstr).

319 Belluco C, Guillem JG, Kemeny N *et al.* p53 nuclear protein overexpression in colorectal cancer: a dominant predictor of survival in patients with advanced hepatic metastases. *J Clin Oncol* 1996;**14**:2696–701.

320 Paradiso A, Maiello E, Ranieri G *et al.* Topo-isomerase-1 and thymidylate synthase primary tumour expression as prognostic and predictive factors for response to CPT-11 in advanced colorectal cancer patients. *Eur J Cancer* 2001;**37**(Suppl. 6):1140(abstr).

321 Temple WJ, Saettler EB. Locally recurrent rectal cancer: Role of composite resection of extensive pelvic tumours with strategies for minimizing risk of recurrence. *J Surg Oncol* 2000;**73**:47–58.

322 Lopez-Kostner F, Fazio VW, Vignali A, Rybicki LA, lavery IC. Locally recurrent rectal cancer: predictors and success of salvage surgery. *Dis Colon Rectum* 2001;**44**:173–8.

323 Estes NC, Thomas JH, Jewell WR, Beggs D, Hardin CA. Pelvic exenteration: a treatment for failed rectal cancer surgery. *Am Surg* 1993;**59**:420–2.

324 Salo JC, Paty PB, Guillem J, Minsky BD, Harrison LB, Cohen AM. Surgical salvage of recurrent rectal carcinoma after curative resection: a 10-year experience. *Ann Surg Oncol* 1999;**6**:171–7.

325 Wanebo HJ, Doness J, Vezeridis MP *et al.* Pelvic resection of recurrent rectal cancer. *Ann Surg* 1994;**220**:586–95.

326 Lowry AM, Rich TA, Skibber JM *et al.* Preoperative infusional chemoradiation, selective intraoperative radiation, and resection for locally advanced pelvic recurrence of colorectal adenocarcinoma. *Ann Surg* 1996;**223**:177–85.

327 Guiney MJ, Smith JG, Worotniuk V, Ngan S, Blakey D. Radiotherapy treatment for isolated loco-regional recurrence of rectosigmoid cancer following definitive surgery: Peter MacCallum Cancer Institute experience, 1981–1990. *Int J Radiat Oncol Biol Phys* 1997;**38**:1019–25.

328 Arnott SJ. The value of combined 5-fluorouracil and x-ray therapy in the palliation of locally recurrent and inoperable rectal carcinoma. *Clin Radiol* 1975;**26**:177–82.

329 Crane CH, Janjan NA, Abbruzzese JL *et al.* Effective pelvic symptom control using initial chemoradiation without colostomy in metastatic rectal cancer. *Int J Radiat Oncol Biol Phys* 2001;**49**:107–16.

330 Hodson DI, Malaker K, McLellan W, Meikle AL, Gillies JM. Hypofractionated radiotherapy for the palliation of advanced pelvic malignancy. *Int J Radiat Oncol Biol Phys* 1983;**9**:1727–9.

331 Allum WH, Mack P, Priestman TJ, Fielding JW. Radiotherapy for pain relief in locally recurrent colorectal cancer. *Ann R Coll Surg Engl* 1987;**69**:220–1.

332 Frykholm GJ, Pahlman L, Glimelius B. Treatment of local recurrences of rectal carcinoma. *Radiother Oncol* 1995;**34**:185–94.

333 Lingareddy V, Ahmad NR, Mohiuddin M. Palliative reirradiation for recurrent rectal cancer. *Int J Radiat Oncol Biol Phys* 1997;**38**:785–90.

334 Garcia-Aguilar J, Cromwell JW, Marra C, Lee SH, Madoff RD, Rothenberger DA. Treatment of locally recurrent rectal cancer. *Dis Colon Rectum* 2001;**44**:1743–8.

335 Tan CC, Iftikhar SY, Allan A, Freeman JG. Local effects of colorectal cancer are well palliated by endoscopic laser therapy. *Eur J Surg Oncol* 1995;**21**:648–52.

336 Gevers AM, Macken E, Hiele M, Rutgeerts P. Endoscopic laser therapy for palliation of patients with distal colorectal carcinoma: analysis of factors influencing long-term outcome. *Gastrointest Endosc* 2000;**51**:580–5.

337 Farouk R, Nelson H, Gunderson LL. Aggressive multimodality treatment for locally advanced irresectable rectal cancer. *Br J Surg* 1997;**84**:741–9.

338 Schulze S, Lyng KM. Palliation of rectosigmoid neoplasms with Nd: YAG laser treatment. *Dis Colon Rectum* 1994;**37**:882–4.

339 Tranberg KG, Moller PH. Palliation of colorectal carcinoma with the Nd-YAG laser. *Eur J Surg* 1991;**157**:57–60.

340 Harris GJ, Senagore AJ, Lavery IC, Fazio VW. The management of neoplastic colorectal obstruction with colonic endolumenal stenting devices. *Am J Surg* 2001;**181**:499–506.

341 Dohmoto M, Hunerbein M, Schlag PM. Application of rectal stents for palliation of obstructing rectosigmoid cancer. *Surg Endosc* 1997;**11**:758–61.

342 Tack J, Gevers AM, Rutgeerts P. Self-expandable metallic stents in the palliation of rectosigmoidal carcinoma: a follow-up study. *Gastrointest Endosc* 1998;**48**:267–71.

343 Repici A, Reggio D, Angelis C *et al.* Covered metal stents for management of inoperable malignant colorectal strictures. *Gastrointest Endosc* 2000;**52**:735–40.

344 Law WL, Chu KW, Ho JW, Tung HM, Law SY, Chu KM. Self-expanding metallic stent in the treatment of colonic obstruction caused by advanced malignancies. *Dis Colon Rectum* 2000;**43**:1522–7.

# 29 Treatment of anal cancer

*John H Scholefield*

## Background

Anal cancer is a rare tumour, accounting for only 3–5% of all large bowel malignancies.[1] Since anal cancer is a rare tumour, large randomised trials are difficult, and consequently the evidence base for its management is largely based on large series of cases with a few recent trials.

Over 80% of anal cancers are of squamous origin arising from the squamous epithelium of the anal canal and perianal area; 10% are adenocarcinomas arising from the glandular mucosa of the upper anal canal, the anal glands and ducts. A very rare and particularly malignant tumour is anal melanoma.[1]

This chapter will deal primarily with anal squamous carcinomas as the evidence base for the management of the adenocarcinoma or melanoma is miniscule. For anal squamous carcinomas there is some evidence that its incidence is increasing, particularly in women who have had vulval or cervical cancer (including high grade intraepithelial neoplasia), and also in the immunosuppressed.[2]

Most anal cancers arise from the squamous epithelium of the anal margin or anal canal, although a few arise from anal glands and ducts.[3] Traditionally the anal region is divided into the anal canal and the anal margin or verge. There has been controversy regarding the exact definition of the anal canal. This argument has become less important as surgery plays a smaller role in treatment, but reports of surgical results from past decades are confused by this variation in definition.

## Aetiology and pathogenesis

Anal squamous cell carcinomas are relatively uncommon tumours; there are between 250 and 300 new cases per year in England and Wales.[4] Based on these figures each consultant general surgeon might expect to see one anal carcinoma every three to four years. However, anal cancers are probably underreported since some anal canal tumours are misclassified as rectal tumours and some perianal tumours as squamous carcinomas of skin.

The Office of Population Censuses and Surveys' Cancer Statistics for England and Wales,[3] recorded 289 cases of anal cancer in 1988.[4] The average age is 57 years for both sexes but canal tumours are more common in women whereas margin tumours are more common in men. However, these figures must be interpreted with caution since the distinction between anal canal and anal margin is poorly defined.

There is wide geographic variation in the incidence of anal cancers around the world,[5] but again these figures must be interpreted with caution for reasons given above. Nevertheless, a low incidence (0·2 cases per 100 000 of population) is reported by Rizal in the Philippines; and the highest incidence (3·6 cases per 100 000 of population) is reported in Geneva, Switzerland. Other areas of high incidence are Poland (Warsaw) and Brazil (Recife). It is notable that these areas also have a high incidence of cervical, vulval and penile tumours (possibly reflecting the common proposed aetiological agent – papillomaviruses). The UK incidence of anal cancer lies between these extremes.

The increasing incidence of HIV infection in the United States has resulted in an increase in the incidence of anal cancer.[6] Areas such as San Francisco with a large gay population have reportedly seen a dramatic increase in the prevalence of anal cancers. A recent study from Denmark has reported a doubling in the incidence of anal cancer, particularly in women over the past 10 years.[2] No other countries have reported similar increases to date, but the Cancer Registry data in Denmark are renowned for their remarkable accuracy and completeness.

Recent epidemiological evidence has suggested that anal cancer may be associated with anal sexual activity; Cooper *et al.*[7] observed four cases of anal cancer arising in homosexual men with long histories of anoreceptive intercourse. The occurrence of a disproportionately high incidence of anal cancer among male homosexual communities was reported from San Francisco and Los Angeles. Daling *et al.*[8] identified risk factors for the development of squamous cell carcinoma of the anus, a history of receptive anal intercourse in males increasing the relative risk of developing anal cancer by 33 times compared with controls with colon cancer. A history of genital warts also increased the relative risk of developing anal cancer (27-fold in men and 22-fold in women). These studies suggest that a sexually transmissible agent may be an aetiological factor in anal squamous cell carcinoma.

Similarly, epidemiological data and molecular biological data have shown an association between a sexually transmissible agent and female genital cancer. With the use of nucleic acid hybridisation techniques, human papillomavirus (HPV) type 16 DNA, and less commonly types 18, 31 and 33 DNA, were consistently found to be integrated into the genome in genital squamous cell carcinomas.[9] Recently the same HPV DNA types have also been identified in a similar proportion of anal squamous cell carcinomas.[10] Human papillomaviruses are DNA viruses, of which there are more than 60 HPV types capable of causing a wide variety of lesions on squamous epithelium. Common warts can be found on the hands and feet of children and young adults and are caused by the relatively infectious HPV types 1 and 2. Anogenital papillomaviruses are less infective than types 1 and 2 and are exclusively sexually transmissible. The epidemiology of genital papillomavirus infection is poorly understood, largely because of the social and moral taboos surrounding sexually transmissible infections. Anogenital papillomavirus-associated lesions range from condylomata to intraepithelial neoplasia to invasive carcinoma. The most common HPV types causing genital warts are types 6 and 11. HPV types 6 and 11 may also be isolated from low grade intraepithelial neoplasia. HPV types 16, 18, 31 and 33 are much less commonly associated with genital condylomas but are more commonly found in high grade intraepithelial neoplasias and invasive carcinomas. Once one area of the anogenital epithelium is infected, spread of papillomavirus infection throughout the rest of the anogenital area probably follows, but remains occult in the majority of individuals.[11] Therefore the commonly held belief that anal cancer only occurs in individuals who practise anal intercourse is probably unfounded.

## Histological types

Included within the category of epidermoid tumours are squamous cell, basaloid (or cloacogenic) carcinomas and mucoepidermoid cancers. The different morphological types of anal cancer do not appear to have different prognoses.[12] Tumours arising at the anal margin tend to be well differentiated and keratinising, whereas those arising in the canal are more commonly poorly differentiated. Basaloid tumours arise in the transitional zone around the dentate line and form 30–50% of all anal canal tumours.

## Patterns of spread

Anal canal cancer spreads locally, mainly in a cephalad direction, so that the tumour may appear to have arisen in the rectum. The tumour also spreads outwards into the anal sphincters and into the rectovaginal septum, perineal body, and the vagina in more advanced cases. Lymph node metastases occur frequently, especially in tumours of the anal canal.[13] Spread occurs initially to the perirectal group of nodes and thereafter to inguinal, haemorrhoidal and lateral pelvic lymph nodes. The frequency of nodal involvement is related to the size of the primary tumour together with its depth of penetration.[14] Approximately 14% of patients will present with inguinal lymph node involvement but this rises to approximately 30% when the primary tumour is greater than 5 cm in diameter.[15,16] Only in 50% of patients with enlarged nodes at presentation will the nodes subsequently be shown to contain tumour. Synchronously involved nodes carry a particularly poor prognosis whereas, when metachronous spread develops, the salvage rate is much higher.

Haematogenous spread tends to occur late and is usually associated with advanced local disease. The principal sites of metastases are the liver, lung and bones.[17] However, metastases have been described in the kidneys, adrenals and brain.

## Clinical presentation

Since anal cancer is rare but anal and rectal bleeding are common symptoms, it is not surprising that 75% of anal cancers are misdiagnosed as benign conditions initially.[18] The predominant symptoms of epidermoid anal cancer are pain and bleeding, which are present in about 50% of cases.[19] The presence of a mass is noted by a minority of patients, around 25%. Pruritus and discharge occur in a similar proportion. Advanced tumours may involve the sphincter mechanism causing faecal incontinence. Invasion of the posterior vaginal wall may cause a discharging fistula through the vagina.

Cancer of the anal margin usually has the appearance of a malignant ulcer, with a raised, everted and indurated edge. Lesions within the canal may not be visible, though extensive lesions spread to the anal verge, or can extend via the ischiorectal fossa to the skin of the buttock.[20] Digital examination of the anal canal is usually painful, and may reveal the distortion produced by the tumour. Since anal cancer tends to spread upwards, there may be involvement of the distal rectum, perhaps giving the impression that the lesion has arisen there. Involvement of the perirectal lymph nodes may be palpable on digital examination, rather more than may be apparent in disseminating rectal cancer. If the tumour has extended into the sphincter muscles, the characteristic induration of a spreading malignancy may be felt around the anal canal.

Although up to one third of patients will have enlarged inguinal lymph nodes, biopsy will confirm metastatic spread in only 50% of these – the rest are due to secondary infection.[19] Biopsy or fine needle aspiration is recommended by many to confirm involvement of the groin nodes if radical block dissection is contemplated. Distant spread is unusual in anal cancer, so hepatomegaly, although it must be looked for, is very uncommon. Frequently other benign perianal conditions will exist in association with anal cancer, such as fistulae, condylomas or leukoplakia.

## Investigation

The most important investigation in the management of anal cancer is examination under anaesthesia. Ideally this should be carried out jointly by the surgeon and radiotherapist. Examination under anaesthesia permits optimum assessment of the tumour in terms of size, involvement of adjacent structures, nodal involvement and also provides the best opportunity to obtain a biopsy for histological confirmation. Sigmoidoscopic examination is probably best performed at this examination.

## Clinical staging

No one system of staging for anal tumours has been adopted universally. However, that of the UICC[21] is the one most widely used. For anal canal lesions this system has been criticised as it has required assessment of involvement of the external sphincter. To overcome this a system has been suggested by Papillon[22] (Box 29.1).

---

**Box 29.1 Clinical staging of anal tumours[22]**

| | |
|---|---|
| T1 | < 2 cm |
| T2 | 2–4 cm |
| T3 | > 4 cm, mobile |
| T4a | invading vaginal mucosa |
| T4b | extension into structures other than skin, rectal or vaginal mucosa |

---

Although insertion of the probe may be difficult or impossible because of the discomfort, ultrasound scanning can provide accurate information regarding sphincter involvement.[23] CT and MRI may provide information on spread beyond the anal canal.

Serum tumour markers and other measures of biological activity such as DNA ploidy are generally unhelpful as they do not provide reliable information.

## Treatment options

### Historical

The initial treatment for anal cancer was radiotherapy as the mortality and morbidity of surgical treatment of anal carcinoma were unacceptable. By the 1930s, however, it was recognised that the low voltage radiotherapy used frequently produced severe radionecrosis. As surgery became safer, abdominoperineal excision for invading lesions, and local excision for small growths, became the standard treatment for the next four decades.

More recently the development of equipment that could deliver high energy irradiation in the 1950s by the cobalt source generator, or more recently by linear accelerators, enabled radiotherapists to deliver higher penetrating doses to deeper placed structures with less superficial expenditure of energy. Radiation damage to surrounding tissues was consequently reduced whilst simultaneously delivering an enhanced tumouricidal effect. Interstitial irradiation alone may produce local tumour control rates of 47%.[24] Improved results have been described with a technique of external beam irradiation, combined with interstitial therapy[25] – two-thirds survived for 5 years, the majority maintaining adequate sphincter function. An alternative is high dose external beam radiotherapy alone, for which 5-year survival rates of 75% at 3 years have been described.[26]

Ironically it was a surgeon, Norman Nigro, reporting the use of combined chemotherapy and radiotherapy to try to turn inoperable cases into candidates for surgical salvage, who began to turn surgeons away from operation as first choice therapy.[27] Over the past 10 years treatment of this condition has been transformed by the use of chemoirradiation and this has been supported by the result of a large randomised trial.

## What is the role of chemoirradiation therapy (combined modality therapy)?

Combined modality therapy for anal cancer was championed by Norman Nigro. Nigro chose to use 5-fluorouracil (5-FU) and mitomycin C empirically as a preoperative regimen aimed at improving the results of radical surgery.[27] The radiotherapy then consisted of 30 Gy of external beam irradiation over a period of 3 weeks. A bolus of mitomycin C was given on day 1 of treatment, and 5-FU was delivered in a synchronous continuous 4-day infusion during the first week of radiotherapy. After the completion of radiotherapy, a further infusion of 5-FU was administered and patients later proceeded to abdominoperineal excision. It was evident to Nigro that the majority had quite dramatic tumour shrinkage – in his 1974 publication the tumour was reported to have disappeared completely in all three patients. No tumour was found in the surgical specimen in both the patients who underwent abdominoperineal excision; the third refused surgery. Nigro's experience over the ensuing 10 years bore out his early enthusiasm. As he became more confident, he no longer routinely pressed his patients to undergo radical surgery, initially confining himself to excising the site of the primary tumour after combined modality therapy. Later he dropped even this relatively minor surgical step if the primary site looked and felt normal after treatment.[28]

A variety of similar techniques have subsequently been described. With wider experience, it became clear that higher doses of radiotherapy (45–60 Gy) could be applied, usually split into two courses to minimise morbidity.

Chemotherapy comprised intravenous infusion of 5-FU at the beginning and end of the first radiotherapy course, and a single bolus of mitomycin C given on the first day of treatment. Modifications of chemotherapy dosage and prophylactic antibiotic therapy were necessary in elderly or frail patients, and those with extensive ulcerated tumours.

All the above are non-randomised studies and, although they describe excellent results, it has yet to be determined whether similar levels of local tumour control and survival can be achieved without chemotherapy, perhaps thereby avoiding some morbidity.

## What do the trials in anal squamous carcinoma show?

The only analysis comparing patients who have been treated with the combined regimen and those receiving radiotherapy alone has suggested that initial local tumour control may be achieved in about 90% of patients receiving various combined treatment protocols compared to 56% with radiotherapy alone.[29] This retrospective review (hence, non-randomised) compared patients who had received a combined treatment programme with historical controls treated by radiotherapy alone in the same institution. The overall uncorrected 5-year survival of the two groups of patients was similar at 58%. This group also looked at the role of mitomycin C in the treatment regimen and concluded from non-controlled data that this contributes to optimum local tumour control.[30]

The most recent data on combined modality therapy came from a randomised multicentre study called ACT I. This trial compared chemoirradiation with radiotherapy alone[31]: 585 patients were randomised making it the largest single trial in anal cancer. At a median follow up of 42 months there was a 42% (95% CI 0·42–0·69) reduction in the risk of local treatment failure in the combined modality group (5FU + mitomycin C + radiotherapy) compared with radiotherapy alone. There was also a reduced risk of death from anal cancer (RR 0·71; 95% CI 0·53–0·95) and a non-significant overall survival advantage (RR 0·86; 95% CI 0·67–1·11). Analysis of quality-of-life data showed that the addition of chemotherapy did not adversely affect the patients' quality of life.[31]

A similar randomised study by the EORTC randomised 110 patients and showed similar results.[32] As a result of this trial it seems that the standard treatment for anal squamous carcinoma should be a combination of radiotherapy and intravenous 5-fluorouracil with mitomycin. Surgery may then be reserved for those who fail.[31] New trials using alternative chemotherapeutic regimes including cisplatin instead of mitomycin C are currently under discussion.[33]

## What is the role of surgery in the treatment of anal cancer?

There are no randomised trials of surgical treatment for anal cancer. The available evidence is from personal series of cases often pooled over several years due to the rarity of the tumour.

Overall the results of surgery for anal cancer are disappointing for what is traditionally thought of as a locoregional disease.

For decades radical *abdominoperineal excision* of the rectum and anus was the preferred method of treatment at most centres around the world. Abdominoperineal excision for anal canal cancer differs little from the procedure used for rectal cancer, but particular care is taken to clear the space below the pelvic floor. Although extended pelvic lymphadenectomy in addition to abdominoperineal excision has been practised, such extensive operations did not appear to improve 5-year survival rates.[33] Compared with anal margin cancers, anal canal cancer is more likely to be locally advanced at presentation, and to be associated with subsequent metastasis,[34] perhaps explaining the general preference for radical surgery in the literature.

Around 20% of anal squamous cancers are incurable surgically at presentation. Results published since the mid 1980s reporting series collected over the previous several decades have varied widely in their survival outcome; on average the 5-year survival has been around 55–60%.[13,19,35] Most post-surgical relapses occur locoregionally.

Around 75% of cancers at the anal margin have been treated in the past by *local excision*.[19,36] The rationale for this was based on the perception that margin lesions rarely metastasise, although this has not always been confirmed by prolonged follow up. Given the rather disappointing 5-year survival rates – around 50–70% – one may speculate that radical surgery may have led to better results.

Whilst the role of surgery in the management of anal cancer may have diminished in the wake of the results of chemoirradiation strategies and their success in enabling patients to avoid colostomies, surgery still has an important contribution to make in the management of these cancers.

### Initial diagnosis

Most patients present to surgeons who are best suited to perform examination under anaesthesia to confirm diagnosis and assess local extent.

### Local excision for anal margin lesions

Small lesions (usually 2 cm across) at the anal margin may still best be treated by local excision alone, obviating the need for protracted courses of non-surgical therapy. There is some evidence that the risk of regional lymph node metastasis is not related to primary tumour size, which may explain the disappointing results sometimes reported after local excision; this conflicts with the view that tumour size is related to stage, which explains the excellent results of local excision in small tumours.[13]

## Surgery for salvage

Surgeons retain an important role in treatment of anal cancer after failure of primary non-surgical treatment, either early or late.[38] Four situations may require surgery after primary non-surgical treatment:

● residual tumour
● complications of treatment
● incontinence or fistula after tumour resolution
● subsequent tumour recurrence.

The appearance of the primary site is often misleading after radiotherapy. In most patients complete remission is indicated by the tumour disappearing completely. In some, however, a lump may remain, occasionally looking like an unchanged primary tumour. Only generous biopsy will reveal whether the residual lump contains tumour or consists merely of inflammatory tissue.[39] Thus histological proof of residual disease is mandatory before radical surgery is recommended to the patient.

Complications of non-surgical treatment for anal cancer do occur in a proportion of patients, which may range from radionecrosis, fistula, or incontinence. Severe anal pain from radionecrosis of the anal lining may necessitate either a colostomy, in the hope that the lesion will heal after faecal diversion, or radical anorectal excision.

Occasionally a tumour is so locally extensive that the patient will be rendered incontinent as a consequence of primary tumour shrinkage. Although rectovaginal fistula may be amenable to repair, sphincter damage is unlikely to improve with local surgery, therefore necessitating abdominoperineal excision of the anorectum. In the author's experience abdominoperineal excision of the rectum under these circumstances is usually best undertaken in conjunction with a rectus abdominis myocutaneous flap to aid perineal wound revascularisation and facilitate healing of the perineal wound.

Should clinical evidence of recurrent disease develop after initial resolution, biopsy is again mandatory prior to surgical intervention. These biopsies need to be of reasonable size, number, and depth as the histological appearances following radiotherapy can make histopathological interpretation difficult. If high dose radiotherapy was used for primary treatment, further non-surgical therapy for recurrence is usually contraindicated, therefore making radical surgical removal necessary.

## Inguinal metastases

Inguinal lymph nodes are enlarged in 10–25% of patients with anal cancers. Although inguinal lymph node involvement may be treated by radiotherapy, some argue that this should be treated surgically; histological confirmation is advisable before radical groin dissection as up to 50% of cases of inguinal lymphadenopathy may be due to inflammation alone.[19] Enlargement of groin nodes some time after primary therapy is most likely to be due to recurrent tumour; radical groin dissection is indicated in this situation, with up to 50% 5-year survival.[17]

## Rarer tumours

### Adenocarcinoma

Adenocarcinoma in the anal canal is usually simply a very low rectal cancer that has spread downwards to involve the canal, but true adenocarcinoma of the anal canal does occur, probably arising from the anal glands, which arise around the dentate line and pass radially outwards into the sphincter muscles. This is a very rare tumour, quite radiosensitive, but usually still treated by radical surgery. There are no randomised or non-randomised trials of the management of this tumour.

### Malignant melanoma

This tumour is very rare, accounting for just 1% of anal canal malignant tumours. As it is so rare, there are no large studies in the management of this tumour. The lesion may mimic a thrombosed external pile owing to its colour, although amelanotic tumours also occur. It has an even worse prognosis than at other sites. As the chances of cure are minimal, radical surgery as primary treatment has been all but abandoned at some centres.[40] Chemoirradiation has little role in the management of anal melanoma as the tumour is not radiosensitive.

## Conclusions

The mainstay of treatment of anal squamous carcinoma is combined modality therapy. At present the evidence would suggest that use of 5-FU and mitomycin C should be given in combination with 30 cGy of radiotherapy. With combined modality therapy, more than 50% of patients will avoid a colostomy **Evidence level Ib**.

Patients with anal cancers often present to surgeons and examination under anaesthesia may be required to allow confirmation of the diagnosis, assessment of the extent of the tumour, and biopsy of the lesion.

Whilst the primary therapy may have become chemoirradiation for these tumours, surgery may still be required for salvage in those cases where combined modality treatment fails. Salvage surgery usually requires abdominoperineal resection. Primary reconstruction of the (irradiated) perineal defect using a myocutaneous flap is advised by many experts.

For small localised anal margin tumours, local excision may be appropriate but adjuvant combined modality therapy can be used as an adjuvant if there is doubt about the completeness of excision.

## References

1 Morson B, Dawson I. In: *Morson and Dawson's gastrointestinal pathology.* Oxford: Blackwell, 1990.

2 Frische M, Melbye M. Trends in the incidence of anal carcinoma in Denmark. *BMJ* 1993;**306**:419–22.

3 Fenger C. The anal transitional zone. Location and extent. *Acta Pathol Microbiol Immunol Scand* 1979;**87**:379–86.

4 Office of Population Censuses and Surveys (1988). *Cancer Statistics Registrations.* London: HMSO.

5 Muir C, Waterhouse J. *Cancer in five continents (V).* Lyons, France: IARC Scientific Publications, Lyons, 1987.

6 Wexner S, Milsom J, Dailey T *et al.* The demographics of anal cancers are changing. Identification of a high risk population. *Dis Colon Rectum* 1987;**30**:942–6.

7 Cooper H, Patchefsky A, Marks G. Cloacogenic carcinoma of the anorectum in homosexual men: an observation of four cases. *Dis Colon Rectum* 1979;**22**:557–8.

8 Daling J, Weiss N, Hislop T *et al.* Sexual practices, sexually transmitted diseases and the incidence of anal cancer. *N Engl J Med* 1987;**317**:973–7.

9 zur Hausen H. Papilloma viruses in human cancers. *Mol Carcinogen* 1989;**1**:147–50.

10 Palmer JG, Scholefield JH, Shepherd N *et al.* Anal cancer and human papillomaviruses. *Dis Colon Rectum* 1989;**32**:1016–22.

11 Syrjanen K. Human papillomavirus in genital carcinogenesis. *Sex Transm Dis* 1994;**21**(Suppl.2):S86–S89.

12 Morson B. The pathology and results of treatment of squamous cell carcinoma of the anal canal and anal margin. *Proc R Soc Med* 1960;**53**:22–6.

13 Boman B, Moertel C, O'Connell M *et al.* Carcinoma of the anal canal. A clinical and pathologic study of 188 cases. *Cancer* 1984;**54**:114–25.

14 Loygue J, Laugier A. Cancer epidermoide de l'anus. *Chirurgie* 1980;**6**:710–16.

15 Klotz R, Pamukcoglu T, Souillard D *et al.* Transitional cell cloacogenic carcinoma of the anal canal. *Cancer* 1967;**20**:1724–45.

16 Stearns M, Urmacher C *et al.* Cancer of the anal canal. *Curr Probl Cancer* 1980;**4**:1–44.

17 Greenall M, Magill G, Quan S *et al.* Recurrent epidermoid cancer of the anus. *Cancer* 1986;**57**:1437–41.

18 Edwards A, Morus L *et al.* Anal cancer: the case for earlier diagnosis. *J R Soc Med* 1991;**84**:395–7.

19 Pintor MP, Northover JM, Nicholls J *et al.* Squamous cell carcinoma of the anus at one hospital from 1948 to 1984. *Br J Surg* 1989;**76**:806–10.

20 Nelson R, Prasad M, Abcarian H *et al.* Anal carcinoma presenting as a perirectal abscess or fistula. *Arch Surg* 1985;**120**:632–5.

21 UICC. *TNM classification of malignant tumours, 4th edn.* [World Health Organization] Geneva, Heidelberg: Springer-Verlag, 1985.

22 Papillon J, Mayer M, Mountberon J *et al.* A new approach to the management of epidermoid carcinoma of the anal canal. *Cancer* 1987;**51**:1830–7.

23 Goldman S, Norming U, Svenson C *et al.* Transanorectal ultrasonography in the staging of anal epidermoid carcinoma. *Int J Colorectal Dis* 1991;**6**:152–7.

24 James R, Pointon R, Martin S *et al.* Local radio-therapy in the management of squamous carcinoma of the anus. *Br J Surg* 1985;**72**:282–5.

25 Papillon J. *Rectal and anal cancers.* Berlin: Springer-Verlag, 1982.

26 Green J, Schaupp W, Cantrill S *et al.* Anal carcinoma: therapeutic concepts. *Am J Surg* 1980;**140**:151–5.

27 Nigro N. Treatment of squamous cell cancer of the anus. *Cancer Treat Res* 1984;**18**:221–42.

28 Nigro N, Vaitkevicius V *et al.* Combined therapy for cancer of the anal canal. A preliminary report. *Dis Colon Rectum* 1974;**27**:354–6.

29 Cummings B, Keane T, O'Sullivan B *et al.* Epidermoid anal cancer: treatment by radiation alone or by 5-fluorouracil with or without mitomycin C. *Radiat Oncol* 1991;**21**:1115–25.

30 Cummings B, Keane T, O'Sullivan B *et al.* Mitomycin in anal canal carcinoma. *Oncology* 1993;**50**(Suppl. 1):63–9.

31 UKCCCR Anal Cancer Trial Working Party. Epidermoid anal cancer: results from the UKCCCR randomised trial of radiotherapy alone versus radiotherapy, 5 fluouracil, and mitomycin. *Lancet* 1996;**348**:1049–54.

32 Bartelink H, Roelofson F, Eschwege F *et al* Concomitant radiotherapy and chemotherapy is superior to radiotherapy alone in the treatment of locally advanced anal cancer. Results of a phase III randomised trial by the EORTC. *J Clin Oncol* 1997;**15**:2040–9.

33 Klas JV, Rothenberger DA, Wong WD, Madoff RD. Malignant tumours of the anal canal. *Cancer* 1999;**85**:1686–93.

34 Paradis P, Douglass HJ, Hoylake E *et al.* The clinical implications of a staging system for carcinoma of the anus. *Surg Gynecol Obstet* 1975;**141**:411–16.

35 Jensen S, Hagen K, Harling H *et al.* Long term prognosis after radical treatment for squamous call carcinoma of the anal canal and anal margin. *Dis Colon Rectum* 1988;**31**:273–8.

36 Greenall M, Quan S, Stearns M *et al.* Epidermoid cancer of the anal margin. Pathologic features, treatment and clinical results. *Am J Surg* 1985;**149**:95–101.

37 Greenall M, Quan S, Urmacher C *et al.* Treatment of epidermoid carcinoma of the anal canal. *Surg Gynecol Obstet* 1985;**161**:509–17.

38 Salmon R, Zafrani B, Habib A *et al.* Prognosis of cloacogenic and squamous cancers of the anal canal. *Dis Colon Rectum* 1986;**29**:336–40.

39 Northover J. The non-surgical management of anal cancer. *Br J Radiol* 1988;**61**:755.

40 Quan S. Anal cancers. Squamous and melanoma. *Cancer* 1992;**70**(Suppl.5):1384–9.

# Section VI

## Treating tumours of the urogenital system

*Malcolm Mason, Editor*

# Levels of evidence and grades of recommendation used in *Evidence-based Oncology*

Levels of evidence and grades of recommendation appear within the text in the clinical chapters, for example, **Evidence Level Ia** and **Grade A**.

## Levels of evidence

Ia    Meta-analysis of randomised controlled trials (RCTs)
Ib    At least 1 RCT
IIa   At least 1 non-randomised study
IIb   At least 1 other well designed quasi-experimental study
III   Non-experimental, descriptive studies
IV   Expert committee reports or opinions/experience of respected authorities

## Grades of recommendations

A    At least one RCT as part of body of literature of overall good quality and consistency addressing recommendation **Evidence levels Ia, Ib**
B    No RCT but well conducted clinical studies available **Evidence levels IIa, IIb, III**
C    Expert committee reports or opinions/experience of respected authorities in the absence of directly applicable good quality clinical studies **Evidence level IV**

From *Clinical Oncology* (2001)**13**:S212
Source of data: MEDLINE, *Proceedings of the American Society of Medical Oncology* (ASCO).

# 30 Kidney cancer

*Chris Coppin, Franz Porzsolt*

Is there evidence that systemic treatment can prolong survival in patients with renal cell cancer, and if so what is the optimal proven therapy and what are the resulting toxicities and effects on symptoms? This question will be considered primarily in the setting of advanced disease and briefly in the adjuvant setting.

## Background

### Definition and magnitude of the problem of advanced kidney cancer

Several excellent and comprehensive general reviews of kidney cancer are available.[1-3] Renal cell cancer constitutes the large majority of primary kidney cancers in adults and is the only specific cancer diagnosis that will be considered here.

Kidney cancer, mostly renal cell carcinoma, accounts for about 3% of cancer incidence and cancer deaths in industrialised countries.[4] The term "advanced disease" is used to refer to metastases detected at diagnosis or after nephrectomy for an operable primary, as well as a technically inoperable primary. By frequency, the commonest advanced situations are lung metastases or lytic bone metastases, with or without the primary in place, locally advanced disease, miscellaneous other metastatic sites, or, uncommonly, local recurrence in the renal bed.[5] These groups are combined because most patients with advanced renal cancer are not generally considered curable and are treated with palliative intent, with the possible exception of clinically solitary metastasis.

### Natural history and prognostic factors

In the absence of particularly effective therapy of advanced renal cancer as will be discussed, for most patients the prognosis is dominated by the natural course of the disease, which therefore deserves consideration in some detail. The clinical picture of advanced renal cell cancer is characterised by variety – of presentation, metastatic sites, and subsequent course. A number of paraneoplastic syndromes have given the disease a reputation as a mimic.[6] Although clinically significant in only a minority of patients, these syndromes can be confusing as the presenting feature and they may respond to treatment such as nephrectomy. The untreated natural history of advanced disease is exceptionally variable and the disease may be clinically stable for many months or sometimes years without therapy, although very rapidly growing disease is also seen. Therefore a brief period of observation can be very helpful to establish the natural history of disease in the asymptomatic or minimally symptomatic individual with incurable advanced disease.

A number of unexplained "spontaneous" complete (CR) or partial (PR) remissions of metastases have been observed in untreated patients, with the best available data coming from two prospective studies. Oliver[7] followed 73 consecutive untreated patients with advanced disease and observed three CRs and two PRs (standard criteria, 7% objective remission rate) lasting 3–84+ months, as well as four patients stable for over 12 months. The spontaneous remissions in this series appear to be in patients with metastatic disease confined to lung. The only published placebo-controlled trial[8] in this condition observed remissions in 6% of patients in the placebo arm, lasting for 2–31+ months.[9]

These observations on untreated advanced disease have substantial implications for patient management and for clinical trial interpretation. In such a variable disease, patient selection should be considered a potential explanation for differences in outcome unless proved otherwise in a randomised controlled trial. Prevalent patients with indolent advanced disease may be rapidly recruited into phase II clinical trials that accrue intermittently, whereas large phase III randomised studies have prolonged accrual of incident patients with a potentially different spectrum of disease dependent on the degree of patient selection. Furthermore, the occasional remissions seen with many types of systemic therapy might have occurred without treatment intervention.

Prognostic factors at diagnosis include TNM stage[10] that can be combined with tumour grade and patient performance status to provide prognostic strata,[11] potentially useful for patient selection and stratification in future adjuvant trials. Recently, a multifactorial nomogram has been proposed for predicting postoperative prognosis.[12] Prognostic factors for survival in patients with advanced renal cell carcinoma have usually been examined retrospectively, an approach limited to factors that can be readily extracted from records of patients treated in a variety of ways. The largest reported series[13] of 670 patients identified five independent factors, namely prior nephrectomy, performance status, haemoglobin, serum calcium and LDH, from which three prognostic strata could be constructed with median survivals of 4, 10 and 20 months. This report also summarises independent prognostic factors reported by other authors, including interval from diagnosis to detection of metastasis, weight loss, sedimentation rate, and the site and number of metastases. It should be emphasised that the range of survival is very wide. Patients who undergo removal or radioablation of a clinically solitary metastasis, with removal of the primary if present, may do well[14] but it is unclear if this is attributable to the therapy or the natural history of the condition.

Prognostic factors are also available on a prospective basis from some randomised controlled trials. A comprehensive survey is beyond the scope of this review. Performance status has been the most consistently reported prognostic factor for survival. Two studies have reported multivariate analyses. Witte *et al.*[15] found low performance status, weight loss, and multiple sites of involvement to be adverse. Lung as sole site of disease appears favourable.[16]

## Treatment approaches for advanced renal cell cancer

The many types of therapy that have been used to treat advanced renal cell carcinoma underscore the general lack of resulting success, while around 5% of patients in clinical trials experience survival over 5 years regardless of the type of systemic therapy.[17] The three main eras of systemic therapy have been with hormones, chemotherapy and biologic therapy. Progestogens may be associated with transient weight gain and improved wellbeing but the introduction of objective criteria showed that objective response was rare. Phase II trials of chemotherapy of many types have been consistently followed by temporary improvement in 0–10%, probably consistent with the natural course of the disease. None of these agents has gone on to phase III trials and it is therefore not possible to state the efficacy of agents such as medroxyprogesterone acetate (MPA) or vinblastine that have most commonly been used as control treatments in the trials of biotherapy to be discussed below.

Because of the observation of spontaneous metastatic regression in some patients, the possibility of a host versus tumour effect has raised the prospect that immune enhancement with biological therapy might be beneficial. At this time, high dose interleukin-2 is the specific biotherapy approved by the US Federal Drug Administration.

Elsewhere, interferon alfa and/or interleukin-2 are in common and approved use. The next section of this review will therefore examine the evidence underlying these treatments. The biologic actions of these agents are complex and will not be discussed here.

## Review of evidence

### Biologic therapy of advanced renal cell carcinoma

Two published meta-analyses of biologic therapy for advanced renal cell carcinoma are available[18,19] and are summarised in Table 30.1. No meta-analysis of individual patient data is available. Hernberg and colleagues[18] conducted a review of published randomised controlled trials that compared an interferon alfa (IFNα)-containing regimen with a non-IFNα control in advanced renal cell carcinoma. In our own work,[19] published randomised controlled trials that included any biotherapy component were reviewed. We used the Cochrane Collaboration methodology that requires an *a priori* protocol before conducting a systematic review and quantitative meta-analysis. Cochrane reviews are published electronically thereby permitting more detail, manipulation of statistical view and periodic updates. The previous review[19] serves as the basis for this section, updated with repeat electronic and hand searches to April 2001. Phase I randomised trials and those that failed to meet essential quality criteria (Table 30.2) were excluded. More detailed information regarding methods is available[19] including search strategy and meta-analytic technique. Our Cochrane review was intended to be as comprehensive as possible, whereas here we have focused on fully published studies reporting survival. Unless specified otherwise, results in the present meta-analysis use a random effects model in view of the heterogeneous nature of the studies.

Response rates to biotherapy are generally low in the phase III setting, averaging 13% though still higher than 3% for non-biotherapy controls (pooled OR 3·5, 95% CI 1·7–7·4).[19] The clinical significance of "response" is unclear, although objective response is commonly considered a *sine qua non* for benefit from cancer therapy. Response rate does not correlate with median survival from randomisation,[19] hardly surprising in view of the low response rates seen. However, there is some correlation of response rate increment with longer median survival in a pooled analysis of randomised trials,[19] not necessarily causal. Except for objective toxicity, the most clinically relevant outcome of quality of life by formal assessment during and after biotherapy has been infrequently documented. Overall survival will therefore be used as the primary endpoint for this section.

**Table 30.1   Published meta-analyses of biotherapy in advanced renal cell carcinoma**

| Quality criterion | Hernberg[18] | Coppin[19] |
|---|---|---|
| Systematic review | Yes | Yes |
| Published protocol | No | Yes (Cochrane) |
| Treatments | IFNα vs no IFNα | Any biotherapy |
| Major outcomes | Response (CR, PR) | Response (CR, PR) |
| | 1-year survival | 1-year survival |
| | | Hazard ratio (IFNα studies) |
| Included studies | | |
|   Randomised phase II/III | 8 | 42 |
|   Other | 0 | 0 |
|   Fully published | 6 | 37 |
|   Abstract only | 2 | 5 |
|   Unpublished data | 0 | 0 |
| Excluded RCTs | 0 | 16 |
| Total included patients | 525 | 4216 |

**Table 30.2   Quality parameters used in this review**

| Parameter | Comment |
|---|---|
| *Essential* | *Required for inclusion in this review* |
| Research design | Randomised controlled trials, excluding phase I |
| Database | MEDLINE, EMBase, and *Cochrane Library* (selects for better quality journals with higher rejection rates for studies with negative results) |
| Hand searching | Abstracts of cancer and urology meetings; references of study reports |
| Publication | Peer-reviewed published studies, required to evaluate other parameters |
| Language | No language restriction (some language bias inherent in databases) |
| Review protocol | Published *a priori* protocol to establish hypothesis, study criteria, methods |
| Randomisation | Adequate randomisation method assumed unless contrary evidence |
| Concealed allocation | Assumed unless evidence to the contrary |
| Intent to treat | Patient exclusions by authors were ignored as far as practicable |
| Primary outcome | Overall survival (at least median or 1-year survival) |
| *Highly desirable* | *Used to evaluate quality of included studies* |
| Stratification | Adequate control for major prognostic factors |
| Blinding | Studies distinguished by double blinding, single blinding, or none |
| Control group | Placebo control, control of known efficacy, or neither |
| Outcome evaluation | Independent blinded review, blinded investigator, or unblinded |
| Palliative benefit | Formal quality-of-life assessment during therapy and any remission |
| Other outcomes | Full survival curve or not; objective partial or complete response |

### Quality parameters used in the systematic review (Table 30.2)

The main attributes of a high quality systematic review are transparency and reproducibility. The strength of the conclusions are dependent on both the quality of identified studies and their reporting in sufficient detail to permit the exclusion of studies that would contribute biased data. The precise application of the quality parameters in Table 30.2 was often compromised by lack of information in published reports so that only the more flagrant breaches of appropriate trial method and analysis could be identified. Another serious issue was the lack of double-blind and preferably placebo-controlled studies of which there was only one[8] in advanced renal cell cancer. Outcomes evaluated by unblinded observers are likely to be biased by expectations in favour of the experimental arm.[20] These readily influenced outcomes include subjective toxicity and formal quality-of-life (QOL) assessments by patients, which can only be addressed by blinding, as well as "objective" measurements by investigators, which can be independently reviewed. The importance and value of an independent monitoring committee has been documented in the Cancer Renal Cytokine (CRECY) study in which major disagreement concerning response occurred in 40% of cases.[21]

### Interferon alfa (IFNα)

Studies using partially purified human leucocyte interferon, IFNα, began in the 1970s.[22] Recombinant techniques later allowed the production of large amounts of pure IFNα suitable for phase III trials. The two published meta-analyses[18,19] including IFNα for advanced renal cell cancer used similar criteria and methods, and came to similar conclusions. Hernberg[18] accessed the databases of the US National Cancer Institute, Schering-Plough (Kenilworth, NJ, USA) and Hoffman-LaRoche (Basel, Switzerland) up to February 1997, but did not identify any truly unpublished trials (two were available only in abstract at that time). Table 30.3 summarises fully published randomised controlled trials reporting survival that included at least one arm that contained IFNα compared with a non-biotherapy control arm. These controls were single agent medroxyprogesterone acetate (MPA), tamoxifen, or vinblastine. No clear effect on survival has been demonstrated for vinblastine,[16,23] or for MPA in the advanced or adjuvant settings,[24,25] although weak effects cannot be excluded. Although MPA has been sometimes regarded as equivalent to oral placebo,[18] it may cause significant adverse effects.[26] Studies that included both interleukin-2 as well as IFNα are considered later. There may be unpublished studies of IFNα versus control therapy and any resulting publication bias would be expected to exaggerate the benefits described below.

Four fully published survival studies of IFNα versus a non-biotherapy control were identified and included 631 patients (Table 30.3). The studies are somewhat heterogeneous in nature, but the clinical effects were consistent in direction. Complete or partial responses were seen more often in IFNα-treated patients compared with controls (40/317 [12·6%] *v* 5/314 [1·6%]; OR 7·5, 95% CI 3·0–18·9). The chance of death in the first year from randomisation was less for IFNα than for controls (OR 0·55, 95% CI 0·39–0·77). The weighted median survival gain was 3·3 months in favour of IFNα but the confidence interval cannot be reliably estimated. The survival experience for these studies was further examined by data extraction from published survival curves,[27] a technique that requires some assumptions regarding censoring.[19] The resulting hazard ratio over 2 years from randomisation for these four studies is 0·74 (95% CI 63–88) (Table 30.3; Figure 30.1).

The optimum subtype, route, dose, schedule and duration of IFNα has not been established. Comparative studies of interferon alfa subtype are not available but benefit has been associated with recombinant IFNα subtype 2a[28,29] and with subtype 2b,[30,31] as well as with administration by the subcutaneous or intramuscular routes. No information is available concerning the possible relationship of IFNα dose with survival. The dose–tumour response relationship of IFNα has been examined in four small prospective studies (Table 30.4). In three of these studies,[33–35] the dose of IFNα was the only variable. With large dose ratios of 3:1 or 10:1, there appears to be a weak dose–response effect if study homogeneity is assumed (Peto OR for response 3·70; 95%CI 1·17–11·67; *P* = 0·03). The fourth study[36] compared high dose intravenous with low dose subcutaneous IFNα and the lack of increased response in the high dose arm could be attributable to the intravenous route of administration.

An adequate duration of a trial of IFNα is important as response may not be seen until the third month of therapy.[30] The optimum duration of therapy in responders is unknown. In the MRC study,[31] therapy duration was nominally for 12 weeks but some patients continued beyond that. The other studies continued therapy until disease progression, patient intolerance, or to 12 months/ 3 months beyond complete remission.[29] This is an important issue since patients do not usually feel well on IFNα therapy at the doses of 8–18 MU used in the validating studies. The clinical significance of stable disease cannot be evaluated unless a baseline observation period preceded therapy.

Interferon alfa is generally very safe but has a substantial adverse effect on patient wellbeing during therapy. The main toxicity is a 'flu-like syndrome with fatigue, anorexia, fever and myalgia. The severity and duration of these symptoms vary substantially between patients from very mild to incapacitating, and therapy is usually better tolerated by patients with good initial performance status. The toxicity can be mitigated by bedtime administration, by prophylactic acetaminophen, and by use of a thrice weekly schedule which allows some recovery between doses whilst maintaining tachyphylaxis.[33] Toxicity is dose-dependent[34] but typically lessens during the first few weeks of therapy,[33] and is ameliorated by 50% dose reductions according to individual tolerance. Toxicity as well as interferon levels diminish in patients who develop interferon antibodies.[34]

Few studies have conducted formal quality-of-life assessment. The MRC trial[31] of IFNα versus MPA used the Rotterdam Symptom checklist and found multiple symptoms from IFNα at 4 weeks; anorexia was the main symptom persisting to the end of the 12 weeks of therapy, but no difference between arms persisted at 6 months. In the Motzer trial[37] of IFNα with or without 13-*cis*-retinoic acid discussed below, a specific instrument was developed, which supplemented the FACT tool[38] with 16 additional validated questions to assess toxicities characteristic of

**Table 30.3** Randomised studies comparing survival with interferon alfa therapy and a non-biotherapy control.

| Study | No. of patients | IFNα arm | v | Non-biotherapy arm | Stratified | Blinded review | Other assessment | OR-RR | OR-death 1 yr (95% CI) | HR (95% CI) |
|---|---|---|---|---|---|---|---|---|---|---|
| *IFNα v control* | | | | | | | | | | |
| Steineck[28] | 60 | IFNα 10#MU s.c. tiw | v | MPA | No | No | Pharm, Ab | 2·07 | 0·85 (0·28–2·61) | 1·05 (0·64–1·72) |
| MRC[31,32] | 335 | IFNα 10MU s.c. tiw | v | MPA | Yes | IMC | QoL | 8·79 | 0·64 (0·42–0·98) | 0·74 (0·60–0·92) |
| *Control ± IFNα* | | | | | | | | | | |
| Pyrhonen[29] | 160 | + IFNα 18MU s.c. tiw | v | VLB | No | Responses | Prog./pred. | 7·78 | 0·49 (0·26–0·93) | 0·65 (0·47–0·91) |
| *IFNα + other vs control* | | | | | | | | | | |
| Kriegmair[30] | 76 | IFNα 8MU i.m. tiw + VLB | v | MPA | No | No | Toxicity | 20·7 | 0·32 (0·12–0·86) | 0·67 (0·37–1·22) |
| *Total:* | 631 pts | | | | | | *Summary statistic:* | 7·48 | 0·55 (0·39–0·77) | 0·74 (0·63–0·88) |

Abbreviations: MPA, medroxyprogesterone acetate; VLB, vinblastine; Ab, anti-interferon antibodies; OR-RR, odds ratio for response; OR-Death1Yr, odds ratio for death by 1 year; HR, hazard ratio for death in first 2 years; IMC, independent monitoring committee; QoL, quality of life; Prog./pred., factors prognostic for survival and predictive of survival benefit; #, escalating dose to 50 MU;

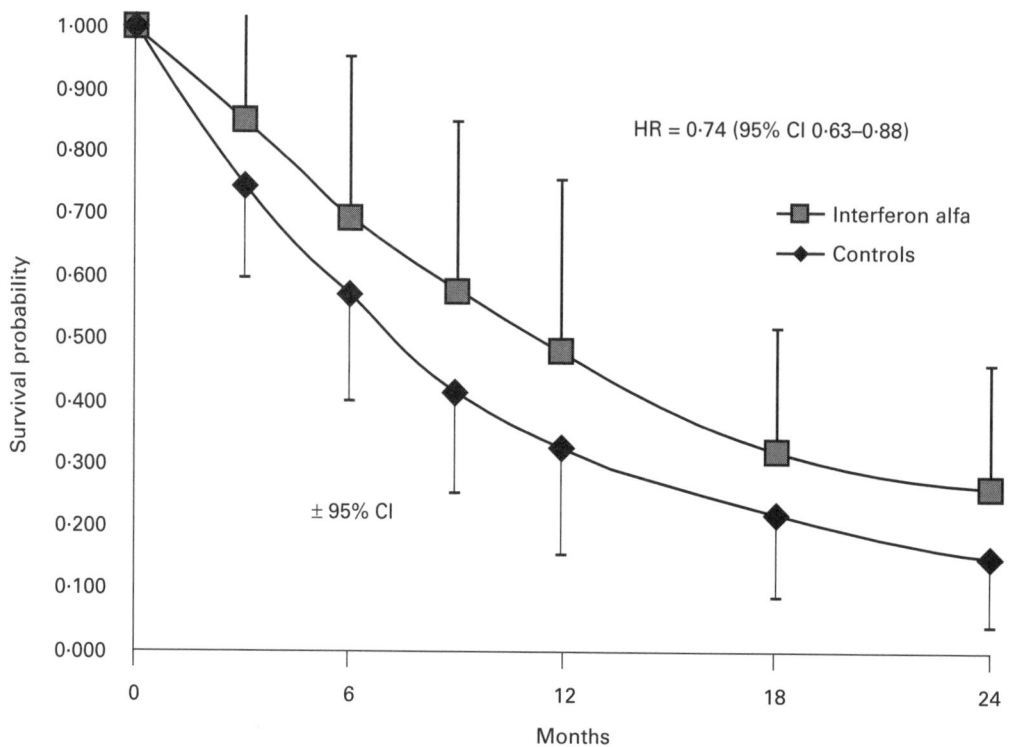

**Figure 30.1** Overall survival from Pamar[27] meta-analysis of four studies of interferon alfa versus non-biotherapy control

**Table 30.4   Interferon alfa dose–response studies**

| Study | IFNα | Route/schedule | Daily dose<br>Arm 1 v 2 | Responses CR+PR<br>Arm 1 v arm 2 | Peto odds ratio<br>Response rate<br>(95% CI) |
|---|---|---|---|---|---|
| *Same Route* | | | | | |
| Kirkwood[33] | Leucocyte | i.m. daily | 10 v 1 MU | 2/16 v 0/14 | 6·97 (0·41–117·8) |
| Quesada[34] | Recombinant 2a | i.m. daily | 20 v 2 MU | 4/15 v 0/15 | 9·31 (1·17–73·7) |
| Fujita[35] | Lymphoblastoid | i.m. daily | 3 v 1 MU | 5/16 v 3/15 | 1·77 (0·36–8·60) |
| | | | | *Summary statistic: | 3·70 (1·17–11·67) |
| *Different route* | | | | | |
| Muss[36] | Recombinant 2b | i.v. x 5 v s.c. tiw | 40 v 2 MU | 3/54 v 5/58 | 0·63 (0·15–2·65) |

*Peto odds ratio, a fixed effects model, has been used in view of the homogeneous nature of the first three trials. If a random effects model is used, the result is no longer statistically significant.

biotherapies. A summary score showed a marked decrease in physical and functional wellbeing for both study arms that persisted with minor recovery through 34 weeks and was worse for the retinoid arm and in patients with poor prognosis disease. However, this study used a more intensive IFNα regimen than the MRC study with daily treatment and dose escalation, and also continued therapy to disease progression or intolerance.

### Interferon-β (IFNβ) and interferon-γ (IFNγ)

IFNβ has been tested in a randomised trial of two dose levels: no remissions were seen.[39] IFNγ has been shown to be inactive in a well conducted double-blind placebo-controlled trial of 197 patients.[8] Remissions were seen in both arms and survival was very similar. Studies which have used IFNγ as a control may therefore be reasonably considered as equivalent to placebo-controlled though not blinded.[40]

**Table 30.5** **Examples of response rates from phase III and preceding phase ii studies.**

| | | | Response Rate (CR+PR) | |
|---|---|---|---|---|
| Intervention | Phase II Reference | Phase III Reference | Phase II | Phase III* |
| Interferon alfa | Quesada[59] | Coppin[19] (pooled) | 26% | 10% |
| IFNα + VLB | Fossa[60] | Neidhart[16] Fossa[23] | 33% | 13% |
| IFNα + ASA | Creagan[61] | Creagan[62] | 34% | 4% |
| Interferon-γ | Aulitsky[63] | Gleave[8] | 30% | 6% |
| HD-IL2 | Lotze[64] | Yang[65] McDermott[46] | 22% | 21% |
| HD-IL2 + LAK | Rosenberg[66] | Law[42] | 33% | 3% |
| IL2+ IFNa+5FU | Kirchner[50] | Negrier[49] | 33% | 15% |

*weighted average; VLB, vinblastine; ASA, aspirin; LAK, lymphokine activated killer cells

## High dose interleukin-2 (HD-IL2)

High dose interleukin-2 (HD-IL2) was developed in the mid 1980s.[41] Here we use the term "high dose" as the use of intravenous bolus IL2 at a dose of at least 600 000 U kg$^{-1}$ every 8 hours.[42] Phase II studies suggested that complete responses to HD-IL2 may sometimes be durable. On this basis, the US Federal Drug Administration licensed HD-IL2 and this remains the sole FDA-indicated biotherapy for advanced renal cell carcinoma in the USA. Updated results from combined US phase II trials of HD-IL2 in 255 patients found 14 (5·5%) still to be in continuous remission for a median of 90+ months.[43] Complete responders often relapse at previously uninvolved sites.[44] Although the high dose treatment is exceptionally toxic[45] owing primarily to capillary leak syndrome, treatment-related mortality is now very low in experienced hands.[41] Our previously published systematic review[19] failed to identify any randomised controlled trials of HD-IL2 that reported a survival outcome by intention to treat. The Cytokine Working Group has recently reported their preliminary results for HD-IL2 versus subcutaneous IL2 plus IFNα in 193 patients.[46] The response rate for HD-IL2 was 25% versus 12% for subcutaneous combination biotherapy, and the median survival was 10 months versus 7 months respectively. Further results are awaited with interest, especially concerning the durability of remissions.

## Reduced dose IL2 regimens

Because of the toxicity of HD-IL2, several investigators have evaluated lower dose IL2 schedules given by an intravenous or subcutaneous route. No randomised controlled trials of such reduced dose IL2 programs versus a non-biotherapy control have been identified. However one large[47] and one small[48] randomised study compared subcutaneous or intramuscular IFNα with reduced dose IL2 given by continuous intravenous infusion. Both studies found greater toxicity with IL2 but without better response or survival than with IFNα. In the CRECY study, two-thirds

of IL2 patients experienced hypotension resistant to vasopressor agents.[47]

## Combination biotherapy/non-biotherapy programmes

Most attempts to improve the efficacy of IFNα and of IL2 regimens with a variety of combinations and enhancers have been disappointing with little evidence of clinical or statistical benefit.[19] Only exceptions to this negative conclusion are discussed here as well as studies reported since our previous review. A large phase III trial[37] of IFNα with or without oral 13-*cis*-retinoic acid found a trend to improved response rate for the combination arm (12% v 6%, P = 0·14) but inferior quality of life by formal assessment; survival was the same overall, but there is a tantalising divergence in the later progression-free and overall survival curves, which will be statistically weak even with additional follow up. The combination of modified schedule IL2 plus IFNα has been compared with either agent alone in two three arm studies mentioned above.[47,48] Assuming study homogeneity, the combination showed a trend to a greater chance of response (17% v 8%; Peto OR 2·48; 95%CI 1·37–4·5) but there was no difference in survival.[19] Toxicity was greater in the combined biotherapy arm. This information will be relevant to the interpretation of the HD-IL2 versus IL2/IFNα study.[46] A substantial phase III study[49] of the addition of 5-fluorouracil chemotherapy to combined biotherapy with IL2 and IFNα has failed to confirm encouraging expectations.[50]

## Autolymphocyte therapy

In 1990, Osband and colleagues reported a randomised controlled unblinded study with better survival and quality of life for autolymphocyte therapy plus oral cimetidine compared with oral cimetidine alone in 90 patients with advanced renal cell carcinoma.[51] Mononuclear cells were harvested from patients and then incubated with a mitogen, stored, and reinfused monthly for 6 months. Toxicity was quite mild. Subsequent publications have updated the outcome of the experimental arm but not the control arm. An independent replication of these results is needed.

### Predictive factors for biotherapy benefit

Given the low frequency of response and the toxicity of a trial of biotherapy for advanced renal cell carcinoma, factors are needed that could define patient groups much more or less likely to benefit than average. We use the term predictive factor in relation to treatment benefit as distinct from prognostic factors associated with the natural history of the disease. Limited information is available regarding factors predictive for survival gain from biotherapy. In the Pyrhonen study[29] of IFN$\alpha$, there was an association between factors prognostic for an adverse survival outcome and those factors predicting for better survival improvement with IFN$\alpha$, especially age over 60 years, high sedimentation rate, and male gender. In other words, IFN$\alpha$ tended to neutralise the adverse association of these prognostic factors, a somewhat unexpected observation that should be regarded as a hypothesis requiring validation. For IL2 therapy, candidate factors include favourable survival associated with development of thyroid antibodies,[52] increased response rate with treatment-related thrombocytopenia,[53] and lack of response in patients with regional node involvement.[54] With regard to response status from prior biotherapy, repeat treatment with HD-IL2 or crossover between IFN$\alpha$ and IL2 are rarely useful.[44,55] Another predictive factor deserving further investigation is erythropoietin production[56] for which haemoglobin level might be a surrogate (Oliver RTD, personal communication, 2000).

### Non-randomised versus randomised trial results

The concept[57] that observational studies tend to exaggerate intervention effects has been challenged[58] for several types of medical interventions reported since 1984. We have conducted a preliminary survey of this question in the context of biotherapy for advanced renal cell carcinoma. For a range of biotherapies, response rates from phase III studies were compared with the response rates from the corresponding early phase II study (Table 30.5). Except for HD-IL2 monotherapy, the response rates were generally much lower in the phase III setting. Potential explanations include differences in the patients, differences in the treatment, and differences in the setting.[67] At this point, phase II results in this condition should be regarded with the usual caution.

### Nephrectomy in advanced renal cell carcinoma

In patients found to have metastases at the time of diagnosis of a technically operable primary kidney cancer, the question of palliative or cytoreductive nephrectomy arises. Until recently, the answer to this question has been largely a matter of opinion and case selection.[68] The preliminary results of two identical randomised trials were recently published.[69,70] These studies examined the role of initial cytoreductive nephrectomy prior to IFN$\alpha$ 5 MU/m$^{-2}$ three times a week for metastases in patients with very good performance status. A statistically significant improvement in overall survival for the nephrectomy arm was seen in both the larger study conducted by the Southwest Oncology Group (median survival 11·1 $v$ 8·1 months, $P = 0.05$, stratified log-rank test) and the smaller EORTC study (median survival 17 $v$ 7 months, log-rank $P = 0.04$). The median survival benefit weighted by study size is 4·8 months. An excellent critique of these studies is available,[71] and concludes that it is now appropriate to recommend nephrectomy before IFN$\alpha$ as an option for selected patients with metastatic renal cancer and high performance status.

### Adjuvant therapy of renal cell carcinoma

At least 10 published randomised trials of adjuvant therapy have attempted to improve outcome following nephrectomy for clinically localised renal cell carcinoma. No published systematic review is available. Interventions have included preoperative radiotherapy,[72] postoperative radiotherapy,[73] medroxyprogesterone acetate,[26] autologous tumour cells,[74,75] keyhole limpet haemocyanin,[76] or interferon alfa,[24,25,77] all with essentially negative results. In addition, autolymphocyte therapy has been used with encouraging preliminary results[78] and a full report is awaited with interest.

### Conclusions

- Advanced renal cell carcinoma is a condition in which the natural history of the disease is very variable and a small proportion of study patients, perhaps 5%, survive 5 years or more. Prognostic factors, especially patient performance status, are powerful compared to therapy. A period of observation is appropriate in patients with minimal symptoms and can provide useful information on the natural history of disease in the individual patient for determining the timing and impact of any subsequent therapy **Evidence level III, Grade B**.
- Remission rates with a variety of interventions have generally been much lower in randomised trials following encouraging results in prospective non-randomised case series (Table 30.5). Patient selection is likely to be the main reason for this observation. Consequently, randomised controlled trials must be considered the required standard of evidence **Evidence level IV, Grade C**.

- Randomised trials of IFNα therapy have consistently shown a greater chance of remission and of 1-year survival compared to oral hormone therapy or when added to intravenous vinblastine (see Table 30.3)[19] **Evidence level Ia, Grade A** . The optimal dose and schedule of recombinant IFNα have not been defined. The current best evidence suggests giving IFNα three times weekly by the subcutaneous route at a target dose of 8–18 MU **Evidence level Ib, Grade A** . Downward adjustment of dose according to individual tolerance is a good principle of palliative therapy rather than a matter of evidence, although toxicity often decreases with time alone. Based on weak evidence, the dose–response slope for IFNα appears relatively flat; dose–survival data is not available. The optimal duration of therapy is unknown but delayed response may be seen so that 3 months of therapy has been regarded a reasonable trial of IFNα therapy in patients with stable disease **Evidence level IV, Grade C** . The addition to IFNα of interleukin-2 or 13-*cis*-retinoic acid may increase the chance of remission, but these agents increase toxicity and have not been shown to improve survival. However, initial cytoreductive nephrectomy prior to IFNα is an option for patients with very good performance status with metastases at diagnosis since this procedure has reproducibly resulted in longer survival **Evidence level Ib, Grade A** . The preponderance of evidence supports a statistically significant benefit of IFNα but because of adverse effects, the clinical utility remains debatable.[71] It is still possible that clinical benefits credited to IFNα are actually due to detrimental effects of inadequately studied control therapies but the consistency of effect provides some reassurance in this regard. Not surprisingly at this level of efficacy, IFNα given adjuvantly after nephrectomy does not improve survival **Evidence level Ib, Grade A** .

- Claims of efficacy of high dose interleukin-2 (HD-IL2) have been based primarily on non-randomised trials. Durable complete remissions have been observed infrequently **Evidence level IIa, Grade B** . In a recent preliminary report[46] of a randomised study of HD-IL2 versus low dose IL2 and IFNα, a higher response rate and longer median survival was seen with the high dose arm. Given the toxicity and potential for treatment-related mortality with HD-IL2, the durability of remissions will be crucial and applicability confined to the fittest patients. The use of moderate to low doses of IL2 yields similar survival to IFNα but with greater toxicity and cannot be recommended **Evidence level Ib, Grade A** .

- In considering the validity of these results, available randomised trials are mostly unblinded and small (average 39 patients per arm), limiting the strength of the conclusions to be drawn. The conclusions of this meta-analysis of published reports are weak compared to a meta-analysis based on individual patient data (IPD). In addition, IPD would potentially identify factors predictive of intervention benefit.

- The applicability of clinical trials results is limited by patient selection, especially with more toxic therapies. For example in the CRECY trial which included moderate dose IL-2, only four of every 19 referred patients were actually enrolled.[49] It should not be assumed that any benefits of therapy demonstrated in a high performance status patient population may be extrapolated to other patient subsets.

- A reinterpretation of these conclusions is presented in Chapter 4.

## Case scenarios

### Case 1

*A 66-year-old man presented in April 1997 with gross painless haematuria. Ultrasound revealed a mass in the right kidney. Nephrectomy showed an 18 cm clear cell carcinoma invading perinephric fat and renal vein, classified as Fuhrman grade IV, stage pT3b.*

Q1.1  What is risk of relapse over five years?

A1.1  70–75% using a published nomogram.[12]

Q1.2  What can be done to reduce this risk?

A1.2  There is no adjuvant therapy of proven benefit.

Q1.3  Is there evidence to support survival benefit from screening for asymptomatic relapse?

A1.3  No evidence is available.

Nine months after nephrectomy, he underwent routine abdominal ultrasound to check the contralateral kidney for a potential second primary. This unexpectedly showed numerous liver metastases up to 9 cm in diameter. He had lost 7 kg over 6 months but was normally active with effort (KPS 80%). Blood showed Hb 94 g litre$^{-1}$ (N ≥ 135), creatinine 267 μ mol litre$^{-1}$ (N ≤ 130), γGT 90 U litre$^{-1}$ (N ≤ 49), LDH 421 U litre$^{-1}$ (N ≤ 415), calcium 2·63 mmol litre$^{-1}$ (N ≤ 2·60). Small lung metastases were observed on chest *x* ray.

Q1.4  What is the prognosis in terms of median and two 2-year survival?

A1.4  With two risk factors (low haemoglobin and high calcium), approximate median survival in clinical trials without cytokine therapy is 7 months and 2-year survival 10%.[13,17]

Q1.5  What proven impact can treatment make to these figures?

A1.5 Interferon alfa is associated with improved median survival by 4 months based on meta-analysis of four randomised clinical trials (Figure 30.1). Two-year survival increases from 11% to 20%. Liver metastasis is an adverse prognostic factor for both survival without interferon and for interferon benefit.[29]

A short period of observation was recommended. Unknown to his physicians, he began taking milk thistle as recommended for liver disease by his grandfather, a German faith healer who trained under Father Kneip. The patient's wife became distressed and obtained a second opinion, after which interferon alfa 5 MU s.c. three times weekly was initiated. After 2 months of interferon, he was anorexic with 5 kg weight loss and rising γGT, but typical interferon toxicity such as fluctuating fatigue and fever were not noted. Cancer cachexia was suspected but at 3 months the liver ultrasound was still unchanged. In the absence of a baseline growth rate, it was unclear if interferon was changing the course of the disease. After 4 months of interferon, he had lost a further 4 kg in weight, Hb was 78, LFTs showed minor deterioration, and one lung lesion was slightly larger; interferon was continued mainly because of lack of alternatives. Therapy was completed at 6 months according to local practice.

Q1.6 Are there firm data to indicate how long interferon alfa therapy should be continued (a) in the absence of response, and (b) in the event of response?

A1.6 No. Most studies have treated to disease progression or patient refusal. Responses may be delayed several months. One study[31] treated for only 12 weeks with similar results to the other trials.

Re-evaluation was carried out shortly after completion of therapy and periodically thereafter. The patient's anorexia cleared soon after discontinuing interferon and lost weight was regained. Hb and LFTs returned to normal. Serial abdominal ultrasounds showed progressive decrease in size and number of metastases. Complete hepatic remission was reached in August 2000 and continues. The chest *x* ray shows a small residual opacity (technical partial remission). No further treatment has been given since October 1998 and he remains well over 3 years later, enjoying travel and fishing trips. His wife developed metastatic cancer and died rapidly in 1999, a sad reversal of fortune.

Q1.7 What is his prognosis now?

A1.7 There are no long-term data for IFNα trials and durable remissions are anecdotal. About 10% of patients treated on various cytokine protocols experience prolonged survival.[17]

Q1.8 To what do you attribute his exceptional outcome?

A1.8 Possible reasons include spontaneous remission, a very high proportion of interferon sensitive cells, unusual host–interferon synergy, or use of alternative therapies. After 3 months of interferon, this patient thought he was dying of cancer but one day he awoke with an inner determination to fight and believes this was the turning point. His anorexia responded to marijuana.

### Case 2

*A 56-year-old man presented with a 5-week history of left flank pain, weight loss and dyspnoea. Imaging showed a renal mass and multiple lung metastases. After 2 weeks, the lung lesions had tripled in size. He died 1 week later.*

### Case 3

*A 76-year-old man presented with a mild but persistent cough. Chest x ray showed numerous round opacities up to 2·5 cm in both lungs typical of metastases. CT chest also showed moderate mediastinal lymphadenopathy. Abdominal ultrasound and CT scan demonstrated a 12 cm mass in the left kidney and a 4 cm pre-aortic mass. A radiologic diagnosis of metastatic kidney cancer was made. He was completely asymptomatic apart from mild cough, playing a full round of golf three times a week with a low and improving golf handicap. Hb was 117 (N ³ 135), chemistry was normal.*

Q3.1 Is a histologic diagnosis mandatory?

A3.1 No histologic confirmation has been obtained in this patient. A biopsy would commonly be recommended, reasons including participation in a clinical trial, and local pattern of practice for medicolegal or other reasons. Risks include bleeding, pneumothorax and seeding of the needle track.

Q3.2 What is the prognosis?

A3.2 Two risk factors are present (anaemia, no nephrectomy) (see A1.3).

Q3.3 Is there data on which to base a recommendation on the timing of any therapy?

A3.3 No, except that performance status should not be permitted to decline and delay would be unwise in patients with paraneoplastic syndromes. A common pattern of practice is immediate biopsy, staging and treatment. Observation has the advantage of establishing a baseline for refining prognosis, and especially to estimate the duration of cytokine therapy before disease progression could be expected in non-responders.

He agreed to a period of observation. After 6 months, there was a slight increase in size of the lung metastases. A follow up CT scan showed the abdominal disease to be unchanged. He remained in excellent health with negligible symptoms and was referred to a urologist for an opinion concerning debulking nephrectomy prior to interferon. A case conference was convened.

Q3.4 What therapy options are available and what are the advantages and disadvantages of each?

A3.4 The main considerations in a good performance status patient are debulking nephrectomy and/or a trial of cytokine therapy. Nephrectomy may be associated with usual operative risks especially in locally advanced disease. Interleukin-2 may result in fatal toxicity in inexperienced hands. Interferon alfa is generally safe but carries chronic morbidity, especially fatigue.

Q3.5 On what basis would you make the decision if you were the patient and which option would you choose?

A3.5 The decision is very personal and depends considerably on the manner of presentation of information. The main factors in fit patients are non-medical and depend on philosophic state of mind and on the relative weight given to immediate health versus toxicity, and to medium- versus long-term outcomes. Cost is also a consideration. After extensive discussion, this patient has declined therapy and remains well.

## Commentary

Clinical trials statistics are good at describing average outcomes, but exceptional outcomes are better illustrated by case scenarios. The first case illustrates a point further elaborated by the personal experience of Stephen Jay Gould, Harvard palaeontologist and popular science writer.[79] The second case is at the other end of the scale and such a patient would not be a participant in a clinical trial. Case 3 illustrates the importance of exploring the values of the individual patient when making decisions about non-curative treatments.

## References

1 Vogelzang NJ, Stadler WM. Kidney cancer. *Lancet* 1998;**352**:1691–6.
2 Bukowski RM, Novick AC, eds. *Renal cell carcinoma: molecular biology, immunology, and clinical management.* Totowa NJ: Humana Press, 2000.
3 Motzer RJ, ed. Renal cell carcinoma. *Semin Oncol* 2000;**27**(2).
4 Greenlee RT, Hill-Harmon MB, Murray T, Thun M. Cancer statistics, 2001. *CA Cancer J Clin* 2001;**51**:15–36.
5 Itano NB, Blute ML, Spotts B, Zincke H. Outcome of isolated renal cell carcinoma fossa recurrence after nephrectomy. *J Urol* 2000;**164**:322–5.
6 Papac RJ, Poo-Hwu W-J. Renal cell carcinoma: a paradigm of Lanthanic disease. *Am J Clin Oncol* 1999;**22**:223–31.
7 Oliver RTD, Nethersell ABW, Bottomley JM. Unexplained spontaneous regression and alpha-interferon as treatment for metastatic renal carcinoma. *Br J Urol* 1989;**63**:128–31.
8 Gleave ME, Elhilali M, Fradet Y *et al.* Interferon gamma-1b compared with placebo in metastatic renal-cell carcinoma. *N Engl J Med* 1998;**338**:1265–71.
9 Elhilali MM, Gleave M, Fradet Y *et al.* Placebo-associated remissions in a multicentre, randomised, double-blind trial of interferon γ-1b for the treatment of metastatic renal cell carcinoma. *BJU Int* 2000;**86**:613–18.
10 Tsui K-H, Shvarts O, Smith RB, Figlin RA, deKernion JB, Belldegrun A. Prognostic indicators for renal cell carcinoma: a multivariate analysis of 643 patients using the revised 1997 TNM staging criteria. *J Urol* 2000;**163**:1090–5.
11 Zisman A, Pantuck AJ, Weider J *et al.* Risk group assessment and clinical outcome algorithm to predict natural history of patients with surgically resected renal cell carcinoma. *J Clin Oncol* 2001;**20**:4559–66.
12 Kattan MW, Reuter V, Motzer RJ, Katz J, Russo P. A postoperative prognostic nomogram for renal cell carcinoma. *J Urol* 2001;**166**:63–7.
13 Motzer RJ, Mazumdar M, Bacik J, Berg W, Amsterdam A, Ferrara J. Survival and prognostic stratification of 670 patients with advanced renal cell carcinoma. *J Clin Oncol* 1999;**17**:2530–40.
14 Dinney CPN, Slaton JW, Perroutte PC, Ellerhorst J, Swanson DA. The effect of organ site on survival after resection of a solitary renal cell carcinoma metastasis. *J Urol* 1999;**161**(4 Suppl.):A737.
15 Witte RS, Leong T, Ernstoff MS *et al.* A phase II study of interleukin-2 with and without beta-interferon in the treatment of advanced renal cell carcinoma. *Invest New Drugs* 1995;**13**:241–7.
16 Neidhart JA, Anderson SA, Harris JE *et al.* Vinblastine fails to improve response of renal cancer to interferon alfa-n1: high response rate in patients with pulmonary metastases. *J Clin Oncol* 1991;**9**:832–6.
17 Motzer RJ, Mazumdar M, Bacik J, Russo P, Berg WJ, Metz EM. Effect of cytokine therapy on survival for patients with advanced renal cell carcinoma. *J Clin Oncol* 2000;**18**:1928–35.
18 Hernberg N, Pyrhonen S, Muhonen T. Regimens with or without interferon-α as treatment for metastatic melanoma and renal cell carcinoma: an overview of randomised trials. *J Immunother* 1999;**22**:145–54.
19 Coppin C, Porzsolt F, Kumpf J, Coldman A, Wilt T. Immunotherapy for advanced renal cell cancer. In: *Cochrane Library*, Issue 3. Oxford: Update Software, 2000.
20 Devereaux PJ, Manns BJ, Ghali WA *et al.* Physician interpretations and textbook definitions of blinding terminology in randomised controlled trials. *JAMA* 2001;**285**:2000–3.
21 Thiesse P, Ollivier L, Di Stefano-Louineau D *et al.* Response rate accuracy in oncology trials: reasons for interobserver variability. *J Clin Oncol* 1997;**15**:3507–14.
22 Kirkwood JM, Ernstoff MS. Interferons in the treatment of human cancer. *J Clin Oncol* 1984;**2**:336–52.
23 Fossa SD, Martinelli G, Otto U *et al.* Recombinant interferon alfa-2a with or without vinblastine in metastatic renal cell carcinoma: results of a European multi-center phase III study. *Ann Oncol* 1992;**3**:301–5.
24 Porzsolt F. Adjuvant therapy of renal cell cancer with interferon alpha-2a. *Proc Ann Meet Am Soc Clin Oncol* 1992;**11**:A622.
25 Pizzocaro G, Piva L, Colavita M *et al.* Interferon adjuvant to radical nephrectomy in Robson stages II and III renal cell carcinoma: a multicentric randomised study. *J Clin Oncol* 2001;**19**:425–31.
26 Pizzocaro G, Piva L, Di Fronzo G *et al.* Adjuvant medroxyprogesterone acetate to radical nephrectomy in renal cancer: 5-year results of a prospective randomised study. *J Urol* 1987;**138**:1379–81.
27 Parmar MKB, Torri V, Stewart L. Extracting summary statistics to perform meta-analyses of the published literature for survival endpoints. *Stat Med* 1998;**17**:2815–34.
28 Steineck G, Strander H, Carbin B-E *et al.* Recombinant leukocyte interferon alpha-2a and medroxyprogesterone in advanced renal cell carcinoma. A randomised trial. *Acta Oncol* 1990;**29**:155–62.

29  Pyrhonen S, Salminen E, Ruutu M *et al.* Prospective randomised trial of interferon alfa-2a plus vinblastine versus vinblastine alone in patients with advanced renal cell cancer. *J Clin Oncol* 1999;**17**:2859–67.

30  Kriegmair M, Oberneder R, Hofstetter A. Interferon alfa and vinblastine versus medroxyprogesterone acetate in the treatment of metastatic renal cell carcinoma. *Urology* 1995;**45**:758–62.

31  Medical Research Council Renal Cancer Collaborators. Interferon-α and survival in metastatic renal cell carcinoma: early results of a randomised controlled trial. *Lancet* 1999;**353**:14–17.

32  Hancock B, Griffiths G, Ritchie A *et al.* Updated results of the MRC randomised controlled trial of alpha interferon vs MPA in patients with metastatic renal carcinoma. *Proc Ann Meet Am Soc Clin Oncol* 2000;**19**:A1336.

33  Kirkwood JM, Harris JE, Vera R *et al.* A randomised study of low and high dose of leucocyte α-interferon in metastatic renal cell carcinoma: the American Cancer Society collaborative trial. *Cancer Res* 1985;**45**:863–71.

34  Quesada JR, Rios A, Swanson D, Trown P, Gutterman JU. Antitumor activity of recombinant-derived interferon alpha in metastatic renal cell carcinoma. *J Clin Oncol* 1985;**3**:1522–8.

35  Fujita T, Inagaki J, Asano H *et al.* Effects of low-dose interferon-alpha (HLBL) following nephrectomy in metastatic renal cell carcinoma. *Proc Ann Meet Am Soc Clin Oncol* 1992;**11**:A685.

36  Muss HB, Costanzi JJ, Leavitt R *et al.* Recombinant alfa interferon in renal cell carcinoma: a randomised trial of two routes of administration. *J Clin Oncol* 1987;**5**:286–91.

37  Motzer RJ, Murphy BA, Bacik J *et al.* Phase III trial of interferon alfa-2a with or without 13-cis-retinoic acid for patients with advanced renal cell carcinoma. *J Clin Oncol* 2000;**18**:2972–80.

38  Cella DF, Tulsky DS, Gray G *et al.* The Functional Assessment of Cancer Therapy scale: development and validation of the general measure. *J Clin Oncol* 1993;**11**:570–9.

39  Borden EC, Rinehart JJ, Storer BE, Trump DL, Paulnock DM, Teitlbaum AP. Biological and clinical effects of interferon-β_{ser} at two doses. *J Interferon Res* 1990;**10**:559–70.

40  Lummen G, Goepel M, Mollhoff S, Hinke A, Otto T, Rubben H. Phase II study of interferon-γ versus interleukin-2 and interferon-α2b in metastatic renal cell carcinoma. *J Urol* 1996;**155**:455–8.

41  Rosenberg SA. Interleukin-2 and the development of immunotherapy for the treatment of patients with cancer. *Cancer J Sci Am* 2000;**6**(Suppl. 1):S2–S7.

42  Law TM, Motzer RJ, Mazumdar M *et al.* Phase III randomised trial of interleukin-2 with or without lymphokine-activated killer cells in the treatment of patients with advanced renal cell carcinoma. *Cancer* 1995;**76**:824–32.

43  Fisher RI, Rosenberg SA, Fyfe G. Long-term survival update for high-dose recombinant interleukin-2 in patients with renal cell carcinoma. *Cancer J Sci Am* 2000;**6**(Suppl.1):S55–S57.

44  Lee DS, White DE, Hurst R, Rosenberg SA, Yang JC. Patterns of relapse and response to retreatment in patients with metastatic melanoma or renal cell carcinoma who responded to interleukin-2-based immunotherapy. *Cancer J Sci Am* 1998;**4**:86–93.

45  Siegal JP, Puri RK. Interleukin-2 toxicity. *J Clin Oncol* 1991;**9**:694–704.

46  McDermott D, Flaherty L, Clark J *et al.* A randomised Phase III trial of high-dose interleukin-2 versus subcutaneous Il2/interferon in patients with metastatic renal cell carcinoma. *Proc Ann Meet Am Soc Clin Oncol* 2001;**20**:A685.

47  Negrier S, Escudier B, Lasset C *et al.* Recombinant human interleukin-2, recombinant human interferon alfa-2a, or both in metastatic renal-cell carcinoma. *N Engl J Med* 1998;**338**:1272–8.

48  Boccardo F, Rubagotti A, Canobbio L *et al.* Interleukin-2, interferon-α and interleukin-2 plus interferon-α in renal cell carcinoma. A randomized Phase 2 trial. *Tumori* 1998;**84**:534–9.

49  Negrier S, Caty A, Lesimple T *et al.* Treatment of patients with metastatic renal carcinoma with a combination of subcutaneous interleukin-2 and interferon alfa with or without fluorouracil. *J Clin Oncol* 2000;**18**:4009–15.

50  Kirchner H, Buer J, Probst-Kepper M *et al.* Risk and long-term outcome in metastatic renal cell carcinoma patients receiving sc interleukin-2, sc interferon-alfa2a and iv 5-fluorouracil. *Proc Ann Meet Am Soc Clin Oncol* 1998;**17**:A1195.

51  Osband ME, Lavin PT, Babayan RK *et al.* Effect of autolymphocyte therapy on survival and quality of life in patients with metastatic renal-cell carcinoma. *Lancet* 1990;**335**:994–8.

52  Franzke A, Peest D, Probst-Kepper M *et al.* Autoimmunity resulting from cytokine treatment predicts long-term survival in patients with metastatic renal cell cancer. *J Clin Oncol* 1999;**17**:529–33.

53  Royal RE, Steinberg SM, Krouse RS *et al.* Correlates of response to IL-2 therapy in patients treated for metastatic renal cancer and melanoma. *Cancer J Sci Am* 1996;**2**:91–8.

54  Pantuck AJ, Zisman A, Chao D *et al.* Regional lymphadenopathy during cytoreductive nephrectomy predicts IL-2 failure in patients with metastatic renal cell cancer. *Proc Ann Meet Am Soc Clin Oncol* 2001;**20**:A686.

55  Escudier B, Chevreau C, Lasset C *et al.* Cytokines in metastatic renal cell carcinoma: is it useful to switch to interleukin-2 or interferon after failure of a first treatment? *J Clin Oncol* 1999;**17**:2039–43.

56  Janik JE, Sznol M, Urba WJ *et al.* Erythropoietin production. A potential marker for interleukin-2/interferon-responsive tumors. *Cancer* 1993;**72**:2656–9.

57  Kunz R, Oxman AD. The unpredictability paradox: review of empirical comparisons of randomised and non-randomised clinical trials. *BMJ* 1998;**317**:1185–90.

58  Benson K, Hartz AJ. A comparison of observational studies and randomised, controlled trials. *N Engl J Med* 2000;**342**:1878–86.

59  Quesada JR, Swanson DA, Gutterman JU. Phase II study of interferon alpha in metastatic renal-cell carcinoma: a progress report. *J Clin Oncol* 1985;**3**:1086–92.

60  Fossa SD, de Garis ST, Heier MS *et al.* Recombinant interferon alfa-2a with or without vinblastine in metastatic renal cell carcinoma. *Cancer* 1986;**57**:1700–4.

61  Creagan ET, Buckner JC, Hahn RG, Richardson RR, Schaid DJ, Kovach JS. An evaluation of recombinant leukocyte A interferon with aspirin in patients with metastatic renal cell cancer. *Cancer* 1988;**61**:1787–91.

62  Creagan ET, Twito DI, Johansson SL *et al.* A randomised prospective assessment of recombinant leukocyte A human interferon with or without aspirin in advanced renal adenocarcinoma. *J Clin Oncol* 1991;**9**:2104–9.

63  Aulitzky W, Gastl G, Aulitzky WE *et al.* Successful treatment of metastatic renal cell carcinoma with a biologically active dose of recombinant interferon-gamma. *J Clin Oncol* 1989;**7**:1875–84.

64  Lotze MT, Chang AE, Seipp CA, Simpson C, Vetto JT, Rosenberg SA. High-dose recombinant interleukin 2 in the treatment of patients with disseminated cancer. Responses, treatment-related morbidity, and histologic findings. *JAMA* 1986;**256**:3117–24.

65  Yang JC, Rosenberg SA. An ongoing prospective randomised comparison of interleukin-2 regimens for the treatment of metastatic renal cell cancer. *Cancer J Sci Am* 1997;**3**:S79–S84.

66  Rosenberg SA, Lotze MT, Muul LM *et al.* A progress report on the treatment of 157 patients with advanced cancer using lymphokine-activated killer cells and interleukin-2 or high-dose interleukin-2 alone. *N Engl J Med* 1987;**316**:889–97.

67  Porzsolt F. Kumpf J, Coppin C, Pöppel E. Stringent application of epidemiologic criteria changes the interpretation of the effects of immunotherapy in advanced renal cell cancer. In *Evidence-based Oncology*. Williams C, ed. London: BMJ Books, 2003.

68  Sawczuk IS, Pollard JC. Renal cell carcinoma: should radical nephrectomy be performed in the presence of metastatic disease? *Curr Opin Urol* 1999;**9**:377–381.

69  Flanigan RC, Salmon S, Blumenstein BA, *et al.* Nephrectomy followed by interferon alfa-2b compared with interferon alfa-2b alone for metastatic renal-cell cancer. *N Engl J Med* 2001;**345**:1655–9.

70  Mickisch GH, Garin A, van Poppel H *et al.* Radical nephrectomy plus interferon-alfa-based immunotherapy compared with interferon alfa alone in metastatic renal-cell carcinoma: a randomized trial. *Lancet* 2001;**358**:966–70.

71  Tannock IF. Commentary on "cytoreduction nephrectomy in metastatic renal cancer: the results of Southwest Oncology Group trial 8949". *J Clin Oncol* 2000;**18**(21 Suppl.):39S–42S.

72  Juusula H, Malmio K, Alfthan O *et al.* Preoperative irradiation in the treatment of renal adenocarcinoma. *Scand J Urol Nephrol* 1977;**11**:277–81.

73  Kjaer M, Iversen P, Hvidt V *et al.* A randomised trial of postoperative radiotherapy versus observation in stage II and III renal adenocarcinoma. A study by the Copenhagen Renal Cancer Study Group. *Scand J Urol Nephrol* 1987;**21**:285–9.

74  Galligioni E, Quaia M, Merlo A *et al.* Adjuvant immunotherapy treatment of renal carcinoma patients with autologous tumor cells and Bacillus Calmette-Guerin. *Cancer* 1996;**77**:2560–6.

75  Adler A, Gillon G, Lurie H *et al.* Active specific immunotherapy of renal cell carcinoma patients: a prospective randomised study of hormono-immuno- versus hormonotherapy. Preliminary report of immunological and clinical aspects. *J Biol Response Mod* 1987;**6**:610–24.

76  Jurincic-Winkler CD, Horlbeck R, von der Kammer H, Scheit KH, Klippel KF. Adjuvant immunotherapy with keyhole limpet hemocyanin in category pT2 N+ and pT3–4, N0-N+, M0 renal cell carcinoma. *Wien Klin Wochenschr* 1994;**106**:455–8.

77  Trump DL, Elson P, Propert K *et al.* Randomised, controlled trial of adjuvant therapy with lymphoblastoid interferon in resected, high-risk renal cell carcinoma. *Proc Ann Meet Am Soc Clin Oncol* 1996;**15**:A648.

78  Sawczuk IS, Graham SD Jr, Miesowicz F, and the ALT Adjuvant Study Group. Randomised, controlled trial of adjuvant therapy with ex vivo activated T cells (ALT) in T1–3a,b,c or T4N+, M0 renal cell carcinoma. *Proc Ann Meet Am Soc Clin Oncol* 1997;**16**:A1163.

79  Gould SJ. The median isn't the message. [http://cancerguide.org/median_not_msg.html]

# 31 Cancer of the bladder

*Mike Shelley, Howard Kynaston, Trevor Roberts, Jim Barber*

Over 11 000 new cases of bladder cancer are diagnosed each year in England and Wales with an incidence of 33 per 100 000 for men and 13 per 100 000 for women.[1] Cancer of the urinary bladder accounts for approximately 2% of all malignant disease and is the fourth most common cancer in men and the ninth in women. Approximately 60–80% of newly diagnosed cases are non-invasive (superficial) confined to the mucosa (Ta tumours) or lamina propria (T1 tumours). Treatment for this category of patients aims to reduce tumour recurrence within the bladder and prevent progression to a more advanced stage of disease. About 20% of patients will present with tumours that have invaded the muscle layer and beyond the bladder (T3–T4 tumours) and these have a poorer prognosis than early stage tumours. Superficial tumours can also progress to invasive tumours. The goal of therapy is to decide which bladders should receive radical radiotherapy with salvage cystectomy for relapse, and which bladders need to be removed surgically (cystectomy).

It is uncommon to diagnose bladder cancer in men or women below the age of 40 and since the average age is over 60 years, management may be complicated by treatment for comorbidities. The most common symptom of bladder cancer is haematuria, although urinary frequency is sometimes present as a consequence of irritation or reduced bladder capacity. Patients with suspected bladder tumours undergo cystoscopy and transurethral resection (TUR) to confirm diagnosis and if possible, completely excise the tumour. Treatment options then consist of instillation of agents directly into the bladder for superficial disease (intravesical therapy), and surgery, radiotherapy, or systemic chemotherapy for more advanced disease.

## What is the most effective treatment for superficial bladder tumours?

Superficial bladder cancers (Ta, T1 and Tis) are treated by transurethral resection and for some low grade Ta tumours (Ta G1) this may be the only treatment indicated. Unfortunately, 20% of patients with low risk superficial tumours and 40% of patients with medium risk tumours, will develop tumour recurrence within 1 year. This compares with 90% of patients with high risk tumours

recurring within 1–2 years.[2] In an attempt to delay or prevent tumour recurrence, intravesical therapy is often used as an adjunct to transurethral resection, but there is controversy regarding the optimum intravesical agent. A number of meta-analyses have evaluated the role of intravesical therapy in the treatment of early stage bladder cancer (Table 31.1), **Evidence level Ia**.

The first meta-analysis compared intravesical therapy with transurethral resection alone in preventing tumour recurrence in patients with superficial bladder cancer.[3] Published randomised studies, in English, were retrieved from only three literature searches including MEDLARS, CancerLit, and Current Contents. No search strategy was given and only one investigator screened each search. Out of an initial yield of 1672 citations, 11 randomised trials comparing TUR alone with intravesical therapy and containing data on 3703 patients with newly diagnosed superficial bladder cancer were included in the analysis. Four studies compared a single intravesical agent with TUR alone, five studies compared two agents and two studies compared three agents. Intravesical adriamycin was the most commonly used cytotoxic agent (eight treatment arms) followed by mitomycin-C (seven treatment arms). Other cytotoxics used in the trials were thiotepa, epirubicin, peplomycin, neocarzinostat and mitoxantrone. A combined analysis of all 11 trials showed that intravesical therapy was associated with a 44% reduction in tumour recurrence at 1 year (OR 0·56; 95% CI 0·48–0·65, $P < 0·00001$). In a sub-analysis on the duration of intravesical therapy, short-term (1258 patients), 1-year (1721 patients), and 2-year schedules were associated with a significant reduction in tumour recurrence at 2 years of 32%, 31% and 75%, respectively. Mitomycin-C was the only drug to show a statistically significant reduction in tumour recurrence in the absence of heterogeneity. Disease progression and survival were not evaluated in this study **Evidence level Ia**.

A separate meta-analysis assessed the benefit of intravesical Bacillus Calmette–Guerin in combination with transurethral resection versus transurethral resection alone.[4] A comprehensive search of seven electronic databases was performed, searching for randomised trials in any language. Six randomised trials were eligible for analysis, and included one German, one Greek, one Japanese, one Spanish and two Amerian studies. Patients

**Table 31.1   Meta-analyses of intravesical therapy for superficial bladder cancer**

| Study reference/aims | Included studies | Results |
| --- | --- | --- |
| (Ref 3) Determine impact of intravesical therapy on tumour recurrence following complete TUR in newly diagnosed patients with superficial bladder cancer. Published RCTs analysed | 3730 patients from 11 RCTs with Ta/T1 GI–G3 tumours. Intravesical therapy consisted of doxorubicin, metomycin, thiotepa, epirubicin, peplomycin, neocarbarzine or mitoxantrone. Treatment varied from a single instillation to a 2-year schedule | There was a significant reduction in tumour recurrence at 1 year with intravesical therapy. Sub analysis indicated improved effect with longer schedules |
| (Ref 4) A meta-analysis of published RCTs to compare incidence of tumour recurrence following TUR alone with intravesical BCG | 585 patients from 6 RCTs (281 TUR alone, 304 BCG). Four different strains of BCG included, with doses of 78–180 mg instilled over 1–2 hours. | Tumour recurrence was significantly less in patients receiving BCG |
| (Ref 5) To make practice recommendations for non-muscle invasive bladder cancer using a statistical approach (bayesian) | Trials comparing TUR alone with TUR plus intravesical therapy or comparing agents following TUR. Data extracted from 181 reprots | All intravesical agents studied resulted in a lower probability of recurrence compared with TUR alone. No evidence that intravesical therapy affects long-term progression |
| (Ref 6) Compare the efficacy of intravesical BCG with mitomycin C (MMC) | A meta-analysis of published data from 1527 Ta/T1 patients in six RCTs (693 MMC *v* 834 BCG) | Pooled analysis shows no difference in recurrence between BCG and MMC. Subanalysis indicates that in high risk patients recurrence is significantly reduced with BCG |
| (Ref 7) To evaluate the impact of prophylactic chemotherapy agents following primary resection, on disease recurrence, progression and survival. An individual patient data meta-analysis | Four EORTC and two MRC (2535 patients) prophylactic RCTs in primary or recurrent Ta/T1 patients assessing TUR with (1629) or without (906) intravesical chemotherapy (thiotepa, VM-26, doxorubicin, epodyl, epirubicin, mitomycin C and oral pyridoxine) | Adjuvant therapy significantly reduced the risk the recurrence and increased the disease-free interval. There was no advantage for adjuvant therapy in terms of disease progression or survival |

Abbreviations: BCG, Bacillus Calmette–Guerin; RCT, randomised controlled trial; TUR, transurethral resection

with Ta and T1 bladder cancer of medium or high risk of tumour recurrence,[2] were eligible for analysis. The total number of patients from the six trials was 586, and of these 281 received TUR alone compared to 304 for BCG. There were no TaG1 patients included in the analysis. The studies investigated three different strains of BCG (Pasteur, Connaught and Tokyo) at doses ranging from 75 mg to 150 mg, instilled for 1 to 2 hours and with varying schedules of therapy. The results of the meta-analysis indicated that transurethral resection plus Bacillus Calmette–Guerin significantly reduced the recurrence rate at 12 months compared with transurethral resection alone (OR 0·3; 95% CI 0·21–0·43). The overall log hazard ratio for recurrence (−0·83, variance 0·03) indicated a significant benefit of Bacillus Calmette–Guerin treatment in reducing tumour recurrence. Complications associated with Bacillus Calmette–Guerin consisted of cystitis (67%), haematuria (23%), fever (25%) and increased urinary frequency (71%).

No toxicity data for transurethral resection alone were reported **Evidence level Ia** . Although Bacillus Calmette–Guerin significantly reduced tumour recurrence, it was not possible to evaluate the impact of this agent on disease progression and survival in the included studies. This was because control patients originally randomised to transurethral resection were given intravesical Bacillus Calmette–Guerin at various times throughout their clinical management.

A bayesian approach was utilised in a meta-analysis comparing intravesical therapy with transurethral resection alone in the management of Ta, T1 and Tis bladder cancer.[5] The aim of this study was to make practice policy recommendations for non-muscle invasive bladder cancer based on published methods **Evidence level Ia** . A search of MEDLINE from 1966 to 1998 was undertaken; however, no other searches were performed and only English articles retrieved. Data were extracted from 181 articles, including

30 randomised trials and 151 case–control studies. The confidence profile method was used for the meta-analysis, which determines the probability of tumour recurrence, tumour progression and complications of treatment. Intravesical therapy with thiotepa, doxorubicin, Bacillus Calmette–Guerin and mitomycin-C decreased the recurrence probability of bladder cancer compared with TUR alone. The calculated number of patients "needed to treat" ranged from 3·3 for Bacillus Calmette–Guerin to 10 for doxorubicin. However, there was no evidence that the rate of progression to muscle-invasive disease was altered by intravesical therapy. It was concluded that intravesical Bacillus Calmette–Guerin or mitomycin-C should be used to treat high grade Ta and T1 tumours following transurethral resection, but guidance on which was the most appropriate was lacking.

This latter point was addressed in a recent meta-analysis comparing intravesical BCG with intravesical mitomycin-C.[6] Seven databases were searched, and hand searching of relevant journals identified 27 randomised studies, six of which were eligible for meta-analysis and comprised of two Dutch, one American, one Norwegian, one Finnish and one German. Patients with Ta or T1 bladder cancer (1527) were randomised to either intravesical mitomycin-C (693) or intravesical Bacillus Calmette–Guerin (834). Doses of mitomycin-C ranged from 20 to 50 mg per instillation and those for BCG ranged from 50 to 150 mg. The patients in each trial were categorised according to their risk of tumour recurrence as defined previously.[2] The overall log hazard ratio (variance) for recurrence was −0·02 (0·005) indicating no difference between Bacillus Calmette–Guerin and mitomycin-C ($P = 0·76$). A subgroup analysis of only high risk patients (three trials) gave a log hazard ratio (variance) for recurrence of −0·371 (0·012), with no evidence of heterogeneity ($P = 0·25$), and was significantly in favour of intravesical Bacillus Calmette–Guerin. This translates into a 31% reduction in the probability of tumour recurrence per unit time associated with Bacillus Calmette–Guerin compared to mitomycin C. Although the recurrence-free survival was significantly prolonged with intravesical Bacillus Calmette–Guerin in high risk patients, there was no difference in terms of disease progression ($P = 0·16$) and survival ($P = 0·5$). Local toxicities (dysuria, cystitis, frequency and haematuria) were associated with both MMC (34%) and BCG (27%), as were systemic toxicities, such as chills, fever and malaise, although skin rash was more common with MMC **Evidence level Ia**.

A combined individual patient data meta-analysis of four EORTC and two MRC randomised trials evaluated the benefits of immediate adjuvant intravesical chemotherapy versus transurethral resection alone on tumour recurrence, disease progression, and survival.[7] Intravesical agents administered in these trials were thiotepa, epirubicin, doxorubicin, mitomycin-C, and oral pyridoxine, and included a total of 2535 patients with primary or recurrent Ta and T1 bladder cancer, 906 patients randomised to TUR alone and 1629 to postoperative intravesical chemotherapy. Analysis was conducted on an "intention-to-treat" basis and indicated that adjuvant therapy significantly prolonged the disease-free interval (log-rank $P < 0·01$) with a hazard ratio of 0·8, equivalent to a 20 + 6% decrease in the risk of recurrence in the treated group compared to the no treatment group. The estimate of the average absolute benefit in the percentage of patients disease-free at 8 years for those randomised to receive adjuvant therapy was 8%. In many cases, patients who did not receive adjuvant chemotherapy proceeded to receive chemotherapy on recurrence, which complicates the analysis of time to progression data and survival. However, after a median follow up of 7·8 years, there was no advantage for adjuvant therapy in delaying progression to muscle-invasive disease, time to appearance of distant metastases, or prolonging survival. These results support the favourable impact of adjuvant prophylactic treatment on the disease-free interval in patients with Ta and T1 bladder cancer. Intravesical Bacillus Calmette–Guerin was not evaluated in this meta-analysis because this agent cannot be used immediately after transurethral resection due to the risk of systemic infection.

## How effective are surgery and radiotherapy for muscle-invasive bladder cancer?

Approximately 20% of patients with bladder cancer will have muscle-invasive disease at the time of presentation. Others will develop invasive disease during the course of their clinical management. These tumours are generally of high grade and originate in the bladder mucosa and progressively extend into the lamina propria, perivesical fat, and contiguous pelvic structures. The prognosis for invasive bladder cancer is poor with 5-year survival ranging between 20% and 50%. The management of these patients consists of either radical cystectomy, considered as standard therapy in the USA, or the approach of radical radiotherapy followed by surgical salvage historically favoured in the UK and Canada. There is a clear need to establish which is the most beneficial in terms of patient survival, or whether a combination is more efficacious (Table 31.2).

There are no randomised trials comparing surgery with radiotherapy alone in muscle-invasive bladder cancer. However, a recent meta-analysis compared preoperative radiotherapy plus radical cystectomy versus radical radiotherapy with salvage cystectomy.[8] Three randomised trials were considered eligible for inclusion and consisted of 439 patients with T2–T4a stage disease. The radical radiotherapy doses and schedules ranged from 40 Gy over 4 weeks with a 20 Gy boost, to 70 Gy in 35 fractions over 7 weeks; those for the preoperative radiotherapy were

**Table 31.2   Meta-analyses and randomised trials in muscle-invasive bladder cancer**

| Study reference/aims | Included studies | Results |
|---|---|---|
| (Ref 8) To compare preoperative radiotherapy plus radical surgery with radical radiotherapy plus salvage cystectomy | Meta-analysis of three RCTs, including 439 patients with T2–T4a tumours (221 surgery, 218 radiotherapy). Analysis carried out on published data | Significant survival benefit with preoperative radiotherapy plus radical surgery |
| (Ref 9) To compare preoperative radiation plus cystectomy with cystectomy alone | Meta-analysis: four RCTs had 5-year survival data and five RCTs had 3-year data | Non-significant benefit with preoperative radiation |
| (Ref 11) Determine whether neoadjuvant or concurrent chemotherapy improves survival | Meta-analysis: individual patient data from four of five RCTs | No evidence that chemotherapy improves survival compared to local therapy alone |
| (Ref 13) RCT to investigate neoadjuvant cisplatin-based chemotherapy and radical surgery or radiotherapy | 976 patients (491 neoadjuvant therapy, 485 no adjuvant therapy) | CR higher with neoadjuvant chemotherapy but no evidence of significant survival benefit |
| (Ref 14) RCT to determine efficacy of neoadjuvant M-VAC plus cystectomy versus cystectomy alone | 307 eligible patients (158 cystectomy alone, 159 three cycles of M-VAC prior to cystectomy) | Neoadjuvant therapy associated with a significant survival advantage |
| (Ref 15) RCT to assess the efficacy of neoadjuvant MCV in patients receiving concurrent chemotherapy and radiotherapy | 123 patients randomised to neoadjuvant chemotherapy (61) or standard therapy alone (62) | No survival benefit to neoadjuvant chemotherapy. Toxicity was greater with neoadjuvant therapy |
| (Ref 16) RCT to see if the addition of concurrent cisplatin to preoperative or definitive radiotherapy improved local control and survival | 99 eligible patients randomised to receive concurrent cisplatin (51) or no cisplatin (48). Local therapy was either preoperative radiotherapy followed by cystectomy or definitive radiotherapy | CR, progression-free survival significantly better with cisplation but no difference in overall survival. |

Abbreviations: CR, complete response; RCT, randomised controlled trial

40–50 Gy in 4–5 weeks. An intention-to-treat analysis of data for overall survival from three trials published in 1976, 1977 and 1991 indicated a significant advantage of preoperative radiotherapy plus radical cystectomy at 3 years (OR 1·19; 95% CI 1·30–2·82) and at 5 years (OR 1·76; 95% CI 1·16–2·67). The mean overall survival rates at 3 and 5 years were 45% and 36% for preoperative radiotherapy plus radical cystectomy, and 28% and 20% for radical radiotherapy with salvage cystectomy **Evidence level Ia** . These results suggest an overall survival benefit with surgery; however, the included trials were small and many advances in both radiotherapy and surgery have taken place since the initiation of these studies, it is therefore highly questionable whether these results can be reliably extrapolated to modern practice.

Radiotherapy prior to cystectomy compared to cystectomy alone has been investigated in an attempt to reduce local failure/recurrence and improve overall survival in patients with muscle-invasive disease. A meta-analysis of five randomised trials compared preoperative radiotherapy at a dose range of 20–54 Gy, followed by cystectomy with

cystectomy alone.[9] A total of 796 randomised patients were included in the analysis, although there was no information on the T-stage of participating patients. Three-year survival data were available from the five studies and meta-analysis indicated no significant difference in survival (OR 0·91; 95% CI 0·64–1·30). Four trials included 5-year survival data and an intention-to-treat analysis indicated no significant benefit of preoperative radiotherapy (OR 0·71; 95% CI 0·48–1·06). No presentation or analysis of morbidity was conducted in this study. These data do not support the use of preoperative radiotherapy in muscle-invasive disease; however, the quality of the included studies was poor **Evidence level Ia** .

## What is the role of neoadjuvant chemotherapy in muscle invasive bladder cancer?

The 5-year survival rates for patients with muscle invasive bladder cancer treated with surgery, radiotherapy or a combination of the two, is about 30%. Occult disseminated disease may be present in approximately 50% of these patients, which limits the clinical outcome of local modalities alone. Frequently, dissemination has occurred before initiation of local therapy and it is therefore reasonable to suggest that these patients may benefit from systemically administered chemotherapy prior to local treatment. The rationale for this is that chemotherapy, with active agents such as cisplatin[10] would reduce the extent of metastatic disease as well as decreasing the volume of the primary tumour, enabling local treatment to be more effective.

The survival benefit of neoadjuvant platinum-based chemotherapy prior to definitive local therapy (radiotherapy or cystectomy) in patients with locally advanced bladder cancer has been the subject of two meta-analyses.[11,12] The Cochrane review[11] was an individual patient data meta-analysis of four randomised trials, including 479 patients **Evidence level Ia** . Three trials completed chemotherapy before starting local therapy and one gave chemotherapy simultaneously with radiotherapy or radiotherapy and cystectomy. Individual patient data analysis suggests a small non-significant benefit of local therapy alone with a hazard ratio of 1·02 (95% CI 0·81–1·26; $P = 0·8$). Supplementation of these data with published data from a fifth trial still showed no significant advantage with chemotherapy ($P = 0·3$). The updated systematic review by Parmar *et al.*[12] confirmed that there was no good evidence that neoadjuvant chemotherapy improves survival. However, neither were able to include full updated results of the largest neoadjuvant chemotherapy study performed by the MRC/EORTC.[13] In this trial, 976 patients, from 106 institutions in 20 countries, undergoing curative cystectomy or full dose external beam radiotherapy were randomly assigned three cycles of neoadjuvant chemotherapy (cisplatin, methotrexate and vinblastine) or no chemotherapy **Evidence level Ib** . Patients then continued to their preplanned cystectomy or radiotherapy. At a median follow up of 4·0 years, 485 patients had died, 78·6% of these were due to bladder cancer. The median survival for the chemotherapy group was 44 months compared to 37·5 months for those not receiving chemotherapy. There was a small but non-significant improvement in 3-year survival with an absolute difference of 5·5% (50% in the chemotherapy group, 55·5% in the no chemotherapy group (95% CI 0·5–11·0; $P = 0·075$). The slight improvement in survival was judged to be too small to support the use of neoadjuvant chemotherapy in this setting. The SWOG 8710 phase III trial **Evidence level Ib** , randomised 317 patients with T2–4a,N0,M0 tumours with locally advanced bladder cancer to neoadjuvant M-VAC (methotrexate, vinblastine, doxorubicin, and cisplatin) plus cystectomy or cystectomy alone.[14] Grade 4 toxicities occurred in 55 of 150 (37%) of patients receiving M-VAC but no chemotherapy-associated deaths. At a median follow up of 7·1 years, 128 patients remain alive with 85 and 94 deaths on the M-VAC and no

M-VAC arms, respectively. The corresponding median survivals were 6·2 and 3·8 years with a hazard ratio of 0·74 (95% CI 0·55–0·99; $P = 0·27$). These data suggest that neoadjuvant M-VAC improves patient survival, although the analysis was based on a one-sided test of significance. Another randomised trial assessed the efficacy of neoadjuvant MCV (methotrexate, cisplatin, vinblastine) chemotherapy in patients with muscle-invasive bladder cancer[15]: 123 patients with T2 to T4aNXM0 tumours were randomised to receive two cycles of MCV (N = 61) before pelvic irradiation (39·6 Gy) with concurrent cisplatin 100 mg m$^{-2}$ for two courses 3 weekly, or the same with no MCV (N = 2). The complete response rate was 61% for patients in the neoadjuvant arm and 55% for those in the control arm, with respective actuarial 5-year overall survival rates of 48% and 49%, respectively. The trial was prematurely closed owing to the high rate of severe neutropenia and sepsis, and failed to show any significant benefit of two cycles of neoadjuvant chemotherapy with MCV **Evidence level Ib** .

Finally, concurrent chemoradiotherapy is the subject of several current studies, but only one randomised trial has been published.[16] Ninety-nine patients with T2 to T4b tumours were selected for definitive radiotherapy or precystectomy radiotherapy and randomised to cisplatin 100 mg m$^{-2}$ at 2-week intervals for three cycles concurrent with radiotherapy, or to no chemotherapy **Evidence level Ib** . The pelvic relapse rate was significantly reduced in the cisplatin treated patients ($P = 0·038$). However, there was no improvement in overall survival or the rate of metastases.

## How effective are radiotherapy and systemic chemotherapy for advanced or metastatic bladder cancer?

A multicentre randomised study was undertaken to evaluate two schedules of palliative radiotherapy for bladder cancer patients who were unfit, or with disease too far advanced for curative treatment.[17] Patients were randomised to 35 Gy in 10 fractions over 2 weeks (N = 248) or 21 Gy in three fractions on alternate weekdays over 1 week (N = 251): 71% and 64% achieved symptomatic improvement in the 35 Gy arm and 21 Gy arm, respectively, with no evidence for a difference in efficacy or toxicity. There was no difference in overall survival with a median for both arms of 7·5 months (hazard ratio 0·99; 95% CI 0·82–1·21; $P = 0·9$). Complete data were not obtained from all patients because of the the palliative nature of this study, consequently modest differences in survival, symptomatic improvement rates, and toxicity cannot be ruled out.

A number of randomised trials have evaluated the benefit of systemic platinum-based chemotherapy in advanced

**Table 31.3   Randomised trials of systemic chemotherapy in disseminated bladder cancer**

| Study reference/comparison | Patients | Results |
| --- | --- | --- |
| (Ref 18) Cisplatin alone *v* cisplatin and cyclophosphamide | 109 patients with metastatic or regionally advanced disease. 50 randomised to cisplatin and 59 to combination chemotherapy | No significant difference in response or progression |
| (Ref 19) Cisplatin compared with cisplatin, doxorubicin, cyclophosphamide | 135 patients with disseminated bladder cancer | Greater toxicity with combination chemotherapy with no significant improvement in survival |
| (Ref 20) Cisplatin monotherapy compared with cisplatin plus methotrexate | 108 patients, 53 randomised to the combination regime and 55 to cisplatin alone | No significant difference in response or survival |
| (Ref 21) Cisplatin *v* cisplatin, methotrexate, vinblastine, doxorubicin (M-VAC) | 225 assessable patients: 122 randomised to cisplatin alone and 133 to M-VAC | With long-term follow up of 6 years, M-VAC significantly superior to cisplatin in terms of survival |
| (Ref 22) Compare M-VAC with cisplatin, cyclophosphamide and doxorubicin (CisCA) | 110 patients recruited | M-VAC significantly superior in terms of response and survival. Minimal difference in side effects |
| (Ref 23) Methotrexate plus vinblastine (MV) compared to cisplatin, methotrexate, vinblastine (CMV) | 214 patients entered, 108 randomised to CMV and 106 to MV | Overall clinical response and survival significantly improved with CMV |
| (Ref 24) Gemcitabine plus cisplatin (GC) *v* M-VAC | 203 patients randomised to GC and 202 to M-VAC | No difference in response rates and survival. M-VAC more toxic |

or metastatic urothelial cancers (not confined solely to bladder). Four randomised trials have evaluated the efficacy of single-agent cisplatin versus combination chemotherapy **Evidence level Ib** . (Table 31.3).

A prospective, multi-institutional trial compared cisplatin $(70 \, mg \, m^{-2})$ with the combination of cisplatin plus cyclophosphamide $(750 \, mg \, m^{-2})$ in 109 patients with advanced bladder cancer.[18] The response rates were not significantly different with 20% for cisplatin compared with 12% for the combination. Of those who responded, 64% progressed at 3 months with cisplatin and 57% in the combination group. Survival was not an endpoint in this small study. A second trial, randomised 135 patients to cisplatin $(60 \, mg \, m^{-2})$ or cisplatin plus cyclophosphamide and doxorubicin given every 3 weeks.[19] Of those patients receiving combination chemotherapy, 34% developed grade 3 or 4 haematological toxicity compared to 3% for those on cisplatin alone; 17% had a partial or complete remission with cisplatin compared with 33% for the combination chemotherapy group. The median overall survival of patients on cisplatin was 6 months compared with 7·3 months in patients receiving the combination $(P = 0·17)$.

One trial randomised patients to cisplatin monotherapy $(80 \, mg \, m^{-2})$ every 4 weeks or a combination cisplatin plus methotrexate.[20] Complete response was seen in 9%

of patients in each arm, with overall response rates of 45% for the combination and 31% for cisplatin $(P = 0·18)$. The median survival among patients treated with the combination was 8·7 months compared with 7·2 months for patients treated with cisplatin $(P = 0·7)$. Haematological toxicity, mucositis, nausea and vomiting were significantly more severe with the combination therapy.

The fourth trial randomised 122 patients to cisplatin alone and 133 to combination chemotherapy with M-VAC (methotrexate, vinblastine, doxorubicin, cisplatin) with repeat courses every 28 days.[21] M-VAC significantly increased response rates, 65% compared with 46% $(P < 0·05)$ and the median survival, 48·3 weeks compared with 36·1 weeks $(P = 0·003)$. However, the evidence suggests that patients with prognostic factors such as non-transitional cell histology, poor performance status and bone metastases are unlikely to benefit significantly.

M-VAC also appears to be superior to CisCA (cisplatin, cyclophosphamide, doxorubicin) in terms of response rates and survival. In a randomised study, 110 patients with metastatic disease were randomised to receive either CisCA or M-VAC.[22] Overall response was significantly better with M-VAC (46% compared with 65%, $P < 0·05$) and median survival (48·3 weeks compared with 36·1 weeks). No randomised studies have compared CMV (cisplatin, methotrexate, vinblastine) with M-VAC; however, a Medical Research Council randomised trial reported superior results for CMV when compared with MV (methotrexate and vinblastine).[23] The overall clinical response for CMV (108 patients) was 46% compared with 19% for MV (106 patients). Survival was significantly improved with CMV (HR 0·68; 95% CI 0·51–0·90; $P=0·0065$).

The combination of gemcitabine and cisplatin (GC) appears to be equivalent to M-VAC in terms of response and survival but is less toxic. In a trial of 405 patients randomised to either GC or M-VAC overall response rates were 54·3% for CG and 55% for M-VAC.[24] The respective time to progressive disease was similar (HR 1·05; 95% CI 0·85–1·30; $P=0·66$) as was overall survival (HR 1·04; 95% CI 0·82–1·32; $P=0·75$). However, M-VAC resulted in more cases of grade 3 and 4 neutropenia, mucositis, infection and diarrhoea.

It appears that combination chemotherapy has an important role in the management of advanced or metastatic bladder cancer. Combination chemotherapy has been shown to be superior to single agent therapy. The combination of cisplatin and gemcitabine is well tolerated and its efficacy appears to be comparable to the best reported regimes.

## Implications for practice and research

It is clear that adjuvant intravesical chemotherapy for superficial bladder cancer is effective in reducing tumour recurrence, and that intravesical Bacillus Calmette–Guerin is the agent of choice for high risk patients, although the optimum schedule needs to be defined. However, the evidence for an impact on disease progression and survival is lacking. There is a need to address the relationship between tumour recurrence and progression both mechanistically and pharmacologically.[25] Preliminary results from a MRC randomised trial suggest that bladder irrigation with glycine may provide a non-toxic procedure to prevent tumour recurrence following TUR.[26] These results are encouraging and merit further study. The controversy between cystectomy and radiotherapy, or a combination of both, in the treatment of invasive bladder cancer requires further investigation. Although the evidence supports preoperative radiotherapy plus cystectomy, a comparison between modern methods of practice would be informative. There is also a need to identify patients that will benefit from bladder preservation strategies. To improve the clinical outcome in patients with advanced bladder cancer, new agents, such as gemcitabine, taxanes and camptothecin analogues, need to be evaluated in randomised trials.[27,28]

## References

1 Coleman M, Babb P, Harris S, Quinn M, Sloggett A, De Stavola B. Cancer survival in England and Wales, 1991–98. In: *Health Statistics Quarterly*. London: Office of National Statistics, 2000.

2 Hall RR, Parmar MK, Richards AB, Smith PH. Proposal for changes in cystoscopic follow up of patients with bladder cancer and adjuvant intravesical chemotherapy. *BMJ* 1994;**308**:257–60.

3 Huncharek M, Geschwind JF, Witherspoon B, McGarry R, Adcock D. Intravesical chemotherapy prophylaxis in primary superficial bladder cancer: a meta-analysis of 3703 patients from 11 randomized trials *J Clin Epidemiol* 2000;**53**:676–80.

4 Shelley MD, Kynaston H, Court J et al. A systematic review of intravesical bacillus Calmette–Guerin plus transurethral resection vs transurethral resection alone in Ta and T1 bladder cancer. *BJU Int* 2001;**88**:209–16.

5 Smith JA, Labasky RF, Cockett ATK, Fracchia JA, Montie JE, Rowland RG. Bladder cancer clinical guidelines panel summary report on the management of nonmuscle invasive bladder cancer (stages Ta, T1 and TIS). *J Urol* 1999;**162**:1697–701.

6 Shelley M, Court J, Burgon K et al. Meta analysis of intravesical therapy for superficial bladder cancer; superiority of Bacillus Calmette–Guerin may be confined to high risk patients. *Br J Cancer* 2001;**85**(Suppl. 1):P79.

7 Pawinski A, Sylvester R, Kurth KH et al. A combined analysis of European Organization for Research and Treatment of Cancer, and Medical Research Council randomized clinical trials for the prophylactic treatment of stage TaT1 bladder cancer. European Organization for Research and Treatment of Cancer Genitourinary Tract Cancer Cooperative Group and the Medical Research Council Working Party on Superficial Bladder Cancer. *J Urol* 1996;**156**: 1934–40, 1940–1.

8 Shelley MD, Barber J, Wilt T, Mason MD. Surgery versus radiotherapy for muscle invasive bladder cancer. In: Cochrane Collaboration, *Cochrane Library*. Oxford: Update Software, 2002.

9 Huncharek M, Muscat J, Geschwind JF. Planned preoperative radiation therapy in muscle invasive bladder cancer; results of a meta-analysis. *Anticancer Res* 1998;**18**:1931–4.

10 Yagoda A, Watson RC, Gonzalez-Vitale JC, Grabstald H, Whitmore WF. Cis-dichlorodiammineplatinum(II) in advanced bladder cancer. *Cancer Treat Rep* 1976;**60**:917–23.

11 Advanced Bladder Cancer Overview Collaboration. Neoadjuvant cisplatin for advanced bladder cancer. In: Cochrane Collaboration, *Cochrane Library*. Oxford: Update Software, 2002.

12 Parmar MK, Burdett S. Commentary. In: Hall RR, ed. *Clinical Management of Bladder Cancer*. London: Arnold, 1999.

13 International Collaboration of Trialists. Neoadjuvant cisplatin, methotrexate, and vinblastine chemotherapy for muscle-invasive bladder cancer: a randomised controlled trial. International collaboration of trialists. *Lancet* 1999;**354**:533–40.

14 Natale RB, Grossman HB, Blumenstein B et al. SWOG 8710; Randomised Phase III trial of neoadjuvant MVAC + cystecomy versus cystectomy alone in patients with locally advanced bladder cancer. *Proc Ann Meet Am Soc Clin Oncol* 2001; Abstr. 3.

15 Shipley W, Winter K. Phase III trial of neoadjuvant chemotherapy in patients with invasive bladder cancer treated with selective bladder preservation by combined radiation therapy and chemotherapy; Initial results of radiation therapy oncology group 89–03. *J Clin Oncol* 1998;**16**:3576–83.

16 Coppin CM, Gospodarowicz MK, James K et al. Improved local control of invasive bladder cancer by concurrent cisplatin and preoperative or definitive radiation. The National Cancer Institute of Canada Clinical Trials Group. *J Clin Oncol* 1996;**14**:2901–7.

17 Duchesne G, Bolger J. A randomised trial of hyperfractionated schedules of palliative radiotherapy in the management of bladder carcinoma; results of medical research council trial BA09. *Int J Radiat Oncol Biol Phys* 2000;**47**:379–88.

18 Soloway MS, Einstein A, Corder MP, Bonney W, Prout GR, Jr, Coombs J. A comparison of cisplatin and the combination of cisplatin and cyclophosphamide in advanced urothelial cancer. A National Bladder Cancer Collaborative Group A Study. *Cancer* 1983;**52**:767–72.

19 Khandekar JD, Elson PJ, DeWys WD, Slayton RE, Harris DT. Comparative activity and toxicity of cis-diamminedichloroplatinum (DDP) and a combination of doxorubicin, cyclophosphamide, and DDP in disseminated transitional cell carcinomas of the urinary tract. *J Clin Oncol* 1985;**3**:539–45.

20 Hillcoat BL, Raghavan D, Matthews J *et al.* A randomized trial of cisplatin versus cisplatin plus methotrexate in advanced cancer of the urothelial tract. *J Clin Oncol* 1989;**7**:706–9.

21 Saxman SB, Propert K, Einhorn LH *et al.* Long-term follow-up of phase III intergroup study of cisplatin alone or in combination with methotrexate, vinblastine, and doxorubicin in patients with metastatic urothelial carcinoma: A Cooperative Group Study. *J Clin Oncol* 1997;**15**:2564–9.

22 Logothetis CJ, Dexeus FH, Finn L *et al.* A prospective randomized trial comparing MVAC and CISCA chemotherapy for patients with metastatic urothelial tumors. *J Clin Oncol* 1990;**8**:1050–5.

23 Mead GM, Russell M, Clark P *et al.* A randomized trial comparing methotrexate and vinblastine (MV) with cisplatin, methotrexate and vinblastine (CMV) in advanced transitional cell carcinoma: results and a report on prognostic factors in a Medical Research Council study. MRC Advanced Bladder Cancer Working Party. *Br J Cancer* 1998;**78**:1067–75.

24 von der Maase H, Hansen SW, Roberts JT *et al.* Gemcitabine and cisplatin versus methotrexate, vinblastine, doxorubicin, and cisplatin in advanced or metastatic bladder cancer: results of a large, randomized, multinational, multicenter, phase III study. *J Clin Oncol* 2000;**18**:3068–77.

25 Au JL, Badalament RA, Wientjes MG *et al.* Methods to improve efficacy of intravesical mitomycin C: results of a randomized phase III trial. *J Natl Cancer Inst* 2001;**93**:597–604.

26 Whelan P, Griffiths G, Stower M *et al.* Preliminary results of a MRC randomized controlled trial of post-operative irrigation of superficial bladder cancer. *ASCO* 2001 (Abstr.708).

27 Albers P, Siener R, Michael R *et al.* Randomised phase II trial of gemcitabine and paclitaxel with or without maintenance treatment in patients with cisplatin refractory transitional cell carcinoma. *ASCO* 2002;79.

28 Khaled HM, Zaghloul MS, Ghoneim M *et al.* A randomized phase III study of neoadjuvant chemotherapy for invasive bladder cancer with gemcitabine and cisplatin. *ASCO* 2002;2421.

# 32 Cancer of the prostate

*Malcolm Mason, Mike Shelley*

An autopsy series of men dying of other causes reported that 40% of men over 50 years and 80% of men over 80 years have tumours arising in the prostate gland.[1] That the majority of these tumours will not have been diagnosed prior to death demonstrates that a significant number of men are alive with prostate cancer and asymptomatic. Prostate cancer is often diagnosed in men undergoing clinical investigations for lower urinary tract symptoms and is rare before the age of 40 years, but the incidence rises sharply with increasing age. It is now the second most commonly diagnosed cancer in men, although there is a wide variation in the incidence of clinically evident prostate cancer. The highest rates, of over 100 per 100 000 population, are found in African–Americans, whilst the lowest rates of less than 10 per 100 000 are seen in Asian countries, with European men being intermediate.[2]

Prostate cancer can be detected by PSA testing, digital rectal examination and transrectal ultrasound. Tumour may also be found by pathological examination of tissues after transurethral resection of the prostate carried out to relieve urinary obstruction. The disease generally progresses slowly, but the prognosis depends heavily on the grade of the tumour. Treatment for early stage disease confined to the prostate may consist of active monitoring, radical prostatectomy, brachytherapy, or external beam radiotherapy. The choice of treatment will depend on the extent of the disease and the consent of the patient.

Androgen deprivation has been the prevailing treatment for advanced prostate cancer since the pioneering work of Huggins in 1941 demonstrating that prostate cancer cells require androgenic stimulation for growth.[3] Androgen deprivation is achieved clinically by orchidectomy or hormone manipulation: the most commonly used agents being luteinising hormone-releasing hormone (LHRH) agonists (leuprolide, gorserelin acetate) and the non-steriodal anti-androgens (flutamide, nilutamide, bicalutamide). About 70% of men with advanced disease will respond initially to hormone therapy; however, the majority will eventually develop androgen-independent tumours and relapse.[4] In patients with locally advanced or asymptomatic prostate cancer, controversy exists concerning the ideal time to initiate hormone therapy. Patients with symptomatic disease should be treated immediately, but for asymptomatic disease the situation is less clear. Owing to the protracted course of

well-differentiated prostate cancer, many men with asymptomatic disease may die of other causes before disease progression requires intervention, and treating such patients with immediate hormone therapy would expose them to unnecessary treatment-related side effects such as gynaecomastia and erectile impotence. In addition, early hormone therapy could theoretically select for androgen-independent cells and prematurely cause a condition to develop that has no viable treatment options. Delaying hormone treatment could provide an effective treatment when disease progresses rather than being palliative to asymptomatic disease. Alternatively, experimental evidence from androgen-dependent tumours suggests that androgen deprivation is more effective when the tumour burden is low,[5] and, clinically, a more favourable response is likely to occur in smaller tumours.[6] Further, early hormone intervention may reduce the need for ancillary procedures, such as TURP, and delay the development of serious complications.

This chapter reviews the evidence comparing immediate hormone therapy, including adjuvant and neoadjuvant therapy, with delayed hormone therapy in men with locally advanced or asymptomatic prostate cancer undergoing primary hormone treatment or in those receiving radiotherapy. Included is the large multinational randomised study of immediate bicalutamide therapy versus placebo in men receiving either active monitoring, radiotherapy, or surgery.[7]

## Are clinical outcomes superior when androgen deprivation is initiated at diagnosis or deferred until clinical signs of disease progression are evident?

The treatment of men with locally advanced or asymptomatic metastatic prostate cancer is controversial and may range from initial aggressive local treatment, with either surgery or radiotherapy, to following the patient closely and reserving treatment until the tumour progresses with symptoms. The deferred treatment is usually hormone therapy and is palliative, and controversy exists as to whether it is more beneficial to initiate adjuvant hormone therapy or delay until disease progression. There have been four randomised trials that have compared the clinical value of giving immediate or delayed androgen deprivation therapy in patients with advanced prostate cancer **Evidence level Ib**.

Between 1960 and 1975 the Veterans Administration Cooperative Urological Research Group (VACURG) conducted a series of randomised trials of various treatments for patients with newly diagnosed prostate cancer.[8–10] The first such trial (1960–66), relevant to this review, and sometimes referred to as VACURG 1, randomised 1903 stage III and IV patients to one of the following groups: placebo, orchidectomy plus placebo, diethylstilbestrol (DES, 5 mg), or orchidectomy plus DES.[8–10] The staging system used by the VACURG was: Stage III (local spread) and Stage IV (distant metastases and/or elevated acid phosphatase). Those patients in the placebo group received hormone therapy with DES or DES plus orchidectomy at the discretion of the clinician when the disease had progressed, and can thus be considered as receiving deferred hormone therapy. Therefore, data from the placebo group (stage III [262], IV [223]) and the orchidectomy group (stage III [266], IV [203]) are relevant to this review. For stage III patients, there were 177 and 184 totals deaths with deferred (placebo) and immediate (orchidectomy) groups, respectively, with the corresponding values for stage IV patients of 189 and 182. There was no significant difference in overall survival between immediate or deferred treatment for both stage III and stage IV patients. It should be noted that only 44% of patients assigned to placebo progressed and actually had their treatment changed.[9]

The second VACURG study (1967–1975), randomised 508 newly diagnosed patients with advanced or metastatic prostate cancer to placebo, 0·2 mg DES, 1·0 mg DES, or 5 mg DES.[6–8] Data pertinent to this review are stage III and IV patients randomised to placebo (deferred N = 128) and the DES 1 mg group (immediate N = 128). There was no indication of the subsequent treatments in the deferred group on disease progression. The DES 5 mg study arm was stopped early because of excess cardiovascular deaths. The results of the study indicated that immediate androgen deprivation (DES 1 mg), beginning at diagnosis, increased overall survival in stages III and IV compared with deferred treatment. However, no statistical $P$ values were reported. These studies have been criticised for a number of reasons including the low number of patients recruited and the fact that bone scans and pelvic lymphadenectomy were not included in the staging process.[10]

A Medical Research Council trial randomised 934 men with histologically confirmed adenocarcinoma of the prostate to receive either immediate (N = 469) or deferred (N = 465) androgen deprivation hormone therapy.[11] Patients had either local disease considered to far advanced for curative treatment (T2–T4) or asymptomatic metastatic

disease and a life expectancy of 12 months or more. Hormone treatment consisted of orchidectomy or an LHRH analogue with an anti-androgen for flare, although alternative hormone therapies were permitted if these became inappropriate. Hormone therapy commenced either immediately at the time of diagnosis or was deferred until the disease had progressed sufficiently to warrant clinical intervention. Significantly fewer men (N = 65) in the immediate arm underwent TURP for local progression compared to the deferred arm (N = 141, $P < 0·001$). In patients with M0 disease, 96 in the immediate arm and 144 patients in the deferred arm developed metastatic disease ($P < 0·001$). In total, 121 (26%) and 211 (45%) of patients in the immediate and deferred arms, respectively, developed pain from metastatic disease ($P < 0·001$), suggesting a significant advantage to patients treated immediately. In terms of mortality, 203 men (43·3%) in the immediate arm and 257 men (55·3%) in the deferred arm died of prostate cancer ($P = 0·001$), and for those patients with M0 disease the respective values were 81 of 256 (31·6%) and 119 of 244 (48·8%, $P = 0·003$). In men with metastatic disease at randomisation, there was no significant difference in survival between the two arms. Overall, significantly more men receiving deferred hormone therapy ($P < 0·05$) developed complications, such as pathological fractures, spinal cord compression, ureteric obstruction, and extraskeletal metastases, although in each complication subset not all comparisons were significant. The results of this study consistently favour immediate hormone therapy. However, a recent review of the data after a longer follow up, indicates that there is no significant difference in overall survival between patients treated immediately and those receiving deferred hormone therapy.[12]

A systematic review and meta-analysis of immediate versus deferred hormone therapy included the three trials discussed above.[13] This analysis was performed on 5-year hazard rates and used a random effect model that reduces to a fixed effect model when the studies were homogeneous. The combined hazard ratio (95% CI) was 0·91 (0·815–1·026) where a ratio of less than 1 indicates that immediate therapy is superior, although statistical significance was not reached (Table 32.1) **Evidence level Ia**.

A further randomised trial to determine the efficacy of immediate hormone therapy compared with observation after radical prostatectomy and pelvic lymphadenectomy in 98 men with node-positive prostate cancer has recently been reported.[14] Immediate anti-androgen therapy (N = 47) consisted of either goserelin or bilateral orchidectomy. Out of the 51 patients in the observational group, 37 received hormone therapy for local or systemic recurrence. After a median follow up of 7·1 years, recurrence was seen in 15% of patients in the immediate group and 82% in the deferred group, with 76% and 18% alive and disease-free,

**Table 32.1** Published meta-analysis[13] of survival at 5 years from three randomised trials comparing immediate versus deferred hormone therapy in prostate cancer

| Included studies | Intervention | No. of patients | Hazard ratio* (95% CI) |
|---|---|---|---|
| VACURG 1[7–9] | Deferred (placebo) | 485 | Stage III 1·0 (0·78–1·29) |
| | Immediate (orchidectomy) | 469 | Stage IV 1·0 (0·79–1·27) |
| VACURG 2[7–9] | Deferred (placebo) | 128 | Stages III and IV |
| | Immediate (diethylstilboestrol 1 mg) | 128 | 0·72 (0·52–0·99) |
| MRC[10] | Deferred | 465 | 0·89 (0·76–1·06) |
| | Immediate (orchidectomy or LHRH) | 469 | |
| | Combined analysis | | 0·91 (0·82–1·03) |

*A hazard ratio of less than 1·0 favours immediate hormone therapy.

respectively (hazard ratio 9·7; 95% CI 4·5–21·0; $P < 0.001$). Death from prostate cancer was recorded in 6·4% for the immediate group compared to 31·4% in the deferred group (hazard ratio 9·7; 95% CI 1·8–21·5; $P < 0.01$), whereas the corresponding deaths from other causes were 7·8% and 3·9% respectively. These data suggest that immediate anti-androgen therapy improves survival and reduces recurrence in patients with node-positive prostate cancer; however, this was a small study **Evidence level Ib**.

A systematic review and meta-analysis (Table 32.2) **Evidence level Ia**, that includes all four of the above studies has been published on the *Cochrane Library*.[15] A comprehensive search strategy did not find any additional studies. The analysis included 2167 patients and highlighted the variability between studies with regard to treatments used and the requirements for initiating treatments. The per cent overall survival at 1, 2, 5 and 10 years for the immediate therapy group was 88%, 73%, 44% and 18%, compared with

86%, 71%, 37% and 12%, respectively, for the deferred group. The pooled estimate for the difference in overall survival consistently favoured immediate treatment but was significant only at 10 years (OR 1·50; 95% CI 1·04–2·16). It is important to note that this review did not have the most recent updated MRC data available for analysis.[12] The pooled estimate of prostate cancer-specific survival also favoured early therapy but the results were not statistically significant. Reporting of complications in the included studies was limited, but there tended to be more adverse advents with early treatment. The limitations of the included studies were discussed including variability in trial design, staging system of prostate cancer, hormone interventions and definitions and reporting outcomes. With these limitations in mind, it was concluded that early androgen suppression may provide some benefit in reducing disease progression and associated complications. A small, but significant, advantage in overall survival may be apparent on long-term follow up.

**Table 32.2** Summary results of a Cochrane systematic review[15] and meta-analysis of four randomised trials comparing immediate with deferred hormone therapy in prostate cancer

| Year | Per cent overall survival | | Pooled OR (95% CI) |
|---|---|---|---|
| | Immediate | Deferred | |
| 1 | 88 | 86 | 1·16 (0·9–1·49) |
| 2 | 73 | 71 | 1·08 (0·89–1·33) |
| 5 | 44 | 37 | 1·19 (0·95–1·50) |
| 10 | 18 | 12 | 1·50 (1·04–2·16) |

Trials included for analysis were references 8–12. A pooled OR < 1 favours immediate hormone therapy.

## Does adjuvant androgen suppression with radiotherapy improve clinical outcomes compared to radiotherapy with androgen suppression deferred until clinical evidence of disease progression?

A number of randomised trials have reported on the adjuvant use of androgen deprivation in local advanced or asymptomatic metastatic prostate cancer **Evidence level Ib**. One small trial randomised 43 previously untreated, stage C patients to receive radiotherapy alone and 39 to receive radiotherapy plus immediate hormone therapy with DES.[16] Patients receiving DES were initially treated with 5 mg daily but the dose was reduced to 2 mg daily and continued indefinitely. Patients in the radiotherapy group alone received deferred hormone therapy, consisting of DES and/or orchidectomy, at relapse. At a median follow up of 14·5 years, disease-free survival was significantly higher in the immediate adjuvant hormone group, with rates of 71%, 63% and 63% at 15 years, respectively, compared with 49%, 42% and 35% for the radiotherapy alone group ($P = 0·008$). However, this benefit was not translated into an improvement in overall survival.

Another randomised trial compared external beam irradiation alone with the same plus the gonadotrophin-releasing hormone agonist gorserelin[17]: 415 previously untreated patients, with locally advanced disease, were randomised to receive pelvic radiotherapy, with 50 Gy in five weeks plus a 20 Gy boost over 2 weeks, or radiotherapy plus 3·6 mg goserelin, given subcutaneously every 4 weeks immediately following radiotherapy, and continuing for 3 years. In the radiotherapy group, treatment at disease progression (deferred) included goserelin and/or orchidectomy. At a median follow up of 45 months, the overall survival at 5 years was significantly better in the adjuvant hormone group: 79% compared with 62% in the deferred group ($P = 0·001$). Disease-free survival was also significantly improved in the adjuvant group, with respective values of 85% and 48% ($P < 0·001$). These data support the use of anti-androgen therapy immediately following radiotherapy for locally advanced prostate cancer.

In a smaller study performed in Sweden,[18] 91 patients with T1–4, pathologically confirmed N0-3, M0 prostate cancer were randomised to radiotherapy alone or radiotherapy plus orchidectomy. Benefits to combined modality therapy were seen in terms of disease progression (61% v 31%; $P = 0.005$), cause-specific survival (44% v 27%; $P = 0·06$), and overall survival (mortality 61% v 38%; $P = 0·02$). These results suggest that early androgen ablation is superior to deferred treatment in these patients.

Improvements in overall survival are also reported on analysis of RTOG 85–31, but this was a subgroup analysis and not a primary endpoint of the study.[19] In this study, 977 patients with non-bulky but locally advanced, or lymph node, metastases (pelvic or para-aortic) were randomised to radiotherapy alone with hormones initiated at relapse or radiotherapy plus indefinite hormone therapy, beginning in the last week of radiotherapy. Improvements were seen with immediate hormone therapy in local failure rates (23% v 37%; $P < 0·0001$), distant metastasis rate (27% v 37%; $P < 0·0001$), and survival with no evidence of disease (35% v 13%; $P < 0·001$). However, overall and cause-specific survival benefits were restricted to a subset of patients with Gleason sum scores of 8–10 ($P = 0·036$ and 0·019, respectively). This study suggests that long-term adjuvant androgen ablation is associated with significant improvements in local control and freedom from metastatic disease, although no toxicity data were presented.

A meta-analysis of the above four randomised trials, but using less recent data from the RTOG 85–31 study,[20] reports on the pooled overall 5-year survival (Table 32.3) **Evidence level Ia**.[13] The analysis of 1565 patients found a significant reduction in mortality associated with immediate androgen deprivation as an adjunct to radiotherapy when compared with deferred hormone treatment (hazard ratio 0·63; 95% CI 0·48–0·83).

**Table 32.3** Meta-analysis[13] of survival at 5 years from four randomised trials comparing immediate versus deferred hormone therapy as adjuvant to radiotherapy (RT) in patients with prostate cancer

| Included studies | Intervention | No. of patients | Hazard ratio* (95% CI) |
|---|---|---|---|
| Zagars *et al.*[16] | Immediate (RT + Diethylstilboestrol) | 38 | 0·76 (0·34–1·71) |
| | Deferred (RT alone) | 40 | |
| Bolla *et al.*[17] | Immediate (RT + goserelin) | 207 | 0·49 (0·34–0·72) |
| | Deferred (RT alone) | 208 | |
| Granfors *et al.*[18] | Immediate (RT + orchidectomy) | 46 | 0·50 (0·33–0·75) |
| | Deferred (RT alone) | 45 | |
| RTOG 85–10[19] | Immediate (RT + goserelin) | 477 | 0·84 (0·66–1·08) |
| | Deferred (RT alone) | 468 | |
| | | Combined analysis | 0·63 (0·48–0·83) |

*A hazard ratio of < 1·0 favours immediate hormone therapy.

The RTOG 86–10 trial has recently been reported.[21] In this study, 477 patients with bulky primary tumours, with or without lymph node metastases, but without distant metastases, were randomised to radiotherapy alone, or radiotherapy plus hormone therapy with goserelin commencing 2 months prior to radiotherapy and continuing until the end of radiotherapy. Those patients receiving radiotherapy alone were followed until local failure, regional failure, or metastases were observed, at which time they received deferred goserelin. In this trial improvements have been seen in local control (42% $v$ 30%; $P = 0.016$), in a reduction in the incidence of distant metastases (34% $v$ 45%; $P = 0.04$), disease-free survival (33% $v$ 21%; $P = 0.004$), biochemical disease-free survival (PSA < 1.5; 24% $v$ 10%; $P < 0.0001$), and cause-specific mortality (23% $v$ 31%; $P = 0.05$) for patients treated with hormone therapy plus radiotherapy. However, subset analysis suggested that in patients with Gleason scores 2–6 there was a highly significant improvement in survival (70% $v$ 52%; $P = 0.015$). In contrast, in patients with Gleason 7–10 tumours, no benefits were seen in local control or survival.

A large, multinational, randomised study reported on bicalutamide as immediate or adjuvant therapy in 8113 men with localised or locally advanced prostate cancer.[7] Patients were randomised to receive either bicalutamide (150 mg per day, N = 4052) or placebo, in addition to standard therapy of radical prostatectomy, radiotherapy, or watchful waiting. At a median follow up of 3 years, bicalutamide significantly reduced the risk of disease progression by 42% compared to placebo (HR 0.58; 95% CI 0.51–0.66; $P = 0.0001$). The reduced risk was seen with all three standard therapies and, overall, 363 patients in the bicalutamide arm had objective progression compared to 559 in the placebo arm. The main side effects observed with bicalutamide were gynaecomastia and breast pain. The results of this trial to date are encouraging, although it is too early to make a statement regarding survival.

## Conclusions and future directions

The studies included in this review were all randomised controlled trials, and the majority documented withdrawal rates and used an intention-to-treat analysis. As such, they were considered of acceptable quality. Some of these trials have been criticised with regard to a number of issues, including the small number of patients recruited, lack of data on patients' comparability, poor reporting of adverse events, the limited duration of hormone therapy, inadequate follow up procedures to identify disease progression and the low percentage of patients in the deferred arms receiving

hormone therapy.[22] However, many of these issues have been recently addressed although the debate continues.[23–25]

With these limitations in mind, the weight of current evidence from two meta-analyses, and recent randomised trials, supports the use of immediate rather than deferred hormone therapy in men with active, progressive disease, but this conclusion must be reviewed as more evidence accumulates over the next few years. The EORTC 30846 prospective randomised trial comparing immediate versus deferred hormone therapy in lymph node positive, non-metastatic patients has been completed, but the results are not yet available. However, in a preliminary analysis of 82 of 412 patients, the time to distant metastases was significantly longer in the immediately treated patients ($P = 0.0001$) compared to those receiving deferred hormone therapy.[26] The full results of this trial are eagerly awaited.

In the early hormone studies with oestrogens, morbidity was severe with potentially fatal cardiovascular complications.[8] Today, hormone therapy with for example, bicalutamide, is better tolerated and may lead to an improved quality of life for prostate cancer patients, especially for younger men in whom sexual potency may be maintained. The very large study of immediate or adjuvant bicalutamide[7] is worthy of further comment. This study, showing a highly significant reduction in disease progression with bicalutamide, although survival data are immature, indicates the value of well-coordinated, multinational trials to recruit large numbers of prostate cancer patients.

Quality-of-life issues are important as they will influence both the choice and timing of hormone therapy, and should be assessed in all trials comparing immediate versus deferred treatment. Future studies should strive to find alternative therapies or schedules that offer effective control of tumour progression but are less toxic. Intermittent androgen suppression, using PSA to indicate when to commence and stop hormone therapy, may allow clinicians to evaluate the value of immediate androgen ablation therapy while reducing side effects and cost.

## References

1 Sakr WA, Grignon DJ, Haas GP, Heilbrun LK, Pontes JE, Crissman JD. Age and racial distribution of prostatic intraepithelial neoplasia. *Eur Urol* 1996;**30**:138–44.
2 Dijkman GA, Debruyne FM. Epidemiology of prostate cancer. *Eur Urol* 1996;**30**:281–95.
3 Huggins C, Hodges C. Studies on prostatic cancer: the effect of castration, of estrogen and of androgen injection on serum phosphatases in metastatic carcinoma of the prostate. *Cancer Res* 1941;**1**:293–7.
4 Scher HI, Sternberg CN. Chemotherapy of urologic malignancies. *Semin Urol* 1985;**3**:239–80.

5   Bruchovsky N, Rennie PS, Coldman AJ, Goldenberg SL, To M, Lawson D. Effects of androgen withdrawal on the stem cell composition of the Shionogi carcinoma. *Cancer Res* 1990;**50**:2275–82.

6   Van Cangh PJ, Gala JL, Tombal B. Immediate vs. delayed androgen deprivation for prostate cancer. *Prostate* 2000;**10**(Suppl.):19–25.

7   Wirth *et al. ASCO,* 2001;(Abstr. 705).

8   Byar DP. Proceedings: The Veterans Administration Cooperative Urological Research Group's studies of cancer of the prostate. *Cancer* 1973;**32**:1126–30.

9   Byar DP, Corle DK. Hormone therapy for prostate cancer: results of the Veterans Administration Cooperative Urological Research Group studies. *NCI Monogr* 1988(7):165–70.

10  Christensen MM, Aagaard J, Madsen PO. Reasons for delay of endocrine treatment in cancer of the prostate (until symptomatic metastases occur). *Prog Clin Biolog Res* 1990;**359**:7–24.

11  Medical Research Council Prostate Cancer Working Party Investigators Group. Immediate versus deferred treatment for advanced prostatic cancer; initial results of the Medical Research Council trial. *Br J Urol* 1997;**79**:235–46.

12  Kirk D. Immediate vs. deferred hormone treatment for prostate cancer: how safe is androgen deprivation? *BJU Int* 2000;**86**(Suppl. 3):220.

13  Agency for Health Care Research and Quality (AHRQ). *Relative effectiveness and cost-effectiveness of methods of androgen suppression in the treatment of advanced prostate cancer.* Report No. 4. Rockville, Maryland: Agency for Health Care Research and Quality (AHRQ), 1999.

14  Messing EM, Manola J, Sarosdy M, Wilding G, Crawford ED, Trump D. Immediate hormonal therapy compared with observation after radical prostatectomy and pelvic lymphadenectomy in men with node-positive prostate cancer. *N Engl J Med* 1999;**341**:1781–8.

15  Nair B, Wilt T, MacDonald R, Rutks I. Early versus deferred androgen suppression in the treatment of advanced prostate cancer. In: Cochrane Collaboration, *Cochrane Library.* Oxford: Update Software, 2002.

16  Zagars GK, Johnson DE, von Eschenbach AC, Hussey DH. Adjuvant estrogen following radiation therapy for stage C adenocarcinoma of the prostate: long-term results of a prospective randomized study. *Int J Radiat Oncol Biol Phys* 1988;**14**:1085–91.

17  Bolla M, Gonzalez D, Warde P *et al.* Improved survival in patients with locally advanced prostate cancer treated with radiotherapy and goserelin. *N Engl J Med* 1997;**337**:296–300.

18  Granfors T, Modig H, Damber JE, Tomic R. Combined orchiectomy and external radiotherapy versus radiotherapy alone for nonmetastatic prostate cancer with or without pelvic lymph node involvement: a prospective randomized study. *J Urol* 1998;**159**:2030–4.

19  Lawton C, Winter K, Murray K. Updated results of the phase III Radiation Therapy Oncology Group (RTOG) trial 85–31 evaluating the potential benefit of androgen suppression following standard radiation therapy for unfavorable prognosis carcinoma of the prostate. *Int J Radiat Oncol Biol Phys* 2001;**49**:937–46.

20  Pilepich MV, Caplan R, Byhardt RW *et al.* Phase III trial of androgen suppression using goserelin in unfavourable-prognosis carcinoma of the prostate treated with definitive radiotherapy; report of Radiation Therapy Oncology Group Protocol 85–31. *J Clin Oncol* 1997;**15**: 1013–21.

21  Pilepich MV, Winter K, John MJ *et al.* Phase III radiation therapy oncology group (RTOG) trial 86–10 of androgen deprivation adjuvant to definitive radiotherapy in locally advanced carcinoma of the prostate. *Int J Radiat Oncol Biol Phys* 2001;**50**:1243–52.

22  Walsh PC, DeWeese TL, Eisenberger MA. A structured debate: immediate versus deferred androgen suppression in prostate cancer-evidence for deferred treatment. *J Urol* 2001;**166**:508–16.

23  Messing EM. Editorial comment: Deferred androgen suppression for prostate cancer. *J Urol* 2001;**166**:515–16.

24  Fourcade RO. Re: A structured debate: immediate versus deferred androgen suppression in prostate cancer-evidence for deferred treatment. *J Urol* 2002;**167**:651–3.

25  Kirk D. Re: A structured debate: immediate versus deferred androgen suppression in prostate cancer – evidence for deferred treatment. *J Urol* 2002;**167**:652–3.

26  Newling D. Advanced prostate cancer: immediate or deferred hormone therapy? *Eur Urol* 2001;**39**(Suppl. 1):15–21.

# 33 Cancer of the penis

*Mike Shelley, Malcolm Mason*

Penile cancer is very rare accounting for less than 1% of all cancers in men. In England and Wales there are about 300 cases per year,[1] and in the USA the number of new cases for the year 2000 is estimated to be 1100.[2] When diagnosed early (stages I and II) penile cancer is curable with 5-year survival rates of about 70%[1] but curability decreases with increasing stage.

Because of the rarity of penile cancer, clinical trials, dealing specifically with this disease are limited. There are no randomised controlled trials of penile cancer and the reports that are available vary in the number of patients included. Small trials can obviously lead to erroneous conclusions, so for the purpose of this review we will confine our discussion to those that included 50 or more patients. The evidence for the treatment of penile cancer is based entirely on observational, and usually retrospective studies; as a result, it is of low grade **Evidence level III**. The studies included here are indicative of a principle, rather than representing an exhaustive literature synthesis.

## How effective is penis-conserving surgery as a curative option in patients with penile cancer?

Total or partial penile amputation is the most common treatment for penile cancer. One study analysed the results of 83 patients with squamous cell carcinoma of the penis followed for at least 3 years or until death.[3] Of these, 61 had Jackson stage I (UICC – Tcis, T1N0M0 and T2N0M0), 11 stage II (T3–4N0M0) and 11 stage III (T1–4N1–3M0). In patients with low stage disease, partial penectomy was employed on 35, partial penectomy plus delayed ilioinguinal lymph node dissection owing to late inguinal metastases on six, and partial penectomy plus immediate ilioinguinal lymph node dissection on another six. The other stage I patients received local excision, with or without partial or total penectomy, circumcision, or topical 5-FU. The 22 high stage patients received partial or total penectomy followed by either inguinal lymph node irradiation or immediate dissection. Forty-one patients with early stage cancer survived at least 3 years and were considered cured. Of the other 20, 12 died of cancer and eight of other causes giving a corrected 5-year survival of 77%. Two out of nine patients with stage II or III disease receiving partial or total

penectomy with or without irradiation survived 3 years or longer, and 11 of 13 having early extended excision of the primary lesion and lymph nodes. The recommendations from this study are that local excision is only appropriate for carcinoma *in situ*, partial penectomy with intense follow up for patients with small, well-differentiated tumours, and partial or total penectomy and immediate ilioinguinal lymphdenectomy for patients with large or moderately to poorly differentiated primary tumours.

The records of 219 patients with proven squamous carcinoma were retrospectively analysed.[4] In this study, there were 129 stage I patients, 24 stage II and 60 stage III. Of these, 160 had partial penectomy, 21 had total penectomy and 42 underwent lymphadenectomy. In patients with tumour confined to the foreskin, circumcision was considered adequate treatment with no need for penectomy. Circumcision was the choice of treatment for 20 such patients, but 10 needed partial amputation because of recurrence. Patients surviving greater than 3 years for stages I, II and III were, respectively, 94, 13 and 12; 65% of patients with no palpable lymph nodes survived 6 years or more, whereas 28% with palpable lymph nodes survived 3–5 years. Survival data were reported only in relation to stage and it was not possible to determine the relative roles of treatment on survival. However, the majority of stage I patients had penis-conserving therapy (N = 101) and had the highest survival rates, although this may be a reflection of stage rather than treatment.

A South African study reviewed the management of 50 patients attending Tygerberg Hospital.[5] The mean patient age was 54 years with 40 of mixed race, eight Caucasian and two Black. Partial penectomy was performed in 29 patients and radical penectomy in 20. The pathological T stage in the partial penectomy group was T1 in four, T2 in 18 and T3 in seven cases, and the stage for the total penectomy group was T2 in seven, T3 in 10 and T4 in three cases. Complications of penectomy occurred in nine patients (20%) and consisted of wound sepsis, bleeding, wound dehiscence and meatal stenosis. Lymphadenectomy was performed in 34 patients, 26 of these experienced postoperative complications such as wound sepsis, dehiscence, lymphocele and wound abscess. The overall incidence of local recurrence was 22%, and the incidence of recurrence or metastases were significantly higher (71%) when the surgical margins were involved with carcinoma. At a mean follow up of 22 months, 62% of patients were alive without disease, 23% were alive with disease and 15% had died. Death and recurrence or metastases were significantly more common in patients with T3–4 compared with T1–2 tumours, and in those with N1–3 compared to N0 disease.

## How effective is prophylactic lymph node dissection in the management of penile cancer?

Lymph node dissection is an effective method to eradicate small metastatic tumours and may be most effective the earlier the surgery is implemented. However, in patients with clinically non-palpable or palpable but non-metastatic penile cancer, the choice of treatment is unclear. In a prospective non-randomised, three arm study, 64 patients with carcinoma of the penis and negative lymph nodes (N0) or palpable nodes (N1–2A), had either bilateral groin node dissection (n = 27), radiotherapy (n = 18) or surveillance (n = 19).[6] Bilateral lymph node dissection was performed 3 weeks after treatment of the primary using a skin bridge technique followed by complete ilioinguinofemoral node dissection. Those receiving radiotherapy had a dose of 50 Gy over 5–6 weeks to the inguinofemoral region, whilst those on surveillance had expectant therapy only. Patients were followed every 3–6 months for at least 2 years, then at 1 year intervals for 5 years. The overall 5-year survival rates were 74% for bilateral lymph node dissection, 66% for the radiotherapy group and 63% for the surveillance group. Subanalysis indicated that N0 patients had a significantly higher survival rate with bilateral groin node dissection compared to radiotherapy and surveillance. The results of this study suggest that lymphadenectomy in this group of penile cancer patients is effective.

A Dutch study retrospectively analysed the management of regional lymph nodes in 110 patients with squamous cell carcinoma of the penis.[7] The management of 66 stage N0 tumours was surveillance of the inguinal region in 57, lymph node dissection in five, adjuvant radiotherapy in one, and external beam radiation therapy (EBRT) in four. The management of 40 patients with positive node patients (N+), consisted of lymph node dissection in 27 with adjuvant radiotherapy in 11, biopsy only in four, EBRT in four and surveillance in five. All those found to have no evidence of lymph node invasion (pN0) were cured; of 21 with positive node metastases, 11 were cured and 10 relapsed, nine of whom subsequently died. The efficacy of regional lymph node dissection was dependent not only on the localisation of the metastases, but also on the number of nodes involved and the grade of the primary tumour.

A retrospective study reported on 350 patients referred to the Brazilian National Cancer Centre who underwent surgical treatment for penile cancer (56 T1, 203 T2, 92 T3, 15 T4 and 48 TX).[8] In 244 patients (64%), resection, partial, or total penectomy was performed as the initial form of treatment, while 102 (29%) underwent amputation and lymphadenectomy, and 24 (27%) underwent palliative surgery for advanced squamous cell carcinoma. The 5-year disease-free survival rate for patients undergoing lymphadenectomy concomitantly with penile surgery was 62%, whereas for those who underwent delayed lymphadenectomy after lymph nodes became clinically suspicious, it was 8% ($P < 0.001$). The 5-year disease-free survival rates for those patients with negative and positive systematic lymphadenectomy were 87% and 29%, respectively ($P < 0.001$). These results suggest better 5-year survival rates for patients concomitantly undergoing lymphadenectomy with penile surgery.

The management of node-negative patients with invasive penile cancer is unclear, with options of prophylactic lymphadenectomy and expectant management with selective node biopsies as a third approach. In a study of 423 patients with invasive penile carcinoma (T2–T4) and clinically negative groin nodes, patients were subjected to prophylactic inguinal lymphadenectomies (N = 113), observation (N = 258), or inguinal biopsies (N = 52).[9] There were 233 T2, 181 T3 and 19 T4 lesions. Positive nodes were found in 20 (18%) of patients who had inguinal lymphadenectomies who subsequently underwent pelvic lymphadenectomy and remained free of disease. In the observation group, inguinal recurrences were seen in 21 (8%) who then underwent illioinguinal block dissection, as did five patients with positive nodes in the inguinal biopsy group. The overall 5-year disease-free survival rates for the prophylactic inguinal lymphadenectomy, observation, and inguinal biopsies groups were 94%, 93% and 85%, respectively, and were not statistically significant. It was concluded that the substantial morbidity associated with prophylactic inguinal lymphadenectomy does not justify its use in node-negative patients, and a strictly enforced observation protocol would be more appropriate.

## How effective is radiotherapy for penile carcinoma?

A retrospective study of 101 men with invasive squamous cell carcinoma of the penis attending the Royal Marsden Hospital was performed to assess the treatment outcome.[10] There were 79 stage T1 patients, 82 were node-negative and two had distant metastases at presentation. Fifty-nine patients had external beam radiation (60 Gy in 2 Gy fractions over 46 days) for the primary tumour, 13 had interstitial brachytherapy, and 29 had total or partial penectomy. At a median follow up of 5·2 years, the 10-year overall and cause-specific survival rates were 39% and 57%, respectively. Adverse prognostic factors were G3, ulcerative/ fungating or T2/T3 tumours, positive lymph nodes, Jackson's stage 2/3/4 and surgical treatment of the primary. Thirty-six out of 98 evaluable patients had recurrences giving a 10-year local failure rate of 45%; 26 of these patients were successfully salvaged with radiotherapy or surgery. This study suggests that radiotherapy may be given as the initial treatment for organ preservation, with surgery reserved for salvage of residual or recurrent disease.

Patients (N = 101) with carcinoma of the penis seen at the Peter MacCallum Cancer Institute, Melbourne have been reviewed.[11] Radical treatment of the primary was by partial penectomy or external beam radiotherapy. Nodal treatment ranged from observation to hind-quarter amputation, but most had some form of radiotherapy either alone or before or after surgery. The 5-year disease-free survival for T1, N0 and T2, N0 primary tumours was 90% for those receiving surgery alone (N = 11) and 60% for those having radiotherapy alone (N = 26). The 10-year overall survival by T stage was T1 90% T2 70% and T3 30%; all T4 patients died within 1 year. The 5-year overall survival by nodal status was N0 80%, N1 68%, N2 25% and N3 18%.

Iridium[192] implant was used as a conservative approach to the management of 165 patients with penile tumours at the Institut Gustave Roussy.[12] Primary lesions were seen in 145 patients and recurrent tumours in 20 patients; 140 patients were node negative and two had distant metastases at presentation. Circumcision was performed with interstitial radiation therapy using $^{192}$Ir at a mean dose of 68 Gy. Node-positive tumours were treated with inguinal and/or pelvic lymphadenectomy, eventually followed by external beam radiotherapy: 111 patients remained free of disease, 27 had local recurrence and 30 patients had lymph node relapse. The 5-year actuarial rate of local control was 83% with an overall 5-year survival of 76%. Penile preservation was achieved in 81%, although late complications of necrosis (23%), urethral stenosis (27%), and penile sclerosis (14%) were encountered. The conservative approach adopted provides good survival and local control but is associated with substantial local complications.

In one multicentre, retrospective study, 259 patients with epidermoid carcinoma of the penis were treated with interstitial implantation using an iridium afterloading technique.[13] In some of these patients interstitial implantation was combined with circumcision, either to expose the glans or excise tumour: 75 of the patients had interstitial implantation combined with surgery, and sometimes with external beam radiotherapy. Most patients had T1N0 or T2 N0 disease. The respective 5- and 10-year overall survival rates were 66% and 52%, and the corresponding rates for

cause-specific survival were 88% and 88%, respectively. There was no significant difference between the patients treated exclusively by implantation (90 patients), implantation and circumcision (94 patients), implantation and radiotherapy (20 patients), implantation and surgery (49 patients), and implantation, surgery and radiotherapy (six patients); 191 patients avoided surgical mutilation of the penis suggesting that interstitial brachytherapy provides a good method of conservative treatment.

Penile conservation with radiotherapy does cure certain patients and, therefore, is an important clinical option, but further studies are needed.

## What factors affect the clinical outcome in the treatment of patients with penile carcinoma?

A Brazilian study evaluated the clinical and pathological factors involved in lymph node metastases in 154 previously untreated patients with penile carcinoma.[14] A total of 88 patients underwent amputation and lymphadenectomy concurrently, whereas 57 underwent amputation with antibiotic therapy for 10 days followed by lymphadenectomy 4–8 weeks later. Of these, 98 (67·6%) underwent total and 47 (32·4%) underwent partial penectomies. The 5-year disease-specific and overall survival rates were 45·3% and 54·3%, respectively. Disease-free survival was significantly influenced by the presence of metastatic lymph nodes ($P = 0·0003$) and clinical N stage ($P = 0·0091$), and overall survival by metastatic lymph nodes ($P = 0·0007$), eosinophilic infiltrate ($P = 0·0072$), N stage ($P = 0·0076$), and patient age ($P = 0·0556$). Metastatic lymph nodes and clinical N stage were the most relevant prognostic factors for risk of recurrence, whereas lymph node metastases, clinical T stage, and eosinophilic infiltrate were relevant risk factors for death. When left untreated, patients with metastatic disease die within 2 years.

A retrospective review of records from 59 patients with penile cancer attending the Kobe University Hospital, Japan, was undertaken to determine factors predictive of survival.[15] Most patients had T1 (N = 32) or T2 (N = 19) stage disease, 16 had lymph node metastases and three had distant metastases. Partial or total penectomy was chosen depending on the site of the primary lesion. At a median follow up of 109 months, the 5- and 10-year cause-specific survival rates were 75·9% and 73·8%, respectively. Lymph node involvement, tumour stage and differentiation were independent risk factors for survival as determined by multivariate analysis. None of the stage I or II patients treated with lymphadenectomy developed recurrence in the inguinal region, whereas four (27%) out of 15 without lymphadenectomy had recurrences suggesting that this procedure improves outcome.

In a Spanish study of 81 patients, retrospective pathological review indicated a significant correlation between lymph node involvement and local extension ($P = 0.004$) and cell grade and local extension ($P = 0.04$).[16] Those patients with negative lymph nodes had significantly improved survival rates compared to those with positive nodes ($P = 0.00001$). In addition, significant differences in survival rates were shown between vertically and superficially spreading tumour growth patterns determined histologically, superficial having the better prognosis ($P = 0.004$). It was recommended that prophylactic lymph node dissection is indicated for tumours of vertical growth and conservative management considered for verrucous growth.

## Conclusion and future direction

The optimal treatment for squamous cell carcinoma of the penis should aim to eradicate the tumour with organ preservation and sexual function, without compromising survival. In many of the cited studies patients were managed in a variety of ways making comparisons difficult. In addition, several were reports of the experience of a single institution which may have involved many clinicians over a number of years.

With conservative therapy for penile cancer, partial penectomy alone might be possible in some selected patients with surgical margins less than 1 cm.[17] No direct comparison between partial or total amputation can be made, although non-randomised studies have suggested the possibility of higher local failure rates with conservative therapy; with salvage therapy ultimate survival rates are similar. Alternative options for primary treatment of penile cancer include external beam radiotherapy, brachytherapy, and laser treatment.[10–13] Penile conservation should be offered routinely, since survival rates with radiotherapy may well be comparable to partial or total penectomy. These modalities need to be compared in randomised clinical trials.

No randomised trials of prophylactic lymph node dissection have been identified and no conclusions can be made regarding the efficacy of this procedure compared to surveillance and therapeutic lymph node dissection for relapse. However, several descriptive, retrospective studies have indicated successful outcomes for some men managed by either of these strategies.[6,7,9,14–16] It is unknown whether prophylactic lymph node dissection and radiotherapy are better than surveillance and salvage lymph node dissection plus radiotherapy. Again these alternatives need to be compared in randomised trials.

As with penis-conserving therapy, there is evidence from non-randomised reports that some patients with clinically or pathologically involved inguinal lymph nodes can be cured by therapeutic lymph node dissection. However, no recommendations can be made regarding technique or extent of surgery.

Patients with metastatic disease have a poor prognosis, although some may respond to chemotherapy with cisplatin, bleomycin and methotrexate. However, there have been no large scale studies of chemotherapy in late stage disease, and there are minimal data regarding the optimum regimen or schedule or regarding the combination of chemotherapy and radiotherapy for primary disease.[17]

The rarity of penile cancer has led to difficulties in setting up randomised studies and in arriving at a consensus for the optimum treatment for this disease. It would be advantageous to have specialised cancer centres run by multidisciplinary teams to manage such patients. In this way clinical experience could be gained and patients channelled into randomised clinical trials. Quality-of-life issues need to be evaluated in such randomised trials.

## References

1 Office for National Statistics. *Mortality statistics – cause, England and Wales, 1999.* Report No.: DH2 no.26. London: The Stationery Office 2000.
2 Woolam GL. Cancer statistics, 2000: a benchmark for the new century. *CA: Cancer J Clin* 2000;**50**:6–33.
3 Fraley E, Zhang G, Sazama R, Lange P. Cancer of the penis – prognosis and treatment plans. *Cancer* 1984;**55**:1618–24.
4 Narayana A, Olney L. Carcinoma of the penis – analysis of 219 cases. *Cancer* 1981;**49**:2185–90.
5 Heyns CF, VanVollenhoven P, Steenkamp JW, Allen FJ. Cancer of the penis – a review of 50 patients. *SA J Surg* 1997;**35**:120–4.
6 Kulkarni JN, Kamat MR. Prophylactic bilateral groin node dissection versus prophylactic radiotherapy and surveillance in patients with N0 and N1–2A carcinoma of the penis. *Eur Urol* 1994;**26**:123–8.
7 Horenblas S. Squamous cell carcinoma of the penis III. Treatment of regional lymph nodes. *J Urol* 1993;**149**:492–7.
8 Ornellas A, Sexias A. Surgical treatment of invasive squamous cell carcinoma of the penis; retrospective analysis of 350 cases. *J Urol* 1993;**151**:1244–9.
9 Ravi R. Prophylactic lymphadenectomy vs observation vs inguinal biopsy in node-negative patients with invasive carcinoma of the penis. *Jap J Clin Oncol* 1993;**23**:53–8.
10 Sarin R, Norman AR, Steel GG, Horwich A. Treatment results and prognostic factors in 101 men treated for squamous carcinoma of the penis. *Int J Rad Oncol Biol Phys* 1997;**38**:713–22.
11 Sandeman TF. Carcinoma penis. *Australas Radiol* 1990;**34**:12–16.
12 Khanfir K, Perez A, Haie-Meder C *et al.* Conservative approach for the management of penile tumours: Experience of the Institut Gustave Roussy (IGR) in about 165 patients. New Orleans, LA: American Society of Clinical Oncology, 2000.
13 Rozan R, Albuisson E, Giraud B *et al.* Interstitial brachytherapy for penile carcinoma – a multicentric survey. *Radiother Oncol* 1995;**36**:83–93.
14 Lopes A, Hildago G. Prognostic factors in carcinoma of the penis; Multivariate analysis of 145 patients treated with amputation and lymphadectomy. *J Urol* 1996;**156**:1637–42.

15  Yamada Y, Gohji K, Hara I, Sugiyama T, Arakawa S, Kamidono S. Long-term follow-up study of penile cancer. *Int J Urol* 1998;**5**: 247–51.

16  Villavicencio H, Rubio-Briones J, Regalado R *et al.* Grade, local stage and growth pattern as prognostic factors in carcinoma of the penis. *Eur Urol* 1997;**32**:442–7.

17  Haas G, Blumenstein B. Cisplatin, methotrexate and bleomycin for the treatment of carcinoma of the penis; a South West Oncology Group study. *J Urol* 1999;**161**:1823–5.

# 34 Testicular germ cell cancer

*Mike Shelley, Tim Oliver, Malcolm Mason*

In 1997 there were 1440 new cases of testicular cancer in England and Wales resulting in an incidence of 5·6 per 100 000 men.[1] Although this is a relatively rare cancer, representing around 1% of all male cancers, it is the most common cancer in young men. Approximately 95% of malignant tumours arising in the testes originate from primordial germ cells, and are accordingly termed germ cell tumours. These tumours are classified as seminomas or non-seminomas and can be present as one tumour type or as a mixture of both. They have different clinical outcomes and require different clinical management. Patients with a suspected testicular tumour most commonly present with a testicular lump and are immediately referred for urological assessment. Once diagnosis is made, orchidectomy is usually performed and further investigations are undertaken to ascertain the extent of the disease, which will determine the subsequent clinical management. Early stage disease (stage I) is confined to the testis, whereas stage II disease extends to the infradiaphragmatic lymph nodes. Later stages of testicular cancer will have spread either to more distant lymph nodes (stage III) or to visceral sites (stage IV). The treatments for testicular cancer are constantly being refined, and following initial orchidectomy may range from radiotherapy for stage I seminoma or surveillance for stage I non-seminoma, to complex polychemotherapy and surgery for metastatic disease. This chapter reviews current treatment of testicular cancer with particular emphasis on high grade evidence from randomised trials. These are limited to randomised trials of first-line therapy; no randomised trials of second-line/salvage therapy appear to have ever been performed, and this is surely a priority for the future.

## What is the optimum curative treatment for stage I testicular seminoma?

Seminomas represent about 50% of all germ cell tumours and are most prevalent in the fourth decade of life. Stage I seminoma is defined as no residual disease following orchidectomy with no evidence of dissemination, normal CT scans, and normal postoperative tumour markers. Treatment options for stage I seminoma include surveillance, adjuvant radiotherapy, or adjuvant chemotherapy, with cure rates reported to be between 96% and 100%, irrespective of the treatment used. No meta-analyses have been identified that address the management of stage I seminoma and no randomised comparisons of the three treatment options have yet been published; however, a number of observational studies **Evidence level III** report on patients with stage I disease followed by surveillance only.[2-6] These studies comprised a total of 547 patients with stage I testicular seminoma followed for a median duration of 23–48 months. Relapse rates of 13–19% were reported with 4-year and 5-year relapse-free survival rates of 80% and 81%, respectively.[2,3] The para-aortic lymph nodes appear to be the main site of relapse and a number of factors, such as age at diagnosis,[3] tumour size,[2] and rete testis invasion[7,8] have been reported to be significant prognostic indicators for relapse during surveillance.

Adjuvant radiotherapy to the subdiaphragmatic lymph nodes is the standard treatment for stage I testicular seminoma since 10–15% of patients will harbour subclinical disease at these sites. An MRC randomised study **Evidence level Ib** evaluated the efficacy of dose reduction in 478 patients with stage I disease and compared relapse rates and toxicities associated with para-aortic (PA) or "dogleg" (DL, that is, para-aortic and ipsilateral pelvic nodes fields).[9] At a median follow up of 4·5 years, nine patients had relapsed in each arm resulting in 3-year relapse-free survival rates of 96% and 96·6% for PA and DL fields, respectively. The survival at 3 years was similar in both arms (99·9% and 100%). During radiotherapy acute toxicity was significantly greater with the DL field and included nausea and vomiting ($P = 0.08$) and leukopenia ($P < 0.001$). This study suggests that reducing the radiotherapy field from a DL to a PA field does not compromise outcomes, and is less toxic. Further reductions in radiotherapy treatment intensity also appear to be possible, as the preliminary results of an MRC randomised trial **Evidence level Ib** comparing a dose of 30 Gy with a dose of 20 Gy has recently been presented.[10] In this trial of over 600 patients, the preliminary results suggest that 20 Gy in 10 fractions is unlikely to produce relapse rates more than 2% higher than for standard 30 Gy radiotherapy, and reductions in morbidity, such as lethargy, enable patients to return to work earlier.

The acute toxicities of adjuvant radiotherapy include nausea and vomiting, and there is Grade Ib evidence from two randomised trials to suggest that this can be reduced by administering antiemetics. The first trial evaluated the efficacy and side effects of prophylactic tropisetron compared to metoclopramide in 23 patients receiving 30 Gy over 3 weeks.[11] Nausea, vomiting, and diarrhoea were significantly lower with tropisetron compared to metoclopramide, although more constipation was seen with tropisetron. In the second trial,[12] 10 stage I patients receiving PA and ipsilateral pelvic nodal radiotherapy provided baseline toxicity data, whilst 20 stage I patients were randomised to DL or PA radiotherapy (10 in each group). The latter were further randomised to receive either prophylactic ondansetron or expectant therapy with metoclopramide. The ondansetron group experienced less nausea ($P = 0.02$) and less vomiting ($P = 0.06$), whilst patients receiving a reduced field size plus ondansetron had less diarrhoea ($P = 0.06$). The number of patients in this study is too small to make any definitive statement but the results suggest that the gastrointestinal toxicity associated with adjuvant radiotherapy is reduced with prophylactic antiemetics.

The excess risk of developing second malignancies in stage I seminoma patients treated with adjuvant radiotherapy is well described and probably translates into a two- to three-fold excess relative risk.[13] This has stimulated interest in the use of single agent carboplatin, or two cycles of adjuvant carboplatin as an alternative to radiotherapy,[6] and carboplatin is now being compared with adjuvant radiotherapy in an MRC randomised trial which should report in 2–3 years time.

## What is the optimum curative treatment for clinical stage I and pathological stage II testicular non-seminoma?

Non-seminomas are most prevalent in men aged between 20 and 30 years, and cure rates for patients managed by surveillance alone are reported to be between 95% and 100%, owing to the effective salvage of the 25% of patients who relapse.[14] The addition of abdominal radiotherapy to surveillance was tested in a randomised trial of 150 patients.[15] Of the 77 patients randomised to surveillance, 23 relapses occurred compared with 11 of 73 patients on radiotherapy (40 Gy in 25 fractions). Based on long-term toxicity and no improvement in survival, abdominal radiotherapy following orchidectomy was not recommended as routine therapy **Evidence level Ib**. In the USA, where retroperitoneal lymph node dissection has been employed more than in the UK, two randomised trials **Evidence level Ib** have evaluated the role of two cycles of chemotherapy in patients with pathological stage II disease (that is, positive para-aortic nodes). One study randomised 213 patients to

two cycles of PVB (cisplatin, vinblastine and bleomycin) or VAB-6 (cisplatin, vinblastine, bleomycin, cyclophosphamide, dactinomycin) versus surveillance.[16] At a median follow up of 4 years, six out of 97 patients receiving adjuvant chemotherapy had tumour recurrence compared with 48 of 98 on observation ($P < 0.001$), although there was no difference in overall survival. The second randomised trial compared two cycles and four cycles of adjuvant PVB in pathological stage II patients, and showed no significant difference in overall survival.[17] This rationale was transferred in the MRC studies **Evidence level IIa** of two cycles of adjuvant BEP (bleomycin, etoposide, cisplatin) or BOP (bleomycin, vincristine, cisplatin) in patients with stage I non-seminomatous germ cell tumours, deemed to be at high risk of recurrence, which reported substantially reduced recurrence rates (from 45% to around 2%) compared with historical controls, albeit not in randomised controlled trials.[18,19] However, it is unlikely that this impacts on the overall survival rates.

## What is the optimum curative chemotherapy for metastatic disease?

Patients with metastatic germ cell tumours are generally stratified into prognostic subgroups, based on retrospective analyses such as that of the International Germ Cell Cancer Collaborative Group.[20] This is the largest retrospective study, based on an international collaboration, which assembled a database of over 6000 patients treated with chemotherapy in the cisplatin era, resulting in the definition of good (90% cure), intermediate (80% cure), and poor (45% cure) prognostic groups. Randomised trials are generally now restricted to one or more specified prognostic group. Some trials classified patients according to one of the then prevailing prognostic classification systems, and there may, therefore, be differences in the case mix between studies.

The drug combination of cisplatin, bleomycin and vinblastine (PVB) was rapidly established in the 1970s as an effective, curative regimen for metastatic germ cell tumours. Bleomycin, etoposide and cisplatin (BEP) were introduced as an alternative to PVB, and reported to be superior in terms of survival and toxicity in a randomised trial.[21] Since then, it has become the most commonly used regimen, hence its use as a control arm in randomised trials.[22,23] The long-term results of BEP chemotherapy have been reported for 121 men with good prognosis treated at the Royal Marsden Hospital.[24] Long-term follow up (median 65 months) showed an overall 5-year survival of 87·2% (95% CI 81·1%–93·3%); 79 men (62%) had a complete radiological and serum marker response to chemotherapy alone, and residual masses post chemotherapy were resected in

**Table 34.1  Randomised trials evaluating the exclusion of bleomycin**

| Trial reference/no. of patients | Comparison | Results |
|---|---|---|
| (25) 419 good risk non-seminoma | 4×BEP v 4×EP | CR significantly better with BEP (P=0·007) |
| (26) 178 good risk GCT | 3×BEP v 3×EP | Toxicities comparable but survival significantly better with BEP |
| (27) 222 good risk GCT | 3×PVB v 3×PV | Toxicities worse with PVB but significantly fewer deaths from progressive disease (P=0·02) |
| (28) 250 good risk non-seminoma | 3×BEP v 4×EP | Response, adverse event frequency and overall survival similar in both arms |

Abbreviations: CR, complete response; GCT, germ cell tumours (seminoma and non-seminoma)

39 patients (31%), showing undifferentiated tumour in only six (15%); 23 of the 127 patients (18%) failed to respond or developed recurrent disease after BEP and only five of these were successfully salvaged. Bleomycin pneumonitis developed in 13% of cases with one death. Twenty-one men had children following chemotherapy, but semen analysis 12 months or more (median 36 months) after treatment showed azoospermia in 11 out of 54 (20%).

## Can other drugs replace bleomycin in BEP in the treatment of metastatic disease?

Bleomycin, although very active in the treatment of disseminated germ cell tumours, can induce fatal lung fibrosis in a small number of patients. This has stimulated clinical research to identify less toxic agents than bleomycin without compromising survival. Several randomised trials have compared regimens that varied only by the inclusion or exclusion of bleomycin (Table 34.1) **Evidence level Ib**. Three trials report inferior results when bleomycin was omitted. The first study compared EP (etoposide, cisplatin) with BEP in 419 patients with good prognosis metastatic non-seminomatous germ cell cancer.[25] Complete response was significantly more frequent in patients receiving BEP (95%) compared to those on EP (87%, P=0·007), although there was no significant difference in the time to progression (HR 1·70; 95% CI 0·85–3·39; P=0·13) or overall survival (HR 1·67; 95% CI 0·68–4·11; P=0·26). A second trial also compared BEP with EP in good risk patients and reported complete remission in 77% of patients on BEP compared to 71% on EP, with respective overall disease-free values of 94% and 88%.[26] The EP arm had significantly worse overall adverse outcomes, such as treatment failure, drug-related mortality, intolerance, and relapse (38% v 17%, respectively; P=0·04). The failure-free survival (86% v 69%; P=0·01) and overall survival (95% v 86%; P=0·01) were significantly inferior with EP. The third trial compared three cycles of cisplatin and vinblastine (PV) with the same plus bleomycin

(PVB) in good prognosis patients.[27] Toxicities such as leucopenia, thrombocytopenia, anaemia, and renal and pulmonary toxicities were significantly worse with PVB. The complete response rate was slightly higher for PVB (89% v 94%; P=0·29), and after a minimum of 4 years follow up relapses were seen in 7% for the PV arm compared to 5% for the PVB arm. Deaths from progressive disease were significantly less with PVB (15% v 5%; P=0·02). These three randomised trials suggest that, although toxicity may be greater with the inclusion of bleomycin, deletion of this drug compromises therapeutic efficacy.

However, a fourth randomised trial,[28] also in good prognosis patients, compared three cycles of BEP with four cycles of EP and showed equivalence in terms of clinical response, (92% v 91%), adverse event occurrence (15 v 19), and overall survival (97% v 96%).

## Are there any alternative chemotherapeutic regimens to BEP?

As an alternative approach to replacing bleomycin, a number of randomised trials have substituted other drug regimens for BEP (Table 34.2) **Evidence level Ib**. One study compared four cycles of BEP with four cycles of alternating PVB and BEP in 250 patients with poor prognosis.[29] The complete response rate was 72% and 76% for the BEP and PVB/BEP arms, respectively (P=0·58), and after an average follow up of 6 years there was no difference in relapse rates (16% v 12%, respectively). There was no significant difference in time to progression (P=0·27) or overall survival (P=0·32), although PVB/BEP was significantly more myelosuppressive (leucopenia P=0·001; leucocytopenic fever P=0·006; thrombocytopenia P=0·001) and neurotoxic (P=0·001). Two randomised trials have compared BEP with VIP (etoposide, ifosfamide, cisplatin). The first study reported on 304 men with poor risk germ cell tumours and found no significant difference in complete response, 31% with BEP and 37% with VIP, and no

**Table 34.2   Randomised trials of alternative chemotherapeutic regimes to BEP**

| Trial reference/no. of patients | Comparison | Results |
| --- | --- | --- |
| (29) 250 poor risk non-seminoma | 4 × BEP v 4 × alternating PVB and BEP | No difference in CR, relapse rates, time to progression or overall survival. PVB/BEP significantly more myelosuppressive and neurotoxic |
| (30) 304 poor risk GCT | 4 × BEP v 4 × VIP | No difference in CR or overall survival but VIP significantly more myelotoxic ($P = 0.001$) |
| (22) 84 intermediate risk non-seminoma | 4 × BEP v 4 × VIP | No difference in CR, relapse rate or 5-year progression-free survival. VIP more myelosuppressive ($P = 0.001$) |
| (31) 190 poor risk non-seminoma | 4 × BEP v 4–6 × CISCA/VB | No difference in response, adverse events, event-free and overall survival. CISCA/VB more myelotoxic |
| (23) 380 poor risk non-seminoma | BOP/VIP-B v BEP/EP | CR, failure-free and overall survival similar in both arms. BOP/VIP-B more toxic |
| (33) 160 (46 minimal/114 maximum disease) GCT | PVB v PVE | No difference in disease-free status, relapse rate or survival, Toxicities similar in both arms |
| (34) 164 good risk | 3 × VAB-6 v 4 × EP | CR and event-free survival similar but VAB-6 significantly more toxic |

Abbreviations: CR, complete response; GCT, germ cell tumours (seminoma and non-seminoma)

difference in overall survival ($P = 0.78$).[30] However, Grade 3 or worse toxicity, particularly haematological ($P = 0.001$) and genitourinary ($P = 0.036$), was significantly more common with VIP. The second trial in patients classified as intermediate prognosis using a previous EORTC definition,[22] again found similar response rates (79% with BEP and 74% with VIP), relapse rates (18% and 11%), and progression-free survival (83% and 85%) between the two regimens, and concurred with the previous trial that VIP was more myelosuppressive ($P = 0.001$).

Preliminary results of a randomised trial comparing BEP with the combination of cisplatin, doxorubicin, cyclophosphamide, vinblastine and bleomycin (CISCA/VB) have been reported, with greater haematological toxicity for the CISCA/VB regimen but with no difference in response rates or survival.[31]

A randomised study has assessed the efficacy of intensive induction-sequential chemotherapy with BOP/VIP-B (bleomycin, vincristine, cisplatin/etoposide, ifosfamide, cisplatin-bleomycin) compared with BEP/EP in poor prognosis patients.[23] Complete response rates were 57% for

BEP/EP and 54% for BOP/VIP-B ($P = 0.68$), with the respective failure-free survival at 1 year of 60% and 53%. There was no difference in overall survival with a HR of 1·30 (95% CI 0·88–1·92; $P = 0.19$), although myelosuppression, febrile neutropenia, and weight loss were greater with BOP/VIP-B. In a second randomisation component of this study, the use of GSCF led to more patients receiving full dose-intensity chemotherapy, although this was not associated with an improvement in either failure-free or overall survival.[32]

One randomised trial compared PVB (cispatin, vinblastine, bleomycin) with PVE (cisplatin, vinblastine, etoposide) and reported both regimens to be equivalent in efficacy and toxicities.[33] Finally, a randomised trial in good prognosis patients compared EP (with an etoposide dose of 500 mg m$^{-2}$) with VAB-6 (vinblastine, bleomycin, cisplatin, cyclophosphamide and dactomycin), a regimen believed[34] to be equivalent to BEP. Complete response and event-free survival were similar with both regimens but toxicity was significantly less with EP (emesis $P = 0.06$; mucositis $P = 0.09$; WBC nadir $P = 0.06$; platelet nadir $P = 0.01$). No

**Table 34.3** Randomised trials varying the number of BEP treatment cycles

| Trial reference/no. of patients | Comparison | Results |
|---|---|---|
| (36) 184 minimal/moderate GCT | 3×BEP *v* 4×BEP (etoposide 500 mg m$^{-2}$) | No difference in disease-free status, relapse rate or overall survival |
| (37) 812 good risk GCT | 3×BEP for 3 days 3×BEP for 5 days 3×BEP+1×EP 3 days 3×BEP+1×EP 5 days (etoposide 485–500 mg m$^{-2}$) | Disease-free status and progression-free survival similar between 3 and 4 cycles. 3- and 5-day schedules equivalent |
| (38) 166 good risk GCT | 4×BEP (etoposide 360 mg m$^{-2}$) 3×BEP (etoposide 500 mg m$^{-2}$) | Overall survival superior with 3×BEP |

Abbreviation: GCT, germ cell tumours (seminoma and non-seminoma)

randomised study has yet demonstrated superior efficacy to BEP, although other regimens where encouraging phase II data have been reported include C-BOP/BEP.[35]

## What is the optimum number of treatment cycles with BEP?

For patients in the "good risk" group, randomised trials have investigated the feasibility of reducing the amount of treatment without reducing its efficacy. Two randomised trials have compared three and four cycles of BEP, both using etoposide at a dose of 500 mg m$^{-2}$ (Table 34.3) **Evidence level Ib**. The first study compared four courses of BEP over 12 weeks with three courses of BEP over 9 weeks, and reported a disease-free status of 98% with four cycles and 97% with three cycles, and corresponding overall survival rates of 97% and 93%.[36] The second and most recent comparison of three cycles with four cycles of BEP, randomised 812 patients in a 2 × 2 factorial design comparing the number of cycles and also a 3-day versus a 5-day version of the regimens (at equivalent doses).[37] The 2-year progression-free survival was 90·4% with three cycles and 89·4% with four cycles. There was no difference in efficacy between the 3-day and the 5-day schedules, but the 3-day schedule was associated with more toxicity.

There have been no randomised comparisons of the "US BEP regime" (based on an etoposide dose of 500 mg m$^{-2}$ per cycle) with the "European" BEP regimen (based on an etoposide dose of 360 mg m$^{-2}$), but a study comparing 3 cycles of BEP using etoposide at a dose of 500 mg m$^{-2}$, cycled 3-weekly, against four cycles of BEP using 360 mg m$^{-2}$ cycled 3-weekly, showed superior overall survival (three *v* 13 deaths, HR 0·22; 95% CI 0·06–0·77; *P*= 0·008) for the shorter, more intensive regimen.[38] In addition, an updated report suggests that the three-cycle regimen may be associated with an equivalent or better quality of life.[39]

## Can carboplatin substitute for cisplatin in the treatment of metastatic germ cell tumours?

The main focus of current treatment strategies in good prognosis patients is to reduce the treatment-induced toxicities. Cisplatin was incorporated into the BEP regimen in the 1970s for the treatment of testicular germ cell tumours and has made a considerable impact on patients' outcome. However, cisplatin is associated with substantial side effects including nausea and vomiting, nephrotoxicity, neurotoxicity, and ototoxicity. Carboplatin was developed as a less toxic alternative to cisplatin and has demonstrated activity in a number of cancers, including testicular germ cell tumours, with reduced toxicity.[40] Consequently, a number of randomised trials have evaluated the feasibility of substituting carboplatin for cisplatin for the treatment of this disease (Table 34.4) **Evidence level Ib**.

Two randomised trials have compared BEP with CEB (carboplatin, etoposide, bleomycin) and both reported inferior results for carboplatin-based chemotherapy in terms of response and survival.[41,42] In the MRC trial,[41] 598 patients were randomised between BEP and CEB. Failure-free survival rates at 1 year were 91% with BEP and 77% with CEB (*P*= 0·009), with 3-year survival rates of 97% and 90%, respectively (*P*= 0·003). In the other study,[42] 54 patients were randomised between BEP and CEB: the deaths of four patients in the CEB arm compared with one in the BEP arm led to early closure of the trial. A third randomised study compared etoposide with either cisplatin or carboplatin in "good risk" patients, and this, too, reported inferior results using carboplatin.[43] This multicentre trial randomised 270 patients to receive four cycles of either EP or EC: 32 patients (24%) who received carboplatin experienced an incomplete response or relapse compared with 17 of 134 patients (13%) who received cisplatin (*P*= 0·02). No difference in overall survival was evident

**Table 34.4   Randomised trials substituting carboplatin (C) for cisplatin (P)**

| Trial reference/no. of patients | Comparison | Results |
| --- | --- | --- |
| (41) good risk non-seminomas | $4 \times BEP$ $v$ $4 \times CEB$ | CR worse with CEB. Significantly more treatment failures and deaths with CEB |
| (42) 54 good risk non-seminomas | $3 \times BEP$ $v$ $4 \times CEB$ | CR similar between regimes. Relapse rate and deaths greater with CEB. Negative event analysis significantly in favour of BEP |
| (43) 270 good risk GCT | $4 \times EC$ $v$ $4 \times EP$ | No difference in CR. Relapse rate greater with EC. No difference in overall survival |
| (44) 130 metastatic seminoma | $4 \times C$ $v$ $4 \times EP$ | Progression-free and overall survival better with EP |
| (45) 251 metastatic seminoma | $4–6 \times C$ $v$ $4–6 \times PEI$ | Relapse rate greater with C. No difference in overall survival. Thrombocytopenia greater with C |

Abbreviations: CR, complete response; GCT, germ cell tumours (seminoma and non-seminoma)

($P = 0.52$). A fourth study, in metastatic seminoma, compared etoposide/cisplatin (EP) with single-agent carboplatin.[44] In the light of inferior progression-free survival in the carboplatin arm, and of the results of the other studies, this trial was discontinued early by the Data Monitoring Committee, although the difference between the two arms was not statistically significant.[44] A second randomised trial has also shown no significant survival difference in patients with metastatic seminoma treated with either single agent carboplatin, or cisplatin, etoposide plus ifosfamide.[45]

The evidence from randomised trials indicates that carboplatin is less active than cisplatin and should not replace cisplatin in the routine treatment of testicular germ cell tumours.

### How effective is high dose chemotherapy in metastatic germ cell tumours?

About 85% of patients with metastatic disease will be cured by combination chemotherapy and salvage surgery for residual disease. For those patients who fail to respond, the main aim of therapy is to improve treatment efficacy and a number of new agents and dose-intensity schedules have been investigated. Six randomised trials have evaluated the benefit of high dose chemotherapy in patients with poor prognosis (Table 34.5) **Evidence level Ib** with two further trials in progress. Two trials comparing high dose regimens to PVB have reported a benefit,[46,47] while two trials evaluating high dose cisplatin[48,49] and two other trials, evaluating high dose combination chemotherapy plus bone marrow transplantation or stem cell support, have reported no benefit.[50,51] Of the two positive trials, one randomised

114 patients to either high dose cisplatin, plus vincristine and bleomycin (N = 56) or low dose cisplatin (N = 58) cycled every 4 weeks.[46] The overall response rate was significantly higher in patients treated with the higher doses of cisplatin (63%) compared with the low doses (43%, $P = 0.03$). A significant survival advantage was also observed for those receiving high dose therapy ($P = 0.009$). However, the doses do not conform to modern definitions of high dose.

The second trial randomised 52 patients to receive either three cycles of PVBE (34 patients) or four cycles of PVB (18 patients), each given at 3-weekly intervals.[47] The relapse rate for patients treated with PVBE was 17% compared with 41% for those patients treated with PVB regimen ($P = 0.2$), with respective 5-year survival rates of 78% and 48% ($P = 0.06$). Myelosuppression was seen in 91% of patients treated with the PVBE regimen and in 50% of patients receiving the PVB regimen ($P = 0.05$). Ototoxicity was diagnosed in 12 patients given PVBE compared with two on PVB.

The results of these randomised trials do not allow a definitive conclusion to be made concerning the role of high dose chemotherapy in poor prognosis patients. Neither of the two trials showing a benefit with high dose chemotherapy permits a reliable comparison with modern, effective BEP therapy, with the use of older and lower dose regimens.

### How does the treatment for testicular cancer affect the patient's quality of life?

Few studies have examined the quality of life of patients with testicular cancer; however, a recent systematic review

**Table 34.5** Randomised trials of high dose chemotherapy in poor risk patients

| Trial reference/ no. of patients | Comparison | Results |
|---|---|---|
| (48) 45 | (a) CAVB + P (cisplatin 20 mg m$^{-2}$) *v* same but cisplatin 40 mg m$^{-2}$<br>(b) responders: VAP *v* AVP + CAP + VAP | Overall CR was 36%. No differences in haematological or renal toxicities<br>Sub-protocol: No significant difference in response rates |
| (49) 159 | 4 × BEP (cisplatin 20 mg m$^{-2}$/day, days 1–5) *v* 4 × BEP (cisplatin 40 mg m$^{-2}$/day, days 1–5) | No difference in response or overall survival. High dose significantly more toxic |
| (50) 115 | 3–4 × VEP + B (30 mg weekly × 3) *v* 2 × VEP + B (20 mg/day × 5 + high dose PEC and Au BMT) | No difference in CR or 2-year overall survival. Toxicity was greater with high dose regime |
| (51) 280 | 4 × VIP/VeIP cisplatin, ifosfamide + either etoposide or vinblastine *v* 3 × VIP/VeIP + 1 × CARBOPEC (high dose arm) | More toxic deaths with high dose (9 *v* 2). No difference in response, 1-year event-free survival or 3-year overall survival |
| (46) 114 | 4 × VB + P (120 mg m$^{-2}$/month) *v* 4 × VB + P (15 mg m$^{-2}$/day, days 1–5) | Overall response rate higher with high dose P (63% *v* 43%, *P* = 0·03). Significant 5-year survival advantage with high dose regime (*P* = 0·009) |
| (47) 52 | 3 × PVBE *v* 4 × PVB | CR and relapse rates similar between arms. 5-year survival rates were better with PVBE (78% *v* 48%, *P* = 0·06). Toxicity greater with PVBE |

Abbreviations: CAVB + P, cyclophosphamide, dactinomycin, vinblastine, cisplatin; CARBOPEC, carboplatin, etoposide, cyclophosphamide, plus autologous stem cell support; CR, complete response; PEC and Au BMT, cisplatin, etoposide, cyclophosphamide plus autologous bone marrow transplantation

and meta-analysis reported on sexual dysfunction in men following treatment.[52] The meta-analysis of six controlled studies indicated significantly reduced or absent orgasm (OR 4·62; 95% CI 2·47–8·63), erectile dysfunction (OR 2·47; 95% CI 1·54–3·96), and ejaculatory function (OR 28·57; 95% CI 1·75–464·78) up to 2 years after treatment **Evidence level IIa** . Whether post-treatment sexual dysfunction is due to biological or psychological causes or a combination is unclear, but it appears common and serious, since it affects the masculinity of a relatively young male population. Further studies are required to develop strategies that will minimise its impact.

Long-term effects of treatment for testicular cancer, including chemotherapy, have not been extensively studied. However, a review of sexual functioning suggested significant morbidity after chemotherapy and radiotherapy, based on a search of MEDLINE and PsycLIT, yielding data on 2775 patients, from 29 retrospective and seven prospective studies.[53] This study did not give any quality-assessment criteria, and the statistical methodology was unclear. A more recent study on the long-term effects of treatment, suggests that the cisplatin-based chemotherapy, and possibly abdominal radiotherapy, are associated with

a slight but permanent reduction in renal function.[54] An additional randomised trial suggests that adjuvant psychological therapy appears to be of little benefit compared with standard medical care in newly diagnosed men with testicular cancer.[55]

## Conclusions

Survival for patients with stage I seminoma following orchidectomy is likely to be similarly high whether they are managed by surveillance or adjuvant radiotherapy and the advantages and disadvantages of each approach need to be weighed. Adjuvant carboplatin is conceptually unlikely to be associated with inferior survival, but the outcome of current studies is awaited. Surveillance remains a satisfactory option for patients with stage I non-seminoma, and adjuvant chemotherapy for patients at high risk of relapse is an alternative option.

Current research aims to clarify the optimum chemotherapeutic regimen for advanced germ cell tumours that maximise survival rates whilst minimising toxicities. BEP chemotherapy remains the standard primary treatment option for all patients with metastatic germ cell tumours following orchidectomy, although the schedule may differ according to the patient's prognostic risk category. Adverse effects of bleomycin may be minimised by the use of three rather than four cycles of BEP. Alternatives to BEP do exist and are used in some centres, but, for the most part, should be evaluated in clinical trials. The toxic and long-term effects of treatment need to be better defined and strategies developed to minimise these. Health awareness programmes should be a high priority, educating young men in testicular self-examination, which may avoid delays in presentation and possibly have an impact on clinical outcomes.

## References

1   Office for National Statistics. *Cancer statistics – registrations, England, 1995–1997*. Report No. MB1 no.28. London: The Stationery Office 2001.

2   von der Maase H, Specht L, Jacobsen GK *et al*. Surveillance following orchidectomy for stage I seminoma of the testis. *Eur J Cancer* 1993;**29A**:1931–4.

3   Warde PR, Gospodarowicz MK, Goodman PJ *et al*. Results of a policy of surveillance in stage I testicular seminoma. *Int J Radiat Oncol Biol Phys* 1993;**27**:11–15.

4   Peckham MJ, Hamilton CR, Horwich A, Hendry WF. Surveillance after orchiectomy for stage I seminoma of the testis. *Br J Urol* 1987;**59**:343–7.

5   Duchesne GM, Horwich A, Dearnaley DP *et al*. Orchidectomy alone for stage I seminoma of the testis. *Cancer* 1990;**65**:1115–18.

6   Oliver RT, Edmonds PM, Ong JY *et al*. Pilot studies of 2 and 1 course carboplatin as adjuvant for stage I seminoma: should it be tested in a randomized trial against radiotherapy? *Int J Radiat Oncol Biol Phys* 1994;**29**:3–8.

7   Warde P, von de Maase H, Horwich A, Gospodarowicz M, Panzarella T, Specht L. Prognostic factors for relapse in stage I seminoma managed by surveillance. In: *Proc Ann Meet Am Soc Clin Oncol* ASCO; 1998;Abstr.1188.

8   Horwich A, Alsanjari N, A'Hern R, Nicholls J, Dearnaley DP, Fisher C. Surveillance following orchidectomy for stage I testicular seminoma. *Br J Cancer* 1992;**65**:775–8.

9   Fossa SD, Horwich A, Russell JM *et al*. Optimal planning target volume for stage I testicular seminoma: a medical research council randomized trial. *J Clin Oncol* 1999;**17**:1146–54.

10  Jones WG, Fossá SD, Mead GM *et al*. Preliminary results of a international randomised trial of radiotherapy at two dose schedules of 20 Gy versus 30 Gy (at 2 Gy/day) as adjuvant treatment of stage 1 seminoma testis, including morbidity and quality of life data (MRC study TE18). In: *Fifth International Germ Cell Tumour Conference 2001*. Leeds: University of Leeds, 2001.

11  Aass N, Hatun DE, Thoresen M, Fossá SD. Prophylactic use of tropisetron or metoclopramide during adjuvant abdominal radiotherapy of seminoma stage I: a randomised, open trial in 23 patients. *Radiother Oncol* 1997;**45**:125–8.

12  Khoo VS, Rainford K, Horwich A, Dearnaley DP. The effect of antiemetics and reduced radiation fields on acute gastrointestinal morbidity of adjuvant radiotherapy in stage I seminoma of the testis: a randomized pilot study. *Clin Oncol* 1997;**9**:252–7.

13  Bokemeyer C, Schmoll HJ. Treatment of testicular cancer and the development of secondary malignancies. *J Clin Oncol* 1995;**13**: 283–92.

14  Read G, Stenning S. Medical Research Council prospective study of surveillance for stage I testicular teratome. Medical Research Council testicular tumours working party. *J Clin Oncol* 1992;**10**:1762–8.

15  Rorth M, Jacobsen GK, Von der Maase H *et al*. Surveillance alone versus radiotherapy after orchidectomy for clinical stage I nonseminomatous testicular cancer. *J Clin Oncol* 1991;**9**:1543–8.

16  Williams SD, Stablein DM, Einhorn LH *et al*. Immediate adjuvant chemotherapy versus observation with treatment at relapse in pathological stage-II testicular cancer. *N Engl J Med* 1987;**317**: 1433–8.

17  Weissbach L, Hartlapp JH. Adjuvant chemotherapy of metastatic stage II nonseminomatous testis tumor. *J Urol* 1991;**146**:1295–8.

18  Cullen MH, Billingham LJ, Cook J, Woodroffe CM. Management preferences in stage I non-seminomatous germ cell tumours of the testis: an investigation among patients, controls and oncologists. *Br J Cancer* 1996;**74**:1487–91.

19  Dearnaley DP, Stenning SP. Management of clinical stage 1 nonseminomatous germ cell tumours (NSGCT): influence of prognostic factors on choice of treatment. In: Jones WG, Appleyard I, Harnden P, Joffe JK, eds. *Germ Cell Tumours IV*. London: John Libbey & Co. Ltd, 1998.

20  International Germ Cell Cancer Collaborative Group. International germ cell consensus classification; a prognostic factor based staging system for metastatic germ cell cancers. *J Clin Oncol* 1997;**15**: 594–603.

21  Williams SD, Birch R, Einhorn LH *et al*. Treatment of disseminated germ-cell tumors with cisplatin, bleomycin, and either vinblastine or etoposide. *N Engl J Med* 1987;**316**:1435–40.

22  de Wit R, Stoter G, Sleijfer D *et al*. Four cycles of BEP vs four cycles of VIP in patients with intermediate-prognosis metastatic testicular non seminoma: a randomized study of the EORTC Genitourinary Tract Cancer Cooperative Group. *Br J Cancer* 1998;**78**:828–32.

23  Kaye SB, Mead GM, Fossá S *et al*. Intensive induction-sequential chemotherapy with BOP/VIP-B compared with treatment with BEP/EP for poor-prognosis metastatic nonseminomatous germ cell tumor: a Randomized Medical Research Council/European Organization for Research and Treatment of Cancer study. *J Clin Oncol* 1998;**16**: 692–701.

24  Dearnaley DP, Horwich A, A'Hern R *et al*. Combination chemotherapy with bleomycin, etoposide and cisplatin (BEP) for metastatic testicular teratoma: long-term follow-up. *Eur J Cancer* 1991;**27**:684–91.

25  de Wit R, Stoter G, Kaye SB *et al*. Importance of bleomycin in combination chemotherapy for good-prognosis testicular nonseminoma: A randomized study of the European Organization for Research and Treatment of Cancer Genitourinary Tract Cancer Cooperative Group. *J Clin Oncol* 1997;**15**:1837–43.

26  Loehrer PJ, Sr, Johnson D, Elson P, Einhorn LH, Trump D. Importance of bleomycin in favorable-prognosis disseminated germ cell tumors: an Eastern Cooperative Oncology Group trial. *J Clin Oncol* 1995;**13**:470–6.

27  Levi JA, Raghavan D, Harvey V *et al*. The importance of bleomycin in combination chemotherapy for good-prognosis germ cell carcinoma. Australasian Germ Cell Trial Group. *J Clin Oncol* 1993;**11**:1300–5.

28  Culine P, Kerbrat J, Bouzy C. Are 3 cycles of bleomycin, etoposide and cisplatin (3BEP) or 4 cycles of etoposide and cisplatin (4EP) equivalent regimens for patients (pts) with good-risk metastatic non seminomatous germ cell tumors (NSGCT)? Preliminary results of a randomized trial. In: *ASCO abstracts online*. 1999;Abstr.1188.

29  de Wit R, Stoter G, Sleijfer DT *et al*. Four cycles of BEP versus an alternating regime of PVB and BEP in patients with poor-prognosis metastatic testicular non-seminoma; a randomised study of the EORTC Genitourinary Tract Cancer Cooperative Group. *Br J Cancer* 1995;**71**:1311–14.

30  Nichols CR, Catalano PJ, Crawford ED, Vogelzang NJ, Einhorn LH, Loehrer PJ. Randomized comparison of cisplatin and etoposide and either bleomycin or ifosfamide in treatment of advanced-disseminated germ cell tumors: An eastern cooperative oncology group, southwest oncology group, and cancer and leukemia group B study. *J Clin Oncol* 1998;**16**:1287–93.

31  Droz J-P, Culine S, Bouzy J *et al*. Preliminary results of a randomized trial comparing bleomycin, etoposide, cisplatin (BEP) and cyclophosphamide, doxorubicin, cisplatin/vinblastin, bleomycin (CISCA/VB) for patients (Pts) with intermediate- and poor-risk metastatic non seminomatous germ-cell tumors (NSGCT). In: *Proc Ann Meet Am Soc Clin Oncol* 2001;Abstr. 690.

32  Fosså SD, Kaye SB, Mead GM *et al.* Filgrastim during combination chemotherapy of patients with poor-prognosis metastatic germ cell malignancy. European Organization for Research and Treatment of Cancer, Genito-Urinary Group, and the Medical Research Council Testicular Cancer Working Party, Cambridge, United Kingdom. *J Clin Oncol* 1998;**16**:716–24.

33  Wozniak AJ, Samson MK, Shah NT *et al.* A randomized trial of cisplatin, vinblastine, and bleomycin versus vinblastine, cisplatin, and etoposide in the treatment of advanced germ cell tumors of the testis: A Southwest Oncology Group study. *J Clin Oncol* 1991;**9**:70–6.

34  Bosl GJ, Geller NL, Bajorin D *et al.* A randomized trial of etoposide + cisplatin versus vinblastine + bleomycin + cisplatin + cyclophosphamide + dactinomycin in patients with good-prognosis germ cell tumors. *J Clin Oncol* 1988;**6**:1231–8.

35  Horwich A, Mason M, Fosså SD *et al.* Accelerated induction chemotherapy (C-BOP-BEP) for poor and intermediate prognosis metastatic germ cell tumours (GCT). In: *Proc Ann Meet Am Soc Clin Oncol* 1997;Abstr. 1137.

36  Einhorn LH, Williams SD, Loehrer PJ *et al.* Evaluation of optimal duration of chemotherapy in favorable-prognosis disseminated germ cell tumors: a Southeastern Cancer Study Group protocol. *J Clin Oncol* 1989;**7**:387–91.

37  de Wit R, Roberts JT, Wilkinson PM *et al.* Equivalence of three or four cycles of bleomycin, etoposide, and cisplatin chemotherapy and of a 3- or 5-day schedule in good-prognosis germ cell cancer: a randomized study of the European Organization for Research and Treatment of Cancer Genitourinary Tract Cancer Cooperative Group and the Medical Research Council. *J Clin Oncol* 2001;**19**:1629–40.

38  Toner G, Stockler M. Comparison of two standard chemotherapy regimens for good prognosis germ cell tumours; a randomised trial. *Lancet* 2001;**357**:739–45.

39  Stockler M, Toner GC, Lewis C *et al.* Health-related quality of life (HRQL) in a randomised trial of two standard chemotherapy regimens for good-prognosis germ cell tumours: the ANZ germ cell trials group good prognosis trial. In: *Proc Ann Meet Am Soc Clin Oncol,* 2002.

40  O'Reilly SM, Rustin GJ, Smith DB, Newlands ES. Single agent activity of carboplatin in patients with previously untreated non-seminomatous germ cell tumours. *Ann Oncol* 1992;**3**:163–4.

41  Horwich A, Sleijfer DT, Fosså SD *et al.* Randomized trial of bleomycin, etoposide, and cisplatin compared with bleomycin, etoposide, and carboplatin in good-prognosis metastatic nonseminomatous germ cell cancer: a Multiinstitutional Medical Research Council/European Organization for Research and Treatment of Cancer Trial. *J Clin Oncol* 1997;**15**:1844–52.

42  Bokemeyer C, Kohrmann O, Tischler J *et al.* A randomized trial of cisplatin, etoposide and bleomycin (PEB) versus carboplatin, etoposide and bleomycin (CEB) for patients with "good-risk" metastatic non-seminomatous germ cell tumors. *Ann Oncol* 1996;**7**:1015–21.

43  Bajorin DF, Sarosdy MF, Pfister DG *et al.* Randomized trial of etoposide and cisplatin versus etoposide and carboplatin in patients with good-risk germ cell tumors: a multiinstitutional study. *J Clin Oncol* 1993;**11**:598–606.

44  Horwich A, Oliver RTD, Wilkinson PM *et al.* A Medical Research Council randomized trial of single agent carboplatin versus etoposide and cisplatin for advanced metastatic seminoma. *Br J Cancer* 2000;**83**:1623–9.

45  Clemm C, Bokemeyer C, Gerl A *et al.* Randomised trial comparing cisplatin/etoposide/ifosfamide with carboplatin monochemotherapy in patients with advanced metastatic seminoma. In: *Proc Ann Meet Am Soc Clin Oncol* 2000;Abstr. 1293.

46  Samson MK, Rivkin SE, Jones SE *et al.* Dose-response and dose-survival advantage for high versus low-dose cisplatin combined with vinblastine and bleomycin in disseminated testicular cancer – a Southwest Oncology Group Study. *Cancer* 1984;**53**:1029–35.

47  Ozols RF, Ihde DC, Linehan WM, Jacob J, Ostchega Y, Young RC. A randomized trial of standard chemotherapy *v* a high-dose chemotherapy regimen in the treatment of poor prognosis nonseminomatous germ-cell tumors. *J Clin Oncol* 1988;**6**:1031–40.

48  DeWys WD, Begg C, Slayton R, Hahn RG, Brodsky I. Chemotherapy for advanced germinal cell neoplasms: preliminary report of an Eastern Cooperative Oncology Group Study. *Cancer Treat Rep* 1979;**63**:1675–80.

49  Nichols CR, Williams SD, Loehrer PJ *et al.* Randomized study of cisplatin dose intensity in poor-risk germ-cell tumors – a Southeastern-Cancer-Study-Group and Southwest- Oncology-Group Protocol. *J Clin Oncol* 1991;**9**:1163–72.

50  Chevreau C, Droz JP, Pico JL *et al.* Early intensified chemotherapy with autologous bone-marrow transplantation in 1st line treatment of poor risk nonseminomatous germ-cell tumors – preliminary results of a French randomized trial. *Eur Urol* 1993;**23**:213–18.

51  Rosti G, Pico J-L, Wandt H *et al.* High-dose chemotherapy (HDC) in the salvage treatment of patients failing first-line platinum chemotherapy for advanced germ cell tumours (GCT); first results of a prospective randomised trial of the European Group for Blood and Marrow Transplantation (EBMT): IT-94. In: *Proc Ann Meet Am Soc Clin Oncol,* 2002.

52  Nazareth I LJ, King M. Sexual function after treatment for testicular cancer A systematic review. *J Psychosom Res* 2001;**51**:735–43.

53  Jonker-Pool G, Van de Wiel HB, Hoekstra HJ *et al.* Sexual functioning after treatment for testicular cancer-review and meta-analysis of 36 empirical studies between 1975–2000. *Arch Sex Behav* 2001;**30**:55–74.

54  Fosså S, Aass N, Winderen M, Börmer O. Long-term reduction of renal function (RF) in patients (Pts) with testicular cancer (TC). In: *Proc Ann Meet Am Soc Clin Oncol,* 2001;Abstr. 771.

55  Moynihan C, Bliss JM, Davidson J, Burchell L, Horwich A. Evaluation of adjuvant psychological therapy in patients with testicular cancer: randomised controlled trial. *BMJ* 1998;**316**:429–35.

# Section VII

## Treating gynaecological tumours

*David Guthrie, Editor*

# Levels of evidence and grades of recommendation used in *Evidence-based Oncology*

Levels of evidence and grades of recommendation appear within the text in the clinical chapters, for example, **Evidence Level Ia** and **Grade A**.

---

**Levels of evidence**

---

Ia   Meta-analysis of randomised controlled trials (RCTs)
Ib   At least 1 RCT
IIa   At least 1 non-randomised study
IIb   At least 1 other well designed quasi-experimental study
III   Non-experimental, descriptive studies
IV   Expert committee reports or opinions/experience of respected authorities

**Grades of recommendations**

---

A   At least one RCT as part of body of literature of overall good quality and consistency addressing recommendation **Evidence levels Ia, Ib**
B   No RCT but well conducted clinical studies available **Evidence levels IIa, IIb, III**
C   Expert committee reports or opinions/experience of respected authorities in the absence of directly applicable good quality clinical studies **Evidence level IV**

---

From *Clinical Oncology* (2001)**13**:S212
Source of data: MEDLINE, *Proceedings of the American Society of Medical Oncology* (ASCO).

# 35 Ovarian and fallopian tube cancers

*Paul A Vasey*

In the United Kingdom, cancer of the ovary is the fourth commonest malignancy, occuring in almost 7000 patients yearly (5%), and represents the commonest cause of death from gynaecologic malignancy and the fourth commonest cause of death from cancer in women.[1] The median age at diagnosis is 63 years and the incidence increases with age and peaks in the eighth decade. Between the age of 70 and 74 years the age-specific incidence is 57 cases/100 000 women per year.

The definitive diagnosis of epithelial ovarian cancer requires a surgical specimen, and pathological diagnosis should be made according to the WHO classification. Established subtypes are: serous, mucinous, endometrioid, clear cell, Brenner, mixed and undifferentiated carcinomas. Surgical staging requires a laparotomy with thorough examination of the abdominal cavity and, where possible, surgery should be performed by an experienced gynaecological oncologist **Evidence level III, Grade B** .

Fallopian tube cancer is the least common gynaecological malignancy and the pathological criteria for distinguishing these tumours from those of the ovary are imprecise. Chemotherapy experiences are limited to small series and case reports, and survival appears to be similar to that in patients with ovarian carcinomas following treatment with platinum-based regimens.[2] For this reason, treatment recommendations for ovarian and fallopian tube cancers are given collectively **Evidence level III, Grade B** .

## In the platinum-taxane era, is initial cytoreductive surgery of benefit in advanced ovarian cancer?

The theoretical benefits of cytoreductive surgery in ovarian cancer have been summarised by many authors[3] and include:

- more favourable growth kinetics owing to improved perfusion, with higher growth fraction being available to cell-cycle dependent cytotoxic drugs;
- removal of phenotypically resistant cells;
- prevention of complications arising from tumour bulk, for example bowel obstruction;
- enhancement of the immunological competence of the patient;
- psychological benefit of tumour resection.

Indirect evidence of a beneficial outcome for cytoreduction was first suggested in 1967 when Long reported improved survival for patients treated by radiotherapy and radical surgery compared with only oophorectomy and radiotherapy.[4] Among the first observational studies to document an outcome benefit for cytoreductive surgery was Griffiths' pivotal study in 1975, where the survival of 102 patients was shown to be related to the largest diameter of residual disease, with survival increasing as the volume of residuum decreased.[5] Since then, there have been many studies in which the effect of cytoreduction has been evaluated retrospectively within a trial of chemotherapy, but no directly comparative randomised trials have been designed to specifically address this issue. This is unfortunate, given that all non-randomised data will undoubtably be confounded by variables, such as the skill of the operating surgeon, choice of postoperative chemotherapy and subsequent treatments. Meta-analyses of many of these studies have described an outcome benefit for optimal cytoreduction, and the more recent analyses attempted to isolate the effect of surgery, controlling for platinum-based chemotherapy. Hunter *et al.* analysed 58 studies with 6962 patients and demonstrated a median survival benefit for maximum debulking surgery of 4·1% (95% CI −0·6–9·1).[6] However, this study included patients in the pretaxane and even some from the preplatinum era, and therefore many patients did not have access to what would now be considered optimal non-surgical therapies. This is demonstrated by a much larger effect of platinum chemotherapy compared with surgery in the same analysis (53%; 95% CI 35–73). Most recently, the results of another meta-analysis looking at the effects of cytoreductive surgery were presented at the 2001 American Society of Clinical Oncology (ASCO) meeting.[7] From studies identified from a MEDLINE literature search, 6885 patients were identified with FIGO stage III/IV ovarian cancer enrolled in 53 studies involving platinum-based chemotherapy. Parameters included the proportion in each cohort undergoing optimal cytoreductive surgery, the platinum dose intensity (mg m$^{-2}$ per week), the proportion of stage IV patients, the median age and the publication date. Simple and multiple linear regression analyses were used to assess the overall effects of such variables on survival. The results demonstrated that maximum or optimal cytoreductive surgery, as a primary procedure, correlated with log median survival, even when controlling for all other variables. Surgical procedures resulting in greater than 75% tumour cytoreduction – what specialist gynaecological oncologists could be expected to achieve – were associated with a weighted median survival time of 37 months compared with 23 months for cohorts with less than 25% cytoreduction, a difference of approximately 60%. Each 10% increase in cytoreduction achieved was associated with an increase in median survival of 6%, and these results were more or less consistent when multiple regression analysis was performed. It also emerged that neither platinum dose intensity or cumulative dose had any effect on log median survival time in either type of analysis – a finding correlating with other analyses of platinum dose intensity.[8] These results suggest that even with platinum-based chemotherapy, cytoreductive surgery is one of the most important and powerful determinants of survival.

In addition, it has been observed that, if stage IV patients are taken out of the Hunter analysis, there is further improvement in outcome for optimal surgery.[9] The effect of cytoreductive surgery in stage IV patients is not clear, but an overview of the published data for these patients suggests that a benefit from surgery may still accrue for certain patients with single sites of disease (for example, pleural cytology, single hepatic metastasis) and good organ function and performance status.[10]

## Can interval cytoreductive surgery improve outcomes for patients not maximally cytoreduced at initial operation and what is the best timing for interval cytoreduction?

Many patients are not maximally cytoreduced at primary surgery for various reasons (for example, skill of surgeon, tumour biology, comorbid medical problems). The ability of chemotherapy to produce significant cytoreduction was first noted in 1970,[11] and subsequently Lawton and colleagues demonstrated an ability to maximally chemically cytoreduce 75% of patients initially only suboptimally surgically cytoreduced.[12] Further evidence as to a potential benefit for this "interval surgery" was demonstrated by Neijt *et al.* in 1991.[13] Here, the survival of patients optimally cytoreduced at primary surgery was identical to that of patients treated by chemotherapy followed by interval surgery, which produced optimal cytoreduction. The European Organisation of Research and Treatment of Cancer (EORTC) Gynaecological Cancer Co-operative Group performed the only randomised trial on interval surgery published to date.[14] In this study, 319 women unable to be optimally

cytoreduced at primary surgery received three initial cycles of cisplatin-cyclophosphamide chemotherapy. Then, those women in whom no progressive disease was documented were randomised to either a further three cycles (N = 138), or an exploratory laparotomy with a view to cytoreduction (N = 138), followed by three more cycles of cisplatin-cyclophosphamide. A 33% (95% CI 10–50) reduction in risk of death at 2 years in the interval cytoreductive group was demonstrated, with significant improvements in progression-free and overall survival ($P = 0.01$). A further trial of interval debulking was carried out by the Gynecologic Oncology Group (GOG Protocol 152) between June 1994 and January 2001. This study utilised a paclitaxel-based regimen as initial chemotherapy, prior to interval surgical cytoreduction for patients suboptimally cytoreduced at first operation. The first results of this trial were presented in 2002[15]; 550 patients with suboptimally cytoreduced advanced stage ovarian cancer (predominantly FIGO stage IIIC) were randomised to receive three cycles of chemotherapy with paclitaxel-cisplatin (as per GOG 111) following initial surgery. Patients not progressing at this stage were then randomised either to continue with three further cycles, or to have a further attempt at debulking (interval debulking surgery/IDS), followed by three cycles of chemotherapy. Treatment arms were well balanced with respect to factors such as the type of surgeon (for example board certified gynaecologic oncologist), and compliance with randomised arm was equally balanced. The results, in contrast to the European study, demonstrated that patients randomised to IDS had a median progression-free survival of 10·5 months versus 10·8 months and likewise there were no differences in median survival with 32 months for the chemotherapy plus IDS arm compared with 33 months for those receiving chemotherapy alone. A similar trial in the UK, Medical Research Council (MRC) Trial OV06, has had problems with patient accrual, and is currently undergoing a redesign, in order to incorporate elements of the timing of such surgery and the extent of initial debulking (that is, differentiating true interval debulking from delayed primary surgery).

Neoadjuvant chemotherapy ("chemical cytoreduction") followed by definitive surgery has been offered to many patients thought to be either initially inoperable or a poor surgical risk, without any prospective randomised clinical trial demonstrating equivalent efficacy with the standard approach of primary surgery followed by chemotherapy. However, many retrospective studies have suggested that this is a feasible option for such patients, with encouraging survivorships.[16,17] The EORTC are conducting a study comparing neoadjuvant chemotherapy and "interval" debulking surgery – actually delayed primary surgery – with maximal initial debulking followed by chemotherapy in the standard fashion.

## Recommendations

- No prospective randomised trials have been performed to evaluate survival in optimal (< 1 cm) versus suboptimal (≥ 1 cm) debulked patients, and it is unethical now to perform such a study. There is overwhelming indirect evidence that cytoreduction is of benefit, a fact acknowledged by the US National Institutes of Health (NIH) in 1994 (NIH Consensus statement, 1994). An attempt should therefore be made at initial laparotomy to remove as much tumour as possible (maximum cytoreduction, aim for < 1 cm nodules) **Evidence level IIa, Grade B**.

- Women should have access to centres where surgical debulking can be performed by expert surgeons for whom optimal cytoreduction can be anticipated in at least 75% of patients **Evidence level III, Grade B**.

- One published randomised trial has shown that interval debulking surgery for patients not cytoreduced at primary surgery who respond after three courses of cisplatin-cyclophosphamide chemotherapy improves progression-free survival and overall survival. Although a further trial using paclitaxel-platinum chemotherapy did not confirm this finding, analysis of these trials suggests that the most likely reason for this discrepancy is that tumour biology and surgical skill are interlinked. If an initial attempt was made by an experienced surgeon, it may be that no further surgical intervention is likely to improve survival. A second attempt at cytoreduction should be considered after three cycles of chemotherapy in patients in whom optimal cytoreduction was not possible at initial surgery **Evidence level Ib, Grade A**.

- It is not clear whether a survival benefit can be shown for cytoreduction in FIGO stage IV patients, but consideration should be given to surgery in fit patients with limited metastatic sites **Evidence level III, Grade C**.

- Selected patients may benefit from neoadjuvant chemotherapy and delayed primary surgery, but randomised studies are needed to establish its role **Evidence level III, Grade B**.

## Is chemotherapy of value in early ovarian cancer?

Only approximately 20% patients with ovarian cancer present with early stage (FIGO I–IIA) disease, and studies evaluating the appropriate management strategy for this group have historically run into problems because of:

- slow recruitment
- lack of statistical power
- insufficient follow up because of infrequent recurrence
- inadequate surgical staging
- lack of a "no-treatment" control arm, and
- lack of proper pathological review processes.

Contamination of studies with occult stage III patients will make outcomes appear worse than actual, whereas contamination with "borderline" tumours will falsely enhance survival curves. Various independent prognostic factors have been identified which predict for relapse and survival, and a meta-analysis of five studies comprising 1545 patients with stage I ovarian cancer demonstrated that degree of differentiation was the strongest prognostic indicator of disease-free survival, followed by presurgical capsular rupture.[18] In addition, the importance of thorough staging procedures is highlighted by a report by Li *et al.*, wherein out of 91 patients thought to be stage I, bilateral abdominopelvic lymph node sampling demonstrated occult metastatic disease in 14 (15%).[19] However, many other factors are likely to be operational including DNA ploidy and newer markers such as *p53* and *VEGF*, but none have yet proven discriminatory or are able to drive treatment strategies and aid subgrouping into low or high risk categories. Most studies consistently define well-differentiated tumours without capsular extension (FIGO stage IA/B, G1) as low risk, as the 5-year survival is greater than 90%. There remains debate over what exactly constitutes high risk and what is the most appropriate treatment. The risk assignment of moderately well-differentiated (G2) histology is controversial. Generally accepted high risk features are capsular or pelvic extension (FIGO stages IC–II), clear cell histology, and poor differentiation (G3); the relapse rate for these patients is over 30%, and 5-year survival approximates 75%. Because of this poorer outcome, many clinicians choose to treat with the same chemotherapy as in advanced disease, although there are no data to define the appropriate drugs, doses or duration of treatment.

**Table 35.1   Five-year survival in early ovarian cancer. Results from Bolis *et al.*, 1995[20]**

**Intermediate risk (stage IA/B; G1/2)**

|  | Cisplatin (%) | No treatment (%) |
| --- | --- | --- |
| DFS | 83 | 64 |
| OS | 87 | 81 |

**High risk (stage IC)**

|  | Cisplatin | IP$^{32}$P |
| --- | --- | --- |
| DFS | 81 | 66 |
| OS | 81 | 79 |

Abbreviations: DFS, disease-free survival; OS, overall survival

**Table 35.2   Eligibility criteria for ICON1/ACTION trials**

| Trial | ICON1 | ACTION |
|---|---|---|
| Eligibility criteria | "Uncertain benefit" for adjuvant chemotherapy | FIGO IA–B, grades 2/3 |
| | | FIGO IC, IIA, all grades |
| | | FIGO I–IIA, all clear cell histology |

The importance of a no-treatment control group was highlighted in an Italian study,[20] which randomised 271 patients with stage I disease and categorised them into two groups, "intermediate risk" (stage I A/B; G1/2) or "high risk" (stage IC). Intermediate risk patients were randomised to either intravenous cisplatin chemotherapy, or no treatment, whereas high risk patients were treated with either cisplatin or intraperitoneal (IP) $^{32}$P, 15 mCi. The results are shown in Table 35.1. Overall survival was not affected in any arm, although there were improvements in disease-free survival for cisplatin over both no treatment and IP$^{32}$P.

Without a control group, if both treatments have the same outcome, the value of each therapy may be no better than no therapy, and treatment can be selected only on the basis of therapeutic index. Experience with IP $^{32}$P suggests an estimated 20% incidence of chronic bowel toxicity,[21] and, in addition, cisplatin can be shown to be associated with a risk of acute leukaemia, which may be as high as 5%. In this particular study, Gynecologic Study Group (GOG) 95, three cycles of cisplatin-cyclophosphamide were compared with IP $^{32}$P in patients with FIGO stage I/II and, although again there was a reduction in recurrence risk with chemotherapy (31%, $P = 0.08$), no difference in survival was observed. In addition, a recently completed GOG trial (GOG 157) has compared three cycles versus six cycles of carboplatin-paclitaxel chemotherapy. Results are awaited, but again the lack of a no-treatment control arm dilutes any conclusions to be made from this study, and there are no data defining specifically which agent(s) to use and how much to give in early stage disease. The same is true of the recently initiated GOG 175, which treats all patients with three cycles of carboplatin-paclitaxel, and then randomises to either no further treatment or 26 weeks of low dose paclitaxel. This means that half these women will receive nearly 1 year of treatment, without any clear clinical evidence base for adjuvant treatment with carboplatin-paclitaxel or continued exposure to "low doses" (with anti-angiogenic properties) of paclitaxel in this situation.

The EORTC and the MRC independently developed clinical trials designed to explore the role of adjuvant chemotherapy for early ovarian cancer patients. These studies were called ACTION (Adjuvant Treatment in Ovarian Neoplasm) and ICON1 (International Collaboration on Ovarian Neoplasms), and common to both trials was a surgery only and a surgery plus platinum-based chemotherapy arm. In ACTION, patients received either no therapy or at least four cycles of generally non-taxane-containing platinum chemotherapy, which was mainly cisplatin-cyclophosphamide. In ICON1, most patients randomised to chemotherapy received single agent carboplatin (and 80% received six cycles). For both studies, survival was to be the primary endpoint. Differences in eligibility (Table 35.2) between the two studies are evident; ACTION strictly defined "high risk" whereas ICON1 patients were entered on the principle that the randomising clinician was uncertain as to the benefit of adjuvant treatment in a particular patient. Recruitment to both trials was slow, and in June 1999, the steering groups agreed that the sample size combined across both trials could be reduced to 900 patients with approximately 450 patients to be recruited in each trial. This allowed a combined analysis providing sufficient events to detect an increase in absolute 3-year survival from 85% to 91% (with 90% power and 5% significance level).

The results of these trials, reporting on a combined total of 925 patients from both studies – making this easily the largest randomised trial in early stage disease to date – were published in January 2003.[22] The median follow up for the combined analysis was 5·5 years and compliance to treatment allocation was 94%. For relapse-free survival (RFS), there was an advantage for patients treated with chemotherapy whether the trials were analysed separately or together. Overall, there was an improvement in 5-year RFS of 11% (62–73%), with a $P$ value of 0·001. In addition, there was an improvement seen in overall survival in the combined analysis in favour of chemotherapy of 8% at 5 years ($P = 0.01$) making this the first study to demonstrate an effect of a treatment on survival in early stage ovarian cancer. Subgroup analysis failed to demonstrate any advantage or disadvantage for chemotherapy by age, stage, cell type, or grade. However, the comprehensiveness of surgical staging was found to be a significant prognostic factor for tumour recurrence in the observation arm, with stage being highly statistically significant ($P = 0.008$) in multivariate analysis in the ACTION trial.

When the data are analysed, it is evident that only approximately one in six patients could be said to have received adequate surgical staging. In the ACTION trial only 34% patients were properly staged, whereas the other 66% were deemed to have had non-optimal surgical procedures. The data collection on ICON 1 was insufficient to capture surgical staging details, but the incidence of optimal surgical staging in this study is unlikely to be any better.

The reason completeness of surgical staging is important emerges when the survival curves analysing the effect of chemotherapy in truly optimally staged patients are examined. In these patients, the benefits of adjuvant chemotherapy are less certain, with wide confidence intervals. There are probably too few events in this subgroup to state conclusively whether or not chemotherapy is of benefit to these patients.

What can we conclude from this combined analysis? The question as to whether chemotherapy is capable of "correcting" for suboptimal staging (by treating occult stage III disease) is suggested, but not answered by this analysis. The importance of these trials is that a significant survival benefit can been shown for adjuvant chemotherapy in early stage ovarian cancer, and therefore a strong argument can be put forward for offering all patients chemotherapy. The argument is less robust for patients optimally surgically staged; however, there are not enough events to conclude that there will definitely not be a benefit to this group also. Moreover, as over 75% of these patients can expect to be cured with surgery alone, late toxicities of chemotherapy (for example, second malignancies) must be considered.

## Recommendations

- Staging procedures in apparent early stage ovarian cancer should involve:

  - total abdominal hysterectomy and bilateral salpingo-oophorectomy
  - random omental and peritoneal biopsies, and
  - pelvic node sampling.

- Node sampling should also involve para-aortic nodes unless pelvic nodes are positive, and bilateral pelvic sampling unless ipsilateral pelvic nodes are positive **Evidence level Ib, Grade A**.
- All patients with early stage, high risk ovarian cancer should be considered for platinum-based chemotherapy **Evidence level Ib, Grade A**.
- The anticipated 5-year survival for properly staged "low risk" FIGO stage I ovarian cancer is > 90% and no study has shown any survival advantage with any form of postoperative therapy. These patients are likely to be surgically cured, and could be followed expectantly **Evidence level Ib, Grade A**.

## What is "standard chemotherapy" for advanced ovarian cancer in 2002?

An updated meta-analysis of first-line chemotherapy based on individual patient data by the Advanced Ovarian Cancer Trialists' Group has been published, succeeding a previous meta-analysis.[23] This analysis recruited 5667 patients in 37 randomised controlled trials. The main conclusions were:

- combination chemotherapy was associated with a better outcome compared with single agent, but results were not significant (hazard ratio 0·93; 95% CI 0·83–1·05; $P = 0·23$) producing a possible benefit in absolute survival of 25% to 28% at 5 years; and
- carboplatin is equivalent to cisplatin either in combination (hazard ratio 1·02; 95% CI 0·92–1·13; $P = 0·66$) or as single agents (hazard ratio 1·01; 95% CI 0·81–1·26; $P = 0·92$).

Further evidence that carboplatin is as efficacious as cisplatin in ovarian cancer comes from three prospective, randomised trials comparing cisplatin-paclitaxel with carboplatin-paclitaxel[24–26] (Table 35.3). Preliminary results from these studies suggest that there is no significant difference in outcome (AGO median progression-free survival 18 *v* 17 months; GOG 158 median time to progression 22 *v* 22 months; Danish–Dutch study 17 *v* 17 months). Overall survival is not mature for the larger studies, but early analysis suggests a trend to improved overall survival in GOG 158 for the carboplatin-paclitaxel arm. Toxicities certainly favour carboplatin-paclitaxel.

The taxane era began in the mid 1990s with the publication of GOG trial 111, which demonstrated a significant survival advantage for the combination of cisplatin and paclitaxel in patients suboptimally debulked, compared with the previous standard treatment, cyclophosphamide and cisplatin.[27] Since then, there have been three further reported prospective randomised trials that have tested a combination of platinum and paclitaxel versus platinum (not incorporating paclitaxel) -based chemotherapy (Table 35.4).

Trial OV.10 essentially replicated the results from GOG 111, with regard to all efficacy parameters (response rates, progression-free survival, overall survival), despite a different patient population in that a third of patients in OV.10 had optimally debulked disease, compared with none in GOG 111.[28] In addition, trial OV.10 gave a 3-hour infusion of 175 mg m$^{-2}$ paclitaxel compared with a 24-hour infusion of 135 mg m$^{-2}$ in trial GOG 111. High levels of neurotoxicity were evident in the European trial, suggesting that the combination of a 3-hour infusion of paclitaxel with cisplatin should not be used.

**Table 35.3  Cisplatin versus carboplatin in combination with paclitaxel**

| Trial | No. of patients | Inclusion | Comparison | Median PFS (months) |
|---|---|---|---|---|
| Danish–Dutch[24] | 196 | IIb–IV Any | Cisplatin 75 mg m$^{-2}$ + paclitaxel 175 mg m$^{-2}$ q3 h | 17 |
| | | | v | |
| | | | carboplatin AUC 5 + paclitaxel 175 mg m$^{-2}$/3 h | 17 |
| AGO[25] | 776 | IIb–IV Any | Cisplatin 75 mg m$^{-2}$ + paclitaxel 185 mg m$^{-2}$/3 h | 18 |
| | | | v | |
| | | | Carboplatin AUC 6 + paclitaxel 185 mg m$^{-2}$ q3 h | 17 |
| GOG 158[26] | 840 | III < 1 cm | Cisplatin 75 mg m$^{-2}$ + paclitaxel 135 mg m$^{-2}$ q24 h | 22 |
| | | | v | |
| | | | Carboplatin AUC 7·5 + paclitaxel 175 mg m$^{-2}$ q3 h | 22 |

Abbreviation: PFS, progression-free survival

**Table 35.4  First-line prospective randomised trials of paclitaxel-platinum versus platinum-based (non-paclitaxel)**

| Comparison | Trial | No. of patients | Reference | Result |
|---|---|---|---|---|
| Paclitaxel 135 mg m$^{-2}$ q24 h + cisplatin 75 mg m$^{-2}$ v Cytoxan 750 mg m$^{-2}$ + cisplatin 75 mg m$^{-2}$ | GOG 111 | 410 | 27 | PFS and OS favours paclitaxel arm |
| Paclitaxel 175 mg m$^{-2}$ q3 h + cisplatin 75 mg m$^{-2}$ v Cytoxan 750 mg m$^{-2}$ + cisplatin 75 mg m$^{-2}$ | OV.10 | 680 | 28 | PFS and OS favours paclitaxel arm |
| Paclitaxel 135 mg m$^{-2}$ q24 h + Cisplatin 75 mg m$^{-2}$ v Cisplatin 100 mg m$^{-2}$ v Paclitaxel 200 mg m$^{-2}$ | GOG 132 | 424 | 29 | No difference in OS all three arms |
| Carboplatin AUC 5/6 + paclitaxel 175 mg m$^{-2}$ q3 h v Carboplatin AUC 5/6 or CAP* | ICON 3 | 2074 | 30 | No difference in PFS or OS |

*Cisplatin 50 mg m$^{-2}$ + adriamycin 50 mg m$^{-2}$ + cytoxan 500 mg m$^{-2}$; centres could choose whether to use CAP or carboplatin as control arm.
Abbreviations: OS, overall survival; PFS, progression-free survival

Another study, trial GOG 132, randomised paclitaxel-cisplatin against either single agent paclitaxel or cisplatin.[29] No difference was demonstrated between the three treatment arms with respect to overall survival, but it was evident that a significant proportion of patients crossed over to the other treatments prior to clinical progression, and therefore essentially received a form of sequential chemotherapy. However, the paclitaxel-cisplatin combination was preferred by the investigators owing to decreased overall toxicity and duration of therapy.

The International Collaborative Ovarian Neoplasm group (ICON3) study randomised 2074 patients to either paclitaxel-carboplatin, single agent carboplatin or the combination cisplatin-adriamycin-cyclophosphamide (CAP).[30] These two control arms were allowed because the mature results of trial ICON2[31] showed no differences in progression-free survival or overall survival between carboplatin and CAP. ICON3 was essentially run as four parallel trials, with four independent randomisation centres. Ratios differed between these four groups, with the MRC and Italian centres randomising 2:1 in favour of the control arm, while the Swiss and Nordic groups randomised 1:1. With data secure to 3 years, no convincing differences in progression-free survival or overall survival are evident. The absolute difference in 2-year overall survival is 1% in favour of paclitaxel-carboplatin, and no statistically significant differences were found between subgroups defined by age, stage, residuum, histological grade or histology, randomisation group, number of patients entered by a centre, or choice of control arm (Parmar, personal communication).

These apparently contradictory results are the subject of much discussion internationally. There is debate as to whether the sequential administration of platinum and paclitaxel prior to progression is responsible for the similar overall survival for all three arms in GOG 132. Of patients initially randomised to single agent cisplatin, 48% received some form of additional chemotherapy before progression (mostly given as "consolidation" after an incomplete response to six cycles of initial chemotherapy); 32% received paclitaxel in this way. In the paclitaxel-only arm, which demonstrated inferiority (based on response rates and progression-free survival) in comparison with the two cisplatin-containing arms, 50% received additional treatment before progression; 48% receiving cisplatin. This study is widely interpreted as a comparison of sequential single agents versus their combination, although it was clearly not designed with this in mind.

ICON3 has been criticised for the non-random allocation of the control arm, the different ratios of randomisation across the randomisation groups, and the presence of > 20% early stage disease patients. Furthermore, a trend of decreased overall survival (not progression-free survival) for centres treating fewer patients (the majority, $P = 0.05$) (Parmar, personal communication) has emerged. It has also been suggested that a more rigorous examination, or formal audit, of the ICON3 data is required, in order for the data to be comparable with GOG studies, and also of the EORTC trials, some of which are also audited. However, the ICON3 Independent Trial Steering Committee have reviewed the data carefully and have concluded an audit is unnecessary because an existing systematic bias of overwhelming scale would be required to change the results, and this was considered to be virtually inconceivable.

ICON3 is an important trial, and the simple fact that over 2000 patients were randomised in a prospective manner is a very powerful argument for its validity. Certainly, the control arm survivorship for single agent carboplatin of 36 months is comparable with any other treatment outcomes for this heterogeneous patient mix, and this may be the most pertinent feature of this analysis. As suggested by Parmar and colleagues (personal communication, unpublished), the fact that the single agent platinum arms of ICON3 and GOG 132 gave overall survival equal to the combination of platinum-paclitaxel, and superior to that of the combination cisplatin-cyclophosphamide in both GOG 111 and OV.10 (Table 35.5) makes a strong case for platinum monotherapy being the most appropriate control arm for randomised studies. The fact that many patients receiving carboplatin in ICON3 were able to receive individualised "dose-tailoring" may indeed have contributed to their excellent outcome. Although such cross-trial comparisons are fraught with difficulties in interpretation, the possibility of an inadequate control arm in GOG 111 and OV.10 is very intriguing. Many of these points will be discussed in the definitive publication of ICON3; however, the ICON3 collaborators have emphasised that paclitaxel should remain an important option at some stage of the patient journey.

As a potential alternative to paclitaxel, docetaxel (Taxotere) has demonstrated single agent efficacy at least equivalent to paclitaxel, with an overall response rate of 28% in 155 platinum-refractory ovarian cancer patients.[32] There is documented activity in ovarian cancer patients who have failed prior paclitaxel,[33] and moreover, docetaxel is generally delivered as a convenient 1-hour infusion, suitable for outpatient administration. Phase II trials of docetaxel-carboplatin have been performed, demonstrating activity and safety,[34,35] and early results of a randomised trial comparing this regimen with paclitaxel-carboplatin has been presented.[36] This trial (Scottish Randomised Trial in Ovarian Cancer; SCOTROC) demonstrated differences in toxicity between the two regimens, with more neurotoxicity seen in paclitaxel-carboplatin, and more myelosuppression in docetaxel-carboplatin ($P < 0.001$). Although mature survival data are awaited, these regimens appear to be equally efficacious.

**Table 35.5    Control arms: median survival (months)**

| Parameter | GOG 111 | OV.10 | ICON3 | GOG 132 |
|-----------|---------|-------|-------|---------|
| PFS | 12·9 | 11·5 | 16·2 | 16·4 |
| OS | 24·4 | 25·9 | 36·0 | 30·2 |

Abbreviations: OS, overall survival; PFS, progression-free survival

The incorporation of a new, potentially non-cross-resistant agent into first-line therapy can give rise to greater toxicity resulting in dose reductions of other active agents. Furthermore, scheduling all agents in the most effective way is often not straightforward. Currently, there are no data supporting the routine incorporation of additional agents into the first-line treatment of ovarian cancer. The results of two large meta-analyses (from the AOCTG and OCMP groups) using data from over 1700 untreated patients demonstrated that the addition of an anthracycline to platinum chemotherapy (not containing taxanes) significantly improved survival (HR 0·85; $P = 0·003$).[37] However, four randomised trials comparing cisplatin-cyclophosphamide with and without doxorubicin did not separately demonstrate a convincing survival advantage for the addition of the anthracycline,[38–41] but when the data were combined in a meta-analysis, they showed a statistically significant 7% increase in overall survival at 6 years in favour of the addition of the anthracycline.[42] In addition, the ICON2 trial showed no difference in time to progression or overall survival when single agent carboplatin was compared with CAP and, as anticipated, toxicity was greater for the anthracycline-containing regimen.

The Arbeitsgemeinschaft Gynakologische Onkologie (AGO) group have now completed a randomised trial comparing carboplatin-paclitaxel (TC) with carboplatin-paclitaxel-epirubicin (TEC) as first-line treatment for FIGO stages IIB–IV ovarian cancer[43]: 1281 patients were randomised, and there was no difference in response rates between TEC and TC (75% *v* 69%; $P = 0·122$). For survival, no apparent differences between TEC and TC for progression-free survival (18 months *v* 17 months, $P = 0·104$) were noted and, although overall survival data were relatively immature, no differences were apparent for suboptimally debulked or stage IV patients (28 *v* 26 months; $P = 0·565$). There was a trend to an improvement in patients optimally surgically cytoreduced and not with stage IV disease (26 *v* 21 months; $P = 0·064$). The three-drug combination produced a markedly higher myelotoxicity (grade 3/4 neutropenia 74% *v* 54% $P < 0·001$), which produced an increased demand on supportive care, more dose reductions, and treatment delays. In addition, this arm

was associated with more emesis (10% *v* 4%; $P < 0·001$). The triple therapy of gemcitabine-paclitaxel-carboplatin produced a response rate of 100% (CR 60%; PR 40%) in 25 evaluable previously treated ovarian cancer patients, but produced grade IV haematological toxicity in most patients, and many dose reductions were required.[44]

Although such triple drug combinations have the advantage of exposing all tumours to the three agents simultaneously, thereby theoretically abrogating the emergence of drug-resistant clones, doses of the most important agent – in this case, platinum – are often compromised by myelosuppression and other toxicities, which result in both dose delays and dose reductions. One alternative is to administer sequential or alternating doublets for as many as eight cycles of treatment – this potentially retains the concept of preventing drug resistance while introducing new agents in a less toxic way. A five arm, prospective randomised trial is in progress by the SWOG, GOG, EORTC and NCIC groups, with an accrual goal of over 5000 patients. This study, GOG 182, is comparing

- four cycles of gemcitabine-carboplatin followed by four cycles of paclitaxel-carboplatin versus
- eight cycles of liposomal doxorubicin/paclitaxel/carboplatin versus
- four cycles of topotecan-carboplatin followed by four cycles of paclitaxel-carboplatin versus
- eight cycles of gemcitabine-paclitaxel-carboplatin versus
- eight cycles of paclitaxel-carboplatin (control arm).

### Recommendations

- Suitable alternatives for the first-line chemotherapy for advanced ovarian cancer are six courses of carboplatin plus paclitaxel **Evidence level Ib, Grade A** or carboplatin as a single agent **Evidence level Ib, Grade A**. Carboplatin plus docetaxel may also be a viable alternative, but mature survival results are awaited. Cisplatin-paclitaxel could also be considered, but paclitaxel must be given by 24-hour infusion because of the increased neurotoxicity.

- To date, there is no evidence base for the off-protocol addition of a third drug to a concurrent combination of a platinum analogue and a taxane in first-line chemotherapy of ovarian cancer. Many randomised trials are in progress, and results are eagerly awaited.

## Does intraperitoneal chemotherapy have a place in the treatment of ovarian cancer?

Direct administration of cytotoxic agents into the peritoneal cavity is a strategy designed to enhance locoregional drug delivery to tumours assumed to be confined there, whilst concurrently reducing dose-limiting toxicities normally associated with systemic use. This method of administration allows concentrations many times higher than would be tolerated in the systemic circulation to be attained at the site of the tumour, and can easily exceed concentrations shown *in vitro* to be required to overcome clinical drug resistance. It has been also demonstrated *in vitro* for many cytotoxic agents that the size of their therapeutic effect is both time- and concentration-dependent. Link *et al.*,[45] using two human colorectal carcinoma cell lines, demonstrated that the cytotoxicity of drugs such as 5-fluorouracil, cisplatin and anthracyclines could be significantly increased with higher concentrations and longer exposure times. However, the problem with extrapolating these studies to the clinical situation lies with the capability to deliver the drug in high therapeutic concentrations into tumour nodules. Using rat peritoneal tumour nodules, Los *et al.* compared the concentration of cisplatin at the periphery of the tumour ($\le 1 \cdot 5$ mm from tumour surface) with the concentration of cisplatin at the centre of the tumour, following both intravenous and intraperitoneal administration. Cisplatin was shown to be present at higher concentration at the tumour periphery when given

intraperitoneally, but there was no difference in the concentration at the tumour centre for both intraperitoneal and intravenous administration.[46] This work suggested that any major therapeutic benefit from intraperitoneal delivery was likely to be restricted to small tumour nodules.

Two sufficiently large prospective randomised trials investigating the benefits of intraperitoneal chemotherapy in maximally cytoreduced ovarian cancer have been published (Table 35.6). The first study, reported in 1996, randomised 546 eligible patients cytoreduced to $\le 2$ cm to receive six cycles of intravenous cytoxan 600 mg m$^{-2}$ in combination with either intravenous or intraperitoneal cisplatin 100 mg m$^{-2}$.[47] Patients obtaining a complete remission underwent a second-look laparotomy. Surgically defined complete responses were seen in 47% in the intraperitoneal arm and 36% in the intravenous arm. Toxicity was reduced for patients receiving intraperitoneal cisplatin, and survival was significantly better for this group (49 months *v* 41 months; $P < 0 \cdot 02$).

In the second study, 462 evaluable patients with disease surgically cytoreduced to $\le 1$ cm were randomised to six cycles of the GOG 111 protocol of intravenous cisplatin 75 mg m$^{-2}$ and paclitaxel 135 mg m$^{-2}$ every 24 hours, or a regimen consisting of two cycles of intravenous carboplatin AUC 9 followed by six cycles of intraperitoneal cisplatin 75 mg m$^{-2}$ and intravenous paclitaxel 135 mg m$^{-2}$.[48] This research arm was significantly more toxic, with approximately one-fifth of patients actually receiving up to two cycles of intraperitoneal cisplatin, largely because of persistent toxicity from carboplatin. Despite this, median progression-free survival favoured the intraperitoneal arm (28 months *v* 22 months; $P = 0 \cdot 01$), as did overall survival (63 months *v* 52 months; $P = 0 \cdot 05$).

Taken at face value, these trials seem to indicate that the new standard of care for optimally cytoreduced ovarian

**Table 35.6** Randomised trials of intraperitoneal versus intravenous chemotherapy

| Trial | No. of patients and size of tumour | Regimens | Overall survival |
|---|---|---|---|
| 1[47] | 546 $\le 2$ cm | Intravenous cisplatin 100 mg m$^{-2}$ + intravenous cytoxan 600 mg m$^{-2}$ *v* intraperitoneal cisplatin 100 mg m$^{-2}$ + intravenous cytoxan 600 mg m$^{-2}$ | 41 *v* 49 months; $P < 0 \cdot 02$ |
| 2[48] | 462 $\le 1$ cm | Intravenous cisplatin 75 mg m$^{-2}$ + intravenous paclitaxel 135 mg m$^{-2}$ *v* intravenous carboplatin AUC 9 + intraperitoneal cisplatin 75 mg m$^{-2}$ + intravenous paclitaxel 135 mg m$^{-2}$ | 63 *v* 52 months; $P = 0 \cdot 05$ |

**Table 35.7** Trials examining duration of first-line chemotherapy

| Trial | No. of patients | Regimens/cycles |
|---|---|---|
| MSKCC[50] | 84 | Cisplatin 100 mg m$^{-2}$ + adriamycin 40 mg m$^{-2}$ + cytoxan 600 mg m$^{-2}$ 5 *v* 10 |
| DACOVA[51] | 202 | Cisplatin 60 mg m$^{-2}$ + adriamycin 40 mg m$^{-2}$ + cytoxan 500 mg m$^{-2}$ 6 *v* 12 |
| North Thames[61] | 233 | Cisplatin 75 mg m$^{-2}$ or carboplatin 400 mg m$^{-2}$ 5 *v* 8 |

cancer patients should be intraperitoneal chemotherapy. However, this is not yet the case. In trial 1, accrual was extended to include more patients with residuum ≤ 0·5 cm, the investigators rationalising that this group would benefit most from intraperitoneal chemotherapy. Counterintuitively, there turned out to be no statistically significant survival benefit for this group. In addition, as the intravenous cisplatin-cytoxan combination has been shown to be inferior to cisplatin-paclitaxel in two randomised studies in both suboptimal (GOG 111) and optimal patients (mix in OV.10), it is not considered an appropriate control arm from which to gauge any new therapy.

Trial 2 suffers from a number of design flaws, not least of which is the fact that delivering two cycles of carboplatin at AUC 9 in addition to six cycles of cisplatin-paclitaxel adds a longer duration of chemotherapy and increased cumulative dose of platinum, thus unbalancing the trial in favour of the research arm, irrespective of the mode of administration. In addition, timing of salvage therapies is not known, and may have influenced the progression-free survival endpoint if administered before progression (and salvage therapies are also likely to have influenced overall survival, and were not controlled). Furthermore, both haematological and non-haematological toxicities were worse in the research arm.

Despite these caveats, the positive results of both trials require that a proper, "correct" study be conducted to once and for all demonstrate whether intraperitoneal therapy has a role in the management of optimally debulked ovarian cancer. GOG Protocol 172 randomised patients cytoreduced to ≤ 1 cm residual disease to receive either six cycles of intravenous cisplatin plus intravenous paclitaxel as per the GOG 111 Protocol or a research arm of six cycles of a three-weekly regimen consisting of intravenous paclitaxel 135 mg m$^{-2}$ (day 1), intraperitoneal cisplatin 100 mg m$^{-2}$ (day 2) and intraperitoneal paclitaxel 80 mg m$^{-2}$ (day 8). The study was powered to detect a 50% increase in progression-free survival.

At the American Society of Clinical Oncology (ASCO) meeting in 2002, data were presented on 416 randomised and eligible patients, and 213 out of 208 required events were available.[49] The intraperitoneal research arm was significantly more toxic, with greater grade 3–4 metabolic, infection, neurologic and GI toxicities. In addition, more haematologic toxicity was also present with more thrombocytopenia and neutropenia. Despite this, the intraperitoneal regimen was feasible and there was a significant advantage in progression-free survival for intraperitoneal chemotherapy (24 *v* 19 months, $P = 0·029$, one-tailed test, hazard ratio 0·73). This advantage also persisted for patients with gross residual disease (21 *v* 16 months). No data for progression-free survival for the subgroup with truly microscopic residual disease were available, and in addition, no data on overall survival were available.

Despite the lack of overall survival data for GOG 172, it is difficult to completely dismiss the fact that there are now three consecutive phase III trials that have all documented outcome advantages for intraperitoneal therapy. However, it is evident that the increased organ toxicities with the intraperitoneal research arm reflect a significant contribution from the systemic administration of chemotherapy.

### Recommendations

- Intraperitoneal chemotherapy in ovarian cancer remains investigational and should not be routinely administered outside of a research protocol **Evidence level Ib, Grade A** .

### How many cycles of chemotherapy are required after primary cytoreductive surgery?

Three randomised trials have been reported, which examined the duration of chemotherapy (that is, different

**Table 35.8  Randomised trials of increased platinum dose intensity**

| Study reference [ ] and year ( ) | Drug | Patient selection | No. of eligible patients | Regimen | Higher cumulative platinum dose | Dose intensity | Overall response | Median survival | Comments |
|---|---|---|---|---|---|---|---|---|---|
| [52] (1989) | C | Unclear | 65 | 120 v 60 mg m$^{-2}$ q3–4wk | Yes, ×2 | ×2 | 55 v 30 | 60% v 30% at 3 years | Significantly increased myelotoxicity in HD arm |
| [53] (1995) | C (+cyclo) | Bulky, suboptimal | 485 | 100 v 50 mg m$^{-2}$ q3wk | No | ×2 | 55 v 60 | 21·3 v 19·5 months | No difference, also increased cyclophosphamide dose intensity |
| [54] (1996) | C | IC–IV | 165 | 100 v 50 mg m$^{-2}$ q3wk | Yes, ×2 | ×2 | 61 v 34 | 28·5 v 17·5 months | Significant difference in median survival but overall survival 32% v 27% |
| [55] (1993) | C | III/IV | 306 | 75 mg m$^{-2}$ q3 ×6 v 50 mg m$^{-2}$ q3wk ×8 | No | ×2 | 66 v 61 | 36 v 33 months | No difference |
| [56] (1997) | Cb | II–IV | 222 | AUC 8 v 4 | Yes, ×2 | ×2 | 16 v 15 (CR) | 19 v 19 months | No difference |
| [57] (1998) | Cb | II–IV | 241 | AUC 12 v 6 | Yes, ×1·22 | ×2 | 63 v 57 | 34 v 31% at 5 years | No difference plus greater toxicity in HD |
| [58] (1983) | C | III/IV | 56 | 100 mg m$^{-2}$ q4wk × v 50 mg m$^{-2}$ q3wk ×6 | No | ×1·5 | 86 v 75 | 27·5 v 23·5 months | Not significant, combination with cyclo and doxorubicin |
| [59] (1994) | C | III/IV | 101 | 100 mg m$^{-2}$ q3wk ×6 v 100 mg m$^{-2}$ q1wk ×6 (5 wk between wk 3 and 4) | No | ×2 | 69 v 65 | 31% v 13% at 4 years | Significant difference in survival maintained at 8 years |

(Continued)

**Table 35.8** *(Continued)*

| Study reference [ ] and year ( ) | Drug | Patient selection | No. of eligible patients | Regimen | Higher cumulative platinum dose | Dose intensity | Overall response | Median survival | Comments |
|---|---|---|---|---|---|---|---|---|---|
| [60] (1996) | C | Bulky, residual | 133 | 50 mg m$^{-2}$ q4wk × 6 v 100 mg m$^{-2}$ q4wk | Yes, × 2 | × 2 | 57 v 61 | 29 v 24 months | No difference combination with cyclo and epirubicin PFS 18 v 13 months |
| [61] (1997) | C/Cb | III/IV | 233 | 75/400 mg m$^{-2}$ q4wk × 5 v 75/400 mg m$^{-2}$ q4wk × 8 | Yes, × 1·6 | × 1 | – | 24 v 24 months | No difference |

Abbreviations: AUC, area under curve; C, cisplatin; Cb, carboplatin; CR, complete response; HD, higher dose; PFS, progression-free survival

number of cycles) in advanced ovarian cancer[50,51,61] (Table 35.7). None of these studies demonstrated a difference in median survival, but longer durations were associated with more toxicity, especially neuropathy.

Any discussion regarding the duration of chemotherapy in ovarian cancer needs to include the possible impact of dose intensity and cumulative dose on outcome. Ten published randomised prospective trials of platinum dose intensification not requiring colony-stimulating factor support are shown in Table 35.8.[52–61] It is clear from these trials that increasing the dose intensity of platinum two-fold – a level achievable without resort to myelogenous growth factor support or incurring unacceptable toxicities – is only of limited long-term benefit in the chemotherapy of advanced ovarian cancer. Indeed, within this range of dose intensity the total dose of platinum may be at least as important a factor in determining outcome. In the 10 studies described here, eight had a planned two-fold increase in dose intensity of cisplatin or carboplatin, but only three demonstrated a beneficial outcome for this therapeutic manoeuvre. Interestingly, two out of these three studies[52,54] had actually also administered a significantly increased total cumulative dose of platinum to the patients randomised to the high dose arm, suggesting that the relative dose intensity of platinum in itself may not be the major determinant of treatment response, but that the total dose actually received could be at least as important. This may not necessarily be the case if higher levels of dose intensification are achieved and, although this should be the subject of further trials, the advent of the taxane era is unlikely to allow this to happen.

It is now feasible to safely deliver four- or five-fold increases in dose (of carboplatin) compared to conventional doses using myeloprotective peripheral blood stem cells, and an important issue will therefore be the number of very high dose treatments given. As mentioned, the *in vitro* models would predict that these are the levels of dose intensification that will be required for platinum compounds if a meaningful impact on drug resistance is to be made. Moreover, further preclinical work has indicated that in order to overcome relative drug resistance *in vitro*, drug concentrations need to be in excess of five-fold higher than the usual cytotoxic range.[62] Extrapolation to the clinical situation suggests that, if the benefit from dose intensification lies in circumventing drug resistance, then dose escalations of this magnitude may also be required. As usual, large, adequately powered randomised clinical trials are needed to evaluate this approach fully and, until results are available, high dose chemotherapy should remain investigational.

Finally, randomised clinical trials investigating the duration of chemotherapy following the attainment of a complete response to initial platinum-based chemotherapy

**Table 35.9  Effect of platinum-free interval on response rate[65]**

| Platinum-free interval (months) | No. of patients | Overall response rate (%) |
|---|---|---|
| 5–12 | 51 | 27 |
| 12–24 | 29 | 33 |
| >24 | 46 | 59 |

are currently being analysed. One trial (AGO-GINECO study OVAR-7) entered over 1300 patients with FIGO IIB–IV disease and randomised those in complete radiological and biochemical remission after six cycles of paclitaxel-carboplatin to either four cycles of topotecan or observation. First results are expected in 2003. GOG Protocol 178/SWOG 9701 randomised patients achieving a complete response to five to six cycles of carboplatin-paclitaxel at standard doses to further cycles of paclitaxel 175 mg m$^{-2}$ given four-weekly for either 3 or 12 months. The primary endpoint, progression-free survival, was achieved early in 2001, after a planned interim efficacy analysis was reported by the data monitoring committee.[63] With 54 events – 34 in the 3-month arm and 20 in the 12-month arm – a statistically significant difference in PFS was observed at 28 versus 21 months ($P = 0.0035$, one-sided; adjusted Cox model analysis $P = 0.0023$). The hazard ratio was 2·31 with 99% CI of 1·08–4·94. The study was therefore closed with 262 randomised and eligible patients. At the time of this analysis, a secondary endpoint, overall survival, did not demonstrate a similar advantage, although with only 17 deaths on the trial in total – eight on the 3-month arm, nine on 12-month arm, $P = 0.63/0.7$ unadjusted/adjusted – robust conclusions are impossible to draw. With regard to toxicity, overall reported levels by NCIC-CTC grades were considered acceptable. Despite this significant advantage in progression-free survival for 1 year of monthly paclitaxel, this trial has not so far achieved widespread adoption and continues to be hotly debated. Confirmatory studies are needed before such approaches are adopted as standard treatment.

## Recommendations

- The evidence from studies using platinum-based (non-taxane-containing) chemotherapy demonstrates that there is no benefit from continuing chemotherapy beyond six cycles **Evidence level Ib, Grade A**. Until the mature results of ongoing trials examining longer duration of therapy are reported, six cycles remains the standard of care.

## How effective is salvage chemotherapy?

Despite the initial chemosensitivity of ovarian cancer, and a high rate of complete responses to first-line treatment, up to 70% of patients suffer recurrences. Unfortunately, few if any of these patients are cured with current "salvage" chemotherapeutic agents, and therefore the underlying principle of chemotherapy in this situation is that all treatment is given with palliative intent.

In general, chemotherapeutic options for relapsed disease falls into one of three categories:

- single agent platinum retreatment
- platinum combinations
- non-platinum-based treatments.

The response rates to chemotherapy in recurrent disease were first noted to be related to the "treatment-free interval" by Blackledge in 1989.[64] Patients with a treatment-free interval of less than 6 months were found to have a response rate of around 10%, compared with a rate of around 90% for patients relapsing more than 18 months after first-line treatment. This finding was confirmed for platinum chemotherapy by Markman and colleagues in 1991[65] (Table 35.9).

In addition to this treatment-free interval, other factors have been identified and associated with a better outcome for relapsed patients. In a multivariate analysis of 704 individual patient data, Eisenhauer and colleagues[66] identified three independent factors predictive for response:

- number of disease sites (< 2 or > 2)
- maximum diameter of largest metastasis/recurrent lesion (< 5 cm or > 5 cm)
- histology (serous *v* others).

Treatment-free interval (< 6 months or > 6 months) was noted to correlate with tumour size.

The use of cisplatin- or carboplatin-based chemotherapy to "rechallenge" potentially chemosensitive disease (for example, response to first-line chemotherapy, treatment-free interval > 18 months) will therefore have an anticipated response rate of over 50%. Late relapsed ovarian cancer such as this is occasionally treated by surgery, but its role in this situation is not clear. There is reason to believe that the longer the disease-free interval after primary therapy the better the survival after secondary cytoreduction. Furthermore, although most reports are from small series, there is generally thought to be a clinical benefit if the disease is cytoreduced, in a salvage setting, to ≤ 2 cm.[67-69] However, in practice, most gynaecological oncologists limit such surgery to patients with a potentially resectable pelvic mass. No randomised trials have yet been reported in this setting,

**Table 35.10  Activity of non-platinum agents in recurrent ovarian cancer***

| Treatment | No. of studies | No. of patients | ORR (%) |
|---|---|---|---|
| Paclitaxel[†] | 12 | 1580 | 22 |
| Topotecan[†] | 10 | 882 | 17 |
| Caelyx[†](Doxil) | 4 | 428 | 18 |
| Altretamine[†] | 6 | 235 | 18 |
| Etoposide | 7 | 234 | 22 |
| Gemcitabine | 6 | 181 | 18 |
| Docetaxel | 4 | 166 | 31 |
| Epirubicin | 6 | 132 | 14 |
| Oxaliplatin | 3 | 118 | 23 |
| Vinorelbine | 2 | 71 | 23 |

*Table from Gore, 2001 with permission.[72]
[†]Licensed in UK for second-line use (also: treosulfan, chlorambucil).
ORR, overall response rate.

although there is an ongoing European Trial called LAROCSON (Late Relapse Ovarian Cancer Surgery Or Not), which may provide some guidance in this area.

In phase II studies, combination chemotherapy is generally associated with higher response rates than single agents, but toxicities are greater. Rose and colleagues have reported a response rate of 89% for carboplatin-paclitaxel in 25 patients who relapsed a median of 10 months from first-line cisplatin-paclitaxel therapy.[70] However, robust evidence for a survival benefit from this approach is lacking. Bolis and colleagues recently reported the results of a randomised trial comparing single agent carboplatin 300 mg m$^{-2}$ with the same dose of carboplatin plus epirubicin 120 mg m$^{-2}$ in 190 patients with potentially platinum-sensitive recurrent disease.[71] This study demonstrated that carboplatin-epirubicin was associated with increased haematological and non-haematological toxicity, but no statistically significant improvement in progression-free survival or overall survival (3 years) compared with carboplatin monotherapy. This trial was statistically underpowered, as the patient numbers were only sufficient to detect a difference of 20% in response, this being used as a surrogate for survival. Further, larger randomised studies addressing this relevant clinical issue are required, which should include endpoints such as quality of life to ensure that any differences in survival are meaningful. Such a study, run by the Medical Research Council (MRC), and known as ICON4, is well under way in the UK, and randomises patients with a progression-free interval of at least 6 months from initial platinum-based chemotherapy to receive either platinum-based (non-taxane-containing) retreatment, or carboplatin-paclitaxel. A target of approximately

800 patients has been set and, as most patients in the control arm are receiving single agent carboplatin, this study is essentially testing carboplatin versus carboplatin-paclitaxel in chemosensitive relapse. The trial has now closed to recruitment and results are eagerly awaited.

In the management of resistant relapse (for example, no response to primary chemotherapy, relapse < 6 months), virtually no relevant randomised studies of combination chemotherapy have been conducted, and single agent chemotherapy is usually chosen because of toxicity. Many agents, novel and established, have demonstrated activity in sensitive and resistant disease, and some of the more important agents are shown in Table 35.10.[72] These data are from individual phase II (some phase III) trials in patients relapsing within 12 months of first-line treatment. Specifically for resistant disease, the most active agents (for example, topotecan, liposomal doxorubicin) all indicate similar response rates (10–20%) and duration of responses (4–9 months).

Again, non-randomised phase I–II combination studies suggest that higher response rates may be possible, but at the expense of higher toxicity. Different schedules of established agents are also being actively investigated, both to abrogate toxicity and perhaps to improve outcomes. Weekly administration of the taxanes, paclitaxel and docetaxel, has been shown to be feasible and active, although no direct efficacy comparisons with the more conventional 3-weekly schedules have been reported. In general, toxicity favours the weekly schedules, with reduced emesis, myelosuppression, neuropathy and hypersensitivity reactions. Other toxicities particular to the weekly schedules appear to be dose limited such as asthenia and cutaneous reactions.

Treating patients with resistant or relatively resistant disease (that is, relapse-ree interval < 12 months) with non-platinum agents is appropriate, and in responding patients may in fact prolong the platinum-free interval, such that the chance of a further response to subsequent platinum is improved. Such an approach may also have the advantage of allowing recovery of cumulative toxicity from platinum with or without paclitaxel first-line chemotherapy, especially neurotoxicity. The potential for non-platinum agents to be successful in this application can be seen from a GOG study in which topotecan $1.5$ mg m$^{-2}$ days 1–5, 3-weekly, was given to patients relapsing with potentially platinum-sensitive disease.[73] Here, 46 patients with a median progression-free interval of 9·6 months were treated with topotecan at first or second recurrence and demonstrated an overall response rate of 33% with a duration of 11 months, disease stabilisation in 48% and median time to progression of nearly 10 months. Overall survival was nearly 2 years.

The possibility of using non-platinum chemotherapy to increase the platinum-free interval in this way has been reported by a group from the MD Anderson Cancer Center.[74] In this study, 30 patients who had previously received a platinum-based regimen and relapsed with either "refractory" (progressed during first-line chemotherapy; 12 patients) or "resistant" (recurrence within 6 months; 18 patients) disease were firstly treated with a paclitaxel-based regimen, and subsequently, on second recurrence, with platinum-based chemotherapy. In patients in whom a response to paclitaxel was demonstrated, and the platinum-free interval was lengthened beyond 12 months, the response to platinum retreatment was 27%. No patients with a platinum-free interval of less than 12 months responded. What is not clear from this approach is whether the response to subsequent platinum rechallenge is maintained; there are also theoretical concerns that more resistant cell populations are selected for in this way.

To conclude, the "ideal" salvage treatment for recurrent ovarian cancer should be:

- active and able to control the rate of tumour progression
- well tolerated with no cumulative toxicity and able to maintain the patient's quality of life
- cost-effective.

The latter point is important because, although some treatments have been compared pharmacoeconomically – for example, liposomal doxorubicin (Caelyx) appears significantly cheaper overall than topotecan[75] – other, much cheaper agents such as etoposide have not been compared for efficacy with the newer generation of agents. Is there an ideal second-line agent? Probably not, and therefore choices of therapy should be mindful of all the factors outlined in this section, but also involve careful consideration of the patient's wishes.

## Recommendations

Treatment recommendations in recurrent disease are difficult to make, as physicians must individualise each patient accordingly, using the above section as a guide to making a decision.

- Patients relapsing with platinum-sensitive disease (> 18 months; over half expected to respond) should be offered chemotherapy with single agent carboplatin until results of randomised trials comparing monotherapy with combination therapy demonstrate unequivocal advantages for combination therapy **Evidence level Ib, Grade A** .
- Patients relapsing 12–18 months after primary chemotherapy fall into a category of potential chemosensitivity, in whom the evidence suggests

that approximately one-third will respond. In these patients, it is acceptable to re-treat with either single agent carboplatin or consider treatment with a non-cross-resistant, non-platinum chemotherapy in an attempt to prolong the platinum-free interval.

- Patients relapsing within 12 months of primary therapy can be predicted to have a low chance of responding to retreatment with platinum and as such it would be again appropriate to offer treatment with non-platinum therapies.

## References

1 The Cancer Research Campaign 2001.

2 Markman M, Zaino R, Fleming P *et al.* Carcinoma of the fallopian tube. In: Hoskins WJ, Perez CA, Young RC, eds. *Principles and Practice of Gynecologic Oncology, 2nd edn.* Philadelphia: Lippincott-Raven Publishers, 1997.

3 Pecorelli S, Odicino F, Favalli G. Ovarian cancer: Best timing and applications of debulking surgery. *Ann Oncol* 2000;**11**(S3):141–4.

4 Long RTL, Johnson RE, Sala JM *et al.* Variations in survival among patients with carcinoma of the ovary. *Cancer* 1967;**20**:1195–202.

5 Griffiths CT. Surgical resection of tumour bulk in the primary treatment of ovarian carcinoma. *Natl Cancer Inst Monogr* 1975;**42**:101–4.

6 Hunter RW, Alexander NDE, Soutter WP *et al.* Meta-analysis of surgery in advanced ovarian carcinoma: Is maximum cytoreductive surgery an independent determinant of prognosis? *Am J Obstet Gynecol* 1992;**166**:504–11.

7 Bristow RE, Tomacruz RS, Armstrong DK *et al.* Survival impact of maximum cytoreductive surgery for advanced ovarian carcinoma during the platinum-era: A meta-analysis of 6,848 patients. *Proc Am Soc Clin Oncol* 2001;**20**:202a(Abstr. 807).

8 Vasey PA and Kaye SB. Dose intensity in ovarian cancer. In: Gershenson DM, McGuire WP, eds. *Ovarian Cancer Controversies in Management.* London: Churchill Livingstone, 1997.

9 Ozols RF. Treatment of ovarian cancer: Current status. *Semin Oncol* 1994;**21**(S2):1–9.

10 Vasey PA, Kaye SB. Stage IV Ovarian cancer: clinical presentation and management. In: Ledermann JA, Vergote I, Kaye SB, Hoskins WJ, eds. *Clinical Management of Ovarian Tumours.* London: Martin Dunitz, 2000.

11 Smith JP, Rutledge F. Chemotherapy in the treatment of cancer of the ovary. *Am J Obstet Gynecol* 1970;**107**:691–703.

12 Lawton FG, Redman CW, Leusley DM *et al.* Neoadjuvant (cytoreductive) chemotherapy combined with intervention debulking surgery in advanced unresected epithelial ovarian cancer. *Obstet Gynecol* 1989;**73**:61–5.

13 Neijt JP, ten Bokkel Huinink WW, van der Burg MEL *et al.* Long term survival in ovarian cancer. *Eur J Cancer* 1991;**27**:1367–72.

14 van der Berg MEL, van Lent M, Buse M *et al.* The effect of debulking surgery after induction chemotherapy on the prognosis in advanced epithelial ovarian cancer. *N Engl J Med* 1995;**332**:629–34.

15 Rose PG, Nerenstone S, Brady M *et al.* A phase III randomised study of interval cytoreduction in patients with advanced stage ovarian carcinoma with suboptimal residual disease; a Gynecologic Oncology Group Study. *Proc Am Soc Clin Oncol* 2002;**21**:201a (Abst. 802).

16 Onnis A, Marchetti M, Padovan P *et al.* Neoadjuvant chemotherapy in advanced ovarian cancer. *Eur J Gynaecol Oncol* 1996;**17**:393–6.

17 Chambers JT, Chambers SK, Voynick IM *et al.* Neoadjuvant chemotherapy in stage X ovarian cancer. *Gynaecol Oncol* 1990;**37**: 327–31.

18 Vergote I, De Brabanter J, Fyles A *et al.* Prognostic importance of degree of differentiation and cyst rupture in stage I invasive epithelial ovarian carcinoma. *Lancet* 2001;**357**:159–60.

19 Li AJ, Cass K, Otero F *et al.* Pattern of lymph node metastases in apparent stage IA invasive epithelial ovarian carcinomas. *Gynecol Oncol* 2000;**76**:239(Abstr.).

20 Bolis G, Colombo N, Pecorelli S *et al.* Adjuvant treatment for early epithelial ovarian cancer: Results of two randomised clinical trials comparing cisplatin to no further treatment or chromic phosphate ($^{32}$P). *Ann Oncol* 1993;**6**:887–93.

21 Young RC, Brady MF, Neiberg RM et al. Randomised clinical trial of adjuvant treatment of women with early (FIGO I-IIA high risk) ovarian cancer. *Proc Am Soc Clin Oncol* 1999;**18**:357a(Abstr.).

22 International Collaborative Ovarian Neoplasm Trial I and Adjuvant Chemotherapy in Ovarian Neoplasm Trial. Two Parallel randomized phase III trials of adjuvant chemotherapy in patients with early-stage ovarian carcinoma. *J Natl Cancer Inst* 2003;**95**:105–12.

23 Advanced Ovarian Cancer Trialists' Group. Chemotherapy in advanced ovarian cancer: four systematic meta-analyses of individual patient data from 37 randomised trials. *Br J Cancer* 1998;**78**:1479–87.

24 Neijt JP, Engelholm SA, Tuxen MK *et al.* Exploratory phase III study of paclitaxel and cisplatin versus paclitaxel and carboplatin in advanced ovarian carcinoma. *J Clin Oncol* 2000;**18**:3084–92.

25 du Bois A, Lueck HJ, Meier W *et al.* Cisplatin/paclitaxel vs. carboplatin/paclitaxel in ovarian cancer: Update of an Arbeitsgemeinshaft Gynaekologishe Onkologie (AGO) Study Group Trial. *Proc Am Soc Clin Oncol* 1999;**18**:356a(Abstr. 1374).

26 Ozols RF, Bundy BN, Fowler J *et al.* Randomised phase III study of cisplatin(CIS)/paclitaxel(PAC) versus carboplatin(CARBO)/PAC in optimal stage III epithelial ovarian cancer (OC): A Gynecologic Oncology Group Trial (GOG 158). *Proc Am Soc Clin Oncol* 1999;**18**:356a(Abstr. 1373).

27 McGuire WP, Hoskins WJ, Brady MF *et al.* Cyclophosphamide and cisplatin compared with paclitaxel and cisplatin in patients with stage III and stage IV ovarian cancer. *N Engl J Med* 1996;**334**:1–6.

28 Piccart MJ, Bertelsen K, James K *et al.* Randomised intergroup trial of cisplatin-paclitaxel versus cisplatin-cyclophosphamide in women with advanced epithelial ovarian cancer: Three year results. *J Natl Cancer Inst* 2000;**92**:699–702.

29 Muggia FM, Braly PS, Brady MF *et al.* Phase III randomised study of cisplatin versus paclitaxel versus cisplatin and paclitaxel in patients with suboptimal stage III or IV ovarian cancer: A Gynecologic Oncology Group Study. *J Clin Oncol* 2000;**18**:106–15.

30 International Collaborative Ovarian Neoplasm (ICON) Group. Paclitaxel plus carboplatin versus standard chemotherapy with either single agent carboplatin or cyclophosphamide, doxorubicin and cisplatin: in women with ovarian cancer: the ICON 3 randomised trial. *Lancet* 2002;**360**:505–15.

31 ICON Collaborators. ICON2: A randomised trial of single agent carboplatin against the 3-drug combination of CAP (cyclophosphamide, doxorubicin and cisplatin) in women with ovarian cancer. *Lancet* 1998;**352**:1571–6.

32 Kaye SB, Piccart M, Aapro M *et al.* Phase II trials of docetaxel (Taxotere) in advanced ovarian cancer – an updated overview. *Eur J Cancer* 1997;**33**:2167–70.

33 Vershraegen CF, Sittisomwong T, Kudelka AP *et al.* Docetaxel for patients with paclitaxel-resistant Mullerian carcinoma. *J Clin Oncol* 2000;**18**:2733–9.

34 Vasey PA, Atkinson R, Coleman R *et al.* Docetaxel-carboplatin as first-line therapy for epithelial ovarian cancer. *Br J Cancer* 2001;**84**:170–8.

35 Markman M, Kennedy A, Webster K *et al.* Combination chemotherapy with carboplatin and docetaxel in the treatment of cancers of the ovary and fallopian tube and primary carcinoma of the peritoneum. *J Clin Oncol* 2001;**19**:1901–5.

36 Vasey P. Preliminary results of the SCOTROC Trial: A phase III comparison of paclitaxel-carboplatin (PC) and docetaxel-carboplatin (DC) as first-line chemotherapy for stage IC-IV epithelial ovarian cancer. *Proc Am Soc Clin Oncol* 2001;**20**:202a(Abstr. 804).

37 A'Hern RP and Gore ME. Impact of doxorubicin on survival in advanced ovarian cancer. *J Clin Oncol* 1995;**13**:726–32.

38 Gruppo Interregionale Cooperativo Oncologico Ginecologia: Randomized comparison of cisplatin with cyclophosphamide/cisplatin and cyclophosphamide/doxorubicin/cisplatin in advanced ovarian cancer. *Lancet* 1987;**2**:353–9.

39  Conte PF, Bruzzone M, Chiara S *et al.* A randomized trial comparing cisplatin plus cyclophosphamide versus cisplatin, doxorubicin and cyclophosphamide in advanced ovarian cancer. *J Clin Oncol* 1986;**4**:965–71.

40  Omura GA, Bundy BN, Berek JS *et al.* Randomized trial of cyclophosphamide plus cisplatin with or without doxorubicin in ovarian carcinoma: A Gynecologic Oncology Group study. *J Clin Oncol* 1989;**7**:457–65.

41  Bertelsen K, Jakobsen A, Andersen JE *et al.* A randomized study of cyclophosphamide and cisplatinum with or without doxorubicin in advanced ovarian carcinoma. *Gynecol Oncol* 1987;**28**:161–9.

42  Ovarian Cancer Meta-Analysis Project. Cyclophosphamide plus cisplatin versus cyclophosphamide, doxorubicin, and cisplatin chemotherapy of ovarian carcinoma: a meta-analysis. *J Clin Oncol* 1991;**9**:1668–74.

43  du Bois A, Weber B, Pfisterer J *et al.* Epirubicin/paclitaxel/ carboplatin (TEC) vs. paclitaxel/carboplatin (PC) in first-line treatment of ovarian cancer FIGO Stages IIb-IV. Interim results of an AGO-GINECO Intergroup Phase III Trial. *Proc Am Soc Clin Oncol* 2001;**20**:202a (Abstr. 805).

44  Hansen SW. Gemcitabine in the treatment of ovarian cancer. *Int J Gynaecol Cancer* 2001;**11**(S1):39–41.

45  Link KH. In vitro pharmocologic rationale for regional chemotherapy. In; Sugarbaker PH ed. *Peritoneal Carcinomatosis: Principles of Management.* Boston: Kluwer Academic Publishers, 1996.

46  Los G, Mutsaers PH, van der Vijgh WJ *et al.* Direct diffusion of cis-diamminedichloroplatinum(II) in intraperitoneal rat tumours after intraperitoneal chemotherapy: A comparison with systemic chemotherapy. *Cancer Res* 1989;**49**:3380–4.

47  Alberts DS, Liu PY, Hannigan EV *et al.* Intraperitoneal cisplatin plus intravenous cyclophosphamide versus intravenous cisplatin plus intravenous cyclophosphamide for stage III ovarian cancer. *N Engl J Med* 1996;**335**:1950–5.

48  Markman M, Bundy BN, Alberts DS *et al.* Phase III trial of standard-dose carboplatin followed by intravenous paclitaxel and intraperitoneal cisplatin in small volume stage III ovarian carcinoma: An intergroup study of the Gynecologic Oncology Group, Southwestern Oncology Group and Eastern Cooperative Oncology Group. *J Clin Oncol* 2001;**19**:1001–7.

49  Armstrong DK, Bundy BN, Baergen R *et al.* Randomised phase III study of intravenous paclitaxel and cisplatin versus IV paclitaxel, intraperitoneal cisplatin and IP paclitaxel in optimal stage III epithelial ovarian cancer (OC): A Gynecologic Oncology Group Trial (GOG 172). *Proc Am Soc Clin Oncol* 2002;**21**:201a(Abst.803).

50  Hakes TB, Chalas E, Hoskins WJ *et al.* Randomised prospective trial of 5 versus 10 cycles of cyclophosphamide, doxorubicin and cisplatin in advanced ovarian carcinoma. *Gynecol Oncol* 1992;**45**:284–9.

51  Bertelsen K, Jacobsen A, Stroyer J *et al.* A prospective randomised comparison of 6 and 12 cycles of cyclophosphamide, adriamycin and cisplatin in advanced epithelial ovarian cancer: A Danish Ovarian Cancer Study Group Trial (DACOVA). *Gynecol Oncol* 1993;**49**:30–6.

52  Ngan HYS, Choo YC, Cheung M *et al.* A randomised study of high dose versus lowdose cisplatin combined with cyclophosphamide in the treatment of advanced ovarian cancer. *Chemotherapy* 1989;**35**:221–7.

53  McGuire WP, Hoskins WJ, Brady MF *et al.* Assessment of dose-intensive therapy in suboptimally debulked ovarian cancer: a Gynecologic Oncology group study. *J Clin Oncol* 1995;**13**:1589–99.

54  Kaye SB, Paul J, Cassidy J *et al.* Mature results of a randomised trial of two doses of cisplatin for the treatment of ovarian cancer. *J Clin Oncol* 1996;**14**:2113–19.

55  Colombo N, Pittelli MR, Parma G *et al.* Cisplatin dose intensity in advanced ovarian cancer: A randomised study of conventional dose versus dose intensive cisplatin monotherapy. *Proc Am Soc Clin Oncol* 1993;**12**:255.

56  Jakobsen A. A dose intensity study of carboplatin in ovarian cancer. *Int J Gynaecol Cancer* 1995;**5**(Suppl. 5):11.

57  Gore ME, Mainwaring PN, Macfarlane V *et al.* A randomised study of high versus standard dose carboplatin in patients with advanced epithelial ovarian cancer. *Proc Am Soc Clin Oncol* 1996;**15**:284.

58  Ehrlich CE, Einhorn L, Stehman FB *et al.* Treatment of advanced epithelial ovarian cancer using cisplatin, adriamycin and cytoxan – the Indiana University experience. *Clin Obstet Gynaecol* 1983;**10**:325–35.

59  Bella M *et al.* Mature results of a prospective randomised trial comparing two different dose intensity regimens of cisplatin in advanced ovarian carcinoma. *Ann Oncol* 5 1994;**5**(Suppl. 8):2.

60  Conte PF, Bruzzone M, Gadducci A *et al.* High doses versus standard doses of cisplatin in combination with epidoxorubicin and cyclophosphamide in advanced ovarian cancer patients with bulky residual disease: A randomised trial. *Proc ASCO* 1993;**12**:273.

61  Lambert HE, Rustin GJ, Gregory WM *et al.* A randomised trial of five versus eight courses of cisplatin or carboplatin in advanced epithelial ovarian carcinoma. A North Thames Ovary Group Study. *Ann Oncol* 1997;**8**:327–33.

62  Behrens BC, Hamilton TC, Masuda H *et al.* Characteristics of cis-diamminedichloroplatinum(II)-resistant human ovarian cancer cell line and the evaluation of platinum analogues. *Cancer Res* 1987; **47**:414–18.

63  Markman M. Paclitaxel consolidation therapy for advanced ovarian cancer: Preliminary findings from GOG 178. SGO 33rd Annual Meeting, March 16–20, 2002.

64  Blackledge G, Lawton F, Redman C *et al.* Response of patients in phase II studies of chemotherapy in ovarian cancer: Implications for patient treatment and the design of phase II trials. *Br J Cancer* 1989;**59**:650–3.

65  Markman M, Rothman R, Hakes T *et al.* Second-line platinum therapy in patients with ovarian cancer previously treated with cisplatin. *J Clin Oncol* 1991;**9**:389–93.

66  Eisenhauer EA, Vermorken JB, Van Glabbeke M. Predictors of response to subsequent chemotherapy in platinum pretreated ovarian cancer: an analysis of 704 patients. *Ann Oncol* 1997; **8**:963–8.

67  Janicke F, Holscher M, Kuhn W *et al.* Radical surgical procedure improves survival time in patients with recurrent ovarian cancer. *Cancer* 1992;**70**:2129–36.

68  Eisenkop SM, Freidman RL, Wang HJ *et al.* Secondary cytoreductive surgery for recurrent ovarian cancer. *Cancer* 1995;**76**:1606–14.

69  Segna RA, Dottino PR, Mendeli JP *et al.* Secondary cytoreduction for ovarian cancer following cisplatin therapy. *Int J Gynecol Cancer* 1997;**7**(S2):9(Abstr. 023).

70  Rose PG, Fusco N, Fluellen L *et al.* Secondline therapy with paclitaxel and carboplatin for recurrent disease following firstline therapy with paclitaxel and cisplatin in ovarian or peritoneal carcinoma. *J Clin Oncol* 1998;**16**:1494–7.

71  Bolis G, Scarfone S, Giardina G *et al.* Carboplatin alone vs carboplatin plus epidoxorubicin as secondline therapy for cisplatin- or carboplatin-sensitive ovarian cancer. *Gynecol Oncol* 2001;**81**:3–9.

72  Gore M. Treatment of relapsed epithelial ovarian cancer. In: *ASCO Educational Book* 2001.

73  McGuire WP, Blessing JA, Bookman MA *et al.* Topotecan has substantial antitumour activity as first-line salvage therapy in platinum-sensitive epithelial ovarian cancer: A Gynecologic Oncology Group Study. *J Clin Oncol* 2000;**18**:1062–7.

74  Kavanagh J, Tresukosol D, Edwards C *et al.* Carboplatin re-induction after taxane in patients with platinum-refractory epithelial ovarian cancer. *J Clin Oncol* 1995;**13**:1584–8.

75  Smith Dh, Johnston SR, Gordon AN *et al.* Economic evaluation of Doxil/Caelyx vs Topotecan for recurrent epithelial ovarian carcinoma: The UK perspective. *Proc Am Soc Clin Oncol* 2001;**20**:3a(Abstr. 808).

# 36 Cancer of the uterine corpus

*Rebecca L Faulkner, Henry C Kitchener*

## Endometrial carcinoma

Cancer of the endometrium is the second commonest gynaecological cancer in England and Wales. The age-standardised incidence has been approximately 12/100 000 since the early 1970, with a decline in incidence in women aged less than 54 years and a rise in women aged over 54 years. The overall 5-year survival is 70%.[1] The median age of patients with endometrial carcinoma is 61 years with 75–80% being postmenopausal and 5% being less than 40 years old. It is generally considered to be a treatable cancer as presentation is early and early stage disease is curable by surgical means. However, there is still a 30% death rate from endometrial carcinoma and suboptimal management of later stage disease. A brief review of the pathology of endometrial carcinoma and management options are discussed below.

Preparation for this chapter included a broad-based electronic database search of PubMed, the *Cochrane Library*, and several relevant websites such as the meta Register of Controlled Trials (mRCT). This was not a systematic review as criteria for included trials were not predetermined nor was the search exhaustive. Cancer of the uterus has not been subjected to a large number of randomised controlled trials. We do not think any have been missed.

## Background

### Aetiology

Several risk factors are known to be associated with endometrial carcinoma. Increased unopposed oestrogen is a significant cause and in younger women is associated with anovulation and nulliparity (for example, polycystic ovarian syndrome). In postmenopausal women the major source of unopposed oestrogen is oestrone converted from androgen in peripheral fat. This explains the increased risk in obese women. There is an association between diabetes mellitus and endometrial cancer, but this is probably due to the common factor of obesity rather than an aetiological association. Unopposed exogenous oestrogen administration increases the risk of endometrial cancer from seven to ten times that of the general population.[2,3] Women who take tamoxifen are also at risk of uterine side effects owing to its oestrogen agonist effect. Risk of neoplasia increases with duration of use and comparison of tamoxifen use or not in

Box 36.1 WHO classification of endometrial cancer

- Endometrioid adenocarcinoma, NOS
    variants
    ciliated cells
    secretory cells
- Adenocarcinoma, NOS, with squamous differentiation
- Mucous adenocarcinoma
- Serous adenocarcinoma
- Clear cell carcinoma
- Squamous carcinoma
- Undifferentiated carcinoma (large and small cell type)
- Mixed carcinoma
- Metastatic carcinoma

women with breast cancer shows an increase in the annual risk of endometrial cancer from 0·2 per 1000 women to 1·6 per 1000 women. Women with a previous history of breast or colon cancer are at increased risk of developing endometrial cancer. Ovarian stromal tumours can secrete oestrogen and 10% of granulosa-thecal cell tumours are associated with concomitant endometrial cancer and 50% with endometrial hyperplasia.

Women who have ever used the combined oral contraceptive pill have a substantially reduced risk of developing uterine carcinoma especially after 10 or more years of use.

### Pathology

The World Health Organization (WHO) and FIGO classifications for endometrial carcinoma are in Boxes 36.1 and 36.2. The latter was developed for endometrial carcinoma, but can be applied to sarcoma also.

In addition to staging there should be verification of the grade of disease. This takes into account the degree of differentiation of the adenocarcinoma as follows:

- G1: ≤ 5% of non-squamous or non-morular solid growth pattern
- G2: 6–50% of a non-squamous or non-morular solid growth pattern
- G3: > 50% of a non-squamous or non-morular solid growth pattern.

Notable nuclear atypia raises the grade by one.

**Box 36.2 FIGO surgicopathological staging for carcinoma of the uterus**

**Stage I**   Tumour is confined to the corpus uteri

    Stage IA:   Tumour limited to endometrium
    Stage IB:   invasion to less than half of the myometrium
    Stage IC:   invasion to greater than half of the myometrium

**Stage II**   Tumour involves the corpus and the cervix, but has not extended outside the uterus

    Stage IIA:   endocervical glandular involvement only
    Stage IIB:   cervical stromal invasion

**Stage III**   Tumour extends outside of the uterus but is confined to the true pelvis

    Stage IIIA:   Tumour invades serosa and/or adnexae and/or positive peritoneal cytology
    Stage IIIB:   vaginal metastases
    Stage IIIC:   metastases to pelvic and/or para-aortic lymph nodes

**Stage IV**:   Tumour invades bladder or bowel mucosa or metastasis to distant sites

    Stage IVA:   Tumour invasion of bladder and/or bowel mucosa
    Stage IVB:   distant metastases, including intra-abdominal and/or inguinal lymph nodes

## Preoperative assessment

### Clinical

As diabetes, hypertension and obesity are known risk factors for endometrial carcinoma, concurrent disease is common. Incidence also increases with age contributing to medical comorbidity. A detailed clinical review is necessary in preoperative assessment and should include cardiorespiratory examination, ECG, chest *x* ray as well as FBC, U&E, LFTs, urine dipstick and plasma glucose if indicated.

Specific investigations are used to make a preoperative diagnosis and to determine extent of tumour spread thus directing management.

### Endometrial sampling

Most women present with irregular or postmenopausal vaginal bleeding. Dilatation and curettage (D&C) historically has been the mainstay of investigation, but this has now been superseded by outpatient investigation. This has economic advantage and avoids anaesthetic risk.

Outpatient hysteroscopy using a rigid hysteroscope is a well-tolerated procedure in the investigation of abnormal uterine bleeding.[4] There have been no randomised controlled trials to study its effectiveness compared to other techniques. In one study 20% of endometrial cancers were diagnosed as such and all other cases were recognised as abnormal.[5] In another study 95% of all pathological conditions were detected by hysteroscopy.[6]

Various devices are available to sample the endometrium and studies have compared them. Randomised trials have shown the Pipelle and Vabra aspirators to give equal diagnostic accuracy. The Pipelle causes less discomfort.[7,8] In general the Pipelle provides less endometrial sample, but is more acceptable and there are no adverse clinical outcomes from the smaller sample. The Novak and Vabra aspirators perform as well as D&C in diagnostic accuracy[9] **Evidence level Ib**.

### Imaging

Transvaginal ultrasound scan has a negative predictive value approaching 100% for the exclusion of endometrial cancer. Sensitivity depends on the cut-off used for normal endometrial thickness, which is usually set at 4 mm or less for the double layer. Endometrial biopsy validation of ultrasound findings has confirmed its use as an effective means of excluding significant endometrial pathology. Reserving biopsy for those with abnormal ultrasound significantly reduces the need for endometrial biopsy.

Having diagnosed endometrial cancer, the next step is to determine the extent of lymph node involvement and invasion of the primary tumour.

Magnetic resonance imaging (MRI) is the optimum modality for assessing myometrial invasion and cervical involvement. It also allows assessment of the pelvic and para-aortic lymph nodes. MRI appears to be superior to CT scanning in detecting stage and myometrial invasion[10,11] **Evidence level IIa**. Neither CT nor MRI can replace surgical sampling in the diagnosis of nodal metastases.

The risk of positive nodes in endometrial carcinoma increases with histological grade, depth of myometrial invasion and radiological suspicion. Accurate preoperative staging assists in determining optimal management for an individual patient.

In a frequently cited surgicopathological study, 12% of 621 women with FIGO stage 1 disease were found to have lymph node metastases: 6% in the pelvic lymph nodes, 4% in the pelvic and para-aortic nodes, and 2% in the para-aortic nodes alone. With poorly differentiated tumours the frequency of positive nodes was 18% ($P = 0.0007$) and in those with deep myometrial invasion it was 22% ($P = 0.0001$). These parameters can therefore be used as preoperative indicators of nodal involvement[12] **Evidence level III**.

In summary the diagnosis of endometrial carcinoma should be made by a combination of transvaginal ultrasound scan and endometrial biopsy. Outpatient hysteroscopy may be of value. In order to determine further management an assessment of risk of lymph node involvement is necessary; this requires consideration of tumour grade, radiological imaging by CT or MR and assessment of myometrial involvement.

## Surgical management

### *Is there evidence that node dissection improves survival in endometrial carcinoma?*

There is no clear international consensus in the management of early stage endometrial cancer. Peritoneal washings, total abdominal hysterectomy and bilateral salpingo-oophorectomy is the treatment of choice, but the practice of lymph node dissection has been variable. This ranges from none at all to periaortic, and selective pelvic node sampling to pelvic clearance. The current FIGO staging is based upon findings at surgery, including the presence or absence of disease in the pelvic and para-aortic lymph nodes.

Lymphadenectomy may have a therapeutic effect, but this is not yet known. It does achieve surgical staging and may reduce morbidity by reducing the need for adjuvant radiotherapy. However, lymph node sampling has been reported to increase the risk of severe radiotherapy complications from 1% to 7% and it may increase operative morbidity because of vascular injury, ureteric injury, pelvic abscess, lymphoedema and pseudocyst formation.[13] In skilled surgical hands morbidity is infrequent and no increase in severe complications was reported by the COSA-NZ-UK study of adjuvant hormone treatment in 1996.[14] In this prospective international study a subset of women had external beam radiotherapy only if nodes were positive following complete pelvic lymphadenectomy. They noted a reduction in severe radiotherapy complications from 4·4% to 1·6% in women who underwent complete pelvic lymphadenectomy as some women were spared radiotherapy. However, the trial was not randomised and the women selected for lymphadenectomy were younger and lighter than the other trial participants.

The effect of lymphadenectomy on survival is uncertain and no prospective randomised controlled trials have yet been reported.

*Retrospective studies.* One retrospective study of 425 cases of endometrial cancer concluded that selective pelvic lymphadenectomy was useful for prognostic purposes, but did not confer a 5-year survival advantage.[15] The COSA-NZ-UK study came to the same conclusion.

A retrospective study of 649 women surgically managed for endometrial adenocarcinoma over a 21-year period found a significant survival advantage for patients having multiple site node sampling. This was overall and in high and low risk groups, strongly suggesting a therapeutic advantage to lymphadenectomy. Overall 5-year survival improved from around 70% to 90% with multiple node sampling.[16] Case mix could confound interpretation of such results.

There are at present no clear factors pre- or intraoperatively to identify which patients require lymph node dissection. If routine lymph node dissection were to be advocated, over 90% of women may have unnecessary removal of lymph nodes with subsequent additional morbidity. The standard approach is to identify patients at high risk of node involvement, (that is, deep myometrial invasion, cervical extension, clear or serous papillary cell types and poorly differentiated tumours) and to perform pelvic lymphadenectomy in these patients. If pelvic nodes are obviously involved then a para-aortic node dissection is undertaken, but women with positive para-aortic nodes almost always die.[17]

Retrospective review of all FIGO stages I and II endometrial cancers diagnosed over a 5-year period showed a significant survival advantage for lymph node sampling in stage I grade 3 disease only.[18] In his discussion Trimble suggests that to clarify the issue would require a large prospective randomised trial with effective surgical and pathological quality control. He asks whether women or their doctors would be willing to cooperate in a trial in which randomisation was between lymph node sampling or no sampling at the time of hysterectomy or between lymph node sampling and complete dissection. Use of adjuvant therapy would also confound the results of the trial.

The MRC ASTEC randomised trial is comparing survival following lymphadenectomy or no lymphadenectomy for stage I disease. Importantly adjuvant radiotherapy, which is also randomised, is given independent of lymph node status. Data from this important trial will not be available until around 2006.

Lymphadenectomy should therefore be considered for high risk endometrial cancer, but cannot yet be recommended routinely in low risk cases, unless as part of a randomised trial **Grade B**.

### *Should surgery always be performed by an oncological specialist?*

In the UK, the time-honoured strategy for managing endometrial cancer has been simple hysterectomy and BSO. Adjuvant radiotherapy has been used for higher risk tumours based on pathological findings. There is now a widely held view among gynaecological oncologists that a pelvic lymphadenectomy should be performed to achieve surgical staging and to better select those women who do not require adjuvant radiotherapy by virtue of negative nodes. Such surgery should be performed by a gynaecologist trained in this technique. Careful preoperative planning is required to identify high risk patients who should therefore be referred to a subspecialist. This should include assessment of tumour grade, myometrial invasion and pelvic MRI or CT.

There have been no randomised studies addressing the issue of surgeon-dependent outcome in uterine cancer. It is now accepted that those requiring lymphadenectomy on the basis of preoperative assessment should be referred to a subspecialist who can perform appropriate surgery. Triaging women into low and high risk categories is a practical basis for selecting those requiring more complex surgery. Low risk women can safely be operated on by a general gynaecologist.

## Laparoscopic surgery

### Is there a place for laparoscopic surgery?

Laparoscopic-assisted vaginal hysterectomy (LAVH) and if required, lymphadenectomy, can be performed, particularly for low risk endometrial cancer. There have been no randomised controlled trials comparing this procedure with open surgery, but there are expert centres pursuing this approach. It will be important to monitor outcomes in these women to ensure that there is no unexpected increase in vault recurrence, for example, or port metastases.

A recently published retrospective review concluded that treatment of low risk endometrial cancer by LAVH is associated with a significantly increased incidence of positive peritoneal cytology. The clinical significance of such findings is undetermined.[19]

## Adjuvant radiotherapy

### What is the place of adjuvant radiotherapy in endometrial cancer?

Since the 1950s radiotherapy has been widely used in women considered to be at increased risk of vault or pelvic recurrence. Increased risk of recurrence is known to be related to poor differentiation, deeply invasive tumours, cervical involvement and lymph node involvement.

Although irradiation will reduce the incidence of local and regional recurrence, improved survival has not been proven.[20–22] To date, randomised phase III trials have failed to demonstrate a survival advantage associated with adjuvant treatment in women with stage I and stage II endometrial cancer **Evidence level Ib**.

Aalders *et al.* reported a seminal study in Norway in 1980 that showed improved pelvic control, but no increased survival in women randomised to external beam radiotherapy (DXT). All received brachytherapy. More recently the PORTEC Study Group in the Netherlands reported a prospective randomised trial that aimed to determine whether postoperative radiotherapy improved locoregional control and survival for patients with stage I endometrial cancer.[22] In this trial, patients with stage I endometrial cancer (grade 1 with deep [≥ 50%] myometrial invasion, grade 2 with any invasion, or grade 3 with superficial [< 50%] invasion) were enrolled. After total abdominal hysterectomy and bilateral salpingo-oophorectomy, without lymphadenectomy, 715 patients from 19 centres were randomised to pelvic radiotherapy or no further treatment. The primary study endpoints were locoregional recurrence and death, with treatment-related morbidity and survival after relapse as secondary endpoints. Median duration of follow up was 52 months.

The 5-year locoregional recurrence rates were 4% in the radiotherapy group and 14% in the control group ($P < 0.001$). Actuarial 5-year survival rates were similar in the two groups: 81% radiotherapy and 85% controls ($P = 0.31$). Endometrial cancer related deaths were 9% in the radiotherapy group and 6% in controls ($P = 0.37$). Treatment-related complications occurred in 25% of radiotherapy patients and in 6% of controls ($P < 0.0001$). Age less than 60 years was associated with a significantly better prognosis than age over 60 years.

They concluded that postoperative radiotherapy in stage I disease reduces locoregional recurrence, but has no impact on overall survival. Locoregional recurrence is often amenable to salvage by radiotherapy particularly with mucosal and vault recurrence. Routine adjuvant radiotherapy increases treatment-related morbidity and is not indicated in patients with stage I endometrial carcinoma below 60 years, and in patients with grade 2 tumours and superficial invasion.

In the MRC ASTEC trial, one aim is to determine the benefit or otherwise of postoperative adjuvant external beam radiotherapy in women with endometrial cancer including high risk pathology. This includes patients in whom the lymph node status is both known and not known. Radiation randomisation involves external beam only; brachytherapy is optional. As previously stated, adjuvant radiation is based purely on endometrial characteristics and not on lymph node status.

## Hormone and chemotherapy

### Is systemic therapy effective in the treatment of endometrial cancer?

The occurrence of distant recurrence in high risk endometrial carcinoma suggests that systemic adjuvant treatment may be of use.[23] Advanced disease is not always amenable to surgery and chemotherapeutic agents have been assessed. So far neither chemotherapy nor hormone therapy have been demonstrated to improve survival.

*Hormone therapy.* A published meta analysis of six randomised controlled trials showed no survival benefit for routine adjuvant progestogen therapy in endometrial cancer.[24] A subsequent randomised controlled trial of 1012 women also showed no overall survival benefit for adjuvant progestogen therapy[25] **Evidence level Ia** .

Progestogen therapy is only beneficial in histologically well-differentiated tumours and/or oestrogen or progesterone receptor-positive tumours. It has been associated with thromboembolic or cardiovascular side effects. High grade tumours have a poorer prognosis and are less likely to be receptor positive.

Other hormone therapies considered have been LHRH agonists[26] and aromatase inhibitors (anastrozole).[27]

Most authorities would, however, agree that medroxyprogesterone acetate should be prescribed for recurrent disease and in the palliative setting.

*Chemotherapy.* Cytotoxic agents do have activity in endometrial cancer although the response rates are not nearly as high as for ovarian cancer. Chemotherapy is not used generally as an adjuvant therapy and its use as a primary therapy would be confined to those women with unresected para-aortic adenopathy or other distal metastases.

Doxorubicin and cisplatin are the most active agents with response rates of 20–40%.[28,29] Paclitaxel also has activity. Further trials are required to determine the most effective use of chemotherapy in advanced and recurrent disease.

Paclitaxel and cisplatin have been used in combination in ovarian carcinoma and show no clinical cross-resistance. A phase II multicentre trial of paclitaxel and cisplatin for use in recurrent or advanced endometrial disease has reported a 67% objective response rate and in these 29% had a complete response **Evidence level IIa** . The combination of paclitaxel and cisplatin with G-CSF support appears active in patients with metastatic or recurrent carcinoma of the endometrium. Neurotoxicity was a significant side effect and is of concern.[30] The response data were similar to those reported by Lissoni *et al.*[31] Improved response rate may not correlate with improved overall survival, and quality-of-life issues become important because median survival is less than 1 year irrespective of treatment.

## Locally advanced disease

### What is the best management for locally advanced disease?

Patients with advanced endometrial cancer represent only 10–15% of newly diagnosed cases, but account for up to 54% of disease-related deaths. These women require to be managed by expert subspecialist teams.

If involvement of the cervix is suspected prior to surgery (stage II), this should be confirmed by MRI, and radical hysterectomy is the recommended treatment together with pelvic and, if indicated, para-aortic lymphadenectomy. This may be a curative procedure and, with good margins and negative nodes, radiotherapy may be avoided.

Stage III disease may be diagnosed at surgery when ovaries or tubes are involved, or even postoperatively by the pathologist. Such disease should be treated with total abdominal hysterectomy and bilateral salpingo-oophorectomy with lymphadenectomy if possible. Postoperative radiotherapy should be offered.

If a patient presents with obvious clinically advanced disease, initial debulking surgery may be possible but, if there is a frozen pelvis or obvious bladder involvement, initial treatment should be by radiotherapy. Consideration can be given to surgery following radiotherapy if there has been a response, but obvious residual disease.[32,33]

In advanced disease there is no standard management protocol and treatment requires to be individualised. High dose progestogen and chemotherapy need to be considered particularly for extra-pelvic disease.

## Recurrent disease

### What is the management of recurrent endometrial carcinoma?

The prognosis for recurrent disease is very dependent on the location of recurrence and whether prior radiotherapy has been prescribed. In women with apparently isolated pelvic recurrence, not previously irradiated, radiotherapy can achieve salvage rates of 50% overall and almost 80% for disease confined to the mucosa.[34] Exenteration can be considered for isolated central pelvic recurrence in previously irradiated patients.

The situation is totally different for sidewall recurrence in previously irradiated patients where the prospect for cure is remote. Chemotherapy can be offered, but a good response is unlikely. For distant metastases, radiotherapy may have a role in local control and chemotherapy can be offered. Prospects for palliation and extending survival need to be balanced against quality of life. Survival is rarely improved by such combination therapy and the toxicity associated with such regimens makes them unappealing in terminally ill women.

## Uterine sarcoma

Uterine sarcomas comprise less than 1% of gynaecological malignancies and 2–5% of all uterine malignancies. The tumours arise primarily from myometrium (leiomyosarcoma), mesodermal elements (müllerian) and endometrial stroma (sarcomas).

One documented aetiological factor in 10–25% of these malignancies is prior pelvic radiation, often administered for benign uterine bleeding 5–25 years earlier.

More recently reports suggest an association between carcinosarcoma and tamoxifen therapy.[35]

The prognosis for uterine sarcoma is primarily dependent on the extent of disease at the time of diagnosis.

The most common histological types of uterine sarcomas are carcinosarcoma (mixed mesodermal sarcomas or MMMT – 50%), leiomyosarcoma (30%) and endometrial stromal tumours (15%), which are divided into endometrial stromal sarcoma (previously designated low grade – LGESS) and high grade sarcoma (previously high grade – HGESS). Tumour cell necrosis and cellular pleomorphism are the histological factors taken into consideration when designating high or low grade. The two tumour types have very different prognoses; that of high grade sarcoma is dismal.[36]

## Treatment

Surgery alone can be curative if the malignancy is contained within the uterus. Metastatic disease is usually incurable as chemo- and radiosensitivities are very limited.

Current studies consist primarily of phase II chemotherapy trials for advanced disease. Adjuvant chemotherapy for stage I and stage II disease is not effective in any randomised trial.[37] Reports of non-randomised trials have claimed improved survival following adjuvant chemotherapy with or without radiation therapy.[38–40]

### *What is the place for adjuvant chemotherapy and radiotherapy in uterine sarcoma?*

Uterine sarcomas comprise a mixed group of tumours, some of which are indolent in nature (endometrial stromal sarcoma) and other more aggressive types (leiomyosarcoma, carcinosarcoma and high grade sarcoma). Stages I–III are routinely treated surgically, but even when disease is confined to the uterus recurrence is in the region of 75% demonstrating the need for an effective adjuvant therapy.[36] Whatever additional treatment is used, stage at presentation is the most consistent predictor of outcome, and adjuvant therapies to date have shown a questionable impact on the natural history of disease.[37,41,42]

*Radiotherapy.* Radiotherapy has been extensively studied. The results are variable with many authors showing no benefit to therapy[41,43] and others claiming decreased rates of local recurrence or even improved survival.[42,44] Sorbe reported on 59 patients with stage I or II disease and concluded that adjuvant radiotherapy decreased the incidence of pelvic recurrence with no impact on survival.[45] Sarcomas generally recur at distant sites and the use of chemotherapy in preference to radiotherapy therefore appears to make more sense.

*Chemotherapy – ifosfamide and doxorubicin:* The Gynecologic Oncology Group has evaluated the activity of the alkylating agent ifosfamide in the management of patients with metastatic or recurrent endometrial stromal sarcomas.[46] Patients with histologically proven advanced or recurrent endometrial stromal sarcomas were given an intravenous course of ifosfamide with Mesna to protect the urothelium. Of the 21 evaluable patients, three (14%) had complete responses and four (19%) had partial responses (median response 3·7 months) giving an overall response rate of 33%. They concluded that the agent was active in the therapy of women with endometrial stromal sarcoma. This has been reinforced by other GOG studies that have shown that ifosfamide induced substantial responses in nine (32%) of 28 women and five (18%) of 28 women with metastatic carcinosarcoma of the uterus.[47] In women with metastatic or recurrent uterine leiomyosarcomas, six (17%) of 35 patients responded to ifosfamide alone and 10 (30%) of 33 responded to treatment with the combination of ifosfamide and doxorubicin.[48,49]

In another recent study ifosfamide was used as adjuvant treatment in 13 patients with completely resected moderate or high grade uterine sarcomas.[50] They found a striking difference between the recurrence rates of carcinosarcoma and leiomyosarcoma. The natural recurrence rates of these two variants have been shown to be quite similar.[37,42] Early stage carcinosarcoma had a 2-year progression-free survival of 100% versus 33% in leiomyosarcoma patients.

Several other studies have also suggested that ifosfamide is more active in carcinosarcoma than LMS.[51] The authors concluded that adjuvant ifosfamide appeared to be safe and well tolerated in patients with completely resected uterine sarcoma. The regimen used was suitable for outpatient treatment. This study was neither randomised nor prospective and is subject both to selection and bias.

The Sarcoma Meta-analysis Collaboration have analysed 1568 patients with localised resectable soft tissue sarcoma from 14 trials of doxorubicin-based adjuvant chemotherapy.[52] They found good evidence that adjuvant doxorubicin improved time to local and distant recurrence and overall recurrence-free survival. There was a trend towards improved overall survival. The effect on survival was independent of doxorubicin being administered alone or in combination with other drugs.

The GOG trial of adjuvant doxorubicin in patients with completely resected uterine carcinosarcoma and leiomyosarcoma was included in the above meta-analysis.[37] The recurrence rate was 47% with doxorubicin whether or not the patient also received radiotherapy. The 2-year progression-free survival was 62%. The numbers were not significantly different from progression rates in women not receiving chemotherapy. The results of this study are to be evaluated with caution as the patient group was heterogeneous and prior radiation therapy was allowed. The study did not contain the power to evaluate different histologies.

### Endometrial stromal sarcoma

Endometrial stromal sarcoma is a rare and indolent tumour. Recurrence is characteristically years after initial surgery. This disease course makes it difficult to conduct a randomised clinical trial or to develop a consensus regarding its management. Recurrence after radical surgery followed by radiotherapy, hormone therapy and eventually surgically uncontrollable recurrent tumour is the usual course of events. Recommended treatment varies according to the extent and location of tumour. Repeated tumour reduction by surgery is the mainstay of treatment.[53] Radiation or chemotherapy is used for palliation only.

The evidence appears to be that there is no effective chemotherapy to treat endometrial stromal sarcoma and, as the disease course is indolent, the emphasis should be on maintaining quality of life.

### Prognosis

The prognosis for sarcomas generally has not improved significantly over the past 30 years and uterine sarcomas are not an exception. There is a need for randomised trials to evaluate the effectiveness of chemotherapy. Comparisons of chemotherapy versus best supportive care are difficult, but may be relevant. Because of the variety of these tumours international cooperation is required to recruit sufficient patients, but would be worthwhile for those women who are unfortunate enough to acquire this dangerous disease.

## Conclusions

It is clear that much of the current management of uterine cancer is not firmly evidence based, because of a lack of randomised controlled trial data. There are some statements that can be made, based on evidence, and currently conducted trials may clarify other issues over the next five years.

- Total abdominal hysterectomy and bilateral salpingo-oophorectomy is highly effective for low and moderate risk stage I endometrial cancer **Grade B**.
- Lymphadenectomy is recommended by FIGO as part of staging, but as yet has not been shown to be therapeutically effective. It may reduce the need for adjuvant radiotherapy by excluding extra-uterine disease **Grade B**.
- Adjuvant radiotherapy has not been shown to confer a survival advantage, but it does reduce pelvic recurrence. It cannot be recommended routinely in cases of moderate risk stage I disease in women below 60 years of age **Grade A**.
- In uterine sarcoma there is no evidence of benefit for adjuvant radiotherapy. There is some evidence that chemotherapy may be of benefit in a small proportion of women with carcinosarcoma **Grade B**.

## References

1 Office for National Statistics. *Cancer trends in England and Wales 1950–1999*. Hardcopy publication. London: Office for National Statistics.
2 Mack TM, Pike MC, Henderson BE *et al.* Estrogens and endometrial cancer in a retirement community. *N Engl J Med* 1976;**294**: 1262–1268.
3 Weiss NS, Szerely DR, English DR, Schweid AI. Endometrial cancer in relation to patterns of menopausal estrogen use. *JAMA* 1979;**242**:261–4.
4 Downes E, Al-Azzawi F. How well do perimenopausal women accept out patient hysteroscopy? Visual analogue scoring of acceptability and pain in 100 women. *Eur J Obstet Gynecol Reprod Biol* 1993;**48**:37–41.
5 Ben-Yehuda OM, Kim YB, Leutcher RS. Does hysteroscopy improve on the sensitivity of dilation and curettage in the diagnosis of endometrial hyperplasia or carcinoma? *Gynecol Oncol* 1998;**68**:4–7.
6 Haller H, Matejcic N, Rukavina B *et al.* Transvaginal ultrasonagraphy and hysteroscopy in women with post menopausal bleeding. *Int J Gynecol Obstet* 1996;**54**:155–9.
7 Eddowes HA, Read MD, Codling BW. Pipelle: a more acceptable technique for outpatient endometrial biopsy. *Br J Obstet Gynaecol* 1990;**97**:961–2.
8 Kaunitz AM, Masciello A, Ostrowski M *et al.* Comparison of endometrial biopsy with the endometrial Pipelle and Vabra aspirator. *J Reprod Med* 1998;**33**:417–31.
9 Stovall TG, Solomon SK, Ling FW. Endometrial sampling prior to hysterectomy. *Obstet Gynecol* 1989;**73**:405–9.
10 Kim SH, Kim HD, Song YS *et al.* Detection of deep myometrial invasion in endometrial carcinoma: comparison of TV ultrasound, CT and MRI. *J Comput Assist Tomogr* 1995;**19**:766–72.
11 Varpula MJ, Kleimi PJ. Staging of uterine endometrial carcinoma with ultra-low field (0·02T) MRI: a comparative study with CT. *J Comput Assist Tomogr* 1993;**17**:641–7.
12 Creasman WT, Morrow CP, Bundy BN *et al.* Surgical pathological spread patterns of endometrial cancer. *Cancer* 1987;**60**:603–41.
13 Corn BW, Lanciano RM, Greven KM *et al.* Impact of improved irradiation technique, age and lymph node sampling on the severe complication rate of surgically staged endometrial cancer patients: a multivariate analysis. *J Clin Oncol* 1994;**12**:510–15.
14 COSA-NZ-UK Endometrial cancer Study groups 1996. Pelvic lymphadenectomy in high risk endometrial cancer. *Int J Gynecol Cancer* 1996;**6**:102–7.
15 Candiani GB, Belloni C, Maggi R, Colombo G, Frigoli A, Carinelli SG. Evaluation of different surgical approaches in the management of endometrial cancer at FIGO Stage 1. *Gynecol Oncol* 1990;**37**:6–8.
16 Kilgore LC, Partridge EE, Alvarez RD *et al.* Adenocarcinoma of the endometrium: survival comparisons of patients with and without pelvic node sampling. *Gynecol Oncol* 1995;**56**:29–33.
17 Belinson JL, Lee KR, Badger GJ, Pretorius RG, Jarrell MA. Clinical stage 1 adenocarcinoma of the endometrium-analysis of recurrences and the potential benefit of staging laparotomy. *Gynecol Oncol* 1992;**44**:17–23.
18 Trimble EL, Kosary C, Park R. Lymph node sampling and survival in endometrial cancer. *Gynecol Oncol.* 1998;**71**:340–3.
19 Sonoda Y, Zerbe M, Smith A, Lin O, Baraket RR, Hoskins WJ. High incidence of positive peritoneal cytology in low risk endometrial cancer treated by laparoscopically assisted vaginal hysterectomy. *Gynecol Oncol* 2001;**80**:378–82.

20  Creutzberg CL, van Putten WLJ, Koper PCM *et al.* Surgery and post operative radiotherapy versus surgery alone for patients with stage-I endometrial carcinoma: multicentre randomised trial. *Lancet* 2000; **355**:1404–11.

21  Aalders J, Abler V, Kolstad P, Onsrud M. Post-operative external irradiation and prognostic parameters in Stage I endometrial carcinoma: a clinical and histopathologic study of 540 patients. *Obstet Gynecol* 1980;**56**:419–27.

22  Roberts JA, Brunetto VL, Keys HM *et al.* A phase III randomised study of surgery vs. surgery plus adjunctive radiation therapy in intermediate risk endometrial adenocarcinoma (GOG). Presented at the 29th annual meeting of the Society of Gynecological Oncologists. *Gynecol Oncol* 1998;**68**:135(Abstr. 258).

23  Jerezek-Fossa B, Badizio A, Jassem J. Surgery followed by radiotherapy in endometrial cancer: analysis of survival and patterns of failure. *Int J Gynecol Cancer* 1999;**9**:285–94.

24  Martin-Hirsch PL, Lilford RJ, Jarvis GJ. Adjuvant progestagen therapy for the treatment of endometrial cancer; a review and meta-analysis of published randomised controlled trials. *Eur J Obstet Gynecol Reprod Biol* 1996;**65**:201–7.

25  COSA-NZ-UK Endometrial cancer study groups. Adjuvant medroxyprogesterone acetate in high risk endometrial cancer. *Int J Gynecol Cancer* 1998;**8**:387–91.

26  Lhomme C, Vennin P, Callet N *et al.* A multicentre phase II study with Triptorelin (sustained release LHRH Agonist) in advanced or recurrent endometrial carcinoma: A French anti-cancer federation study. *Gynecol Oncol* 1999;**75**:187–93.

27  Rose P, Brunetto VL, Van Le L, Bell J, Walker JL, Lee RB. A phase II trial of anastrozole in advanced recurrent or persistent endometrial carcinoma. A GOG study. *Gynecol Oncol* 2000;**78**:212–16.

28  Thigpen JT, Buschsbaum HJ, Mangan C, Blessing JA. Phase II trial of adriamycin in the treatment of advanced or recurrent endometrial carcinoma: a GOG study. *Cancer Treat Rep* 1979;**63**:21–7.

29  Thigpen JT, Blessing JA, Homesley HD, Creasman WT, Sutton G. Phase II trial of cisplatin as first line chemotherapy in patients with advanced or recurrent endometrial carcinoma. A GOG study. *Gynecol Oncol* 1989;**33**:68–70.

30  Dimopoulos MA, Papadimitriou CA, Georgoulias V *et al.* Paclitaxel and cisplatin in advanced or recurrent carcinoma of the endometrium. Long term results of a phase II multicentre study. *Gynecol Oncol* 2000;**78**:52–7.

31  Lissoni A, Gabriele A, Gorga G *et al.* Cisplatin, epirubicin and paclitaxel-containing chemotherapy in uterine adenocarcinoma. *Ann Oncol* 1997;**8**:969–72.

32  Munkarah A. Editorial. Is there a role for surgical cytoreduction in stage IV endometrial cancer? *Gynecol Oncol* 2000;**78**:83–4.

33  Bristow RE, Zerbe MJ, Rosenshein NB, Grumbine FC, Montz FJ. Stage IVB endometrial carcinoma: The role of cytoreductive surgery and determinants of survival. *Gynecol Oncol* 2000;**78**:85–91.

34  Ackerman I, Malone S, Thomas G, Franssen E, Balough J, Dembo A. Endometrial carcinoma – relative effectiveness of adjuvant irradiation vs. therapy reserved for relapse. *Gynecol Oncol* 1996;**60**:177–83.

35  Mccluggage WG, Abdulkader M, Price JH *et al.* Uterine carcinosarcomas in patients receiving tamoxifen. A report of 19 cases. *Int J Gynecol Cancer* 2000;**10**:280–4.

36  Rose PG, Boutselis JG, Sachs L. Adjuvant therapy for stage I uterine sarcoma. *Am J Obstet Gynecol* 1987;**156**:660–2.

37  Omura GA, Blessing JA, Major F *et al.* A randomized clinical trial of adjuvant adriamycin in uterine sarcomas: a Gynecologic Oncology Group study. *J Clin Oncol* 1985;**3**:1240–5.

38  Piver MS, Lele SB, Marchetti DL *et al.* Effect of adjuvant chemotherapy on time to recurrence and survival of stage I uterine sarcomas. *J Surg Oncol* 1988;**38**:233–9.

39  Van Nagell JR, Hanson MB, Donaldson ES *et al.* Adjuvant vincristine, dactinomycin, and cyclophosphamide therapy in stage I uterine sarcomas. A pilot study. *Cancer* 1986;**57**:1451–4.

40  Peters WA, Rivkin SE, Smith MR *et al.* Cisplatin and adriamycin combination chemotherapy for uterine stromal sarcomas and mixed mesodermal tumors. *Gynecol Oncol* 1989;**34**:323–7.

41  Olah KS, Gee H, Blunt S, Dunn JA, Kelly K, Chan KK. Retrospective analysis of 318 cases of uterine sarcoma. *Eur J Cancer* 1991;**27**: 1095–9.

42  Knocke TH, Kucera H, Dorfler D, Pokrajac B, Potter R. Results of post operative radiotherapy in treatment of sarcoma of the corpus uteri. *Cancer* 1998;**83**:1972–9.

43  Hornback NB, Omura G, Major FJ. Observations on the use of adjuvant radiation therapy in patients with stage I and II uterine sarcoma. *Int J Radiat Oncol Biol Phys* 1986;**12**:2127–30.

44  Gerszen K, Faul C, Kounelis S, Huang Q, Kelly J, Jones MW. The impact of adjuvant radiotherapy on carcinosarcoma of the uterus. *Gynecol Oncol* 1998;**68**:8–13.

45  Sorbe B. Radiotherapy and/or chemotherapy as adjuvant treatment of uterine sarcomas. *Gynecol Oncol* 1985;**20**:281–9.

46  Sutton G, Blessing J, Park R, DiSiaa P, Rosenshein N. Ifosfamide treatment of recurrent or metastatic endometrial stromal sarcomas previously unexposed to chemotherapy; a study of the Gynecologic Oncology Group. *Obstet Gynecol* 1996;**87**:747–50.

47  Sutton GP, Blessing JA, Rosenshein N, Photopulos G, DiSaia PJ. Phase II trial of ifosfamide and mesna in mixed mesodermal tumors of the uterus: A Gynecologic Oncology Group study. *Am J Obstet Gynecol* 1989;**161**:309–12.

48  Sutton GP, Blessing JA, Barrett RJ, McGehee R. Phase II trial of ifosfamide and mesna in leiomyosarcoma of the uterus: a Gynecologic Oncology Group study. *Am J Obstet Gynecol* 1992;**166**:556–9.

49  Sutton G, Blessing JA, Malfetano JH. Ifosfamide and doxorubicin in the treatment of advanced leiomyosarcomas of the uterus: a Gynecologic Oncology Group study. *Gynecol Oncol* 1996;**62**:226–9.

50  Kushner DM, Webster KD, Belinson JL, Rybicki LA, Kennedy AW, Markman M. Safety and efficacy of adjuvant single agent ifosfamide in uterine sarcoma. *Gynecol Oncol* 2000;**78**:221–7.

51  Hawkins RE, Wiltshaw E, Mansi JL. Ifosfamide with and without adriamycin in advanced uterine leiomyosarcoma. *Cancer Chem Pharm* 1990;S26–S29.

52  Sarcoma Meta-analsis Collaboration. Adjuvant chemotherapy for localised resectable soft-tissue sarcoma of adults: meta-analysis of individual data. *Lancet* 1997;**350**:1647–54.

53  Krieger PD, Gusberg SB. Endolymphatic stromal myosis A grade I endometrial sarcoma. *Gynecol Oncol* 1973;**1**:299–313.

# 37 Cancer of the cervix and vagina

*RP Symonds*

Sixty years ago, cervical cancer was the most common cause of death from cancer in American women. Screening and other measures have dramatically reduced both incidence and mortality in the USA (13 700 new cases in and 4900 deaths in 1998).[1] In Britain, following the overhaul of the screening programme, incidence fell by 50% and mortality by 35% between 1988 and 1997.[2]

Worldwide, however, cervical cancer is second to breast cancer in incidence and mortality with an estimated incidence of 500 000 cases annually. The incidence is particularly high in South and South East Asia, South America, and sub-Saharan Africa where this disease is the major cause of female cancer deaths.[3]

Molecular and epidemiological studies have demonstrated a strong relationship with infection with human papilloma virus and both premalignant disease and invasive cancer.[4] The most common histological type is squamous (80%) followed by adeno- and adenosquamous carcinoma (10–15%). There is evidence that the incidence of adenocarcinoma is increasing, particularly in younger women.[5]

Primary vaginal cancer is defined as a malignant lesion of the vagina with no involvement of cervix or vulva.[6] In comparison with cervical cancer, cancer of the vagina is rare and accounts for only 1–2% of all female malignancies. In the 1980s, two British series gave an incidence of about 35 cases of cervical cancer to each case of primary carcinoma of vagina.[7,8]

Squamous cancer is the most common histological type. In the past it was a disease of the elderly associated often with chronic irritation of the vaginal mucosa secondary to prolapse and the use of ring pessaries.[7] In the past 20 years, more cases have been seen in young women associated with HPV infection and the premalignant lesion, vaginal intraepithelial neoplasia (VAIN). A proportion of cases of clear cell carcinoma of vagina were associated with diethylstilbestrol (DES) injections in the past.[9]

The chemoradiotherapy section below is based upon the results of a Cochrane review.[10]

## Carcinoma of the cervix

### Has the FIGO staging system for cervical cancer survived the test of time?

A uniform staging system for cervical cancer was first suggested by the Cancer Commission of the League of

---

**Box 37.1 FIGO staging rules for carcinoma of cervix 1994**

**Stage 0:** Carcinoma *in situ*, cervical intraepithelial neoplasia grade III

**Stage I:** The carcinoma is strictly confined to the cervix (extension to the corpus would be disregarded)

   **Ia:** Invasive carcinoma, which can be diagnosed only by microscopy. All macroscopically visible lesions – even with superficial invasion – are allotted to stage 1b carcinomas. Invasion is limited to a measured stromal invasion with a maximal depth of 5·0 mm and a horizontal extension of not more than 7·0 mm. Depth of invasion should not be over 5·0 mm in tissue taken from the base of the epithelium of the original tissue – superficial or glandular. The involvement of vascular spaces – venous or lymphatic – should not change the stage allotment

      **Ia$_1$:** Measured stromal invasion of not more than 3·0 mm in depth and extension of not more than 7·0 mm

      **Ia$_2$:** Measured stromal invasion of more than 3·0 mm and not more than 5·0 mm with an extension of not more than 7·0 mm

   **Ib:** Clinically visible lesions limited to the cervix uteri or preclinical cancers greater than stage 1a

      **Ib$_1$:** Clinically visible lesions not more than 4·0 cm

      **Ib$_2$:** Clinically visible lesions more than 4·0 cm

**Stage II:** Cervical carcinoma invades beyond the uterus but not to the pelvic wall or to the lower third of the vagina

   **IIa:** Involvement of upper third of vagina
   **IIb:** Obvious parametrial involvement

**Stage III:** The carcinoma has extended to the pelvic wall. On rectal examination there is no cancer-free space between the tumour and the pelvic wall. The tumour involves the

*(Continued)*

---

Box 37.1 *(Continued)*

> lower third of the vagina. All cases with hydronephrosis of non-functioning kidney are included, unless they are known to be due to other causes
>
> **IIIa:** Tumour involves lower third of the vagina with no extension to the pelvic wall
>
> **IIIb:** Extension to the pelvic wall and/or hydronephrosis or non-functioning kidney

**Stage IV:** The carcinoma has extended beyond the true pelvis, or has involved (biopsy-proven) the mucosa of the bladder or rectum. Bullous oedema, as such, does not permit a case to be allotted to stage IV

> **IVa:** Spread of the growth to adjacent organs
> **IVb:** Spread to distant organs

Table 37.1  Carcinoma of the cervix. Patients treated in 1990–92. Survival by FIGO stage[11]

| Stage | Patients (N = 11 945) | Overall 5-year survival (%) |
|---|---|---|
| Ia1 | 518 | 95·1 |
| Ib2 | 384 | 94·9 |
| Ib | 4657 | 80·1 |
| IIa | 813 | 66·3 |
| IIb | 2251 | 63·5 |
| IIIa | 180 | 33·3 |
| IIIb | 2350 | 38·7 |
| IVa | 294 | 17·1 |
| IVb | 198 | 9·4 |

Nations in 1928 and with modifications this became the basis of the first staging system of the International Federation of Gynaecology and Obstetrics in 1950.[11] The latest revision of the scheme was in 1994 and is listed in Box 37.1.

The basis of this staging system is essentially clinical and the only mandatory investigations are examination under anaesthetic, cystoscopy, chest $x$ ray and urography. More sophisticated imaging such as computed tomography (CT scanning) and medical resonance imaging (MRI) are not compulsory. This means that cancer of the cervix can be staged in a District General Hospital in virtually any part of the world.

The purpose of any cancer staging scheme is to facilitate comparison of the results of treatment and to act as a prognostic discriminator. This essentially empirical clinical staging system still fulfils these criteria. It allows the clinician to choose whether the patients should have non-radical or radical surgery, radiotherapy, or chemoradiotherapy. The stage categories fit into broad prognostic bands each with a survival difference of roughly 15–20%. This can be seen in the results of patients treated between 1990 and 1992 as reported to the International Federation of Gynecology and Obstetrics[11] (Table 37.1) **Evidence level III, Grade B** .

## Can microinvasive carcinoma be treated by less than radical means?

The term microinvasive carcinoma was first defined in 1947 to include a group of patients who perhaps could be treated by less than radical means. Since 1961, the definition of microinvasive cancer has undergone a number of changes. The current classification (see Box 37.1) has two groups: stage Ia$_1$ and stage Ia$_2$.

There are no randomised trials in the treatment of stage Ia carcinoma of cervix but retrospective series seems to indicate that stage Ia$_1$ can be managed by less than radical means, but more extensive treatment is more effective in stage Ia$_2$.

### Management of stage Ia$_1$

Large retrospective population-based studies indicate that prognosis for this cancer stage is excellent and radical surgery is not required. A 100% 5-year survival was reported for patients treated in Dundee[12] and in the west of Scotland.[13] The very large American SEER study of 10% of all patients treated for gynaecological cancer in the United States between 1973 and 1987 reported a 97% 5-year survival.[14] The large series of 309 patients reported from Graz[15] suggests that simple hysterectomy or cone biopsy is as effective as either radical vaginal or abdominal hysterectomy if there is less than 3 mm stromal invasion **Evidence level III, Grade B** .

### Treatment of stage Ia$_2$

Again, there are no prospective randomised studies to guide us in the management of stage Ia$_2$. The FIGO definition of this disease seems to be valid as both depth of stromal invasion, surface horizontal spread and lymph vascular space invasion (not included in the FIGO definition) are predictors of outcome. Spread to regional lymph nodes is a major predictor for both recurrence and survival in cervical cancer. Patients with stromal invasion between 3 and 5 mm have a reported incidence of lymph node metastasis in the order of 7% and an overall recurrence rate of about 5%. Vascular space involvement is a useful predictor of possible nodal metastasis. In a retrospective series of about 94 patients[16] the incidence of lymph node metastasis with or without lymph vascular space invasion was 16·1% and 3·2%, respectively. It is more difficult to measure the horizontal surface dimension of a tumour compared to the depth of stromal invasion. A stage Ia$_2$ lesion must extend less than 7 mm horizontally. The most important aspect of this measurement is to distinguish patients with microinvasive tumours from those where the staging is frankly stage 1b (and usually visible to the naked eye) who unequivocally require radical treatment.

Owing to the small risk of recurrence and pelvic lymph node metastasis, the consensus is that the majority of patients with stage Ia$_2$ should be treated by extra fascial modified radical hysterectomy and pelvic lymphadenectomy, although there are few prospective data to support this point of view. Large retrospective series such as those of Burghardt *et al.*[15] certainly do suggest that more extensive treatment is more effective than simple hysterectomy or conisation, but even so the number of deaths associated with conservative treatment are small **Evidence level III, Grade B** .

## Radiotherapy or radical hysterectomy for stage Ib–IIa carcinoma of cervix?

Population-based retrospective studies show very similar results for radical surgery or radical radiotherapy in the treatment of potentially operable cervical cancer.[13] This may explain the lack of clinical trials over the years.

In 1975, Newton and colleagues[17] reported a randomised study of 119 patients, randomised to receive either radical hysterectomy or radical surgery. The 10-year survival rates favoured surgery (75%) rather than radiotherapy (65%) but were not statistically different. It is noteworthy that six out of 12 patients whose cancer recurred after surgery were successfully cured by radiotherapy.

The definitive modern randomised study was carried out in North Italy,[18] 343 patients with stage Ib or IIa tumours fit for either modality were randomised to either radical surgery or radical radiotherapy: 5-year overall and disease-free survival was identical for both surgical and radiotherapy groups (83% and 74%, respectively) (Figures 37.1–37.4).

A surprisingly large percentage of patients (64%) had postoperative radiotherapy following radical surgery for adverse pathological findings. This high frequency of postoperative radiotherapy does not explain the increased morbidity in patients treated by surgery. Of those treated by surgery alone 31% had grade 2–3 morbidity. By comparison, only 12% of patients treated by radiation had grade 2–3 morbidity. The combination of both treatments produced a grade 2–3 morbidity of 29%. In this study, although the frequency of serious complications was greater in the surgical arm, these complications were easier to correct than those secondary to radiation.

The conclusion of this study is that the optimum candidates for primary radical surgery were women with normal ovarian function and cervical diameters of 4 cm

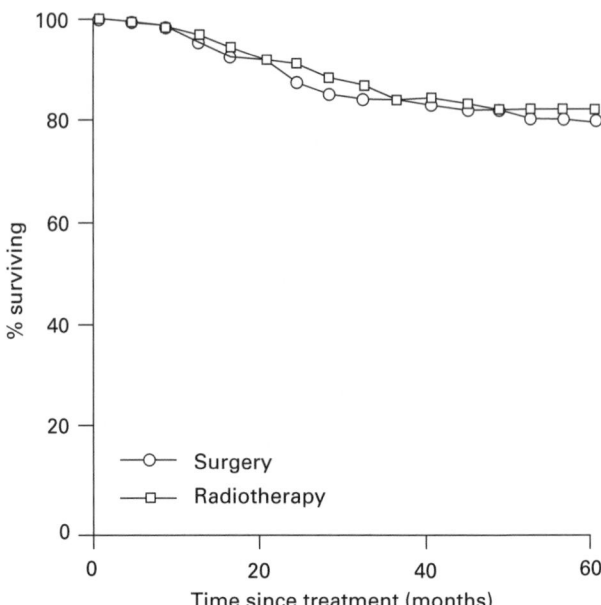

**Figure 37.1**  Overall actuarial survival by treatment group. Adapted with permission from Landoni *et al. Lancet* 1997;**350**:28–33)

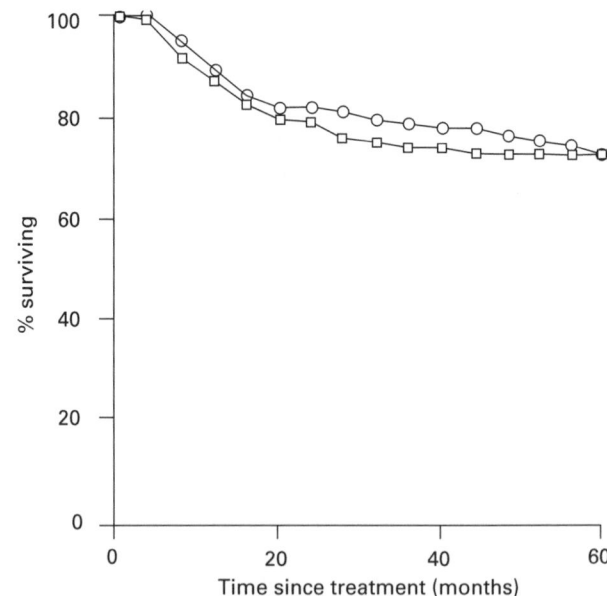

**Figure 37.2**  Disease-free actuarial survival by treatment group. Adapted with permission from Landoni *et al. Lancet* 1997;**350**:28–33)

or smaller, whereas radiotherapy was preferable for postmenopausal women. It is noteworthy in this series that 88% of patients with tumours greater than 4 cm treated by primary surgery, required postoperative radiotherapy **Evidence level Ib, Grade A** .

It is commonly said that radical surgery preserves sexual function compared to irradiation in the treatment of

**Table 37.2** Five of the most influential trials of radiotherapy and cisplatin-based chemotherapy.

| Trial | No. of patients | Stage | External beam R/T | LDR brachytherapy dose to point A | Chemotherapy | Survival | Reduction in risk of death | P |
|---|---|---|---|---|---|---|---|---|
| GOG 85[23] | 368 | IIb, III, IVa | As GOG 120 | As GOG 120 | Hydroxyurea or hydroxyurea cisplatin and 5-FU | 43% 55% | 0·74 | 0·018 |
| GOG 120[24] | 575 | IIb, III, IVa | 40·8 Gy in 24 fractions (stage IIb) 51·0 Gy in 30 fractions (stage III, IVa) | 40 Gy (stage IIb) 30 Gy (III or IVa) in 1 or 2 insertions | Hydroxyurea or hydroxyurea cisplatin and 5-FU or weekly cisplatin | 47% 65% at 3 years 65% | 0·58 0·61 | 0·004 0·002 |
| RTOG 9001[25] | 403 | IIb III, IVa, or Ib IIa >5 cm or +ve pelvic nodes | Pelvic and para-aortic 45 Gy in 25 fractions or pelvic 45 Gy in 25 fractions | 40 Gy (minimum total dose 85 Gy) in 1 or 2 insertions | None or cisplatin and 5-FU | 58% at 5 years 73% | 0·52 | 0·004 |
| GOG 123[26] | 374 | Bulky Ib (>4 cm) | 45 Gy in 25 fractions | 30 Gy | None or weekly cisplatin | 74% at 3 years 83% | 0·54 | 0·008 |
| SWOG 8797[27] | 243 | Ia$_2$, Ib, IIa p.o. adverse path finding | 49·3 Gy in 29 fractions | No brachytherapy | None or cisplatin 5-FU | 71% at 4 years 81% | 0·50 | 0·007 |

operable cervical cancer. There are no randomised trials to support this claim. A Swedish study comparing sexual function of women treated with early stage cervical cancer, compared with a control group randomly selected for age and region of residence, found that persistent vaginal changes compromised sexual activity and resulted in considerable distress.[19] The authors found treatment with surgery alone was associated with increased risks of insufficient vaginal lubrication, vaginal shortness and reduced vaginal elasticity. As compared with surgery alone, intracavity or external beam therapy, or both, in addition or instead of surgery, had a small effect, if any, on the risks of reduced vaginal lubrication, reduced genital swelling, vaginal shortness, or vaginal inelasticity. The effect of treatment upon sexual function is a very poorly investigated topic and requires further study **Evidence level IV, Grade C** .

### What is the best treatment for stages II, III and IVa cervical cancer?

Radiotherapy is the treatment of choice for more advanced stage cancer. Treatment is usually a combination of external beam megavoltage radiotherapy to the pelvis plus a local boost to the pelvis using brachytherapy. There is no consensus on the best technique of brachytherapy or even where and how to measure the radiation dose given to the tumour.[20]

One reason may be that in skilled hands the 5-year survival at various stages is remarkably similar with the use of conceptually different external beam schedules and types of brachytherapy. Typical results appear in Table 37.1. Recently the fashion has been to treat fitter patients with chemotherapy along with radiotherapy **Evidence level III, Grade B** .

### What is the value of combined chemoradiotherapy?

Both clinical studies and animal experiments have shown that radiation doses that will consistently eradicate small tumours will be only effective in a minority of large lesions. The maximum radiation dose that can be given to patients with carcinoma of cervix is limited by the tolerance of surrounding organs such as bladder or bowel. Even employing what is considered optimal external beam

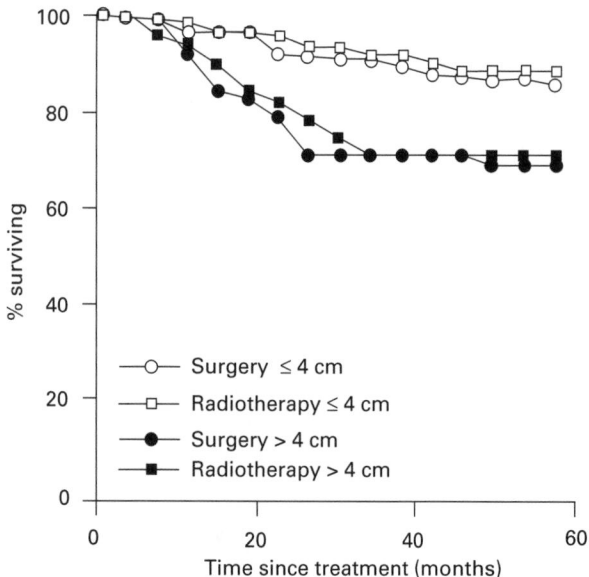

**Figure 37.3** Overall actuarial survival by treatment group and cervical diameter. Adapted with permission from Landoni *et al. Lancet* 1997;**350**:28–33)

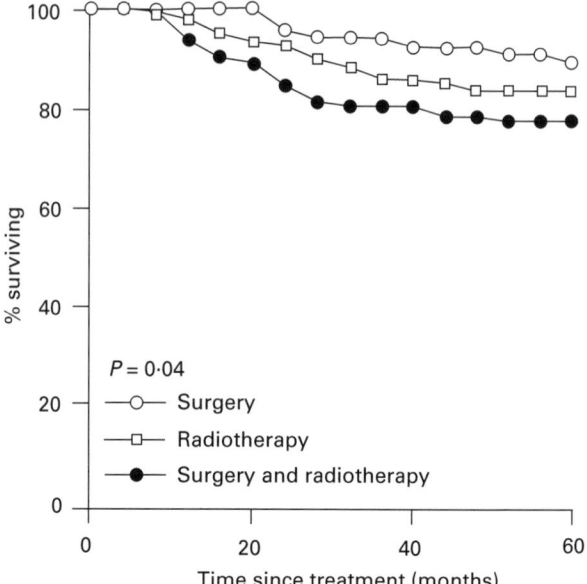

**Figure 37.4** Overall actuarial survival by treatment group. Adapted with permission from Landoni *et al. Lancet* 1997;**350**:28–33)

fractionation in combination with intracavity treatment, local control is seen in only approximately half of patients with stage III and stage IVa tumours.

Theoretically, chemotherapy combined with radiotherapy may increase the therapeutic ratio by producing a greater tumour regression than either component alone without any increase in toxicity. Chemotherapy may act as a cytotoxic within its own right, killing cells within the irradiated pelvis and by acting upon distant metastases. Chemotherapy can also act as a radiation sensitiser leading to superadded cell kill.

Cisplatin is the most effective cytotoxic agent in the treatment of cervical cancer. Response rates of up to 72% have been seen in previously untreated patients when cisplatin-based chemotherapy has been given before radiotherapy,[21] but a meta-analysis of chemotherapy given before radiotherapy has not shown a consistent survival advantage.[22] However, chemotherapy given along with radiotherapy seems to be much more effective.

The magnitude of this effect led the National Cancer Institute of the United States in February 1999 to consider that all patients with cervical cancer should be considered for concomitant chemoradiotherapy. This view was based on results of five of the then unpublished randomised clinical trials that showed a reduction of between 30% and 50% in the odds of mortality.

Five of the most influential studies are listed in Table 37.2. A meta-analysis has been carried out of 19 trials (17 published, two unpublished) performed between 1981 and 2000 using the Cochrane collaborative methodology.[28] These trials included 4580 randomised patients although, owing to patient exclusion and differential reporting, between 2865 and 3611 patients were available for different analyses. The trials differed in size, design, accrual period, and anticancer agent and schedule, cisplatin being the most commonly employed agent. The review strongly suggests that chemoradiation improves overall survival (HR 0·71; $P < 0.00001$) whether platinum was used (HR 0·70; $P < 0.00001$) or not (HR 0·81; $P = 0.20$) (Figure 37.3).

These effects were not modulated by the use of sequential chemotherapy, use of hydroxyurea in the control arm, or the timing of chemotherapy. There was some evidence that the beneficial effect was greater in trials including a higher proportion of stage I and stage II patients ($P = 0.009$). These relative effects translated into an absolute benefit of 16% (95% CI 13–19%) and 12% (95% CI 8–16%) in progression-free survival and overall survival respectively. There is evidence that chemotherapy reduced both local recurrence (OR 0·61; $P < 0.0001$) and also distant metastases. In addition to the expected improvement in local control, there was a highly significant reduction in the rate of distant metastases (OR 0·57; $P < 0.0001$) in patients treated with platinum or non-platinum based chemotherapy, an effect that was not apparent in individual trials (see Figure 37.4). This reduction was achieved with relatively

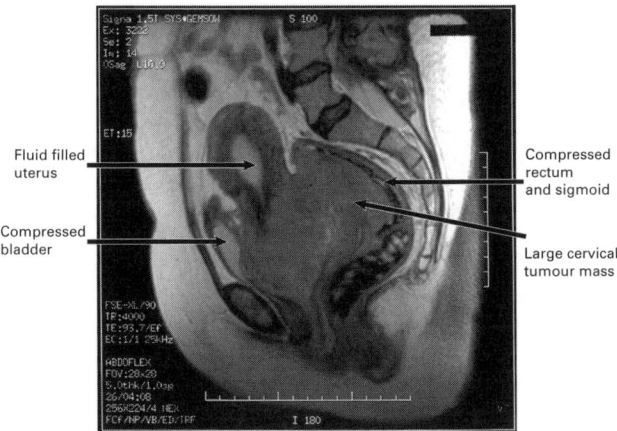

**Figure 37.5**   MRI scan of a patient with a stage III poorly differentiated cervical carcinoma before treatment

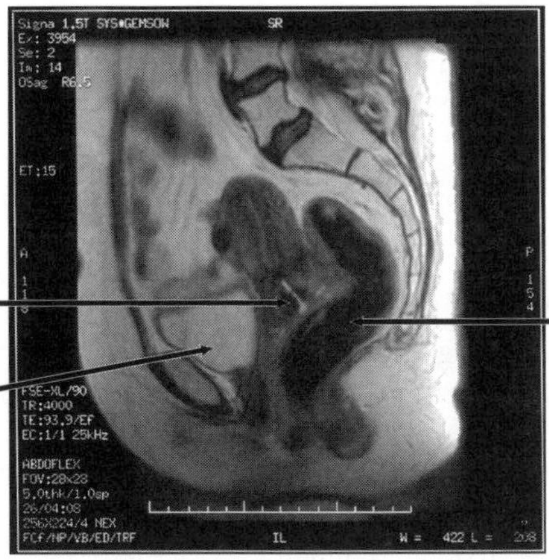

**Figure 37.6**   MRI scan of a patient with a stage III poorly differentiated cervical carcinoma after treatment

short courses of chemotherapy combined with local treatment, yet currently there is no evidence that chemotherapy given before radiotherapy reduces the incidence of distant metastases.

Combined chemoradiotherapy seems to improve the therapeutic ratio. However, acute toxicity, particularly leucopenia and gastrointestinal effects, was increased in the combined arms of all trials. Acute side effects are generally of short duration and resolve with medical management, whilst the late complications of radiotherapy lead to damage, which can be difficult to reverse, and may permanently impair quality of life. Unfortunately, late toxicity was recorded systematically in only three studies and the details of late morbidity reported in other studies were sparse. Published information so far would indicate that there is no apparent increase in late complications but this question has not been fully answered.

Combined chemoradiotherapy has become the current standard of care but there still remains a number of outstanding issues, particularly the impact of radiation dose and the treatment duration plus the role of other cytotoxics in addition to cisplatin and drug scheduling **Evidence level Ia, Grade A** .

Figure 37.5 is an MRI scan of a patient with a stage III poorly differentiated cervical carcinoma filling the pelvis, compressing both the bladder and the rectosigmoid colon. She was treated with six pulses of cisplatin ($40 \text{ mg m}^{-2}$) given weekly during pelvic radiotherapy; 45 Gy was given to the pelvic tumour using four 10 Mv *x* ray beams. This was followed by a single Selectron insertion of 26 Gy to point A at 1·46 Gy per hour. An MRI scan 2 months after treatment (Figure 37.6) showed no evidence of tumour.

This was confirmed by examination under anaesthetic, laparoscopy and biopsies of the cervix.

## What is the role of chemotherapy for stage IVb or recurrent disease?

Chemotherapy is rarely curative when given either to treat stage IVb disease or for recurrence after radiotherapy or surgery. This treatment is palliative in nature and should be used only to treat symptomatic disease. It is therefore surprising that no studies have looked at the impact of chemotherapy upon quality of life. Response to chemotherapy is usually associated with a statistically significant increase in survival. However, no studies have been carried out with a no treatment or best supportive care arm. Such trials are difficult to conduct, as patients are reluctant to be randomised to no anticancer treatment. There is a perception that they may miss the chance of living longer.

Most published studies are of the phase II type often containing at most 30–40 patients. There are few published phase III trials. The reason why response rates vary markedly between series may be due to patient variability between studies. The highest response rates are seen in previously untreated patients. The worst response rates are seen in patients with recurrence in previously irradiated sites. Obstructive uropathy is common and this may compromise the administration of the most effective drugs, which are renally excreted. Similarly, if there has been extensive radiotherapy, bone marrow reserves may be depleted and only lower drug doses can be given.

Cisplatin is the most effective agent.[29] There is evidence of a dose–response relationship. A comparison of 50 mg m$^{-2}$ and 100 mg m$^{-2}$ given 3 weekly demonstrated 21% and 31% response rates, but there was only a minimal increase in complete response rate (CR) from 10% to 13%, as well as no significant improvement in response duration, progression-free interval or survival.[30]

Scheduling may be important. The response rate to cisplatin 50 mg m$^{-2}$ given weekly was 47% with a response rate of 56% in previously irradiated sites. Interestingly any response was seen within 1 month of starting treatment. However, the mean survival of all treated patients was only 32 weeks, but there were a small number of long-term survivors (13%) at 18 months.[31]

The platinum analogues carboplatin and iproplatin are generally viewed as inferior to cisplatin with response rates of 15% and 11%, respectively. Amongst other drugs, only ifosfamide and anthracyclines have reproducible response rates above 15%.[29]

The message from published phase III trials seems clear. Response rates from combination chemotherapy are higher than those seen after single agent cisplatin but survival is not enhanced. Typical results were seen in a large prospective randomised Gynecological Oncology Group trial. A combination of cisplatin and ifosfamide had a higher response rate (31·1%) compared to cisplatin alone (17·8%). Overall survival time was not increased – 8·3 and 8 months respectively.[32]

The dilemma currently faced by clinicians is that the most effective drug, cisplatin, is now frequently used along with radiation therapy as initial treatment. On relapse, there is no obvious drug of choice. A number of new drugs have shown modest activity of 15–20% including paclitaxel,[33] docetaxel,[34] vinorelbine[35] and gemcitabine.[36] Trials need to be conducted to find the optimum combination. Weekly docetaxel and gemcitabine looks promising. A major problem is that unlike cisplatin these drugs are very expensive. As the bulk of this disease is seen in the developing world, most patients will not be able to afford these treatments **Evidence level Ib, Grade A** .

## Carcinoma of vagina

### What is the best treatment for vaginal cancer?

As vaginal cancer is rare, the literature is all retrospective series with no phase III trials. The outstanding questions are the best management of vaginal intraepithelial neoplasia and the role of surgery and radiotherapy.

### *Staging*

The staging of vaginal cancer is largely by clinical examination, cystoscopy, and proctoscopy and is listed in

---

**Box 37.2 FIGO staging of vaginal cancer**

**Stage 0:** Carcinoma *in situ*, vaginal intraepithelial neoplasia (VAIN)
**Stage 1:** Carcinoma confined to the vaginal wall
**Stage II:** Carcinoma involves the subvaginal tissue but has not extended to the pelvic wall
**Stage III:** Carcinoma extends to the pelvic wall
**Stage IV:** Carcinoma extends beyond the true pelvis or involves mucosa of bladder or rectum

    **IVa:** Spread to adjacent organs
    **IVb:** Spread to distant organs

---

Box 37.2. The results of treatment tend to be slightly worse than cervical cancer and the 5-year survival compiled from six published series[6] is listed in Table 37.3.

### *Vaginal intraepithelial neoplasia (VAIN)*

VAIN is an asymptomatic pathological finding in the vaginal mucosa with histological changes identical to cervical intraepithelial neoplasia. Most patients with VAIN have a history of previous dysplasia or carcinoma of the cervix or vulva. As with CIN, VAIN is graded according to the severity of histological change. Approximately 50% of cases are VAIN 1, 20% are VAIN 2, and 30% are VAIN 3. Unlike CIN, VAIN has been studied less intensively and its natural history is not well defined. However between 20% to 36%[37,38] of high grade lesions progress to invasive cancer.

The uncertainty about the natural history makes management strategies difficult to justify, particularly in terms of intensity and toxicity. Successful treatment of VAIN is difficult and there is no general agreement on the most appropriate management. Good short-term results have been reported following $CO_2$ laser vaporisation[39] but other series have reported 50–70% incidence of treatment failure.[40] One reason for failure after laser therapy is that atypical epithelia may be inaccessible to the laser in the vault suture line or hidden in the angles of the vaginal vault. The reported incidence of recurrence after partial or total

**Table 37.3 Primary vaginal cancer: stage distribution and 5-year survival[6]**

| Stage | Per cent distribution | Percent 5-year survival |
|---|---|---|
| I | 27 | 73 |
| II | 39 | 49 |
| III | 20 | 27 |
| IV | 14 | 17 |

vaginectomy is 4–17%.[41] This operation is difficult to perform and sequelae include vagina shortening, stenosis and bladder hypotonia.

Intracavity radiotherapy is a highly effective treatment with 83–100% of patients remaining free of disease. Side effects can include vaginal adhesions, shortening and stenosis. Concerns have been raised about the risks of radiation-induced cancer.[39] Little is known of this risk of treatment. However, a multinational study of 182 040 patients treated by radiation for cervical cancer showed that the risk of secondary cancer was very low[42] **Evidence level III, Grade B** .

### Surgery

Surgery as primary treatment has a limited role. Suitable patients would be young and fit, and have a stage I cancer involving the upper posterior vagina. The patient would require a radical hysterectomy (if the uterus was still present), a partial vaginectomy and lymphadenectomy.

More advanced staged tumours are best treated by radiotherapy. The alternative is pelvic exenteration, which is an extensive and mutilating operation involving the creation of one or two permanent stoma, loss of sexual function and considerable change in body image. The place of this operation has been well explored in the treatment of cervical cancer[43] but not in the management of this disease. Exenteration has been used as a palliative measure in the face of overwhelming symptoms in the management of recurrent vaginal cancer[44] **Evidence level IV, Grade C** .

### Radiotherapy

Radiotherapy is the treatment of choice in most cases, as patients tend to be elderly and unfit. Small superficial lesions can be treated by brachytherapy only, but a combination of external beam and interstitial therapy is the treatment of choice in most cases.[7] The results of external beam treatment alone are inferior to combination treatment.[45] The most appropriate brachytherapy technique depends on the tumour site. Those in the upper third of the vagina are treated with the same techniques used in cervical cancer. Either a vaginal tube or interstitial implant can be used in the mid-third. Interstitial implantation is the boost technique of choice in the lower third of the vagina.

Analysis of a series of 40 patients treated over a 12-year period, suggested that radiotherapy was more effective in the treatment of tumours in the proximal part of the vagina (actuarial overall survival 81%) compared with the distal group (41%)[46] **Evidence level III, Grade B** .

### Chemoradiotherapy

There is no available information about the value of concomitant chemotherapy and radiation treatment in this rare disease. However, as the tumour behaves very similarly to cervical cancer, concomitant therapy should be considered for suitable fit patients **Evidence level IV, Grade C** .

## References

1  Shoell WMJ, Janicek MF, Mirhashemi R, Epidemiology and biology of cervical cancer. *Semin Surg Oncol* 1999;**16**:203–11.
2  Quinn M, Babb P, Jones J *et al.* Effects of screening on incidence of and mortality from cancer of the cervix in England: evaluation based on routinely collected statistics. *BMJ* 1999;**318**:904–8.
3  Pisani P, Parkin DM, Bray F, Ferlay J. Estimates of the world wide mortality from 25 cancers in 1990. *Int J Cancer* 1999;**83**:18–29.
4  Visscher DW, Lawrence WD. Human papilloma virus and cervical cancer. In: Hillier SG, Kitchener HC, Neilson JP, eds. *Scientific essentials of reproductive medicine.* London: WB. Saunders, 1996.
5  Sasieni P, Adams P. Changing rates of adenocarcinoma and adenosquamous carcinoma of the cervix in England. *Lancet* 2001;**357**:1490–3.
6  Goodman A. Primary vaginal cancer. *Surg Oncol Clin North Am* 1998;**7**:347–61.
7  MacNaught R, Symonds RP, Hole D, Watson ER. Improved control of primary vaginal tumours by combined external beam and interstitial radiotherapy. *Clin Radiol* 1986;**37**:29–32.
8  Al-Kurdi M, Monaghan JM. Thirty two years experience in the management of primary tumours of the vagina. *Br J Obstet Gynaecol* 1981;**88**:1145–50.
9  Herbst AL, Ulfelder H, Poskanzer DC. Adenocarcinoma of the vagina: association of maternal stilbestrol therapy with tumour appearance in young women. *N Engl J Med* 1971;**284**:878–81.
10  Green J, Kirwan J, Tierney J *et al.* Survival and recurrence after concomitant chemotherapy and radiotherapy for cancer of the uterine cervix: a systemic review and meta-analysis. *Lancet* 2001;**358**:781–6.
11  Benedet J, Odicino F, Maisonneuve P *et al.* FIGO 1990–92 annual report: results of treatment of carcinoma of the cervix uteri. *J Epidemiol Biostat* 1998;**3**:5–34.
12  Duncan ID, Walker J. Microinvasive squamous carcinoma of cervix in the Tayside region of Scotland. *Br J Obstet Gynaecol* 1977;**84**:67–70.
13  Bisset D, Lamont DW, Nwabineli NJ, Brodie MM, Symonds RP. The treatment of Stage I carcinoma of cervix in the west of Scotland 1980–1987. *Br J Obstet Gynaecol* 1994;**101**:615–20.
14  Kosary CL. FIGO Stage, histology, histologic grade, age and race prognostic factors in determining survival for cancers of the female gynecological system: an analysis of 1973–1987 SEER cases of cancers of the endometrium, cervix, ovary, vulva and vagina. *Semin Surg Oncol* 1994;**10**:31–46.
15  Burghardt E, Giradi F, Lahousen M, Pickel H, Tamussino K. Microinvasive carcinoma of the uterine cervix (International Federation of Gynaecology and Obstetrics Stage IA) *Cancer* 1991;**67**:1037–45.
16  Buckley SL, Tritz DM, Van Le L *et al.* Lymph node metastases and prognosis in patients with Stage Ia₂ cervical cancer. *Gynecol Oncol* 1996;**63**:4–9.
17  Newton M. Radical hysterectomy or radiotherapy for Stage I cervical cancer: A prospective comparison with 5 and 10 year follow up. *Am J Obstet Gynecol* 1975;**123**:535–42.
18  Landoni F, Maneo A, Colombo A *et al.* Randomised study of radical surgery versus radiotherapy for Stage Ib-IIa cervical cancer. *Lancet* 1997;**350**:28–33.
19  Bergmark K, Avall-Lundquist E, Dickman PW, Henningsohn L, Steineck G. Vaginal changes and sexuality in women with a history of cervical cancer. *N Engl J Med* 1999;**340**:1383–9.
20  Visser AG, Symonds RP. Dose and volume specification for reporting gynaecological brachytherapy: time for a change. *Radiother Oncol* 2001;**58**:1–4.
21  Sundfor K, Trope CG, Hogberg T *et al.* Radiotherapy and neoadjuvant chemotherapy for cervical carcinoma. *Cancer* 1996;**77**:2371–8.
22  Tierney JF, Stewart LA, Parmar MK. Can the published data tell us about the effectiveness of neoadjuvant chemotherapy for locally advanced cancer of the uterine cervix? *Eur J Cancer* 1999;**35**:406–9.

23  Whitney CW, Sause W, Bundy BN *et al.* Randomised comparison of Fluourouracil plus Cisplatin versus Hydroxyurea as an adjunct to radiation therapy in Stage IIb–IVa carcinoma of cervix with negative para-aortic nodes; A Gynecologic Oncology Group and South West Oncology Group study. *J Clin Oncol* 1999;**17**:1339–48.

24  Rose PG, Bundy BN, Watkins EB *et al.* Concurrent cisplatin based radiotherapy and chemotherapy for locally advanced cervical cancer. *N Engl J Med* 1999;**340**:1144–53.

25  Morris M, Eiffel PJ, Lu JD *et al.* Pelvic radiation with concurrent chemotherapy compared with pelvic and para-aortic radiation for high risk cervical cancer. *N Engl J Med* 1999;**340**:1137–43.

26  Keys HM, Bundy BN, Stehman FB *et al.* Cisplatin, radiation and adjuvant hysterectomy compared with radiation and adjuvant hysterectomy for bulky Stage Ib cervical carcinoma. *N Engl J Med* 1999;**340**:1154–61.

27  Peters WA, Liu PY, Barrett RJ *et al.* Concurrent chemotherapy and pelvic radiation therapy compared with pelvic radiation therapy alone as adjuvant therapy after radical surgery in high risk early stage cancer of the cervix. *J Clin Oncol* 2000;**18**:1606–13.

28  Green JA, Kirwan JM, Tierney JF *et al.* Systematic review and meta-analysis of randomised trials of concomitant chemotherapy and radiotherapy for cancer of the uterine cervix: better survival and reduced distant recurrence rate. *Lancet* 2001;**358**:781–6.

29  Omura GA. Chemotherapy for Stage IVb or recurrent cancer of uterine cervix. *J Natl Cancer Inst Monogr* 1996;**21**:123–6.

30  Bonomi P, Blessing JA, Stehman EF *et al.* Randomised trial of three Cisplatin dose schedules in squamous cell carcinoma of the cervix: a Gynecologic Oncology Group study. *J Clin Oncol* 1985;**3**:1079–85.

31  Daly M, Cowie VJ, Davis JA *et al.* A short and intensive single agent cisplatin regimen for recurrent carcinoma of the uterine cervix. *Int J Gynecol Cancer* 1996;**6**:61–7.

32  Omura GA, Blessing JA, Vaccarello L *et al.* Randomised trial of cisplatin versus cisplatin plus mitolactol versus cisplatin plus ifosfamide in advanced squamous carcinoma of the cervix: A Gynecologic Oncology Group study. *J Clin Oncol* **15**:165–71.

33  Thigpen T, Vance R, Khansur T, Malamud F. The role of paclitaxel in the management of patients with carcinoma of the cervix. *Semin Oncol* 1997;**24**(Suppl. 2):451–6.

34  Kudelka AP, Verschraegen CF, Levy T *et al.* Preliminary report of the activity of Docetaxel in advanced or recurrent squamous cancer of the cervix. *Anti Cancer Drugs* 1996;**7**:398–401.

35  Morris M, Brader KR, Levenback C *et al.* Phase II study of Vinorelbine in advanced and recurrent squamous carcinoma of cervix. *J Clin Oncol* 1998;**16**:1094–8.

36  Burnett AF, Roman LD, Garcia AA *et al.* Phase 2 study of Gemcitabine and Cisplatin in patients with advanced persistent or recurrent squamous carcinoma of the cervix. *Gynecol Oncol* 2000;**76**:63–6.

37  Aho M, Vesterinen E, Meyer B *et al.* Natural history of vaginal intraepithelial neoplasia. *Cancer* 1991;**68**:195–7.

38  McIndoe WA, McLean MR, Jones RW *et al.* The invasive potential of carcinoma *in situ* of the cervix. *Obstet Gynecol* 1984;**64**:451–8.

39  Campagnutta E, Parin A, De Piero G *et al.* Treatment of vaginal intraepithelial neoplasia (VAIN) with the carbon dioxide laser. *Clin Exp Obstet Gynec* 1999;**26**:127–30.

40  Ogino I, Kitamura T, Okajima H, Matsubara S. High dose rate intracavity brachytherapy in the management of cervical and vaginal intraepithelial neoplasia. *Int. J Radiat Oncol Biol Phys* 1998;**40**:881–7.

41  Ireland D, Monaghan JM. The management of the patient with abnormal vaginal cytology following hysterectomy. *Br J Obstet Gynaecol* 1992;**95**:973–5.

42  Boice JD, Day NE, Andersen A *et al.* Second cancers following radiation treatment for cervical cancer. An international collaboration among cancer registries. *J Natl Cancer Inst* 1985;**74**:955–75.

43  Monaghan JM. Surgical management of advanced and recurrent cervical carcinoma: the place of pelvic exenteration. *Clin Obstet Gynecol* 1985;**12**:169–82.

44  Woodhouse CRJ, Plail RO, Schlesinger PE *et al.* Exenteration as palliation for patients with advanced pelvic malignancy. *Br J Urol* 1995;**76**:315–20.

45  Dixit S, Singhal S, Baboo HA. Squamous carcinoma of the vagina; a review of 70 cases. *Gynecol Oncol* 1993;**48**:80–7.

46  Ali MM, Huang DT, Goplerud DR *et al.* Radiation alone for carcinoma of the vagina: variation in response related to the location of the primary tumour. *Cancer* 1996;**77**:1934–9.

## Acknowledgements

I would like to thank Mrs J Symonds for typing the manuscript and the Editor of the *Lancet* for permission to reproduce Figures 37.1, 37.2, 37.3 and 37.4.

# 38 Treating vulval cancer

*Anca Ansink, Jacobus van der Velden, Lena van Doorn*

Vulval cancer is a disease of elderly women with a mean age at diagnosis of approximately 70 years. The incidence in industrialised countries is two per 100 000 per year.[1] According to population-based studies, about 75% of vulvar malignancies are squamous cell carcinomas.[1,2] The tumour metastasises primarily to the inguinal lymph nodes.[3]

Standard treatment for patients with cT1-2N0-1M0 tumours is primary surgery, followed by radiotherapy if indicated.[4] Surgery consists of radical excision of the tumour and bilateral femoroinguinal lymph node dissection. This treatment policy results in excellent survival figures, but also high complication rates. Wound healing problems are observed in a large proportion of patients and, in the long term, psychosexual complications and lymphoedema are frequently seen. Because of high complication rates, a more individualised approach has been developed in recent years in order to reduce complications without compromising survival.[4] Currently, patients with small tumours undergo less extensive surgery. In this chapter, we will discuss whether this less extensive surgery is as effective as the previously applied extensive procedure (see the first four questions).

The role of radiotherapy in the treatment of vulval cancer has become more prominent over the past two decades. Primary groin irradiation has been proposed as an alternative to primary groin dissection as it is anticipated that this treatment modality will induce less morbidity than primary surgery. The role of adjuvant radiotherapy in patients with positive groin nodes will be discussed (questions five and six).

In patients with T3 and T4 tumours, there is no such thing as a widely accepted standard treatment. Local control is difficult to achieve by surgery alone. Tumours are either unresectable or resection would result in considerable mutilation. Therefore, the role of chemoradiation, either as sole treatment or as a neoadjuvant approach will also be discussed (questions seven and eight).

Finally the potential role of adjuvant chemotherapy in node-positive patients is addressed in the last question.

## Criteria for studies used

### Types of studies

Studies regarding patients with histologically proven squamous cell carcinoma of the vulva are considered. Only

---

**Box 38.1 FIGO staging for carcinoma of the vulva (1995)**

**Stage 0:**  Carcinoma *in situ* (preinvasive carcinoma)

**Stage I:**  Tumour confined to vulva or vulva and perineum, 2 cm or less in greatest dimension. Inguinofemoral lymph nodes negative

**IA:**  Tumour confined to vulva or vulva and perineum, 2 cm or less in greatest dimension and with stromal invasion no greater than 1·0 mm*

**IB:**  Tumour confined to vulva or vulva and perineum, 2 cm or less in greatest dimension and with stromal invasion greater than 1·0 mm*

**Stage II:**  Tumour confined to the vulva or vulva and perineum, more than 2 cm in greatest dimension. Inguinofemoral lymph nodes negative

**Stage III:**  Tumour invades any of the following: lower urethra, vagina, anus and/or unilateral inguinofemoral lymph node metastases

**Stage IV:**

**IVA:**  Tumour invades any of the following: bladder mucosa, rectal mucosa, upper urethral mucosa, or is fixed to bone, and/or bilateral inguinofemoral lymph node metastases

**IVB:**  Any distant metastasis including pelvic lymph nodes

*The depth of invasion is defined as the measurement of the tumour from the epithelial-stromal junction of the adjacent most superficial dermal papilla, to the deepest point of invasion

---

studies on the effectiveness of treatment are incorporated. Because only a small number of randomised controlled trials have been conducted on the treatment of vulval cancer, observational studies, case–control studies and studies with historical controls have also been considered in this chapter.

### Types of participants

The current FIGO staging system for vulval cancer is based on surgical and pathological data (Box 38.1). It is therefore not possible to use this system for pretreatment assessment. When pretreatment staging is relevant, the clinical TNM system is applied (Box 38.2).

---

> **Box 38.2 TNM classification for carcinoma of the vulva**
>
> **T1:** Tumour confined to the vulva, maximum diameter 2 cm
> **T2:** Tumour confined to the vulva, diameter larger than 2 cm
> **T3:** Tumour extending into the distal vagina, distal anal mucosa, and/or distal urethral mucosa
> **T4:** Tumour extending into the proximal vagina, urethra, or anal mucosa
>
> **N0:** No clinically suspicious lymph nodes
> **N1:** Palpable but clinically non-suspicious inguinofemoral lymph nodes
> **N2:** Suspicious inguinofemoral lymph nodes
> **N3:** Fixed/ulcerated inguinofemoral lymph nodes
>
> **M0:** No clinical suspicion of distant metastases
> **M1:** Distant metastasis including clinically suspicious pelvic lymph nodes

For questions one to five, only those studies on patients with early vulval cancer were considered (cT1–2N0–1M0). In question three, a lateral tumour is defined as a tumour that is localised at least 1 cm from the mid-line of the vulva, at least 1 cm below the urethra and at least 1 cm above the posterior fourchette. Studies relating to patients with all stages of vulval cancer are included when considering the efficacy of chemoradiation as neoadjuvant or sole treatment (questions seven and eight). For the questions on adjuvant treatment for those with positive groin nodes, only studies with patients having positive nodes are considered (questions six and nine).

## Types of interventions

Radical vulvectomy is defined as excision of the complete vulval skin and subcutaneous tissue. A radical local excision is defined as an excision of the tumour with a margin of 1 cm, horizontally as well as vertically.

Inguinal and femoral lymphadenectomy is defined as removal of all lymph node-bearing fatty tissue between the inguinal ligament, the sartorius muscle and the adductor longus muscle, and dissection of the femoral lymph nodes located in the fossa ovalis medial to the femoral vein.

Inguinal lymphadenectomy is defined as removal of all lymph node-bearing fatty tissue between the inguinal ligament, the sartorius muscle and the adductor longus muscle above the level of the fascia lata.

Pelvic lymph node dissection is defined as removal of the lymph node-bearing tissue along the distal part of the external iliac artery and vein, and along the obturator nerve.

Radiotherapy to the groin is defined as radiotherapy to a volume including the inguinal and femoral lymph nodes. This volume is limited cranially by the inguinal ligament, medially by the fossa ovalis up to 2 cm lateral to the mid-line, laterally by the superior iliac spine and caudally by the crossing of the sartorius and adductor longus muscle (which should be 6 cm caudal to the middle of the inguinal ligament). The level of the femoral vessels limits this volume dorsally.

Chemoradiation is defined as radiotherapy with concurrent chemotherapy. The respective chemotherapy agents and dosages are described in detail in the section on question eight.

## Types of outcome measurements

- Overall survival, disease-specific survival and disease-free interval.
- Complications of treatment: treatment-related mortality, toxicity, wound healing, lymphoedema, psychosexual problems.
- Specific to question eight: conversion of surgical therapy to less radical procedures, or surgery made possible in previously inoperable tumours.

## Search strategy for identification of studies

The literature search was carried out according to the criteria set by the Cochrane Gynaecological Cancer Group and is described in more detail in a systematic review on the surgical treatment of vulval cancer.[5]

## Selection criteria for studies used to answer the questions

- All participants to have histologically proven squamous cell carcinoma of the vulva. For questions one to five, only studies that allowed separate analysis of early stages (cT1–2N0–1M0) were included.
- Interventions are defined adequately.
- For studies with (non-randomised) controls, interventions should be the same in each group, apart from the experimental intervention.

These criteria are not very strict but, if commonly used criteria had been applied, not a single study would have been selected, resulting in no answers to any of the questions asked.

## Is radical local excision as effective as radical vulvectomy?

### Background

In most patients with T1–2 tumours, radical vulvectomy is replaced by a radical local excision of the tumour.

### Evidence found

Two studies were found to be suitable to answer the question. Both were observational studies.[6,7] A methodological limitation of both studies is that radiotherapy interventions were not sufficiently defined. Furthermore, description of common complications (wound complications, voiding problems, cellulitis, lymphoedema) was not stated in one study.[7] The grade of complications was not defined in either study. In only one study were sexual problems (briefly) addressed.[7]

### Conclusion

Ninety-four patients were included in the two studies. In nine (10%), a local recurrence occurred, but none of the patients with a local recurrence died of vulval cancer. The conclusion is that radical local excision is a safe alternative to radical vulvectomy. It is unlikely that an RCT on this issue will be initiated as, in most referral centres, radical local excision instead of radical vulvectomy has become standard treatment in patients with T1–T2 tumours Evidence level III, Grade B .

## Is the triple incision technique as effective as *en bloc* dissection?

### Background

In current practice, patients with T1–T2 tumours and no clinical suspicion of groin node involvement, undergo a triple incision groin node dissection and radical vulvectomy instead of an *en bloc* dissection of nodes and vulva.

### Evidence found

Four observational studies were identified that could potentially answer the question.[8–11] However, when the selection criteria as described above were applied strictly, not a single study was found to be suitable to answer the question due to heterogeneity of the study populations. It was felt that it could not be left there, as the question addresses an important clinical issue because of the potential occurrence of skin bridge recurrences when the triple incision technique is used. It was therefore decided to pool all triple incision cases and calculate the incidence of these recurrences. Within this heterogeneous group of 303 patients, three (1%) skin bridge recurrences were detected.

### Conclusion

Based on the available evidence, it is concluded that the triple incision technique is safe. It is unlikely that an RCT on this issue will be initiated as, in most referral centres, the triple incision technique has replaced the *en bloc* resection in patients with T1–T2 tumours Evidence level III, Grade B .

## Is ipsilateral groin node dissection alone as effective as bilateral groin node dissection in patients with a lateral tumour?

### Background

In the lateral part of the vulva, lymph drainage is ipsilateral.[12] For this reason, performing only an ipsilateral lymph node dissection was introduced for patients with lateral tumours.

### Evidence found

Only one study[6] that may answer this question was selected. Recurrent disease in a previously undissected contralateral groin occurred in one out of 51 patients with a lateral tumour. She was salvaged by groin dissection and radiotherapy.

### Conclusion

Based on the limited evidence available, the omission of a contralateral groin node dissection appears to be safe Evidence level III, Grade B .

## Is a superficial groin node dissection as effective as a femoroinguinal groin node dissection?

### Background

It has been presumed that the omission of a femoral lymph node dissection is safe in patients with T1–2N0M0 tumours, and that morbidity would be reduced by this omission.

### Evidence found

Two studies were selected to answer the question. Groin recurrences did not occur in the (highly selected) 18 patients studied by DiSaia *et al.*[7] but did occur in three (4%) of the 76 patients studied by Burke *et al.*[6] All three groin recurrences occurred in previously tumour-negative groins.

## Conclusion

It is not safe to omit femoral node dissection Evidence level III, Grade B .

## Is primary groin irradiation as effective as primary groin node dissection?

### Background

The morbidity of primary radiotherapy to the groin is anticipated to be considerably less than that of surgery. The effectiveness with respect to tumour control by radiotherapy or surgery is addressed.

### Evidence found

Three studies were selected to answer the question[13–15] The first study was an RCT that compared primary radiotherapy to the groin with surgery.[13] The groin recurrence rate after surgery was 0/25. This was significantly lower compared with the 5 out of 27 (18·5%) groin recurrences after radiotherapy and the study was closed early. Overall survival and progression-free survival were significantly lower in the radiotherapy arm compared with the surgery arm ($P = 0.04$ and $P = 0.03$, respectively). In a case–control study on patients with clinical T1N0 vulval cancers, primary groin irradiation was compared with a "wait and see" policy. The groin recurrence rate after irradiation was 4·6%.[14] In the third study (observational), two out of 19 patients with T1–2N0–1 vulval cancer showed groin recurrences after primary groin irradiation.[15]

### Discussion

After publication of the study by Stehman,[13] there has been ample discussion regarding the adequate depth of the groin irradiation.[16–19] It is obvious that the irradiation technique in the RCT by Stehman was not adequate, as the radiotherapy dose was delivered at 3 cm below the skin instead of between 4·5 and 6 cm.

However, this does not imply that an adequate dose of radiotherapy is as effective as surgery. From an extensive literature review on surgical treatment, we know that the incidence of groin recurrences after surgery in patients with early vulval cancer is low and does not exceed 2%.[20] The incidence of groin recurrences after primary radiotherapy in the two observational studies included in this review using sufficient depth is higher in both studies (4·6% and 10%).[14,15]

## Conclusion

There is insufficient evidence to prove that radiotherapy is as effective as surgery in groin node control. In the only randomised study, both groin control and survival were better in the surgery arm. In the remaining observational studies groin recurrences occurred more frequently after radiotherapy when compared with what would be expected after surgical treatment as reported in the literature Evidence level Ib, Grade A .

## Is postoperative radiotherapy of any benefit to patients with positive nodes?

### Background

There are no randomised studies on the efficacy of adjuvant radiotherapy to the groin where positive lymph nodes have been found. Nevertheless, it is widely accepted, and indeed recommended, in various textbooks that adjuvant groin and pelvic radiotherapy should be administered when more than one or two positive groin nodes are found.[21]

### Evidence found

The evidence for this recommendation is based on a randomised study where the aim of the study was to compare pelvic node dissection with pelvic irradiation in patients in whom positive inguinofemoral lymph nodes were found at primary surgery.[22] In this study the 2-year survival in the group of patients treated with radical vulvectomy and groin node dissection followed by groin and pelvic radiotherapy was significantly better (68%) than that in the patients who were treated by surgery alone (54%). It was not better pelvic tumour control in the radiotherapy arm that was responsible for the survival benefit but better tumour control in the groin (5% groin recurrences with radiotherapy *v* 24% without radiotherapy). Furthermore, radiotherapy was only of benefit when more than one groin node was involved with tumour.

Apart from the results of the RCT published by Homesley, which does not directly address the question posed, five observational studies were selected to deal with the current question.[23–27] In two studies[23,24] consisting of 66 patients, all patients with positive nodes were irradiated. After a sufficient follow up period, only one groin recurrence was observed.

The incidence of groin recurrence is obviously higher when radiotherapy is given only to patients with more than three positive nodes, as was shown in two studies (128 patients) where 14 (11%) groin recurrences were observed.[25,26] When radiotherapy is omitted altogether in patients with positive groin nodes, the incidence of groin recurrence can be as high as 20%.[27]

## Conclusion

Based on the evidence of one RCT and five observational studies, it is justifiable to administer radiotherapy to patients with positive nodes **Evidence level III, Grade B** .

## Is (chemo)radiotherapy justified as sole treatment for carcinoma of the vulva?

### Background

From the answer to a previous question, it is obvious that radiotherapy is not the first choice for treatment of groin lymph nodes. Does the same hold true for the primary tumour?

### Evidence found

On this issue, only studies with considerable heterogeneity with respect to participants as well as interventions were identified. As it was felt that the current question is an important one, the data from all seven observational studies[28–34] is presented in Table 38.1. It is emphasised that drawing conclusions from these data is hazardous.

From this table it appears that (chemo)radiation as sole treatment results in complete local control in 60% of patients. During follow up local tumours had recurred in at least another 20% of patients who had had a clinical complete remission. This resulted in 48% of patients with local control of the primary vulval cancer when treated by (chemo)radiation alone with a follow up from 2 to over 60 months.

## Conclusion

The aforementioned data regarding local control and the data from the section on the previous question on primary groin irradiation versus groin node dissection suggest that (chemo)radiation as sole treatment for vulval cancer cannnot be advocated in general. It can be justified only as sole treatment for the primary when the morbidity from surgery is likely to outweigh the possible benefits **Evidence level III, Grade B** .

## Is neoadjuvant chemoradiotherapy of value for patients with large tumours?

### Background

A standard radical vulvectomy is usually insufficient to obtain tumour-free margins in patients with T3–4 tumours. Primary surgical treatment would imply that large and mutilating procedures should be performed. In recent years, neoadjuvant treatment has become an alternative to extensive primary surgery in order to reduce tumour size and improve resectability. The question as to whether neoadjuvant chemoradiotherapy improves locoregional tumour resectability and survival in patients who present with a large carcinoma of the vulva is discussed in this section.

### Evidence found

Only studies that include surgery as part of the primary treatment after induction with chemoradiation were considered to answer the question. Three suitable studies[35–37] were identified and are presented in Table 38.2.

**Table 38.1   (Chemo)radiation as sole treatment for carcinoma of the vulva**

| First author | TNM | Dose (Gy) | Chemo | CR | Local recurrence | Survival | Follow up |
|---|---|---|---|---|---|---|---|
| Eifel[28] | T2–3, N2 | 40 | 5-FU/P | 2/3 | 01/02 | 01/03 | 6–28 |
| Pirtoli[29] | T1–3, N0–3 | 45–85 | | 12/19 | 3/12* | 5/19 | >60 |
| Thomas[30] | Med 4 cm | 45–60 | 5-FU/MMC | 6/9 | 3/6 | 6/9† | 5–43 |
| Wahlen[31] | T3–4, N0–1 | 45–51 | 5FY/MMC | 10/19 | 1/10 | 17/19 | 11–56 |
| Russel[32] | T2–4, N0–2 | 34–72 | 5-FU/P | 16/18 | 2/16 | 14/17 | 2–52 |
| Cunningham[33] | T3–4 | 50–65 | 5-FU/P | 9/14 | 1/9 | ? | 7–81 |
| Sebag-Montefiore[34] | T3–4, N2–3 | 45 | 5-FU/MMC | 7/16 | 30%‡ | 33%‡ | 6–36 |
| Total | T1–T4 | 34–85 | | 60% | 20% | 58% | 2–60 |

Abbreviations: CR, complete response; 5-FU, 5-fluorouracil; MMC, mitomycin C; P, cisplatin
*Data not complete, extrapolated from paper: > 3/12
†Three patients remain alive after radiotherapy alone, all others had salvage surgery
‡Percentage of total group (primary and recurrent tumours)

**Table 38.2   Is neoadjuvant chemoradiotherapy of value for patients with large tumours?**

| Study and treatment details | First author/year | | |
|---|---|---|---|
| | Lupi 1996[35] | Montana 2000[36] | Moore 1998[37] |
| Type of study | Prospective | Phase II GOG | Phase II GOG |
| No. of patients | 31 | 46* | 73* |
| Extent of tumour | Primary = 24 | Primary + fixed or | Primary, T3 and T4 |
| | Recurrent = 7† | ulcerated nodes | |
| *Radiotherapy* | | | |
| Vulva | 54 Gy | 47·6 Gy | 47·6 Gy |
| Groin nodes | 36 Gy | 47·6 Gy | 47·6 Gy (N+ ) |
| Pelvic nodes | 36 Gy | 47·6 Gy | 47·6 Gy (N+) |
| Fraction size | 1·8 Gy | 1·7 Gy | 1·7 Gy |
| Interval (weeks) | 1–2 | 1–3 | 1–3 |
| *Chemotherapy* | | | |
| 5-Fluorouracil | 750×5 | 1000×4 | 1000×4 |
| Cisplatin | – | 50 | 50 |
| Mitomycin C | 1 | – | – |
| Frequency (wks) | 1 and 6 or 7 | 1 and 5 | 1 and 5 |
| *Surgery* | | | |
| Local excision vulva | See below | Yes | Yes |
| Radical vulvectomy | Yes | No | No |
| Bilateral inguinal LA | Yes | Yes | Yes |
| Bilateral pelvic LA | If groins positive | No | No |
| **Complications of treatment** | | | |
| Type of study | Postoperative | Phase II GOG | Phase II GOG |
| No. of cases | 31 | 46* | 71* |
| Recording system | Not specified | GOG standard | GOG standard |
| *Complications* | | | |
| Grade 3 or 4 | – | 49 | 64 |
| Acute | Myelotoxicity (18) | Skin problems (36) | Skin problems (39) |
| Postoperative | Sepsis (2), wound and lymph problems (18), sepsis (2) | Wound breakdown (7/38) | Death (1), fistula (1), sepsis (2), others (12) |
| Long-term | – | Hip fracture (1) | Hip fracture (1), fistula (1) |
| **Outcome** | | | |
| Type of study | Prospective | Phase II GOG | Phase II GOG |
| No. of patients | 31 | 46* | 73* |
| Median follow up | 34 | 78 | 50 |
| plus range (months) | 22–90 | 56–89 | 22–72 |
| NED | 15 | 12 | 40 |
| DOD | 6 | 14 | 22 |
| DOC | 0 | 8 | 5 |
| TRD | 3 | 2 | 4 |
| Alive with disease | – | 10 | 2 |

*(Continued)*

**Table 38.2** *(Continued)*

| Study and treatment details | First author/year | | |
| --- | --- | --- | --- |
| | Lupi 1996[35] | Montana 2000[36] | Moore 1998[37] |
| *Local control* | | | |
| Pathological CR | V 36% | V 20/38 (53%) | 22/71 (31%) |
| | | G 15/37 (41%) | |
| Unresectable | – | Nodes (2) | Tumour (2) |
| Local recurrence | 7/22 | 11/38 | V 11/71, G 3/71 |
| Time to recurrence (months) | 18 (5–48) | – | – |
| *Feasibility* | | | |
| CRT | 24 | 42/46 | 71/73 |
| Surgery | 22 (92%) | 38 (92%) | 67 (83%) |

Abbreviations: CR, complete remission; DOC, dead, other causes; DOD, dead of disease (ca vulva); GOG, Gynecological Oncology Group; LA, lymphadenectomy; NED, no evidence of disease; TRD, treatment related death
*The same GOG protocol: 23 patients had unresectable groin lymph nodes and unresectable vulval tumours and as a result they are included in both studies
†Primary tumours were: T1 + T2 N2 (5); T3 (17), T4 (2)

More than 90% of the eligible patients were treated with chemoradiation according to the protocol. In 72–92% of cases, surgery followed the induction therapy according to schedule. Protocol violations were due to patients' refusal, deteriorating medical condition, inoperable residual tumour, or death. Chemotherapy and radiotherapy was given uniformly within each study. Complications were reported in all studies. The majority of patients showed adverse skin effects. Myelotoxicity necessitating adjustment of treatment was reported by Lupi *et al.*[35] Prolonged wound healing, lymphoedema, lymphorrhoea, and lymphoceles were reported in 18–71%. Treatment-related death occurred in 4–12·5% of the patients.

In the study by Moore *et al.*,[37] 50 patients would have required exenteration surgery for adequate excision if treated by surgery alone. After neoadjuvant chemotherapy, continence could be preserved in 47 of them. In 96% of Montana *et al.*'s patients the lymph nodes became resectable after induction therapy.

Histopathological complete remission was achieved in 31–53% of patients. Locoregional relapses occurred in 20–32% of patients; 26–63 % of the patients showed no evidence of disease after median follow up of 34–78 months. Although the follow up period is rather short, death due to disease and treatment-related deaths were as high as 35%.

### Conclusion

The available evidence shows that preoperative chemoradiotherapy reduces the tumour size and improves operability. However, serious complications are observed.

Patients with inoperable primary tumours or lymph nodes do benefit from this treatment when resectability is achieved. In patients with large tumours that can only be treated with anterior and/or posterior exenteration complications of neoadjuvant therapy may outweigh the sequelae of exenteration surgery. With the current knowledge neoadjuvant therapy is not justified in patients with tumours that can be adequately treated with radical vulvectomy alone **Evidence level IIa, Grade B** .

### Is there evidence of benefit for adjuvant chemotherapy in node-positive patients?

#### Background

Whether adjuvant chemotherapy in high risk patients with vulval cancer is of benefit is unknown.

#### Evidence found

There are no data in the literature to support or refute this. From a theoretical point of view it would be of interest to study the effect of adjuvant chemotherapy in patients with vulval cancer.

It was shown in the section dealing with the previous question that a considerable response to neoadjuvant chemotherapy can be achieved.

### General recommendations for further studies on the treatment of vulval cancer

From this chapter is has become obvious that most studies on the treatment of vulval cancer are of mediocre quality at best. Cancer of the vulva is a rare disease. Therefore, RCTs are not easy to conduct. However, observational studies can also help to increase the amount of evidence. Until now, the great majority of published observational studies do not meet the minimum criteria set by the Cochrane Collaboration and there is therefore considerable room for improvement.

Future observational studies on the effectiveness of treatment of vulval cancer should at least meet the following criteria:

- clear definitions of the type of participants and type of interventions
- uniform interventions
- clearly stated follow up time
- clearly account follow up status for all participants
- definition of type, incidence and grade of complications.

## References

1 Platz CE, Benda JA. Female genital tract cancer. *Cancer* 1995;**75**:270–94.
2 Van der Velden J, Van Lindert ACM, Gimbrere CHF, Oosting J, Heintz APM. Epidemiologic data on vulvar cancer: comparison of hospital with population based data. *Gynecol Oncol* 1996;**62**:379–83.
3 Morley GW: Infiltrative carcinoma of the vulva: results of surgical treatment. *Am J Obstet Gynecol* 1976;**124**:874–88.
4 Hacker NF: Vulvar cancer. In: Berek JS, Hacker NF, eds. *Practical gynecologic oncology. 2nd edn.* Baltimore: Williams and Wilkins, 1994.
5 Ansink AC, Van der Velden J. Surgical interventions for early squamous cell carcinoma of the vulva. In: Cochrane Collaboration, *Cochrane Library*, Issue 2. Oxford: Update Software, 2000.
6 Burke TW, Levenback C, Coleman RL, Morris M, Silva EG, Gershenson DM. Surgical therapy of T1 and T2 vulvar carcinoma: further experience with radical wide excision and selective inguinal lymphadenectomy. *Gynecol Oncol* 1995;**57**:215–20.
7 DiSaia PJ, Creasman WT, Rich WM. An alternate approach to early cancer of the vulva. *Am J Obstet Gynecol* 1979;**133**:825–30.
8 Farias-Eisner R, Crisano FD, Grouse D *et al.* Conservative and individualized surgery for early squamous carcinoma of the vulva: the treatment of choice for stage I and II (T1-2N0-1M0) disease. *Gynecol Oncol* 1994;**53**:55–8.
9 Grimshaw RN, Murdoch JB, Monaghan JM: Radical vulvectomy and bilateral inguinal-femoral lymphadenectomy through separate incisions – experience with 100 cases. *Int J Gynecol Cancer* 1993;**3**:18–23.
10 Hacker NF, Leuchter RS, Berek JS *et al.* Radical vulvectomy and bilateral inguinal lymphadenectomy through separate groin incisions. *Obstet Gynecol* 1981;**8**:574–9.
11 Helm CW, Hatch K, Austin JM *et al.* A matched comparison of single and triple incision techniques for the surgical treatment of carcinoma of the vulva. *Gynecol Oncol* 1992;**46**:150–6.
12 Iversen T, Aas M. Lymph drainage of the vulva. *Gynecol Oncol* 1983;**16**:179–89.
13 Stehman FB, Bundy BN, Thomas GT *et al.* Groin dissection versus radiation in carcinoma of the vulva: a Gynecologic Oncology Group study. *Int J Radiat Oncol Biol Phys* 1992;**24**:389–96.
14 Manavi M, Berger A, Kucera E *et al.* Does T1, N0-1 vulvar cancer treated by vulvectomy but not lymphadenectomy need inguinofemoral radiation? *Int J Radiat Oncol Biol Phys* 1997;**38**:749–53.
15 Perez CA, Grigsby PW, Clifford Chao KS *et al.* Irradiation in carcinoma of the vulva: factors affecting outcome. *Int J Radiat Oncol Biol Phys* 1998;**42**:335–44.
16 Petereit DG, Mehta MP, Buchler DA *et al.* Inguinofemoral radiation of N0,1 vulvar cancer may be equivalent to lymphadenectomy if proper radiation technique is used. *Int J Radiat Oncol Biol Phys* 1993;**27**:963–7.
17 Lanciano RM, Corn BW: Groin node irradiation for vulvar cancer: treatment planning must do more than scratch the surface. *Int J Radiat Oncol Biol Phys* 1993;**27**:987–9.
18 McCall AR, Olson MC, Potkul RK. The variation of inguinal lymph node depth in adult women and its importance in planning elective irradiation for vulvar cancer. *Cancer* 1995;**75**:2286–8.
19 Koh WJ, Chiu M, Stelzer KJ, Greer BE, Mastras D, Comsia N, Russell KJ, Griffin TW. Femoral vessel depth and the implications for groin node radiation. *Int J Radiat Oncol Biol Phys* 1993;**27**:969–74.
20 Van der Velden J, Hacker NF. Update on vulvar carcinoma. In: Rothenberg ML, ed. *Gynecologic oncology: controversies and new developments.* Boston: Kluwer Academic Publishers, 1994.
21 Berek JS, Hacker NF. *Practical Gynecologic Oncology, 3rd edn.* Philadelphia: Lippincott, Williams & Wilkins, 2000.
22 Homesley H, Bundy BN, Sedlis A., Adcock L. Radiation therapy versus pelvic node resection for carcinoma of the vulva with positive groin nodes. *Obstet Gynecol* 1986;**68**:733–40.
23 Burger MPM, Hollema H, Emanuels AG, Krans M, Pras E, Bouma J. The importance of the groin node status for the survival of T1 and T2 vulvar carcinoma patients. *Gynecol Oncol* 1995;**57**:327–34.
24 Mariani L, Lombardi A, Atlante M, Atlante G. Radiotherapy for vulvar carcinoma with positive inguinal nodes. Adjunctive treatment. *J Reprod Med* 1993;**38**:429–36.
25 Paladini D, Cross P, Lopes A, Monaghan JM. Prognostic significance of lymph node variables in squamous cell cancer of the vulva. *Cancer* 1994;**74**:2491–6.
26 Curry SL, Wharton JT, Rutledge F. Positive lymph nodes in vulvar squamous carcinoma. *Gynecol Oncol* 1980;**9**:63–7.
27 Hacker NF, Berek JS, Lagasse LD, Leuchter RS, Moore JG. Management of regional lymph nodes and their prognostic influence in vulvar cancer. *Obstet Gynecol* 1983;**61**:408–12.
28 Eifel PJ, Morris M, Burke TW, Levenback C, Gershenson DM. Prolonged continuous infusion cisplatin and 5-fluorouracil with radiation for locally advanced carcinoma of the vulva. *Gynecol Oncol* 1995;**59**:51–6.
29 Pirtoli L, Rottoli ML. Results of radiation therapy for vulvar carcinoma. *Acta Radiol Oncol* 1982;**21**:45–8.
30 Thomas G, Dembo A, DePetrillo A *et al.* Concurrent radiation and chemotherapy in vulvar carcinoma. *Gynecol Oncol* 1989;**34**:263–7.
31 Wahlen SA, Slater JD, Wagner RJ *et al.* Concurrent radiation therapy and chemotherapy in the treatment of primary squamous cell carcinoma of the vulva. *Cancer* 1995;**75**:2289–94.
32 Russell AH, Mesic JB, Scudder SA *et al.* Synchronous radiation and cytotoxic chemotherapy for locally advanced or recurrent squamous cancer of the vulva. *Gynecol Oncol* 1992;**47**:14–20.
33 Cunningham MJ, Goyer RP, Gibbons SK, Kredentser DC, Malfetano JH, Keys H. Primary radiation, cisplatin, and 5-fluorouracil for advanced squamous carcinoma of the vulva. *Gynecol Oncol* 1997;**66**:258–61.
34 Sebag-Montefiore DJ, McLean C, Arnott SJ *et al.* Treatment of advanced carcinoma of the vulva with chemoradiotherapy- can exenterative surgery be avoided? *Int J Gynecol Cancer* 1994;**4**:150–5.
35 Lupi G, Raspagliesi F, Zucali R *et al.* Combined preoperative chemoradiotherapy followed by radical surgery in locally advanced vulvar carcinoma. *Cancer* 1996;**77**:1472–8.
36 Montana GS, Thomas GM, Moore DH *et al.* Preoperative chemoradiation for carcinoma of the vulva with N2/N3 nodes: a gynecological oncological group study. *Int J Radiat Oncol Biol Phys* 2000;**48**:1007–13.
37 Moore DH, Thomas GM, Montana GS, Saxer A, Gallup DG, Olt G. Preoperative chemoradiation for advanced vulvar cancer: a phase II study of the Gynecological Oncology Group. *Int J Radiat Oncol Biol Phys* 1998;**42**:79–85.

# 39 Gestational trophoblastic disease

*ES Newlands*

The development of the treatment for gestational trophoblastic disease has been rather different from other gynaecological malignancies. In the late 1950s assays for the pregnancy hormone human chorionic gonadotrophin (hCG) were developing and moved on from mouse uterine weight assays to radioimmunoassays in 1960s. At the same time Li and Hertz[1] identified that the antifolate methotrexate was highly active in a small number of patients with trophoblastic disease. Although gestational trophoblastic disease (GTD) is rare, the ability to monitor tumour growth by rising hCG values and tumour response by falling hCG values allows clinicians to see, with a remarkable degree of accuracy, whether their treatment is effective or not. Combining the ability to accurately monitor the effect of any individual treatment, together with the fact that GTD is nearly always initially chemosensitive, has allowed effective treatment to develop largely in the absence of randomised controlled clinical trials. It is interesting to speculate how the management of other gynaecological malignancies might have developed if we had this combination of the ability to see the effect of a treatment and having a very chemosensitive disease. The use of both hCG and alpha-fetoprotein (AFP) together with CA-125 and LDH in ovarian germ cell tumours has to some extent been comparable to the development of treatment for this rare disease.[2] If one clinically has those two key parameters – a sensitive ability to monitor disease activity and effective treatment – the role of randomised clinical trials really is relegated to the minor refinement of treatments in areas where there is still therapeutic difficulty.

## When to suspect GTD

By definition GTD results from a normal or abnormal pregnancy (Table 39.1). The commonest presentation of a patient with GTD is where a patient has a complete or partial molar pregnancy. The majority of these women present between 6 and 8 weeks after their last period with a positive pregnancy test and no evidence of fetus in the uterus and, if the molar pregnancy is sufficiently well developed, molar vesicles can be seen on ultrasound. The presentation of GTD can be much more difficult where either the patient has had a previous full-term pregnancy or the obstetric history is uncertain or completely obscure.

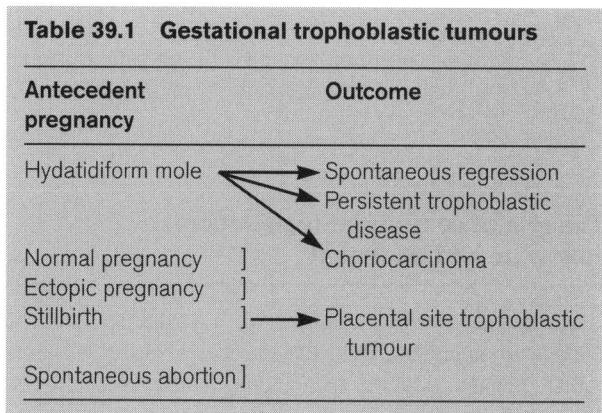

**Table 39.1  Gestational trophoblastic tumours**

| Antecedent pregnancy | Outcome |
|---|---|
| Hydatidiform mole | Spontaneous regression |
| | Persistent trophoblastic disease |
| Normal pregnancy ] | Choriocarcinoma |
| Ectopic pregnancy ] | |
| Stillbirth ] | Placental site trophoblastic tumour |
| Spontaneous abortion ] | |

Most women with GTD will have varying amounts of irregular vaginal bleeding. In this context a woman with a raised hCG in the serum or urine and the absence of either an intra- or extrauterine pregnancy on ultrasound raises the suspicion of the patient having GTD. Where there is no histological evidence of a molar pregnancy initially, it may well be appropriate to exclude an ectopic pregnancy by laparoscopy.

Diagnosis of a patient with a molar pregnancy is usually relatively straightforward as outlined above. The suspicion of the presence of GTD should occur in any women of child bearing age who has a raised hCG value in the serum or urine and no evidence of an intra- or extrauterine pregnancy. Sometimes patients present with widely metastatic disease; measuring the serum or urine hCG in women of child-bearing age should be routinely considered – if the hCG is normal then the patient will not have typical GTD.

## What is the correct initial management?

Patients presenting with molar pregnancies as indicated above usually present to their antenatal clinic after 6–8 weeks of amenorrhoea and varying amounts of vaginal bleeding. Ultrasound, which shows no evidence of pregnancy and usually some evidence of molar vesicle formation, immediately raises the suspicion of the patient having a molar pregnancy. The initial management is evacuation of the uterine cavity, usually by suction evacuation, to minimise the chance of uterine perforation.

The molar pregnancy should be confirmed on histology but it should be noted that, with the much earlier evacuation of molar pregnancies at 6–8 weeks, pathologically there is less vesicle formation and there may even be the presence of fetal red cells in the blood vessels.[3,4] The majority of complete moles can usually be recognised by an expert pathologist at this stage. However, the more common partial moles can be very difficult to distinguish from hydropic abortions.[5] Cases of doubtful histology should be sent for expert review.

Once the diagnosis of a molar pregnancy has been made or a patient is suspected of having GTD, the patient should be registered with the appropriate trophoblastic disease centre.

## The role of centralised registration, follow up and treatment

Since GTD is a rare condition with a wide spectrum of biological expression, from the majority of patients whose molar pregnancy remits spontaneously after evacuation of the uterine cavity, to highly aggressive tumours, there is a national service in the UK based on three reference laboratories in Dundee, Sheffield and the Charing Cross Hospital in London. These three centres register between 1300 and 1400 women per annum for serial hCG estimations (Table 39.2). In the UK there are treatment centres at Sheffield and Charing Cross and only those

patients whose disease is causing problems, either with persistent vaginal bleeding or non-remitting disease (confirmed by a plateau on serial hCG values), or the disease is growing (shown by rising hCG values), are selected for treatment.

## Who needs chemotherapy?

The criteria for selecting patients for chemotherapy are shown in Box 39.1.[6] Patients with an hCG greater than 20 000 IU l$^{-1}$ more than 4 weeks after evacuation of the molar pregnancy are at risk of uterine perforation and therefore they are brought in for chemotherapy. Since GTD is so vascular, it is not always possible to oversew the bleeding point of a perforated uterus and emergency hysterectomy is necessary in some of these cases. GTD consists of a pathological spectrum from molar pregnancies, which are premalignant conditions, to frank choriocarcinoma. Choriocarcinoma is an established malignancy and will need treatment if it has not been completely resected. Clinical evidence of widely metastatic disease strongly implies that the patient has choriocarcinoma. Persistent uterine haemorrhage from GTD can usually be controlled within 48–72 hours by a combination of bed rest and effective chemotherapy. Many patients on the post-mole registration scheme are selected for treatment on the basis of plateau or rising hCG values. The last main indication for treating a patient with GTD is

**Table 39.2  Hydatidiform mole registration centres (no. of patients registered)**

| Year | London | Sheffield | Dundee | Total |
|------|--------|-----------|--------|-------|
| 1981 | 548 | 289 | 59 | 896 |
| 1982 | 644 | 280 | 66 | 990 |
| 1983 | 678 | 327 | 76 | 1081 |
| 1984 | 566 | 374 | 83 | 1023 |
| 1985 | 626 | 358 | 98 | 1082 |
| 1986 | 676 | 356 | 90 | 1122 |
| 1987 | 663 | 390 | 78 | 1131 |
| 1988 | 637 | 413 | 82 | 1132 |
| 1989 | 583 | 358 | 75 | 1016 |
| 1990 | 688 | 377 | 89 | 1154 |
| 1991 | 692 | 404 | 77 | 1173 |
| 1992 | 693 | 383 | 97 | 1173 |
| 1993 | 761 | 384 | 93 | 1238 |
| 1994 | 789 | 365 | 102 | 1256 |
| 1995 | 810 | 391 | 111 | 1312 |
| 1996 | 780 | 426 | 93 | 1299 |
| 1997 | 927 | 421 | 93 | 1441 |
| 1998 | 883 | 446 | 115 | 1444 |
| 1999 | 835 | 438 | 101 | 1374 |

## Box 39.1 Indications for chemotherapy

- Serum hCG above 20 000 IU litre$^{-1}$ more than 4 weeks after evacuation, because of the risk of uterine perforation
- Histological evidence of choriocarcinoma
- Evidence of metastases in brain, liver, or gastrointestinal tract, or radiological opacities > 2 cm on chest *x* ray
- Long-lasting uterine haemorrhage
- Rising hCG values (or static hCG values on repeated samples)
- hCG in body fluids 4–6 months after evacuation

## Box 39.2 1992 Revised FIGO staging system for gestational trophoblastic tumour

### Stage

- **I:** Disease confined to the uterus
- **II:** Disease extending outside the uterus but limited to the genital structures (adnexa, vagina, broad ligament)
- **III:** Disease extending to the lungs, with or without known genital tract involvement
- **IV:** Disease at other metastatic sites

### Substage

- **A:** No risk factor
- **B:** One risk factor
- **C:** Two risk factors

### Risk factors

- **1:** hCG > 100 000 IU litre$^{-1}$
- **2:** Duration from termination of the antecedent pregnancy to diagnosis > 6 months

whether the hCG is still raised 6 months after evacuation of the uterus, and this is because the longer the disease remains in the body the more resistant it tends to become to chemotherapy.

## Is anatomical staging relevant or is identifying prognostic factors more important in management of GTD?

In Box 39.2 is the FIGO classification of GTD. Like most FIGO classifications for gynaecological malignancy, the disease is categorised as stages 1–4. Unfortunately this anatomical approach does not identify the main prognostic variables in GTD.[7] These are shown in the WHO scoring system in Table 39.3. Here the concept is the higher the score that a patient achieves on the prognostic variables, the higher the risk of drug resistance and the higher the risk of mortality. In the WHO scoring system patients are categorised into low, medium and high risk. The most important prognostic variables in this table are the antecedent pregnancy: trophoblastic tumours occurring after a term pregnancy are always choriocarcinoma and are frequently aggressive. The interval from the known antecedent pregnancy is an adverse prognostic variable increasing the risk of drug resistance, particularly if the interval is more than 12 months. An hCG value of over $10^5$ IU l$^{-1}$ correlates with relatively large volume disease in the patient and this tends to be associated with multiple metastases in a number of different sites. In the WHO scoring system brain metastases, as expected, are an adverse prognostic variable

**Table 39.3   WHO prognostic scoring system for gestational trophoblastic tumour**

| Parameter | Score* | | | |
|---|---|---|---|---|
| | 0 | 1 | 2 | 4 |
| Age in years | < 39 | > 39 | | |
| Antecedent pregnancy | Mole | Abortion | Term | |
| Interval in months† | < 4 | 4–6 | 7–12 | >12 |
| Pretreatment hCG, log | < 3 | < 4 | < 5 | >5 |
| ABO group | | A×O | AB | |
| (female × male) | | O×A | B | |
| Largest dimension in cm | | 3–5 | > 5 | |
| Site of metastases | | Spleen, Kidney | GI, Liver | Brain |
| No. of metastases identified | | 1–4 | 4–8 | >8 |
| Prior chemotherapy failed | | | Single | >2 |

Abbreviations: GI, gastrointestinal; hCG, human chorionic gonadotrophin; WHO, World Health Organization
*The total score for a patient is obtained by adding the individual scores for each prognostic factor. Total score < 5, low risk; 5–7, medium risk; > 7, high risk.
†Time between the end of the antecedent pregnancy and the start of chemotherapy.

**Table 39.4 Proposed changes to WHO scoring system based on prognostic factors 1998**

| Prognostic factors* | Score[†] | | | |
|---|---|---|---|---|
| | 0 | 1 | 2 | 4 |
| Age in years | < 39 | > 39 | | |
| Antecedent pregnancy | Mole | Abortion | Term | |
| Interval[‡] | < 4 | 4–6 | 7–12 | > 12 |
| hCG (IU litre$^{-1}$) | < $10^3$ | $10^3$–$10^4$ | $10^4$–$10^5$ | > $10^5$ |
| Largest tumour (cm) | | 3–5 | > 5 | |
| Site of metastases | | Spleen, Kidney | GI tract, | Brain, Liver |
| No. of metastases identified | | 1–4 | 5–8 | > 8[d] |
| Prior chemotherapy failed | | | Single | > 2 |

Abbreviation: GI, gastrointestinal
*Placental site trophoblastic tumours are excluded from this table.
[†]The total score for a patient is obtained by adding the individual scores for each prognostic factor. Total score ≤ 6, low risk; ≥ 7, high risk.
[‡] "Interval" is the time (in months) between the end of the antecedent pregnancy and the start of chemotherapy.
[§]If all the metastases are in the lung, two or more of these should measure > 2 cm on a chest x ray or CT scan to score 4.

but subsequent analysis of patients with liver metastases are also categorised in the highest risk group.[8] Failure of multiple prior chemotherapy increases the chance of drug resistance developing and this also is clearly an adverse prognostic variable.

In discussion with FIGO a modification of the WHO scoring system has been proposed and is shown in Table 39.4. Here the main changes are that placental site trophoblastic tumours (PSTT) are excluded from this classification since the management is different. Since everybody's data on the ABO blood groups are incomplete and this is a minor prognostic variable, this has been omitted. Recognition that liver metastases are a major adverse prognostic variable has also been recognised. Analysis of patients treated at the Charing Cross Hospital confirms that treating patients to methotrexate resistance does not compromise their subsequent successful treatment with combination chemotherapy. Therefore the patient categories have been simplified to just have two risk categories, low and high risk.[9]

## Why is GTD inherently chemosensitive?

It is widely recognised that GTD tends to remain highly chemosensitive and develops drug resistance at a later stage than most other adult malignancies. The biological features underlying this are poorly understood. One possibility is that in established trophoblastic tumours such as choriocarcinoma there are stem cells (the cytotrophoblastic cells), and there are end-stage cells (the syncytiotrophoblastic cells). A biological feature of chemotherapy may be to force all the stem cells into syncytiotrophoblasts so that the tumour cannot repopulate itself. Another feature that may well be relevant in explaining the inherent chemosensitivity of GTD is evidence that *p53* is usually intact in cell lines from trophoblastic tumours in culture. It may be the continuing ability of trophoblastic cells to switch on apoptosis that accounts for their remarkable chemosensitivity to DNA damaging agents.[10]

## Why does GTD only grow clinically with detectable hCG production?

hCG is produced throughout a normal pregnancy. Initially the majority of the hCG produced is intact hCG and, as pregnancy progresses, it becomes increasingly nicked, which reduces the biological activity of the molecule. The function of hCG during normal pregnancy is very poorly understood. It may be that hCG is a growth-modulating and possibly growth-stimulating molecule. In patients with GTD, hCG is nearly always measurable if the disease is causing clinical problems, provided that the hCG is measured on a sensitive assay such as a radioimmunoassay. Even patients with the rare variant of GTD, PSTT, produce enough hCG to be measured, even though the concentrations of hCG may be quite low in relation to the volume of disease.

One of the features of the management of patients with GTD is that one can rely on the serial measurements of hCG in a way that one cannot entirely rely on other serum tumour markers in managing diseases such as germ cell tumours and ovarian adenocarcinoma. Patients are monitored after the initial diagnosis on serial hCG values to identify whether the disease is regressing or progressing. hCG is used to monitor the key treatment decisions in patients on chemotherapy or in the minority requiring surgery. hCG is key to the follow up of patients in picking up relapses. hCG needs to be measured again after each subsequent normal pregnancy as patients who have had a prior trophoblastic tumour have a statistically increased chance of having a further trophoblastic disease event after each subsequent normal pregnancy.[11]

## Why are the molecular genetics of GTD relevant?

GTDs are unique in cancer biology since all types of GTD contain paternal genes unlike the rest of oncology where the disease is the product of the patient's own disordered genes.

Molar pregnancies consist of two different genetic origins in the majority of cases. Complete moles are the product of either mono- or sometimes di-spermic fertilisation of an ovum in which the maternal genes have been deleted. Complete moles are androgenetic conceptuses in the majority of cases.[12]

Partial moles, in contrast to complete moles, are the product of di-spermic fertilisation of an ovum, and these conceptions are triploid with two paternal haplotypes and one maternal haplotype. The biological behaviour of complete and partial moles is different. Approximately 15% of patients with complete moles will need chemotherapy in contrast to 0.5% of partial moles requiring chemotherapy.[13] However, it is well recognised that complete moles can modulate to choriocarcinoma with a frequency probably of the order of 3%. Occasionally partial moles can transform to choriocarcinoma and triploid choriocarcinoma has been genetically confirmed.[14]

Tumours following a term pregnancy are histologically choriocarcinoma and the majority of these are bi-parental in origin and in most cases are presumed to derive from the recent term pregnancy. Occasionally patients can have reactivation of trophoblastic disease presumably after the hormonal surge associated with a subsequent normal pregnancy. In a few cases we have been able to prove that the choriocarcinoma following the subsequent pregnancy actually came from a previous mole and the choriocarcinoma was androgenetic in origin.[15]

A recent syndrome has been identified in a small number of families where there has been a history of inbreeding. In these cases some of the women have had repeat molar pregnancies and some of these have been bi-parental in origin. In these cases it would appear that the women concerned have inherited a defect in the ova, which allows either all or the majority of their pregnancies to develop as complete molar pregnancies.

The relevance of being able to detect the presence of paternal genes in a tumour can be important clinically. A range of tumours arising at other sites can differentiate down trophoblastic lineage and appear histologically as choriocarcinoma. The primary sites of these tumours in descending order of frequency are carcinoma of the bronchus, carcinoma of the gastrointestinal tract and bladder cancer, and it is important to recognise that atypical presentations of a trophoblastic tumour can be due to this event. Genetic analysis on these patients' tumours confirms that there is no evidence of paternal genes.[16] From the patient's point of view the prognosis is radically different from that of a patient with GTD. Nearly all the patients with choriocarcinoma presenting without paternal genes in the tumour die from their disease. This is in contrast to women with paternal genes in their GTD where the survival is over 90%.

## Why is stratification of treatment by prognostic variables important?

Nearly all patients with GTD can achieve complete remission and probable long-term cure. In Tables 39.3 and 39.4 are the WHO and most recently proposed classification of prognostic variables for patients with GTD. The treatment of choice for patients with low risk disease is methotrexate and folinic acid in a well-established schedule shown in Box 39.3.[17,18] Provided that patients have normal renal function and have a relatively high fluid intake (urine output of $> 2 \, l$ per 24 hours), this schedule has few side effects, does not induce alopecia, and there is no evidence of late sequelae in terms of second tumour induction. However, approximately 25% of patients will become resistant to methotrexate and folinic acid, and our policy is currently for those patients whose tumour becomes resistant at an hCG value of 150 IU $l^{-1}$ or less to be switched to single agent actinomycin D, and patients in whom the tumour becomes resistant at an hCG value greater than 150 IU $l^{-1}$ to be switched to the high risk regimen EMA/CO (Box 39.3). The results of 476 patients managed in this way are shown in Box 39.4. All patients achieved complete remission and only a small number of patients needed salvage treatment. This policy exposes the minimum number of patients to combination chemotherapy, which does have a slight increase in incidence of second tumours.

Patients presenting with high risk disease need combination chemotherapy from the outset. Since 1979 we have used EMA (etoposide, methotrexate and actinomycin D), alternating at weekly intervals with CO (cyclophosphamide and vincristine [Oncovin]) (Box 39.3). This schedule is generally reasonably well-tolerated but patients will need 5HT$_3$ antagonists (such as ondansetron and granisetron) as antiemetics. The majority of patients will also require granulocyte colony stimulating factor given for between 3 and 5 days between each course of treatment to maintain a reasonable granulocyte count. We have published the results of 272 patients treated with the EMA/CO schedule in 1997 and the cumulative 5-year survival rate was 86%.[19] The EMA/CO schedule has been widely adopted worldwide as the first-line treatment for patients with high risk GTD. It appears that the intensity of

chemotherapy and also its frequency is important in maximising the complete remission rate. Traditional chemotherapy given on a 3-weekly schedule for GTD appears to have a high relapse rate, although this has not been the subject of a randomised study.

## Why is salvage treatment for GTD so effective?

Drug resistance develops late in most cases of GTD and, even where relative drug resistance has developed, it is rarely complete. By combining the introduction of additional new chemotherapeutic agents together with surgery, a surprisingly high proportion of patients can be salvaged after failure of their initial therapy. Our main relapse schedule has been introducing cisplatinum in the EP regimen (etoposide and cisplatinum), alternating with a shortened EMA schedule (omitting day 2) and the results were published in 2000.[20] The majority (30/34 [88%]) of patients with typical GTD can be salvaged using either EP/EMA alone or with selective surgery to the main sites of metastatic disease. The main subgroup of GTD where we still have problems are those patients with PSTT. There is a curious phenomenon with PSTT in that, if the last known pregnancy is within 2 years, these tumours can be cured either by hysterectomy or by EP/EMA chemotherapy. However, in patients with PSTT developing more than 2 years from the last known pregnancy, the tumour can have complete drug resistance and, if the patient cannot be salvaged with surgery, there is as yet no satisfactory salvage treatment for this extremely rare subgroup of GTD.

Several new agents have come into oncology over the past decade and include the taxanes, paclitaxel and docetaxel, and also gemcitabine. These agents are active in the salvage treatment for patients with germ cell tumours and are likely to be active also in patients with refractory GTD. Integrating these newer agents into salvage treatment, possibly also with high dose chemotherapy with autologous bone marrow support, is an experimental procedure that needs to be studied to identify whether it is effective in eliminating GTD refractory to standard treatments.

## Why is centralising treatment important for outcome?

As has been indicated in the previous sections, patients with GTD form a spectrum from post-molar trophoblastic disease, where the disease remits spontaneously after evacuation of the uterine cavity, to highly aggressive tumours that are widely metastatic and occasionally, in the case of PSTT, also highly drug resistant. By centralising the management of these patients with this rare disease, experience is accumulated to optimise the treatment for patients with problematic variants of this disease. This is illustrated by the management of PSTT, where at the Charing Cross Hospital, which has the largest series of any trophoblastic disease centre, we have only admitted 36 patients with PSTT. This small number for a tumour that is clearly heterogeneous is an inadequate database from which to draw definitive conclusions.

Another important reason for centralising the management of patients with GTD is that patients are reassured by having contact with the full range of staff who are familiar with this disease and can support them through sometimes lengthy and toxic treatments.

## Survival, quality-of-life issues and late side effects of treatment

Survival for most patients with GTD is excellent. As illustrated in Box 39.4 patients with low risk GTD have 100% survival and no patient has died of their disease in the past decade at the Charing Cross Hospital. In patients with high risk disease, there is still a small mortality and this is principally in two different subgroups:

- patients presenting with widely metastatic disease such as brain, lung and liver disease who succumb from disease extent before adequate therapy can be administered;
- patients with PSTT developing more than 2 years after the last known pregnancy.

The survival of patients treated at the Charing Cross Hospital between 1958 and 1992 is shown in Figure 39.1. This shows that, even with relatively simple treatment in the 1950s and 1960s, the outcome for the majority of patients was good. Between 1974 to 1978 patients were stratified by prognostic category from the start of their treatment with the use of essentially the same scoring system as the WHO scoring system.[7] The patients treated from 1979 to 1992 have had the benefit of the introduction of etoposide, cisplatinum, and the improvements in CT scanning and MRI scanning, which have facilitated the selection of patients for surgery.

Following completion of chemotherapy patients get back to normal activity in 2–4 months. In patients treated when they are under 40 years, menstruation restarts between 2 and 6 months after completing chemotherapy with EMA/CO, and usually more rapidly after methotrexate therapy. Most patients who want to have subsequent normal pregnancies succeed in doing so. Interestingly 83% of patients treated with methotrexate alone and 83% of patients treated with combination chemotherapy (mainly

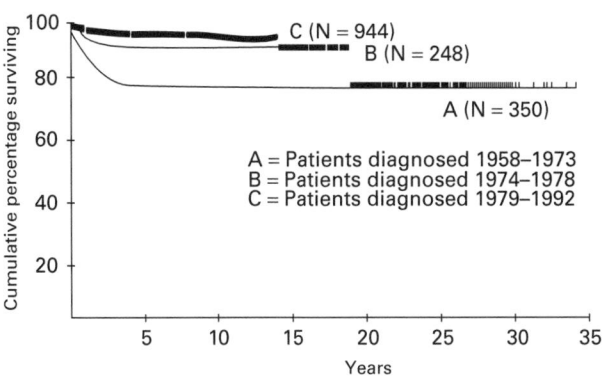

**Figure 39.1** Survival of patients treated at the Charing Cross Hospital since the original cohort A starting in 1958 through 1973, cohort B dating from 1974 through 1978, and cohort C dating from 1975 through 1992. (For details of treatments see text)

EMA/CO chemotherapy) had a normal pregnancy post chemotherapy.[21] Patients receiving combination chemotherapy do have a small increase in second tumours but shortening the duration of their intensive chemotherapy to a maximum of 6 months has meant that we have not had a further case of acute myeloid leukaemia in patients treated in the past decade.[22] However, it should be noted that methotrexate, to a lesser extent, and combination chemotherapy, to a greater extent, will bring forward the age of the menopause from a mean of 52–53 years in patients with molar pregnancies who have never received chemotherapy, to around 47 years in patients who received EMA/CO chemotherapy.[23] Clearly, these patients need to be assessed for hormone replacement therapy as and when they develop premature menopause.

## Why have randomised clinical trials made little contribution to the development of treatment?

The combination of having a tumour marker hCG, which is an accurate reflection of disease progression or regression, together with effective chemotherapy has meant that clinicians can modify their treatment to adjust to unexpected tumour behaviour, such as the development of drug resistance. By centralising the management of patients with this rare disease in trophoblastic disease centres, experience has accumulated to optimise treatment and to minimise toxicity to cover the spectrum of disease expression. In a sense the need for randomised clinical trials reflects the inability to see the biological effect of individual treatments and also in many malignant diseases the treatment itself is relatively ineffective.

## Conclusions

The learning curve for treating patients with trophoblastic tumours spans just over 40 years. In that period the outlook for patients with this rare tumour has probably become the most successful outcome of any adult tumour treated primarily by chemotherapy. By studying the disease closely and identifying a range of prognostic variables, experience has been developed, largely in the absence of randomised trials, to cure most of these patients. Three keys to this success are:

- the ability to monitor disease progression/regression by serial hCG estimations;
- the inherent chemosensitivity of the disease to DNA damaging agents;
- centralising the management of these patients so that expertise can be developed as rapidly as possible.

The level of evidence of the main recommendations is **Evidence level IIa, Grade B** .

## References

1  Li MC, Hertz R, Spencer DB. Effect of methotrexate therapy upon choriocarcinoma and chorioadenoma. *Proc Soc Exp Biol Med* 1956;**43**:361–9.

2  Dark GG, Bower M, Newlands ES, Paradinas F, Rustin GJS. Surveillance policy for stage I ovarian germ cell tumors. *J Clin Oncol* 1997;**15**:620–4.

3  Paradinas FJ. Pathology of trophoblast. In: Hancock BW, Newlands ES, Berkowitz RS, eds. *Gestational Trophoblastic Disease*. London: Chapman and Hall Medical, 1997.

4  Paradinas FJ, Fisher RA, Browne P *et al.* Diploid hydatidiform moles with fetal red blood cells in molar villi: I. Incidence, pathology and prognosis. *J Pathol* 1997;**181**:183.

5  Paradinas FJ, Browne P, Fisher RA *et al.* A clinical, histopathological and flow cytometric study of 149 complete moles, 146 partial moles and 107 non-molar hydropic abortions. *Histopathology* 1996;**28**:101.

6  Newlands E. Presentation and management of persistent gestational trophoblastic disease and gestational trophoblastic tumors in the UK. In: Hancock BW, Newlands ES, Berkowitz RS, eds. *Gestational Trophoblastic Disease*. London: Chapman and Hall Medical, 1997.

7  Bagshawe KD. Risk and prognostic factors in trophoblastic neoplasia. *Cancer* 1976;**38**:1373–85.

8  Crawford RA, Newlands E, Rustin GJS, Holden L, A'Hern R, Bagshawe KD. Gestational trophoblastic disease with liver metastases: the Charing Cross experience. *Br J Obstet Gynaecol* 1997;**104**:105–9.

9  Kohorn EI, Goldstein DP, Hancock BW *et al.* Combining the staging system of the International Federation of Gynecology and Obstetrics with the scoring system of the World Health Organization for Trophoblastic Neoplasia. Report of the Working Committee of the International Society for the Study of Trophoblastic Disease and the International Gynecologic Cancer Society. *Int J Gynecol Cancer* 2000;**10**:84–8.

10  Fulop V, Mok SC, Genest DR *et al.* p53, p21, Rb and mdm2 oncoproteins. Expression in normal placenta, partial and complete mole and choriocarcinoma. *J Reprod Med* 1998;**43**:119.

11  Newlands ES. Investigation and treatment of patients with persistent gestational trophoblastic disease and gestational trophoblastic tumors in the UK. In: Hancock BW, Newlands ES, Berkowitz RS, eds. *Gestational Trophoblastic Disease*. London: Chapman and Hall Medical, 1997.

12  Fisher RA. Genetics of gestational trophoblastic disease. In: Hancock BW, Newlands ES, Berkowitz RS, eds. *Gestational Trophoblastic Disease*. London, Chapman and Hall Medical, 1997.

13  Paradinas FJ. The histological diagnosis of hydatidiform moles. *Curr Diagn Pathol* 1994;**1**:24.

14  Seckl MJ, Fisher RA, Salerno G, Rees H, Paradinas FJ, Foskett M, Newlands ES. Choriocarcinoma and partial hydatidiform moles. *Lancet* 2000;**356**:36–9.

15  Fisher RA, Soteriou B, Meredith L *et al.* Previous hydatidiform mole identified as the causative pregnancy of choriocarcinoma following birth of normal twins. *Int J Gynecol Cancer* 1995;**5**:64.

16  Fisher RA, Newlands ES, Jeffreys AJ *et al.* Gestational and non-gestational trophoblastic tumours distinguished by DNA analysis. *Cancer* 1992;**69**:839.

17  Berkowitz RS, Goldstein DP, Bernstein MR. Ten years experience with methotrexate and folinic acid as primary therapy for gestational trophoblastic disease. *Gynecol Oncol* 1986;**23**:111–18.

18  Bagshawe KD, Dent J, Newlands ES *et al.* The role of low-dose methotrexate and folinic acid in gestational trophoblastic tumours (GTT). *Br J Obstet Gynaecol* 1989;**96**:795–802.

19  Bower M, Newlands ES, Holden L *et al.* EMA/CO for high-risk gestational trophoblastic tumors: Results from a cohort of 272 patients. *J Clin Oncol* 1997;**15**:2636–43.

20  Newlands ES, Mulholland PJ, Holden L, Seckl, MJ, Rustin GJS. Etoposide and Cisplatin/Etoposide, Methotrexate and Actinomycin D (EMA) chemotherapy for patients with high-risk gestational trophoblastic tumors refractory to EMA/Cyclophosphamide and Vincristine chemotherapy and patients presenting with metastatic placental site trophoblastic tumors. *J Clin Oncol* 2000;**18**:854–9.

21  Woolas RP, Bower M, Newlands ES, Seckl M, Short D, Holden L. Influence of chemotherapy for gestational trophoblastic disease on subsequent pregnancy outcome. *Br J Obstet Gynaecol* 1998;**105**: 1032–5.

22  Rustin GJS, Newlands ES, Lutz J-M *et al.* Combination but not single-agent methotrexate chemotherapy for gestational trophoblastic tumors increases the incidence of second tumors. *J Clin Oncol* 1996;**14**:2769–73.

23  Bower M, Rustin GJS, Newlands ES *et al.* Chemotherapy for gestational trophoblastic tumours hastens menopause by 3 years. *Eur J Cancer* 1998;**34**:1204–7.

# Section VIII

## Treating breast cancer

*John F Forbes, Editor*

# Levels of evidence and grades of recommendation used in *Evidence-based Oncology*

Levels of evidence and grades of recommendation appear within the text in the clinical chapters, for example, **Evidence Level Ia** and **Grade A**.

---

**Levels of evidence**

---

Ia    Meta-analysis of randomised controlled trials (RCTs)
Ib    At least 1 RCT
IIa   At least 1 non-randomised study
IIb   At least 1 other well designed quasi-experimental study
III   Non-experimental, descriptive studies
IV    Expert committee reports or opinions/experience of respected authorities

**Grades of recommendations**

---

A    At least one RCT as part of body of literature of overall good quality and consistency addressing recommendation **Evidence levels Ia, Ib**
B    No RCT but well conducted clinical studies available **Evidence levels IIa, IIb, III**
C    Expert committee reports or opinions/experience of respected authorities in the absence of directly applicable good quality clinical studies **Evidence level IV**

---

From *Clinical Oncology* (2001)**13**:S212
Source of data: MEDLINE, *Proceedings of the American Society of Medical Oncology* (ASCO).

# 40 Breast cancer

*John F Forbes*

## Background

Breast cancer is the third most frequent cancer worldwide (796 000 cases, 1990) but the most common cancer in women (21% of total). The mortality/incidence ratio is about 0·6 worldwide, but less than 0·3 in developed countries (for example, USA, Australia), where early diagnosis with screening and effective treatments are widely available. Breast cancer caused 314 000 deaths in 1990, 14·1% of all cancer deaths in women.[1]

Incidence is highest in developed countries, (USA 86·3%/100 000/year, age-standardised, Australia, 71·7%) and lowest in China (11·8%), and middle Africa (13·6%).[1]

Five-year survival rates are highest in Japan (74%), USA (73%), and Australia/New Zealand (68%), and lower in Europe (53–63%) and developing countries (55%). These figures are dependent on stage at diagnosis and are improved when effective early detection programmes are widely available.[1]

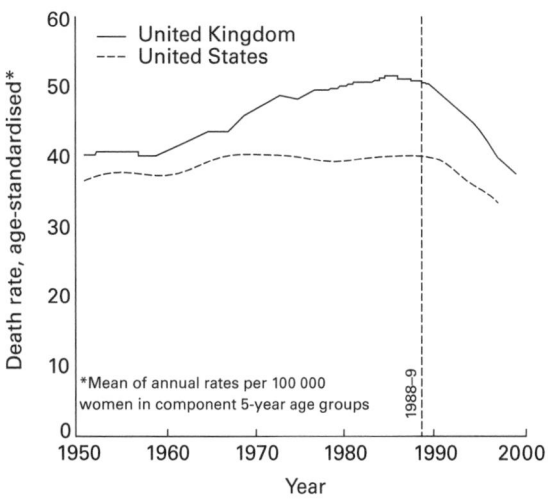

**Figure 40.2**  Recent decrease in breast cancer mortality at ages 20–69 years in UK/USA, 1950–1999[3]

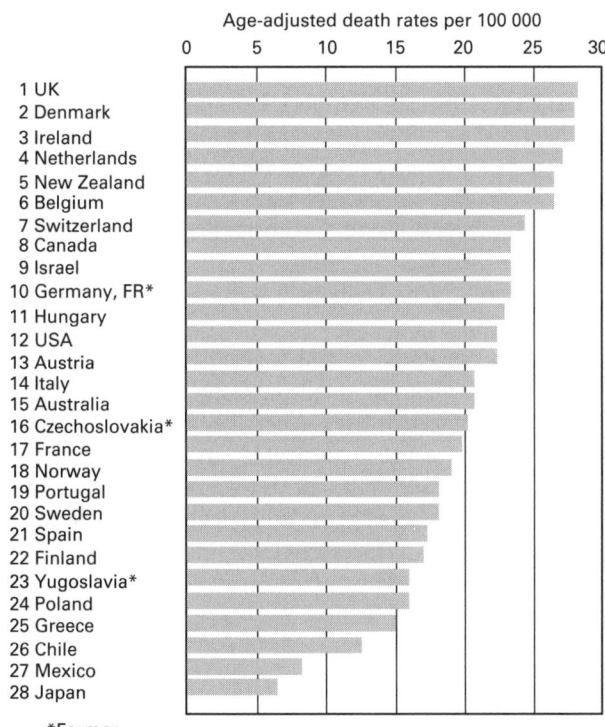

*Former

**Figure 40.1**  Cancer of the breast – female, 1988–1992[139]

Mortality rates have been falling since the late 1980s (about 30% in the UK since 1989).[2,3] Prior to this fall, age-adjusted death rates per 100 000 were highest in the UK (26%) and Denmark (25·5%), lower in the USA (23%) and Australia (21%), and lowest in Japan (6·5%), (Figure 40.1). With current trends it is predicted that there will be 1·35–1·45 million new cases of breast cancer in 2010, depending on the increase in China and East Asia, which may be around 5% per year. The incidence may double from 1990 to 2015.[1]

Mortality, which has fallen in the UK and US (Figure 40.2) and other developed countries, is likely to continue to fall. This is because the lead time from wide availability of new effective treatments to an impact on mortality is several years. Current treatments are superior to those used in the early 1980s, which in turn would likely have contributed to the fall in the mortality a decade later. Hence future falls in mortality are likely.

More than 90% of women will not get breast cancer. Factors increasing risk are summarised in Table 40.1. Models to predict risk in terms of robust data have been developed and include age, number of first-degree female relatives, age of menarche, age of first live birth, number of

**Table 40.1  Established and probable risk factors for breast cancer[5,140]**

| Factor | Relative risk | High risk group |
|---|---|---|
| Age | >10 | Elderly |
| Geographical location | 5 | Developed country |
| Age at menarche | 3 | Menarche before age 11 |
| Age at menopause | 2 | Menopause after age 54 |
| Age at first full pregnancy | 3 | First child in early 40s |
| Family history | ≥2 | Breast cancer in first-degree relative when young |
| Previous benign disease | 4–5 | Atypical hyperplasia |
| Cancer in other breast | >4 | |
| Socioeconomic group | 2 | Groups I and II |
| Diet | 1·5 | High intake of saturated fat |
| Body weight: | | |
|    premenopausal | 0·7 | Body mass index >35 |
|    postmenopausal | 2 | Body mass index >35 |
| Alcohol consumption | 1·3 | Excessive intake |
| Exposure to ionising radiation | 3 | Abnormal exposure in young females after age 10 |
| Taking exogenous hormones: | | |
|    oral contraceptives | 1·24 | Current use |
|    hormone replacement therapy | 1·35 | Use for ≥ 10 years |
|    diethylstilbestrol | 2 | Use during pregnancy |

previous breast biopsies and the presence of atypical hyperplasia in a previous biopsy specimen.[4] The Gail Model may underestimate risk for women with a genetically determined risk (it omits history of associated cancers, such as ovarian cancer, bilateral disease, age of onset for relatives and paternal relatives), but has been shown to be a reliable predictor of risk in some populations.[5] Other models estimate risk in the presence of a family history of breast cancer.[6]

Prognosis depends on extent of disease at diagnosis, patient characteristics, tumour characteristics and availability of effective treatment.

Breast cancer may be staged by the TNM (tumour, nodes, metastases) system, which has recently been updated.[7] This is more valuable for populations than for individual patients, where additional characteristics including hormone receptor status (oestrogen receptor, ER) and tumour grade are important for clarifying diagnosis, selecting treatments and determining prognosis. Categories of risk for node-negative (N-) patients (who may benefit from adjuvant systemic treatment) have been defined by an international panel after consideration of available evidence. They include, minimal/low risk (ER- and/or PgR-positive, and size ≤ 2 cm, grade 1 and age ≥ 35 years). Average/high risk

N- patients include ER- and/or PgR-positive, with at least one of: size > 2 cm, or grade 2–3, or age < 35 years.[8]

Breast cancer has been the subject of more clinical trials than any other cancer and this has contributed to the fall in mortality. Between 1985 and 2000, four overviews of available clinical trials' data have been conducted by the Early Breast Cancer Trialists' Collaborative Group (EBCTCG).[9–16]

The EBCTCG Overviews and additional overviews of trials' data on breast cancer prevention, radiotherapy and systemic treatment of advanced breast cancer form the main basis of this review. Data from prospective randomised trials addressing specific additional questions, for example treatment of duct carcinoma *in situ* (DCIS), are also considered.

Consensus conferences and panels have been convened in St Gallen (Seventh International Conference on Adjuvant Therapy of Primary Breast Cancer),[9] and in Washington.[17] These expert panels considered available data and commented on issues relevant to treatment of early breast cancer. Data considered were largely published subsequent to the 1995 EBCTCG Overviews.

This review considers prevention of breast cancer, treatment of DCIS, early invasive breast cancer and advanced breast cancer.

# Prevention

*John F Forbes, Jack Cuzick*

### Can tamoxifen prevent breast cancer?

The potential for tamoxifen to prevent breast cancer was recognised in 1985 after it was noted that tamoxifen reduced the rate of contralateral breast cancer when used as adjuvant treatment of early breast cancer.[18,19] Subsequently, a pilot tamoxifen prevention trial was commenced in women at increased risk.[20] Two other tamoxifen trials for women at increased risk – the International Breast cancer Intervention Study (IBIS-I),[21] which commenced in 1992, and the National Surgical Breast & Bowel Project (NSABP) P1 trial soon followed.[22] A fourth tamoxifen prevention trial involved women at normal risk, who had had a hysterectomy (Table 40.2).[23]

An overview of all four prospective, randomised, double-blind trials of tamoxifen versus placebo has been published.[20–26] This included the published IBIS-I and NSABP P-1 trials and updated data provided from the other two trials. Data from the EBCTCG 2000 Overview (unpublished) were provided on contralateral breast cancer rates in trials of adjuvant tamoxifen treatment. The overview also included data from a trial of the selective oestrogen receptor modulator (SERM) raloxifene ("MORE" trial[27] – see below) (Table 40.2). The planned tamoxifen regimen was 20 mg per day for 5 years for each trial. Three trials were confined to women at increased risk of breast cancer and one[23] included women at normal risk, who had a hysterectomy. These trials included 28 406 women. Total follow up for all four trials was more than 70 000 women-years for each of the tamoxifen and placebo arms (Table 40.3).[24]

Overall, tamoxifen reduced the incidence of breast cancer by 38% (28–46%, $P < 0.001$), without evidence of heterogeneity between the four trials (Figure 40.3, Table 40.3).[24] **Evidence level Ia**.

### Which women benefit?

The reduction in breast cancer was similar for both invasive breast cancer and duct carcinoma *in situ* (DCIS) (Table 40.3), but was confined to reduction of hormone receptor-positive tumours (ER+), (48%, 36–58%; $P < 0.01$) rather than ER-negative tumours, which were increased, but not significantly (hazard ratio 1·22, 0·89–1·67) (Figures 40.3–40.5). There was no evidence of any significant effect on the magnitude of breast cancer reduction by age,[21,22] prior or current use of hormone replacement therapy (HRT),[21] or level of risk at entry.[22] In the P-1 trial, the largest risk reduction was seen in women who had a history of atypical hyperplasia.[22]

**Table 40.2   Breast cancer prevention trials**

| Trial (entry dates) | Population | No. Randomised | Agents (*v* placebo) and daily dose | Intended duration of treatment |
|---|---|---|---|---|
| Royal Marsden (1986–1996) | High risk Family history | 2471 | Tamoxifen 20 mg | 5–8 years |
| NSABP-P1 (1992–1997) | >1·6% 5y risk | 13 388 | Tamoxifen 20 mg | 5 years |
| Italian (1992–1997) | Normal risk hysterectomy | 5408 | Tamoxifen 20 mg | 5 years |
| IBIS-I (1992–2001) | >2-fold relative risk | 7139 | Tamoxifen 20 mg | 5 years |
| MORE (1994–1999) | Normal risk post-menopausal women with osteoporosis | 7705 | Raloxifene 60 or 120 mg (3 arm) | 4 years |
| Adjuvant overview (1976–1995) | Women with ER+ operable breast cancer in 14 trials | ~15 000 | Tamoxifen 20–40 mg with or without chemotherapy in both arms | 3 years or more (average ~5 yrs) |

Table 40.3 Major events according to age at randomisation

| | Royal Marsden | NSABP-P1 | Italian | IBIS-I | All tamoxifen prevention trials | Adjuvant (5 years tamoxifen) | MORE (60 v 120 v placebo) |
|---|---|---|---|---|---|---|---|
| **Breast cancer** | 62 v 75 | 124 v 244 | 34 v 45 | 69 v 101 | 289 v 465 | 109 v 198 | 31/2 v 43 |
| Invasive | 54 v 64 | 89 v 175 | 28 v 40 | 64 v 85 | 233 v 359 | 109 v 198 | 22/2 v 39 |
| DCIS | 7 v 7 | 35 v 69 | 5 v 4 | 5 v 16 | 53 v 98 | N/A | 9/2 v 4 |
| Unknown | 1 v 4 | — | 1 v 1 | — | 3 v 8 | — | – |
| **ER status (invasive only)** | | | | | | | |
| ER+ (invasive only) | 31 v 44 | 41 v 130 | 19 v 30 | 44 v 63 | 134 v 265 | N/A | 10/2 v 31 |
| ER– (invasive only) | 17 v 10 | 38 v 31 | 14 v 12 | 19 v 19 | 88 v 70 | N/A | 9/2 v 4 |
| **Endometrial cancer** | 6 v 2 | 36 v 15 | –† | 11 v 5 | 53 v 22 | 44 v 14 | 5 v 4 v 5 |
| **Thromboembolic events** | | | | | | | |
| Venous thromboembolic event (excluding superficial) | 12 v 8 | 53 v 28 | 9 v 7 | 43 v 17 | 117 v 60 | | 31 v 35 v 12 |
| Superficial thrombophlebitis | 8 v 5 | — | 27 v 9 | 27 v 9 | 62 v 23 | | |
| **Cardiovascular** | | | | | | | |
| Myocardial infarction | 6 v 3 | 31 v 28 | 5 v 5 | 5 v 5 | 47 v 41 | NA | |
| Cerebrovascular | 9 v 17 | 57 v 49 | 15 v 9 | 15 v 18 | 96 v 93 | 11 v 14* | NA |
| CVA/stroke | 4 v 7 | 38 v 24 | 5 v 0 | 12 v 8 | 59 v 39 | | |
| TIA only | 5 v 10 | 19 v 25 | | 3 v 10 | 27 v 45 | | |
| Women-years of follow up | 12 211 v 12 169 | 26 154 v 26 247 | 18 270 v 18 324 | 14 998 v 14 969 | 71 633 v 71 709 | 32 227 v 31 908 | 16 958/2 v 8357 |

*Mortality
†All women in Italian trial had a hysterectomy before randomisation

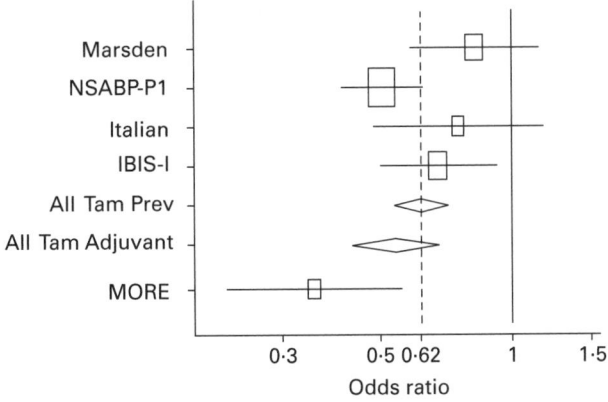

**Figure 40.3** Breast cancer incidence (including DCIS). Abbreviations: Prev, previous; Tam, tamoxifen[24]

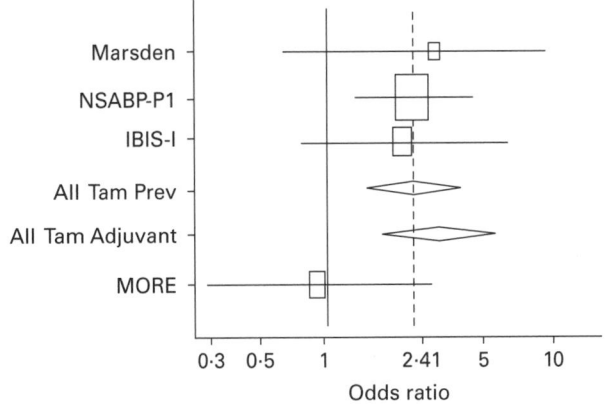

**Figure 40.6** Endometrial cancers. Abbreviations: Prev, previous; Tam, tamoxifen[24]

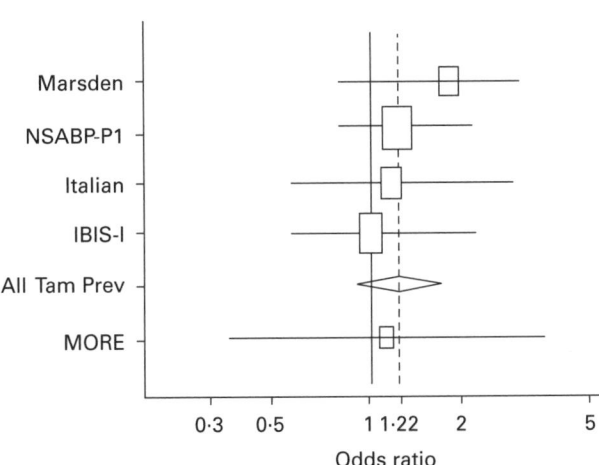

**Figure 40.4** ER-negative breast cancer. Abbreviations: Prev, previous; Tam, tamoxifen[24]

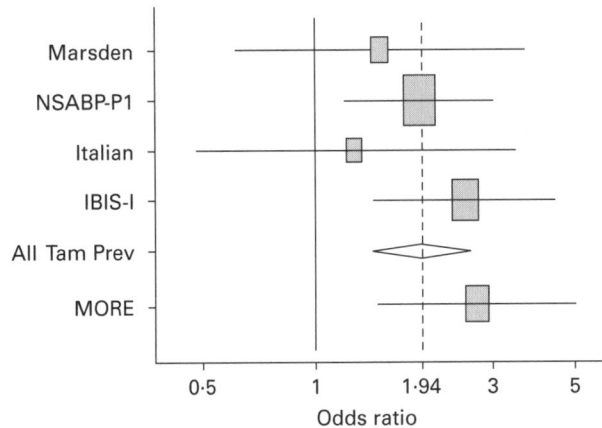

**Figure 40.7** Venous thromboembolic risk. Abbreviations: Prev, previous; Tam, tamoxifen[24]

## What serious side effects are caused by tamoxifen?

Serious events were more common with tamoxifen. Endometrial cancer rates were increased in each tamoxifen trial (overall RR 2·4, 1·5–4·0), but the increase was largely confined to women aged 50 years or more[24] (Figure 40.6).

All four trials reported an increased rate of venous thromboembolic disease: overall relative risk 1·9 (1·4–2·7). This risk was reported in younger (premenopausal) and older women, and was greater when other risk factors such as prolonged immobilisation were present in IBIS-I (Figure 40.7).[22–24]

The P1 trial, found a small increased risk of cataracts on tamoxifen. This was not evident in IBIS-I.[20,21]

No significant effect on breast cancer mortality has been reported to date, although follow up still remains relatively short at the times of analyses in the two larger trials. The overview found a 10% (NS) reduction in all-cause mortality

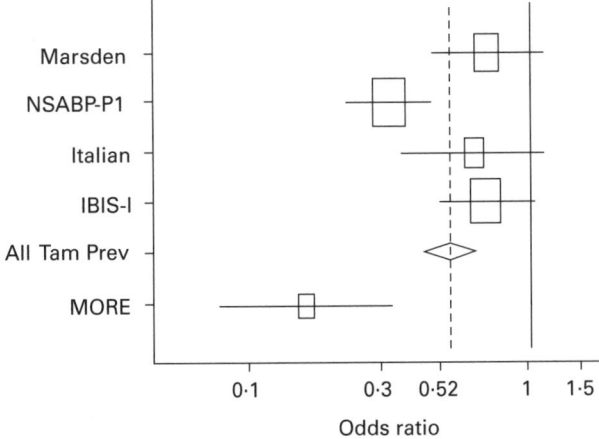

**Figure 40.5** ER-positive invasive breast cancer. Abbreviations: Prev, previous; Tam, tamoxifen[24]

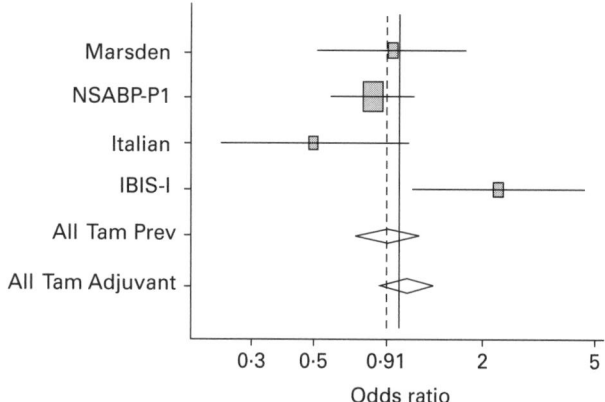

**Figure 40.8** Death from any cause (except breast cancer for adjuvant trials). Abbreviations: Prev, previous; Tam, tamoxifen[24]

(112 *v* 123), with one trial (IBIS-I) reporting a significant increase in all-cause mortality (25 *v* 11 deaths).[21] There was substantial heterogeneity (*P* = 0·026) across the trials (Figure 40.8).[21] As there was no significant increase of other cancers or serious cardiac events on tamoxifen in IBIS-I, it is plausible that the increased mortality is due to the play of chance.

## How long should tamoxifen be given for?

Tamoxifen use was planned for 5 years and compliance was close to 70% at 5 years. There was no evidence of significant variation of risk reduction with time on tamoxifen. Sufficient data are not yet available to determine breast cancer event rates after tamoxifen is stopped. Such data may help clarify whether tamoxifen delays or prevents breast cancer. The IBIS-I trial is continuing to collect unbiased data on these late breast cancer events, but, unbiased follow up of women on NSABP-P1 is not possible since this trial was stopped when results became available.

## How many breast cancer deaths could be avoided with tamoxifen?

It has been estimated that 1000 high risk women treated for 5 years with tamoxifen would have 18% fewer breast cancer deaths within 10 years (17·25–14·1, that is, reduction of 3·15 per 1000).[24]

## Other tamoxifen data

The Early Breast Cancer Trialists' Collaborative Group (EBCTCG) overviews of adjuvant tamoxifen treatment for early breast cancer trials have measured the effect of

tamoxifen on the incidence of new, contralateral breast cancers[14] with a similar tamoxifen regimen (20–40 mg per day, for an average of 5 years). The risk reduction was 46% (29–63%). The endometrial cancer rate was increased by tamoxifen, HR 3·1 (1·7–5·7) almost entirely in women aged 50 years or more. There was no difference for non-breast cancer deaths in these adjuvant trials.[24]

## Should tamoxifen be offered to all women?

It remains too soon to draw conclusions about the overall risk–benefit ratio of tamoxifen in individual women at increased risk of breast cancer. A young woman, for example, aged 38, with a very high risk of breast cancer (such as known positive for the breast cancer susceptibility gene *BRCA2*), might have more to gain. Risk of uterine cancer would be very low but risk of thromboembolic events would probably be increased, but partly avoidable. Tamoxifen could reduce breast cancer risks substantially and hence be an option. Alternatively an older women (aged 65 for example), with an intact uterus, no additional risk factors and a past history of stroke or thrombosis, should avoid tamoxifen.

Rather than simple assessment of risk, what is required is assessment of risk for hormone-sensitive breast cancer. Use of the Gail Model[4] and measurement of breast density and oestrogen levels, may contribute to this. The overview data show an increased risk of ER-negative tumours (22%, NS). If women at risk for ER-negative tumours could be identified, they should, at present, avoid tamoxifen.[24]

## What other agents might prevent breast cancer?

The selective oestrogen receptor modulator (SERM), raloxifene, was found to reduce the risk of breast cancer when evaluated in a prospective randomised clinical trial, as a treatment for osteoporosis in postmenopausal women (64% reduction) (Figures 40.3–40.7).[27] The risk reduction was greatest in women with higher levels of oestrogen. This effect was also confined to a reduction in ER-positive tumours, and raloxifene also significantly increased venous thromboembolic events, but had no apparent effect on the incidence of endometrial cancer in this population.[24] Breast cancer was not a primary endpoint in this trial.

A randomised trial that compared the aromatose inhibitor, anastrozole, with tamoxifen as adjuvant therapy in postmenopausal women with hormone-responsive breast cancer, found a 58% reduction in contralateral invasive breast cancer for women on anastrozole (anastrozole 27 *v* tamoxifen 9, *P* < 0·0068), after 33 months median follow up.[28]

## What other prevention trials are being conducted?

The NSABP is conducting the "STAR" trial, comparing tamoxifen with raloxifene in a prospective double-blind trial in postmenopausal women at high risk. The IBIS-II trial is comparing anastrozole with placebo in postmenopausal women at increased risk, and anastrozole with tamoxifen in women with locally excised DCIS. These trials will take several years to complete.

## Does ovarian ablation reduce new breast cancer risk?

The EBCTCG overview[13] of ovarian ablation, used as adjuvant treatment for early breast cancer, contained insufficient information to draw conclusions on the effect on contralateral breast cancer (30 contralateral breast cancers as first event among 712 women allocated ablation, *v* 32 among 679 controls in trials with data; log-rank 0-E – 2·8, variance 15·1, NS). A randomised trial comparing chemical ovarian ablation by the luteinising hormone releasing hormone (LHRH), goserelin (Zoladex), for 3 years, plus tamoxifen for 5 years versus six cycles of cyclophosphamide, methotrexate and fluorouracil (CMF), reported a significant reduction in contralateral breast cancer events in the endocrine treatment arm (3 *v* 12, *P* < 0·0001).[29]

A prospective randomised trial comparing adjuvant ovarian suppression in premenopausal women by goserelin with no suppression in women with early breast cancer noted a reduction in contralateral breast cancer rates. As most women also received tamoxifen, the reduction reported with goserelin may be important.[30]

Indirect evidence comes from 43 women with *BRCA1* mutations who had prophylactic bilateral oophorectomy and who had not had breast cancer, ovarian cancer, or prophylactic bilateral mastectomy. When these women were compared with 79 matched controls who had not had surgery, a significant reduction in breast cancer risk was noted, most evident in women followed for 5–10 years, or at least 10 years after surgery. There was no evidence that exposure to hormone replacement therapy compromised the risk reduction.[31]

Taken together, these data are consistent with a role for ovarian ablation in preventing new breast cancer. Prospective clinical trials are required in premenopausal women at increased risk.

## How effective is mastectomy in preventing breast cancer?

There are no data from prospective randomised clinical trials. The value of prophylactic surgery to reduce breast cancer risk, based on uncontrolled data has been reviewed.[32] A retrospective study of 639 women with a family history of breast cancer, who had undergone a prophylactic bilateral mastectomy between 1960 and 1993, found a risk reduction of 89·5% (37·4 expected, four observed; *P* < 0·001) and the risk reduction was similar for high risk women (3/214) when compared with their sisters (156/403).[33] **Evidence level IIa**.

Women with *BRCA1* or *BRCA2* mutations who had prophylactic bilateral mastectomy (76 women) had no breast cancer observed after mean follow up for 2·9 years, compared with eight breast cancers in women having surveillance without prophylactic bilateral mastectomy, after 3 years mean follow up.[34]

## What strategies of "risk management" could a woman at high risk choose?

Options include regular mammography screening, bilateral oophorectomy, bilateral mastectomy and tamoxifen.

Screening is essential for all women with breast tissue. For women at high risk, 12-month mammography screening is associated with high interval cancer rates and a high risk of node-positive disease. If the interval cancer rate reflected rapid growth, more frequent mammography would be appropriate. If mammography was not sufficiently sensitive then alternatives such as MRI screening might be required.

Bilateral oophorectomy reduces the risk of both breast cancer and cancer of the ovary, which may be associated and has no reliable screening method to detect it early. It may also have an effect on breast density (lowering), which may enhance mammography sensitivity. Bilateral mastectomy is effective but disfiguring. Individual women must balance their risk against the value and shortcomings of these strategies, and tamoxifen.

### Duct carcinoma *in situ*

Duct carcinoma *in situ* (DCIS) is non-invasive and hence non-metastatic and is usually cured by local treatment. The small number of patients found to have involved lymph nodes or distant metastases have presumably had undetected invasive breast cancer. Total mastectomy without axillary dissection is associated with excellent long-term survival.

With the use of mammography for screening well women, subclinical DCIS can be detected by radiological localisation methods and may be treated by wide excision of the lesion with breast preservation. This procedure would be curative if all of the DCIS was removed, and if there was no other associated DCIS or invasive disease in other parts of the breast. Such patients would still be at risk of new DCIS or invasive breast cancer, ipsilateral or contralateral.

Prior to the wide use of mammography screening, DCIS was an uncommon diagnosis and usually treated by mastectomy. Uncontrolled follow up studies of treatment with mastectomy have documented breast cancer recurrence rates of 0·2%, with follow up of 5·5–20 years. Mastectomy may, however, be considered as overtreatment for some patients. Multidiscipline guidelines for diagnosis and management of DCIS have been produced including technical aspects.[35] This section focuses on evidence from randomised trials that can be a basis for treatment.

## Does radiotherapy reduce local recurrence rates after breast preservation?

Radiotherapy produces a substantial relative reduction in recurrences in the preserved breast. Absolute reductions are smaller. **Evidence level Ib**

Two randomised clinical trials have compared breast preservation with and without radiotherapy for local treatment of DCIS. Each has shown substantial reduction in ipsilateral local recurrence rates, with radiotherapy. In the NSABP B-17 trial, for DCIS (80% detected by mammographic screening), radiotherapy produced a significant reduction in both ipsilateral invasive (13.4% $v$ 3·9%; $P < 0·005$) and *in situ* recurrence (13.4% $v$ 8·2%; $P < 0·007$) with mean of 90 months follow up (range 67–130 months).[36,37]

Of those patients with 8 or more years of follow up, the reduction in recurrence was 61%, (94/303; 31% $v$ 43/320; 13%; $P < 0·0001$). Of several pathological features examined, reoccurrence in the non-irradiated group was associated with moderate or severe comedo necrosis (40% risk compared with 23% risk if comedo necrosis was absent or minimal). The width of excision margins was not reliably documented.[38,39]

A similar trial was conducted by the European Organisation for Research and Treatment of Cancer (EORTC). Patients with DCIS up to 5 cm in diameter were randomised to breast preservation surgery, with or without radiotherapy. Most lesions were detected on mammography (71%).[40] Breast cancer recurrence rates were 9% (radiotherapy) versus 16% (no radiotherapy) (log-rank $P = 0·005$) after a median follow up of 4·25 years. Risk reduction was significant and similar for both subsequent invasive disease and DCIS. There were no differences in distant disease rates or survival.[40]

Hence, it is concluded that breast preservation by surgical excision followed by radiotherapy to the breast, is an acceptable alternative to mastectomy for DCIS.

## Is radiotherapy always required for breast preservation in DCIS?

There are no published data available from randomised trials.

Radiotherapy provides a substantial risk reduction for ipsilateral breast events, but no apparent survival gain. If woman have a low risk of ipsilateral recurrence of breast cancer, for example 5–10%, they will have little gain from radiotherapy, despite the cost and morbidity, as even with a 60% risk reduction, this reduces to 2–4%, for example. It has been suggested that a low risk population might include small, low grade DCIS excised with clear margins.[35] This requires testing in prospective randomised trials. Radiotherapy is associated with a relative risk reduction, but the absolute benefit will be small for some women. Individual women and doctors must consider risk and benefits in considering whether radiotherapy should be used.

## What is the role of tamoxifen in treating DCIS?

Tamoxifen reduces both the ipsilateral and contralateral breast cancer event rate. A prospective randomised clinical trial has evaluated the role of tamoxifen in women with DCIS treated by breast preserving surgery. In the NSABP B-24 trial, women with DCIS had excision and radiotherapy and were randomised to tamoxifen 20 mg per day or placebo for 5 years. Women on tamoxifen experienced 37% fewer breast cancer events, 13·4% versus 8·2% ($P < 0·0009$) after 74 months median follow up. The reduction was significant both for invasive breast cancer (43%, $P < 0·004$); and DCIS (31%, $P < 0·40$) and for ipsilateral and contralateral events. The tamoxifen effect was greater for women under 50 (38%) than for women 50 and over (22%), and the latter was not significant. Most women in this study were in the younger age group. Tamoxifen was associated with an increased risk of endometrial cancer (in older women) and deep vein thrombosis. Hence, the overall risk–benefit is more favourable in younger women who obtain a greater benefit with less risk of serious side effects.[41]

# Early invasive breast cancer

Early invasive breast cancer is confined to the breast and axillary lymph nodes. It does not include breast cancer with local signs of advanced disease in the breast (large, fixed tumour, skin involvement, peau d'orange, inflammatory breast cancer) or nodes (large, matted, or fixed nodes).

Treatments are local (surgery and radiotherapy) or systemic (endocrine treatments or cytotoxic chemotherapy). Endocrine treatments include ovarian ablation (and tamoxifen) in women with functioning ovaries, and tamoxifen in postmenopausal women. Recently data suggest that a new type of endocrine therapy – aromatase inhibition – may be superior to tamoxifen in postmenopausal women with hormone-sensitive tumours.

This section considers surgery first and then the role and cost-benefit of radiotherapy. Systemic treatments, ovarian ablation, tamoxifen and chemotherapy follow.

## Surgery

Surgery for early breast cancer has involved total mastectomy (TM), radical mastectomy (RM), dissection of axillary nodes (AD), extended radical mastectomy (ERM), and less than mastectomy, that is, breast preservation (BP) with complete local excision of the primary tumour (CLE). Randomised clinical trials have compared more with less surgery, and surgery with the same surgery plus radiotherapy (see the section below on radiotherapy).

## Is more surgery beyond mastectomy better?

There is no evidence that more surgery than mastectomy is beneficial. An EBCTCG overview,[12] (Table 40.4), included 10 trials, which commenced prior to 1985 comparing more with less surgery. Nine trials involving 3400 women compared mastectomy (TM or RM) with more extensive surgery. After 10 years' follow up no significant difference was found for survival (mortality: more extensive surgery 48%, less extensive surgery 50·1%) overall, or separately for node-positive or node-negative cancer, and the small (1·5%) difference in rates of recurrence in favour of more extensive surgery (48·8% v 50·3%; odds ratio; ·98 ± 0·05) was not significant (Figures 40.9 and 40.10).[12] **Evidence level Ia**

The NSABP have published 25-year follow up data from trial NSABP-04. This trial randomised women with invasive breast cancer and "clinically negative" axillary nodes (1079) to RM or TM and regional radiotherapy, or TM and AD only if nodes became positive. Women with "clinically positive" axillary nodes (1586) were randomised to RM or TM plus regional radiotherapy. After follow up to 25 years, there were no differences in disease-free survival, relapse-free survival, distant disease-free survival, or overall survival in either stratum.[42]

**Table 40.4    Randomised trials of local therapy for early breast cancer.[12]**

| Type of comparison | No. of trials | No. of women | No. of deaths |
|---|---|---|---|
| Radiotherapy plus surgery *v* the same surgery alone | | | |
| Common surgery *v* mastectomy alone | 5 | 4541 | 2642 |
| Common surgery *v* mastectomy plus axillary sampling | 4 | 3286 | 817 |
| Common surgery *v* mastectomy plus axillary clearance | 23 | 6378 | 2936 |
| Common surgery *v* breast conservation plus axillary clearance | 4 | 3068 | 629 |
| Subtotal | 36 | 17 273 | 7024 |
| More-extensive surgery *v* less extensive surgery | | | |
| Less extensive *v* radical or total mastectomy | 5 | 2090 | 1062 |
| Less extensive *v* simple mastectomy | 4 | 1296 | 805 |
| Less extensive *v* breast-conserving surgery | 1 | 1432 | 497 |
| Subtotal | 10 | 4818 | 2364 |
| More-extensive surgery  *v*  less extensive surgery plus radiotherapy | | | |
| Mastectomy *v* breast conservation plus radiotherapy | 9 | 4891 | 1120 |
| Axillary clearance *v* radiotherapy | 8 | 4370 | 2396 |
| Mastectomy plus axillary clearance *v* conservation plus radiotherapy | 1 | 630 | 428 |
| Subtotal | 18 | 9891 | 3944 |
| Total available for analyses of mortality* | 58 | 28 405 | 11 834 |
| Total not yet available† | 5 | 770 | – |

*This total (58 trials, not 64) avoids double counting and excludes the other comparisons of local therapy, which involved an additional 3358 women, of whom 1131 died, in 15 trials.

†The numbers known not to be available were as follows: mastectomy plus axillary clearance, with or without radiotherapy, two trials with a total of about 600 women; radical mastectomy *v* simple mastectomy, one trial with 15 women; mastectomy versus breast-conserving surgery, one trial with 16 women; and mastectomy *v* breast-conserving surgery plus radiotherapy, one trial with about 10 women.

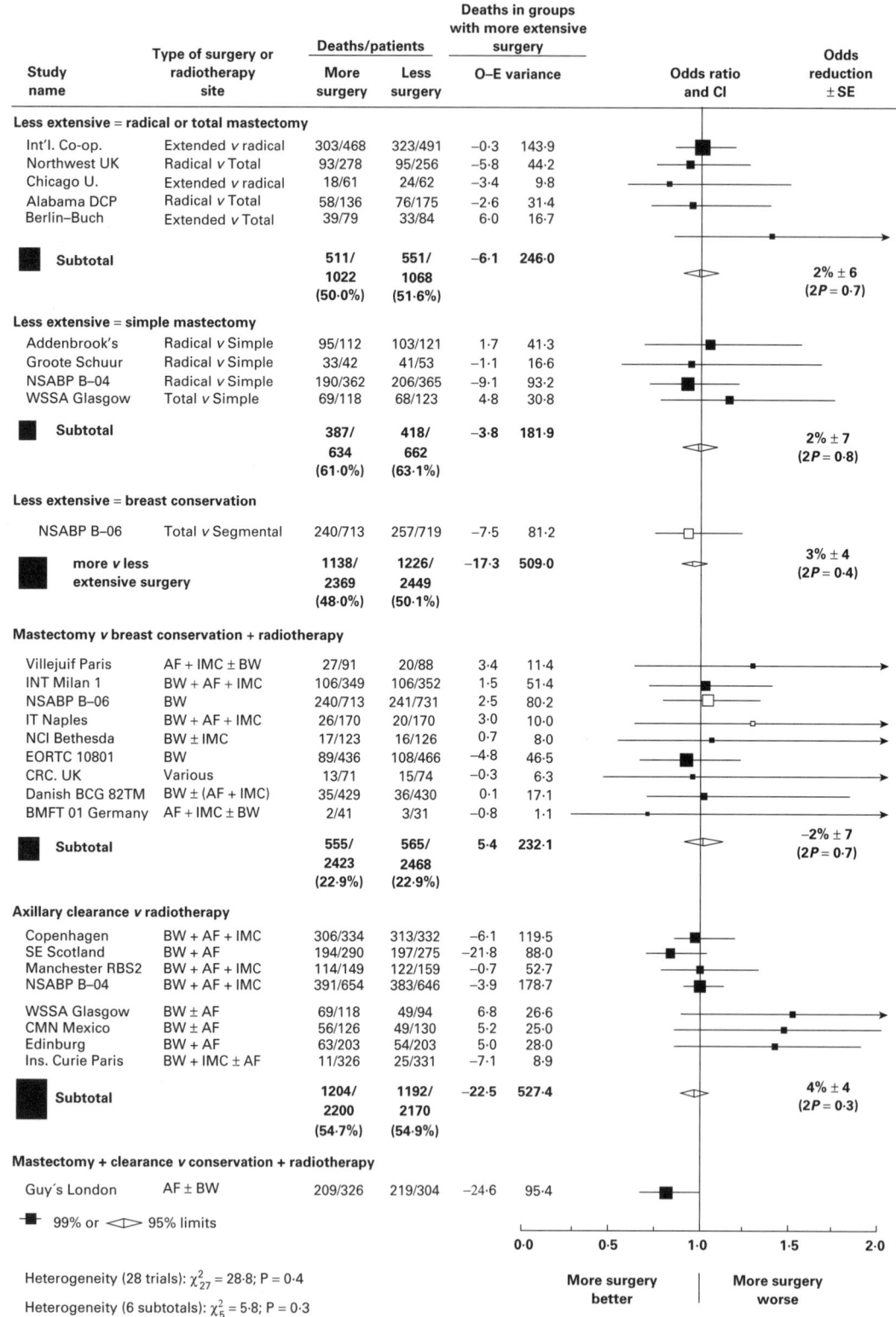

**Figure 40.9** Mortality among women in 10 trials comparing more extensive surgery with less extensive surgery and 18 trials comparing more extensive surgery with less extensive surgery plus radiotherapy[12]

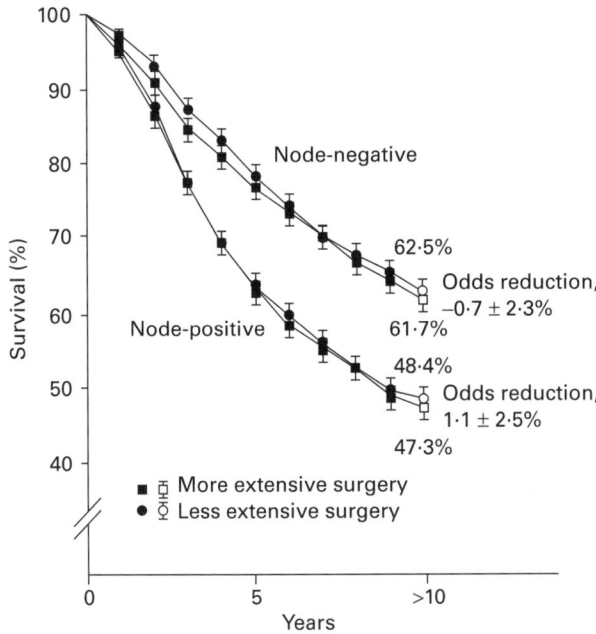

**Figure 40.10** Ten-year survival among approximately 3400 women in nine randomised trials comparing more extensive surgery with less extensive surgery, with neither conserving the breast[12]

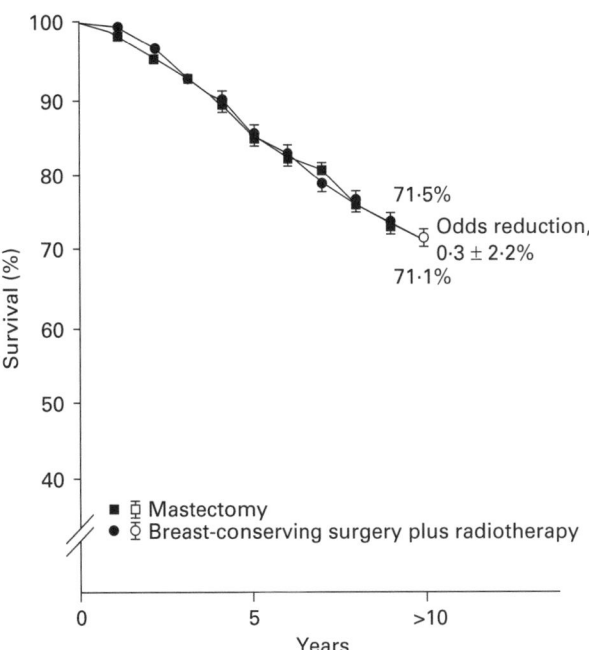

**Figure 40.11** Ten-year survival among approximately 3100 women in seven randomised trials comparing mastectomy with breast-conserving surgery plus radiotherapy[12]

There can be no doubt that surgery beyond total mastectomy is not required for early breast cancer.

### Is radiotherapy better than surgery for treating axillary nodes?

In eight trials of axillary clearance versus radiotherapy there was no difference in total mortality (54·7% v 54·9%), or in recurrence as first event. Radiotherapy was associated with fewer isolated local recurrences (odds reduction $15 \pm 8\%$, $P = 0.06$).[12]

One of these trials[42] has now published data from follow up to 25 years, with no significant differences in regional recurrence or overall survival. No patients received systemic adjuvant therapy. About 10% of the group with clinically negative nodes who had TM and AD had involved nodes, so a substantial number in the TM alone group would have had untreated axillary nodes. Despite this, and without any systemic treatment, survival at 25 years was the same for each group.[42]

### Is breast preservation with radiotherapy a safe alternative to mastectomy for early invasive breast cancer?

The EBCTCG overview (1995) considered nine trials of mastectomy versus breast-conserving surgery plus radiotherapy for early breast cancer.[12,43–51] Overall there was no difference in total mortality (22·9% v 22·9%) after

10 years, or for node-positive or node-negative tumours.[12] There were no data available on cause of death. Six trials (3107 women) with data on recurrences showed fewer recurrences after mastectomy (OR $0.96 \pm 0.08$, NS). Local recurrence rates were 6·2% (mastectomy) and 5·9% (preservation)[12] (Figure 40.11).

Two of these trials had substantially higher local recurrence rates,[51,52] which have been attributed to incomplete tumour removal, as the aim was only "gross tumour removal" and margins were not always clear. This suggests that the extent of residual disease after surgery may influence the efficacy of control by radiotherapy, but clinical trials have not directly tested this important question.

Two of these trials have now reported 20-year follow up data. The National Surgical Breast and Bowel Project (NSABP) Protocol B-06 is the largest such trial, involving 1851 women.[45] Information from B-06 was only partly included in the EBCTCG overview. Women were randomised to TM, "lumpectomy" alone, or "lumpectomy" plus breast irradiation. All women had axillary nodes removed from the lower part of the axilla (levels I and II) and tumours were 4 cm or less in size. With follow up to 20 years, there were no significant differences for disease-free survival, distant disease-free survival, or overall survival. In the two breast preservation groups, radiotherapy produced a substantial reduction in ipsilateral breast recurrence as the first event (39·2% v 14·3%, $P < 0.001$); and this was significant both for women with negative nodes (36·2% *v* 17·0%, *P* < 0·001) and with positive nodes (44·2% *v* 8·8%, *P* < 0·001). Survival rates at 20 years were TM, 47 ± 2%; "lumpectomy" alone, 46 ± 2%; "lumpectomy" plus irradiation, 46 ± 2%).

The second trial with 20-year follow up compared RM with "quadrantectomy" followed by ipsilateral breast irradiation, in 701 women with tumours 2 cm or less in size.[47] Women in the RM group had significantly less local (breast) recurrences (2·3% *v* 8·8%, *P* < 0·001). There were no significant differences for rates of distant metastases, contralateral breast cancer, or second primary cancers. At 20 years, death rates for all causes and for breast cancer were RM 41·2% and 24·3%, and breast preservation, 41·7% and 26·1%.[48]

It is clear that mastectomy and breast preservation with radiotherapy are comparable in terms of efficacy **Grade A**.

Mastectomy remains an important treatment for these woman who cannot have all the tumour excised with an acceptable cosmetic result (for example, large tumour and small breast, extensive or multifocal cancer, some invasive lobular cancers) or those who prefer to have a mastectomy after informed discussion.

## Is radiotherapy essential for breast preservation?

In the EBCTCG overview[12] four trials comparing preservation with and without radiotherapy were included. Overall there was a non-significant reduction in mortality in favour of breast preservation plus radiotherapy (odds reduction 12% ± 9, 2*P* = 0·2). Radiotherapy produced a significantly lower breast recurrence rate.[12]

Several additional trials have compared breast-conserving surgery with and without breast irradiation. Although these trials differ in populations treated and treatments studied (patient selection, type and extent of surgery and radiotherapy, and use of adjuvant systemic therapies), all showed a significant reduction in breast recurrence in the irradiated groups.[45,53,54–59]

Subgroup analyses have identified patients for whom the risk reduction is sufficiently small for patients and clinicians to consider whether they wish radiotherapy to be added or not. In a Swedish trial[56] breast recurrence rates were 11% and 6% without and with radiotherapy, respectively, for women aged over 55 with small invasive ductal tumours. Hence 95% of patients in this group might receive irradiation unnecessarily and the 5% avoiding recurrence had no apparent survival gain. In a Milan trial[47,54] comparing quadrantectomy alone with quadrantectomy and radiotherapy, the advantage for radiotherapy in women 60 and over was also very small, without any survival advantage.

Women having radiotherapy could avoid radiotherapy if the absolute risk of breast recurrence was already low.

## Does tamoxifen reduce local recurrence rates for small invasive tumours?

Other trials[57,58] evaluated whether the addition of tamoxifen to breast preservation without radiotherapy would provide local control comparable to radiotherapy. NSABP-21[57] included women with tumours up to 1 cm in size that were lymph node negative. After "lumpectomy", women were randomised to radiotherapy alone, tamoxifen alone, or radiotherapy plus tamoxifen. With a follow up through 8 years cumulative, breast recurrence rates were 16·5% (tamoxifen), 9·3% (radiotherapy) and 2·8% (radiotherapy plus tamoxifen), respectively. Radiotherapy alone was superior to tamoxifen alone in reducing breast cancer recurrence, regardless of ER status. There were no differences in overall or cause-specific survival.[57] Tamoxifen is unlikely to be as effective as radiotherapy in controlling local breast recurrence unless excision is wide and clear.

# The benefits and side effects of radiotherapy in early breast cancer

*Jack Cuzick*

The use of radiotherapy in the treatment of breast cancer was the first question to be addressed in cancer treatment by a randomised trial[60] which began in 1948. However, controversy remains to this day about its role. Over 50 randomised trials have been conducted throughout the intervening years and a substantial evidence base now exists on its use in various circumstances. Radiotherapy techniques have changed substantially in the past five decades, as has surgical technique, and the use of adjuvant hormonal and chemotherapy, and radiotherapy needs to be viewed in the context of other available treatments. Interactions between treatments, changes in the way radiotherapy is given, its side effect profile and the long natural history of breast cancer have all contributed to the need to continue to evaluate its role in treatment of early breast cancer today.

Most of the evidence on the effect on mortality and local control from randomised trials has been summarised in a series of overviews.[12,16,61,62] The last of these was published in 2000 and provided 10-year and 20-year results from 40 trials that had commenced before 1990. These trials involved 20 000 women, 178 000 women-years of follow up, almost 10 000 deaths and more than 2700 isolated local recurrences.

Most of these trials evaluated radiotherapy following mastectomy with axillary clearance (23 trials, 6379 women, 3585 deaths), but there were also trials of irradiation following mastectomy with axillary sampling (six trials, 3901 women, 2106 deaths), mastectomy alone (five trials, 5125 women, 3125 deaths), and breast conservation with axillary clearance (six trials, 4177 women, 1022 deaths).[13,16] There are a number of trials where the results are not yet available involving breast conservation with or without axillary clearance, and the data on this issue are substantially less mature.

Other more clinically orientated reviews of selected subsets of trials have also been conducted.[63–67]

## Results: benefits and side effects

The relevant outcomes of breast irradiation can be grouped into four separate categories:

- local control
- breast cancer mortality
- mortality from other causes
- non-fatal side-effects.

The context in which it is offered for curative effect can be usefully divided into three groups:

- post-mastectomy
- following complete local excision (CLE) for invasive disease
- following CLE for DCIS.

## What is the overall benefit of radiotherapy for local control?

The trials are very consistent regarding the effect of radiotherapy on local-regional breast cancer recurrence. The data from individual trials are summarised in Figure 40.12 and further evaluated by type of treatment and patient/tumour characteristics in Figure 40.13. Overall the use of radiotherapy is associated with a two-thirds reduction in local recurrence (8·8% v 27·2% at 10 years). Some of the more recent trials suggest that a higher reduction of 75% can now be achieved, especially if radiotherapy is used in conjunction with chemotherapy or tamoxifen.[12,16]

No significant interaction was seen with type of surgery, nodal status of the patient, age, type, dose, or fields of radiotherapy; use of systemic therapy, time period of trial commencement, or trial size, although there was a non-significant difference in favour of greater effects in the more recent trials and in patients with node-positive tumours.[12,16]

## Does radiotherapy improve overall survival?

Somewhat surprisingly this large effect on local recurrence had no effect on overall survival (Figure 40.14). However, this comparison is overly simplified, as there are differences in breast cancer and non-breast cancer death rates, which cancel each other out, and it is more informative to look at these two types of death separately.

## Does radiotherapy affect breast cancer mortality

Long-term breast cancer mortality appears to be reduced by about 5% (Figure 40.15). None of these effects is seen within the first 5 years after treatment and the majority of this benefit appears to occur in the 5–15 year period. Some of the more recent trials suggest that a larger effect may be obtainable, especially in conjunction with chemotherapy[64,69] but this requires further confirmation.

## Does radiotherapy affect non-breast cancer mortality?

Much of the benefit obtained from reduced breast cancer mortality appears to be counterbalanced by an increase in non-breast cancer deaths, at least for trials with long-term

**Isolated local recurrence**

| Study | Events/women | | Radiotherapy events | | Ratio of annual event rates |
| | allocated radiotherapy | adjusted control | log-rank O–E | variance of O–E | radiotherapy : control |
|---|---|---|---|---|---|
| **Mastectomy alone** | | | | | |
| NSABP B–03 | | | *(no data)* | | |
| Manchester RBS1 | 54/355 | 129/359 | –42·3 | 42·9 | |
| Kings/Cambridge | 144/1376 | 419/1424 | –142·7 | 135·9 | |
| NSABP B–04 | 18/386 | 49/384 | –16·1 | 16·4 | |
| Scottish D | 7/47 | 15/46 | –3·9 | 5·2 | |
| Subtotal | 223/2164 (10·3%) | 612/2213 (27·7%) | –205·0 | 200·4 | 64% (SE 4) reduction 2P < 0·00001 |
| **Mastectomy with axillary sampling** | | | | | |
| Edinburgh I | 13/173 | 50/175 | –19·5 | 15·0 | 77% (SE 4) reduction 2P < 0·00001 |
| Danish BCG 82b | 44/890 | 221/911 | –94·7 | 63·5 | |
| Danish BCG 82c | 30/724 | 203/736 | –89·9 | 56·2 | |
| 3 smaller trials | 21/142 | 59/150 | –20·3 | 17·3 | |
| Subtotal | 108/1929 (5·6%) | 533/1972 (27·0%) | –224·4 | 152·0 | 77% (SE 4) reduction 2P < 0·00001 |
| **Mastectomy with axillary clearance** | | | | | |
| Oslo X–ray | 13/285 | 30/267 | –9·4 | 10·6 | |
| Oslo Co–60 | 7/278 | 19/285 | –5·9 | 6·5 | |
| Stockholm A | 38/639 | 164/642 | –44·7 | 25·1 | |
| SASIB | 18/186 | 42/191 | –12·0 | 14·3 | |
| S Swedish BCG | 15/386 | 43/382 | –14·9 | 14·3 | |
| BCCA Vancouver | 11/164 | 22/154 | –6·2 | 8·0 | |
| ECOG EST3181 | 14/171 | 29/161 | –7·9 | 10·2 | |
| 14 smaller trials | 89/1124 | 199/1145 | –55·9 | 67·3 | |
| Subtotal | 205/3233 (6·3%) | 548/3227 (17·0%) | –156·9 | 156·3 | 63% (SE 5) reduction 2P < 0·00001 |
| **Breast conservation with axillary clearance** | | | | | |
| NSABP B–06 | 47/731 | 108/719 | –33·8 | 38·0 | |
| Uppsala–Örebro | 6/184 | 37/197 | –16·1 | 10·4 | |
| St George's | 25/208 | 59/192 | –20·2 | 19·3 | |
| Ontario COG | 26/416 | 115/421 | –48·8 | 33·4 | |
| Scottish | 16/293 | 77/296 | –31·6 | 22·3 | |
| CRC, UK | 30/259 | 63/261 | –17·8 | 22·3 | |
| Subtotal | 150/2091 (7·2%) | 459/2086 (22·0%) | –168·2 | 145·7 | 68% (SE 5) reduction 2P < 0·00001 |
| Total | 686/9417 (7·3%) | 2152/9498 (22·7%) | –754·5 | 654·4 | 68·4% (SE 2·3) reduction 2P < 0·00001 |

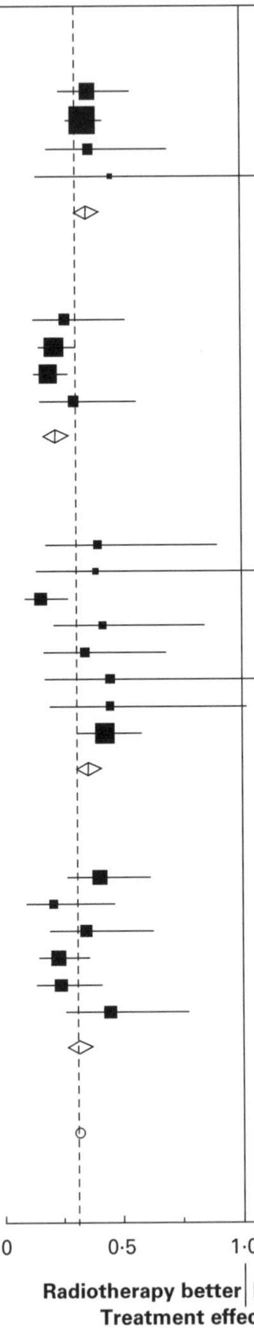

■ 99% or ◁▷ 95% CI

Heterogeneity between 4 subtotals: $\chi^2_3 = 22\cdot8$; $P = 0\cdot00005$

Heterogeneity within subtotals: $\chi^2_{18} = 34\cdot2$; $P = 0\cdot01$

Heterogeneity between 22 strata: $\chi^2_{21} = 57\cdot0$; $P = 0\cdot00004$

0    0·5    1·0    1·5    2·0

**Radiotherapy better | Radiotherapy worse**
Treatment effect 2P < 0·00001

**Figure 40.12** Proportional effects of radiotherapy on isolated local recurrence[16]

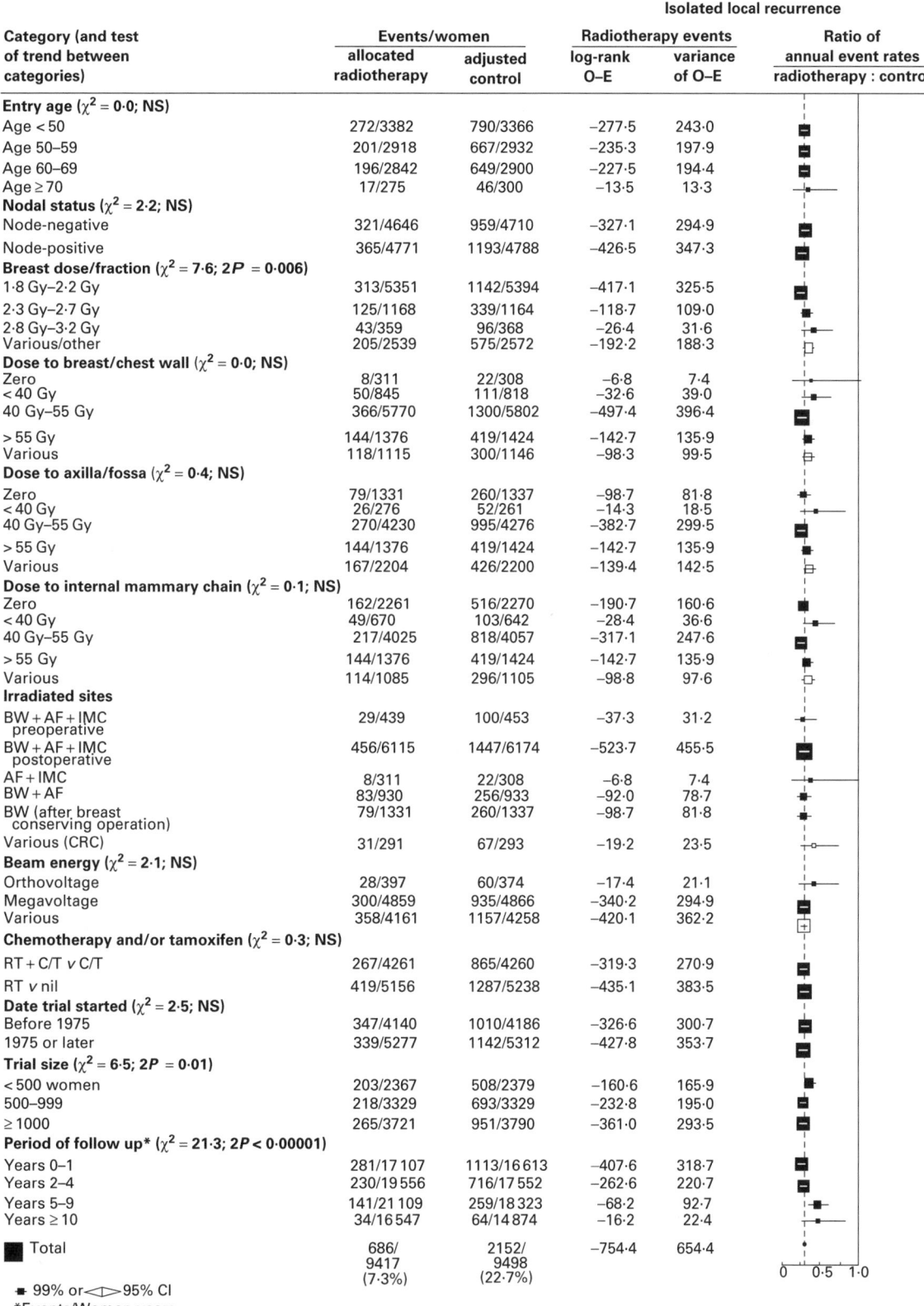

**Isolated local recurrence**

| Category (and test of trend between categories) | Events/women allocated radiotherapy | Events/women adjusted control | Radiotherapy events log-rank O–E | variance of O–E | Ratio of annual event rates radiotherapy : control |
|---|---|---|---|---|---|
| **Entry age ($\chi^2 = 0.0$; NS)** | | | | | |
| Age < 50 | 272/3382 | 790/3366 | −277·5 | 243·0 | |
| Age 50–59 | 201/2918 | 667/2932 | −235·3 | 197·9 | |
| Age 60–69 | 196/2842 | 649/2900 | −227·5 | 194·4 | |
| Age ≥ 70 | 17/275 | 46/300 | −13·5 | 13·3 | |
| **Nodal status ($\chi^2 = 2.2$; NS)** | | | | | |
| Node-negative | 321/4646 | 959/4710 | −327·1 | 294·9 | |
| Node-positive | 365/4771 | 1193/4788 | −426·5 | 347·3 | |
| **Breast dose/fraction ($\chi^2 = 7.6$; $2P = 0.006$)** | | | | | |
| 1·8 Gy–2·2 Gy | 313/5351 | 1142/5394 | −417·1 | 325·5 | |
| 2·3 Gy–2·7 Gy | 125/1168 | 339/1164 | −118·7 | 109·0 | |
| 2·8 Gy–3·2 Gy | 43/359 | 96/368 | −26·4 | 31·6 | |
| Various/other | 205/2539 | 575/2572 | −192·2 | 188·3 | |
| **Dose to breast/chest wall ($\chi^2 = 0.0$; NS)** | | | | | |
| Zero | 8/311 | 22/308 | −6·8 | 7·4 | |
| < 40 Gy | 50/845 | 111/818 | −32·6 | 39·0 | |
| 40 Gy–55 Gy | 366/5770 | 1300/5802 | −497·4 | 396·4 | |
| > 55 Gy | 144/1376 | 419/1424 | −142·7 | 135·9 | |
| Various | 118/1115 | 300/1146 | −98·3 | 99·5 | |
| **Dose to axilla/fossa ($\chi^2 = 0.4$; NS)** | | | | | |
| Zero | 79/1331 | 260/1337 | −98·7 | 81·8 | |
| < 40 Gy | 26/276 | 52/261 | −14·3 | 18·5 | |
| 40 Gy–55 Gy | 270/4230 | 995/4276 | −382·7 | 299·5 | |
| > 55 Gy | 144/1376 | 419/1424 | −142·7 | 135·9 | |
| Various | 167/2204 | 426/2200 | −139·4 | 142·5 | |
| **Dose to internal mammary chain ($\chi^2 = 0.1$; NS)** | | | | | |
| Zero | 162/2261 | 516/2270 | −190·7 | 160·6 | |
| < 40 Gy | 49/670 | 103/642 | −28·4 | 36·6 | |
| 40 Gy–55 Gy | 217/4025 | 818/4057 | −317·1 | 247·6 | |
| > 55 Gy | 144/1376 | 419/1424 | −142·7 | 135·9 | |
| Various | 114/1085 | 296/1105 | −98·8 | 97·6 | |
| **Irradiated sites** | | | | | |
| BW + AF + IMC preoperative | 29/439 | 100/453 | −37·3 | 31·2 | |
| BW + AF + IMC postoperative | 456/6115 | 1447/6174 | −523·7 | 455·5 | |
| AF + IMC | 8/311 | 22/308 | −6·8 | 7·4 | |
| BW + AF | 83/930 | 256/933 | −92·0 | 78·7 | |
| BW (after breast conserving operation) | 79/1331 | 260/1337 | −98·7 | 81·8 | |
| Various (CRC) | 31/291 | 67/293 | −19·2 | 23·5 | |
| **Beam energy ($\chi^2 = 2.1$; NS)** | | | | | |
| Orthovoltage | 28/397 | 60/374 | −17·4 | 21·1 | |
| Megavoltage | 300/4859 | 935/4866 | −340·2 | 294·9 | |
| Various | 358/4161 | 1157/4258 | −420·1 | 362·2 | |
| **Chemotherapy and/or tamoxifen ($\chi^2 = 0.3$; NS)** | | | | | |
| RT + C/T v C/T | 267/4261 | 865/4260 | −319·3 | 270·9 | |
| RT v nil | 419/5156 | 1287/5238 | −435·1 | 383·5 | |
| **Date trial started ($\chi^2 = 2.5$; NS)** | | | | | |
| Before 1975 | 347/4140 | 1010/4186 | −326·6 | 300·7 | |
| 1975 or later | 339/5277 | 1142/5312 | −427·8 | 353·7 | |
| **Trial size ($\chi^2 = 6.5$; $2P = 0.01$)** | | | | | |
| < 500 women | 203/2367 | 508/2379 | −160·6 | 165·9 | |
| 500–999 | 218/3329 | 693/3329 | −232·8 | 195·0 | |
| ≥ 1000 | 265/3721 | 951/3790 | −361·0 | 293·5 | |
| **Period of follow up\* ($\chi^2 = 21.3$; $2P < 0.00001$)** | | | | | |
| Years 0–1 | 281/17 107 | 1113/16 613 | −407·6 | 318·7 | |
| Years 2–4 | 230/19 556 | 716/17 552 | −262·6 | 220·7 | |
| Years 5–9 | 141/21 109 | 259/18 323 | −68·2 | 92·7 | |
| Years ≥ 10 | 34/16 547 | 64/14 874 | −16·2 | 22·4 | |
| ■ Total | 686/9417 (7·3%) | 2152/9498 (22·7%) | −754·4 | 654·4 | |

■ 99% or ◁▷95% CI
\*Events/Women-years

0   0·5   1·0

**Figure 40.13** Proportional effects of radiotherapy on isolated local recurrence, according to characteristics of the patients and type of treatment[16]

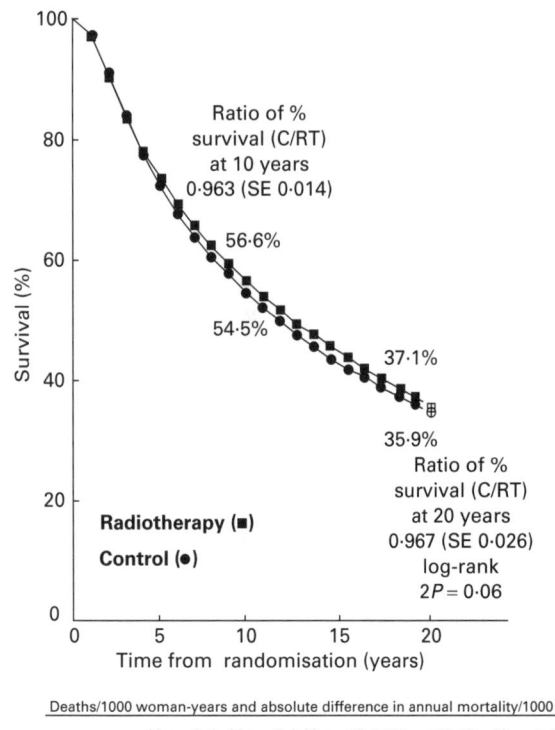

**Figure 40.14** Absolute effects of radiotherapy on 20-year survival in 20 000 breast cancer patients in 40 trials[16]

Deaths/1000 woman-years and absolute difference in annual mortality/1000

| | Years 0–4 | Years 5–9 | Years 10–14 | Years 15–19 | Years ≥ 20 |
|---|---|---|---|---|---|
| Radiotherapy | 2612/42·7 | 1363/26·1 | 584/13·5 | 314/7·4 | 130/2·6 |
| Control | 2599/40·8 | 1371/23·9 | 547/12·1 | 238/6·4 | 80/2·4 |
| Difference | 2·4 (SE 1·7) | 5·2 (SE 2·1) | 2·1 (SE 2·6) | –5·3 (SE 3·4) | –16·4 (SE 5·7) |

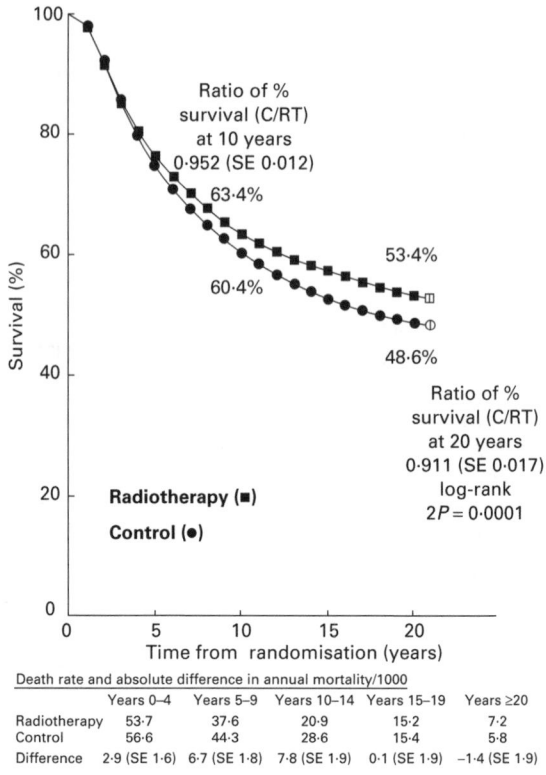

**Figure 40.15** Absolute effects of radiotherapy on cause-specific survival – breast cancer deaths only[16]

Death rate and absolute difference in annual mortality/1000

| | Years 0–4 | Years 5–9 | Years 10–14 | Years 15–19 | Years ≥20 |
|---|---|---|---|---|---|
| Radiotherapy | 53·7 | 37·6 | 20·9 | 15·2 | 7·2 |
| Control | 56·6 | 44·3 | 28·6 | 15·4 | 5·8 |
| Difference | 2·9 (SE 1·6) | 6·7 (SE 1·8) | 7·8 (SE 1·9) | 0·1 (SE 1·9) | –1·4 (SE 1·9) |

follow up (Figure 40.16). The excess mortality occurs rather late and most of it appears after 10 years of follow up, leading to a 4·3% increase in the proportional types of other causes after 20 years of follow up. Most of the effect appears to be associated with vascular disease (Table 40.5), as might be expected if radiation injured cardiac tissue and the great vessels. This effect is likely to be highly technique-dependent and presumably avoidable with appropriate techniques. The effects may not be so great for the more recent trials, where more care has been taken to avoid exposure to the relevant tissues, but follow up is necessarily shorter, so firm conclusions cannot be drawn at this stage.

## What non-fatal effects can result from radiotherapy?

Tiredness, local inflammation and breast oedema are common after radiotherapy but usually resolve rapidly.[63] Breast and chest wall pain is also increased, but this difference only persists for 6–18 months.[68] Axillary radiation can lead to arm and shoulder symptoms, but is much reduced by modern techniques using tangential

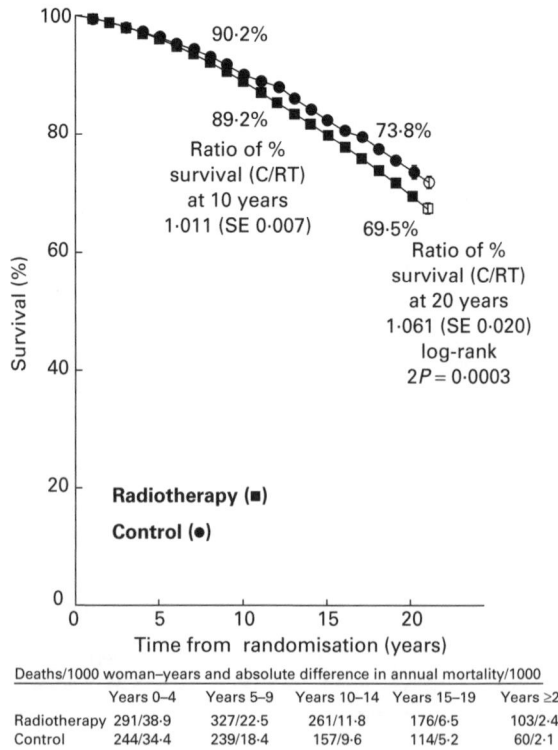

Deaths/1000 woman–years and absolute difference in annual mortality/1000

| | Years 0–4 | Years 5–9 | Years 10–14 | Years 15–19 | Years ≥20 |
|---|---|---|---|---|---|
| Radiotherapy | 291/38·9 | 327/22·5 | 261/11·8 | 176/6·5 | 103/2·4 |
| Control | 244/34·4 | 239/18·4 | 157/9·6 | 114/5·2 | 60/2·1 |
| Difference | –0·4 (SE 0·6) | –1·6 (SE 1·2) | –5·7 (SE 1·9) | –5·2 (SE 2·9) | –14·4 (SE 5·5) |

**Figure 40.16** Absolute effects of radiotherapy on cause-specific survival – non-breast cancer deaths[16]

**Table 40.5  Effects of radiotherapy (RT) allocation on particular causes of death for women dying without any breast cancer recurrence**

| Underlying cause of death without breast cancer recurrence | Number of deaths | | Log-rank analyses (RT events) | | | Ratio of annual death rates (SE) |
|---|---|---|---|---|---|---|
| | Allocated RT | Adjusted control | O−E | Variance of O−E | Log-rank 2P | |
| *Vascular* | 437 | 322 | 43·9 | 169·0 | 0·0007 | 1·30 (0·09) |
| *Non-vascular* | | | | | | |
| Total | 382 | 313 | 21·6 | 156·7 | 0·08 | 1·15 (0·09) |
| Respiratory | 81 | 64 | 5·0 | 34·0 | 0·4 | :: |
| Acute myeloid leukaemia | 5 | 7 | −0·8 | 2·7 | 0·6 | :: |
| Other leukaemia/lymphoma | 32 | 18 | 5·6 | 11·8 | 0·1 | :: |
| Lung cancer | 37 | 22 | 5·2 | 13·5 | 0·2 | :: |
| Other neoplastic* | 139 | 116 | 8·0 | 57·4 | 0·3 | :: |
| Other non-vascular | 88 | 86 | −1·4 | 38·4 | 0·8 | :: |
| *Unknown* | | | | | | |
| Total | 339 | 292 | 12·1 | 141·9 | 0·3 | 1·09 (0·09) |
| Completely unknown† | 162 | 140 | 6·2 | 72·0 | 0·5 | :: |
| Unknown, specified as not breast cancer | 177 | 152 | 5·9 | 69·9 | 0·5 | :: |
| **Total** | 1158 | 927 | 77·6 | 462·7 | 0·0003 | 1·18 (0·05) |
| Follow up duration (1000 woman-years before recurrence) | 82·1 | 74·8 | :: | :: | :: | :: |

Heterogeneity between proportional increases in vascular and in non-vascular mortality: $\chi^2_1 = 1\cdot2$, $2P > 0\cdot1$.

*Includes 17 RT $v$ 14 control from unspecified neoplastic causes.

†Of these, 64 RT $v$ 62 control were in the trials that did not seek causes, and 97 $v$ 105 (log-rank O−E = −5·7 with variance 49·1) were in years 0–9.

fields.[70] Breast and chest wall sarcomas are a very rare outcome of radiotherapy,[63] and leukaemia and cardiac events have also been reported, but usually in conjunction with chemotherapy.[71]

As a general principle, adjuvant radiotherapy is most indicated when the risk of local recurrence is higher. This will depend on the characteristics of the tumour (especially number of positive nodes and tumour size), and the extent of surgical treatment. A threshold for treatment of a predicted 20% chance of locoregional recurrence has been suggested by some groups.[72]

## What is the role of radiotherapy following mastectomy?

Most studies of post-mastectomy radiotherapy have employed chest wall irradiation, axillary irradiation, and often irradiation of the supraclavicular and/or internal mammary fields. Axillary irradiation is most associated with short-term side effects, but the other fields may contribute to an increased rate of vascular events. There is little evidence for deciding which fields to irradiate, but locoregional recurrence rates are high when four or more axillary nodes are involved or the primary tumour exceeds 5 cm in diameter, and most centres recommend radiation in this case. For smaller, node-negative tumours, there is a general consensus that radiation is unnecessary, but uncertainty remains about the usefulness of radiotherapy for smaller tumours with one to three positive nodes. This is currently under further investigation in clinical trials and will depend critically on the ability to limit excess non-breast cancer mortality.

## What is the role of radiotherapy after complete local excision for breast preservation?

Several trials have documented high local recurrence rates after complete local excision (CLE) without radiotherapy, and the benefits of such treatment in terms of local control and breast cancer deaths have been well documented in the overview. However, the follow up of these trials is shorter and little information exists about late non-breast cancer deaths after 15 years of follow up. Thus, there is still some uncertainty about the risk–benefit ratio, especially for very good prognosis tumours (for example ≤ 1 cm, N0, grade 1) which are increasingly being detected by mammography.

## What is the role of radiotherapy after excision of DCIS?

Three trials have reported on the use of radiotherapy after CLE for DCIS (Table 40.6)[16]. All found a substantial effect on local recurrence rates, but no effect on breast cancer

mortality. A debate is currently ongoing concerning the need for radiotherapy in completely excised unifocal tumours. The extent of tumour margins and tumour grade appear to be key factors in determining recurrence.[73]

## What is the role of ovarian ablation in early breast cancer?

Surgical ovarian ablation was first described as a systemic therapy for advanced breast cancer in 1896.[74] Other methods of ablation include irradiation, drug-induced suppression and chemotherapy.

For women aged under 50, an overview was completed by the Early Breast Cancer Trialists' Collaborative Group (EBCTCG) of the 12 available prospective randomised clinical trials, which compared ovarian ablation (surgery or irradiation) against no ablation, which began prior to 1980 and have long follow up.[13] Fifteen-year survival was significantly improved among those allocated ovarian ablation (52·4% v 46·1%, with 6·3 fewer deaths per 100 women, log-rank $2P = 0.001$). Recurrence-free survival was also significantly improved (45·0% v 39·0%, $2P < 0.0007$). Menopausal status was defined incompletely (hence, the analysis was confined to women under 50). Oestrogen receptor measurements were available only from trials where ablation was added to cytotoxic chemotherapy and women with women with overall numbers and events were too small for subgroup analyses (2102 women, 1130 deaths and 153 additional recurrences). Both, women with node-negative and women with node-positive disease had improved survival (6 per 100 and 12 per 100 respectively) in trials not involving chemotherapy.

Benefits were smaller and not significant in the trials where all women also received chemotherapy, and were confined to women with "ER-positive" primary tumours (odds reduction: 13% for recurrence-free survival, 17% overall survival). For those women aged 50 or over, a non-significant benefit was seen in survival and recurrent-free survival (Figures 40.17 and 40.18).[13]

The substantial benefit seen from ovarian ablation for both survival and recurrence-free survival would probably be greater for women with known hormone-sensitive tumours, as was seen for the trials involving chemotherapy. There was no significant difference between treatment groups for vascular deaths, other non-breast cancer deaths, or in all non-breast cancer deaths. **Evidence level Ia**

## What were the other effects of ovarian ablation?

The EBCTCG overview (1996)[13] did not include data from the four available trials that assessed ovarian

**Table 40.6  Summary outcomes in DCIS radiotherapy trials**

| Trial | Any event | Ipsilateral events | Ipsilateral invasive | Contralateral events | Distant recurrence | Breast cancer deaths |
|---|---|---|---|---|---|---|
| NSABP B-17 Fisher et al. 1998 | 35% v 25% 43% reduction P = 0·00003 | 26·8% v 12·1% 59% reduction P ≤ 0·00001 | 13·4% v 3·9% 71% reduction P = 0·00001 | 19 v 20 | 6 v 8 (XRT) | 4 v 9 (XRT) |
| EORTC 10853 Julien et al. 2000 | 18% v 14% 18% reduction P = 0·2 | 16% v 9% 38% reduction P = 0·005 | 8% v 4% 40% reduction P = 0·04 | 8 v 21 2·5-fold increase | 12 v 12 | 12 v 12 |
| UK/ANZ | 16·1% v 7·3% 57% reduction P < 0·0001 | 13·6% v 5·6% 62% reduction P < 0·0001 | 5·9% v 2·9% 55% reduction P = 0·01 | 9 v 11 | n/a | n/a |

Fisher B, Dignam J, Wolmark N et al. Lumpectomy and radiation therapy for the treatment of intraductal breast cancer: findings from National Surgical Adjuvant Breast and Bowel Project B-17. J Clin Oncol 1998;**16**:441–52.

Julien J-P, Bijker N, Fentiman IS et al. Radiotherapy in breast-conserving treatment for ductal carcinoma in situ: first results of the EORTC randomised phase III trial 10853. Lancet 2000;**355**:528–33.

UKCCCR DCIS Working Party. The UK, Australian and New Zealand randomised trial comparing radiotherapy and tamoxifen in women with completely excised ductal carcinoma in situ of the breast. (Submitted for publication).

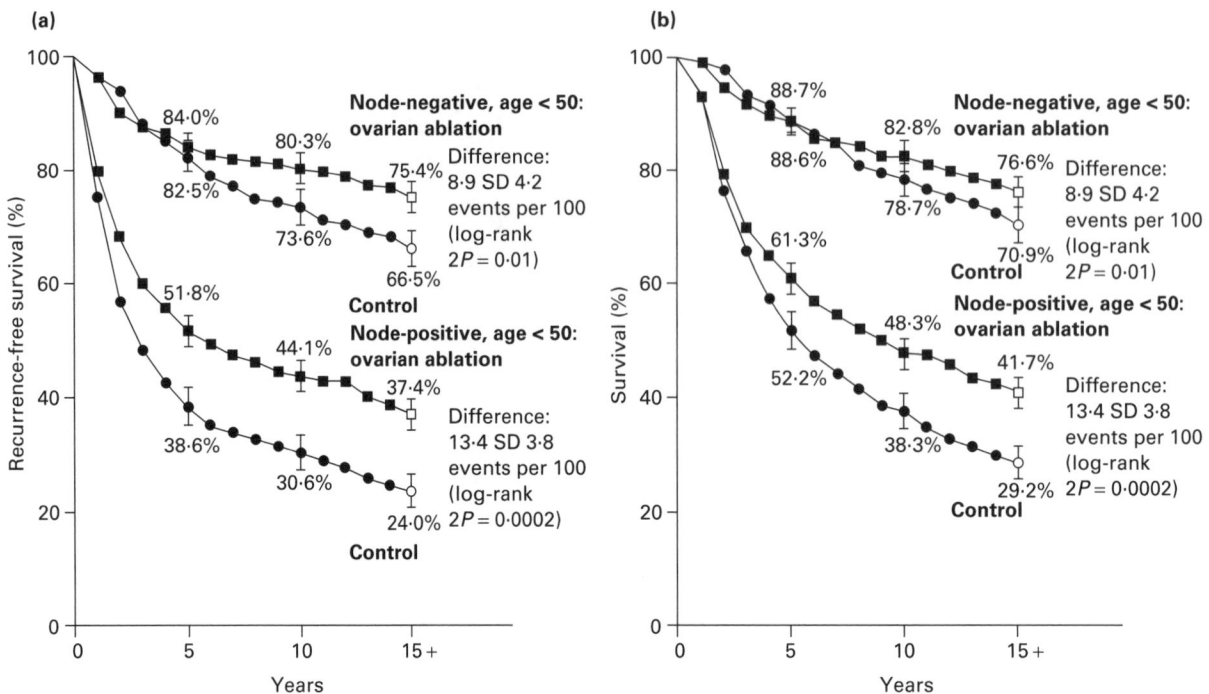

**Figure 40.17**  Absolute effects of ovarian ablation in absence of routine chemotherapy in all trials combined among women aged under 50 at entry. (a) Recurrence-free survival and (b) overall survival[13]

suppression by drugs, as these commenced after 1985, although these were considered in the EBCTCG 2000 overview (unpublished). Several direct comparisons in randomised clinical trials involving drug suppression of the ovaries have been reported, and document the efficacy of this approach, but there have been no direct comparisons of different types of ovarian suppression in early breast cancer. The overview was also unable to provide data on the efficacy of ovarian suppression versus chemotherapy, or versus ovarian suppression plus tamoxifen.

### Is ovarian suppression a comparable treatment to chemotherapy in early breast cancer?

The largest trial (1640 premenopausal women), the Zoladex Early Breast Cancer Research Association (ZEBRA) trial, compared the luteinising hormone-releasing hormone (LHRH), goserelin (monthly subcutaneous injections for 2 years) with oral cyclophosphamide, methotrexate and fluorouracil (CMF) (six cycles). All women had lymph node-positive tumours. With a median follow up of 6 years, women who had ER-positive tumours (80%) had equivalent disease-free survival (DFS) and overall survival (OS) for goserelin treatment. In contrast, for women with ER-negative tumours, CMF produced a significantly better DFS and OS.[75,76]

Both treatments produced amenorrhoea, but close to two-thirds of women on goserelin regained menses on drug

cessation, whereas 80% of women having CMF remained amenorrhoeic at three years. Both treatments caused reduction in bone density, which improved after goserelin was stopped, but persisted longer after CMF. Quality of life was superior at 6 months for women on goserelin (largely because of fewer chemotherapy-induced symptoms, such as nausea and vomiting), and at 3 years women on goserelin had fewer menopause related symptoms.[75,76]

A smaller trial (332 premenopausal women with node-positive breast cancer) failed to find any difference in event-free or overall survival with a maximum follow up of 12 years. A retrospective analysis of 270 women with available data from ER analyses found that the women with more detectable ER (at least 20 fml mg$^{-1}$ protein) had a better outcome after ovarian ablation and those with lower detectable ER concentrations did better on CMF. The "CMF" used was an intravenous regimen (six to eight cycles, with or without prednisone).[77]

### Does tamoxifen improve outcome if added to ovarian ablation?

Five trials have directly compared ovarian ablation, with or without tamoxifen, against chemotherapy.[29,30,78–85] Collectively they suggest that, in premenopausal patients with node-positive ER-positive tumours, the combined endocrine therapy is equivalent to chemotherapy.

(a)

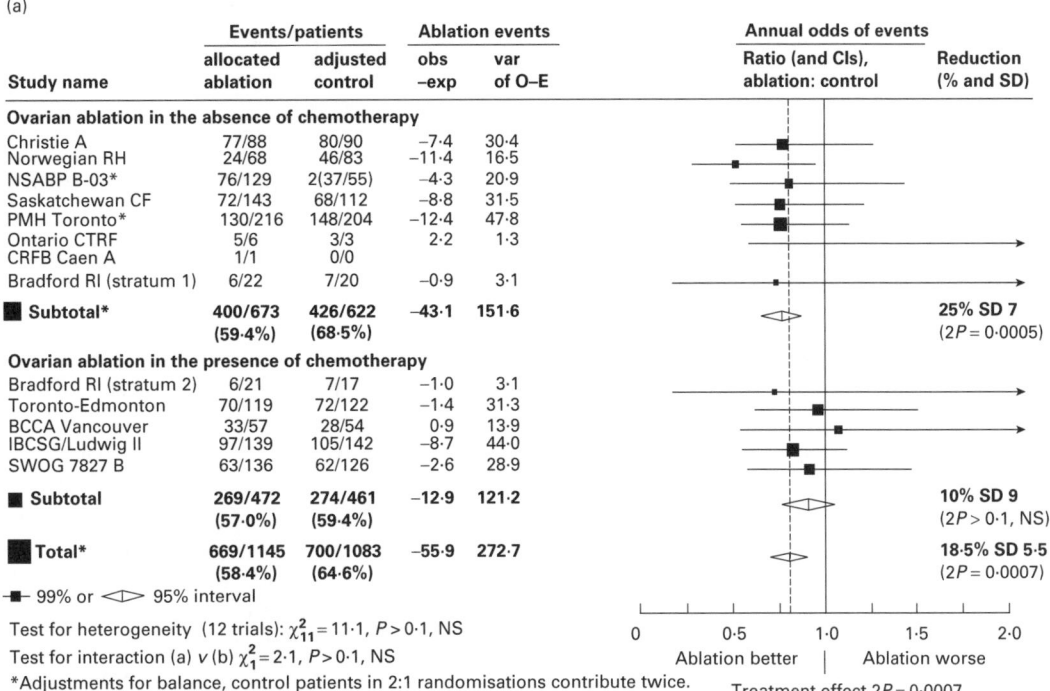

(b)

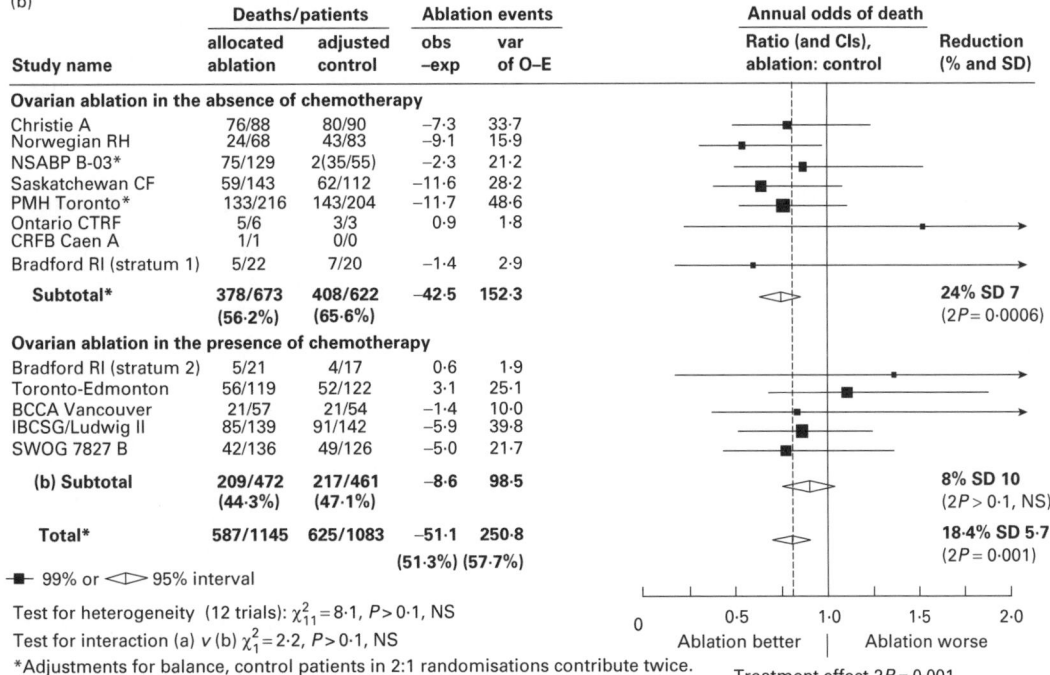

**Figure 40.18** Proportional effects of ovarian ablation in each trial and overall, with subdivisions by absence or presence of chemotherapy, among women aged under 50 years at entry[13] (a) Recurrence-free and (b) overall survival. Each trial, or part of trial, is described by a single line showing numbers of events and patients and summary log-rank statistics. For each subdivision, the ratio of the annual event rate in the ovarian ablation group to that in the control group (odds ratio) is plotted as ■ with 99% CI. For subtotals and total, 95% CIs are represented by ◇. Solid vertical line, odds ratio of 1·0 (that is, no difference between ovarian ablation and control), whereas broken vertical line, "typical odds ratio" in total of all these trials. For balance, control patients in 2:1 randomisations (NSABP and part of PMH) are counted twice in adjusted control totals, but not in statistical calculations. Var, variance; NS, not significant

Chemotherapy regimens have included CMF with either oral or intravenous cyclophosphamide. Two additional trials in women with ER-positive tumours, involving anthracycline-containing chemotherapy, did not find any significant differences between endocrine therapies and chemotherapy. An overview of these trials is needed.

## Is the combination of chemotherapy and ovarian ablation more efficient than single modality therapy?

Direct comparisons involving combination therapy have been reported.

An Intergroup trial (INT 0101), involving 1503 premenopausal women with lymph node-positive, receptor-positive breast cancer, found a significant 5-year DFS advantage for the addition of tamoxifen to the combined therapy of goserelin and chemotherapy (CAF: six cycles of cyclophosphamide, adriamycin and fluorouracil) (77% *v* 70%), but no difference in overall survival. There was no significant advantage found for the addition of goserelin to FAC (DFS or OS).[83]

A randomised clinical trial "ZIPP" (2648 premenopausal women, early breast cancer, any steroid receptor type) tested the addition of goserelin to other adjuvant therapies given based on clinical judgement. These included chemotherapy (43% of patients) and tamoxifen in the majority of patients. Only 56% of patients were known to have ER-positive breast cancer. Overall, patients receiving goserelin had 20% fewer first events with median follow up of 4·2 years (*P* < 0·001). An improvement seen in survival was not significant.[30,84]

A single randomised clinical trial in node-negative breast cancer compared goserelin with CMF and with the combination of CMF and goserelin. There was no advantage for chemotherapy over goserelin alone in patients with ER-positive tumours.[86]

Thus, there is clear evidence that ovarian ablation with goserelin, with or without tamoxifen, has comparable efficacy to chemotherapy in women with hormone-sensitive early breast cancer. There is no clear evidence that the combination of ovarian suppression and chemotherapy is superior to ovarian suppression alone in this population. For women with oestrogen receptor-poor tumour, there is clear evidence that chemotherapy (CMF) is superior to ovarian ablation. **Grade A**

## Adjuvant tamoxifen for early breast cancer

Tamoxifen was one of the earliest systemic treatments used for treating breast cancer and it quickly became widely used because of its efficacy, and general tolerability. It has been shown to be beneficial for treating advanced and early invasive breast cancer, DCIS and for prevention of breast cancer in high risk women. The major source of evidence concerning its use comes from the EBCTCG overviews.[9–11,14]

## What benefit is obtained from tamoxifen for early breast cancer?

About 5 years of adjuvant tamoxifen 20 mg per day substantially improves the 10-year survival and disease-free survival of women with ER-positive tumours or with tumours of unknown ER status. These effects are largely unaffected by other patient characteristics. The EBCTCG overview[14] reported on 55 trials involving 37 000 women, comparing tamoxifen with no tamoxifen. Tamoxifen treatment for about 5 years produced a 26% proportional mortality reduction (SD 4); and a 47% proportional recurrence reduction, during about 10 years follow up, in those women (about 30 000) with known ER-positive tumours, or with untested tumours (estimated two-thirds ER-positive). The proportional mortality reductions were similar for women with node-positive and node-negative disease, thus producing a greater absolute effect on survival in node-positive disease: absolute 10-year survival improvement 10·9% (SD 2·5), (61·4% *v* 50·5%, 2*P* < 0·00001); node-negative disease: absolute 10-year survival improvement 5·6% (SD 1·3), (78·9% *v* 73·3%, 2*P* < 0·00001) (Figures 40.19 and 40.20).[14]

## Which patients benefited from tamoxifen?

Benefit was confined to patients with ER-positive tumours or those women where ER was untested. The benefit was largely independent of age, menopausal status, or daily tamoxifen dose (mostly 20 mg per day) or whether chemotherapy was also given to all patients. Trials in which women who had ER-positive or unknown ER status of tumours were randomised to chemotherapy or the same chemotherapy plus tamoxifen for about 5 years, showed a substantial advantage for the tamoxifen arm: 52% (SD 8) proportional reduction in recurrence and 47% (SD 9) reduction in mortality.[14]

## How long should tamoxifen be given for?

Tamoxifen should be given for 5 years. The EBCTCG overview provides compelling data that 5 years is superior to shorter durations (Figure 40.20).

A review of three trials testing duration of more than 5 years provides inconclusive data.[87–92] These three trials involved different patient populations. For example, the percentage of patients in these trials with ER-positive tumours was NSABP-B14 (100%); ECOG E4181/E5181 (73%), and Scottish (39–78%).[87,89,90] The tamoxifen

(a)

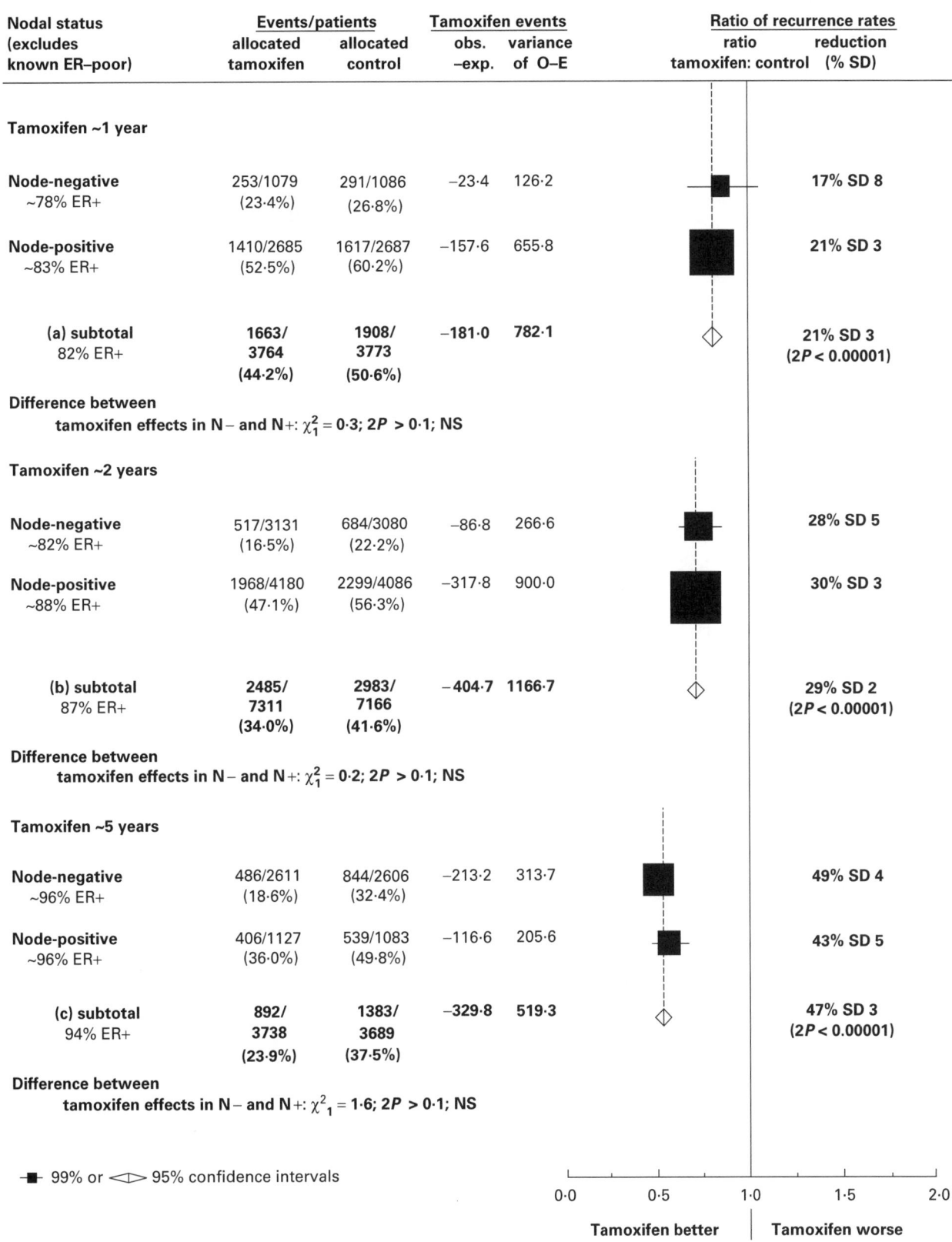

| Nodal status (excludes known ER–poor) | Events/patients | | Tamoxifen events | | Ratio of recurrence rates | |
|---|---|---|---|---|---|---|
| | allocated tamoxifen | allocated control | obs. –exp. | variance of O–E | ratio tamoxifen: control | reduction (% SD) |
| **Tamoxifen ~1 year** | | | | | | |
| Node-negative ~78% ER+ | 253/1079 (23·4%) | 291/1086 (26·8%) | –23·4 | 126·2 | | 17% SD 8 |
| Node-positive ~83% ER+ | 1410/2685 (52·5%) | 1617/2687 (60·2%) | –157·6 | 655·8 | | 21% SD 3 |
| (a) subtotal 82% ER+ | 1663/ 3764 (44·2%) | 1908/ 3773 (50·6%) | –181·0 | 782·1 | | 21% SD 3 (2P < 0.00001) |

Difference between
tamoxifen effects in N– and N+: $\chi^2_1 = 0\cdot3$; $2P > 0\cdot1$; NS

| | | | | | | |
|---|---|---|---|---|---|---|
| **Tamoxifen ~2 years** | | | | | | |
| Node-negative ~82% ER+ | 517/3131 (16·5%) | 684/3080 (22·2%) | –86·8 | 266·6 | | 28% SD 5 |
| Node-positive ~88% ER+ | 1968/4180 (47·1%) | 2299/4086 (56·3%) | –317·8 | 900·0 | | 30% SD 3 |
| (b) subtotal 87% ER+ | 2485/ 7311 (34·0%) | 2983/ 7166 (41·6%) | –404·7 | 1166·7 | | 29% SD 2 (2P < 0.00001) |

Difference between
tamoxifen effects in N– and N+: $\chi^2_1 = 0\cdot2$; $2P > 0\cdot1$; NS

| | | | | | | |
|---|---|---|---|---|---|---|
| **Tamoxifen ~5 years** | | | | | | |
| Node-negative ~96% ER+ | 486/2611 (18·6%) | 844/2606 (32·4%) | –213·2 | 313·7 | | 49% SD 4 |
| Node-positive ~96% ER+ | 406/1127 (36·0%) | 539/1083 (49·8%) | –116·6 | 205·6 | | 43% SD 5 |
| (c) subtotal 94% ER+ | 892/ 3738 (23·9%) | 1383/ 3689 (37·5%) | –329·8 | 519·3 | | 47% SD 3 (2P < 0.00001) |

Difference between
tamoxifen effects in N– and N+: $\chi^2_1 = 1\cdot6$; $2P > 0\cdot1$; NS

■ 99% or ◁▷ 95% confidence intervals

0·0   0·5   1·0   1·5   2·0

Tamoxifen better | Tamoxifen worse

**Figure 40.19** (a) EBCTCG overview of randomised trials: recurrence as first event[14]

(b)

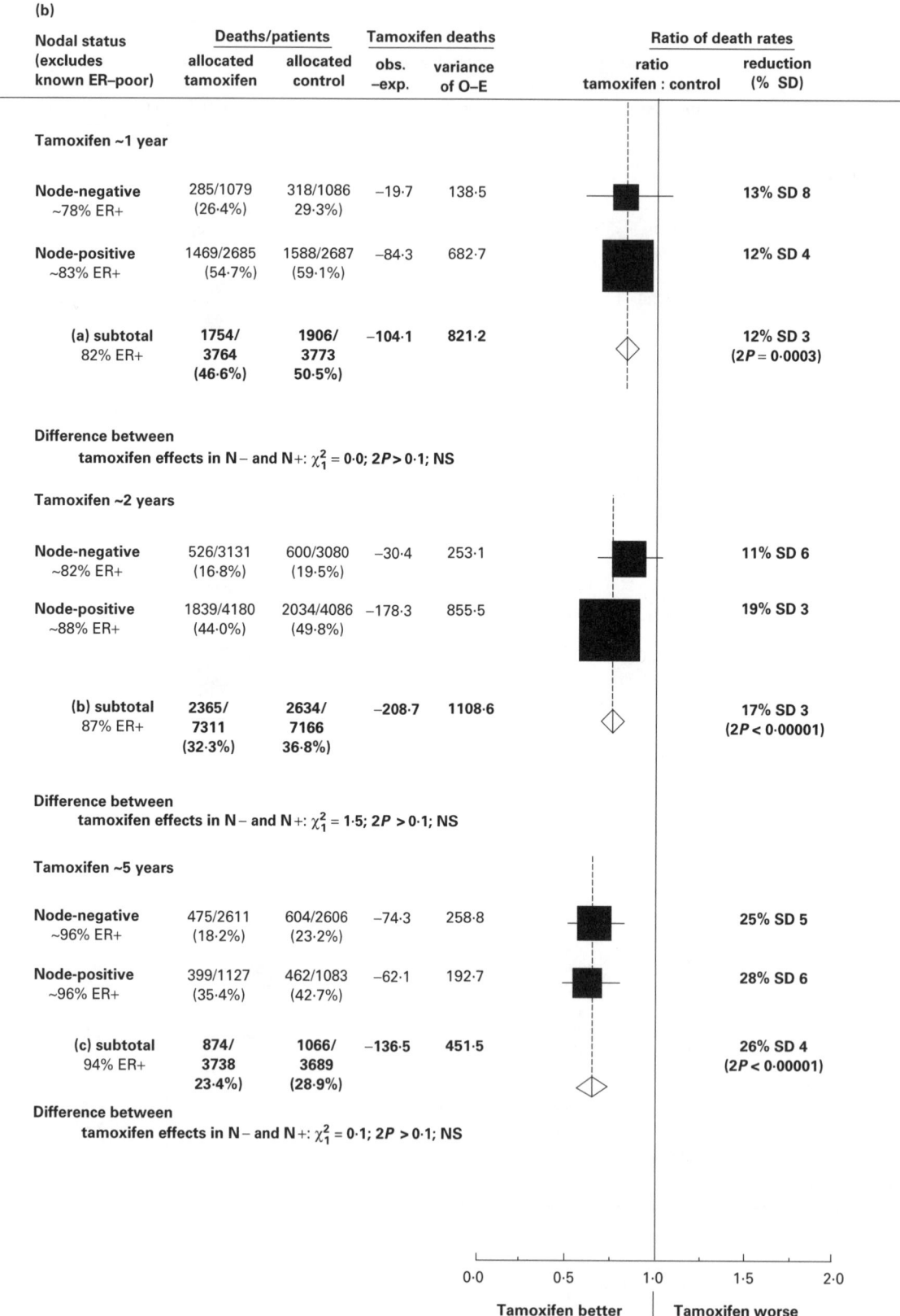

| Nodal status (excludes known ER–poor) | Deaths/patients | | Tamoxifen deaths | | Ratio of death rates | |
|---|---|---|---|---|---|---|
| | allocated tamoxifen | allocated control | obs. –exp. | variance of O–E | ratio tamoxifen : control | reduction (% SD) |
| **Tamoxifen ~1 year** | | | | | | |
| Node-negative ~78% ER+ | 285/1079 (26·4%) | 318/1086 29·3%) | –19·7 | 138·5 | | 13% SD 8 |
| Node-positive ~83% ER+ | 1469/2685 (54·7%) | 1588/2687 (59·1%) | –84·3 | 682·7 | | 12% SD 4 |
| **(a) subtotal** 82% ER+ | **1754/ 3764 (46·6%)** | **1906/ 3773 50·5%)** | –104·1 | 821·2 | | 12% SD 3 (2*P* = 0·0003) |

Difference between
   tamoxifen effects in N– and N+: $\chi_1^2 = 0.0$; 2*P* > 0·1; NS

| | | | | | | |
|---|---|---|---|---|---|---|
| **Tamoxifen ~2 years** | | | | | | |
| Node-negative ~82% ER+ | 526/3131 (16·8%) | 600/3080 (19·5%) | –30·4 | 253·1 | | 11% SD 6 |
| Node-positive ~88% ER+ | 1839/4180 (44·0%) | 2034/4086 (49·8%) | –178·3 | 855·5 | | 19% SD 3 |
| **(b) subtotal** 87% ER+ | **2365/ 7311 (32·3%)** | **2634/ 7166 36·8%)** | –208·7 | 1108·6 | | 17% SD 3 (2*P* < 0·00001) |

Difference between
   tamoxifen effects in N– and N+: $\chi_1^2 = 1.5$; 2*P* > 0·1; NS

| | | | | | | |
|---|---|---|---|---|---|---|
| **Tamoxifen ~5 years** | | | | | | |
| Node-negative ~96% ER+ | 475/2611 (18·2%) | 604/2606 (23·2%) | –74·3 | 258·8 | | 25% SD 5 |
| Node-positive ~96% ER+ | 399/1127 (35·4%) | 462/1083 (42·7%) | –62·1 | 192·7 | | 28% SD 6 |
| **(c) subtotal** 94% ER+ | **874/ 3738 23·4%)** | **1066/ 3689 (28·9%)** | –136·5 | 451·5 | | 26% SD 4 (2*P* < 0·00001) |

Difference between
   tamoxifen effects in N– and N+: $\chi_1^2 = 0.1$; 2*P* > 0·1; NS

**Figure 40.19** (b) EBCTCG overview of randomised trials: mortality (death from any cause)[14]

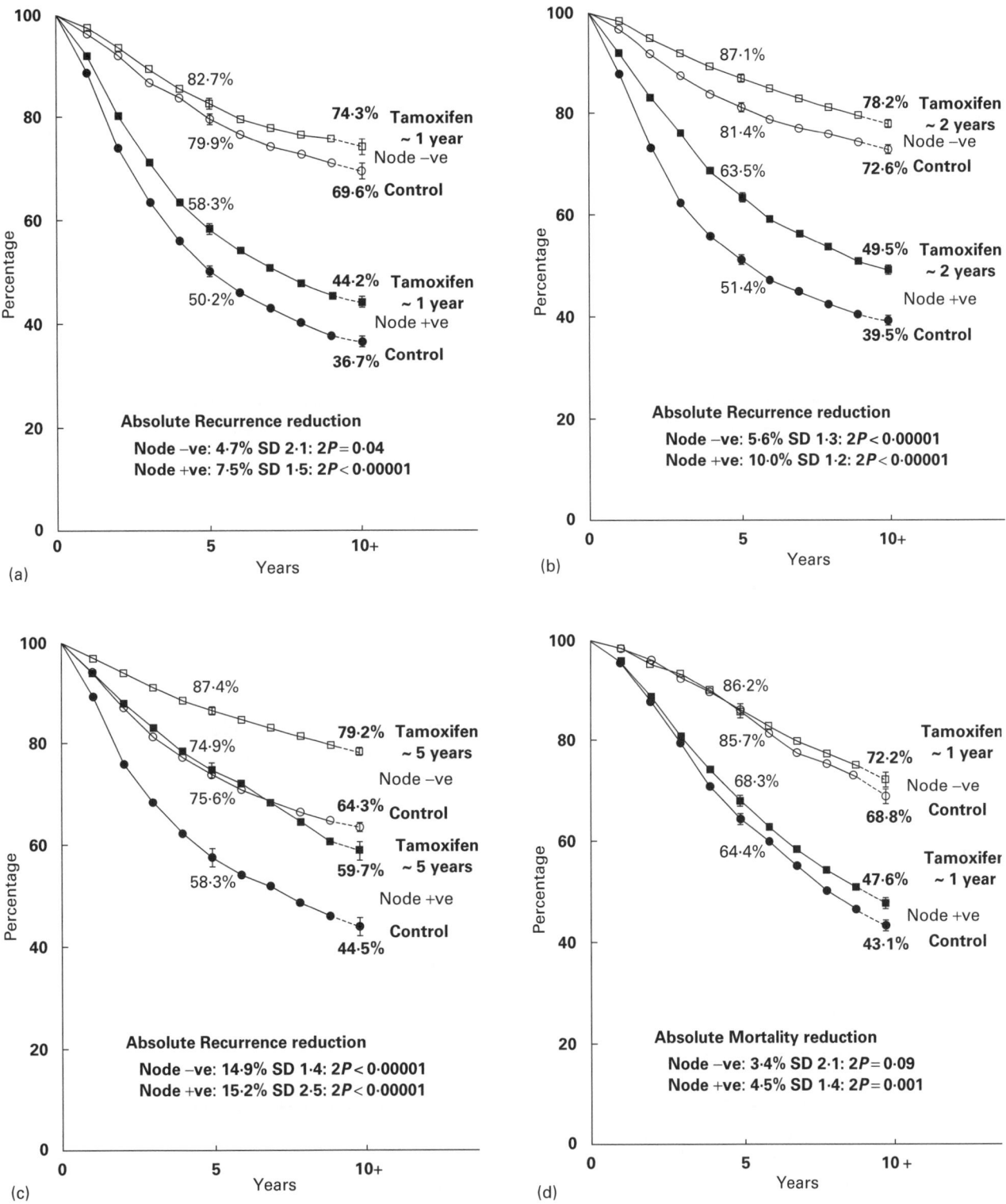

**Figure 40.20** (a–c) Absolute risk reduction during the first 10 years, subdivided by tamoxifen duration and by nodal status (after exclusion of women with ER-poor disease): recurrence as first event[14] *(Continued)*

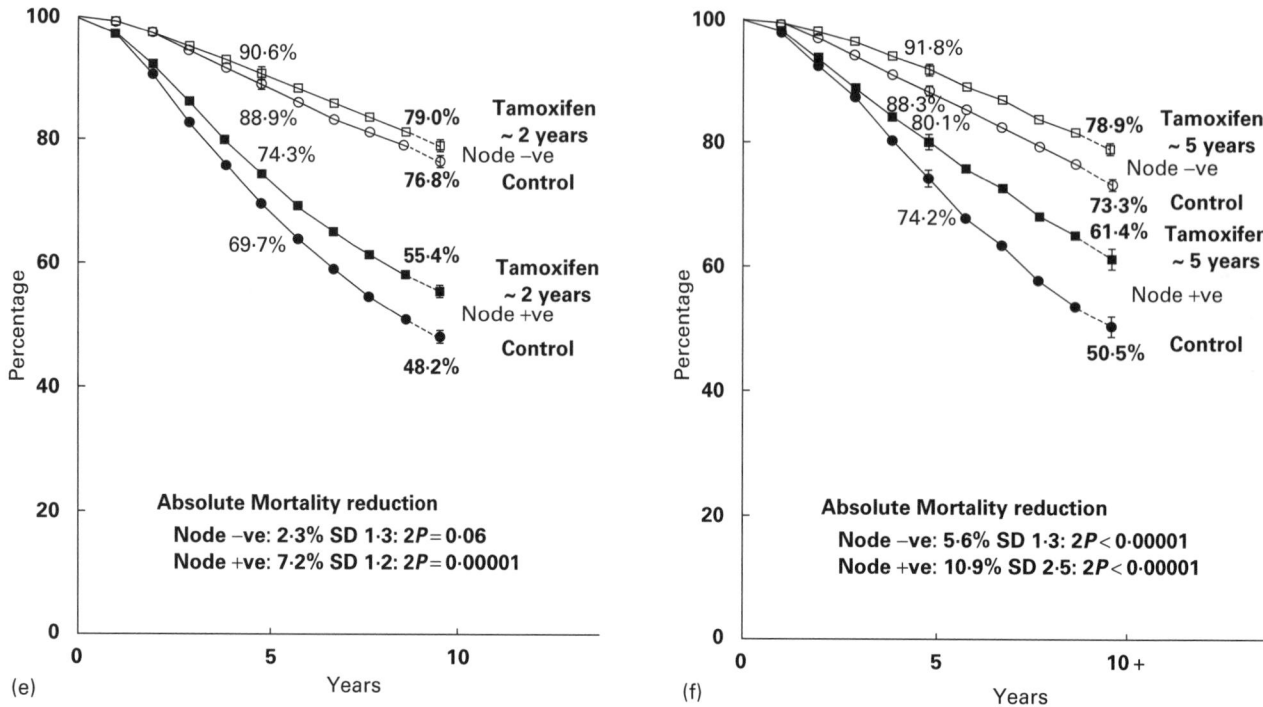

**Figure 40.20** (d–f) Absolute risk reduction during the first 10 years, subdivided by tamoxifen duration and by nodal status (after exclusion of women with ER-poor disease): mortality (death from any cause)[14]

carryover effect noted in the overview, whereby the benefit from tamoxifen continues substantially beyond 5 years of therapy, for example, may require much longer follow up for definite analyses. Two additional large trials, Adjuvant Tamoxifen Longer Against Shorter (ATLAS)[93] and Adjuvant Tamoxifen Treatment Offer More (aTTom)[94] are continuing accrual. Unpublished analysis of all five trials, for patients having at least 4 years of tamoxifen failed to show any statistically significant effect on breast cancer events or mortality, and suggested a (non-significant) benefit in the period after commencement of the longer therapy. Hence, the recommended duration should be 5 years.[92]

The proportional mortality reduction for trials of 1 year, 2 years and about 5 years of adjuvant tamoxifen during 10-year follow up were 12%, 17% and 26%, respectively, with a significant test for trend ($2P = 0.003$). The corresponding proportional recurrence reductions were 21%, 29% and 47%, respectively (test for trend, $2P = 0.003$) (Figure 40.20).[14]

A similar trend was seen for the proportional reductions in contralateral breast cancer with reductions of 13%, 26% and 47% for trials of 1, 2 and about 5 years of adjuvant tamoxifen, respectively.[14] As this analysis also included those women with "ER-poor" tumours, this effect might plausibly be greater for women with known ER-positive tumours. **Evidence level Ia**

## What were the serious side effects of tamoxifen for treatment?

Tamoxifen caused a significant increase in the risk of endometrial cancer: about two-fold for trials of 1- or 2-year tamoxifen, and about four-fold for 5 years of tamoxifen. There was no apparent effect on the incidence of colorectal cancer, or on the main categories of cause of death (excluding deaths from breast or endometrial cancer).

It has been estimated that for 1000 women with early breast cancer treatment with tamoxifen, about 78 breast cancer deaths will be avoided, and up to one death from thromboembolic disease and one death from uterine cancer might be attributable to tamoxifen.[24]

## Adjuvant systemic chemotherapy for early breast cancer

Two trials of adjuvant chemotherapy for early, node-positive breast cancer, one using the single agent L-PAM (phenylalanine mustard)[95] and the other a polychemotherapy regimen "CMF" (oral cyclophosphamide, and intravenous methotrexate and fluorouracil)[96] changed the treatment of early breast cancer. Each showed an early significant benefit from the chemotherapy in terms of disease-free survival (most evident in premenopausal

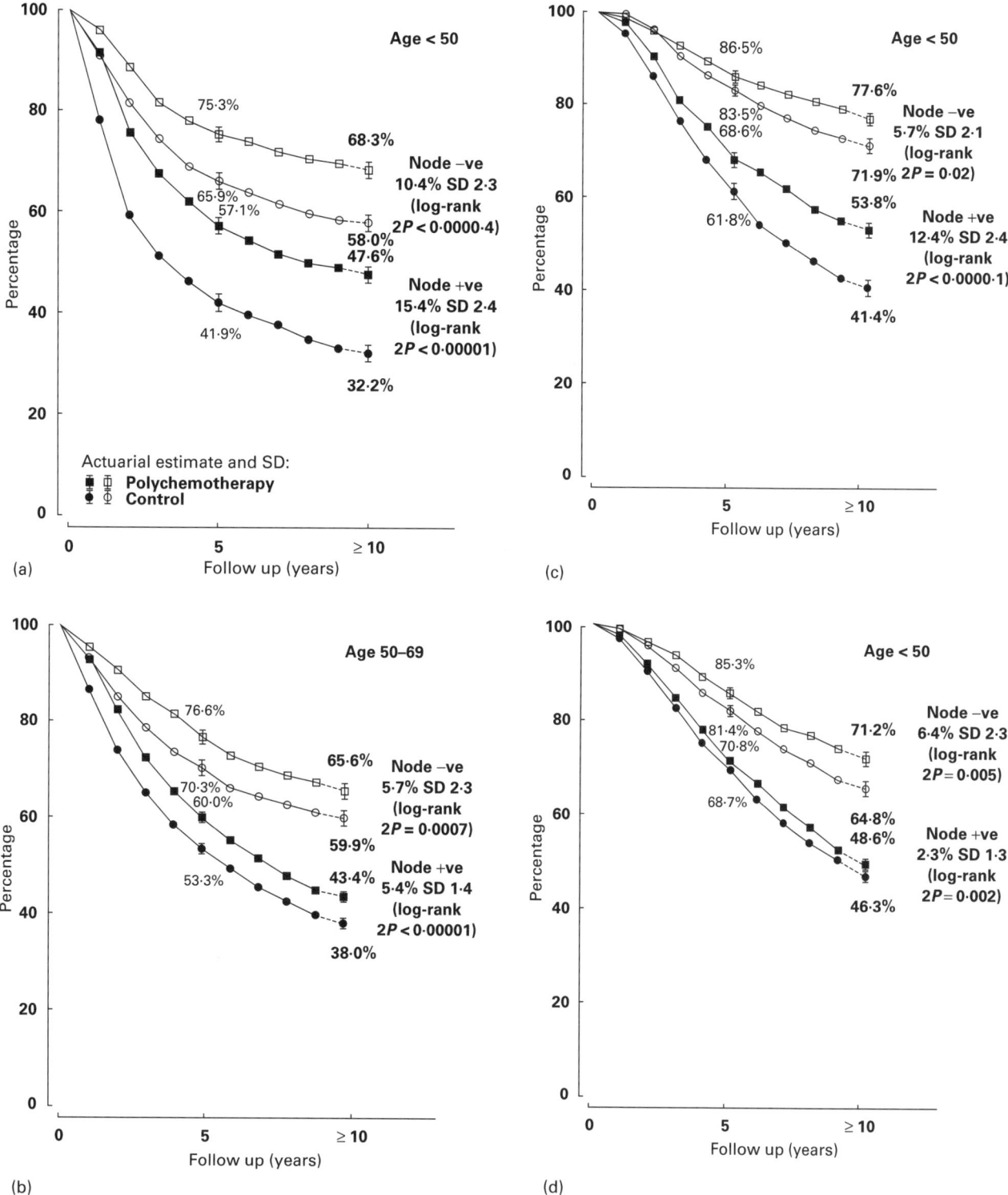

**Figure 40.21** (a, b) Absolute risk reductions with polychemotherapy during the first 10 years of follow up, subdivided by age at randomisation and nodal status: recurrence as first event. (c, d) Absolute risk reductions with polychemotherapy during the first 10 years of follow up, subdivided by age at randomisation and nodal status: mortality (death from any cause)[15]

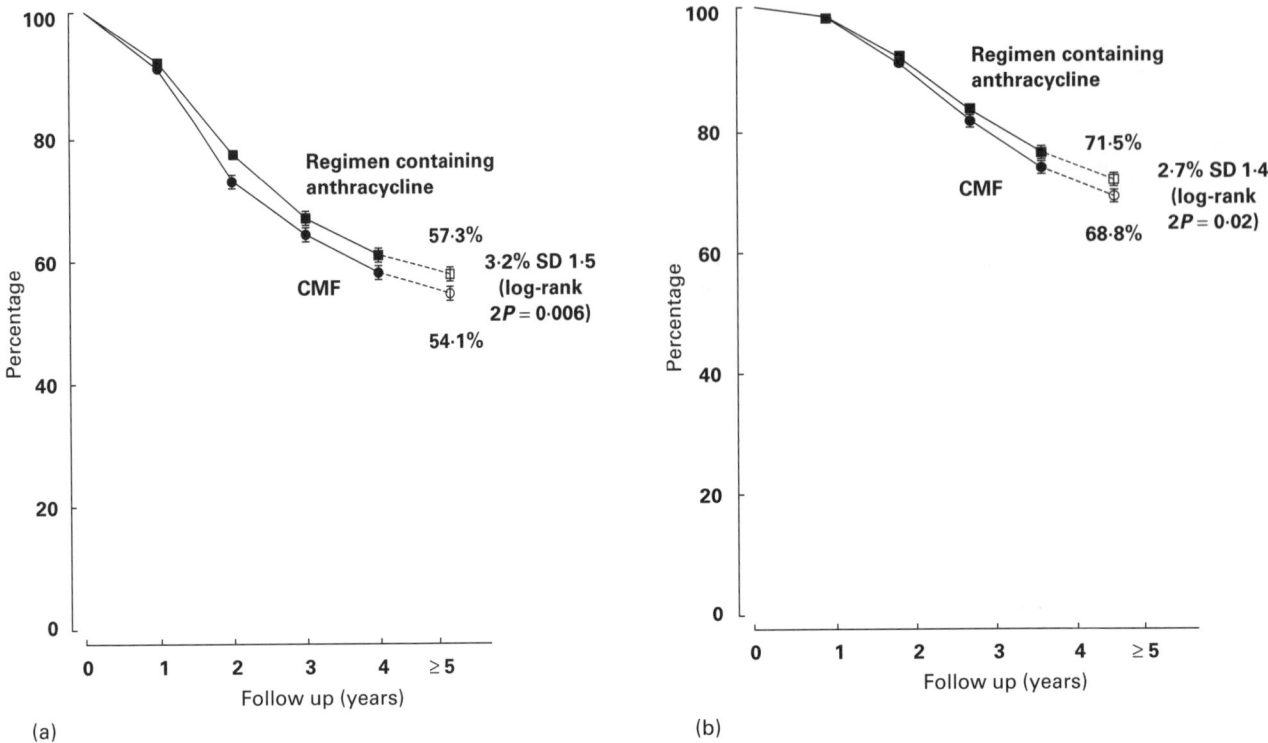

**Figure 40.22** Absolute effects of anthracycline-containing regimens compared with CMF.[15] (a) Recurrence as first event and (b) mortality (death from any cause)

women), and subsequently in terms of survival. Adjuvant therapy using chemotherapy soon became widely accepted. Since then, four EBCTCG overviews have examined the available data on trials including tamoxifen and chemotherapy, the most recent (1995 overview) published in 1998, considered polychemotherapy trials.[15]

Adjuvant chemotherapy trials have also addressed questions of therapy duration, single agent versus polychemotherapy, combined modality therapy and efficacy in different populations of women. More recently, preoperative and high dose therapy, and use of agents such as taxanes have also been considered.

### How much benefit is obtained from adjuvant polychemotherapy in early breast cancer?

The EBCTCG overview (1998)[15] involved about 30 000 women in 69 trials, including 18 000 women in trials involving prolonged polychemotherapy versus no chemotherapy, 6000 women in 11 trials of longer versus shorter polychemotherapy, and about 6000 in 11 trials of anthracycline containing regimens versus CMF.

Polychemotherapy produced significant proportional reduction in mortality for both: women aged under 50

(27%, SD 5 reduction; $2P < 0.00001$) and women aged 50–69 (11%, SD 3 reduction; $2P = 0.0001$). There were proportional reductions in recurrence for women aged under 50 (35%, SD 4 reduction; $P < 0.00001$) and women aged 50–69 (20%, SD 3 reduction; $2P < 0.00001$). There were no data reported for women aged 70 or over. Reductions in recurrence were most evident during the first 5 years of follow up, whereas survival differences increased throughout the first 10 years (Figure 40.21).

The proportional risk reductions were similar for node-negative and node-positive disease, but the absolute difference was greater for node-positive disease. The 10-year survival differences for mortality for women aged under 50 at randomisation were: node-positive patients, 11% (53% *v* 42%); and node-negative patients, 7% (78% *v* 71%). The corresponding absolute differences for women aged 50–69 were: node-positive patients, 3% (49% *v* 46%); and node-negative patients 2%, (69% *v* 67%). No analysis was undertaken specifically for women with ER-poor tumours (Figure 40.21).[15] **Evidence level Ia**

These age-specific benefits of prolonged polychemotherapy were largely irrespective of menopausal status at presentation, or oestrogen receptor status of the primary tumour, and of whether or not adjuvant tamoxifen was also given.

## What else is known about adjuvant polychemotherapy effects?

Polychemotherapy reduced contralateral breast cancer rates by about 20% ($2P = 0.05$). There was no apparent effect on deaths from other causes. There was no additional survival advantage seen for polychemotherapy regimens extending beyond 3–6 months. Regimens containing an anthracycline were superior to non-anthracycline containing regimens for recurrence ($2P = 0.006$), and, possibly for mortality (69% $v$ 72%, 5-year survival log-rank $2P = 0.02$).

Thus, for women with early breast cancer, polychemotherapy with CMF or an anthracycline-containing regimen for several cycles produces an absolute improvement of about 7–11% in 10-year survival for women aged under 50 and about 2–3% in 10-year survival for women aged 50–69 (Figure 40.22).[15] **Evidence level Ia**

## Is preoperative chemotherapy of value?

Randomised clinical trials have evaluated various aspects of preoperative chemotherapy.[97–102] These trials have demonstrated that tumour response (clinical and pathological) can be obtained, that lymph node-positive rates can be reduced, and that breast preservation rates can be increased. They have also documented a close relationship between "responders" and outcomes.[103] They have not, however, shown that these "responders" are in any way different to those patients who have a better outcome from postoperative adjuvant chemotherapy.

What is lacking are trials that identify responders and non-responders to preoperative therapy and then randomise subsequent treatments for each group.

## What is the role of taxanes in adjuvant therapy of early breast cancer?

Taxane-containing regimens are not a standard therapy for early breast cancer. Three published trials have tested the addition of a taxane (paclitaxel or docetaxel) and have failed to demonstrate a clear advantage for taxanes.[104–106]

A substantial number of trials involving a large number of women are in progress, and should be the subject of a future overview analysis.

## Is high dose chemotherapy of value for early breast cancer?

There is no clear evidence from randomised clinical trials that high dose chemotherapy is superior to conventional dose chemotherapy. Six of the published trials have involved women with early breast cancer.[107–112] An additional 10 trials, involving node-positive patients and different strategies are ongoing.[113] Further follow up of these trials is required to determine whether an identifiable population benefits from high dose chemotherapy.

# Systemic therapy for metastatic breast cancer

*Nicholas Wilcken*

Metastatic breast cancer is more heterogeneous in its behaviour than most other metastatic cancers, and hence its management requires flexibility. There are a greater number of active treatments than for other cancers, and patient preference therefore takes on special significance. Also, unlike many other cancers, there are no randomised trials of chemotherapy, endocrine therapy, or biological therapy versus best supportive care. Indirect evidence for beneficial effects of these agents on survival is strong, however, and to an extent this also applies to effects on quality of life. Supportive treatments that do not affect cancer growth are naturally also an important part of the management of this disease.

The Cochrane Collaboration's specialised register of randomised controlled trials in breast cancer contains over 5000 entries, about 1000 of which are randomised controlled trials pertaining specifically to metastatic breast cancer. Two sets of systematic reviews exist. These were both commissioned with the aim of reviewing a number of separate questions based on published randomised controlled trials, one for the British National Health Service in 1996,[114,115] and the other for the National Breast Cancer Centre of Australia in 1997.[116,117] Existing and ongoing Cochrane reviews are updating and expanding this work (www.ctc.usyd.edu.au/cochrane/). The original report to the National Breast Cancer Centre of Australia has been used as the starting point for developing this section, with appropriate updating.

## Does systemic therapy prolong survival in metastatic breast cancer?

No randomised trials directly comparing best supportive care with and without systemic anticancer therapy in metastatic breast cancer have been published. Strong indirect support for the effects of anticancer therapies on survival in metastatic breast cancer comes from two sources. Firstly, there is overwhelming evidence that both endocrine therapy and chemotherapy prolong survival in women with early breast cancer. Secondly, existing randomised trials of endocrine therapy, chemotherapy and trastuzumab in metastatic breast cancer also provide indirect evidence of efficacy as follows.

- Chemotherapy given for a longer duration modestly improves survival compared to treatment given for a shorter duration in a meta-analysis[117,118]

- Chemotherapy at standard doses is associated with longer survival than treatment at less than standard doses in a single trial.[119]
- One chemotherapy regimen can result in better overall survival than another in a single trial.[120]
- Polychemotherapy leads to better survival than single agent chemotherapy in a meta-analysis.[115]
- One endocrine therapy regimen can result in better progression-free survival than another in single trials.[121,122]
- Chemotherapy plus trastuzumab compared to chemotherapy alone gives better progression-free survival and a trend to better overall survival (despite significant crossover) in a single trial.[123]

Thus a number of randomised trials and meta-analyses demonstrate a survival benefit for certain durations, doses, particular agents and regimens over their comparators, strongly suggesting that, if systemic treatments were tested against best supportive care, a survival benefit would also be seen. **Evidence level Ia,b**

## When should treatment start?

There are no randomised trials that have deliberately assessed the effects of delaying treatment on survival or quality of life. However, an ongoing meta-analysis of trials comparing chemotherapy with endocrine therapy does not show a statistically significant difference in survival (see below). Since there was a significant proportion of women with hormone receptor-negative tumours in these trials, the results of the meta-analysis reflect in part a comparison of early and delayed chemotherapy. Thus it would appear that modest delays in initiating treatment do not have a significant impact on overall survival. The question of when to start treatment, particularly in asymptomatic women, is a matter of judgement for the woman and her doctor.

## Should initial treatment be endocrine therapy, cytotoxic therapy or both?

An ongoing systematic review has so far identified 10 randomised trials involving 854 women, comparing chemotherapy with endocrine therapy.[124] Eight trials have information on tumour response rates (817 women) and six trials have information on overall survival (692 women). These trials were generally small and were published between 1963 and 1995. The largest trial involved 339 women and compared endocrine therapy and chemotherapy given sequentially or in combination.[125] Many contained women whose tumours were ER-negative or unknown.

**Table 40.7**   Randomised comparison of tamoxifen, ovarian suppression (OS) or both[127,128]

|  | OS + tam | OS | Fam | *P* |
|---|---|---|---|---|
| RR | 48% | 34% | 28% | *P* = 0·11 |
| PFS (months) | 9·7 | 6·3 | 5·6 | *P* = 0·03 |
| Overall survival (years) | 3·7 | 2·5 | 2·9 | *P* = 0·01 |
| 5-year OS | 34% | 15% | 18% |  |
| (95% CI) | (20–48%) | (4–26%) | (7–30%) |  |

Abbreviations: RR, response rate; PFS, progression-free survival

**Table 40.8**   Efficacy and cardiac toxicity with trastuzumab[123]

|  | CT + trastuzumab | CT alone | *P* |
|---|---|---|---|
| Response rate | 50% | 30% | *P* = 0·001 |
| Progression-free survival (months) | 7·4 | 4·6 | *P* = 0·001 |
| Median survival | 25·1 | 20·3 | *P* = 0·001 |

| | AC + trastuzumab | AC alone | Paclitaxel + trastuzumab | Paclitaxel alone |
|---|---|---|---|---|
| Cardiac toxicity | 27% | 8% | 13% | 1% |

Abbreviations: CT, chemotherapy; AC, adriamycin plus cyclophosphamide

While there was evidence of an increased tumour response rate with chemotherapy (RR 1·26; CI 1·03–1·55; *P* = 0·03), there was no evidence of a significant difference in overall survival (HR 0·94; CI 0·79–1·12; *P* = 0·5). There were no reliable data on toxicity or quality of life.

A 1996 meta-analysis found no survival benefit for the addition of chemotherapy to endocrine therapy (seven trials), and a modest non-significant trend favouring the addition of endocrine therapy to chemotherapy (10 trials).[117] **Evidence level Ia**

Thus there is moderately strong evidence that using endocrine therapy first (in hormone receptor-positive or unknown disease) is reasonable and not disadvantageous. A combination of endocrine and chemotherapy does not appear to be of benefit over either modality alone.[125] It is generally believed that chemotherapy may be preferable to endocrine therapy in the presence of rapidly progressing visceral disease, although this is a policy that falls into the realm of "common sense-based medicine" rather than evidence-based medicine.

## Which endocrine therapy?

Until recently, there has been no reason not to recommend tamoxifen at a dose of 20 mg per day as the ideal initial endocrine therapy. Using overall survival as the endpoint of efficacy, a 1996 meta-analysis found no evidence to favour any one particular class of agent over another, any combination of endocrine agents over single endocrine agents used sequentially, or higher doses of any given agent over lower doses within a standard range.[117]

Since then, the available evidence suggests two modifications to these findings. First, large individual trials have compared tamoxifen with the aromatase inhibitors anastrozole and letrozole in postmenopausal women. While there are minor differences between the trials, they suggest that these aromatase inhibitors are at least as effective and probably slightly more effective than tamoxifen, with a change in toxicity profile.[121,122] This is consistent with a large adjuvant trial with short follow up that showed superior disease-free survival for anastrozole compared with tamoxifen.[126] Apart from some increase in the risk of bone fractures, most side effects were either similar or less frequent in women taking anastrozole.

Second, in premenopausal women there is now evidence that the combination of ovarian suppression and tamoxifen is superior to either agent alone. A single three arm trial compared tamoxifen, ovarian suppression, or both.[127] The combination arm was superior for all measures of tumour efficacy (response rate, progression-free survival, overall survival), but caused more hot flushes than tamoxifen alone (Table 40.7). A meta-analysis[128] identified four randomised trials comparing combined ovarian suppression and tamoxifen with ovarian suppression alone, and also found superior progression-free survival (HR 0·70; $P = 0·0003$) and overall survival (HR 0·78; $P = 0·02$) (Table 40.8).

Thus in postmenopausal women, many would now regard a third generation aromatase inhibitor the best first-line endocrine option. **Grade A** In those premenopausal women not exposed to tamoxifen, combined endocrine therapy should be considered.

### Chemotherapy – how much and for how long?

Systematic reviews dating from the mid 1990s found no strong evidence that, within the range of usual doses, there is any benefit in higher as opposed to lower total doses of chemotherapy. Similarly, increasing dose density has not improved survival, at least for anthracycline, cyclophosphamide combinations, in either advanced disease[129] or the adjuvant setting.[130,131] These questions are the subject of ongoing, updated Cochrane reviews, including an analysis of all the available high dose stem cell support trials.[132] There is, however, some evidence that lower than standard doses may be associated with reduced overall survival and quality of life.[119]

How long to continue chemotherapy will naturally depend on individual patient circumstances and the toxicity associated with treatment. The only systematic review to examine this question was limited to randomised trials that compared different durations of the same chemotherapy regimens (so, for example, a trial where women received six cycles of drug X and were then randomised to no further treatment or six cycles of drug Y would not have qualified). That meta-analysis[117] found a modest prolongation of overall survival associated with a longer duration of treatment (HR 0·77; $P = 0·01$). This evidence of a survival benefit is enhanced by data from the largest of these randomised trials, which found that the use of a greater number of cycles of chemotherapy was also associated with better quality of life.[133]

Of course, modest benefits in overall survival must be weighed against possible toxicity. As a general rule however, trials that have measured quality of life indicate that more effective anticancer therapy also improves quality of life.[119,133,134] Overall, the policy of giving standard doses of combination chemotherapy over several cycles (perhaps six cycles or more) is the best option if overall survival and quality of life are taken as measures of efficacy. **Grade A**

### Which drugs and how many?

As in early breast cancer, the best evidence from systematic reviews is that multiagent regimens are superior to single agent chemotherapy.[115] However, regimens containing anthracyclines were *not* superior to other regimens. These findings may not be expected to remain

static over time, as newer and more active agents appear. However, even a relatively new, highly active drug such as docetaxel yielded better results when combined with capecitabine than when used alone.[120]

Decisions about which particular chemotherapy regimens to use will depend on a number of factors. Only broad statements can be made about the relative efficacy of drug combinations. If an anthracycline combination is taken as a reference point, then taxane-containing regimens are clearly very active.[137] However, the combination of anthracycline and taxane may be associated with significant toxicity. Additionally, there has recently been enthusiasm for taxanes given in a weekly schedule, and whether this is best done alone or in combination has yet to be established. A randomised trial in locally advanced disease suggested that weekly paclitaxel may be superior to three-weekly paclitaxel.[136] Other active, low toxicity drugs include capecitabine, vinorelbine and gemcitabine, but it is not yet clear how their efficacy compares with more conventional regimens.

It is worth noting that numerous studies comparing chemotherapy regimens and schedules are currently underway, and consequently findings in this area are rapidly evolving.

### Biological therapies

At present, there are only mature data about trastuzumab, a humanised monoclonal antibody directed against the extracellular domain of the HER2 (erbB2) receptor. Trastuzumab is active as a single agent in pretreated metastatic breast cancer.[137] The only currently published randomised study compared trastuzumab alone with trastuzumab plus chemotherapy (paclitaxel or AC).[137] Trastuzumab-containing regimens led to superior response rates, progression-free survival, and overall survival (Table 40.8), but an increase in cardiac toxicity. Efficacy is closely linked to receptor expression, and is only seen when there is evidence of amplification of the *HER2* gene. The cardiac toxicity was an unexpected finding and requires prospective investigation. However, in the meantime, it would seem prudent to avoid the *concurrent* administration of trastuzumab and anthracycline.

### Bisphosphonates

A Cochrane systematic review of bisphosphonates in breast cancer identified 19 randomised studies, of which eight included 1962 women with advanced breast cancer and existing bone metastases.[138] Bisphosphonates reduced the risk of developing a skeletal event by 14% (RR 0·86; 95% CI 0·80–0·91; $P < 0·00001$). Significant improvements in pain were reported in four studies, and improvements in quality of life were reported in two studies. Treatment with bisphosphonates does not appear to affect survival in women with advanced breast cancer. In the three studies of bisphosphonates in 320 women with advanced breast cancer *without* clinically evident bone metastases, there was no significant reduction in the incidence of skeletal events (RR 0·99; 95% CI 0·67–1·47; $P > 0·9$).

Figures 40.3–40.8 and 40.12–40.22 reproduced with permission from the *Lancet*. Figures 40.9–40.11 and Table 40.4 reproduced with permission from the *New England Journal of Medicine*.

# References

1    Parkin MD, Pisani P, Ferlay J. Global cancer statistics. *CA Cancer J Clin* 1999;**49**:33064.

2    Peto R. Mortality from breast cancer has decreased suddenly. *BMJ* 1998;**317**:476.

3    Brown P. UK death rates from breast cancer fall by a third. *BMJ* 2000;**321**:849.

4    Gail MH, Brinton LA, Byar DP *et al*. Projecting individualised probabilities of developing breast cancer for white females who are being examined annually. *J Natl Cancer Inst* 1989;**81**:1879–86.

5    Costantino JP, Gail MH, Pee D *et al*. Validation studies for models projecting the risk of invasive and total breast cancer incidence. *J Natl Cancer Inst* 1999;**91**:1541–8.

6    Claus EB, Risch N, Thompson WD. Autosomal dominant inheritance of early-onset breast cancer: Implications for risk prediction. *Cancer* 1994;**73**:643–51.

7    Singletary SE, Allred C, Ashley P *et al*. Revision of the American Joint Committee on Cancer Staging System for Breast Cancer. *J Clin Oncol* 2002;**20**:3628–36.

8    Goldhirsch A, Guck JH, Gelber RD, Coates A. Meeting highlights: International Consensus Panel on the treatment of primary breast cancer. *J Clin Oncol* 2001;**19**:3817–27.

9    Early Breast Cancer Trialists' Collaborative Group. Effects of adjuvant tamoxifen and of cytotoxic therapy on mortality in early breast cancer: an overview of 61 randomised trials among 28,896 women. *N Engl J Med* 1988;**319**:1681–60.

10   Early Breast Cancer Trialists' Collaborative Group. *Treatment of early breast cancer, Vol 1: Worldwide evidence 1985–1990*. Oxford: Oxford University Press, 1990.

11   Early Breast Cancer Trialists' Collaborative Group. Systematic treatment of early breast cancer by hormonal, cytotoxic, or immune therapy: 133 randomised trials involving 31,000 recurrences and 24,000 deaths among 75,000 women. *Lancet* 1992;**339**:1–15, 1–85.

12   Early Breast Cancer Trialiasts' Collaborative Group. Effects of radiotherapy and surgery in early breast cancer: an overview of the randomised trials. *N Engl J Med* 1995;**333**:1444–55.

13   Early Breast Cancer Trialists' Collaborative Group. Ovarian ablation in early breast cancer: overview of the randomised trials. *Lancet* 1996;**348**:1189–96.

14   Early Breast Cancer Trialists' Collaborative Group. Tamoxifen for early breast cancer: an overview of the randomised trials. *Lancet* 1998;**351**:1451–67.

15   Early Breast Cancer Trialists' Collaborative Group. Polychemotherapy for early breast cancer: an overview of the randomised trials. *Lancet* 1998;**352**:930–42.

16   Early Breast Cancer Trialists' Collaborative Group. Favourable and unfavourable effects of long-term survival of radiotherapy for early breast cancer: an overview of the randomised trials. *Lancet* 2000;**355**:1757–70.

17   National Institute of Health Consensus Development Panel, National Institute of Health Consensus Development Conference Statement: Adjuvant therapy for breast cancer, Nov 1–3, 2000. *J Natl Cancer Inst* 2000;**93**:979–89.

18   Cuzick J, Baum M. Tamoxifen and contralateral breast cancer. *Lancet* 1985;**1**:282.

19   Cuzick J, Wong DY, Bulbrook RD. The prevention of breast cancer. *Lancet* 1986;**2**:83–6.

20   Powles TJ, Tillyer CR, Jones AL *et al*. Prevention of breast cancer with tamoxifen: an update on the Royal Marsden Pilot programme. *Eur J Cancer* 1990;**26**:680–4.

21   IBIS Investigators (Writing Committee: Cuzick J, Forbes JF, Edwards R *et al.*). First results from the International Breast cancer Intervention Study (IBIS 1): a randomised prevention trial. *Lancet* 2002;**360**: 817–24.

22   Fisher B, Costantino JP, Wickerham DL *et al*. Tamoxifen for prevention of breast cancer: Report of the National Surgical Adjuvant Breast and Bowel Project P-1 Study. *J Natl Cancer Inst* 1998;**90**:1371–88.

23   Veronesi U, Maisonneuve P, Costa A *et al*. Prevention of breast cancer with tamoxifen: Preliminary findings from the Italian randomised trial among hysterectomied women. *Lancet* 1998;**352**:93–7.

24   Cuzick J, Powles T, Veronesi U *et al*. Overview of the main outcomes in breast cancer prevention trials. *Lancet* 2003;**361**:296–300.

25   Powles T, Eeles R, Ashley S *et al*. Interim analysis of the incidence of breast cancer in the Royal Marsden Hospital Tamoxifen Randomised Chemoprevention Trial. *Lancet* 1998;**352**:98–101.

26   Veronesi U, Maisonneuve P, Sacchini V *et al*. Tamoxifen for breast cancer among hysterectomied women. *Lancet* 2002;**359**:1122–4.

27   Cauley JA, Norton L, Lippman ME *et al*. Continued breast cancer risk reduction in postmenopausal women treated with raloxifene: 4 year results from the MORE trial. *Breast Cancer Res Treat* 2001;**65**: 125–34.

28   The ATAC (Arimidex, Tamoxifen Alone or in Combination) Trialists' Group. Anastrozole alone or in combination with tamoxifen versus tamoxifen alone for adjuvant treatment of postmenopausal women with early breast cancer: first results of the ATAC randomised trial. *Lancet* 2002;**359**:2131–9.

29   Jakesz R, Hausmaninger H, Kubista E *et al*. Randomised adjuvant trial of Tamoxifen and Goserelin versus Cyclophosphamide, methotrexate and fluorouracil: Evidence for the superiority of treatment with endocrine blockade in premenopausal patients with hormone-responsive breast cancer – Austrian Breast & Colorectal Cancer Study Group Trial 5. *J Clin Oncol* 2002;**20**:4621–7.

30   Rutqvist LE. Zoladex and tamoxifen as adjuvant therapy in premenopausal breast cancer: a randomized trial by the Cancer Research Campaign (CRC) Breast Cancer Trials Group, the South-East Sweden Breast Cancer Group, Stockholm Breast Cancer Study Group and the Gruppo Interdisciplinare Valutazione Interventi in Oncologia (GIVIO) [abstract]. *Proc ASCO* 1999;**18**:67a.

31   Rebbeck TR, Levin A, Eisen A *et al*. Breast cancer risk after bilateral prophylactic oophorectomy in BRCA1 mutation carriers. *J Natl Cancer Inst* 1999;**91**:1475–9.

32   Anderson BO. Prophylactic surgery to reduce breast cancer risk: a brief literature review. *Breast J* 2001;**7**:321–30.

33   Hartman LC, Schaid DJ, Woods JE *et al*. Efficacy of bilateral prophylactic mastectomy in women with a family history of breast cancer. *N Engl J Med* 1999;**340**:77–84.

34   Meijers-Heijboer H, van Geel B, van Putten WL *et al*. Breast cancer after prophylactic bilateral mastectomy in women with a BRCA1 or BRCA2 mutation. *N Engl J Med* 2001;**345**:159–64.

35   Morrow M, Strom EA, Bassett LW. Standard for the Management of Ductal Carcinoma In Situ (DCIS). (Report from Advisory Group with representatives from the American College of Radiology, American College of Surgeons, College of American Pathologists, and Society of Surgical Oncology). *CA Cancer J Clin* 2002;**52**:256–76.

36   Fisher B, Costantino J, Redmond C *et al*. Lumpectomy compared with lumpectomy and radiation therapy for the treatment of intraduct breast cancer. *N Engl J Med* 1993;**328**:1581–6.

37   Mamounas E, Fisher B, Dingham J *et al*. Effects of breast irradiation following lumpectomy in intraduct carcinoma (DCIS): Updated results from NSABP B-18. *Proc Soc Surg Oncol* 1997;**50**:7.

38   Fisher ER, Costantino J, Fisher B *et al*. Pathologic findings from the National Surgical Adjuvant Breast Project (NSABP) Protocol B-17, Intraduct Carcinoma (ductal carcinoma in situ). *Cancer* 1995;**75**: 1310–19.

39  Fisher ER, Dignam J, Tan-Chiu F *et al.* Pathologic findings from the National Surgical Adjuvant Breast Project (NSABP) eight-year update of Protocol B-17: Intraduct carcinoma (see comments). *Cancer* 1999;**86**:429–38.

40  Julien JP, Bijker N, Fentiman IS *et al.* Radiotherapy in breast conserving treatment for ductal carcinoma in situ: First results of the EORTC randomised phase III trial 14053. *Lancet* 2000;**355**:528–33.

41  Fisher B, Dignam J, Wolmark N *et al.* Tamoxifen in treatment of intraduct breast cancer: National Surgical Adjuvant Breast & Bowel Project B-24 randomised controlled trial. *Lancet* 1999;**353**:1993–2000.

42  Fisher B, Jeong J-H, Anderson S, *et al.* Twenty-five year follow up of a randomised trial comparing radical mastectomy, total mastectomy, and total mastectomy followed by irradiation. *N Engl J Med* 2002; **347**:567–75.

43  Fisher B, Bauer M, Margolese R *et al.* Five-year results of a randomised clinical trial comparing total mastectomy and segmented mastectomy with or without radiation in the treatment of breast cancer. *N Engl J Med* 1985;**312**:665–73.

44  Fisher B, Redmond C, Poisson R *et al.* Eight-year results of a randomised clinical trial comparing total mastectomy and lumpectomy with or without irradiation in the treatment of breast cancer. *N Engl J Med* 1989;**320**:822–8 (Erratum, *N Engl J Med* 1994;**330**:1467).

45  Fisher B, Anderson S, Bryant J *et al.* Twenty-year follow-up of a randomised trial comparing total mastectomy, lumpectomy, and lumpectomy plus irradiation for the treatment of invasive breast cancer. *N Engl J Med* 2002;**347**:1233–41.

46  Veronesi U, Saccozzi R, Del Vecchio M *et al.* Comparing radical mastectomy with quadrantectomy, axillary dissection, and radiotherapy in patients with small cancers of the breast. *N Engl J Med* 1981;**305**:6–11.

47  Veronesi U, Luini A, Galimberti V *et al.* Conservation approaches for the management of stage I/II carcinoma of the breast: Milan Cancer Institute Trials. *Wld J Surg* 1994;**18**:70–5.

48  Veronesi U, Cascinelli N, Mariani L *et al.* Twenty-year follow-up of a randomised study comparing breast-conserving surgery with radical (Halsted) mastectomy for early breast cancer. *N Engl J Med* 2002; **347**:1227–32.

49  Sarrazin D, Le MG, Arriagada R *et al.* Ten-year results of a randomised trial comparing a conservative treatment to mastectomy in early breast cancer. *Rad Oncol* 1989;**14**:177–84.

50  Blichert-Toft M, Rose C, Andersen JA *et al.* Danish randomized trial comparing breast conservation therapy with mastectomy: Six-years of life – table analysis. In*: Consensus Development Conference on the treatment of early-stage breast cancer.* Monograph No. 11, (NIH Publication No. 90–3187). Bethesda: National Cancer Institute, 1992.

51  Jacobsen JA, Danforth DN, Cowan KH *et al.* Ten-year results of a comparison of conservation with mastectomy in the treatment of stage I and II breast cancer. *N Engl J Med* 1995;**332**:907–11.

52  Van Dongen JA, Voogd AC, Fentiman IS *et al.* Long-term results of a randomized trial comparing breast-conserving therapy with mastectomy: European Organization for Research & Treatment of Cancer 10801 trial. *J Natl Cancer Inst* 2000;**92**:1143–50.

53  Veronesi U, Luini A, Del Vecchio M *et al.* Radiotherapy after breast preserving surgery in women with localised cancer of the breast. *N Engl J Med* 1993;**328**:1587–91.

54  Forrest AP, Stewart JH, Everington D *et al.* Randomised trial of conservation therapy for breast cancer: 6-year anaylsis of the Scottish trial. Scottish Cancer Trials Breast Group. *Lancet* 1996;**348**:708–13.

55  Clark RM, Whelan T, Levine M *et al.* Randomised clinical trial of breast irradiation following lumpectomy and axillary dissection for node-negative breast cancer: An update. *J Natl Cancer Inst* 1996;**88**: 1659–64.

56  Liljegren G, Holmberg L, Bergh J *et al.* 10-year results after sector resection with or without post operative radiotherapy for stage I breast cancer: A randomised trial. *J Clin Oncol* 1999;**17**:2326–33.

57  Fisher B, Bryant J, Dignam JJ *et al.* Tamoxifen radiation therapy, or both for prevention of ipsilateral breast tumour recurrence after lumpectomy in women with invasive breast cancer of one centimetre or less. *J Clin Oncol* 2002;**20**:4141–9.

58  Blamey RW, on behalf of the BASO Breast Group Trialist's. The British Association of Surgical Oncology Trial (BASO II) of the treatment of small differentiated node negative tumours (abstract). *Breast Cancer Treatm* 1999;**47**:50.

59  Spooner D, Morrison JM, Oates GD *et al.* The role of radiotherapy in early breast cancer (stage I): A West Midlands Breast Group prospective randomised collaborative study (BR 3002). *Breast* 1995;**57**:34.

60  Jones JM, Ribeiro GG. Mortality patterns over 34 years of breast cancer patients in a clinical trial of post-operative radiotherapy. *Clin Radiol* 1989;**40**:204–8.

61  Cuzick J, Stewart H, Peto R *et al.* Overview of randomized trials of postoperative adjuvant radiotherapy in breast cancer. *Cancer Treatm Rep* 1987;**71**:15–29.

62  Cuzick J, Stewart H, Rutqvist L *et al.* Cause-specific mortality in long-term survivors of breast cancer who participated in trials of radiotherapy. *J Clin Oncol* 1994;**12**:447–53.

63  Morrow M, Harris JR. Local management of invasive breast cancer. In: *Diseases of the breast.* Harris JR, Lippman ME, Morrow M, Osborne CK, eds. Philadelphia: Lippincott-Raven, 2000.

64  Ragaz J, Jackson SM, Le N *et al.* Adjuvant radiotherapy and chemotherapy in node-positive, pre-menopausal women with breast cancer. *N Engl J Med* 1997;**388**:956–62.

65  Nixon AJ, Manola J, Gelman R *et al.* No long-term increase in cardiac-related mortality after breast-conserving surgery and radiation therapy using modern techniques. *J Clin Oncol* 1998;**16**:1374–9.

66  Recht A, Bartelink H, Forquet A *et al.* Postmastectomy radiotherapy: questions for the twenty-first century. *J Clin Oncol* 1998;**16**:2886–9.

67  Sauer R, Wallgren A, Kurtz JM. Adjuvant radiotherapy after breast conserving surgery for breast cancer. *Eur J Cancer* 2000;**36**:1073–84.

68  Whelan TJ, Levine M, Julian J *et al.* The effects of radiation therapy on quality of life of women with breast carcinoma: results of a randomized trial. *Cancer* 2000;**88**:2260–6.

69  Overgaard M, Hansen PS, Overgaard J *et al.* Postoperative radiotherapy in high-risk postmenopausal women with breast cancer who receive adjuvant chemotherapy. *N Engl J Med* 1997;**337**:949–55.

70  Liljegren G, Holmberg L. Arm morbidity after sector resection and axillary dissection with or without postoperative radiotherapy in breast cancer stage I. Results from a randomised trial. *Eur J Cancer* 1997;**33**:193–9.

71  Shapiro CL, Harrigan Hardenbergh P, Gelman R *et al.* Cardiac effects of adjuvant doxorubicin and radiation therapy in breast cancer patients. *J Clin Oncol* 1998;**16**:3493–501.

72  Kurtz J, for the EUSOMA Working Party. The curative role of radiotherapy in the treatment of operative breast cancer. *Eur J Cancer* 2002 2000;**38**:1961–74.

73  Silverstein MJ, Lagios MD, Groshen S *et al.* The influence of margin width on local control of ductal carcinoma in situ of the breast. *N Engl J Med* 1999;**340**:1455–61.

74  Beatson GT. On the treatment of inoperable cases of carcinoma of the mamma: suggestions for a new method of treatment. *Lancet* 1896;**2**: 104–7.

75  Jonat W. Zoladex (goserelin) vs. CMF as adjuvant therapy in pre/perimenopausal early (node-positive) breast cancer: preliminary efficacy, QOL, and BMD results from the SEBRA study [abstract]. *Breast Cancer Res Treat* 2000;**64**:29.

76  Jonat W, Kaufman M, Sauerbrei W *et al.* Goserelin versus cyclophosamide methotrexate and fluorouracil as adjuvant therapy in premenopausal patients with node-positive breast cancer: The Zoladex Early Breast Cancer Research Association Study. *J Clin Oncol* 2002;**20**:4628–35.

77  Scottish Cancer Trials Breast Group and ICRF Breast Unit, Guy's Hospital, London. Adjuvant ovarian ablation versus CMF chemotherapy in premenopausal women with pathological stage II breast carcinoma: the Scottish trial. *Lancet* 1993;**341**:1293–8.

78  Boccardo F, Rubagotti A, Amoroso D, Mesiti M, Romeo D, Sismondi P *et al.* Cyclophosphamide, methotrexate, and fluorouracil versus tamoxifen plus ovarian suppression as adjuvant treatment of estrogen receptor-positive pre-/perimenopausal breast cancer patients: results of the Italian Breast Cancer Adjuvant Study Group 02 randomized trial. *J Clin Oncol* 2000;**18**:2718–27.

79  Jakesz R, Hausmaninger H, Samonigg H *et al.* Comparison of adjuvant therapy with tamoxifen and goserelin *v* CMF in premenopausal stage I

and II hormone-responsive breast cancer patients: four-year results of Austrian Breast Cancer Study Group (ABCSG) Trial 5 [abst]. *Proc ASCO* 1999;**18**:67a.

80  Jakesz R, Gnant M, Hausmaninger H *et al.* Combination goserelin and tamoxifen is more effective than CMF in premenopausal patients with hormone-responsive tumours in a multi-center trial of the Austrian Breast Cancer Study Group (ABCSG) [abstract]. *Breast Cancer Res Treat* 1999;**57**:25.

81  Roché H, Mihura J, de Lafontan B *et al.* Castration and tamoxifen versus chemotherapy (FAC) for premenopausal, node and receptor positive breast cancer patients: a randomized trial with a 7 year median follow-up [abstract]. *Proc ASCO* 1996;**15**:117.

82  Roché HH, Kerbrat P, Bonneteere J *et al.* Complete hormonal blockage versus chemotherapy in premenopausal early-stage breast cancer patients (Pts) with positive hormone-receptor (HR+) and 1–3 node-positive (N+) tumor, results of the FASG 06 trial [abst]. *Proc ASCO* 2000; **19**:72a.

83  Davidson N, O'Neill A, Vukov A, Osborne CK, Martino S, White D *et al.* Effect of chemohormonal therapy in premenopausal node (+) receptor (+) breast cancer: an Eastern Cooperative Oncology Group Phase III Inter-group Trial (E5188, INT-0101) [abst]. *Proc ASCO* 1999;**18**:67a.

84  Baum M. Adjuvant treatment of premenopausal breast cancer with Zoladex and tamoxifen [abst]. *Breast Cancer Res Treat* 1999;**57**:30.

85  Love RR, Duc NB, Binh NG *et al.* Oophorectomy and tamoxifen adjuvant therapy in premenopausal Vietnamese and Chinese women with operable breast cancer [abst]. *Proc ASCO* 2001;**20**:269.

86  Castiglione-Gertsch M, O'Neill A, Gelber RD *et al.* Is the addition of adjuvant chemotherapy always necessary in node negative (N-) pre/perimenopausal breast cancer patients (pts) who receive goserelin?: first results of IBCSG trial VIII. *Proc ASCO* 2002;**21**:149.

87  Fisher B, Dignam J, Bryant J *et al.* Five versus more than five years of tamoxifen therapy for breast cancer patients with negative lymph nodes and oestrogen-receptor-positive tumours. *J Natl Cancer Inst* 1996;**88**:1529–42.

88  Fisher B, Dignam J, Bryant J. Five versus more than five years of tamoxifen for node-negative breast cancer: updated findings. *J Natl Cancer Inst* 2001;**93**:684–90.

89  Tormey DC, Gray R, Falkson HC. Post-chemotherapy adjuvant tamoxifen therapy beyond five years in patients with lymph node-positive breast cancer. *J Natl Cancer Inst* 1996;**88**:1828–33.

90  Stewart JH, Forrest Ap, Everington D *et al.* for the Scottish Cancer Trials Breast Group. Randomised comparison of 5 years of adjuvant tamoxifen with continuous therapy for operable breast cancer. *Br J Cancer* 1996;**74**:297–9.

91  Stewart JH, Prescott RJ, Forrest AP. Scottish adjuvant tamoxifen trial updated to 15 years. *J Natl Cancer Inst* 2001;**93**:456–62.

92  Bryant J, Fisher B, Dignam J. Duration of tamoxifen adjuvant therapy. *J Natl Cancer Inst Monogr* 2001;**30**:56–61.

93  Clinical Trials Service Unit. *Adjuvant tamoxifen longer against shorter (ATLAS). Protocol. April, 1995.* ATLAS Office, Oxford: Clinical Trials Service Unit, Radcliffe Infirmary, 1995.

94  Cancer Research Campaign Trials Unit. *Adjuvant tamoxifen treatment after more? (aTTom). Protocol.* Birmingham: CRC Trials Unit, Clinical Research Block, Queen Elizabeth Hospital.

95  Fisher B, Carbone P, Economou SG *et al.* 1-Phenylalanine mustard (L-PAM) in the management of primary breast cancer: A report of early findings. *N Engl J Med* 1975;**292**:117–22.

96  Bonadonna G, Brusamolino E, Valagussa P *et al.* Combination chemotherapy as an adjuvant treatment in operable breast cancer. *N Engl J Med* 1976;**294**:405–10.

97  Mauriac L, Durand M, Avril A, Dilhuydy JM. Effects of primary chemotherapy in conservative treatment of breast cancer patients with operable tumours larger than 3 cm. Results of a randomized trial in a single centre. *Ann Oncol* 1991;**2**:347–54.

98  Scholl SM, Fourquet A, Asselain B *et al.* Neoadjuvant versus adjuvant chemotherapy in premenopausal patients with tumours considered too large for breast conserving surgery: preliminary results of a randomised trial: S6. *Eur J Cancer* 1994;**30A**:645–52.

99  Powles TJ, Hickish TF, Makris A *et al.* Randomized trial of chemoendocrine therapy started before or after surgery for treatment of primary breast cancer. *J Clin Oncol* 1995;**13**:547–52.

100  Makris A, Powles TJ, Ashley SE *et al.* A reduction in the requirements for mastectomy in a randomized trial of neoadjuvant chemoendocrine therapy in primary breast cancer. *Ann Oncol* 1998;**9**:1179–84.

101  Fisher B, Brown A, Mamounas E *et al.* Effect of preoperative chemotherapy on local-regional disease in women with operable breast cancer: findings from National Surgical Adjuvant Breast and Bowel Project B-18. *J Clin Oncol* 1997;**15**:2483–93.

102  Fisher B, Bryant J, Wolmark N *et al.* Effect of preoperative chemotherapy on the outcome of women with operable breast cancer. *J Clin Oncol* 1998;**16**:2672–85.

103  Wolmark N, Wang J, Mamounas E *et al.* Preoperative chemotherapy in patients with operable breast cancer: nine-year results from National Surgical Adjuvant Breast and Bowel Project B-18. *J Natl Cancer Inst Monographs*, 2001;**30**:96–102.

104  Henderson IC, Berry D, Demetri G *et al.* Improved disease-free and overall survival from the addition of sequential paclitaxel but not from the escalation of doxorubicin dose level in the adjuvant chemotherapy of patients with node-positive primary breast cancer [abst]. *Proc ASCO* 1998;**17**:101a.

105  Thomas E, Buzdar A, Theriault R *et al.* Role of paclitaxel in adjuvant therapy of operable breast cancer: preliminary results of a prospective randomized clinical trial [abstract]. *Proc ASCO* 2000;**19**:74a.

106  Mamounas EP. Evaluating the use of paclitaxel following doxorubicin and cyclophosphamide in patients with breast cancer and positive axillary nodes. *Proceedings from the NIH Consensus Development Conference on Adjuvant Therapy for Breast Cancer, 2000; Nov 1–3, 2000.* Bethesda (MD): National Institutes of Health, 2000.

107  Rodenhuis S, Bontenbal M, Beex L *et al.* Randomized phase III study of high-dose chemotherapy with cyclophosphamide, thiotepa and carboplatin in operable breast cancer with 4 or more axillary lymph nodes [abst]. *Proc ASCO* 2000;**19**:74.

108  Peters WP, Rosner G, Vredenburgh J *et al.* A prospective, randomized comparison of two doses of combination alkyating agents as consolidation after CAF in high-risk primary breast cancer involving ten or more axillary lymph nodes: preliminary results of CALGB 9402/SWOG 9114/NCIC MA-13 [abstract]. *Proc ASCO* 1999;**18**:1a.

109  Bergh J, Wiklund T, Erikstein B *et al.* Tailored fluorouracil, epirubicin, and cyclophosphamide compared with marrow-supported high-dose chemotherapy as adjuvant treatment for high-risk breast cancer: a randomised trial. Scandinavian Breast Group 9401 study. *Lancet* 2000;**356**:1384–91.

110  Weiss RB, Rifkin RM, Stewart FM *et al.* High-dose chemotherapy for high-risk primary breast cancer: an on-site review of the Bezwoda study. *Lancet* 2000;**355**:999–1003.

111  Rodenhuis S, Richel DJ, van der Wall E *et al.* Randomized trial of high-dose chemotherapy and hematopoietic progenitor-cell support in operable breast cancer with extensive axillary lymph-node involvement. *Lancet* 1998;**352**:515–521.

112  Hortobagyi GN, Buzdar AU, Theriault RL *et al.* Randomized trial of high-dose chemotherapy and blood cess autografts for high-risk primary breast cancrinoma. *J Natl Cancer Inst* 2000;**92**:225–33.

113  Antman KH. *Overview of the Six Available Randomized Trials of High-Dose Chemotherapy With Blood or Marrow Transplant in Breast Cancer. J Natl Cancer Inst Monogr* 2001;**30**:114–16.

114  NHS Executive. *Guidance for Purchasers: Improving Outcomes for Breast Cancer – The Research Evidence.* Leeds: NHS Executive, 1996.

115  Fossati R, Confalonieri C, Torri V *et al.* Cytotoxic and hormonal treatment for metastatic breast cancer. A systematic review of published randomized trials involving 31510 women. *J Clin Oncol* 1998;**10**:3439–60.

116  Stockler M, Wilcken N, Ghersi D, Simes J. *The management of advanced breast cancer: Systematic reviews of randomised controlled trials regarding the use of cytotoxic chemotherapy and endocrine therapy.* Sydney: NHMRC National Breast Cancer Centre, 1997.

117  Stockler MR, Wilcken NRC, Ghersi D, Simes RJ. The use of chemotherapy and endocrine therapy in the management of metastatic breast cancer: a series of systematic reviews. *Cancer Treat Rev* 2000;**26**:151–68.

118 Stockler MR, Wilcken NRC and Coates AS. Chemotherapy for metastatic breast cancer – when is enough enough? *Eur J Cancer* 1997;**33**:2147–8.

119 Tannock IF, Boyd NF, DeBoer G *et al.* A randomized trial of two dose levels of cyclophosphamide, methotrexate and fluorouracil chemotherapy patients with metastatic breast cancer. *J Clin Oncol* 1988;**6**:1377–87.

120 O'Shaughnessy J, Miles D, Vukelja S *et al.* Superior survival with capecitabine plus docetaxel combination therapy in anthracycline-pretreated patients with advanced breast cancer: phase III trial results. *J Clin Oncol* 2002;**20**:2812–23.

121 Mouridsen H, Gershanovich M, Sun Y *et al.* Superior efficacy of letrozole versus tamoxifen as first-line therapy for postmenopausal women with advanced breast cancer: results of a phase III study of the International Letrozole Breast Cancer Group. *J Clin Oncol* 2001;**19**:2596–606.

122 Nabholtz JM, Buzdar A, Pollak M *et al.* Anastrozole is superior to tamoxifen as first-line therapy for advanced breast cancer in postmenopausal women: results of a North American multicenter randomized trial. Arimidex Study Group. *J Clin Oncol* 2000;**18**: 3758–67.

123 Slamon DJ, Leyland-Jones B, Shak S *et al.* Use of chemotherapy plus a monoclonal antibody against HER2 for metastatic breast cancer that overexpresses HER2. *N Engl J Med* 2001;**344**:783–92.

124 Hornbuckle J, Wilcken N, Ghersi D. Chemotherapy alone versus endocrine therapy alone for metastatic breast cancer (Protocol for a Cochrane Review). In: Cochrane Collaboration. *Cochrane Library* Issue 4. Oxford: Update Software, 2000.

125 The Australian New Zealand Breast Cancer Trials Group. A randomized trial in postmenopausal patients with advanced breast cancer comparing endocrine and cytotoxic therapy given sequentially or in combination. *J Clin Oncol* 1986;**4**:186–93.

126 ATAC Trialists' Group (2002). Anastrozole alone or in combination with tamoxifen versus tamoxifen alone for adjuvant treatment of postmenopausal women with early breast cancer: first results of the ATAC randomised trial. *Lancet*;**359**:2131–9.

127 Klijn JGM, Beex L, Mauriac L *et al.* Combined treatment with Buserelin and Tamoxifen in premenopausal metastatic breast cancer: a randomized study. *J Natl Cancer Inst* 2000;**92**:903–11.

128 Klijn JGM, Blamey RW, Boccardo F *et al.* Combined tamoxifen and Luteinizing hormone-release hormone LHRH agonist versus LHRH agonist alone in premenopausal advanced breast cancer: a meta-analysis of four randomised trials. *J Clin Oncol* 2001;**19**:343–53.

129 Ackland SP, Gebski V, Wilson A *et al.* High dose epirubicin and cyclophosphamide with filgrastim versus standard dose epirubicin and cyclophosphamide in advanced breast cancer. *Proc Am Soc Clin Oncol* 2000 (Abstr. 288).

130 Fisher B, Anderson S, DeCillis A *et al.* Further evaluation of intensified and increased total dose of cyclophosphamide for the treatment of primary breast cancer: findings from National Surgical Adjuvant Breast and Bowel Project B-25. *J Clin Oncol* 1999;**17**: 3374–88.

131 Henderson IC, Berry D, Demetri C *et al.* Improved disease free survival and overall survival from the addition of sequential paclitaxel but not from the escalation of doxorubicin dose level in the adjuvant chemotherapy of patients with node-positive primary breast cancer. *Proc Am Soc Clin Oncol* 1999 (Abstr. 390A).

132 Farquhar C, Basser R. High dose chemotherapy and autologous bone marrow or stem cell transplantation versus conventional chemotherapy for women with metastatic breast cancer. In: *Cochrane Database of Systematic Reviews*, Issue 1. Oxford: Update Software, 2003.

133 Coates A, Byrne M, Bishop JF, Forbes JF. Intermittent versus continuous chemotherapy for breast cancer. *N Engl J Med* 1988;**318**:1468.

134 Priestman T, Baum M, Jones V, Forbes J. Treatment and survival in advanced breast cancer. *BMJ* 1978;**2**:1673–4.

135 Mackey JR, Paterson A, Dirix LY *et al.* Final results of the phase III randomised trial comparing TAC to FAC as first line chemotherapy for patients with metastatic breast cancer. *Proc Am Soc Clin Oncol* 2002 (Abstr. 137).

136 Green MC, Buzdar AU, Smith T *et al.* Weekly paclitaxel followed by FAC improves complete remission rates when compared to every three week paclitaxel followed by FAC. *Proc Am Soc Clin Oncol* 2002 (Abstr. 135).

137 Vogel CL, Cobleigh MA, Tripathy D *et al.* Efficacy and safety of trastuzumab as a single agent in first-line treatment of HER2-overexpressing metastatic breast cancer. *J Clin Oncol* 2002; **20**:719–26.

138 Pavlakis N. Stockler M. Bisphosphonates in breast cancer. *Cochrane Database of Systematic Reviews*, Issue 1. Oxford: Update Software, 2002.

139 Tominaga S, Kuroishi T, Aoki K. *Cancer mortality statistics in 33 countries 1953–1992*. Nayoya, Japan: Roppo Shupan Co. Ltd., 1998.

140 McPherson K, Steel Cm, Dixon JM. ABC of breast diseases: breast cancer – epidemiology, risk factors, and genetics. *BMJ* 2000;**321**:628.

# Section IX

## Treating skin cancer

*Hywel C Williams, Editor*

# Levels of evidence and grades of recommendation used in *Evidence-based Oncology*

Levels of evidence and grades of recommendation appear within the text in the clinical chapters, for example, **Evidence Level Ia** and **Grade A**.

## Levels of evidence

| | |
|---|---|
| Ia | Meta-analysis of randomised controlled trials (RCTs) |
| Ib | At least 1 RCT |
| IIa | At least 1 non-randomised study |
| IIb | At least 1 other well designed quasi-experimental study |
| III | Non-experimental, descriptive studies |
| IV | Expert committee reports or opinions/experience of respected authorities |

## Grades of recommendations

| | |
|---|---|
| A | At least one RCT as part of body of literature of overall good quality and consistency addressing recommendation **Evidence levels Ia, Ib** |
| B | No RCT but well conducted clinical studies available **Evidence levels IIa, IIb, III** |
| C | Expert committee reports or opinions/experience of respected authorities in the absence of directly applicable good quality clinical studies **Evidence level IV** |

From *Clinical Oncology* (2001)**13**:S212
Source of data: MEDLINE, *Proceedings of the American Society of Medical Oncology* (ASCO).

# 41 Cutaneous melanoma

*Dafydd Roberts, Thomas Crosby*

## Localised disease

### Background

Malignant melanomas (MM) of the skin arise from melanocytes within the epidermis. After a variable period of time the tumour becomes invasive and penetrates the underlying dermis and subcutaneous fat. Once this occurs the tumour has potential for distant metastatic spread. MM may also rarely arise from other areas of the body including meninges, retina, GI tract, nasopharyngeal epithelium and vagina.

### Incidence

The incidence of cutaneous malignant melanoma, particularly thin curable lesions, has increased steadily over the past 30 years in all Western countries and this has been accompanied by a similar but less marked increase in mortality.[1] Whilst mortality has continued to rise in most countries, recent reports from Scotland, Canada, Australia and Wales suggest that mortality rates may have levelled off or declined in some groups, notably in women.[2-5] This may have resulted from intensive public education campaigns leading to earlier detection of thinner lesions with a better prognosis. The prevention of MM is an important topic and is dealt with other skin cancers in Chapters 9 and 10 of this book. Early recognition of MM and surgical excision present the best opportunity for cure.

### Prognosis

The prognosis of MM is related to a number of factors including sex, tumour site and ulceration, but the single most important guide to prognosis is the Breslow thickness.[6] This is a measure of the depth of invasion of the tumour from the granular layer of the epidermis. Lesions which are confined to the epidermis have no metastatic potential, those which are less than 1 mm in depth have a very good prognosis with 5-year survival rates of approximately 95%, whereas tumours deeper than 4 mm may have survival rates of about 50%. The involvement of regional lymph nodes with metastases at presentation further reduces survival rates to 25–50%.[7]

### Diagnosis

The clinical diagnosis of classical MM is straightforward, but early changes may be subtle. Various clinical guides have been developed such as the ABCDE rule (A = asymmetry, B = irregular border, C = irregular colour, D = diameter > 5 mm and E = elevation), and the seven-point checklist which may be useful as reminders of the main features of MM on clinical examination and history. The main clinical features are of a pigmented lesion with an irregular edge and irregular pigmentation, over 95% of patients giving a history of change in size, shape, or colour, and fewer than 50% describing a change in sensation or bleeding of the lesion.[8,9] Dermatoscopy has gained ground as an aid to diagnosis but training and experience are required to maximise its usefulness.[10]

### Treatment objectives

The main aims of treatment are to detect the lesion as early as possible and to excise it with adequate margins without unnecessarily mutilating the patient. Outcomes measured usually include both disease-free survival (that is, until the first appearance of recurrence of the primary lesion or distant metastatic spread) and overall survival.

### Searches

MEDLINE was searched for the period 1966 to end of 2001. Citations found in review articles and other main articles found were also scrutinised for additional evidence.

### What is the place of a diagnostic incisional biopsy?

Occasionally pigmented lesions clinically suspicious of being an MM may be considered to be too large or in a difficult anatomical site for complete immediate excision without extensive surgery. There is therefore a dilemma for the clinician as to whether or not an incisional biopsy of the lesion may be needed to confirm the diagnosis before more extensive surgery. Also, providing the biopsy is taken from a representative area of the melanoma, an incisional biopsy provides an indication of the depth of invasion of the lesion, thereby assisting the planning of the next course of appropriate treatment. There is some concern based on empirical reasoning, that to take a biopsy of part of a malignant lesion might release some malignant cells into the bloodstream and local tissues, thereby worsening the eventual prognosis for that person.

## Efficacy

There have been no randomised controlled studies of incisional versus excisional surgery. Retrospective studies of large numbers of patients have reported different results. A large study in 1985 of 472 patients with stage I cutaneous MM reported on the survival rate with different modalities of surgery: 119 patients underwent an incisional or punch biopsy initially whereas 353 patients had their lesions excised. Survival in the two groups did not differ, regardless of the depth of invasion. Of 76 patients who had an incisional biopsy of a lesion less than 1·7 mm in depth, none died. In the intermediate thickness group (1·7 mm–3·64 mm) there was a 35% mortality rate compared with 18% in the excision group, and in the thick lesion group (> 3·65 mm) the mortality rates were respectively 64% and 50%. Cox regression analysis showed that the best predictors for outcome were tumour thickness and anatomical location but not biopsy type.[11] In a further study of 1086 patients followed up for 5 years, 96 of the patients underwent an incisional biopsy initially. The mortality was 48·9% in the incisional biopsy group (mean thickness 3·47 mm) and 39·2% in the wide excision group (mean thickness 2·77 mm) compared with 33·9% in the narrow margin group (mean thickness 2·34 mm). After correcting for tumour thickness there was no statistical difference in survival rates or local recurrence between those having an incisional biopsy and those who had their lesions fully excised initially.[12] A more recent and larger case–control study from Scotland of 5727 patients identified 265 patients who had undergone an incisional biopsy. These were matched to 496 controls. The survival analysis of time to recurrence and time to death revealed no difference between the groups.[13]

## Drawbacks

Incisional biopsies run the inherent risk of providing material that is not representative of the whole tumour, therefore errors may occur in assessing the depth of the tumour. One study reported that 38 of the 96 incisional biopsies on patients with cutaneous melanoma (40%) gave insufficient material to provide a full histological assessment of the lesion.[12] On the other hand, excising all pigmented lesions suspected of being a melanoma regardless of their site and size could lead to inappropriate surgery in some cases. One study reported the results of a retrospective series of patients with cutaneous melanoma limited to the head and neck; 159 patients were followed up for a median period of 38 months: 79 patients had their lesions fully excised, 48 had an incisional biopsy, and other procedures such shave excision or cryotherapy were carried out in a further 32; 31% of the patients who underwent an incisional biopsy died and 25% of the other biopsy group died, compared with 9% of those who had their lesions excised initially. As this was a retrospective study the initial surface area of the lesions was not known. There was no significant difference in the depth of invasion of the tumours or the sex of the patients between the three groups, but a significantly higher proportion of the patients in the incisional biopsy and other groups had ulcerated tumours compared with the excision group.[14]

## Comment

The evidence on incisional biopsy in MM remains controversial but the balance of observational evidence suggests that it is unlikely to influence prognosis adversely **Evidence level IIb, Grade B**. Large studies have shown that in general incisional biopsies do not affect prognosis, except for the single study of melanoma of the head and neck, where there was a significant worsening in the survival of patients who underwent an incisional biopsy, compared with those who had their lesions excised initially.[14] This study was, however, retrospective and no adjustment was made for ulceration of the tumours, which is known to worsen prognosis. Any future study should be prospective and the design of the study should ensure that study groups are randomised to balance for the various factors that may influence prognosis.

## What are the surgical recommendations for excision margins for different Breslow thickness tumours?

The Breslow thickness represents the depth of invasion of cutaneous melanoma and is measured histologically from the granular layer to the deepest melanoma cells. It is the single best indicator of prognosis in primary cutaneous malignant melanoma.[6] All of the trials so far performed in patients with malignant melanoma use the Breslow thickness of the tumour to categorise different patient groups. As a result of these trials surgical margins of excision of malignant melanoma have decreased significantly over the past 20 years.

## Efficacy

The recommendations for surgical margins are based on three randomised control trials and have included patients with lesions of Breslow thickness up to 5 mm. The World Health Organization Melanoma Group randomised 612 patients with melanomas less than 2 mm in depth to surgical excision with either 1 cm or 3 cm margins.[15] The mean follow up period was 90 months and there was no difference in overall or disease-free survival between the two groups. A US Intergroup Study randomised 486 patients with intermediate thickness lesions, 1–4 mm in depth, to either 2 cm or 4 cm margins.[16] The median follow up period was 6 years. The local recurrence rate was 0·8% for the 2 cm margin group and 1·7% for the 4 cm group. The overall survival rate over 5 years was 79·5% and 83·7%, respectively. The Swedish Melanoma Study Group randomised 769 patients with lesions of 0·8 mm to 2 mm in depth to either 2 cm or 5 cm margins and they have recently reported their long-term results with a median follow up period of 11 years.[17] The estimated relative hazard ratios for overall survival and relapse-free survival were 0·96 (95% CI 0·75–1·25) and 1·02 (95% CI 0·8–1·30) respectively. There was no significant difference in local recurrence rates or overall survival between the narrower and wider margins of excision in any of the trials.

A retrospective observational study of 278 patients with thick lesions (median thickness 6 mm) suggested that 2 cm margins were adequate and that wider margins did not improve local recurrence rates, disease-free survival, or overall survival rates.[18]

## Drawbacks

Excision with narrow surgical margins can often be performed in an outpatient setting, whereas larger margins may require skin grafting and inpatient treatment. The Word Health Organization study demonstrated that skin grafting could be reduced by 75% with the 1 cm versus the 3 cm margins.[15] Some concern was expressed in the Intergroup trial as three patients developed local recurrence as a first sign of relapse, all of whom had undergone a 1 cm excision margin for primary lesions between 1 and 2 mm in thickness.[16]

## Comment

The evidence that narrow surgical margins are as beneficial in terms of local recurrence and survival compared with more extensive surgical treatment is reasonably strong. The studies have suggested that lesions which are less than 1 mm in depth can be safely treated with surgical margins of 1 cm and those which are between 1 mm and 4 mm in depth can be safely treated with margins of 2 cm **Evidence level Ib, Grade A**. There is also evidence from one observational study that 2 cm margins are also sufficient for thicker tumours **Evidence level III, Grade B**.

Malignant melanomas less than 0·75 mm in depth have not been studied in any controlled trials and neither have thicker lesions greater than 4 mm in depth. Melanoma *in situ*, where the melanoma cells are confined to the epidermis, appear to have no potential for metastatic spread[19] and the current consensus view based on empirical reasoning is that it is safe to excise such lesions with a margin of 5 mm of clinically normal skin to obtain a clear histological margin **Evidence level IV, Grade C**.

## How should patients with lentigo maligna or lentigo maligna melanoma be managed?

Lentigo maligna (LM) is the premalignant phase of lentigo maligna melanoma (LMM) where the malignant melanocytes are entirely confined to the epidermis. These usually occur on sun-exposed sites such as the face and neck. There is usually a prolonged premalignant phase before dermal invasion and the development of LMM. Difficulties in management of these lesions occur for several reasons. Patients with these lesions tend to be elderly, with other comorbidities that may limit extensive surgery; the lesions themselves may be large and occur close to important anatomical structures and therefore full surgical excision with suitable margins may be difficult or even impossible, and histological changes within the epidermis may occur at some distance from the clinically obvious margins.[21]

## Efficacy

LM and LMM will be considered separately.

### Lentigo maligna

*Surgery.* There have been no randomised controlled trials of patients in this category. A comparative study of 42 cases of LM showed a recurrence rate of 9% (2/22) following surgical excision compared with a recurrence rate of 35% (7/20) with other techniques such as radiotherapy, curettage, and cryotherapy surgery, with a mean follow up period of 3·5 years (range 1 month to 11 years).[22] A further retrospective report of 38 cases of LM suggested cure rates of 91% (two recurrences) over a time period of 1–12 years (mean 3 years).[23] Mohs micrographic surgery has also been evaluated in small numbers of patients usually with excellent results being reported: 26 patients with LM were treated in one study with no recurrences after a median follow up of 58 months.[24]

*Cryotherapy.* There have been no randomised controlled trials of cryotherapy for the treatment of LM. One study of 30 patients reported recurrence rates of 6·6% (two patients) in a follow up period of 3 years. Eleven patients who were observed for more than 5 years had no recurrences.[25] A further study of 12 patients showed a recurrence rate of 8·3% over a follow up period of 51 months.[26]

*Radiotherapy.* There have been no randomised controlled trials of radiotherapy for LM. One case series reported two recurrences in 68 patients with a 5-year follow up.[27] A further study showed a cure rate of 94% in 18 patients with a follow up of 3 years in younger patients and a 86% cure rate in 36 patients at 5 years.[28]

*Other treatments.* There have been a few case reports on the use of various lasers in LM but the numbers are too small to be conclusive. A study of 5-fluorouracil cream showed 100% recurrence rate[29] and a similar study on Retin A showed no benefit.[30] Azelaic acid has been reported as giving a recurrence rate of 22% in 50 patients, all of whom subsequently cleared with retreatment.[31]

### Lentigo maligna melanoma

*Surgery.* Patients with LMM have not been included in any of the large randomised trials on surgical margins. However, it has been shown that the prognosis for patients with the invasive LMM is the same as that for any other type of melanoma when matched for thickness.[32] Patients with LMM were included in a case series of Mohs micrographic surgery, which found a 100% cure rate after 29 months and a 97% cure rate after 58 months.[24]

*Radiotherapy.* An uncontrolled follow up study of fractionated radiotherapy in both LM and LMM showed that of 64 patients with LM, none showed any signs of recurrence. Among 22 patients with LMM, who also had the nodular part of the lesion excised, there were two recurrences. The mean follow up period was 23 months.[33]

### Drawbacks

All of the treatment modalities including surgery, cryotherapy, radiotherapy and any other destructive treatment may result in scarring and no studies have compared the long-term scars with any other methods described. Cryotherapy may lead to inadequate destruction of melanocytes extending down hair follicles and there have been subsequent reports of recurrences, sometimes amelanotic in type, after cryotherapy of these lesions. No reports have compared the short-term discomfort, pain, or costs of these treatments.

### Comment

In the absence of any controlled trials, it is not surprising that a recent survey of British dermatologists has shown a wide variation in treatment modalities in use in the UK. An algorithm was devised on the basis of the current treatments for LM suggesting that surgical resection was the initial treatment of choice if possible, and Mohs surgery when the margins were unclear. For those lesions that are not amenable to surgical resection, radiotherapy or cryotherapy may be suitable choices. There is an absence of information on the rate of progression of LM, and in the very old and infirm observation only may be considered appropriate[34] **Evidence level IV, Grade C**. As the prognosis of LMM is the same as any other MM when matched for Breslow thickness the same surgical margins should be advised whenever possible until better evidence becomes available.

## Does elective lymph node dissection improve outcome?

There is some evidence to show that lymph node dissection is beneficial when performed in people with evidence of metastatic spread. However, there is still some controversy about the place of elective lymph node dissection where there are no clinically involved lymph nodes.

### Efficacy

Four randomised controlled trials have compared elective lymph node dissection with primary excision of the cutaneous lesion only. In all 1718 people with no clinical evidence of lymph node metastases have been entered into the studies. None of these studies showed an overall survival benefit in patients receiving elective lymph node dissection. However, an unplanned subset analysis found non-significant trends in favour of elective lymph node dissection in those with intermediate thickness tumours over the age of 60.[35–38]

### Drawbacks

Lymph node dissection is not without risk, lymphoedema being the commonest complication occurring in 20% in one study; temporary seroma occurred in 17%, wound infection in 9%, and wound necrosis in 3%.[39]

### Comment

In view of the lack of any clear benefits for elective lymph node dissection in the RCTs mentioned above, elective lymph node dissection has been largely abandoned in favour of sentinel lymph node biopsy, which is considered separately **Evidence level Ib, Grade A**.

## What is the role of sentinel lymph node biopsy?

The technique of sentinel lymph node biopsy (SLNB) involves the identification and biopsy of the first-station lymph node draining an affected area. It was pioneered in MM by Morton.[40]

The SLN is found by injecting blue dye and/or radiolabelled colloid into the skin surrounding the primary lesion. The technique enables the identification of patients with micrometastases affecting the regional lymph nodes and can successfully identify the sentinel node in up to 97% of cases. Patients so identified as having micrometastases are submitted to a therapeutic lymph node dissection.

The technique is well established and is reproducible.[41] It is now regarded as an excellent indicator of prognosis and has therefore been incorporated into the new American staging system for MM (AJCC staging). Gershenwald *et al.* demonstrated that of 500 patients who underwent SLNB, 85 (15%) were positive and 495 (85%) were negative. This study showed that SLN status was the most significant prognostic factor with respect to disease-free and disease-specific survival. Although tumour thickness and ulceration influenced survival in SLN-negative patients they provided no additional prognostic information in SLN-positive patients.[42] The psychological benefits of accurate staging for a patient have not been studied extensively, but one small questionnaire study of 110 patients did show a slight psychological benefit in those who underwent SNLB regardless of the result of the biopsy.[43]

### Efficacy

No RCTs of sentinel node biopsy accompanied by further treatment such as lymph node dissection or interferon therapy as an intervention (as opposed to SLNB as a pure staging procedure) could be found.

### Drawbacks

Patients who do not undergo SNLB are treated by wide excision of the primary cutaneous melanoma. The additional surgery therefore, entails some risk as general anaesthetic is usually necessary and there are also additional costs, although these are difficult to quantify. About 3% of patients developed a seroma, and a further 3% developed a wound infection in one report of SLNB.[44]

### Comment

SLNB is generally agreed to be useful as a staging procedure in patients with primary cutaneous melanoma, but no randomised trials have yet shown any therapeutic benefit in patients who have undergone SLNB

Evidence level Ib, Grade A. A randomised multicentre trial is now comparing survival after wide excision alone versus wide excision plus SLNB in patients with cutaneous melanoma equal to or greater than 1 mm in depth or Clark level IV. The trial has been underway for 5 years and 11 000 patients had already been recruited by 1999.[41] There are additional potential benefits of accurate staging if adjuvant treatments such as interferon prove to be of value in patients with positive results.

## Are there any effective adjuvant treatments?

Once patients with MM develop distant metastatic disease the prognosis is poor. Therefore there is a need to investigate additional or adjuvant treatments that can be given either after primary tumour resection in those with thicker lesions, who appear to have non-metastatic disease, or after regional lymph node resection in those with established metastatic disease.

The role of adjuvant treatments mainly in the form of interferon alfa is still controversial. Interferon alfa has a biologically modifying effect on MM as shown in several studies, but the effect on overall survival has been variable. Side effects are a major problem with patients receiving high dose interferon alfa.

### Efficacy

Trials have studied the role of interferon alfa in high and low dosage regimens.

#### High dose studies

An early RCT of high dose treatment (20 MU of interferon alfa 2B intravenously daily for 1 month, followed by 10 MU three times weekly for 11 months) in 287 people with lesions greater than 4 mm in depth at presentation showed a significant improvement in disease-free and overall survival compared with those receiving no additional treatment. The overall survival in the treated group was 3·1 years compared with 2·8 years treated with surgery alone.[45] In a second and larger study of 642 patients, however, there was no difference in the overall survival of patients with either high dose or low dose interferon alfa compared with no further therapy.[46] A very recent study from the same authors compared high dose interferon alfa 2B with vaccine treatment (GM2-KLH/QS-21) in patients with resected stage IIB–III melanoma of the skin[47]: 880 patients were randomised equally between the two groups and the trial demonstrated a significant treatment benefit for those receiving interferon alfa 2B in both relapse-free survival (hazard ratio = 1·47; CI 1·14–1·90; $P = 0.0015$) and overall survival (hazard ratio = 1·52; CI 1·07–2·15; *P* = 0·009). There was no control (observation only) arm so a direct comparison with no adjuvant treatment could not be made, but the outcome for patients receiving the vaccine seemed to be no worse than for similar patients receiving observation based on comparisons with the observation arm of previous adjuvant trials carried out. This study therefore seems to have confirmed the relapse-free survival and overall survival benefits of high dose interferon reported earlier.[45]

### Low dose treatment

To date two clinical trials have used low dose interferon (3 MU three times weekly subcutaneously) in patients presenting with lesions greater than 1·5 mm in depth but with negative lymph nodes. In the first trial of 499 patients this regimen was continued for 18 months compared with surgery alone. There was a significant extension of the relapse-free interval and a trend towards extension of overall survival.[48] The second trial randomised 311 patients to receive treatment for 12 months versus observation only, following surgical removal of melanoma. At 41 months relapse-free survival was prolonged but overall survival was not.[49]

## Drawbacks

Toxicity and withdrawal rates have been high in the high dose interferon studies. In one study there were two treatment-related deaths. In the latest study 10% of patients discontinued treatment because of adverse advents, but there were no treatment-related deaths. The commonest side effects in patients receiving interferon alfa 2B at high dosage was fatigue (20%), granulocytopenia/leucopenia (50%), liver abnormalities and neurological toxicity in about 30%.

In the low dose treatment trials about 10% of people suffered significant toxicity as well as the milder nausea and 'flu-like illness experienced by most patients on the day of treatment.

## Comment

From the information provided by the most recent trial, interferon alfa 2B is the most effective adjuvant treatment now available with significantly improved prolongation in relapse-free survival and overall survival compared with vaccine therapy in patients with resected high risk melanoma. The rate of severe or very severe side effects is high, and further studies are now underway combining interferon alfa 2B with other peptide vaccines as well as with polychemotherapy plus interleukin-2. Low dose interferon alfa 2B may also have a disease-modifying effect, but as yet no benefit on overall survival has been shown. Treatment with interferon is expensive and attempts have

been made to perform economic analyses of the different regimens used. In an analysis of the high dose regime the estimated cost per life-year gained was US $13 700 over 35 years and US $32 600 over 10 years, whereas the low dose treatment cost per life-year gained was estimated to be approximately US $1700 over a lifetime and US $6600 over 10 years. These were thought to be comparable costs to many other oncological treatments.[50,51]

### Key points

- The incidence of cutaneous malignant melanoma continues to rise worldwide but there is evidence of a levelling off of mortality in some groups as patients are presenting earlier.
- Incisional biopsy of a melanoma does not in general alter the prognosis adversely but may lead to problems in interpreting the histology.
- The main treatment for primary melanoma of the skin is surgical excision.
- There is good evidence from RCTs that the narrower margins used over the past 20 years are safe.
- All of the treatments used for LM and LMM have poor evidence to support them and well organised RCTs are needed in this area. Surgical excision probably represents the best treatment on current evidence.
- Elective lymph node dissection of uninvolved nodes does not improve prognosis in most patient groups.
- Sentinel lymph node biopsy is a useful staging tool but there is no evidence as yet that it improves overall survival.
- Interferons used as adjuvant treatments can benefit some patient groups with MM, but further information is needed to clarify the optimum usage of this treatment.

## References

1 Armstrong BK, Kicker A. Cutaneous melanoma. *Cancer Surv* 1994;**19–20**:219–40.
2 Mackie RM, Hole D, Hunter JA *et al.* Cutaneous malignant melanoma in Scotland: incidence survival and mortality 1979–1994. *BMJ* 1997;**315**:1117–21.
3 Giles GG, Armstrong BK, Burton RC *et al.* Has mortality from melanoma stopped rising in Australia. Analysis of trends between 1931 and 1994. *BMJ* 1996;**312**:1121–5.
4 National Cancer Institute of Canada. *Canadian Cancer Statistics 1997*. Toronto: NCIC, 1997.
5 Holme SA. Malinovsky K, Roberts DL. Malignant melanoma in South Wales: changing trends in presentation (1986–98). *Clin Exper Derm* 2001;**26**:484–9.
6 Breslow A. Thickness, cross sectional areas and depth of invasion in the prognosis of cutaneous melanoma. *Ann Surg* 1970;**172**:902–8.
7 Balch CM, Soong SJ, Shaw HM *et al.* An analysis of prognostic factors in 8500 patients with cutaneous melanoma. In: Balch CM, Houghton

Anilton GW, Sober AL, Soong S, eds. *Cutaneous Melanoma, 2nd edn.* New York: Ellis Horwood, 1992.

8   Friedmann RJ, RigelDS, Silverman M, Kopf AW. The continued importance of the early detection of malignant melanoma. *CA Cancer J Clin* 1991;**41**:201–2.

9   Healsmith MF, Bourke JF, Osborne JE, Graham Brown RAC. An evaluation of the revised seven-point checklist for the diagnosis of cutaneous malignant melanoma. *Br J Dermatol* 1994;**130**:48–50.

10  Nachbar F, Stolz W, Merkle T *et al.* The ABCD rule of dermatoscopy. High prospective value in the diagnosis of doubtful melanocytic skin lesions. *J Acad Dermatol* 1994;**30**:4:551–9.

11  Lederman JS. Sober AJ. Does biopsy type influence survival in clinical stage I cutaneous melanoma. *J Am Acad Dermatol* 1985;**13**:983–7.

12  Lees VC. Briggs JC. Effect of an initial biopsy on prognosis in stage I invasive cutaneous malignant melanoma; review of 1086 patients. *Br J Surg* 1991;**71**:1108–10.

13  Bong JL, Herd RM, Hunter JAA. Incisional biopsy and melanoma prognosis. *J Am Acad Dermatol* 2002;**46**:690–4.

14  Austin JR, Byers RM, Brown WD. Wolf P. Influence on biopsy on the prognosis of cutaneous melanoma of the head and neck. *Head Neck* 1996;**18**:107–17.

15  Veronesi U, Cascinelli N. Narrow excision (1 cm margin); a safe procedure for thin cutaneous melanoma. *Arch Surg* 1991;**126**:438–41.

16  Balch CM, Urist MM, Karakousis CP *et al.* Efficacy of 2 cm surgical margins for intermediate – thickness melanomas (1–4 mm): result of a multi-institutional randomised surgical trial. *Ann Surg* 1993;**218**:262–7.

17  Cohn-Cedermark G, Rutqvist LE, Andersson R *et al.* Long term results of a randomised study by the Swedish Melanoma Study Group on 2 cm versus 5 cm resection margins for patients with cutaneous melanoma with a tumour thickness of 0·8 mm–2·0 mm. *Cancer* 2000;**89**:1495–501.

18  Heaton KM, Sussman JJ, Gershanwald JE *et al.* Surgical margins and prognostic factors in patients with thick(> 4 mm) primary melanoma. *Ann Surg Oncol* 1998;**5**:322–8.

19  Guerry IV D, Synnestvedt M, Elder DE, Schultz D. Lessons from tumour progression; the invasive radial growth phase of melanoma is common, incapable of metastasis, and indolent. *J Invest Dermatol* 1993;**100**:3428–55.

20  Sober AJ, Tsu-yi Chang, Duvic M *et al.* Guidelines of care for primary cutaneous melanoma. *J Am Acad Dermatol* 2001;**45**:579–86.

21  Mackie RM. Melanocytic naevi and malignant melanoma. In Rook, Wilkinson and Ebling. *Textbook of Dermatology, Vol 2: 6th edn.* Oxford: Blackwell Science 1998.

22  Pitman GH, Kopf AW, Bart RS *et al.* Treatment of lentigo maligna and lentigo maligna melanoma. *J Dermatol Surg Oncol* 1979;**5**:727–37.

23  Coleman WP III, Davis RS, Reed RJ *et al.* Treatment of lentigo maligna and lentigo maligna melanoma. *J Dermatol Surg Oncol* 1980;**6**:476–9.

24  Cohen LM, McCall MW, Zax RH. Mohs' micrographic surgery for lentigo maligna and lentigo maligna melanoma: a follow up study. *Dermatol Surg* 1998;**24**:673–7.

25  Kufflik EG, Gage AA. Cryosurgery for lentigo maligna. *J Am Acad Dermatol* 1994;**31**:75–8.

26  Bohler-Sommerregger K, Schuller-Petrovic S, Knobner R *et al.* Reactive lentiginous hyperpigmentation after cryosurgery for lentigo maligna. *J Am Acad Dermatol* 1992;**27**:523–6.

27  Arma-Szlachcic M, Ott F, Storck H. Zur Strahlentherapie der melanotischen *Pracancerosen. Hautartz* 1970;**21**:505–8.

28  Tsang RW, Liu F, Wells W, Payne DG. Lentigo maligna of the head and neck; results of treatment by radiotherapy. *Arch Dermatol* 1994;**130**:1008–12.

29  Litwin MS, Kremetz ET, Mansell PW, Reed RJ. Topical treatment of lentigo maligna with 5-fluorouracil. *Cancer* 1995;**3**:721–33.

30  Rivers JK, McCarthy WH. No effect of topical tretinoin in lentigo maligna (letter). *Arch Dermatol* 1991;**127**:129.

31  Nazzoro-Porro M, Passi S, Zina G *et al.* Ten years' experience of treating lentigo maligna with topical azelaic acid. *Acta Dermatol Venereol* 1989;**143**(Suppl.):49–57.

32  Cox NH, Aitchision TC, Sirel JM, MacKie RM. Comparison between lentigo maligna melanoma and other histogenic types of malignant melanoma of the head and neck. Scottish Melanoma Group. *Br J Cancer* 1996;**73**:940–4.

33  Schmid-Wendtner MH, Brunner B, Konz B *et al.* Fractionated radiotherapy of lentigo maligna and lentigo maligna melanoma in 64 patients. *J Am Acad Dermatol* 2000;**43**:477–82.

34  Mahendran R, Newton-Bishop JA. Survey of UK current practice in the treatment of lentigo maligna. *Br J Dermatol* 2001;**144**:71–6.

35  Balch CN, Soong SJ, Bartolucci AA *et al.* Efficacy of an elective regional lymph node dissection of 1–4 mm thick melanomas for patients 60 years of age and younger. *Ann Surg* 1996;**224**:225–263.

36  Cascinelli N, Moradite A, Santinorrii M *et al.* Immediate or delayed dissection of regional nodes in patients with melanoma of the trunk: a randomised trial. WHO melanoma programme. *Lancet* 1998;**351**:793–6.

37  Sim PH, Taylor WF, Ivins JC *et al.* A prospective randomised study of the efficacy of routine elective lymphadenectomy in management of malignant melanoma: preliminary results. *Cancer* 1978;**41**:948–56.

38  Veronesi U, Adamus J, Bandiera DC *et al.* Inefficacy of immediate node dissection in stage I melanoma of the limbs. *N Engl J Med* 1977;**297**:627–30.

39  Baas PC, Schrafferdt KH, Koops H *et al.* Groin dissection in the treatment of lower extremity melanoma: short term and long term morbidity. *Arch Surg* 1992;**127**:281–6.

40  Morton DL, Wen D-R, Wong JH *et al.* Technical details of intra-operative lymphatic mapping for early stage melanoma. *Arch Surg* 1992;**127**:392–9.

41  Morton DL, Thompson JF, Essner R *et al.* Validation of the accuracy of intra-operative lymphatic mapping and sentinel lymphadenectomy for early-stage melanoma. *Ann Surg* 1999;**230**:453–65.

42  Gershenwald JE, Thompson W, Mansfield PF *et al.* Multi-institutional melanoma lymphatic mapping experience: the prognostic value of sentinel lymph node status in 612 stage 1 or 11 melanoma patients. *J Clin Oncol* 1999;**17**:976–83.

43  Rayatt SS, Hettiaratchy SP. Having this biopsy gives psychological benefits. *BMJ* 2000;**321**:1285.

44  Jansen L, Nieweg OE, Peterse JL, Hoefnagel CA, Ohnos RA, Kroon BBR. Reliability of sentinel lymph node biopsy for staging melanoma. *Br J Surg* 2000;**87**:484–9.

45  Kirkwood JM, Strawderman MH, Ernstoff MS *et al.* Interferon Alfa-2b adjuvant therapy of high risk resected cutaneous melanoma: The Eastern Co-operative Oncology Group Trial. EST. 1684. *J Clin Oncol* 1996;**14**:7–17.

46  Kirkwood JM, Ibrahim JG, Sondak VK *et al.* High- and low-dose interferon alfa-2b in high-risk melanoma: first analysis of Intergroup trial 1690/S9111/C9190. *J Clin Oncol* 2000;**18**:2444–58.

47  Kirkwood JM, Ibrahim JG, Sosman JA *et al.* High-dose Interferon alfa 2b significantly prolongs relapse-free and overall survival compared with the GM2-KLH/QS-21 vaccine in patients with resected stage IIb-III melanoma: results of Intergroup trial E1694/S9512/C509801. *J Clin Oncol* 2001;**19**:2370–80.

48  Grob JJ, Dreno B, de la Salmoniere P *et al.* Randomised trial of Interferon Alpha–2b as adjuvant therapy in resected primary melanoma thicker than 1·5 mm without clinically detectable node metastases. French Co-operative Group on Melanoma. *Lancet.* 1998;**351**:1905–10.

49  Perhamberger H, Peter Soyer H, Steiner A *et al.* Adjuvant interferon alfa-2b in resected primary stage II cutaneous melanoma. *J Clin Oncol* 1998;**16**:1425–9.

50  Hillner BE, Kirkwood JM, Atkins MB, Johnson ER, Smith TJ. Economic analysis of adjuvant interferon Alfa-2B in high risk melanoma based on projections from Eastern Cooperative Oncology Group 1684. *J Clin Oncol* 1997;**15**:2351–8.

51  Lafuma A, Dreno B, Delauney M *et al.* Economic analysis of adjuvant therapy with interferon alpha-2a in stage II malignant melanoma. *Eur J Oncol* 2001;**37**:369–75.

# Metastatic malignant melanoma

Metastatic, or stage IV, malignant melanoma is a devastating disease. It is defined by dissemination of the cutaneous tumour to other organs or non-regional lymph nodes. The skin, subcutaneous tissues and lymph nodes are the first site of metastatic disease in 59% of patients. When haematogenous spread to liver, bone and brain occurs, the natural history is that of one of the most aggressive of all malignant diseases **Evidence level III** .

Of all patients with metastatic disease, the median survival is approximately 7 months: 25% will be alive after 1 year and only 5% of patients will be alive 5 years after diagnosis. Patients with a higher performance status (a numerical measure of physical fitness) and women have a better prognosis ($P = 0.001$ and $0.056$ respectively)[1,2] **Evidence level III** . Survival is also better in patients with a longer duration of remission after primary disease, fewer metastatic sites involved, and in those with non-visceral disease (Table 41.1) **Evidence level III** .

The intention of treatment remains palliative in all but a few patients. A patient who is fit enough to tolerate systemic therapy will often choose active therapy despite the modest responses seen with such treatment. The aim of therapy should clearly be to optimise a patient's quality of survival, and therefore must take into account the morbidity and convenience of therapy.

## Is there a preferred systemic therapy in metastatic melanoma?

### Efficacy

A systematic review found no RCTs testing systemic therapy against best supportive care.[3] It is doubtful that such a trial will ever be done given that there is great deal of evidence for albeit modest activity in patients with advanced disease.

**Table 41.1  Median survival in patients with metastatic melanoma**

| Prognostic factor | Median survival (months) |
| --- | --- |
| *Number of metastatic sites* | |
| One | 7 |
| Two | 4 |
| Three | 2 |
| *Site of metastatic disease* | |
| Cutaneous, nodes | 12·5 |
| Lung | 11 |
| Brain, liver, bone | 2–6 |

**Box 41.1 Usual schedule for dacarbazine**

- Intravenous 850–1000 mg m$^{-2}$ day 1 every 3 weeks

or

- 200 mg m$^{-2}$ days 1–5 every 4 weeks
- Given with intravenous or oral 5HT–3 antagonists/ dexamethasone as antiemetics

Dacarbazine (DTIC, di-methyl triazeno imidazole carboxamide) has been the most tested single chemotherapeutic agent. With current antiemetics, it is well tolerated and is considered by many to be the "gold standard", against which other therapies should be tested[4–7] **Evidence level IIa** . When used alone it gives partial response rates of ~20% (> 50% regression for at least 4 weeks), complete responses (complete regression of measurable disease for at least 4 weeks) in 5–10%, and long-term remissions in less than 2% of patients. It is usually scheduled as in Box 41.1.

Temozolamide is a novel oral alkylating agent with a broad spectrum of antitumour activity, but with 100% oral bioavailability and good penetration of the blood–brain barrier and CSF. Its efficacy is at least equal to that of dacarbazine in metastatic MM, median survival being 7·7 months with temozolamide and 6·4 months with dacarbazine (hazard ratio 1·18; 95% CI 0.92–1.52), and with improvement in some parameters of quality of life (QoL)[8] **Evidence level Ib** . Given its similar mechanism of action, it is not surprising that response rates are fairly similar but, in a disease with such a poor prognosis, ease of administration and QoL are clearly very important.

### Drawbacks

The dose-limiting toxicities with such regimens are marrow suppression and nausea/vomiting, requiring admission or threatening life, in 20% and 5% of patients, respectively.[9,10] **Evidence level III** .

## Does combination chemotherapy help?

### Efficacy

Many other drugs such as platinum agents, vinca alkaloids, nitrosoureas, and, more recently, taxanes have been tried alone and in various combination regimens. Higher response rates have been claimed for some of these, but it remains unclear whether they offer significant improvement in quantitative or qualitative outcome over single-agent therapy. An example of the false promise of such combinations was seen when a response rate of 55%

**Table 41.2  Survival in patients on dacarbazine compared with Dartmouth regimen**

|  | Response rate (%) | Median survival (months) | 1-year survival (%) |
|---|---|---|---|
| Dacarbazine | 9·9 | 7·7 months (95% CI 6·3–8·9) | 27 |
| Dartmouth regimen | 16·8 | 6·3 months (95% CI 5·4–8·7) | 22 |

was reported for the combination of dacarbazine, cisplatin, carmustine and tamoxifen[11] **Evidence level Ib** . This has become known as the Dartmouth regimen. However a multicentred randomised trial comparing this regimen with single agent dacarbazine found no survival advantage and only a small, non-significant increase in tumour response in an intention-to-treat analysis (Table 41.2)[9] **Evidence level Ib** .

**Drawbacks**

Bone marrow suppression, nausea/vomiting and fatigue were significantly more common with the combined therapy[9] **Evidence level III** .

**Comment**

Combination therapies should not be used routinely outside the context of clinical trials **Grade B** .

**Do hormonal therapies help?**

**Efficacy**

Tamoxifen, an oestrogen receptor blocking agent widely used to treat breast cancer, has also been used, usually together with cytotoxic agents, and may modify the disease response to such drugs. An early study in 117 patients suggested a benefit for the addition of tamoxifen to single agent dacarbazine (response rates 28% $v$ 12%, $P = 0·03$, median survival 48 weeks $v$ 29 weeks, $P = 0·02$)[12] **Evidence level Ia** . Again, this was not confirmed in a four arm study in 258 patients with metastatic malignant melanoma. Response rates for patients receiving tamoxifen were 19% (95% CI 12–26) and 18% in the non-tamoxifen group (95% CI 12–25)[13] **Evidence level Ib** .

**Drawbacks**

Antioestrogens can cause hot flushes, thromboembolic events, pulmonary embolism and endometrial cancer.

**Comment**

There is no consistent evidence to suggest a benefit for hormonal therapy **Grade A** .

**Does immunotherapy help either used alone or with cytotoxic therapy?**

The immune system is important in metastatic melanoma, as evidenced by lymphoid infiltration into tumour and surrounding tissues, and well reported spontaneous remissions[4,5,7,14] **Evidence level III** . This has led to attempts to modulate the immunological environment of tumours, usually by the use of cytokines, especially interferon alfa[15] and interleukin-2,[16] given directly or by gene therapy. This has improved outcomes in other tumours.[17] Such therapy has single agent response rates of 15–20% and it has been suggested that such therapy produces a higher rate of durable remissions[15] **Evidence level III** .

**Efficacy**

One meta-analysis has compared single agent dacarbazine versus combination chemotherapy with or without immunotherapy in metastatic melanoma.[18] Twenty randomised controlled trials were found comprising 3273 patients. Although the addition of interferon alfa increased the response rate by 53% over dacarbazine alone, and dacarbazine combination therapy by 33% over single agent therapy, there was no overall survival advantage for combination treatment.

**Drawbacks**

Interferons commonly cause malaise, fevers and 'flu-like symptoms. High dose interferon alfa causes significant (> grade 3) myelosuppression in 24% of people, hepatotoxicity in 15% (including 2 deaths), and neurotoxicity in 28%.[19] With low dose interferon, 10% of people suffered significant toxicity[20] **Evidence level III** .

**Comment**

Outside clinical trials, it is difficult to justify the additional toxicity with these complex regimens **Grade A** .

**Implications for clinical practice**

Treatment remains unsatisfactory. Response rates, which often appear encouraging in single centre, single arm studies have to date been very disappointing when tested in larger, multicentre randomised trials. Responses are usually partial (approximately 10–25% of patients), rarely complete (less than 10%), and are of short duration (median overall survival approximately 6 months).

Outside clinical trials standard therapy should remain single agent dacarbazine, with temozolamide for selected patients **Grade A** .

## References

1 Balch CM, Reintgen DS, Kirkwood JM *et al.* Cutaneous melanoma. In: DeVita VT Jr, Hellman S, Rosenberg SA, eds. *Cancer: Principles and practice of oncology, 5th edn.* Philadelphia: Lippincot-Raven, 1997.

2 Unger JM, Flaherty LE, Liu PY *et al.* Gender and other survival predictors in patients with metastatic melanoma on Southwest Oncology Group Trials. *Cancer* 2001;**91**:1148–55.

3 Crosby T, Fish R, Coles B *et al.* Systemic treatments for metastatic cutaneous melanoma. *Cochrane Database Syst Rev* Issue 2. 2000;CD001215.

4 Balch CM, Houghton AN, Peters LJ. Cutaneous melanoma. DeVita VT Jr, Hellman S, Rosenberg SA, eds. *Cancer: Principles and practice of oncology, 4th edn.* Philadelphia: Lippincot-Raven, 1993.

5 Cascinelli N, Clemente C and Belli F. Cutaneous melanoma. In: Peckham M, Pinedo HM, Veronesi U, eds. *Oxford Textbook of Oncology.* Oxford: Oxford University Press 1995.

6 Pritchard KI, Quirt IC, Cowman DH *et al.* DTIC therapy in metastatic malignant melanoma: A simplified dose schedule. *Cancer Treat Rep* 1980;**64**:1123–6.

7 Taylor A and Gore M. Malignant melanoma. In: Price P, Sikora K, eds. *Treatment of Cancer, 3rd edn.* London: Chapman and Hall Medical, 1995.

8 Middleton MR, Grob JJ, Aaronson N *et al.* Randomised phase III study of temozolamide versus dacarbazine in the treatment of patients with advanced metastatic malignant melanoma. *J Clin Oncol* 2000; **18**:158–66.

9 Chapman PB, Einhorn LH, Meyers ML *et al.* Phase III multicenter randomised trial of the Dartmouth regimen versus dacarbazine in patients with metastatic melanoma. *J Clin Oncol* 1999;**17**:2745–51.

10 Falkson CI, Falkson G, Falkson HC. Improved results with the addition of interferon alfa-2b to dacarbazine in the treatment of patients with metastatic malignant melanoma. *J Clin Oncol* 1991; **9**:1403–8.

11 Del prete SA, Maurer LF, O'Donnell J *et al.* Combination chemotherapy with cisplatin, carmustine, dacarbazine, and tamoxifen in metastatic melanoma. *Cancer Treat Rep* 1984;**68**:1403–5.

12 Cocconi G, Bella M, Calabresi F *et al.* Treatment of metastatic malignant melanoma with dacarbazine plus tamoxifen. *N Engl J Med* 1992;**327**:516–23.

13 Falkson CI, Ibrahim J, Kirkwood JM, Coates AS, Atkins MB, Blum RH. Phase III trial of dacarbazine versus dacarbazine with interferon-alpha 2b versus dacarbazine with tamoxifen versus dacarbazine with interferon-alpha 2b and tamoxifen in patients with metastatic malignant melanoma: An Eastern Cooperative Oncology Group Study. *J Clin Oncol* 1998;**16**:1743–51.

14 Rosenberg SA, Yang JC, Topalian SL *et al.* Treatment of 283 consecutive patients with metastatic melanoma or renal cell cancer using high-dose bolus interleukin-2. *JAMA* 1994;**271**:907–13.

15 Legha SS. The role of interferon alfa in the treatment of metastatic melanoma. *Semin Oncol* 1997;**24**:S24–31.

16 Legha SS, Gianin MA, Plager C *et al.* Evaluation of interleukin-2 administered by continuous infusion in patients with metastatic melnoma. *Cancer* 1996;**77**:89–96.

17 Atzpodien J, Kirchner H, Franzke A *et al.* Results of a randomised clinical trial comparing SC interleukin-2, SC alpha-2a-interferon, and IV bolus 5-fluorouracil against oral tamoxifen in progressive metastatic renal cell carcinoma patients. *Proc Am Assoc Clin Oncol* 1997; **16**:326.

18 Huncharek M, Caubet JF, McGarry R. Single agent DTIC versus combination chemotherapy with or without imunotherapy in metastatic melanoma: a meta-analysis of 3273 patients from 20 randomised trials. *Melanoma Res* 2001;**11**:75–81.

19 Kirkwood JM, Strawderman MH, Erstoff MS *et al.* Interferon alfa-2b adjuvant therapy of high-risk resected cutaneous melanoma: The Eastern Cooperative Oncology Group trial EST 1684. *J Clin Oncol* 1996;**14**:7–17.

20 Kleeberg UR, Brocker EB, Lejeune F. Adjuvant trial in melanoma patients comparing rIFN-alfa to rIFN-gamma to Iscador to a control group after curative resection high risk primary or regional lymph node metastasis (EORTC 18871). *Eur J Cancer* 1999;**35** (Suppl. 4):S82.

# 42 Treatment of basal cell carcinoma

*Fiona Bath, William Perkins*

## Background

### Definition

Basal cell carcinoma (BCC) is defined as a slow-growing, locally invasive malignant epidermal skin tumour that mainly affects Caucasians.[1]

### Incidence/prevalence

BCC (or rodent ulcer) is the most common malignant cutaneous neoplasm found in humans.[1–3] For example, over 30 000 new cases are reported each year in the UK. This is likely to be an underestimate because of inconsistencies in registration of BCC at Regional Cancer Registries.[4] Many registries only register a person's first skin cancer, thus further underestimating the real burden of the problem. The tumour may occur at any age but the incidence of BCC increases markedly after the age of 40. The incidence of BCC appears to be increasing in younger people, probably as a result of increased sun exposure.[5] The incidence rate (standardised using the European standard population) for new BCCs in the Trent Cancer Registry (UK) increased from 36·8 in 1985 to 71·3 in 2000 for men, and from 25·6 to 52·0 in women (Trent Cancer Registry, written communication, September 2001). A total of 3826 new BCCs were registered in Trent in 2000 (80% of all non-melanoma skin cancers). A sustained rise in the incidence of BCC has been documented using a validated register in South Wales, UK.[6] Reliable national figures for BCC incidence are impossible to obtain because some cancer registries in the UK do not register BCCs. In America, the incidence of BCC has doubled approximately every 14 years[7] and similar changes have occurred in Australia.[8]

### Aetiology

Eighty-five per cent of all BCCs appear on the head and neck region.[9,10] Risk factors are fair skin, tendency to freckle,[11] degree of sun exposure,[12–14] excessive sunbed use, radiotherapy, phototherapy, male gender and a genetic predisposition.[15] Naevoid BCC syndrome (Gorlin syndrome) is an autosomal dominantly inherited condition characterised by developmental abnormalities and the occurrence of

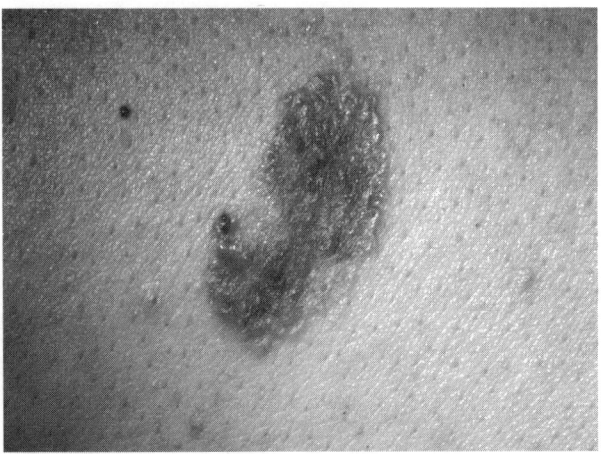

**Figure 42.1** Superficial basal cell carcinoma

multiple BCCs. Mutations in patients with naevoid BCC syndrome has been found on the patched gene located on chromosome 9, which appears to be crucial for proper embryonic development and for tumour suppression.[16]

### Clinical patterns

As shown, clinical appearances and morphology for BCC are diverse. They include superficial (Figure 42.1), nodular (Figure 42.2), cystic, ulcerated (rodent ulcer), morphoeic (scarring) (Figure 42.3), keratotic and pigmented variants. Nodular BCC is the most common type (60%) in the UK. However, in other countries such as Australia, superficial BCC is the most common type.[17] Because BCCs appear on visible areas such as the head and neck region, a good cosmetic and functional result is important.

### Prognosis

Growth of BCC is a localised phenomenon in people with a competent immune system. BCCs tend to infiltrate surrounding tissues in a three-dimensional fashion through the irregular extension of finger-like outgrowths, which may not be apparent clinically.[3,18] If left untreated, or if they are inadequately treated, the BCC can cause extensive local tissue destruction, particularly on the face. Neglected cases

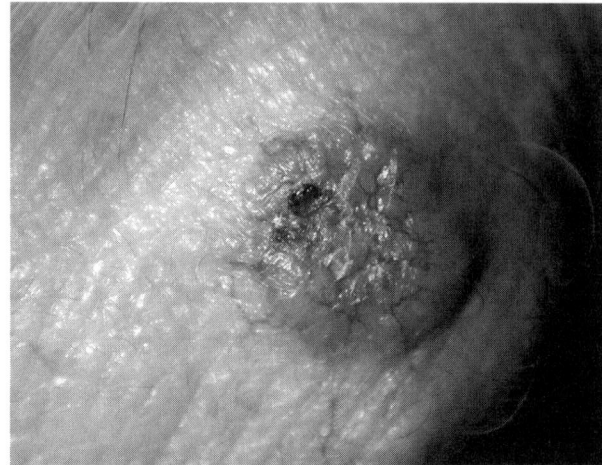

**Figure 42.2**  Nodular basal cell carcinoma

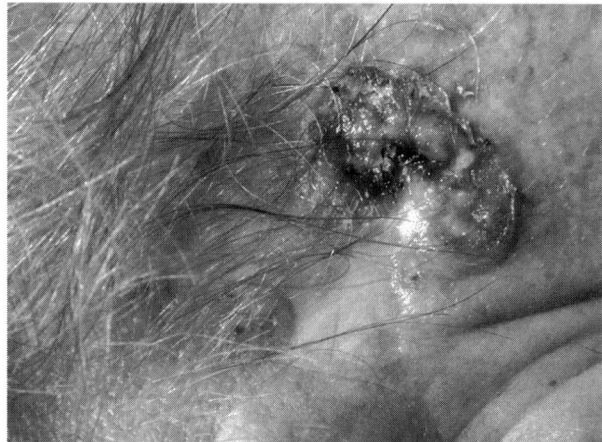

**Figure 42.3**  Morphoeic basal cell carcinoma

may even infiltrate bone and deeper structures such as the brain and cause death.[19] Death from BCC is extremely rare, but may occur in neglected cases and/or those with major underlying immunosuppression. The clinical course of BCC is unpredictable. It can remain small for years with little tendency to grow, it may grow rapidly, or it may proceed by successive spurts of extension of tumour and partial regression.[20] Histological subtype (infiltrative, micronodular, or morphoeic patterns), initial diameter and male sex have recently been shown to be the best independent predictors of BCC invasion.[21] It is unknown whether the phenotypic characterstics of people who present with clusters of BCCs or those who develop BCCs on truncal sites are also associated with increased growth once a BCC has established.

## Diagnostic tests

The diagnosis is usually made clinically with histological confirmation being made at the time of the intended

definitive treatment, often surgical removal. Diagnostic biopsies are usually performed prior to treatments such as radiotherapy.

## Aims of treatment

The three fundamental principles of treatment are to:

- eradicate the tumour
- preserve function
- produce an excellent or acceptable cosmetic result.

From a patient's perspective, the treatment should result in as little distress as possible in terms of pain, number of hospital visits and scarring. From a health provider's perspective, it is important to balance efficacy against cost.

## Relevant outcomes

Clearance of the lesion is measured by early treatment failure within 6 months; long-term recurrence of the lesion is measured at 3–5 years, since this is what would happen in practice. Adverse effects are measured in terms of atrophy, scarring, changes in pigmentation and discomfort to the patient in terms of pain during treatment and afterwards.

## Questions

This chapter addresses the following issues.

- What are the effective therapeutic interventions for BCC of the skin?
- How do the therapeutic interventions for BCC compare to each other?
- How do the cosmetic outcomes for these interventions compare?
- Are these interventions cost-effective?

There are multiple interventions – these are discussed individually together with sections on comparisons of different treatments.

## Treatment

The first-line treatment of BCC is often surgical excision. Numerous alternatives are available and include: curettage, cryosurgery, laser, excision with predetermined margins, excision under frozen section control, Mohs micrographic surgery (the removal of the tumour layer by layer until it has gone as determined histologically), radiotherapy, topical therapy, intralesional therapy, photodynamic therapy (the application of a cream to induce photo damage to the tumour using varying light sources), immunomodulators (agents used to stimulate the immune system and work on eradicating the tumour), and chemotherapy. Surgical treatment requires access to a minor operating theatre and most other treatments are carried out in specialist centres. Although there are wide varieties of treatment modalities used in the management of BCC, and the vast majority of the tumours are probably successfully treated, little research is available accurately comparing these different treatment modalities.

## Is there an optimal method of surgical excision?

There are no large RCTs comparing surgical excision with a predetermined margin with any other intervention for BCC despite this modality being probably the commonest treatment. There are however large case series, which demonstrate excellent "success" rates for this modality.[22]

Mohs micrographic surgery is a technique whereby 100% of the surgical margin is examined by mapping horizontal frozen sections from successive excision layers until clearance is achieved. No RCTs have investigated the margin of excision that would be effective in the removal of BCC by surgical excision with predetermined margins. Proxy measures based on Mohs micrographic surgical margins required to remove BCCs and histopathological studies of excised specimens have suggested that for small nodular or superficial BCC a 4 mm margin of normal skin will clear 95% of tumours.[18,23] Larger margins are required for tumours greater than 20 mm or morphoeic tumours.[18]

### Surgical excision with frozen section margin control

One RCT of 347 patients compared surgical excision with frozen section margin control versus radiotherapy in primary BCC of the face less than 40 mm diameter.[24] As shown in Table 42.1, the main outcome measure was persistent or recurrent disease at 4 years. The secondary endpoint was the cosmetic results assessed by the patient, the dermatologist and three persons not involved in the trial.

*Treatment efficacy.* The 4-year failure rate (95% CI) was 0·7% (95% CI 0·1–3·9%) in the surgery group and 7·5% (95% CI 4·2–13·1%) in the radiotherapy group. Cosmetic outcome as assessed by five observers over the 4 years of the study consistently favoured surgery.[25] At 4 years the patients assessed their cosmetic results as good in 87% after surgery and in 69% after radiotherapy.

*Potential drawbacks.* After radiotherapy dyspigmentations and telangiectasia developed in more than 65% of the patients at 4 years. Radiodystrophy affected 41% of the patients at 4 years.

**Table 42.1 Randomised controlled trial evaluating surgical excision in the treatment of basal cell carcinoma Evidence level Ib, Grade A**

| Study | Method | Participants | Interventions | Outcomes | Notes |
|---|---|---|---|---|---|
| [24]France | Single centre; randomisation by sequential sealed envelopes; ITT | Histologically proven BCCs T1: 174 patients T2: 173 patients. *Histological type* T1: 79 N, 52 ulcerated, 36 superficial pagetoid, 7 sclerosing T2: 74 N, 50 ulcerated, 41 S. pagetoid, 8 sclerosing. *Location* T1: 53 nose, 36 eyelids, 36 forehead, 10 chin, 5 ear T2: 49 nose, 42 cheek, 35 eyelids, 29 forehead, 12 chin, 6 ear | *T1*: surgery – resection of whole tumour with a free margin of at least 2 mm from visible borders *T2*: radiotherapy – Three radiation techniques available: interstitial brachytherapy; superficial contractherapy; conventional therapy. Radiotherapist chose the therapy according to tumour parameters, location on face and patient characteristics | Follow up: at 3, 6, 12 months after end of treatment, then yearly until fourth year Rate of histologically confirmed persistent tumour or recurrence after 4 years Patients were examined by dermatologists and photographs of scar taken at 3 standardised distances | Ex: BCC on scalp or neck; patients who had total removal of BCC at biopsy, with five or more BCCs; life expectancy below 3 years |

Abbreviations (for all tables): 5-FU/epi, 5-fluorouracil/epinephrine; ALA, 5-aminolevulinic acid; BCC, basal cell carcinoma; Ex, exclusion; IFN, interferons; ITT, intention to treat; MOR, morphea-like; MU, megaunits; N, nodular; PC, phosphatidyl choline; PDT, photodynamic therapy; PP, per protocol; S, superficial; T1, treatment group 1; T2, treatment group 2; T3, treatment group 3

**Table 42.2   Randomised controlled trials evaluating cryotherapy in the treatment of basal cell carcinoma Evidence level Ib, Grade A**

| Study | Method | Participants | Interventions | Outcomes | Notes |
|---|---|---|---|---|---|
| [27]UK | Single-centre Method of randomisation not known PP | UK: 105 patients *Biopsy-proven BCCs*: T1: 44 patients T2: 49 patients *Sites*: T1: 30 neck and face, 6 eyelids, 8 trunk T2: 40 neck and face, 3 eyelids, 6 trunk | *T1*: cryotherapy carried out using a Cry-Owen liquid nitrogen spray gun All lesions treated with two freeze–thaw cycles, freezing for 1 min each time, with a thaw time of at least 90 s *T2*: radiotherapy, (130 KV *x* rays) | Follow up: recurrence of tumour and cosmetic appearance noted at 1, 6, 12, 24 months after treatment Tumour identified histologically | 12 excluded: 5 died of other causes, 7 lost to follow up. Ex: recurrent tumours, lesions on nose or pinna, lesion near eye and vision in eye less than 6/18 |
| [28]UK | Single-centre Method of randomisation not known PP | UK: 84 patients Mostly clinically proven BCCs Facial lesions of 1·5 cm or less and not extending more than 3 mm below skin were included T1: 36 patients T2: 48 patients | *T1*: single 30 s freeze–thaw cycles *T2*: double 30 s freeze–thaw cycle *Mean age* T1: 67 years; T2: 69 years | Follow up: T1: period 10 months to 7·1 years; T2: period 1·2 to 6·1 years Lesions assessed clinically | 7 patients were lost to follow up, T1: 2 and T2: 5. |
| [29]Netherlands | Single-centre Method of randomisation not known PP | Netherlands: 103 patients Some biopsy proven BCCs Lesions superficial or nodular, less than 2 cm in diameter localised anywhere on the head and neck area | *T1*: surgery *T2*: cryosurgery (curette no. 3 used to debulk tumour and no. 1 used to remove remainder of BCC around borders Freezing carried out in two freezing periods each lasting 20 s | Follow up: cosmetic and recurrence at 1 year Recurrence assessed clinically | Lost to follow up: 3 patients in control group did not turn up or visits; 1 patient died (unrelated to treatment); 3 patients developed recurrent BCC (all in cryosurgery group) |

Abbreviations: see Table 42.1

*Comment.* Concealment of allocation was clear and the paper showed evidence of an *a priori* sample size calculation; however, analysis was conducted per protocol. Several previous studies have reported cure rates and cosmetic results with surgery and radiotherapy; however, the above study was the first randomised trial giving an unbiased comparison of the two treatments.

*Implications for practice.* The trial shows that the failure rate was significantly lower in surgery than in radiotherapy for the treatment of BCC of the face for lesions of less than 4 cm in diameter. Surgery may also be preferred for its cosmetic result.

### Mohs micrographic surgery

There are no RCTs comparing this with any other intervention although large case series with 5-year follow up suggest that this modality has the highest cure rates for all types of BCC (0·5–1·3%) depending on site.[26]

### Which is the best method of cryotherapy?

Three RCTs were found and are shown in Table 42.2. One study of 93 patients compared radiotherapy with cryotherapy for primary BCC excluding lesions on the nose or pinna.[27] The aims of the study were to compare the control of the tumours with the two treatments, to assess the final cosmetic result and to compare the discomfort and inconvenience experienced by the patient. Cryotherapy consisted of two freeze–thaw cycles, freezing for 1 minute each time.

### Radiotherapy versus cryotherapy

*Treatment efficacy.* Recurrence rates at 1 year were 4% (2/49) in the radiotherapy group and 39% (17/44) in the cryotherapy group. At 2 years no further tumours had recurred in either group. The cosmetic results for the two modes of treatment were not significantly different.

*Potential drawbacks.* The degree of pain, discomfort, discharge and bleeding from the treated areas were the same in both groups. Only one patient from each group was seriously inconvenienced by their treatment. Hypopigmentation was more common than hypergimentation with both modes of treatment (81% of those in the radiotherapy group and 88% of those in the cryotherapy group). Seven patients treated with radiotherapy developed some radiation telangiectasia. Hypopigmentation and telangiectasia tend to be lifelong. Five patients treated with cryotherapy developed milia – these all disappeared by 1 year.

*Comments.* The concealment of allocation was unclear and analysis was conducted per protocol. The paper also gave no indication of the type of lesion.

*Implication for clinical practice.* Cryotherapy, although convenient and less expensive than radiotherapy, does not appear to have better cure rates as compared with radiotherapy (especially for lesions > 2 cm). Cosmetic effect is comparable for radiotherapy.

Variations in technique occur between different physicians and may account for differences in outcome. Lesions bigger than 2 cm diameter treated by cryotherapy recurred, but lesions bigger than 2 cm and treated with radiotherapy were controlled.

It was concluded that cryotherapy does not offer a satisfactory alternative to radiotherapy in the treatment of BCC.

### Varying number of freeze–thaw cycles

In a second study of 84 patients one freeze–thaw cycle of 30 seconds was compared with two freeze–thaw cycles of 30 seconds for low risk facial BCCs.[28]

*Treatment efficacy.* Recurrence rates were significant: 4·7% were observed with 2 freeze–thaw cycles and 20·6% with one cycle at a median time of 18 months.

*Potential drawbacks.* No mention was made of adverse effects of the treatment.

*Comment.* Concealment of allocation was unclear and the analysis was conducted per protocol. Only common

facial lesions of 1·5 cm or less were included and the lesions were not all biopsied. Variations in technique may exist between different physicians and this may account for differences in outcome.

*Implication for clinical practice.* Facial lesions require a double freeze–thaw cycle with liquid nitrogen if they are to achieve high cure rates that are equivalent to many reports of formal excision or radiotherapy.

Although case series suggest that higher clearance rates can be achieved particularly with low risk tumours, more prospective evidence is required.

### Cryotherapy versus surgical excision

In a third study of 96 patients,[29] cryosurgery was compared with surgical excision for BCC of the head and neck. The primary outcome was cosmetic result; however, recurrence rates in both groups was also compared. Recurrences were treated by surgical excision. Cosmetic results were judged by five independent professional observers and by the patients.

*Treatment efficacy.* Recurrence rate for cryosurgery was 3/48 at 1 year. In the surgery group no recurrences developed at 1 year. Cosmetic results after surgical excision generally got significantly higher evaluation compared with cryosurgery for superficial and nodular subtypes localised in the head/neck region.

*Comments.* Concealment of allocation was unclear and the analysis was conducted per protocol; however, the paper showed evidence of an *a priori* sample size calculation.

*Potential drawbacks.* Two patients (4%) developed secondary wound infections in weeks 1 and 2 after surgery for which systemic antibiotics were given. Ninety per cent of patients in the cryotherapy group complained of moderate to severe swelling of the treated area, followed by long-lasting leakage of exudates from the defect. Three cases (6%) had secondary wound infection for which systemic antibiotics were given.

*Implication for clinical practice.* Surgical excision for nodular and superficial lesions smaller than 2 cm is cosmetically more acceptable as compared with cryosurgery. Cryotherapy does not appear to be a satisfactory option to surgery for superficial or nodular lesions in the head and neck area of less than 2 cm in diameter.

### How effective is photodynamic therapy (PDT)?

PDT is a non-ionising radiation treatment modality under development using the interaction between visible light and tumour sensitising agents to generate cell death. Two RCTs were identified and these are shown in Table 42.3. No published trials have compared PDT against the standard treatment of surgical excision.

**Table 42.3    Randomised controlled trials evaluating photodynamic therapy in the treatment of basal cell carcinoma
Evidence level Ib, Grade A**

| Study | Method | Participants | Interventions | Outcomes | Notes |
|---|---|---|---|---|---|
| [31]Sweden | Single-centre Randomised according to stratified randomisation pattern in blocks of 10 patients PP | Histologically proven BCC 88 patients, 44 women and 44 men Age range: 42–88 *Type*: *T1*: 22 S, 25 N *T2*: 17S, 24N *Distribution*: 47 on trunk, 25 on head and neck, 10 on legs and 6 on arms | *T1*: PDT (20% weight-based ALA/water in oil cream applied to lesion and irradiation took place 6 hours later *T2*: cryosurgery – two freeze–thaw cycles given | Follow up 1, 4, 8 weeks and 3 months after treatment; last follow up 12 months after first treatment; at 3 and 12 months punch biopsy taken | Ex: BCC on nose; morphoeic growth; porphyria; abdominal pain of unknown aetiology; photosensitivity; treatment of BCC with topical steroids type III or i.v. within the last month |
| [32]Norway | Single-centre Randomisation numbers in locked envelopes Patients were randomly allocated on treatment day to one of two arms in blocks of four patients ITT | Histological proven BCC 83 patients and 245 lesions | All lesions in both groups treated with same drug (topical application of 20% ALA; 3 hours later cream removed and light source applied *T1*: laser light (630 nm) *T2*: broad band light | Follow up: 3, 6 months after treatment. *Outcomes*: complete, partial or no response; cosmetic outcome and pain intensity during treatment and follow up period | |

Abbreviations: see Table 42.1.

### PDT versus cryotherapy

In a trial of 88 patients, photodynamic therapy was compared with two freeze–thaw cycles of cryotherapy for BCC.[30]

*Treatment efficacy.* There were no statistically significant difference in recurrence rates at 12 months. The PDT group had histological recurrence rates of 25% (11 of 44) compared with 15% (6 of 39) in the cryotherapy group, at 1 year, despite multiple retreatments in the PDT group. Scarring and tissue defect scored significantly better following PDT.

*Potential drawbacks.* More patients indicated pain and discomfort during and after treatment with PDT but the differences were not statistically significant.

*Comments.* Concealment of allocation was clear; however, analysis was conducted per protocol and no sample size calculation was given.

*Implications for clinical practice.* Although patient tolerability was greater and cosmetic outcomes were considered better in the PDT group, the efficacy data do not support the introduction of PDT for the treatment of BCC without further studies demonstrating greater efficacy.

### PDT using laser versus broadband halogen light

A second RCT[31] of 83 patients compared the clinical and cosmetic outcome of superficial BCCs, using either laser or broadband halogen light, in photodynamic therapy with topical 5-aminolevulinic acid (ALA).

*Treatment efficacy.* Eighty-six per cent in the laser group and 82% in the broadband halogen group were evaluated as complete response by both investigators at the end of the study (6 months). The study showed no statistically significant difference in cure rate ($P = 0.49$, 95% CI $-7\%$, $+14\%$) or cosmetic outcome ($P = 0.075$), between light exposure from a simple broad lamp with continuous spectrum (570–740 nm) or from a red-light laser (monochromatic 630 nm).

*Comments.* Although 83 patients were involved, 245 superficial BCCs were included in the study indicating that more than one lesion per patient was included in the study.

Concealment of allocation was clear and analysis was carried out by intention to treat; however, no sample size calculation was included.

*Potential drawbacks.* Eighty-three per cent of patients in the laser light and 76% of those in the broadband halogen light groups reported some discomfort during and after illumination; 68% of the patients in the laser light and 74% in the broadband halogen light reported pain and some burning sensation during the first week after treatment (stinging, itching, pain, headache, sensation of warmth or blushing). No serious adverse events were reported during the 6-month follow up.

*Implications for practice.* The results show that topical ALA-based PDT with a broadband halogen light source gives cure rates and cosmetic outcomes similar to those obtained with a laser light source. Reduced costs, increased safety, as well as the possibility of general use by dermatologists, are other elements in favour of the lamp as a suitable light source.

This remains a technique for BCC in need of further research and or modifications prior to its use due to the poor outcomes reported.

A further randomised trial, although ongoing, aims to compare the efficacy of 5-ALA PDT following minimal debulking curettage with surgery for low risk nodular BCCs, and compare pain and morbidity experienced by each procedure.[32]

## How effective is intralesional interferon therapy?

Interferons are naturally occurring glycoproteins that exhibit antiviral, antitumour and immunomodulatory activities. Four RCTs were found and these are shown in Table 42.4.

### IFNα 2a, 2b or IFNα 2a and 2b

In the first trial 45 patients were randomised to receive 15 or 30 MU of either IFNα 2a, 2b, or both 2a and 2b.[33] The aim of the study was to evaluate the effectivness of the IFNα 2a and 2b, and whether this effect might be increased by their combination.

*Efficacy.* Complete response at 8 weeks was similar at 66–73% in each treatment group. No significant differences were found between the groups in this respect.

*Potential drawbacks.* There was pain at the injection site and all patients had a 'flu-like syndrome (fever, chills, headaches, fatigue, myalgia) especially within the first 2 weeks after the initiation of IFNα therapy.

*Comments.* Concealment of allocation unclear; however, analysis was performed with intention to treat.

*Implication for clinical practice.* Combining IFNα 2a and 2b does not increase their effectiveness.

### IFNα 2b versus vehicle

Another trial of 165 patients[34] compared 1·5 MU IFNα 2b three times weekly for 3 weeks with vehicle in a 3:1 ratio.

*Efficacy.* Eighty-one per cent of interferon-treated patients were clinically and histologically cured at 52 weeks compared with 20% of placebo-treated patients. The cure rate was independent of lesion type or size.

*Potential drawbacks.* 'Flu-like symptoms occurred more commonly in the interferon-treated group.

*Comments.* Concealment of allocation was clear; however, analysis was conducted per protocol. It was interesting that 20% of people treated with vehicle only appeared to have histological cure at 1 year. Longer-term studies are needed to determine whether this is genuine.

*Implications for clinical practice.* IFNα 2b could be considered for patients who are not candidates for simple surgery or desire non-surgical therapy. INFα 2b does not compare with current standards of surgical or radiotherapy cures and so cannot be recommended.

### Number of doses of IFNα 2b

In a third trial, protamine zinc chelate IFNα 2b doses of 10 MU once or weekly for 3 weeks were compared in 65 patients.[35]

*Treatment efficacy.* Histological cure rates at 16 weeks were 52% and 80% for 10 and 30 MU respectively. Cosmetic effect was graded by patients as follows: excellent 51%, very good 22%, good 14%, satisfactory 10% and poor 3%.

*Potential drawbacks.* All patients experienced at least one adverse reaction. Side effects were similar for both single and repeated dosage groups, and were those common to interferon. Adverse reactions occurring in at least 20% of subjects were fever, rigours, myalgia, headache and nausea. Other side effects included arthralgia, malaise, fatigue, diarrhoea, paraesthesias, somnolence, thirst, dizziness, vomiting, rashes and anorexia. Adverse reactions began on the day of treatment and generally lasted 5–8 hours, except for headaches which lasted about 1 day. Mild erythema was often present at the treatment site in week 16 of the study.

*Comments.* Concealment of allocation was unclear and analysis was conducted per protocol. There was also a lack of any other active or standard treatment as comparator.

*Implications for clinical practice.* Refinement of the formulation to improve control of release of interferon in order to help minimise side effects has not been realised. A trial is needed to compare sustained-release formulation of INFα 2b with INFα 2b.

**Table 42.4** Randomised controlled trials evaluating intralesional interferon in the treatment of basal cell carcinomas Evidence level Ib, Grade A

| Study | Method | Participants | Interventions | Outcomes | Notes |
|---|---|---|---|---|---|
| [33]Turkey | Single-centre Method of randomisation not known ITT | 45 patients with histologically proven BCCs T1: 15 patients; T2: 15 patients; T3: 15 patients *Mean age:* T1: 58·7; T2: 63·6; T3: 60·3 *Histological type of BCC:* T1:12 N, 1 S, 2 MOR T2: 11 N, 2 S, 2 MOR; T3: 11 N, 2 S, 2 MOR | T1: IFNα 2a T2: IFNα 2b; T3: IFNα 2a and 2b | Follow up: 8 weeks after completion of therapy, cytologic specimens taken and all cases evaluated clinically and histologically | Ex: recurrent lesions, genetic or nevoid conditons, deep tissue involvement |
| [34]USA | Multicentre (4) Randomisation computer generated. PP | T1: 123 patients; T2: 42 patients with biopsy-proven BCCs *Mean age:* T1: 56; T2: 57 *Histological type:* T1: 57 S, 66 N, ulcerative; T2: 19 S, 23 N | T1: intralesional injections 1·5 MU of IFNα 2b T2: placebo (vehicle for interferon preparation) Rx: T1 and T2 on 3 alternate days per week for 3 consecutive weeks | Follow up: weekly after each of the 3 treatments then at 5, 9, 13 weeks after completion of treatment, then every 3 months to 52 weeks | Ex: previously received therapy to test site, immunosuppressive or cytotoxic therapy (within prior 4 weeks), or exonogous interferon/IFNα 2b (Intron A) Lesion debilitating illness, in perioral or central area of the face or penetrating to deep tissue |
| [35]USA | Single centre Method of randomisation not known PP | 65 patients T1: 33, T2: 32 Biopsy proven BCCs *Age range:* 35–65 *Histological type:* T1: 16 S, 17 N; T2: 15 S, 15 N | T1: single injection of 10 MU zinc chelate IFNα 2b T2: one dose of 10 MU of zinc chelate IFNα 2b per week for 3 weeks | BCC measured, photographed before each treatment and at beginning of the 2nd, 8th, 12th and 16th week after the first injection; biopsy at week 16 | Ex: thromboembolic disease, radiation therapy to the test site area, history of arsenic ingestion, pregnancy, immunosuppression, receiving NSAID, morphoeic BCC, recurrent cancers, deeply invasive lesions, periorificial tumours and central facial BCC |
| [36]Poland | Single centre. Method of randomisation not known ITT | 35 patients T1: 17, T2: 18 | T1: recombinant IFNβ T2: placebo | Follow up: 16 weeks after treatment and 2 years | |

Abbreviations: see Table 42.1.

**Table 42.5   Randomised controlled trial evaluating BEC-5 in the treatment of basal cell carcinoma**
**Evidence level Ib, Grade A**

| Study | Method | Participants | Interventions | Outcomes | Notes |
|---|---|---|---|---|---|
| [37]UK | Multicentre Method of randomisation not known | 94 patients, with biopsy-proven BCCs Age range 32–95 | *T1*: BEC-5 (mixture of 0·005% solasodine) *T2*: vehicle T1 and T2 treated twice daily under occlusion with either BEC-5 or vehicle for 8 weeks | Patients were reviewed every 2 weeks A repeat punch biopsy on 84 patients was performed at 8 weeks | 10 patients in T1 did not complete the study |

Abbreviations: see Table 42.1.

### Recombinant IFNβ

A fourth trial of 35 patients looked at recombinant IFNβ (1 MU) given three times weekly for 3 weeks and compared with placebo.[36]

*Treatment efficacy.* Forty-seven per cent in the treatment group showed complete response compared with none in the placebo group at 2 years follow up.

*Potential drawbacks.* Inflammation at the injection site was found in 11/16 patients in the treatment group and 4/18 receiving placebo.

*Comment.* Analysis was conducted per protocol and concealment of allocation is not known.

*Implications for clinical practice.* The paper suggests recombinant IFNβ as an alternative treatment for BCC. Response rate for this trial is lower compared with others; 47% is not a sufficiently good response rate to recommend a treatment.

### How useful are other drugs in treatment?

#### BEC-5 cream

BEC-5 is a mixture of 0·005% solasodine glycosides found in solanaceous plants (aubergine). BEC-5 cream binds to endogenous ectins and shows preferential cytotoxicity to human cancer cells. A double-blind randomised trial of BEC-5 cream was compared with matching vehicle[37] and is summarised in Table 42.5. Biopsy-proven lesions, excluding morphoeic BCC, were treated twice daily under occlusion with BEC-5 or vehicle for 8 weeks.

*Treatment efficacy.* There was a significant histological cure at week 8, 66% (41/62) for the BEC-5 group and 25% (8/32) for the vehicle group. Cure at 1-year follow up was also significant – 52% (32/62) for the BEC-5 group and 16% (5/32) for the vehicle group.

*Potential drawbacks.* There were no major treatment-related adverse effects.

*Comment.* Concealment of allocation was unclear and analysis was conducted using intention to treat.

*Implications for clinical practice.* Although significant differences were found between the groups, the cure rate is probably not as sufficiently high as compared with other treatments to recommend this method. It was not clear from the published abstract what the proportions of nodular and superficial BCC were – further trials are required to ascertain its true usefulness.

### Fluorouracil (5-FU)

The primary mechanism of action of 5-FU is thought to be inhibition of DNA synthesis by competitive inhibition of thymidylate synthetase.[38] A double-blind randomised pilot study[39] of 5-FU cream 5% in phosphatidyl choline (PC) vehicle was compared with 5-FU 5% in petrolatum. Further details of this study are given in Table 42.6. PC was used as a vehicle to facilitate the penetration of 5-FU.

#### 5-FU in PC versus 5-FU in petrolatum

*Treatment efficacy.* Histological cure at week 16 was 90% for the 5% 5-FU in a PC vehicle group and 57% for those treated with 5% 5-FU in a petrolatum-based cream. (The patients also evaluated the treatment site on each visit for cosmetic appearance.) There was absolutely no difference detected in the clinical appearance and adverse effects between the two therapeutic arms of the study.

*Comments.* The study was not powered to detect any statistically significant differences in outcome between the groups and concealment of allocation was unclear; however, analysis was conducted using intention to treat.

*Potential drawbacks.* Local irritation, erythema, ulceration and tenderness were common but well tolerated

**Table 42.6   Randomised controlled trials evaluating 5-FU in the treatment of basal cell carcinoma**

| Study | Method | Participants | Interventions | Outcomes | Notes |
|---|---|---|---|---|---|
| [39]USA | Single-centre<br>Method of randomisation not known<br>ITT | 13 patients with 17 biopsy proven non-superficial BCCs measuring at least 0·7 cm in greatest diameter | *T1:* 5% 5-FU in PC vehicle<br>*T2:* 5% 5-FU in petrolatum base<br>T1 and T2 applied am and pm for 4 consecutive weeks | Follow up: every 4 weeks for 16 weeks<br>Final visit was biopsy of site | Ex: systemic disease, women of childbearing age, facial BCCs |
| [40]USA | Multicentre<br>Randomised, open-label<br>Method of randomisation not known<br>PP | 122 patients<br>Single biopsy-proven BCCs<br>Mean age 61 yrs<br>97 males and 25 female<br>*Histological type:* 38 S, 85 N<br>*Location:* 9 head, 9 neck, 38 upper extremities, 11 lower extremities, 55 trunk<br>Lesion area median 80 mm$^2$ | 6 treatment regimens:<br>*T1:* 1·0 ml 5-FU/epi gel once weekly for 6 weeks<br>*T2:* 0·5 ml 5-FU/epi gel once weekly for 6 weeks<br>*T3:* 1·0 ml 5-FU/epi gel twice weekly for 3 weeks<br>*T4:* 0·5 ml 5-FU/epi gel twice weekly for 3 weeks<br>*T5:* 0·5 ml 5-FU/epi gel twice weekly for 4 weeks<br>*T6:* 0·5 ml 5-FU/epi gel three times weekly for 2 weeks | Follow up: examinations of patients at 1, 4, 8, 12 weeks after last injection<br>At each visit patient and investigator gave subjective evaluation of cosmetic appearance of lesion | Ex: high risk sites; lesions with deep tissue involvement, basal cell naevus syndrome, hypersensitivities or allergies to 5-FU, sulfites, epinephrine, bovine collagen, history of autoimmune disease, pregnancy<br>Six patients were lost to follow up |

Abbreviations: see Table 42.1.

by the patients. Minimal itching and discomfort were experienced by some of the patients in both treatment arms.

*Implications for clinical practice.* The study could indicate an increase in short-term eradication of BCC using a PC-based vehicle as compared with conventional petrolatum-based formulations. There were excellent cosmetic outcomes in all treatment sites before excision at week 16. Further larger scale double-blind therapeutic trials are necessary to definitively establish the efficacy of this treatment modality.

**Varying treatment regimens of 5-FU/epinephrine (adrenaline) injectable gel**

An open-label randomised study of 122 patients[40] was performed to test the safety, tolerance, and efficacy of six treatment regimens of 5-FU/epinephrine gel (5-FU/epi gel). Two doses and four treatment schedules were used.

*Efficacy.* Overall, the six regimens had an average response rate of 91% as defined by absence of any tumour on the basis of histological analysis of excised specimen. There was 100% complete response rate in patients who received 0·5 ml 5-FU/epi gel twice weekly for 4 weeks. There was a 92% response rate for superficial lesions and a 91% response rate for nodular lesions.

All regimens appeared to work well and there were no statistically significant differences between them. The variable treatment regimens, with increased dose and/or treatment frequency, resulted in higher tumour complete response rate than that obtained in an earlier pilot study.[41]

Cosmetic appearance of lesion site prior to excision at 3 months ranged from good to excellent.

*Potential drawbacks.* All patients had transient, moderate to severe stinging, burning, or pain at the time of injection. Local tissue reactions were confined to the treatment site and included erythema, swelling, desquamation, erosions and eschar in most patients. Hyperpigmentation was observed in 83% of patients but typically cleared up by follow up; 47% of patients had ulcerations at the treatment site. The 0·5ml (5-FU/epi gel) three times per week for 2 weeks produced the lowest incidence and severity of reactions.

*Comments.* Analysis was per protocol. Concealment of allocation was unclear and no sample size calculation was shown.

*Implication for clinical practice.* High local drug concentrations can be maintained longer with 5-FU/epi gel drug delivery. A trial of 5-FU/epi gel versus surgical excision, monitoring adverse effect is required, to confirm the claim that response rates are comparable to surgery.

## Imiquimod

Imiquimod is an immune response modifier that has been shown to induce cytokines that promote a TH1 lymphocyte or cell-mediated immune response.[42–44] These include IFNα, IFNλ, and interleukin-12 (IL-12). In animal studies, imiquimod has demonstrated broad antiviral and antitumor effects that are largely mediated by IFNα.[45] In humans, imiquimod 5% cream has been demonstrated to be safe and effective in the treatment of external anogenital warts.[45–47] We found six RCTs and these are shown in Table 42.7.

### Trial 1

One study of 35 patients has evaluated the safety and efficacy of imiquimod 5% cream in the treatment of superficial and nodular BCC.[48,49]

*Treatment efficacy.* This small trial suggested success rates similar to those of excision surgery with the added advantage of no scarring.

*Potential drawbacks.* Adverse events were predominantly local reactions at the target tumour site, with the incidence and severity of local skin reactions declining in groups dosed less frequently.

### Trial 2

Another phase II dose–response trial tested imiquimod 5% cream applied for 6 weeks in 99 Australian patients with primary superficial BCC, where clearance was defined as patients with no histological evidence of BCC, when the site of the treated lesion was excised 6 weeks after imiquimod treatment.[50]

*Treatment efficacy.* All patients treated with a twice-daily regimen showed histological clearance (3/3); 88% showed clearance on a once-daily day regimen (29/33); 73% showed clearance (22/30) on the 6 × week regimen, and 70% showed clearance (23/33) on the 3 × week regimen.

### Trial 3

Another similar multicentre RCT of 128 patients with superficial BCC compared imiquimod twice daily, once daily, 5 days per week or 3 days per week against vehicle, using the same endpoints.[51]

*Treatment efficacy.* Intention-to-treat analysis showed clearance rates of: 100% (10/10), 87% (27/31), 81% (21/26) and 52% (15/29) for the twice daily, once daily, 5 days a week and 3 days a week groups, respectively. Interestingly, there was a small vehicle response rate of 19% (6/32).

*Potential drawbacks.* Local reactions were common, mostly mild or moderate, and well tolerated by patients.

### Trial 4

Another study[52] of 93 patients with superficial BCC found that occlusion increased the success rate for thrice weekly application of imiquimod.

*Treatment efficacy.* Occlusion increased success rate from 76% (19/25) to 87% (20/23).

*Potential drawbacks.* Local reactions were mild to moderate.

### Trials 5 and 6

Two further industry-sponsored trials conducted in Australia and the US have evaluated 5% imiquimod cream for the treatment of nodular BCC.

*Treatment efficacy.* One of these studies[53] reported histological clearance rates of 71% (25/35) for once daily treatment for 6 weeks.

*Potential drawbacks.* Local reactions were mild to moderate and well tolerated by patients dosing daily or less frequently.

### Trial 7

Another vehicle-controlled RCT[54] consisted of 92 patients with nodular BCC who underwent treatment for 12 weeks using twice daily, once daily, 5 days a week, or 3 days a week.

**Table 42.7   Randomised controlled trials evaluating imiquimod 5% cream in the treatment of basal cell carcinomas Evidence level Ib, Grade A**

| Study | Method | Participants | Interventions | Outcomes |
|---|---|---|---|---|
| [48]USA | Single-centre Randomisation to give 2:1 ratio of imiquimod cream to vehicle cream Method of randomisation not known ITT | Biopsy proven BCCs *T1*: 7 patients *T2*: 4 patients *T3*: 4 patients *T5*: 5 patients *T6*: 11 patients *Age range*: 37–81 *Size range*: 0·5–2 cm$^2$ *Location*: mainly on upper body *Histological type*: T1: 1 N, 2 S; T2: 1 N, 3 S; T3: 4 S; T4: 2 N, 3 S; T5: 2 N, 2 S; T6: 1 N, 10 S | 5 treatment schedules with the imiquimod 5% cream: *T1*: twice/day *T2*: once/day *T3*: three times/week *T4*: twice/week *T5*: once/week *T6*: vehicle | Follow up: 6 weeks after treatment tumour site excised and histologically examined |
| [49]Australia and NZ | Multicentre Method of randomisation not known ITT | 99 patients: 72 male and 27 female Histological proven superficial BCC *Surface area*: 0·5–2 cm$^2$ *Location*: 32% upper limbs, 28% trunk, 40% head and neck | All groups treated with 5% imiquimod: *T1*: twice/day *T2*: once/day *T3*: twice/day for 3 days each week *T4*: once/day for 2 days each week | Follow up: 1, 2, 4, 6 weeks Excision at week 6 *Lost to follow up*: T2: 2 due to pruritus; T3: 1 due to CVA; T4: 1 excision of nearby tumour |
| [51]USA | Multicentre, randomised, blinded, vehicle-controlled dose–response study Method of randomisation not known ITT | Single, primary, biopsy-proven superficial BCC (measuring 0·5–2·0 cm$^2$) | *T1*: imiquimod, twice daily for 12 weeks *T2*: imiquimod, once daily, for 12 weeks *T3*: imiquimod, 5 days per week (Mon–Fri) for 12 weeks *T4*: imiquimod, 3 days per week (Mon-Wed-Fri) for 12 weeks | Follow up: surgical excision 6 weeks after treatment |
| [52]USA | Multicentre, randomised open label, dose–response Method of randomisation not known ITT | 93 patients Single, primary, biopsy-proven superficial BCC (0·5–2 cm$^2$) | *T1*: imiquimod thrice per week for 6 weeks with occlusion *T2*: thrice per week without occlusion for 6 weeks *T3*: twice a week with occlusion for 6 weeks *T4*: twice per week without occlusion for 6 weeks | Follow up: surgical excision 6 weeks after treatment |
| [53]USA | Multicentre, randomised, open label, dose–response study Method of randomisation not known ITT | 99 patients Single, primary, biopsy proven nodular BCC (measuring 0·5–1·5 cm$^2$) | *T1*: imiquimod twice daily for 6 weeks *T2*: once daily for 6 weeks *T3*: twice daily 3 days per week for 6 weeks (6 per week) *T4*: 3 per week for 6 weeks | Follow up: surgical excision 6 weeks after treatment |

*(Continued)*

**Table 42.7** *(Continued)*

| Study | Method | Participants | Interventions | Outcomes |
|---|---|---|---|---|
| [54]USA | Multicentre, randomised, blinded, vehicle-controlled dose-response study<br>Method of randomisation not known<br>ITT | 92 patients<br>Single, primary, biopsy-proven nodular BCC (measuring $0.5–1.5\,cm^2$) | *T1*: imiquimod twice daily for 12 weeks<br>*T2*: imiquimod, once daily for 12 weeks<br>*T3*: imiquimod, 5 days per week (Mon–Fri) for 12 weeks<br>*T4*: imiquimod, 3 days per week (Mon-Wed-Fri) for 12 weeks | Follow up: surgical excision 6 weeks after drug treatment |

Abbreviations: see Table 42.1

*Treatment efficacy.* Intention-to-treat histological clearance rates were 75% (3/4), 76% (16/21), 70% (16/23), and 60% (12/20) for the four groups, respectively, with a vehicle response rate of 13% (3/24).

*Implications for practice.* This study suggested that longer treatment times (that is, 12 weeks as opposed to 6 weeks) are needed to treat nodular tumours. This is what one might anticipate from a treatment that relies on percutaneous penetration, that is tumour depth may be an important predictor of treatment response.

*Potential drawbacks in all trials.* There may be some local skin reaction to the cream including: redness, oedema, skin hardening, vesicles, erosion, ulceration, flaking and scabbing. These brisk inflammatory reactions, at least clinically, would be consistent with an acute immunologic reconstitution of the sun-damaged skin, resulting in an immunologically mediated elimination of malignant and premalignant cells.

*Comment on all trials.* Concealment of allocation is unclear for all of the imiquimod trials; however, analysis is by intention to treat. There was no long-term follow up for recurrence. In all trials, patients were themselves able to apply the cream, a distinct advantage in today's busy dermatology departments.

*Implications for clinical practice.* A long-term randomised controlled trial (RCT) of imiquimod 5% cream versus the best treatment currently available (surgery) needs to be carried out. If successful, topical imiquimod could become a useful treatment for superficial and low risk BCCs. Application of a cream could allow dermatologists more time to concentrate on the high risk BCCs.

**Key points**

- Despite the enormous amount of work involved in the treatment of BCC, there has been very little good quality research on the efficacy of the treatment modalities used.
- Surgery and radiotherapy appear to be the most effective treatments. Other treatments might have some use, but they have all avoided comparison against surgery.
- It should be noted that most studies have been performed on low risk BCCs, the results of which are probably not be applicable to tumours of the morphoeic type shown in Figure 42.3. Specific trials or subgroup analyses are required for morphoeic tumours in future trials.
- Cryotherapy, although convenient and less expensive than surgery or radiotherapy does not have better cure rates than surgery or radiotherapy (especially for lesions > 2 cm). Cosmetic effect is better for surgery and comparable for radiotherapy.
- If cryosurgery is to be used, two freeze–thaw cycles are recommended for nodular and superficial facial lesions (Figures 42.1 and 42.2) if it is to achieve cure rates approaching equivalence to that of formal excision or radiotherapy.
- A randomised controlled trial of photodynamic therapy versus surgery is needed.
- Further studies for all of the interferon treatments and photodynamic therapies that demonstrate greater efficacy are needed before they can be recommended.

- Broadband halogen light source may give cure rates and cosmetic outcomes similar to laser light photodynamic therapy with possible benefits of reduced costs, increased safety, and ease of use.
- The efficacy of IFNα has not been directly compared with standard surgical treatment and is associated with significant side effects, which may overshadow its usefulness especially in the elderly. Interferon therapy requires several clinic visits.
- Increased short-term eradication of BCC using 5-fluorouracil in a phosphatidyl choline-based vehicle to increase permeability should be further investigated with a long-term follow up comparison against surgery.
- Preliminary studies suggest a high success rate (87–88%) for imiquimod for treating superficial BCC using a once daily regimen for 6 weeks, and a useful (76%) treatment response for nodular BCC for 12 weeks. These results need to be confirmed in long-term studies of 3–5 years with excision surgery as a comparator.
- Studies comparing excision with predetermined margins versus Mohs micrographic surgery in high risk tumours would be useful.

# References

1  Telfer NR, Colver GB, Bowers PW. Guidelines for the management of basal cell carcinoma. *Br J Dermatol* 1999;**141**:415–23.

2  Preston DS, Stern RS. Nonmelanoma cancers of the skin. *N Engl J Med* 1992;**327**:1649–62.

3  Miller SJ. Biology of basal cell carcinoma (part1). *J Am Acad Dermatol* 1991;**24**:1–13.

4  Goodwin RG, Roberts DL. Skin cancer registration in the United Kingdom. *Br J Dermatol* 2001;**145**(Suppl. 59):17.

5  Walberg P, Skog E. The increasing incidence of basal cell carcinoma. *Br J Dermatol* 1994;**131**:914–15.

6  Holme SA, Malinovszky K, Roberts DL. Changing trends in non-melanoma skin cancer in South Wales,1988–98. *Br J Dermatol* 2000; **143**:1224–9.

7  Chuang TY, Popescu A, Su WP, Chute CG. Basal cell carcinoma: a population-based incidence study in Rochester, Minnesota. *J Am Acad Dermatol* 1990;**22**:413–17.

8  Marks R, Staples M, Giles GG. Trends in non-melanocytic skin cancer treated in Australia: the second national survey. *Int J Cancer* 1993; **53**:585–90.

9  Roenigk RK, Ratz JL, Bailin PL, Wheeland RG. Trends in the presentation and treatment of basal cell carcinomas. *J Dermatol Surg Oncol* 1986;**12**:860–5.

10  McCormack CJ, Kelly JW, Dorevitch AP. Differences in age and body site distribution of the histological subtypes of basal cell carcinoma: a possible indicator of differing causes. *Arch Dermatol* 1997; **133**:593–6.

11  Gilbody JS, Aitken J, Green A. What causes basal cell carcinoma to be the commonest cancer?. *Aust J Publ Health* 1994;**18**:218–21.

12  Zaynoun S, Ali LA, Shaib J. The relationship of sun exposure and solar elastosis to basal cell carcinoma. *J Am Acad Dermatol* 1985; **12**:522–5.

13  Pearl DK, Scott EL. The anatomical distribution of skin cancers. *Int J Epidemiol* 1986;**15**:502–6.

14  Mackie RM, Elwood JM, Hawk JLM. Links between exposure to ultraviolet radiation and skin cancer. A report of the Royal College of Physicians. *J R Coll Phys Lond* 1987;**21**:91–6.

15  Schreiber MM, Moon TE, Fox SH, Davidson J. The risk of developing subsequent nonmelanoma skin cancers. *J Am Acad Dermatol* 1990;**23**:1114–18.

16  Johnson RL, Rothman AL, Xie J *et al.* Human homolog of patched, a candidate gene for the basal cell nevus syndrome. *Science* 1996;**272**:1668–71.

17  Staples M, Marks R, Giles G. Trends in the incidence of non-melanocytic skin cancer (NMSC) treated in Australia 1985–1995: are primary prevention programs starting to have an effect? *Int J Cancer* 1998;**78**:144–8.

18  Breuninger H, Deitz K. Prediction of subclinical tumour infiltration in basal cell carcinoma. *J Dermatol Surg Oncol* 1991;**17**:574–8.

19  Gussack GS, Schlitt M, Lushington A, Woods KE. Invasive basal cell carcinoma of the temporal bone. *Ear Nose Throat J* 1998;**68**:605–6, 609–11.

20  Franchimont C. Episodic progression and regression of basal cell carcinomas. *Br J Dermatol* 1982;**106**:305–10.

21  Takenouchi T, Nomoto S, Ito M. Factors influencing the linear depth of invasion of primary basal cell carcinoma. *Dermatol Surg* 2001; **27**:393–6.

22  Dubin N, Kopf AW. Multivariate risk score for recurrence of cutaneous basal cell carcinoma. *Arch Dermatol* 1983;**119**:373–7.

23  Wolf DJ, Zitelli JA. Surgicla margins for basal cell carcinoma. *Arch Dermatol* 1987;**123**:340–4.

24  Avril MF, Auperin A, Margulis A et al. Basal cell carcinoma of the face: surgery or radiotherapy? Results of a randomised study. *Br J Cancer* 1997;**76**:100–6.

25  Petit JY, Avrial MF, Margulis A *et al.* Evaluation of cosmetic results of a randomised trial comparing surgery and radiotherapy in the treatment of basal cell carcinoma of the face. *Plast Reconstr Surg* 2000; **105**:2544–51.

26  Rowe DE, Carroll RJ, Day CL, Jr. Long term recurrence rates in previously untreated (primary) basal cell carcinoma: implications for patient follow up. *J Dermatol Surg Oncol* 1989;**15**:315–28.

27  Hall VL, Leppard BJ, McGill J *et al.* Treatment of basal cell carcinoma: Comparison of radiotherapy and cryotherapy. *Clin Radiol* 1986; **37**:33–4.

28  Mallon E, Dawber R. Cryosurgery in the treatment of basal cell carcinoma. *Dermatol Surg* 1996;**22**:854–8.

29  Thissen MRTM, Nieman FHM, Ideler AHLB, Berretty PJM, Neumann HAM. Cosmetic results of cryosurgery versus surgical excision for primary uncomplicated basal cell carcinomas of the head and neck. *Dermatol Surg* 2000;**26**:759–64.

30  Wang I, Bendsoe N, Klinteberg CA *et al.* Photodynamic therapy vs cryosurgery of basal cell carcinomas: results of phase III clinical trial. *Br J Dermatol* 2001;**144**:832–40.

31  Soler AM, Angell-Petersen E, Warloe T *et al.* Photodynamic therapy of superficial basal cell carcinoma with 5-aminolevulinic acid with dimethylsulfoxide and ethylendiaminetetraacitic acid: A comparison of two light sources. *Photochem Photobiol* 2000;**71**:724–9.

32  Clark C. Randomised trial of minimal curettage and topical 5-aminolaevulinic acid (5-ALA) photodynamic therapy (PDT) compared with excision for the treatment of basal cell carcinomas with low recurrence risk. Ongoing trial. Photobiology Unit, Ninewells Hospital and Medical School, Tayside University Hospitals NHS Trust, Dundee, DD1 9SY, Scotland, UK.

33  Alpsoy E, Yilmaz E, Basaran E, Yazar S. Comparison of the effects of intralesional interferon alfa-2a, 2b and the combination of 2a and 2b in the treatment of basal cell carcinoma. *J Dermatol* 1996;**23**:394–6.

34  Cornell RC, Greenway HT, Tucker SB *et al.* Intralesional interferon therapy for basal cell carcinoma. *J Am Acad Dermatol* 1990;**23**:694–700.

35  Edwards L, Tucker SB. The effects of an intralesional sustained release formulation of interferon alfa2b on basal cell carcinomas. *Arch Dermatol* 1990;**126**:1029–32.

36  Rogozinski TT, Jablonska S, Brzoska J, Michalska I, Wohr C, Gaus W. Intralesional treatment with recombinant interferon beta is an effective alternative for the treatment of basal cell carcinoma. Double-blind, placebo-controlled study. *Przeglad Dermatologiczny* 1997;**84**:259–63.

37  Punjabi S, Cook IJ, Kersey P *et al.* A double-blind, multicentric parallel group study of BEC-5 cream in basal cell carcinoma (BCC). *Eur Acad Dermatol Venereol* 2000;**14**(Suppl.1):47–60.

38 Fluorouracil. In: McEvoy GK, ed. *American Hospital Formulacy Service Drug Information*. Bethesda. MD: American Society of Hospital Pharmacists, 1993.

39 Romagosa R, Saap L, Givens M *et al.* A pilot study to evaluate the treatment of basal cell carcinoma with 5-fluorouracil using phosphatidyl choline as a transepidermal carrier. *Dermatol Surg* 2000;**26**:338–40.

40 Miller BH, Shavin JS, Cognetta A *et al.* Nonsurgical treatment of basal cell carcinomas with intralesional 5-fluorouracil/epinephrine injectable gel. *J Am Acad Dermatol* 1997;**36**:72–7.

41 Orenberg EK, Miller BH, Greenway HT. The effect of intralesional 5-fluorouracil therapeutic implant (MPI 5003) for treatment for basal cell carcinoma. *Acad Dermatol* 1992;**27**:723–8.

42 Testerman TL, Gerster JF, Imbertson LM *et al.* Cytokine induction by the immunomodulators imiquimod and S-27609. *J Leukoc Biol* 1995; **58**:365–72.

43 Slade HB, Owens ML, Tomai MA, Miller RL. Imiquimod 5% cream. *Exper Opin Invest Drugs* 1998;**7**:437–49.

44 Imbertson LM, Beaurline JM, Couture AM *et al.* Cytokine induction in hairless mouse and rat skin after topical application of the immune response modifiers imiquimod and S-28463. *J Invest Dermatol* 1998;**110**:734–9.

45 Beutner KR, Spruance SL, Hougham AJ *et al.* Treatment of genital warts with an immune response modifier imiquimod. *J Acad Dermatol* 1998;**38**:230–9.

46 Beutner KR 2, Tyring SK, Trofatter KR *et al.* Imiquimod, a patient applied immune response modifier for treatment of external genital warts. *Antimicrob Agents Chemother* 1998;**42**:798–94.

47 Edwards L, Ferenczy A, Eron L *et al.* Self-administered topical 5% imiquimod cream for external anogenital warts. *Arch Dermatol* 1998;**134**:25–30.

48 Beutner KR, Geisse JK, Helman D, Fox TL, Ginkel A, Owens ML, Therapeutic response of basal cell carcinoma to the immune response modifier imiquimod 5% cream. *J Am Acad Dermatol* 1999; **41**:1002–7.

49 Bavinck JN. Biological treatment of basal cell carcinoma. *Arch Dermatol* 2000;**136**:774–5.

50 Marks R, Gebauer K, Shumak S *et al.* Imiquimod 5% cream in the treatment of superficial basal cell carcinoma: results of a multicenter 6-week dose-response trial. *J Am Acad Dermatol* 2001;**44**:807–13.

51 Geisse JK, Marks R, Owens ML, Andres K, Ginkel AM. Imiquimod 5% cream for 12 weeks treating superficial BCC. 8th World Congress on *Cancers of the Skin*, Zurich, Switzerland 18–21 July 2001, Abstract P58.

52 Sterry W, Bichel J, Andres K, Ginkel AM. Imiquimod 5% cream for 6 weeks with occlusion treating superficial BCC. 8th World Congress on *Cancers of the Skin*, Zurich, Switzerland 18–21 July 2001, Abstract P61.

53 Shumak S, Marks R, Amies M, Andres K, Ginkel AM. Imiquimod 5% cream for 6 weeks treating nodular BCC. 8th World Congress on *Cancers of the Skin*, Zurich, Switzerland 18–21 July 2001, Abstract P55.

54 Robinson JK, Marks R, Owens ML, Andres K, Ginkel AM. Imiquimod 5% cream for 12 weeks treating nodular BCC. 8th World Congress on *Cancers of the Skin*, Zurich, Switzerland 18–21 July 2001, Abstract P57.

# 43 Squamous cell carcinoma

*Nanette J Liégeois, Suzanne Olbricht*

## Background

### Definition

Squamous cell carcinoma (SCC) is a form of skin cancer that originates from epithelial keratinocytes.[1] It is thought to arise as a focal intra-epidermal proliferation from precancerous lesions, including actinic keratoses, SCC *in situ*, Bowen's disease, bowenoid papulosis, erythroplasia of Queyrat, and arsenical keratoses.[2] Without treatment, SCC may continue to grow, invade the dermis or subcutaneous tissues, or metastasise.[3] This chapter focuses on interventions for localised, non-metastatic invasive SCC. Prevention of SCC is dealt with in Chapters 10 and 11.

### Epidemiology

Since the 1960s, the overall incidence of SCC has been increasing annually.[4,5] In 1997, the Rochester Epidemiology Project in the US estimated the overall incidence of invasive SCC to be 106 per 100 000 people.[5] However, several population-based studies have shown that the risk of SCC appears to correlate with geographic latitude. The reported incidence of SCC is higher in tropical regions than in temperate climates, with an annual incidence approaching 1:100 in Australia.[6–9] Regional differences related to latitude have also been noted in the US.[4,10–13]

Sunlight exposure is an established independent risk factor for the development of SCC. SCC arises more commonly in the sun-exposed areas, including the head, neck and arms, but also occurs on the buttocks, genitals, and perineum.[14] Other risk factors for SCC include older age, male sex, Celtic ancestry, increased sensitivity to sun exposure, increased number of precancerous lesions and immunosuppression.[4,15,16] Exposure to oral psoralens, arsenic, cigarette smoking, coal-tar products, UVA photochemotherapy and human papillomavirus (5 and 8) have been associated with SCC. Genetic disorders that predispose to SCC include epidermodysplasia verruciformis, albinism and xeroderma pigmentosum.

Stasis ulcers, osteomyelitic sinuses, scarring processes such as lupus vulgaris, and vitiligo have been reported to increase the risk of SCC, but the underlying process may delay the diagnosis.[15,16]

## Pathogenesis

Several studies have shown that sun exposure, photo irradiation and ionising irradiation play a major role in the pathogenesis of SCC. DNA damage is a fundamental process that occurs in the development of cancer. Both UV light and ionising radiation are potent mutagens. Specifically, UVB light has been shown to produce pyrimidine dimers in DNA; these result in DNA point mutations during keratinocyte replication, which lead to abnormal cell function and replication.

In addition to direct DNA damage, genes involved in DNA repair have been implicated in the pathogenesis of SCC. The *p53* gene is mutated in most SCC cases, disabling normal *p53* function, which is thought to be critical in suppressing the development of SCC by repairing of UV-damaged DNA.[17–20] Keratinocytes with *p53* mutations cannot repair the mutations induced by irradiation and subsequently proliferate to develop cancer.[17] Furthermore, mice with *p53* mutations develop skin tumours more readily. Mutations in *p53* can either be acquired (through multiple pathways including human papillomavirus, UV light, carcinogens) or inherited. People with xeroderma pigmentosum have a defective *p53* pathway and develop numerous skin cancers; they cannot repair mutations induced by irradiation.[21]

Immunological status has also been implicated in the development of SCC. The rate of SCC in transplant recipients is high, particularly in those with a kidney or heart transplant.[22–25] How immunosuppression increases the risk is not known, but decreasing the immunosuppressive therapy helps to reduce the number of SCCs. Further studies are needed to determine how altered immune responses influence the development of SCC.

## Prognosis

The prognosis of local recurrence, metastases and survival in SCC depends on the location of disease and modality of treatment. The term "recurrence rate" at a post-treatment time point is preferable to "cure". The latter term wrongly suggests that no further recurrences occur after that point whereas in fact recurrence rate increases as the length of follow up increases. The overall local recurrence rate after excision of an SCC involving the sun-exposed areas is 8%, while the recurrence rates on the ear and lip are 19% and 11%, respectively.[26] The metastatic rate for primary SCC of the sun-exposed areas is 5%, while the rates for SCC on the external ear, lip and non-sun-exposed areas are 9%, 14% and 38%, respectively.[27] The 5-year overall survival rate associated with metastatic SCC of the skin has been estimated at 34%.[27]

Clinical factors that have been associated with an increased risk of local recurrence or metastases include treatment modality, size greater than 2 cm, depth greater than 4 mm, poor histological differentiation, location on the ear or non-sun-exposed areas, perineural involvement, location within scars or chronic inflammation, previously failed treatment and immunosuppression.[27]

## Diagnostic tests

The diagnosis of SCC relies on the histopathological finding of atypical hyperproliferative keratinocytes compared with adjacent normal epidermis. Common findings include cytological and architectural disorganisation, decreased differentiation and atypical mitoses. SCC *in situ* is diagnosed when atypia is identified only in the epidermal compartment. Invasive SCC is distinguished from SCC *in situ* by the invasion of the dermis by epithelioid cells. SCC may also be classified according to the degree of differentiation, a clinically important specification since more undifferentiated tumours are associated with poor prognosis.

## Aims of treatment and relevant outcomes

Treatment aims to remove or destroy the tumour completely and to minimise cosmetic and functional impairment **Evidence level IIb**. Success should therefore be measured by rates of recurrence or metastasis at fixed time points or survival analyses that document time to first recurrences in groups of patients. The morbidity of the procedure, as measured by short- and longer-term pain, infection, scarring, skin function and overall cosmesis should all be considered when the appropriate treatment modality is being chosen.[28,29] In addition, the cost and tolerance to the specific treatment modalities should be considered.

This chapter will address three main issues pertinent to the 72-year-old man in Figure 43.1. He has an uncomplicated SCC on his leg.

- What are the effective therapeutic interventions for localised invasive SCC of the skin?
- How do the effective therapeutic interventions for SCC compare with each other?
- How do the cosmetic outcomes for these interventions compare?

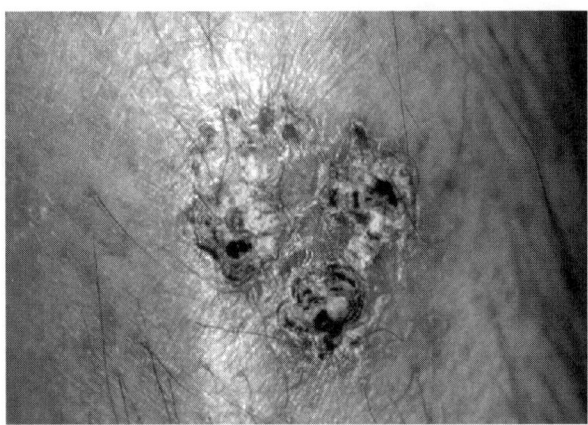

**Figure 43.1** Squamous cell carcinoma arising on the leg of a 72-year-old man

## Treatment options

### Excision

Surgical excision remains the primary treatment for invasive SCC. Surgical excision of SCC is performed in the outpatient setting under local anaesthesia. Standard excision techniques involve the visual estimation of the tumour border and marking a predetermined margin. A steel blade is used to excise the tumour and closure is performed using complex layered, flap, or graft technique. The histology of the tumour is examined in formalin-fixed sections.

#### *Effectiveness*

No large randomised controlled trial (RCT) has compared the effectiveness of surgical excision with any other treatment modality. No RCT has compared predetermined margin widths for the surgical removal of SCC.

Several case series demonstrate an excellent clearance of SCC lesions with surgical excision. Freeman *et al.*[30] reported 91 surgically excised SCC, with a follow up ranging from 1 to 5 years. Metastases developed in three of the 91 patients. The authors did not note the size or location of the tumours. For SCC less than 2 cm in diameter, surgical excision resulted in a 5-year cure rate of 96% (22 of 23 patients). For lesions greater than 2 cm, 83% (10 of 12) of patients were free of disease 5 years later.

While many authors report high cure rates for excision, with variable follow up, the recommendations for the width of the excision margin have ranged from 4 mm to 1 cm. In one prospective study, 141 SCC lesions were excised with incremental 1 mm margins and subclinical extension of tumours was examined using frozen tissue sectioning via Mohs micrographic surgery (MMS).[31] With 4 mm surgical margins tumours less than 2 cm had a greater than 95% clearance, while tumours greater than 2 cm required at least 6 mm excision margins to achieve a greater than 95% clearance.

### Drawbacks

Large tumours, or tumours in cosmetically complex areas such as near the eyelids or ears, often require an involved flap or graft technique for repair. The subsequent scar from surgical excision usually results in a hypopigmented line, and hypertrophic and keloidal changes may occur. SCC excision also requires removal of underlying fat as well as the tumour, which may disrupt normal vasculature, lymphatics, or innervation. Since the surgical site is closed at the time of surgery and histology is performed on fixed tissues, the discovery of residual tumour may necessitate further surgical interventions.

### Comment

Surgical excision remains the main definitive treatment option for SCC less than 2 cm in diameter. Caution is necessary when using this technique for larger SCC or lesions in cosmetically complex areas.

## Mohs micrographic surgery

Mohs micrographic surgery (MMS) is a form of surgery that is performed in stages over several hours. The surgeon functions as a pathologist and extirpates the tumour and immediately evaluates the extirpated tissue, which is processed under frozen section. Before closure, the positive margins are removed in subsequent stages and final closure is performed once the tumour is declared fully removed by the attendant surgeon. MMS is thought to be a highly curative procedure for non-melanoma skin cancers since immediate histopathological evaluation permits further tumour extirpation in successive stages. Although more tumour is removed from the positive margins in these stages, the remaining tissue is spared since only the tumour is removed, limiting potential damage to adjacent tissues.

### Effectiveness

Although MMS is frequently used in the treatment of SCC, there are no RCTs comparing MMS with other treatments.

Mohs reported a 5-year cure rate of 95% for primary SCC.[32] In a case-series analysis, Rowe *et al.* found that MMS resulted in a lower rate of local recurrence compared with other treatment modalities.[27] Holmkvist and Roenigk report a cure rate for primary SCC of the lip of 92% after MMS for 50 patients in a 2·5-year average follow up.[33] Lawrence and Cottel reported only three local recurrences of SCC in 44 patients with perineural invasion treated by

MMS in a 1-year follow up, and further noted that predicted survival was higher than previously published survival rates for surgical excision.[34–36]

### Drawbacks

MMS is expensive and is not accessible to all patients. Full extirpation of the tumour may require multiple stages over a period of many hours. Patients who cannot lie down because of a comorbid condition may not tolerate the potentially lengthy procedure. In addition, the processing of the frozen sections is labour intensive and costs much more than conventional histology.

### Comments

MMS appears to have higher cure rates than other treatment modalities. Because it uses sequential extirpation of tissue, it is more sparing of adjacent tissue. This provides a cosmetic advantage for tumours located in functionally critical areas. The procedure is performed in an outpatient setting and most patients tolerate it.[29] The technique avoids the delay associated with formalin-processed tissues and the need for multiple surgical procedures. For low risk small-diameter SCC (minimally invasive or in a low risk site), other treatment modalities should be considered as there is probably little to be gained in efficacy and much to be lost in terms of cost and time.

## Electrodesiccation and curettage

Electrodesiccation and curettage (ED&C) is frequently used in the treatment of SCC, particularly for *in situ* or minimally invasive lesions on the trunk or limbs. The tumour is prepared for ED&C and margins are marked. To take advantage of the finding that skin tumours are usually more friable than the surrounding normal tissue, the sharp tip of a curette can be used to debulk the tumour. Electric current through a fine-tipped needle is used to desiccate the base and destroy any residual tumour. This sequence is repeated several times and the eschar that remains is left to heal by secondary intention whereby the epidermis is allowed to regrow from the base and edges of the ulcer. Generally, secondary intention takes longer than primary closure and results in a circular rather than linear scar.

### Effectiveness

ED&C is frequently used for SCC, but no RCTs have compared ED&C with other treatments. Several case series have examined the cure rate of ED&C for SCC lesions. Freeman *et al.*[30] treated 407 SCC lesions by ED&C over a 20-year period with follow up ranging from 1 to over 5 years. In patients with a greater than 5-year follow up, they found that ED&C cured 96% (46/48) of SCC less than 2 cm in diameter and 100% (9/9) of SCC greater than 2 cm in diameter. Of the 407 treated SCC lesions, 355 were less than 2 cm, suggesting choice of this technique for smaller SCCs. Knox *et al.*[37] noted that only four SCC lesions recurred in 315 tumours treated with a follow up of 4 months to 2 years. SCC lesions in this study were all less than 2 cm and without significant invasion. Honeycutt and Jansen[38] treated 281 invasive SCC lesions by ED&C and reported three recurrences in a follow up of up to 4 years. Of the patients who developed recurrences, two had had tumours greater than 2 cm.[38] Whelan and Deckers[39] treated 26 SCC lesions and reported a 100% cure rate in a 2–9-year follow up.

## Drawbacks

The high cure rates obtained with ED&C in published case series probably reflect a selection bias for smaller and less invasive lesions. Cosmetically, the scar from ED&C is usually a hypopigmented sclerotic circle, as compared with a thin line from excision. Although the circular scar often contracts, hypertrophic changes can also occur that may make it difficult to recognise recurrent SCC. For SCC lesions on the face, particularly adjacent to critical tissues, contraction of resultant scars may distort or destroy the normal or functional anatomy. In addition, a surgeon performing ED&C at sites adjacent to vital or anatomically complex structures (such as the nose or eye) might limit the margins of destruction or be less aggressive in order to preserve native tissue; this is likely to diminish the effectiveness of this technique. Whelan and Deckers[39] found that 65% of treated wounds took only 4 weeks to heal, while in a separate study they found that the average time for healing was 5·1 weeks.[40]

Prolonged healing compared with surgical excision should be considered, particularly for lesions on the legs. Daily wound care is an essential part of ED&C, and diligence is required to prevent infection.

## Comment

ED&C appears to be effective for minimally invasive SCC lesions less than 2 cm in diameter. One clear advantage of ED&C over other modalities is that it is rapidly and easily performed by the experienced surgical clinician. Although the healing time may be increased, ED&C is an affordable, effective and rapid treatment option for SCC and should be considered for small or less invasive tumours. Adequate follow up is essential to recognise the rare recurrences.

## Cryotherapy

Cryotherapy has been used for decades and is highly effective for treating small or minimally invasive SCC. The standard treatment protocol for cryotherapy consists of two cycles of freezing with liquid nitrogen lasting 1·5 minutes per cycle. The technique takes longer than ED&C but less time than surgical excision.

### Effectiveness

No RCTs have compared the effectiveness of cryotherapy with other treatments. Several case series have examined the cure rate of cryosurgery in SCC. Over an 18-year period, Zacarian[41] treated 4228 skin cancers with cryotherapy, which included 203 SCC lesions. He noted a 97% cure rate in a follow up ranging from less than 3 months to over 10 years. Most recurrences (87%) occurred in the first 3 years. Zacarian further noted a healing time that ranged from 4 to 10 weeks. Kuflik and Gage[42] found a 96% 5-year cure rate for 52 SCC lesions. Holt[10] reported 34 SCC lesions treated with cryotherapy and a 97% cure after follow up ranging from 6 months to 5·5 years.

### Drawbacks

Cryotherapy is usually initially complicated by oedema, followed by blister formation. After rupture, the resultant crust takes 4–10 weeks to heal.[41] Hypopigmentation is universal, with occasional hypertrophic scarring.[41] Atrophic scars can be seen on the face, and neuropathy has been reported.[41] Since cryotherapy rarely destroys deep tissues, significant invasion should be considered a relative contraindication.[41]

Patients with abnormal cold tolerance, cryoglobulinaemia, autoimmune deficiency, or platelet deficiency should not be treated with cryotherapy.[41]

### Comment

Cryotherapy is effective for treating minimally invasive SCC on the trunk or limbs. Caution is needed when treating SCC on the face, particularly near vital structures.

## Other treatment options

Many other treatment modalities such as radiotherapy, photodynamic therapy, oral retinoids and topical imiquimod have been or are being tried for SCC.

## Clinical implications

In relation to the clinical scenario of an uncomplicated small SCC in an immunocompetent man, there is little in the evidence base to suggest that any one of the modalities above is "better" than the others. Choice of treatment will largely depend on the operator's preference, convenience to the patient and cost. Surgical excision has the advantage of offering clear visualisation of the tumour margins whereas ED&C and cryotherapy might be more convenient.

## Key points

- Risk factors for recurrence of cutaneous SCC are treatment modality, size greater than 2 cm, depth greater than 4 mm, poor histological differentiation, location on the ear or non-sun-exposed areas, perineural involvement, location within scars or chronic inflammation, previously failed treatment and immunosuppression.

- The evidence base for treatment of cutaneous SCC is poor **Evidence level IIb**.

- None of the commonly used procedures has been tested in rigorous RCTs.

- Case series which have followed up patients with SCC treated by surgical excision, MMS, ED&C and cryotherapy all suggest 3–5-year success rates of over 90%.

- Comparison of the success rates between the existing main treatments is almost impossible as choice of treatment is probably based on likelihood of success (for example, only people with small uncomplicated SCCs are treated by curettage).

- Based on the available case series, there is no evidence to suggest that any of the commonly used treatments for SCC are ineffective.

- Small (less than 2 cm) tumours at non-critical sites can probably be treated equally well by surgical excision with a 4 mm margin, ED&C, or cryotherapy.

- Larger tumours, especially at sites where tissue sparing becomes vital, are probably best treated by MMS.

- RCTs are needed to inform clinicians about the relative merits of the various treatments currently used for people with SCC.

- Such trials will need to be large to exclude small but important differences, and they will need to describe accurately the sorts of people entered in terms of risk factors for recurrences. Follow up in such studies needs to be 5 years or longer.

## References

1 Kirkham N. Tumors and cysts of the epidermis. In: Elder D, Elenitsas R, Jaworsky C, Johnson B Jr, eds. *Lever's Histopathology of the Skin.* Philadelphia: Lippincott-Raven, 1997.

2 Lohmann CM, Solomon AR. Clinicopathologic variants of cutaneous squamous cell carcinoma. *Adv Anat Pathol* 2001;**8**:27–36.

3 Barksdale SK, O'Connor N, Barnhill R. Prognostic factors for cutaneous squamous cell and basal cell carcinoma. Determinants of risk of recurrence, metastasis, and development of subsequent skin cancers. *Surg Oncol Clin North Am* 1997;**6**:625–38.

4 Preston DS, Stern RS. Nonmelanoma cancers of the skin. *N Engl J Med* 1992;**327**:1649–62.

5 Gray DT, Suman VJ, Su WPD *et al.* Trends in the population-based incidence of squamous cell carcinoma of the skin first diagnosed between 1984 and 1992. *Arch Dermatol* 1997;**133**:735–40.

6 Stenbeck KD, Balanda KP, Williams MJ *et al.* Patterns of treated non-melanoma skin cancer in Queensland – the region with the highest incidence rates in the world. *Med J Aust* 1990;**153**:511–15.

7 Magnus K. The Nordic profile of skin cancer incidence. A comparative epidemiological study of the three main types of skin cancer. *Int J Cancer* 1991;**47**:12–19.

8 Marks R, Staples M, Giles GG. The incidence of non-melanocytic skin cancers in an Australian population: results of a five-year prospective study. *Med J Aust* 1989;**150**:475–8.

9 Giles GG, Marks P, Foley P. Incidence of non-melanocytic skin cancer treated in Australia. *BMJ (Clin Res Ed)* 1988;**296**:13–17.

10 Holt PJ. Cryotherapy for skin cancer: results over a 5-year period using liquid nitrogen spray cryosurgery. *Br J Dermatol* 1988;**119**:231–40.

11 Scotto J, Kopf AW, Urbach F. Non-melanoma skin cancer among Caucasians in four areas of the United States. *Cancer* 1974;**34**:1333–8.

12 Schreiber MM, Shapiro SI, Berry CZ, Dahlen RF, Friedman RP. The incidence of skin cancer in southern Arizona (Tucson). *Arch Dermatol* 1971;**104**:124–7.

13 Serrano H, Scotto J, Shornick G, Fears TR, Greenberg ER. Incidence of nonmelanoma skin cancer in New Hampshire and Vermont. *J Am Acad Dermatol* 1991;**24**:574–9.

14 Dinehart SM, Pollack SV. Metastases from squamous cell carcinoma of the skin and lip. An analysis of twenty-seven cases. *J Am Acad Dermatol* 1989;**21**:241–8.

15 Johnson TM, Rowe DE, Nelson BR, Swanson NA. Squamous cell carcinoma of the skin (excluding lip and oral mucosa). *J Am Acad Dermatol* 1992;**26**:467–84.

16 Kwa REK, Campana K, Moy RL. Biology of cutaneous squamous cell carcinoma. *J Am Acad Dermatol* 1992;**26**:1–26.

17 Ziegler A, Jonason AS, Leffell DJ *et al.* Sunburn and p53 in the onset of skin cancer. *Nature* 1994;**372**:773–6.

18 Taguchi M, Watanabe S, Yashima K *et al.* Aberrations of the tumor suppressor p53 gene and p53 protein in solar keratosis in human skin. *J Invest Dermatol* 1994;**103**:500–3.

19 Campbell C, Quinn AG, Ro YS, Angus B, Rees JL. p53 mutations are common and early events that precede tumor invasion in squamous cell neoplasia of the skin. *J Invest Dermatol* 1993;**100**:746–8.

20 Brash DE, Rudolph JA, Simon JA *et al.* A role for sunlight in skin cancer: UV-induced p53 mutations in squamous cell carcinoma. *Proc Natl Acad Sci USA* 1991;**88**:10124–8.

21 Robbins JH. Xeroderma pigmentosum. Defective DNA repair causes skin cancer and neurodegeneration. *JAMA* 1988;**260**:384–8.

22 Hartevelt MM, Bavinck JN, Kootte AM, Vermeer BJ, Vandenbroucke JP. Incidence of skin cancer after renal transplantation in The Netherlands. *Transplantation* 1990;**49**:506–9.

23 Liddington M, Richardson AJ, Higgins RM *et al.* Skin cancer in renal transplant recipients. *Br J Surg* 1989;**76**:1002–5.

24 Boyle J, MacKie RM, Briggs JD *et al.* Cancer, warts, and sunshine in renal transplant patients. A case-control study. *Lancet* 1984;**8379**:702–5.

25 Dinehart SM, Chu DZ, Maners AW, Pollack SV. Immunosuppression in patients with metastatic squamous cell carcinoma from the skin. *J Dermatol Surg Oncol* 1990;**16**:271–4.

26 Rowe DE, Carroll RJ, Day CL Jr. Long-term recurrence rates in previously untreated (primary) basal cell carcinoma: implications for patient follow-up. *J Dermatol Surg Oncol* 1989;**15**:315–28.

27 Rowe DE, Carroll RJ, Day CL Jr. Prognostic factors for local recurrence, metastasis, and survival rates in squamous cell carcinoma of the skin, ear, and lip. Implications for treatment modality selection. *J Am Acad Dermatol* 1992;**26**:976–90.

28 Drake LA, Dinehart SM, Goltz RW *et al.* Guidelines of care for cutaneous squamous cell carcinoma. *J Am Acad Dermatol* 1993;**28**:628–31.

29 Drake LA, Dinehart SM, Goltz RW *et al.* Guidelines of care for Mohs micrographic surgery. *J Am Acad Dermatol* 1995;**33**:271–8.

30 Freeman RG, Knox JM, Heaton CL. The treatment of skin cancer: A statistical study of 1341 skin tumors comparing results obtained with

irradiation, surgery, and curettage followed by electrodesiccation. *Cancer* 1964;**17**:535–8.

31   Brodland DG, Zitelli JA. Surgical margins for excision of primary cutaneous squamous cell carcinoma. *J Am Acad Dermatol* 1992;**27**: 241–8.

32   Mohs FE. *Chemosurgery: Microscopically controlled surgery for skin cancer.* Springfield: Thomas CC, 1978.

33   Holmkvist KA, Roenigk RK. Squamous cell carcinoma of the lip treated with Mohs micrographic surgery: outcome at 5 years. *J Am Acad Dermatol* 1998;**38**:960–6.

34   Lawrence N, Cottel WI. Squamous cell carcinoma of skin with perineural invasion. *J Am Acad Dermatol* 1994;**31**:303.

35   Goepfert H, Dichtel WJ, Medina JE *et al.* Perineural invasion in squamous cell skin carcinoma of the head and neck. *Am J Surg* 1984;**148**:542–7.

36   Ballantyne AJ, McCarten AB, Ibanez ML. The extension of cancer of the head and neck through peripheral nerves. *Am J Surg* 1963;**106**:651–67.

37   Knox JM, Lyles TW, Shapiro EM, Martin RD. Curettage and electrodessication in the treatment of skin cancer. *Arch Dermatol* 1960;**82**:197–204.

38   Honeycutt WM, Jansen GT. Treatment of squamous cell carcinoma of the skin. *Arch Dermatol* 1973;**108**:670–2.

39   Whelan CS, Deckers PJ. Electrocoagulation for skin cancer: an old oncologic tool revisited. *Cancer* 1981;**47**:2280–7.

40   Whelan CS, Deckers PJ. Electrocoagulation and curettage for carcinoma involving the skin of the face, nose, eyelids, and ears. *Cancer* 1973;**31**:159–64.

41   Zacarian SA. Cryosurgery of cutaneous carcinomas. An 18-year study of 3,022 patients with 4,228 carcinomas. *J Am Acad Dermatol* 1983;**9**:947–56.

42   Kuflik EG, Gage AA. The five-year cure rate achieved by cryosurgery for skin cancer. *J Am Acad Dermatol* 1991;**24**:1002–4.

# 44 Primary cutaneous T-cell lymphoma

*Sean Whittaker*

## Background

### Definition

Primary cutaneous T-cell lymphomas (CTCL) represent a heterogeneous group of extranodal non-Hodgkin's lymphoma of which mycosis fungoides/Sézary syndrome (MF/SS) are the most common clinicopathological subtypes.[1] Mycosis fungoides is characterised by distinct clinical stages of cutaneous disease consisting of patches/plaques, tumours and erythroderma in which the whole skin is involved (Figures 44.1–44.4). Peripheral adenopathy may or may not be present. Sézary syndrome is defined by the presence of erythroderma, peripheral lymphadenopathy, and the presence of a minimum number of Sézary cells within the peripheral blood. These clinicopathological entities are closely related pathogenetically but distinct from other less common types of primary cutaneous T-cell lymphomas.

### Incidence/prevalence

The overall annual incidence of primary CTCL in the US is 0·5–1·0 per 100 000 based on population data in 1988 but the prevalence is much higher because most patients have low grade disease and long-term survival.[2] Males (2:1) and the Black population are affected more commonly.[2,3] The incidence has increased during the past two decades but this almost certainly reflects improved diagnosis of earlier stages and possibly better registration particularly in the USA.[3]

### Aetiology

The underlying aetiology is unknown. There is evidence for inactivation of key tumour suppressor genes and TH2 cytokine production by tumour cells in mycosis

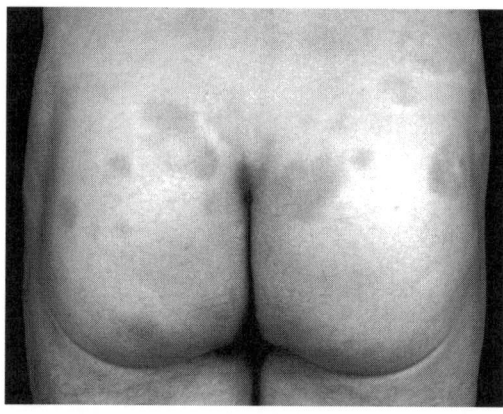

**Figure 44.3** Patch stage mycosis fungoides (IA)

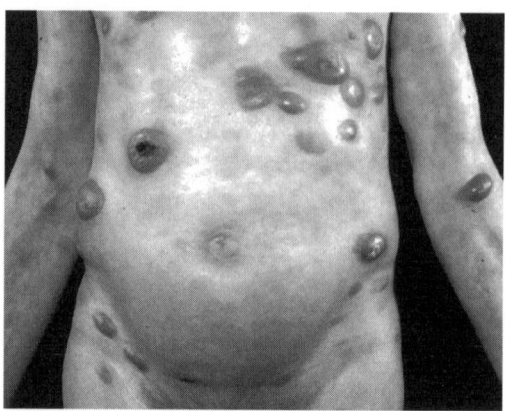

**Figure 44.4** Tumour stage mycosis fungoides (IIB)

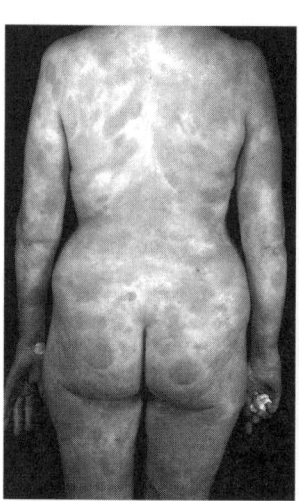

**Figure 44.1** Plaque stage mycosis fungoides (IB/IIA)

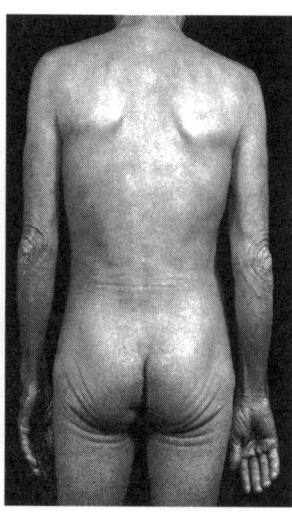

**Figure 44.2** Erythrodermic mycosis fungoides (III)

fungoides/Sézary syndrome but as yet no disease-specific molecular abnormality has been identified.[4] Primary CTCL must be distinguished from human T-lymphotropic virus type-1 (HTLV-I) associated adult T-cell leukaemia lymphoma (ATLL) in which cutaneous involvement often closely mimics the clinicopathological features of MF/SS and may be the presenting feature.[1]

## Prognosis

The majority of cases of primary CTCL are not curable, and independent prognostic features in mycosis fungoides include the cutaneous and lymph node stage of disease and age of onset ($> 60$), while the lymph node status and tumour burden within peripheral blood determine the prognosis in Sézary syndrome.[5,6] Serum LDH and the thickness of the infiltrate in plaque stage mycosis fungoides are also independent markers of prognosis.[3,7] Multivariate analysis indicates that an initial complete response to various therapies is an independent favourable prognostic feature, particularly in early stages of disease.[8–10] For mycosis fungoides two staging systems are in regular use, including a TNM system and a clinical staging specifically designed for CTCL (Box 44.1; Table 44.1).[5] These staging systems can also be applied to Sézary syndrome although neither system provides a quantitative method for assessing peripheral blood disease other than an additional B0 and B1 in the TNM system and this has prompted alternative approaches for Sézary syndrome.[6]

Recent published actuarial survival data for mycosis fungoides are summarised in Table 44.2. The overall 5- and 10-year actuarial survival (OS) in mycosis fungoides is 80% and 57% respectively with disease-specific survival (DSS) rates of 89% and 75% at 5 and 10 years respectively.[8] Patients with very early stage disease (IA) are very unlikely to die of their disease with DSS of 100% and 97–98% at 5 and 10 years respectively and risks of disease progression varying from 0% to 10% over 5 to 20 years.[8–11] In one study of 122 patients with stage IA disease, median survival was not reached at 32·5 years.[9]

---

**Box 44.1 TNM (primary tumour, regional nodes, metastasis) classification for mycosis fungoides (including "B" system for cutaneous T-cell lymphoma [CTCL] to incorporate Sézary syndrome)**

**Skin**

**T1** Limited patches/plaques (< 10% of total skin surface)
**T2** Extensive patches/plaques (> 10% of total skin surface)
**T3** Tumours
**T4** Erythroderma

**Nodes**

**N0** No clinical lymphadenopathy
**N1** Clinically enlarged lymph nodes but histologically uninvolved
**N2** Lymph nodes not enlarged but histologically involved
**N3** Clinically enlarged lymph nodes and histologically involved

**Visceral**

**M0** No visceral involvement
**M1** Visceral involvement

**Blood**

**B0** No peripheral blood Sézary cells (< 5%)
**B1** Peripheral blood Sézary cells (> 5% of total lymphocyte count)

---

Stage IB patients have an OS varying from 73% to 86% at 5 years and 58% to 67% at 10 years, and DSS rates of 96% and 83% at 5 and 10 years respectively.[3,8,10] A median survival of 12·1–12·8 years should be expected for stage IB patients with a risk of disease progression varying from 10% to 39%. The explanation for this marked variation in different studies of stage IB is unclear but it appears that patients with folliculotropic variants of mycosis fungoides have a worse prognosis compared with other patients with stage IB disease, which may reflect the depth of infiltrate and a consequent reduced therapeutic efficacy for skin-directed therapy.[8]

There is limited accurate data regarding stage IIA patients (patches/plaques and clinical adenopathy with no histological

---

**Table 44.1   Clinical staging system for CTCL (mycosis fungoides)**

| Clinical stages | T | N | M |
|---|---|---|---|
| IA | T1 | N0 | M0 |
| IB | T2 | N0 | M0 |
| IIA | T1–2 | N1 | M0 |
| IIB | T3 | N0–1 | M0 |
| III | T4 | N0–1 | M0 |
| IVA | T1–4 | N2–3 | M0 |
| IVB | T1–4 | N0–3 | M1 |

**Table 44.2  Published outcomes according to clinical stage in cutaneous T-cell lymphoma.**

| Parameter | IA | IB | IIA | IIB | III | IVA | IVB | Overall | Reference | No. of patients | Median follow up (years) |
|---|---|---|---|---|---|---|---|---|---|---|---|
| *Overall survival (%)** | | | | | | | | | | | |
| 5 years | 99 | 86 | 49 | 65 | | 40 | 0 | 80 | 8[†] | 309 | 5·2 |
| | 100 | 84 | | 52 | 57 | | | | 3[‡] | 489 | 4·7 |
| | 96 | (78) | | (40) | (40) | | | | 9[§] | 122 | 9·8 |
| | | 73 | 73[ǁ] | | | | | | 10[ǁ] | 176 | 8 |
| | | | | | 45 | 17 | | | 12[¶] | 106 | 10·5 |
| | | | | | | 15 | 15 | | 11[**] | 112 | |
| 10 years | 84 | 61 | 49 | 27 | | 20 | 0 | 57 | 8 | 309 | 5·2 |
| | 100 | 67 | | 39 | 41 | | | | 3 | 489 | 4·7 |
| | 88 | (60) | | (20) | (20) | | | | 9 | 122 | 9·8 |
| | | 58 | 45[ǁ] | | | | | | 10 | 176 | 8 |
| | | | | | | 5 | 5 | | 11 | 112 | |
| *Disease-specific survival (%)* | | | | | | | | | | | |
| 5 years | 100 | 96 | 68 | 80 | | 40 | 0 | 89 | 8 | 309 | 5·2 |
| 10 years | 97 | 83 | 68 | 42 | | 20 | 0 | 75 | 8 | 309 | 5·2 |
| | 98 | | | | | | | | 9 | 122 | 9·8 |
| **Median survival (years)** | NR[§] | 12·1 | | 2·9 | 3·6 | | | | 9 | 556 | 9·8 |
| | | 12·8 | 10·0 | | | | | | 10 | 176 | 8 |
| | | | | | 4·6 | 13 months | | | 12 | 106 | 10·5 |
| | | | | | | 13 months | 13 months | | 11 | 546 | |
| *Disease progression (%)* | | | | | | | | | | | |
| 5 years | 4 | 21 | 65 | 32 | | 70 | 100 | | 8 | 309 | 5·2 |
| 10 years | 10 | 39 | 65 | 60 | | 70 | 100 | | 8 | 309 | 5·2 |
| 20 years | 0 | 10 | | 36 | 41 | | | | 11 | 546 | |
| Overall | 9 | | | | | | | | 9 | 122 | 9·8 |
| | | 20 | 34[ǁ] | | | | | | 10 | 176 | 8 |
| *FFR (%)* | | | | | | | | | | | |
| 5 years | 50 | | | | | | | | 9 | 122 | 9·8 |
| | | 36 | 9 | | | | | | 10 | 176 | 8 |
| 10 years | 25 (50) | | | | | | | | 9 | 122 | 9·8 |
| | | 31 | 3 | | | | | | 10 | 176 | 8 |

*All overall (OS) survival curves were calculated using the Kaplan–Meier method.

[†]In the study by Doorn *et al.*[8] the presence of follicular mucinosis was an independent poor prognostic feature possibly related to depth of infiltrate in patients with stage IB disease (disease-free survival of 81% and 36% and OS of 75% and 21% at 5 and 10 years, respectively). A lack of a complete response to initial therapy was also associated with a poor outcome ($P<0.001$) in a multivariate analysis as well as increasing clinical stage and the presence of extracutaneous disease. A different staging system was used in this study (Hamminga *et al. Br J Dermatol* 1982;**107**:1451–5) but for the purposes of this table the staging has been altered to be consistent. This study is the only one to provide comprehensive disease-specific survival (DSS) data for different stages of mycosis fungoides. Only three patients had stage IVB disease and only 18 patients each had stage IIA and IVA disease. Therefore the results for these stages must be interpreted cautiously.

[‡]In the study by Zackheim *et al.*,[3] Black patients had a relatively more advanced stage of disease than White patients. The TNM classification was used in this study. Lymph node stage had an unfavourable impact on survival but this trend did not reach significance for *each individual* T stage because of a lack of sufficient power (an estimated 1700 subjects required) and

*(Continued)*

**Table 44.2** *(Continued)*

IIA/IVA patients were not designated separately. Similar considerations apply to peripheral blood involvement. Similar outcomes for patients with stage IIB (T3) and III (T4) disease are consistent with other studies but this might reflect a lack of lymph node staging data included in this study.

§The 1996 study by Kim *et al.*[9] primarily included data on 122 patients with stage IA disease, but survival data on 556 patients with all stages were also included to give the values in parentheses. The freedom from relapse (FFR) data at 5 and 10 years are confusing because the text states that the FFR at 10 years was 25% but the figure indicates that it remains at approximately 50%, as for FFR at 5 years. The median survival for stage IA patients was not reached at 32·5 years. NR, not reached.

‖In the 1999 study by Kim *et al.*[10] OS at 20 years for stages IB and IIA patients was 27%. DSS was better for patients <58 years of age (*P*<0·03). In 23 of the 56 patients with palpable lymphadenopathy, no histological assessment was made and these patients were assumed to have reactive/dermatopathic nodes (IIA). This might account for the lack of difference in OS at 5 years between stage IB and IIA patients, although there appears to be a difference in OS at 10 years.

¶In the 1995 study by Kim *et al.*[12] the OS and median survival data was calculated from the date of initial treatment, which was usually within 3 months of diagnosis. This study also stratified patients into three groups according to the presence of none, one, or two, or three poor prognostic parameters, namely: age at presentation (>65 years), the presence of clinical adenopathy, and B1 stage, producing varied median survivals of 10·2 years (no factors), 3·7 years (one factor), and 1·5 years (two or three factors) *P*<0·005.

**The study by Connick *et al.*[11] included 112 patients with extracutaneous disease at presentation or with progression and 434 patients with only cutaneous disease, giving the 546 patients listed in the table for median survival and disease progression.

evidence of lymphoma) but it appears that this stage may be associated with a worse outcome with overall survival rates of 49%, DSS of 68%, and risk of disease progression of 65% at both 5 and 10 years. The lack of difference in outcome at 5 and 10 years in this study is surprising but these data were only based on 18 patients and need confirmation with larger numbers.[8] Of the 176 patients reported by Kim *et al.* (1999) 56 (32%) had peripheral adenopathy (stage IIA) but in 23 of these 56 patients no histological assessment was made and therefore some of these patients could have had stage IVA disease.[10] Nevertheless the OS is similar to stage IB disease at 5 years (73%) with a slight difference at 10 years (45% *v* 58%) associated with a small difference in median survival of 10 years (stage IIA) compared with 12·8 years (stage IB) and overall risk of disease progression of 34% and 20%, respectively. Further studies of larger numbers of patients with stage IIA disease are required to compare outcomes with those of stage IB patients.

Patients with tumour stage disease (stage IIB) have OS varying from 40% to 65% at 5 years and 20% to 39% at 10 years[3,8,9] and a median survival of 2·9 years in one study.[9] In one study DSS of 80% and 42% at 5 and 10 years respectively were reported for patients with stage IIB disease.[8] The survival data for patients with erythrodermic mycosis fungoides, but no evidence of lymph node or peripheral blood involvement (stage III), are broadly similar to those for stage IIB disease, although median survival may be better (4·6 *v* 2·9 years).[3,9,12] In contrast the OS and DSS at 5 and 10 years for stage IVA and IVB patients are poor (15–40% and 5–20% for IVA and 0–15% and 0–5% for stage

IVB at 5 and 10 years respectively) and a median survival of 13 months for both extracutaneous stages.[8,11,12]

The overall survival in CTCL based on stage of disease has led to suggestions that the staging system should be modified with four broad categories[13]:

- stage IA patients have a normal life expectancy, but
- stage IB and IIA disease may have a similar prognosis, although the thickness of the infiltrate is an important prognostic factor in this group.
- Similarly stage IIB and III disease has a similar prognosis, which is better than those patients with nodal or visceral disease (IVA/B). This proposal is similar to that suggested by Sausville *et al.* in 1988.[14]

Patients with Sézary syndrome have an 11% 5-year survival with a median survival of 32 months from diagnosis.[1] In contrast, other clinicopathological variants of CTCL are generally associated with an excellent long-term prognosis (100% 5-year survival in lymphomatoid papulosis and 90% in primary cutaneous CD30+ large cell anaplastic cutaneous lymphoma), with the exception of patients with subcutaneous panniculitis-like T-cell lymphomas and primary cutaneous NK-like T-cell/NK cell lymphomas.[1]

### Diagnostic tests

The diagnosis of different variants of primary CTCL is based on a critical assessment of the clinicopathological features.

Repeated biopsies may be required to establish the diagnosis and correlation between the histology and clinical features is essential. Immunophenotypic studies are required to identify different CTCL variants, and analysis of T-cell receptor genes in DNA extracted from skin biopsies can identify a T-cell clone, which helps to confirm the diagnosis. However T-cell clones are not always detected in early stages of mycosis fungoides owing to a lack of sensitivity. Investigations including a CT scan of the chest, abdomen and pelvis to exclude systemic involvement, and assessment of peripheral blood for Sézary cells and lymphocyte subsets are indicated in all patients with the exception of those with early stages of mycosis fungoides (IA/IB) and lymphomatoid papulosis.[15] Bone marrow aspirate/trephine biopsies are indicated in CTCL variants but rarely in mycosis fungoides and Sézary syndrome.

## Aims of treatment

Treatment is aimed at inducing complete or partial remissions of disease and prolonging disease-free and overall survival while maintaining the patient's quality of life.

## Relevant outcomes

- Severity of symptoms (pruritus, sleep disturbance, pain) and signs (erythema, scaling, fissuring, excoriation, oedema and thickness of plaques, presence of nodules, tumours, peripheral lymphadenopathy)
- Body surface area involvement
- Assessment of overall tumour burden with histological assessment of skin and lymph nodes, staging CT scans, and peripheral blood Sézary cell counts/lymphocyte subsets
- Establishment of molecular remission using TCR gene analysis of skin and peripheral blood
- Quality of life.

Several recent trials have used various scoring systems involving computed measures of the above but most studies included in this review define responses in terms of simple clinical observation with complete responses (CR) defined as complete resolution of clinically apparent disease (usually based in CTCL on cutaneous signs of disease) for at least 4–6 weeks. Partial responses (PR) are usually defined as greater than a 50% reduction of clinical disease or tumour burden, although some studies in CTCL have defined this as more than 25% reduction in tumour burden. More importantly most studies do not include a validated scoring system, which effectively makes any interpretation of PR impossible. Similar considerations apply to assessment of stable disease (SD), defined usually as less than 50% improvement, and progressive disease (PD), defined as over 25% increase in tumour burden. For most studies in CTCL PD is defined as a deterioration in clinical stage of disease.

## What are the effects of topical therapy in mycosis fungoides?

### Topical corticosteroids

#### *Benefits*

No systematic reviews and no RCTs have been identified. One large open uncontrolled study of 79 patients with mycosis fungoides (stage T1/T2) who were treated with class I–III (potent/moderate potency) topical corticosteroids twice daily for 3–4 months and under occlusion showed complete clinical remissions in 63% and partial remissions in 31% of stage T1 patients, and complete and partial responses in 25% and 57% respectively for patients with stage T2.[16] Complete responses were confirmed histologically in seven patients but the median duration of complete response was not documented **Evidence level IIa**.

#### *Drawbacks*

Reversible depression of serum cortisol levels occurred in 13% of patients and skin atrophy in one patient.

#### *Comment*

Lack of controlled studies and short median follow up of 9 months weakens impact of results. There was no evidence of impact on disease-free or overall survival. However, it does appear that topical corticosteroids, especially class 1 (potent) compounds, are effective at temporarily clearing patches and plaques in some patients with early stage IA/IB mycosis fungoides **Grade B**.

### Topical mechlorethamine (nitrogen mustard)

#### *Benefits*

No RCTs were identified. A retrospective review of 123 patients treated at one institution (1969–85) with whole body once daily application of topical mechlorethamine (10–20 mg ml$^{-1}$ aqueous preparation from 1968–1980 and ointment base from 1980–1985) until maximum response reported complete response rates of 51% in IA, 26% in IB, 0% in IIB and 22% in stage III disease.[17] There were no differences in outcome with the aqueous or ointment base. Fifty patients had received total skin electron beam therapy (TSEB) prior to topical mechlorethamine. Relapse occurred in 56% of patients who achieved a complete response despite continued maintenance treatment for 1–2 years[17] **Evidence level III**.

A study of 117 patients reported complete response in 76% for stage I disease, 45% for stage II and 49% for stage III patients within 2 years of therapy (median response duration of 45 months).[18] Patients in this study were allowed local radiotherapy for tumours as well and these were not excluded as responders. Overall 5-year survival for all patients in this study was 89% **Evidence level IIb**.

In a retrospective review of 331 patients (all stages/ 1968–1982), treated with topical mechlorethamine daily and with maintenance therapy daily or on alternate days for at least 3 years for those with a complete response, a complete remission was observed in 20% lasting 4–14 years but was confined to those with stage IA–IB.[19] However, patients in this series were allowed other therapies including radiotherapy, TSEB, phototherapy and methotrexate to achieve a response. Subsequent relapse occurred in only 17% of these patients within 8 years of withdrawing therapy, suggesting that some patients with very early stage disease may have achieved a cure. Response rates were highest in early stages of disease (IA, 80%; IB, 68%; IIA, 61%; IIB, 49%; III, 60%; IVA, 13%; IVB, 11%). Stage-specific 5/10 year survival rates were 94/89% (IA), 85/83% (IB), 82/67% (IIA), 59/31% (IIB), 75/49% (III), 20/13% (IVA) and 11/0% (IVB), respectively[19] **Evidence level III**.

## Drawbacks

Topical mechlorethamine may cause an irritant reaction and contact hypersensitivity develops in up to 40% of patients. This is less common with the ointment (0·01–0·02%) and the aqueous solution (10–20 mg in 40–60 ml of water) is less stable. Mechlorethamine (nitrogen mustard) is carcinogenic and secondary cutaneous malignancies (non-melanoma skin cancer) have been attributed to long-term use of topical mechlorethamine (8·6-fold and 1·8-fold increased risk for SCC and BCC, respectively). Home use is acceptable with patients applying topical treatment overnight, but partners should avoid contact especially when pregnant. Appropriate protection for staff members applying topical therapy in the hospital setting is required, although no toxic effects have been reported.[20]

## Comments

Mechlorethamine is an effective topical therapy for early stage (patches/thin plaques) mycosis fungoides. However, interpretation of these studies is confounded by the use of other therapeutic modalities for most patients and the retrospective nature of these studies. Duration of response varies and the benefits of maintenance therapy (6–18 months) and whole body application remains unclear, but cures may be achieved in some patients with stage IA disease. The survival data reported for topical mechlorethamine are similar to those previously published for patients with early stage disease (Table 44.2). Any clinical benefit of topical mechlorethamine therapy after TSEB has to be confirmed. Almost all patients with stage IA mycosis fungoides have

normal life expectancy and so controlled trials are required **Grade B**.

## Topical carmustine (BCNU)

### Benefits

No RCTs were found. A retrospective review of therapy in 143 patients revealed complete response in 86% stage IA, 47% stage IB, 55% stage IIA, 17% stage IIB, 21% stage III and 0% in stage IV.[21] Median time to complete response was 11·5 weeks. Alternate day or daily treatment with 10 mg of BCNU in dilute (95%) alcohol (60 ml) or 20–40% BCNU ointment can be used **Evidence level III**.

### Drawbacks

Contact hypersensitivity is uncommon (10%) but bone marrow suppression is common (30%). The risk of secondary cutaneous malignancies may be lower than with mechlorethamine. Total doses should not exceed 600 mg per course and repeated courses may be required. Maintenance therapy should be avoided. The ointment is more stable than the alcohol solution (3 months).

### Comments

Although data are limited, topical carmustine appears to be clinically effective but has greater systemic absorption than mechlorethamine and therefore has a significant risk of bone marrow suppression. It may be helpful in patients with early stage disease who show an irritant or allergic contact reaction to mechlorethamine. Appropriate comparative trials are indicated **Grade B**.

## Topical retinoids

### Benefits

No RCTs were found. A phase I/II open study of 0·1–1% bexarotene (Targretin) gel at incremental doses in 67 patients with stage IA/IB/IIA disease (initially alternate day treatment increasing to a maximum of q.i.d. daily treatment if tolerated) showed a response rate of 63%, with 21% of patients showing a complete clinical response.[22] Median time to and duration of response were 20 and 99 weeks, respectively **Evidence level IIa**.

### Drawbacks

1% gel b.d. was well tolerated. Mild/moderate pruritus, burning pain, and rash (12% irritant contact dermatitis) were common.

### Comment

The lack of a placebo control makes interpretation difficult but the Federal Drug Agency (FDA) has approved

1% Targretin gel for the treatment of patients with stage IA/IB disease. Further studies are required **Grade B**.

## Topical peldesine (BCX-34)

Peldesine is an inhibitor of the enzyme purine nucleoside phosphorylase involved in purine degradation within lymphocytes.

### *Benefits*

One RCT has compared topical application of peldesine twice daily to the entire skin surface for 24 weeks with a placebo (vehicle control) in 90 patients with stage IA/IB mycosis fungoides.[23] Partial or complete clinical responses occurred in 28% of patients treated with Peldesine and 24% of patients treated with placebo ($P = 0.677$) **Evidence level Ib**.

### *Drawbacks*

Minor pruritus and rash were noted by a small minority of patients.

### *Comment*

This is the only published placebo-controlled trial in CTCL. Although no significant benefit is apparent, the results indicate a high placebo therapeutic response (mostly PRs) which should be considered when interpreting the efficacy of different topical therapies in early stage mycosis fungoides. This study also emphasises the importance of developing a validated scoring system to assess partial responses **Grade A**.

## What are the effects of phototherapy in MF/SS?

## Phototherapy

### *Benefits*

No RCTs were found. Broadband UVB (290–320 nm) phototherapy with maintenance therapy produced complete responses in 83% of 35 patients with early stage disease (IA/IB) with a median response time of 5 months and median response duration of 22 months[24] **Evidence level IIa**.

Narrow band UVB (TL-01/311–313 nm) also produced complete responses in 75% of patients (six of eight cases with early patch stage IA disease) with a mean duration of response of 20 months[25] **Evidence level IIa**.

High dose UVA1 phototherapy (340–400 nm) has been used in 13 patients (eight stage IB, four IIB, and one III disease) with 100 J cm$^{-2}$ on a 5-day weekly basis until maximal response: 11/13 patients showed a complete

response, defined by a complete resolution of cutaneous lesions (mean number of sessions 22 and cumulative dose 2149 J cm$^{-2}$) and seven patients remained in CR after a mean follow up of 7·2 months.[26] **Evidence level IIa**.

### *Drawbacks*

UV-induced erythema and non-melanoma skin cancer with high cumulative doses were seen.

### *Comments*

UVB phototherapy is an effective therapy for early patch and thin plaques but duration of disease-free remission varies and treatment probably does not affect long-term survival rates. UVA1 has a deeper penetration than both UVB and PUVA but whether this is clinically relevant has not yet been established. No adequate comparative studies between different forms of phototherapy and PUVA have been published **Grade B**.

## PUVA photochemotherapy

### *Benefits*

No RCTs were found. An open study of 82 patients treated with PUVA and followed for up to 15 years reported an overall complete response rate of 65% (79% for stage IA, 59% for stage IB and 83% for stage IIA disease) and mean cumulative doses of 134 J cm$^{-2}$ (IA), 140 J cm$^{-2}$ (IB) and 240 J cm$^{-2}$ (IIA) respectively with a median time to complete response of 3 months.[27] Few patients with more advanced disease were treated making interpretation of results for patients with worse than stage IIA difficult. In this study 67% of stage IA, 41% of stage IB and 67% of stage IIA patients were free of disease at 2 years but maintenance PUVA was given to most patients.[27] Survival rates at 5 and 10 years were 89% for stage IA, 78% for stage IB and, surprisingly, 100% for stage IIA, respectively **Evidence level IIa**.

A further open study of PUVA in 82 patients with CTCL showed complete responses in 62% of patients with 88% CR in stage IA (mean cumulative PUVA dose 160 J cm$^{-2}$), 52% CR in stage IB (mean cumulative PUVA dose 498 J cm$^{-2}$) and 46% in stage III disease (mean PUVA cumulative dose 178 J cm$^{-2}$). No responses were seen in stage IIB patients. The maximum duration of response was 68 months and 38% of complete responders relapsed despite maintenance PUVA[28] **Evidence level IIa**.

Although maintenance therapy has been recommended for responders, a further open study has shown that 56% of stage IA and 39% of stage IB patients with a complete response had no recurrence of CTCL during a maximum period of 44 months follow up despite no maintenance therapy[29] **Evidence level IIa**.

## Drawbacks

Nausea, phototoxic reactions, and skin carcinogenesis are well recognised adverse effects. The risk of non-melanoma skin cancer is directly related to the cumulative dose and total number of sessions.

## Comments

Despite the lack of controlled trials, PUVA remains one of the most useful skin directed therapies for early stages of mycosis fungoides. RCTs comparing PUVA with TL01 and topical mechlorethamine would be helpful in early stage disease (IA/IB). Duration of response and DFS/OS data are also urgently required. The role of maintenance therapy is unclear but high cumulative doses are associated with a significant risk of SCC. A comparison of the disease-free and overall survival rates in patients treated with topical chemotherapy, phototherapy and TSEB is difficult because there are no RCTs, but there appears to be little difference in early stage disease, which emphasises the urgent need for RCTs **Grade B**.

## Combination regimens involving photochemotherapy

### Benefits

An RCT has compared PUVA (2–5 times per week) plus interferon alfa (IFNα) (9 MU × 3 per week) with IFNα plus acitretin (25–50 mg per day) in 98 patients (maximum duration of treatment in both groups 48 weeks).[30] In 82 patients with stage I/II 70% complete responses were observed in the PUVA/IFNα group compared with 38% in the IFNα/acitretin group ($P < 0.05$). Responses were assessed on the basis of clinical observation only. Time to response in the PUVA/IFNα was 18·6 weeks compared with 21·8 weeks in the IFNα/acitretin group ($P = 0.026$) but no data on duration of response were reported. Total cumulative doses of IFNα were similar in both groups **Evidence level IIb**.

An open study of 69 patients has compared PUVA and acitretin with PUVA alone in mycosis fungoides.[31] This showed that the cumulative dose of PUVA to achieve a CR was lower in the combined treatment group although the overall CR (73%/72%) in both groups was similar. No data on duration of response were documented[31] **Evidence level IIa**.

Phase I and II studies of PUVA (3 times a week) combined with variable doses of IFNα (maximum tolerated dose of 12 MU m$^{-2}$ × 3 a week) in 39 patients with mycosis fungoides (all stages) and Sézary syndrome have reported an overall response rate of 90% with 62% showing a complete response and 28% a partial response (CRs of 79% in stage IB, 80% in IIA, 33% in IIB, 63% in III, 40% in IVA).[32] PUVA

was continued as a maintenance therapy indefinitely while IFNα was continued for 2 years or until disease progression or withdrawal owing to adverse effects. The median response duration was 28 months with a median survival of 62 months [32] **Evidence level IIa**.

## Drawbacks

Adverse effects were similar to those with PUVA, IFNα and acitretin alone. In the RCT similar rates of mild/moderate adverse effects were noted in both groups but there were more treatment discontinuations in the IFN/acitretin group because of adverse effects.

## Comments

The RCT comparing PUVA and interferon alfa with PUVA and acitretin is one of very few in CTCL and the data clearly indicate that combined PUVA and IFNα are more effective than IFNα and acitretin in early stage I/II disease **Grade A**. A weakness of this study is the lack of a validated scoring system to assess tumour burden and lack of evidence that outcome was assessed blind to allocation status. In addition data regarding the duration of response and DFS/OS are urgently required.

The PUVA versus PUVA plus acitretin trial suggests a reduction in mean cumulative dose of PUVA to CR, which would be helpful, but disappointingly there is no evidence for increased overall efficacy in the retinoid-PUVA group **Grade B**. The combination of IFNα and PUVA appears to be highly effective in all stages of CTCL, and an RCT comparing PUVA alone with PUVA and IFNα has recently closed but results are awaited.

## What are the effects of immunotherapy in MF/SS?

### IFNα

### Benefits

No RCTs of IFNα have been reported in CTCL except as combination therapy (see above). In an open study 20 heavily pretreated patients (stage IB–III) were given maximally tolerated doses of IFNα (50 MU m$^{-2}$ i.m. × 3 per week) for 3 months.[33] An overall response rate of 45% was reported with a median duration of 5 months **Evidence level IIa**.

A subsequent non-randomised study revealed response rates of 64% in 22 patients (stage IA–IVA) with an overall complete response rate of 27%.[34] Objective responses were greater (78% v 37%) in the group treated with an escalating dose schedule of IFNα (36 MU per day) compared with those on a low dose regimen (3 MU per day) for 10 weeks, but overall numbers were too small for statistical comparison **Evidence level IIa**.

An open study of 43 patients treated with escalating doses (3–18 MU daily) of IFNα showed an overall response rate of 74% with a complete response rate of 26%.[35] Responses were more common in those who had not had prior treatment and in those with stage I/II (88%) compared with those with stage III/IV (63%) disease. Disease-free survival was 21% at 55 months **Evidence level IIa**.

A phase II study of intermittent high dose IFNα 2a given on days 1–5 every 3 weeks (mean dose 65·5 MU m$^{-2}$ per week) showed a response rate of 29% with only one CR in 24 patients with advanced (IVA/B) refractory CTCL.[36] Dose reductions were necessary and no improved responses were seen in those patients receiving dose escalation **Evidence level IIa**.

In an open study 45 patients with CTCL including 13 patients with Sézary syndrome were treated with low dose IFNα (6–9 MU daily) for 3 months and those responding were continued on IFNα alone while non-responders were given a combination of IFNα and acitretin (0·5 mg kg$^{-1}$ per day).[37] After 12 months' therapy 62% achieved a partial or complete response including 11 patients on combined therapy. However, this study design does not exclude the possibility that the response in the IFNα non-responder group was due to a delayed benefit from continued IFNα therapy after 3 months **Evidence level IIa**.

Intralesional IFNα (1–2 MU × 3 per week for 4 weeks) can induce complete regression of individual plaques (10 of 12 sites) compared with placebo-treated sites (1 of 12 sites)[38] **Evidence level IIb**.

### Drawbacks

Dose-limiting toxicity of IFNα includes reversible haematological abnormalities, hepatitis, 'flu-like symptoms consisting of fever, weight loss, myalgia, lethargy, anorexia, headache and depression.

### Comments

The clinical efficacy of IFNα in all stages of CTCL is supported by the complete response rates seen in these uncontrolled studies, and it appears that higher doses are more effective, although dose-limiting toxicity is a problem. Response rates are lower in advanced stages of disease (IVA/B) **Grade B**. Critical questions remain, however, about the effect on disease-free and overall survival and the role of combined therapy with PUVA. RCTs are required to address these issues.

### Interferon gamma

#### Benefits

No RCTs were found. A phase II trial of IFNγ in 16 CTCL patients with escalating doses to a maximum of 0·5 mg m$^{-2}$ intramuscularly daily reported objective partial responses of 31% with a median duration of 10 months[39] **Evidence level IIb**.

### Drawbacks

Adverse effects were similar to those following IFNα.

### Comments

The lack of complete responses is disappointing. Further studies are required but are a low priority **Grade B**.

### Interleukins

#### Benefits

No RCTs were found. Interleukin-2 (20 MU m$^{-2}$ every 2 weeks for 6 weeks and then monthly for 5 months) produced responses in five of seven CTCL patients including three complete responses[40] **Evidence level IIb**.

In a phase I dose escalation trial of subcutaneous interleukin-12 (50–300 ng kg$^{-1}$) twice weekly for up to 24 weeks, objective responses were noted in five CTCL patients (4/5, IB; 1/3, SS).[41] Two patients with stage IB disease had a CR within 7–8 weeks, which was confirmed histologically. Intralesional therapy was also effective for individual tumours in two patients with stage IIB disease, although both developed progressive disease[41] **Evidence level IIb**.

### Drawbacks

There were minor adverse effects including 'flu-like symptoms, mild transient liver function abnormalities and depression.

### Comments

RCTs are required to establish whether interleukin-2 and interleukin-12 have any therapeutic role in CTCL **Grade B**.

### Extracorporeal photopheresis

#### Benefits

No RCTs have been reported. A systematic review (1987–1998) of response rates and outcomes in open non-randomised and mostly retrospective studies of extracorporeal photopheresis (ECP) in erythrodermic CTCL (stage III/IVA) showed an overall response rate of 35–71% with complete response rates from 14% to 26%.[42] Responses have been assessed mostly using a similar scoring system to that devised for the original study[43] **Evidence level IIb**.

A further retrospective study of 34 patients with mostly erythrodermic CTCL (overall 22, IV; 10, III; 2, I) reported an overall response rate of 50% with 18% achieving a CR.[44] Response was restricted to those with erythrodermic disease. This study involved a modified "accelerated" treatment schedule consisting of nine (as opposed to six) collections during each cycle and an increase to twice monthly treatment if there was a lack of response **Evidence level III**.

Other studies have reported minor responses (25–50% improvement) but this would not satisfy accepted criteria for a partial response. ECP is generally administered on two consecutive days (one cycle each month) and it is accepted that at least six cycles are required to assess response. Survival data have been reported in four studies of erythrodermic disease with median survivals of 39 to 100 months from diagnosis.[45–48]

A randomised cross-over study comparing ECP with PUVA in non-erythrodermic (stage IB-IIA) MF patients has shown no increased clinical efficacy for ECP in early stages of mycosis fungoides compared with PUVA, although numbers were small and ECP was only given for 6 months[49] **Evidence level Ib**.

In contrast an uncontrolled study has reported successful responses in patients with non-erythrodermic disease. A 9-year retrospective study of ECP alone in 37 patients (68%, IB; 5%, IIB; 27%, III) showed a CR in 14% and a PR in 41% with an improved response rate in resistant patients with the addition of IFNα[50] **Evidence level III**.

### Combination regimens

A prospective open non-randomised study of 14 patients with non-erythrodermic mycosis fungoides (IIA/IIB) treated with combined IFNα (maximum tolerated dose of 18 MU × 3 weekly) and ECP for 6 months showed a CR in four and a PR in three (overall response of 50%) but this design does not exclude responses to IFNα alone[51] **Evidence level IIa**.

A non-randomised retrospective study in erythrodermic disease (stage III/IVA) (1991–1996) showed that six of nine patients treated with combined IFNα and ECP showed a response with four CRs while only one of 10 patients treated with ECP alone achieved a response (CR). In the patients achieving a complete response lymph node disease also resolved[52] **Evidence level IIb**.

In contrast, combined IFNα and ECP failed to produce significant clinical responses in six patients with Sézary syndrome[53] **Evidence level III** although isolated case reports have described patients with Sézary syndrome in whom complete clinical and molecular remission has been achieved with this combination.[54,55]

A retrospective non-randomised study (1974–1997) has compared DSS and OS in 44 patients with erythrodermic CTCL treated with either TSEB alone or TSEB and adjuvant or neoadjuvant ECP (see later section) **Evidence level III**.

### Drawbacks

ECP is well tolerated. Mild lymphopenia and anaemia can occur with long-term therapy. High cost and lack of availability means that ECP will remain confined to specialist centres.

### Comments

ECP appears to have some efficacy in erythrodermic disease but controlled trials are urgently required to compare ECP to standard single agent chemotherapy regimens in erythrodermic disease and specifically in Sézary syndrome **Grade B**. In addition some previous studies have not clearly defined their diagnostic criteria for erythrodermic CTCL and others have included patients with non-erythrodermic disease.

Combination therapy with ECP and IFNα is frequently used but the existing studies do not exclude a beneficial response to IFNα alone **Grade B**. An RCT is currently addressing this important issue. Studies suggest that ECP requires a minimum tumour burden within peripheral blood[56] and the only RCT of ECP in non-erythrodermic, early stage disease suggests that it is not effective.

## Thymopentin

### Benefits

In a phase II trial 20 patients with Sézary syndrome were treated with 50 mg intravenously of thymopentin (TP-5), a synthetic pentapeptide, three times weekly for a mean of 16 months. The overall response rate was 75% with eight CRs and and seven PRs and a median duration of 22 months. Four-year survival was 54%[57] **Evidence level IIb**.

### Drawbacks

TP-5 is usually well tolerated. Mild hypersensitivity reactions were noted during the infusion.

### Comments

Its mechanism of action remains unclear. Overall response rate is very high but lack of subsequent reports is surprising and further studies are required to confirm this data **Grade B**.

## Ciclosporin

### Benefits

A phase II trial of ciclosporin (15 mg kg$^{-1}$ per day) in 16 patients with refractory T-cell lymphomas including 11 CTCL (all stage IVA/B) revealed only two responses in

CTCL with eight CTCL patients developing progressive disease and one patient dying from drug related causes.[58] The two patients showing a partial response had a rapid relapse of disease when treatment was discontinued **Evidence level IIa**.

### Drawbacks

High doses are poorly tolerated with frequent dose reductions required. Hypertension, renal toxicity and infection were common.

### Comments

This study suggests that ciclosporin is not effective in CTCL and anecdotal reports suggest that ciclosporin can actually cause rapid disease progression in CTCL **Grade B**.

## What are the effects of systemic retinoids in MF/SS?

### Etretinate/acitretin/isotretinoin

#### Benefits

A systematic review (1988–1994) of open studies of oral retinoids in CTCL (MF and SS) showed an overall mean response rate of 58% and a complete response rate of 19% with a median duration of response of 3–13 months[59] **Evidence level IIa**.

A non-randomised study of 68 patients with various stages of mycosis fungoides and Sézary syndrome compared 13-*cis*-retinoic acid with etretinate and showed similar efficacy and toxicity (isotretinoin: CR 21%/PR 38%; etretinate: CR 21%/ PR 46%)[60] **Evidence level IIa**.

A phase II study of isotretinoin in 25 patients with MF (IB–III) showed an overall response of 44% with three patients achieving a CR and a median response duration of 8 months on high doses (2 mg kg$^{-1}$ per day)[61] **Evidence level IIa**.

An RCT comparing PUVA and IFNα with PUVA and acitretin showed a significantly better response rate for PUVA and IFNα[30] (see above).

### Drawbacks

Mucocutaneous erosions and xerosis, hyerlipidaemia, hepatotoxicity and teratogenicity were recorded.

### Comments

Acitretin and etretinate have some efficacy in early stages of disease, but are no better and probably less effective than other modalities such as PUVA and IFNα **Grade B**.

### Bexarotene

Bexarotene is a novel retinoid capable of binding to the RXR as opposed to the RAR retinoid receptor. This drug has antiproliferative and pro-apoptotic properties.

#### Benefits

No RCTs were found. A phase II open trial compared two doses (6·5 mg m$^{-2}$ per day and 650 mg m$^{-2}$ per day) of oral bexarotene in 58 patients with refractory stage IA–IIA CTCL.[62] The optimal dose was 300 mg m$^{-2}$ per day in terms of response and tolerability. Objective responses of 20%, 54% and 67% were noted at the 6·5, 300 and 650 mg m$^{-2}$ doses respectively. Rates of disease progression were 47%, 21% and 13% at the same dose levels. Median duration of response at the high dose level was 516 days **Evidence level IIa**.

In late stages of disease (stages IIB–IVB) overall responses of 45% (at 300 mg m$^{-2}$ per day) and 55% (at doses higher than 300 mg m$^{-2}$ per day) have been reported with a relapse rate of 36% and projected median duration of response of 299 days[63] **Evidence level IIa**.

### Drawbacks

Reversible adverse effects included hyperlipidaemia, central hypothyroidism, leucopenia, headache and asthenia, as well as other retinoid adverse effects.

### Comments

These studies suggest a therapeutic efficacy for bexarotene in all stages of CTCL but comparative studies with other therapies and data on effects on disease-free and overall survival in later stages of disease are required. An EORTC RCT comparing PUVA with PUVA and bexarotene in stage IB/IIA disease is due to start enrolment in 2003 **Grade B**.

## What are the effects of antibody and toxin therapies in MF/SS?

### Anti-CD4 monoclonal antibody

#### Benefits

In a phase I/II trial seven mycosis fungoides patients were treated with a chimeric (murine/human) anti-CD4 monoclonal antibody with successive increasing doses (10, 20, 40 and 80 mg) twice weekly for 3 weeks. All patients showed some clinical response with one CR and two PRs but these were all short-lived (median duration of 2 weeks)[64] **Evidence level IIb**.

A subsequent study from the same group showed partial responses in seven of eight patients receiving higher doses (50–200 mg) with a median freedom from progression of 28 weeks[65] **Evidence level IIb**.

### Drawbacks

The compound is well tolerated with no acute toxicity. There is marked but temporary suppression of T-cell proliferative responses to PHA and no documented depletion of CD4 counts. Immunogenicity of antibody is unclear.

### Comments

Preliminary data suggest some therapeutic efficacy but the effect of neutralising antibodies is unclear and the role of anti-CD4 monoclonal antibody in CTCL has not yet been established **Grade B**.

## CAMPATH-1H (Alemtuzumab)

### Benefits

As part of a phase II trial in advanced low grade NHL, eight patients with MF received 30 mg of CAMPATH-1H intravenously three times a week for a maximum of 12 weeks[66]: 50% of CTCL patients achieved a response with two (25%) showing a complete response. No details of duration of response were provided **Evidence level IIb**.

A retrospective study in a variety of mature post-thymic T-cell malignancies showed 100% responses in three patients with CTCL using 30 mg intravenously three times a week until maximum response with duration up to 4 years[67] **Evidence level III**.

### Drawbacks

Severe neutropenia and opportunistic infections common with viral reactivation are associated with prolonged lymphopenia.

### Comments

CAMPATH-1H (Alemtuzumab) is a humanised anti-CD52 antibody, which binds to all normal and most malignant lymphocytes. This study[67] suggests that patients with CTCL show the highest response rate but infectious complications leading to death do occur **Grade B**. Further studies are justified.

## Denileukin diftitox (diphtheria IL-2 fusion toxin)

### Benefits

A phase III open uncontrolled study of Denileukin diftitox in 71 patients with stage IB–IVA CTCL has shown overall responses of 30% with 10% showing a complete clinical response.[68] Only CTCL cases with biopsies showing over 20% CD25+ (IL-2R) lymphocytes were enrolled. Median duration of response was 6·9 months. No difference in response rates or duration of response noted at doses of 9 micrograms kg$^{-1}$ per day and 18 micrograms kg$^{-1}$ per day. The development of anti-denileukin diftitox antibodies apparently did not affect response rates **Evidence level IIa**.

### Drawbacks

Adverse effects include 'flu-like symptoms, acute infusion related hypersensitivity effects, a vascular leak syndrome and transient elevations of hepatic enzymes.

### Comments

This uncontrolled study suggests that CD25+ CTCL can respond to this novel fusion toxin but the duration of response is short. However, patients recruited for this trial were heavily pretreated, suggesting that this is likely to be a useful additional therapy for CTCL patients with resistant disease despite potential adverse effects **Grade B**. A randomised placebo controlled trial, in stages IB/IIB/III mycosis fungoides patients with less than three previous treatments, is currently ongoing.

## Ricin-labelled anti-CD5 immunoconjugate (H65-RTA)

### Benefits

A phase I trial of H65-RTA in 14 patients with resistant CTCL revealed a maximum tolerated dose of 0·33 mg kg$^{-1}$ per day and partial responses in only four patients of short duration (3–8 months)[69] **Evidence level IIb**.

### Drawbacks

Acute hypersensitivity effects and vascular leak syndrome were noted.

### Comments

Efficacy in this small study is questionable **Grade B**.

## Radioimmunoconjugate (90Y-T101)

### Benefits

A phase I trial of this radioimmunoconjugate (which also targets CD5+ lymphocytes) in 10 patients with (CD5+)

haematological malignancies, of whom 8 patients had CTCL, gave partial responses in three CTCL patients with a median response duration of 23 weeks.[70] Biodistribution studies showed good uptake in skin and involved lymph nodes **Evidence level IIb** .

### Drawbacks

Bone marrow suppression was observed. T-cell recovery occurred within 3 weeks but B-cell suppression persisted after 5 weeks.

### Comments

This is an interesting phase I study because CTCL is a radiosensitive tumour but response rates are disappointing. Further studies are required **Grade B** .

## What are the effects of radiotherapy in MF/SS?

### Superficial radiotherapy

### Benefits

No systematic reviews or RCTs were identified. Dose–response studies have clearly established that localised superficial radiotherapy is an effective palliative therapy for individual lesions in mycosis fungoides.[71] A retrospective study of palliative superficial radiotherapy used to treat 191 lesions from 20 patients with mycosis fungoides showed complete responses in 95% for plaques and small (< 3 cm) tumours and a CR of 93% for large tumours (> 3 cm) irrespective of dose. However, in-field recurrences within 1–2 years were more common for those lesions treated with lower doses (42% for < 1000 cGy, 32% for 1000–2000 cGy, 21% for 2000–3000 cGy, and 0% for those > 3000 cGy) **Evidence level III** .

### Drawbacks

It was normally well tolerated, although there was mild erythema and occasional erosion. Use of low dose/energy (400 cGy in 2–3 daily fractions at 80–150 Kv) is therapeutically effective and allows treatment of overlapping fields and lower limb sites.

### Comments

CTCL is a highly radiosensitive malignancy and localised superficial radiotherapy is an invaluable palliative therapy for patients with all stages of mycosis fungoides. Treatment should be palliative except for patients with solitary localised disease where "cure" is possible. Although in-field recurrence rates were very low for lesions treated with over 3000 cGy, the number of lesions treated with this dose was very low compared with the other groups, and this form of

therapy is only palliative in mycosis fungoides because it is multifocal. Therefore the use of high dose fractionation regimens for individual lesions should be avoided in mycosis fungoides because complete response rates are similar to those for low dose regimens (see above), and recurrent disease adjacent to previously treated fields can be treated with overlapping fields if necessary. However, treatment of disease on the lower legs can be difficult in view of a higher risk of radiation necrosis with repeated treatments **Grade B** .

## Total skin electron beam therapy (TSEB)

### Benefits

A systematic review (meta-analysis) of open uncontrolled and mostly retrospective studies of TSEB as monotherapy for 952 patients with all stages of CTCL has established that the rate of complete response is dependent on stage of disease, skin surface dose and energy, with complete response rates of 96% in stages IA/IB/IIA disease, 36% in stage IIB disease, and 60% in stage III disease.[72] Greater skin surface dose (32–36 Gy) and higher energy (4–6 MeV electrons) were significantly associated with a higher rate of complete responses with 5-year relapse-free survivals of 10–23% noted[72] **Evidence level Ia** .

An RCT has compared TSEB with topical mechlorethamine in 42 patients with similar rates of complete response and duration of response in both groups in early stages of disease, but better overall responses in later stages of disease with TSEB[73] **Evidence level Ib** .

A retrospective study of TSEB (median dose 32 Gy; median treatment time 21 days) as monotherapy for 45 patients with erythrodermic CTCL (28, stage III; 13, stage IVA; 4, stage IVB) showed a 60% complete response rate with 26% disease free at 5 years.[74] Overall median survival was 3·4 years, which was associated significantly with an absence of peripheral blood involvement (stage III disease). Higher rates of complete response (74%) and disease-free progression (36%) were noted in those patients receiving a more intense regimen (32–40 Gy and 4–6 MeV) **Evidence level IIb** .

A retrospective study of 66 CTCL patients (1978–1996) treated with 30 Gy in far fewer fractions (12 fractions over 40 days) showed complete responses of 65% with progression free survival of 30% at 5 and 18% at 10 years, respectively.[75] Responses and specifically overall 5-year survival were highest in those with early stage disease (79–93% for IA/IB/III) compared with late stages (44% for IIB/IVA/B) **Evidence level III** .

Although it has been recommended that TSEB can only be given once in a lifetime several reports have described multiple courses in CTCL.[76,77] A retrospective analysis of 15 patients (1968–1990) with mycosis fungoides who received two courses of TSEB reported a mean dose of 32·6 Gy for the first course and 23·4 Gy for the second, with a mean interval of 41·3 months. No additional toxicities were noted but the complete response rate for the second course was lower (40% compared with 73%).[76] A further retrospective study of 14 patients with CTCL revealed a mean dose of 36 Gy for the first (93% CR) and 18 Gy for the second course (86% CR).[77] In this series five patients received a third course (total doses 12–30 Gy). The median duration of response was 20 months for the first and 11·5 months for the second course. No additional toxicities were reported. In both of these studies, the fractionation regimens employed may have been critical for tolerability (1 Gy per day over 9–12 weeks; 6 MeV electrons) **Evidence level III** .

An EORTC consensus document on the use and clinical indications for TSEB has recently been published.[78]

## Combination TSEB regimens

An RCT in 103 CTCL patients comparing TSEB and multiagent chemotherapy (CAVE) with sequential topical therapy including superficial radiotherapy and phototherapy revealed a higher complete response rate in the TSEB/chemotherapy group (38% compared with 18%; $P = 0.032$) but, after a median follow up of 75 months, there was no significant difference in disease-free or overall survival[79] **Evidence level Ib** .

A retrospective non-randomised study comparing TSEB (32–40 Gy) alone and TSEB followed by extracorporeal photopheresis (ECP given 2 days monthly for a median of 6 months) in 44 patients with erythrodermic CTCL (57% stage III, 30% stage IVA, 13% stage IVB, overall 59% had haematological involvement, B1), has reported an overall complete response rate of 73% after TSEB with a 3-year disease-free survival of 49% for 17 patients who received only TSEB (overall survival 63%) and 81% for 15 patients who received TSEB followed by ECP (overall survival 88%).[80] A multivariate analysis suggested that the combination of TSEB and ECP was significantly associated with a prolonged disease-free and cause-specific survival when corrected for peripheral blood involvement (B1) and stage of disease **Evidence level IIb** .

### Drawbacks

Adverse effects of TSEB include radiation-induced secondary cutaneous malignancies, telangiectasia, pigmentation, anhidrosis, pruritus, alopecia and xerosis. Treatment generally is given only once in a lifetime but several reports suggest that multiple therapies may be tolerated (see above).

### Comments

Although these studies are uncontrolled and mostly retrospective, the response rates indicate that TSEB is a highly effective therapy for all stages of CTCL **Grade B** .

The lack of a long-term response in early stage disease suggests that TSEB should be reserved for later stages of disease particularly as an RCT has indicated that responses are similar for TSEB and topical mechlorethamine. **Grade B** .

Meta-analysis of observational data indicates that higher dose regimens are more effective (32–40 Gy with 4–6 MeV) **Grade A** .

An RCT in CTCL clearly indicates that combined TSEB and chemotherapy is not more effective than sequential skin directed therapy **Grade A** .

A further trial comparing TSEB alone with TSEB and chemotherapy in late stages of disease (stage IIB) would be helpful.

The current data on long-term disease-free and overall survival in erythrodermic CTCL suggest that TSEB is effective, particularly if combined with ECP, but this requires confirmation in an RCT **Grade B** .

## What are the effects of single agent chemotherapy in MF/SS?

### Single agent chemotherapy regimens

#### Benefits

No RCTs have been reported. A systematic review of uncontrolled open studies of single-agent regimens in 526 CTCL patients (1988–1994) revealed overall response rates of 62% with complete responses of 33% and median response durations of 3–22 months.[59] These therapies included alkylating agents (chlorambucil and cyclophosphamide), antimetabolites (methotrexate), vinca alkaloids, and topoisomerase II inhibitors **Evidence level Ia** .

#### Drawbacks

As with all chemotherapy regimens, infection and myelosuppression are significant risks.

#### Comments

The lack of controlled studies makes interpretation difficult but single agent regimens may have similar efficacy to combination regimens (see below) with lower toxicity, and therefore may be preferable as palliative therapy in late stages of mycosis fungoides and Sézary syndrome, especially as durable responses and cures are rarely if ever achieved. RCTs are urgently required **Grade A** .

### Methotrexate

#### Benefits

No RCTs have been identified. A retrospective report of low dose methotrexate in 29 patients with erythrodermic

CTCL (III/IVA) has shown a 41% complete remission rate with an overall response of 58%.[81] Median freedom from treatment failure and overall survival was 31 months and 8·4 years respectively. Weekly doses ranged from 5 to 125 mg for a median duration of 23 months. A majority (62%) of patients satisfied criteria for a diagnosis of SS **Evidence level III**.

## Drawbacks

Adverse effects included reversible abnormalities of liver function, mucositis, cutaneous erosions, reversible leucopenia, thrombocytopenia, nausea and diarrhoea, and in one case pulmonary fibrosis.

## Comments

Although these are uncontrolled data, the overall survival in this cohort is surprisingly good **Grade B**. A randomised study comparing methotrexate with other single-agent chemotherapies in erythrodermic CTCL would be worthwhile.

## Purine analogues

### Benefits

No RCTs were found. A systematic review of purine analogues in CTCL (1988–1994) revealed overall and complete response rates of 41% and 6% for deoxycoformycin (63 patients), 41% and 19% for 2-chlorodeoxyadenosine (27 patients), and 19% and 3% for fludarabine (31 patients) respectively.[59] Most of these studies included some patients with peripheral T-cell lymphomas. No comparative studies are available **Evidence level Ia**.

A prospective open study of deoxycoformycin in 28 heavily pretreated patients of whom 21 had CTCL (14, SS; 7, IIB) revealed an overall response rate of 71% with 25% CR and 46% PR, (OR 10/14 SS – 4 CR; 4/7 stage IIB patients – 1 CR). Response duration was short-lived (median duration of 2 months for stage IIB disease and 3·5 months for SS) except in two cases of SS with remissions for 17 and 19 months. The regimen consisted of starting doses between 3·75 to 5·0 mg m$^{-2}$ per day for 3 days every 3 weeks. A dose escalation to 6·25 mg m$^{-2}$ per day was rarely possible because of toxicity[82] **Evidence level IIa**.

Two recent open studies of deoxycoformycin in CTCL (27 MF and 37 SS patients) have shown overall responses ranging from 35% to 56% with complete responses from 10% to 33%, and a reported median disease-free interval of 9 months in one of the studies[83,84] **Evidence level IIa**. Interestingly, responses are better in Sézary syndrome than in mycosis fungoides. The usual schedule for deoxycoformycin consists of once weekly treatment at a dose of 4 mg m$^{-2}$

intravenously for 4 weeks and then every 14 days for either 6 months or until maximal response.

Combination therapy consisting of deoxycoformycin and IFNα in CTCL has shown overall and complete response rates of 41% and 5% respectively[85] **Evidence level IIa**.

A recent phase II trial of 2-chlorodeoxyadenosine in 21 refractory CTCL patients (MF-IIB/IV and SS) revealed an overall response rate of 28% with 14% CR (median duration of 4·5 months) and 14% PR (median duration of 2 months)[86] **Evidence level IIa**.

## Drawbacks

Side effects include nausea, infections (especially herpetic), CD4 lymphopenia, renal toxicity, hepatotoxicity, and myelosuppresion (especially for 2-chlorodeoxyadenosine and fludarabine).

## Comments

Purine analogues are attractive therapeutic candidates for CTCL because they are potent inhibitors of the enzyme adenosine deaminase, which preferentially accumulates in lymphoid cells, and these drugs therefore exert a selective lymphocytotoxic effect independent of cell division. Although efficacy in CTCL is moderate, most of these patients were heavily pretreated and relatively chemoresistant. Patients with Sézary syndrome appear to respond better than those with late stages of mycosis fungoides. Purine analogues are appropriate options as monotherapy, especially in Sézary syndrome, but response duration may be short **Grade B**. Comparative trials with other single-agent regimens are required in Sézary syndrome.

## Gemcitabine

### Benefits

A phase II prospective trial (1200 mg m$^{-2}$ weekly for 3 weeks each month for a total of three cycles) in 44 previously treated patients with CTCL (30 mycosis fungoides patients with stage IIB or III disease) reported partial responses of 59% and complete responses of 12%, with a median duration of 10 and 15 months respectively[87] **Evidence level IIa**.

### Drawbacks

Gemcitacine is normally well tolerated. Mild haematological toxicity only was noted.

### Comments

Gemcitabine is a novel pyramidine antimetabolite that appears to be well tolerated producing significant responses in heavily pretreated patients with advanced stages of mycosis fungoides **Grade B**. Further trials are required.

## Doxorubicin

### Benefits

An open study of pegylated liposomal doxorubicin (20 mg m$^{-2}$ monthly to maximum of 400 mg or eight cycles) in 10 patients with various stages of mycosis fungoides revealed a complete response in six and a partial response in two patients with a median response duration of 15 months[88] **Evidence level IIb**.

### Drawbacks

Mild haematological toxicity was noted.

### Comments

There are encouraging preliminary data suggesting a significant overall response rate **Grade B**. An EORTC phase II trial in advanced stages of mycosis fungoides ($\geq$ IIB) is due to start enrolment in 2003.

## What are the effects of multiagent chemotherapy regimens in MF/SS?

### Combination chemotherapy

#### Benefits

An RCT in 103 CTCL patients comparing TSEB and multiagent chemotherapy (CAVE) with sequential topical therapy including superficial radiotherapy and phototherapy revealed a higher complete response rate in the TSEB/chemotherapy group (38% compared with 18%; $P = 0.032$ with overall responses of 90% and 65% respectively) but after a median follow up of 75 months there was no significant difference in disease-free or overall survival[79] **Evidence level Ib**.

A systematic review of all systemic therapy in CTCL (MF/SS 1988–1994) showed an overall response rate of 81% in 331 patients treated with various different combination chemotherapeutic regimens with a complete response rate of 38% and response duration ranging from 5 to 41 months with no documented cures for patients with late stages of disease (IIB–IVB)[59] **Evidence level Ia**.

Recent prospective non-randomised studies of different multiagent chemotherapy regimens have revealed similar overall response rates. A third generation anthracycline (idarubicin) was used in combination with etoposide, cyclophosphamide, vincristine, prednisolone and bleomycin (VICOP-B) to treat 25 CTCL patients (8, IIB; 13, IVA; 4,

IVB) for 12 weeks. Overall response rates of 80% with 36% CR were documented, although 10 patients had not received any previous therapy. The two SS patients did not respond and the median duration of response in MF was 8.7 months. Stage IIB patients had a median duration of response of 22 months but four previously untreated patients received additional TSEB therapy after completion of chemotherapy[89] **Evidence level IIa**.

A combination of etoposide, vincristine, doxorubicin, cyclophosphamide, and prednisolone (EPOCH) was used to treat 15 patients with advanced, refractory CTCL (6, SS; 4, IVB-MF; 1, ATLL; 4, LCAL). After a median of 5 cycles 27% had a CR and 53% achieved a PR (overall RR of 80%) with an overall median survival of 13.5 months[90] **Evidence level IIb**.

### Drawbacks

Multiagent chemotherapy regimens are associated with very high rates of toxicity and considerable morbidity including nausea, anorexia, infection, hepatotoxicity, and myelosuppression. Patients with CTCL are at high risk of septicaemia and therapy-related mortality with combination chemotherapy is a significant risk.

### Comments

Although the RCT comparing TSEB and chemotherapy with skin-directed therapy showed a similar OS/DFS, this group of patients included some with early stage disease, and patients with late stages of CTCL (IIB–IVB) will require treatment with a chemotherapy regimen and possibly TSEB because response duration with chemotherapy alone is short **Grade A**.

The individual patient's quality of life should always be considered before embarking on very toxic regimens with limited efficacy. Single agent regimens (see previous section) appear to have similar efficacy, although studies involving a comparison between single agent and multiagent regimens, with or without TSEB, are required. To date there have been no studies assessing the use of biochemotherapy in CTCL although subsequent treatment with immunotherapy for patients achieving a response with chemotherapy should be considered.

## Myeloablative chemotherapy with autologous/allogeneic peripheral blood/bone marrow stem cell transplantation

### Benefits

No systematic reviews or RCTs have been identified. Most studies are based on small numbers of patients. High dose chemotherapy with additional TSEB and TBI in four and three patients (two patients had both TSEB and TBI) respectively in six MF patients (3, IIB; 1, IVA; 2, IVB) followed by autologous bone marrow transplantation produced five complete clinical responses but disease relapse occurred in three patients within 100 days.[91] The other two patients, who had both received a combination of carmustine-etoposide-cisplatin chemotherapy, were disease-free at almost 2 years (666 and 631 days post-transplant) **Evidence level IIb**.

High dose chemotherapy combined with either TSEB or TBI and followed by autologous peripheral blood stem cell transplantation in nine patients with stage IIB/IVA mycosis fungoides revealed complete responses in eight and durable clinical responses in four (median disease free survival 11 months)[92] **Evidence level IIb**.

Isolated case reports of high dose chemotherapy with TBI followed by allogeneic bone marrow or stem cell transplantation have shown excellent long-term complete remissions in both stage IIB mycosis fungoides (CR for 17 months at time of report), Sézary syndrome and stage IV disease (CR for 2 years at time of report)[93–95] **Evidence level IIb**.

### Drawbacks

There was a high incidence of toxicity associated with myeloablative therapy and systemic infections, and significant mortality especially with allogeneic transplantation.

### Comments

The use of autologous or allogeneic transplantation may be appropriate for younger patients with late stage disease who have failed to respond to chemotherapy and/or TSEB, and long-term remissions are possible particularly with allogeneic procedures **Grade B**. However, controlled trials in late stage disease are required comparing autologous transplantation with standard chemotherapy as conducted in systemic follicular B-cell lymphoma. The mortality rate associated with allogeneic transplantation makes this a less attractive approach, but the use of mini-allogeneic procedures to induce a graft versus tumour effect would be worth investigating.

## Conclusions

### Implications for clinical practice

- Although there are few well-designed RCTs in CTCL, there is convincing evidence that several skin directed therapies, namely topical mechlorethamine and phototherapy, have a significant therapeutic effect **Grade B**. However, there is a fundamental lack of data about the impact of different therapies on disease-free and overall survival, which will only become clearer when the results of key RCTs in different stages

of disease become available in the future. In addition patients with early stage disease can have a normal life expectancy, which should always be considered carefully in order to avoid aggressive therapies with a significant mortality and morbidity, especially when the chance of a cure is very low.

- Patients with early stage disease (IA/IB/IIA) should be offered skin-directed therapies such as topical mechlorethamine, phototherapy, PUVA and superficial radiotherapy **Grade A**. IFNα should be considered for patients with persistent or recurrent stage IB/IIA disease **Grade B**. Some patients with stage IA disease may not require any specific therapy **Grade B**.
- Patients with late stages of disease (IIB/IV) should be offered TSEB, single agent palliative chemotherapy and multiagent chemotherapy according to performance status **Grade B**.
- Patients with erythrodermic disease should be offered photopheresis, immunotherapy and single agent chemotherapy as palliative therapy with the intention of improving quality of life **Grade B**. TSEB therapy may be indicated for erythrodermic disease when there is a lack of significant peripheral blood tumour burden **Grade B**.

### Recommendations for the future

- Assessment of novel topical therapies should be in the context of well-designed clinical trials involving a comparison with topical mechlorethamine.
- The role of novel immunotherapies and retinoids in early stage (IB/IIA) disease should involve comparative RCTs with standard therapies such as PUVA.
- TSEB therapy with or without adjuvant immuno- and chemotherapy should be reserved for patients with late stages of disease preferably in the context of clinical trials.
- There is an urgent need for more effective therapy for late stage disease and this should be based on appropriate RCTs involving novel immunotherapies, adjuvants, single and multiagent chemotherapies, and both (mini)allogeneic and autologous transplants in selected individuals.

### References

1   Willemze R, Kerl H, Sterry W *et al*. EORTC classification for primary cutaneous lymphomas: A proposal from the cutaneous lymphoma study group of the European Organisation for Research and Treatment of Cancer. *Blood* 1997;**90**:354–71.
2   Weinstock M, Horm J. Mycosis fungoides in the United States: increasing incidence and descriptive epidemiology. *JAMA* 1988;**260**:42–6.
3   Zackheim H, Amin S, Kashani-Sabet M, McMillan A. Prognosis in cutaneous T-cell lymphoma by skin stage: long term survival in 489 patients. *J Am Acad Dermatol* 1999;**40**:418–25.

4  Siegel R, Pandolfino T, Guitart J, Rosen S, Kuzel T. Primary cutaneous T-cell lymphoma: review and current concepts. *J Clin Oncol* 2000;**18**: 2908–25.

5  Bunn P and Lamberg S. Report of the committee on staging and classification of cutaneous T-cell lymphomas. *Cancer Treat Rep* 1979;**63**:725–8.

6  Scarisbrick J, Whittaker S, Evans A *et al.* Prognostic significance of tumour burden in the blood of patients with erythrodermic primary cutaneous T-cell lymphoma. *Blood* 2001;**97**:624–30.

7  Marti L, Estrach T, Reverter J, Mascaro J. Prognostic clinicopathologic factors in cutaneous T-cell lymphoma. *Arch Dermatol* 1991;**127**: 1511–16.

8  Doorn R, Van Haselan C, Voorst Vader P *et al.* Mycosis fungoides: Disease evolution and prognosis of 309 Dutch patients. *Arch Dermatol* 2000;**136**:504–10.

9  Kim Y, Jensen R, Watanabe G, Varghese A, Hoppe R. Clinical stage IA (limited patch and plaque) mycosis fungoides. *Arch Dermatol* 1996;**132**:1309–13.

10  Kim Y, Chow S, Varghese A, Hoppe R. Clinical characteristics and long-term outcome of patients with generalised patch and/or plaque (T2) mycosis fungoides. *Arch Dermatol* 1999;**135**:26–32.

11  Coninck E, Kim Y, Varghese A, Hoppe R. Clinical characteristics and outcome of patients with extracutaneous mycosis fungoides. *J Clin Oncol* 2001;**19**:779–84.

12  Kim Y, Bishop K, Varghese A, Hoppe R. Prognostic factors in erythrodermic mycosis fungoides and the Sézary syndrome. *Arch Dermatol* 1995;**131**:1003–8.

13  Kashani-Sabet M, McMillan A, Zackheim H. A modified staging classification for cutaneous T-cell lymphoma. *J Am Acad Dermatol* 2001;**45**:700–6.

14  Sausville E, Eddy J, Makuch R, Fischmann A *et al.* Histopathologic staging at initial diagnosis of mycosis fungoides and the Sézary syndrome. Definition of three distinctive prognostic groups. *Ann Intern Med* 1988;**109**:372–82.

15  Bunn P, Huberman M, Whang-Peng J *et al.* Prospective staging evaluation of patients with cutaneous T-cell lymphomas. *Ann Intern Med* 1980;**93**:223–30.

16  Zackheim H, Kashani-Sabet M Amin S. Topical corticosteroids for mycosis fungoides. *Arch Dermatol* 1998;**134**:949–54.

17  Hoppe R, Abel E, Deneau D, Price N. Mycosis fungoides: management with topical nitrogen mustard. *J Clin Oncol* 1987;**5**: 1796–803.

18  Ramsey D, Ed M, Halperin P *et al.* Topical mechlorethamine therapy for early stage mycosis fungoides. *J Am Acad Dermatol* 1988;**19**: 684–91.

19  Vonderheid E, Tan E, Kantor A *et al.* Long term efficacy, curative potential and carcinogenicity of topical mechlorethamine chemotherapy in cutaneous T-cell lymphoma. *J Am Acad Dermatol* 1989;**20**:416–28.

20  Zachariae H, Thestrup-Pedersen K, Sogaard H. Topical nitrogen mustard in early mycosis fungoides. *Acta Derm Venereol* 1985;**65**:53–8.

21  Zackheim H, Epstein E, Crain W. Topical carmustine (BCNU) for cutaneous T-cell lymphoma: a 15-year experience in 143 patients. *J Am Acad Dermatol* 1990;**22**:802–10.

22  Breneman D, Duvic M, Kuzel T, Yocum R, Truglia J, Stevens V. Phase I and I trial of bexarotene gel for skin directed treatment of patients with cutaneous T-cell lymphoma. *Arch Dermatol* 2002;**138**:325–32.

23  Duvic M, Olsen E, Omura G *et al.* A phase III, randomised, double-blind, placebo-controlled study of peldesine (BCX-34) cream as topical therapy for cutaneous T-cell lymphoma. *J Am Acad Dermatol* 2001;**44**:940–7.

24  Ramsey D, Lish K, Yalowitz C, Soter N. Ultraviolet-B phototherapy for early stage cutaneous T-cell lymphoma. *Arch Dermatol* 1992;**128**: 931–3.

25  Clark C, Dawe R, Evans A, Lowe G, Ferguson J. Narrowband TL-01 phototherapy for patch stage mycosis fungoides. *Arch Dermatol* 2000; **136**:748–52.

26  Zane C, Leali C, Airo P *et al.* "High dose" UVA1 therapy of widespread plaque-type, nodular and erythrodermic mycosis fungoides. *J Am Acad Dermatol* 2001;**44**:629–33.

27  Hermann J, Roenigk H, Hurria A *et al.* Treatment of mycosis fungoides with photochemotherapy (PUVA): long term follow-up. *J Am Acad Dermatol* 1995;**33**:234–42.

28  Roenigk H, Kuzel T, Skoutelis A *et al.* Photochemotherapy alone or combined with interferon alpha in the treatment of cutaneous T-cell lymphoma. *J Invest Dermatol* 1990;**95**:198–205S.

29  Honigsmann Brenner W, Rauschmeier W, Konrad K, Wolff K. Photochemotherapy for cutaneous T cell lymphoma. *J Am Acad Dermatol* 1984;**10**:238–45.

30  Stadler R, Otte H, Luger T *et al.* Prospective randomised multicentre clinical trial on the use of interferon alpha-2a plus acitretin versus interferon alpha-2a plus PUVA in patients with cutaneous T-cell lymphoma stages I and II. *Blood* 1998;**10**:3578–81.

31  Thomsen K, Hammar H, Molin L *et al.* Retinoids plus PUVA (RePUVA) and PUVA in mycosis fungoides plaque stage. *Acta Derm Venereol* 1989;**69**:536–8.

32  Kuzel T, Roenigk H, Samuelson E *et al.* Effectiveness of interferon alfa-2a combined with phototherapy for mycosis fungoides and the Sézary syndrome. *J Clin Oncol* 1995;**13**:257–63.

33  Bunn P, Ihde D, Foon K. The role of recombinant interferon alpha-2a in the therapy of cutaneous T-cell lymphomas. *Cancer* 1986;**57**: 1689–95.

34  Olsen E, Rosen S, Vollmer R *et al.* Interferon alfa-2a in the treatment of cutaneous T-cell lymphoma. *J Am Acad Dermatol* 1989;**20**:395–407.

35  Papa G, Tura S, Mandelli F *et al.* Is interferon alpha in cutaneous T-cell lymphoma a treatment of choice? *Br J Haematol* 1991;**79**:48–51.

36  Kohn E, Steis R, Sausville E, Veach S *et al.* Phase II trial of intermittent high-dose recombinant interferon alfa-2a in mycosis fungoides and the Sézary syndrome. *J Clin Oncol* 1990;**8**:155–60.

37  Dreno B, Claudy A, Meynadier J *et al.* The treatment of 45 patients with cutaneous T-cell lymphoma with low doses of interferon-alpha 2a and etretinate. *Br J Dermatol* 1991;**125**:456–9.

38  Vonderheid E, Thompson R, Smiles K, Lattanand A. Recombinant interferon alpha-2b in plaque phase mycosis fungoides. Intralesional and low dose intramuscular therapy. *Arch Dermatol* 1987;**123**:757–63.

39  Kaplan E, Rosen S, Norris D *et al.* Phase II study of recombinant interferon gamma for treatment of cutaneous T-cell lymphoma. *J Natl Cancer Inst* 1990;**82**:208–12.

40  Marolleau J, Baccard M, Flageul B *et al.* High dose recombinant interleukin-2 in advanced cutaneous T-cell lymphoma. *Arch Dermatol* 1995;**131**:574–9.

41  Rook A, Wood G, Yoo E, Elenitsas R, Kao D, Sherman M *et al.* Interleukin-12 therapy of cutaneous T-cell lymphoma induces lesion regression and cytotoxic T-cell responses. *Blood* 1999;**94**:902–8.

42  Russell Jones R. Extracorporeal photopheresis in cutaneous T-cell lymphoma. Inconsistent data underline the need for randomised studies. *Br J Dermatol* 2000;**142**:16–21.

43  Edelson R, Berger C, Gasparro F *et al.* Treatment of cutaneous T-cell lymphoma by extracorporeal photochemotherapy. *N Engl J Med* 1987;**316**:297–303.

44  Duvic M, Hester J, Lemak N. Photopheresis therapy for cutaneous T-cell lymphoma. *J Am Acad Dermatol* 1996;**35**:573–9.

45  Heald P, Rook A, Perez M *et al.* Treatment of erythrodermic cutaneous T-cell lymphoma with extracorporeal photopheresis. *J Am Acad Dermatol* 1992;**27**:427–33.

46  Zic J, Stricklin G, Greer J *et al.* Long term follow up of patients with cutaneous T-cell lymphoma treated with extracorporeal photochemotherapy. *J Am Acad Dermatol* 1996;**35**:935–45.

47  Gottlieb S, Wolfe J, Fox F *et al.* Treatment of cutaneous T-cell lymphoma with extracorporeal photopheresis monotherapy and in combination with recombinant interferon-alpha: a 10 year experience at a single institution. *J Am Acad Dermatol* 1996;**35**:946–57.

48  Fraser–Andrews E, Seed P, Whittaker S, Russell Jones R. Extracorporeal photopheresis in Sézary syndrome: no significant effect in the survival of 44 patients with a peripheral blood T-cell clone. *Arch Dermatol* 1998;**134**:1001–5.

49  Child F, Mitchell T, Whittaker S, Watkins P, Seed P, Russell Jones R. A randomised cross-over study to compare PUVA and extracorporeal photopheresis (ECP) in the treatment of plaque stage (T2) mycosis fungoides. *Br J Dermatol* 2001;**145**(Suppl. 59):16.

50 Bisaccia E, Gonzalez J, Palangio M, Schwartz J, Klainer A. Extracorporeal photochemotherapy alone or with adjuvant therapy in the treatment of cutaneous T-cell lymphoma: A 9 year retrospective study at a single institution. *J Am Acad Dermatol* 2000;**43**:263–71.

51 Wollina U, Looks A, Meyer J *et al.* Treatment of stage II cutaneous T-cell lymphoma with interferon alfa-2a and extracorporeal photochemotherapy: a prospective controlled trial. *J Am Acad Dermatol* 2001;**44**:253–60.

52 Dippel E, Schrag H, Goerdt S, Orfanos C. Extracorporeal photopheresis and interferon-α in advanced cutaneous T-cell lymphoma. *Lancet* 1997;**350**:32–3.

53 Vonderheid E, Bigler R, Greenberg A, Neukum S, Micaily B. Extracorporeal photopheresis and recombinant interferon alfa-2b in Sézary syndrome. *Am J Clin Oncol* 1994;**17**:255–63.

54 Haley H, Davis D, Sams M. Durable loss of a malignant T-cell clone in a stage IV cutaneous T-cell lymphoma patient treated with high-dose interferon and photopheresis. *J Am Acad Dermatol* 1999;**41**:880–3.

55 Yoo E, Cassin M, Lessin S, Rook A. Complete molecular remission during biologic response modifier therapy for Sézary syndrome is associated with enhanced helper T type I cytokine production and natural killer cell activity. *J Am Acad Dermatol* 2001;**45**:208–16.

56 Evans A, Wood B, Scarisbrick J *et al.* Extracorporeal photopheresis in Sézary syndrome: hematologic parameters as predictors of response. *Blood* 2001;**98**:1298–301.

57 Bernengo M, Appino A, Bertero M *et al.* Thymopentin in Sézary syndrome. *J Natl Cancer Inst* 1992;**84**:1341–6.

58 Cooper D, Braverman I, Sarris A *et al.* Cyclosporine treatment of refractory T-cell lymphomas. *Cancer* 1993;**71**:2335–41.

59 Bunn P, Hoffman S, Norris D, Golitz L, Aeling J. Systemic therapy of cutaneous T-cell lymphomas (mycosis fungoides and the Sézary syndrome). *Ann Intern Med* 1994;**121**:592–602.

60 Molin L, Thomsen K, Volden G *et al.* Oral retinoids in mycosis fungoides and Sézary syndrome: a comparison of isotretinoin and etretinate. *Acta Dermatol Venereol* 1987;**67**:232–6.

61 Kessler J, Jones S, Levine N *et al.* Isotretinoin and cutaneous helper T-cell lymphoma (mycosis fungoides). *Arch Dermatol* 1987;**123**:201–4.

62 Duvic M, Martin A, Kim Y *et al.* Phase 2 and 3 clinical trial of oral bexarotene (Targretin capsules) for the treatment of refractory or persistent early stage cutaneous T-cell lymphoma. *Arch Dermatol* 2001;**137**:581–93.

63 Duvic M, Hymes K, Heald P *et al.* Bexarotene is effective and safe for treatment of refractory advanced-stage cutaneous T-cell lymphoma: multinational phase II-III trial results. *J Clin Oncol* 2001;**19**:2456–71.

64 Knox S, Levy R, Hodgkinson S *et al.* Observations on the effect of chimeric anti-CD4 monoclonal antibody in patients with mycosis fungoides. *Blood* 1991;**77**:20–30.

65 Knox S, Hoppe R, Maloney D, Gibbs, Fowler S *et al.* Treatment of cutaneous T-cell lymphoma with chimeric anti-CD4 monoclonal antibody. *Blood* 1996;**87**:893–9.

66 Lundin J, Osterborg A, Brittinger G *et al.* CAMPATH-1H monoclonal antibody in therapy for previously treated low-grade non-Hodgkin's lymphomas: a phase II multicenter study. European study group of CAMPATH-1H treatment in low-grade non-Hodgkin's lymphoma. *J Clin Oncol* 1998;**16**:3257–63.

67 Dearden C, Matutes E, Catovsky D. Alemtuzumab in T-cell malignancies. *Med Oncol* 2002;**19**:S27–32.

68 Olsen E, Duvic M, Frankel A *et al.* Pivotal phase III trial of two dose levels of Denileukin Diftitox for the treatment of cutaneous T-cell lymphoma. *J Clin Oncol* 2001;**19**:376–88.

69 LeMaistre C, Rosen S, Frankel A *et al.* Phase I trial of H65-RTA immunoconjugate in patients with cutaneous T-cell lymphoma. *Blood* 1991;**78**:1173–82.

70 Foss F, Raubitscheck A, Mulshine J *et al.* Phase I study of the pharmacokinetics of a radioimmunoconjugate, 90Y-T101, in patients with CD5-expressing leukaemia and lymphoma. *Clin Cancer Res* 1998;**4**:2691–700.

71 Cotter G, Baglan R, Wasserman T, Mill W. Palliative radiation treatment of cutaneous mycosis fungoides: a dose response. *Int J Radiat Oncol Biol Phys* 1983;**9**:1477–80.

72 Jones G, Hoppe R, Glatstein E. Electron beam treatment for cutaneous T-cell lymphoma. *Haematol Oncol Clin North Am* 1995;**9**:1057–76.

73 Hamminga B, Noordijk E, Van Vloten W. Treatment of mycosis fungoides: total skin electron beam irradiation *v* topical mechlorethamine therapy. *Arch Dermatol* 1982;**118**:150–3.

74 Jones G, Rosenthal D, Wilson L. Total skin electron beam radiation for patients with erythrodermic cutaneous T-cell lymphoma (mycosis fungoides and the Sézary syndrome). *Cancer* 1999;**85**:1985–95.

75 Kirova Y, Piedbois Y, Haddad E *et al.* Radiotherapy in the management of mycosis fungoides: indications, results, prognosis. Twenty years experience. *Radiother Oncol* 1999;**51**:147–51.

76 Becker M, Hoppe R, Knox S. Multiple courses of high dose total skin electron beam therapy in the management of mycosis fungoides. *Int J Radiat Oncol Biol Phys* 1995;**30**:1445–9.

77 Wilson L, Quiros P, Kolenik S *et al.* Additional courses of total skin electron beam therapy in the treatment of patients with recurrent cutaneous T-cell lymphoma *J Am Acad Dermatol* 1996;**35**:69–73.

78 Jones G, Kacinski B, Wilson L *et al.* Total skin electron radiation in the management of mycosis fungoides: Consensus of the European Organization for Research and Treatment of Cancer (EORTC) cutaneous lymphoma project group. *J Am Acad Dermatol* 2002;**10**:1–7.

79 Kaye F, Bunn P, Steinberg S *et al.* A randomised trial comparing combination electron beam radiation and chemotherapy with topical therapy in the initial treatment of mycosis fungoides. *N Engl J Med* 1989;**321**:1748–90.

80 Wilson L, Jones G, Kim D *et al.* Experience with total skin electron beam therapy in combination with extracorporeal photopheresis in the management of patients with erythrodermic (T4) mycosis fungoides. *J Am Acad Dermatol* 2000;**43**:54–60.

81 Zackheim H, Kashani-sabet M, Hwang S. Low dose methotrexate to treat erythrodermic cutaneous T-cell lymphoma: results in twenty-nine patients. *J Am Acad Dermatol* 1996;**34**:626–31.

82 Kurzrock R, Pilat S, Duvic M. Pentostatin therapy of T-cell lymphomas with cutaneous manifestations. *J Clin Oncol* 1999;**17**:3117–21.

83 Deardon C, Matutes E, Catovsky D. Pentostatin treatment of cutaneous T-cell lymphoma. *Oncology* 2000;**14**:37–40.

84 Ho A, Suciu S, Stryckmans P *et al.* Pentostatin in T-cell malignancies. Leukaemia cooperative group and the European Organisation for Research and Treatment of Cancer. *Semin Oncol* 2000;**27**:52–7.

85 Foss F, Ihde D, Breneman D *et al.* Phase II study of pentostatin and intermittent high dose recombinant interferon alfa-2a in advanced mycosis fungoides/Sézary syndrome. *J Clin Oncol* 1992;**10**:1907–13.

86 Kuzel T, Hurria A, Samuelson E *et al.* Phase II trial of 2-chlorodeoxyadenosine for the treatment of cutaneous T-cell lymphoma. *Blood* 1996;**87**:906–11.

87 Zinzani P, Baliva G, Magagnoli M *et al.* Gemcitabine treatment in pretreated cutaneous T-cell lymphoma: experience in 44 patients. *J Clin Oncol* 2000;**18**:2603–6.

88 Wollina U, Graefe T, Kaatz M. Pegylated doxorubicin for primary cutaneous T-cell lymphoma: a report on ten patients with follow-up. *J Cancer Res Clin Oncol* 2001;**127**:128–34.

89 Fierro M, Doveil G, Quaglino P, Savoia P, Verrone A, Bernengo M. Combination of etoposide, idarubicin, cyclophosphamide, vincristine, prednisone and bleomycin (VICOP-B) in the treatment of advanced cutaneous T-cell lymphoma. *Dermatology* 1997;**194**:268–72.

90 Akpek G, Koh H, Bogen S, O'Hara C, Foss F. Chemotherapy with etoposide, vincristine, doxorubicin, bolus cyclophosphamide and oral prednisone in patients with refractory cutaneous T-cell lymphoma. *Cancer* 1999;**86**:1368–76.

91 Bigler R, Crilley P, Micaily B *et al.* Autologous bone marrow transplantation for advanced stage mycosis fungoides. *Bone Marrow Transpl* 1991;**7**:133–7.

92 Olavarria E, Child F, Woolford A, Whittaker S *et al.* T-cell depletion and autologous stem cell transplantation in the management of

tumour stage mycosis fungoides with peripheral blood involvement. *Br J Haematol* 2001;**114**:624–31.

93 Burt R, Guitart J, Traynor A *et al.* Allogeneic hematopoietic stem cell transplantation for advanced mycosis fungoides: evidence of a graft-versus-tumour effect. *Bone Marrow Transpl* 2000;**25**:111–13.

94 Molina A, Nademanee A, Arber D, Forman S. Remission of refractory Sézary syndrome after bone marrow transplantation from a matched unrelated donor. *Biol Blood Marrow Transpl* 1999;**5**:400–4.

95 Masood N, Russell K, Olerud J *et al.* Induction of complete remission of advanced stage mycosis fungoides by allogeneic stem cell transplantation. *J Am Acad Dermatol* 2002;**47**:140–5.

# 45 Kaposi's sarcoma

*Imogen Locke, Margaret F Spittle*

## Background

### Definition

Kaposi's sarcoma (KS), first described by Moritz Kaposi in 1872, is a multifocal vascular tumour. It is characterised histologically by a proliferation of spindle-shaped tumour cells surrounding abnormal slit-like vascular channels with extravasated erythrocytes. It may present with cutaneous or mucosal lesions (mouth, gastrointestinal, bronchial), visceral lesions, or lymphadenopathy.

There are four clinical variants of KS, which appear in specific populations but have identical histological features:

- *Classical KS* (Figure 45.1a). Classical KS typically affects elderly men of Mediterranean or Jewish descent, presenting with purple blue ulcerated plaques on the lower legs, which progress over a period of years.
- *Endemic (African) KS* (Figure 45.1b). Endemic (or African) KS is common in sub-Saharan Africa and in its nodular form may run an indolent course similar to classical KS, with oedema of the lower legs. A more aggressive lymphadenopathic form of disseminated

endemic KS is seen in children and young adults. Florid and infiltrative types of endemic KS affect adults and are locally aggressive.

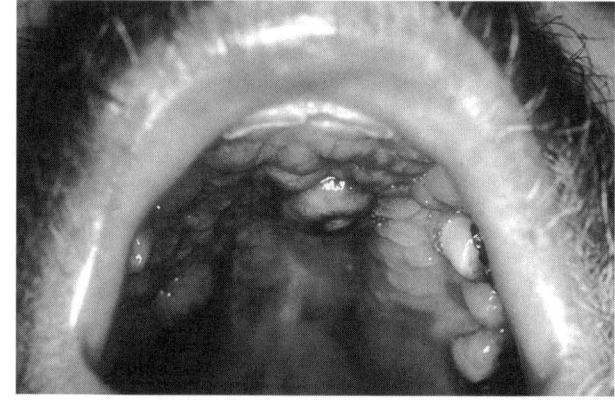

**Figure 45.2** Kaposi's sarcoma of the hard palate in a patient with AIDS

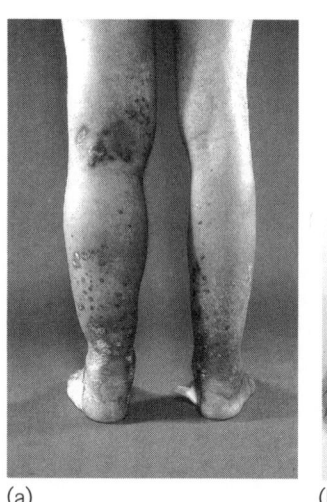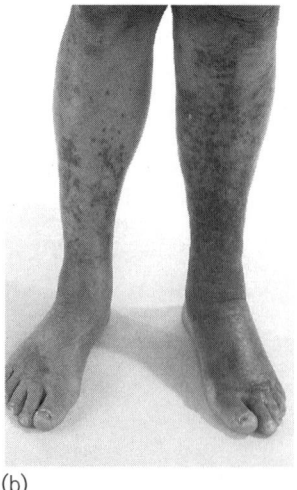

(a)                       (b)

**Figure 45.1** (a) Classical Kaposi's sarcoma with lower limb oedema (b) Endemic (African) Kaposi's sarcoma

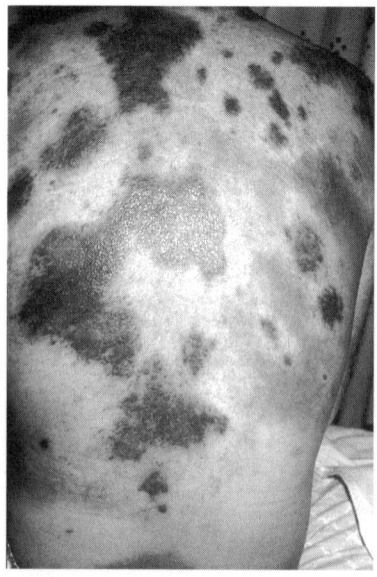

**Figure 45.3** Extensive cutaneous Kaposi's sarcoma in a patient with AIDS

- *Transplant/immunosuppression-related KS.* Transplant recipients and patients receiving immunosuppressive therapy are another group in which KS is seen. The same ethnic groups in which classical KS is seen are at higher risk but the disease tends to run a more aggressive course.
- *AIDS-related KS* (Figures 45.2 and 45.3). In 1981 Friedman-Kien *et al.* reported a cluster of patients with aggressive KS involving lymph nodes and viscera, affecting young homosexual men, in association with a syndrome of opportunistic infections and a defect in cell-mediated immunity, subsequently named the acquired immune deficiency syndrome (AIDS).[1] This aggressive form of KS was seen up to 20 times more frequently in homosexual men with AIDS than in haemophiliac men with AIDS. KS is now an AIDS-defining illness by the Centers for Disease Control guidelines.

## Incidence/prevalence

Classical KS is rare; it is much more common in men than women, with a ratio of up to 15:1. The peak age of onset is 50–70 years. Endemic (African KS) is a common tumour in equatorial Africa and in 1971 comprised up to 9% of all cancers seen in Uganda.[2] Since the beginning of the AIDS epidemic, KS has become the most frequently occurring tumour in central Africa, in HIV-negative and HIV-positive men, accounting for up to 50% in some countries.[3] Since the introduction of highly active antiretroviral therapy (HAART), the proportion of patients with AIDS-related KS is decreasing, but it remains the most common AIDS-associated malignancy, affecting 20–40% of homosexual men with HIV.[4] In published series of organ transplant recipients, between 0·5% and 5·3% have developed KS; in one study the mean period between transplantation and development of KS was 12·5 months (range 1–37 months).[5–7]

## Aetiology

The unusual geographical distribution of KS has long suggested an infective cause. Epidemiological evidence, including the 20 times greater frequency of AIDS-related KS in homosexual men compared with haemophiliacs, suggested a sexually transmitted cofactor. In 1994, Chang *et al.* described the identification of fragments of a novel herpes virus within a biopsy of an AIDS-related KS lesion.[8] KS-associated herpesvirus (KSHV), also known as human herpes virus 8 (HHV8), can be identified in virtually all KS specimens regardless of subtype but is absent from uninvolved skin. The KSHV genome encodes proteins that are homologous to human oncoproteins and have the potential to induce cellular proliferation and inhibit apoptosis. The presence of KSHV seems to be necessary for the development of KS but the role of cofactors such as host immunosuppression, cytokines, and the human immunodeficiency virus (HIV) is unclear.

## Prognosis

Classical KS typically runs an indolent course over years or decades with gradual development of new lesions and complications such as lower limb lymphoedema. An increased risk of developing a second malignancy, usually non-Hodgkin's lymphoma has been reported. Endemic (African) KS may run an indolent course similar to classical KS with nodules and plaques in association with lower limb oedema. The lymphadenopathic form of African KS in children has an aggressive course and carries a poor prognosis. Epidemic AIDS-related KS may be a disseminated and fulminant disease. The prognosis is determined by the extent of tumour (T), severity of immunodeficiency (I) and the presence or absence of systemic illness (S). Each of these variables is independently associated with survival and has resulted in the prospectively validated tumour, immunodeficiency and systemic illness (TIS) staging classification (see Table 45.1).[9] Immune status is the most important prognostic factor and patients with a CD4 count greater than $200 \times 10^6$ cells $l^{-1}$ have a better prognosis. Opportunistic infections are often the cause of death in this group of patients. However, with the advent of HAART and better prophylaxis of opportunistic infections, the prognosis of AIDS-associated KS may be improving, although newer therapies specifically for KS have not been shown to improve overall survival.

## Aims of treatment

In the UK and North America, AIDS-related KS is the most common variant of KS. In this group, where overall prognosis is often determined by other complications such as opportunistic infections, treatment aims to improve the cosmetic appearance of cutaneous disease and palliate symptoms associated with lymph node or visceral disease, such as oedema, bleeding and shortness of breath, with minimal toxicity. However, the introduction of HAART and more effective prophylaxis of opportunistic infections is modifying the natural history of HIV infection and delaying progression to AIDS. Other endpoints such as time-to-treatment failure and overall survival may become more important in the future in this group of KS patients.

**Table 45.1   AIDS Clinical Trials Group staging classification**

| Parameter | Good risk (0) (All of the following) | Poor risk (1) (Any of the following) |
|---|---|---|
| Tumour (T) | Confined to skin and/or lymph nodes and/or minimal oral disease* | Tumour-associated oedema or ulceration Extensive oral KS Gastrointestinal KS KS in other non-nodal viscera |
| Immune system (I) | CD4 count >or = $200 \times 10^6$ litre$^{-1}$ | CD4 count < $200 \times 10^6$ litre$^{-1}$ |
| Systemic illness (S) | No history of opportunistic infections or thrush | History of opportunistic infections and/or thrush |
| | No "B" symptoms† Performance status >or = 70% (Karnofsky) | "B" symptoms present Performance status < 70% Other HIV-related illness (for example neurological disease, lymphoma) |

*Minimal oral disease is non-nodular KS confined to the palate.
†"B" symptoms are unexplained fever, night sweats, > 10% involuntary weight loss or diarrhoea persisting more than 2 weeks.

## Relevant outcomes

Response rate in terms of the number and size of lesions, and flattening and degree of pigmentation, is an important endpoint for systemic therapies in the treatment of cutaneous disease. One of the problems comparing studies of systemic therapy in KS is the subjective nature of the assessment of response. Recent randomised studies of systemic therapies in AIDS-related KS have adopted the AIDS Clinical Trials Group criteria for assessment of response (Box 45.1)[10] The overall cosmetic effect is also an important endpoint particularly for local therapies such as radiotherapy which have long-term effects on normal skin surrounding lesions. Consider, for example, the young homosexual man with telltale purple nodular HIV-associated KS lesions on a highly visible area such as the face. Local radiotherapy to this area, with a margin of normal skin may leave him with an equally unsightly area of residual brown discoloration and a contrasting "halo" of depigmentation. Palliation of associated symptoms such as tumour-associated oedema is another endpoint for which assessment is very subjective.

## Methods of search

MEDLINE was searched from 1966 to 2001. We first performed a highly sensitive search using the truncated term Kaposi* which generated over 8400 abstracts. We then performed a more specific MEDLINE search using "sarcoma, Kaposi" [MeSH Terms] or "Kaposi's Sarcoma" [Text Word] combined with the following interventions AND [surgery, laser*, photodynamic therapy, cryotherapy, cryosurgery, intralesional therapy, intralesional vincristine or vinblastine, radiotherapy, interferon, chemotherapy,

anthracycline, bleomycin, vinca-alkaloid, vincristine, vinblastine, taxane, paclitaxel, liposomal therapy, gemcitabine, navelbine, thalidomide, antiangiogenic agent, retinoids, retinoic acid, antiretroviral therapy, zidovudine, ganciclovir, cidofovir or foscarnet].

The Cochrane Controlled Trials Register and Database of Systematic Reviews was also searched using the search terms "Kaposi" or "Kaposi's sarcoma".

## What are the effects of local therapies in KS (surgical excision, cryotherapy, photodynamic therapy and intralesional chemotherapy)?

### Evidence summary

We found no systematic reviews or randomised controlled trials of local therapies in KS. There were a relatively small number of uncontrolled phase II studies of each of the above interventions.

### Surgical excision

We found no clinical trials.

### Cryotherapy

One uncontrolled phase II study of 20 patients with cutaneous AIDS-related KS, treated with liquid nitrogen cryotherapy, reported a complete response rate of 80% lasting a minimum of 6 weeks.[11] On average each lesion required three treatments at 3-weekly intervals and the main side effects were blistering and local discomfort

**Box 45.1 AIDS Clinical Trials Group (ACTG) response criteria**

**Complete response (CR)**

**Clinical complete response (CCR)**

The absence of any detectable residual disease, including tumour-associated oedema, persisting for at least 4 weeks. In patients in whom pigmented (brown or tan) macular skin lesions persist after apparent CR, biopsy of at least one representative lesion is required to document the absence of malignant cells. In patients known to have had visceral disease, an attempt at restaging with appropriate endoscopic or radiographic procedures should be made. If such procedures are medically contraindicated, the patient may be classified as having a clinical CR (CCR)

**Partial response (PR)**

The absence of new cutaneous or oral lesions, new visceral sites of involvement, or the appearance or worsening of tumour-associated oedema or effusions in addition to at least one of the following:

- a 50% or greater decrease in the number of all previously existing skin lesions (skin, oral, measurable, or evaluable visceral disease)
- a 50% decrease in the size of lesions (includes a 50% decrease in the sum of the products of the largest perpendicular diameters of bi-dimensionally measurable marker lesions and/or complete flattening of at least 50% of the lesions (that is, 50% of previously nodular or plaque-like lesions become macules)
- in those patients with predominantly nodular lesions, flattening to an indurated plaque of 75% or more of the nodules
- patients with residual tumour-associated oedema or effusion who otherwise meet the criteria for CR.

**Stable disease (SD)**

Any response not meeting the criteria for progression or PR

**Progressive disease (PD)**

An increase of 25% or more in the size of previously existing lesions and/or the appearance of new lesions or new sites of disease and/or a change in the character of 25% or more of the skin or oral lesions from macular to plaque-like or nodular. The development of new or increasing tumour-associated oedema or effusion is also considered to represent disease progression

**Evidence level III**. Another uncontrolled study of patients with AIDS-related facial KS found cryosurgery more effective for small lesions measuring less than 1 cm.[12]

### Photodynamic therapy

In one uncontrolled phase I/II study of 348 AIDS-related KS lesions in 25 patients treated with Photofrin photodynamic therapy the maximum tolerated 630 nm light dose was determined to be 300 J cm$^{-2}$ if given with 1·0 mg kg$^{-1}$ of Photofrin 48 hours beforehand.[13] Of 289 evaluable lesions, 33% had a complete clinical response and 63% had a partial response. At light doses of 400 J cm$^{-2}$ full field necrosis and scabbing occurred, whereas at doses of 250 J cm$^{-2}$ side effects were erythema and oedema within the treatment field. Another uncontrolled phase II study found that 2 mg kg$^{-1}$ of Photofrin with 70–120 J cm$^{-2}$ of 630 nm light therapy, for the treatment of 83 evaluable lesions in eight homosexual men with AIDS-related cutaneous KS, resulted in high overall response rates (83–100%). However, acute toxicity was unacceptable and the long-term cosmetic result was poor, with scarring and hyperpigmentation.[14] A further small uncontrolled phase II study treated 30 AIDS-associated KS lesions with indocyanine green ($2 \times 2$ mg kg$^{-1}$ i.v.) followed immediately by 850 nm light therapy (100 J cm$^{-2}$)[15]: 19 lesions resolved completely, leaving an atrophic scar, with no recurrences in 2 years **Evidence level IIb**.

### Intralesional chemotherapy

Two uncontrolled phase II studies have examined the effect of treating intraoral, oropharyngeal, or laryngeal AIDS-related KS by intralesional injection of vinblastine.[16,17] One obtained a 62% complete response rate (16/26 lesions) in 24 patients with AIDS-associated oropharyngeal or laryngeal KS.[16] Lesions were injected with 0·1–0·2 mg ml$^{-1}$ of vinblastine and the injection was repeated 4–5 weekly until complete response or stable disease. Side effects included self-limiting pain and ulceration. In 11 of 24 patients the pain was not relieved by paracetamol **Evidence level IIb**.

A similarly high complete response rate was found in another uncontrolled phase II study of intralesional vinblastine as a local treatment for oral cavity AIDS-associated KS[17]: 144 lesions in 50 patients were injected and the complete response rate was 74%. The most common site of intraoral KS is the hard palate.

Intralesional chemotherapy (vinblastine, vincristine, or bleomycin) has also been used to treat cutaneous KS lesions with overall response rates (CR plus PR) in small uncontrolled studies of 88–100%.[18,19]

### Comment

In the absence of randomised controlled studies, the comparative efficacy of local therapies in the treatment of KS cannot be assessed. High response rates have been described in uncontrolled case series for cryotherapy, photodynamic therapy, and intralesional chemotherapy, but at the expense of troublesome local side effects.

## Is radiotherapy an effective local treatment for cutaneous KS?

### Evidence summary

No systematic reviews were found. Two randomised trials in AIDS-related KS have compared different radiotherapy dose-fractionation schedules.[20,21] There have also been many case series typically using total doses of radiotherapy ranging from 8 Gy to 40 Gy. However, the dose each lesion received in these series was individualised depending on both patient and lesion factors. Conclusions cannot be drawn from these latter non-randomised studies as to the optimum dose-fractionation schedule in AIDS-related KS. No randomised studies of radiotherapy in classical KS, endemic KS, or immunosuppression-related KS were found. Many retrospective case series of radiotherapy as a local therapy for classical KS have been reported suggesting it is a radiosensitive disease, but often criteria for assessment of response are not stated and vary between studies.

### Efficacy

#### AIDS-related KS

A randomised trial of radiotherapy in 71 cutaneous AIDS-associated KS lesions comparing three different dose-fractionation regimens – 8 Gy in a single fraction, 20 Gy in 10 fractions over 2 weeks and 40 Gy in 20 fractions over 4 weeks were found.[20] Lesions were treated using 6 MeV electrons with 0·5 cm skin bolus allowing a 2 cm margin around palpable tumour. An objective response was defined as at least a 50% decrease in palpable tumour area, which was taken as the product of the perpendicular dimensions. Complete response (CR) was defined as resolution of all palpable tumour with or without residual pigmentation. More complete responses were achieved with 40 Gy in 20 fractions (83%) and 20 Gy in 10 fractions (79%) than with an 8 Gy single fraction (50%). A greater proportion of CRs were without residual purple pigmentation in the group who received 40 Gy (53%) compared with those who received 20 Gy or 8 Gy (11% and 17% respectively).[20] The median time to treatment failure (defined as measurable growth in tumour area) for the 40 Gy, 20 Gy and 8 Gy groups were 43 weeks, 26 weeks and 13 weeks, respectively.[20]

Another prospective randomised trial compared 8 Gy in a single fraction with 16 Gy in four fractions over 4 days for the treatment of cutaneous AIDS-related KS[21]; 596 lesions in 57 patients were treated in total of which 172 lesions in

27 patients were treated in a randomised fashion. The method of randomisation was not reported. In a concurrent non-randomised prospective trial, 424 lesions in 49 patients were treated, where the radiotherapy regimen was given according to patient preference. Lesions were treated using 75 or 100 kV superficial radiotherapy with a margin of 3–5 mm.

The overall response rate for the randomised and non-randomised lesions was 79% (465/590), which included complete responses and pigmented complete responses. The overall response rate for lesions treated with a single 8 Gy fraction was 78% (305/392) and 81% (160/198) for the lesions which received 16 Gy in four fractions. The overall response rates for the 172 lesions treated as part of the randomised trial were 71% (57/80) and 82% (75/92) for the 8 Gy and 16 Gy groups, respectively. The two response rates do not differ significantly $(0·25 > P > 0·1)$. Facial lesions had the highest response rate. The response rates for the lesions treated non-randomly were 79% (248/313) for those that received 8 Gy and 80% (85/106) for those in the 16 Gy arm[21] **Evidence level Ib**.

A large retrospective case series of 643 patients with AIDS-related KS treated over a 10-year period (June 1986–December 1996) reported an objective response rate of 92% in 621 evaluable patients.[22] The radiotherapy was delivered as a split course with 20 Gy given in 2·5 Gy fractions over 2 weeks treating four times per week followed by 10 Gy in 1 week after a 2-week rest period. Extended cutaneous fields were treated with 4 MeV or 8 MeV electrons. Localised fields were treated with 45–100 KV superficial $x$ rays.[22]

Another large series, of AIDS-related KS lesions treated with radiotherapy, retrospectively reviewed 375 lesions in 187 patients of which 266 sites were cutaneous.[23] The lesions were treated in a non-randomised fashion with total doses of 2 to 40 Gy in fractions of 1·5 Gy to 8 Gy. Of the 266 cutaneous lesions, 111 received an 8 Gy single fraction and 155 received a more protracted fractionation regimen. In this study a response was defined as complete flattening of a lesion or a decrease in size to at least 50% of its pretreatment size with reduced pigmentation: 93% of the cutaneous lesions, which received an 8 Gy single fraction, responded compared with 96% of the lesions that received a fractionated course of radiotherapy. The response or time to relapse did not differ between the two groups.[23]

Many smaller case series have used a variety of dose-fractionation schedules, which have shown similar high response rates of cutaneous KS to radiotherapy, but criteria used to assess response vary.

#### Classical and endemic (African) KS

We found no randomised studies of radiotherapy in endemic (African) or classical KS. A case series of 82 patients with classical KS treated with radiotherapy between 1972 and 1985 reported a complete response rate of more than 50% with doses ranging from 6·5 Gy in a single fraction to 35 Gy in 10 fractions.[24] Long-term control was greater with doses of 27·5 Gy or more delivered in 10 fractions over a 2-week period.[24] Brenner *et al.* reported a similar complete response rate for radiotherapy in classical KS of 58%.[25] Another case series of 60 patients with classical KS treated with radiotherapy reported an overall response rate of 93%. In this study a variety of radiotherapy techniques were used including megavoltage electrons, megavoltage photons, and a combination of both or total skin electron beam therapy[26] **Evidence level III**.

One retrospective case series of 28 men with endemic (African) KS treated with radiotherapy between 1978 and 1990 reported a complete response rate of 32% and a partial response rate of 54%, but the criteria used to assess response were not stated.[27] Radiotherapy dose ranged from an 8–10 Gy single fraction to 14–24 Gy fractionated over 1 to 3 weeks using orthovoltage, cobalt[60] or 6–8 MeV electrons.

## Drawbacks

In the randomised trial of Stelzer and Griffin, toxicity was graded using the Radiation Therapy Oncology Group scoring system.[20] Grade 1 acute toxicity (skin erythema, dry desquamation, or alopecia) was seen in 3/24 (12%) of the patients who received 8 Gy, 11/24 (46%) of patients who received 20 Gy, and 22/23 (96%) patients who received 40 Gy. No acute toxicity greater than grade 1 was seen. Late toxicity occurred only in the 40 Gy group (6/23 patients) but did not exceed grade 1 (slight hyperpigmentation or alopecia). In a large retrospective case series of 621 evaluable patients, the frequency of grade 1 skin reactions was 7%, grade 2 reactions 69%, and grade 3 reactions 23·4%.[22]

Harrison *et al.* developed a subjective four-point grading system to assess pigmentation in the normal skin surrounding lesions following irradiation as part of overall cosmesis.[21] The scoring system graded cosmesis from grade 0 (no evidence of pigmentation) to grade 3 (severe skin pigmentation or telangiectasia). Of the 172 randomised lesions cosmesis grade 0 or 1 was found in 87% of those who received a single fraction and in 90% of those who received four fractions, a non-significant difference.

## Comment

Radiotherapy gives high response rates in the treatment of cutaneous KS and is an effective local palliative therapy. In the absence of any placebo group, it is difficult to state with certainty that the responses are solely due to the treatment, but inclusion of a placebo or sham radiotherapy group would be ethically unjustifiable. The rates of complete response and duration of lesion control are higher with increasing total doses of radiotherapy in AIDS-related KS.[20] However, in this group of patients prognosis is that of the underlying AIDS diagnosis. In the study of Harrison *et al.*, for example, participating patients survived for a median of 17 months only; with the advent of HAART prognosis for patients with AIDS may be improving.[21] Treatment is given with palliative intent and cosmesis is an important endpoint.

One of the difficulties in comparing trials of radiotherapy in cutaneous KS is variation in the definitions of response and the subjective nature of assessment particularly of lesion colour and nodularity. A lesion may flatten or reduce in size with treatment but haemosiderin within the skin may leave residual brown pigmentation influencing the overall cosmetic outcome. Uniform criteria of response in future trials should include assessment of lesion flatness, size, residual pigmentation, and tumour-associated oedema after therapy. Evaluation of the effect of radiotherapy on the surrounding skin is also important in the overall cosmetic outcome following treatment. Patients should be warned that radiotherapy might lead to depigmentation of the surrounding normal skin, producing a "halo" effect.

## Implication for clinical practice

Radiotherapy can improve the appearance of cutaneous KS lesions and provide temporary local control. In the population with AIDS-related cutaneous KS, a single 8 Gy fraction of radiotherapy with superficial *x* rays or electrons gives a high response rate **Grade A**. Some good evidence indicates that higher response rates and a greater duration of local control are seen with fractionated radiotherapy courses to a higher total dose. However, fractionated regimens more often cause acute toxicity and require more visits to hospital. This matters particularly in a group whose prognosis depends on the course of the underlying AIDS, although with more effective antiretroviral therapy longer term local control may become increasingly important.

## Is interferon alfa an effective systemic treatment for AIDS-related KS alone or in combination with zidovudine?

### Evidence summary

Interferons (IFNs) have multiple effects on immune function and cell proliferation and may act synergistically in the treatment of AIDS-related KS with antiretroviral therapy.

We found no systematic reviews of the use of IFN in AIDS-related KS. Early phase II trials demonstrated activity of IFN as monotherapy for AIDS-related KS before the advent of nucleoside reverse transcriptase inhibitors. One small randomised trial compared two doses of IFNα as monotherapy in AIDS-related KS.[28] On the basis of *in vitro* studies suggesting synergy between IFNα and antiretroviral drugs, multiple subsequent phase II trials have examined the combination of IFNα and zidovudine in the treatment of AIDS-related KS. We found one randomised comparative trial of 108 patients with AIDS-related KS using zidovudine antiretroviral therapy combined with one of two different IFNα dose levels.[29] We found no placebo-controlled trials.

## IFNα alone in AIDS-related KS

### *Efficacy*

One small prospective randomised trial of IFN as monotherapy in AIDS-related KS tested the efficacy of high versus low dose IFNα in AIDS-associated KS[28]: 20 patients were randomised between high dose intravenous IFN (50 MU m$^{-2}$ for 5 days on alternate weeks) and low dose subcutaneous IFN (1 MU m$^{-2}$ for 5 days on alternate weeks) **Evidence level IIb**. A 40% objective response rate was seen in the high dose arm and a 20% objective response rate in the low dose arm.[28] Many uncontrolled phase II studies have been conducted and these have reported higher response rates for patients with CD4 lymphocyte counts of $200 \times 10^6$ cells litre$^{-1}$, higher doses of IFN (> 20 MU per day) and in the absence of previous opportunistic infections. However, most of these individual studies are small and use of a wide variety of IFN doses and schedules makes comparisons difficult. These trials often compare two different doses or preparations of IFN and we found no placebo-controlled randomised trials of IFN in the treatment of KS. In one larger series of 273 patients with AIDS-related KS, CD4 counts of greater than $400 \times 10^6$ cells litre$^{-1}$ were associated with response rates of 45% whereas the response rate for patients with CD4 counts of less than $200 \times 10^6$ cells litre$^{-1}$ was only 7%.[30] Another series of uncontrolled phase II trials with a total of 114 patients given IFNα 2b demonstrated higher response rates with high dose (50 MU m$^{-2}$ i.v.) than low dose IFN (1 MU m$^{-2}$ s.c.).[31] Patients with early stage disease and without "B" symptoms were more likely to respond.[31]

### *Drawbacks*

Almost all patients experienced 'flu-like symptoms with IFNα and in the study of Volberding *et al.* 6% of patients discontinued therapy owing to adverse reactions.[31] In addition to 'flu-like symptoms, adverse events included haematological toxicity and abnormalities in liver function tests. In the randomised study of Groopman *et al.* mild

haematological and hepatic toxicity were seen at both high and low dose levels of IFNα.[28]

## IFNα (low versus high dose) plus zidovudine in AIDS-related KS

### *Efficacy*

We found one randomised study comparing two dose levels of IFNα combined with zidovudine. In this study of 108 patients with AIDS-related KS, patients received zidovudine 500 mg per day and were randomised to low (1 MU per day) or intermediate dose (8 MU per day) of subcutaneous IFNα.[29] Response rates for the 54 patients randomised to 8 MU per day were significantly greater than for the 53 patients who received 1 MU per day, 31% and 8% respectively ($P = 0.0011$) **Evidence level Ib**. Time to progression was longer for intermediate dose IFN (18 weeks) than for low dose IFN (13 weeks) ($P = 0.002$). Response rates were higher for patients who had a CD4 count above $150 \times 10^6$ cells litre$^{-1}$.[29] Other phase I/II trials in AIDS-related KS using doses of IFNα ranging from 4·5 MU per day to 27 MU per day combined with zidovudine 500 mg per day to 1200 mg per day have achieved objective response rates of 5% to 47%.[32–38]

### *Drawbacks*

In the largest of the above randomised studies comparing two dose levels of IFNα combined with zidovudine in the treatment of AIDS-related KS, both haematological and non-haematological toxicities were higher for 8 MU daily than 1 MU daily resulting in dose reductions for 50 of 54 patients receiving the higher dose.[29]

## IFN versus bleomycin

A small randomised study compared IFNα 2a plus zidovudine with bleomycin plus zidovudine in 26 patients with AIDS-related KS, of which 22 were evaluable for response[39]: 2 of 10 (20%) assessable patients, who received bleomycin 15 mg every 2 weeks plus zidovudine 250 mg twice daily, had an objective response to treatment after 5·3 months on treatment compared with 1 of 12 (8%) evaluable patients who received IFNα 2a 9 MU per day plus zidovudine 250 mg twice daily after 4·7 months on treatment.[39]

## IFN combined with cytotoxic chemotherapy

One small uncontrolled study of 24 patients with AIDS-related KS treated with IFNα 2b and etoposide found an objective response rate of 38% (8/21 evaluable patients).[40] Another small study combined intermediate dose IFNα with combination chemotherapy with actinomycin D, vinblastine and bleomycin in 13 patients with AIDS-related KS **Evidence level IIb** . There was one complete response and four partial responses but four patients required hospital admission for febrile neutropenia.[41]

## Comment

Zidovudine alone is no longer standard therapy for HIV infection and the advent of HAART has changed the clinical course of AIDS-related KS. The effectiveness of IFN combined with HAART is unknown. No randomised trials have compared liposomal anthracyclines with IFN in early AIDS-related KS. IFN combined with cytotoxic chemotherapy is of unknown effectiveness. All of the above trials compared two or more active or different doses of IFN and therefore may be comparing several ineffective treatments. None of these trials was placebo-controlled.

## Implications for practice

Patients with early stage disease, CD4 counts greater than 200 cells $\times$ 106 litre$^{-1}$, no "B" symptoms, and no previous opportunistic infections are more likely to respond to IFN$\alpha$ **Evidence level Ib** . Response rates are greater with higher doses of IFN whether given alone or in combination with zidovudine. A disadvantage of IFN in the treatment of KS is the need for frequent subcutaneous injections. The development of pegylated IFN requiring less frequent administration may be an advantage.

## What are the effects of systemic chemotherapy in KS and do liposomal anthracyclines produce higher response rates (by AIDS Clinical Trials Group criteria), with less toxicity, than conventional combination chemotherapy in advanced AIDS-related KS?

## Evidence summary

We found no systematic reviews of chemotherapy in KS. The majority of the randomised evidence base is in the treatment of advanced AIDS-related KS. We found three small randomised trials of chemotherapy in African KS. Several drugs have been found to have single agent activity in uncontrolled phase II studies, the most active of which include paclitaxel, liposomal anthracyclines, vinca alkaloids, and bleomycin. Two commonly used combination cytotoxic regimens in the treatment of AIDS-related KS are bleomycin plus vincristine (BV) and doxorubicin plus bleomycin plus vincristine (ABV), which have been compared in randomised studies with single agent chemotherapy, including newer drugs such as liposomal anthracyclines. We found no randomised placebo-controlled trials and all the

trials compared two or more actives apart from a small randomised cross-over comparison of liposomal daunorubicin versus observation for early KS.

## Single agent chemotherapy

### Bleomycin

We found three small uncontrolled phase II trials of bleomycin as single agent therapy in the treatment of AIDS-related KS and one small non-randomised study comparing single agent bleomycin with combination ABV chemotherapy (doxorubicin plus bleomycin plus vincristine).[42–45] In one non-randomised phase II study of single agent bleomycin, 30 patients received intramuscular bleomycin (5 mg per day for 3 days every 14–21 days) and another 30 patients received bleomycin by infusion (6 mg m$^{-2}$ per day for 4 days every 28 days) **Evidence level IIb** . The overall partial response rate for the combined groups was 48% (29/60) and the response rate in the intramuscular group and the continuous infusion group were similar (although the groups were not randomly assigned).[42] Mean duration of bleomycin therapy was 5 months; 19 patients died during the treatment and four patients after withdrawal of bleomycin. Opportunistic infections were the cause of death in 18 of the 23 patients who died.[42] In another small uncontrolled study 17 patients with AIDS-related KS were treated with infusional bleomycin at 20 mg m$^{-2}$ per day for 3 days every 21 days and the partial response rate by ACTG criteria (see Box 45.1) was 65%.[43] Three of five previously treated patients also had a partial response. Median survival was 7 months.[43] In a third uncontrolled phase II study 70 patients with AIDS-related mucocutaneous KS were given 5 mg per day of intramuscular bleomycin for 3 days every 2 weeks: two patients had a complete response and 50 patients had a partial response giving an overall response rate of 74%.[44] The median time to relapse was 10 weeks.

In a small non-randomised study comparing bleomycin with ABV combination chemotherapy in 24 patients with extensive AIDS-related KS, there were no complete or partial responses in 12 patients who received bleomycin alone but four out of 12 patients who received ABV chemotherapy had a partial response.[45]

### Vinca alkaloids

We found one randomised study comparing oral etoposide with vinblastine in the treatment of classical KS in elderly Mediterranean patients.[46] We found no randomised evidence for the use of single agent vinca alkaloids in AIDS-related KS. Several uncontrolled phase II studies used single agent vinblastine in the treatment of both classical and AIDS-related KS.[25,47–52]

In one study, 65 elderly patients with classical KS were randomised between oral etoposide and intravenous vinblastine[46] **Evidence level IIb**. Etoposide was given 3-weekly at a dose of 60 mg m$^{-2}$ days 1–3 for the first cycle, days 1–4 for the second cycle and days 1–5 for the third cycle. Vinblastine was given intravenously at a dose of 3 mg m$^{-2}$ weekly for the first 3 weeks then 6 mg m$^{-2}$ every 3 weeks. The overall response rate to etoposide was 73% and 58% for vinblastine ($P = 0.3$). An uncontrolled phase II study of single agent vinblastine in 38 patients with AIDS-related KS reported an overall response rate of 26% with weekly vinblastine 4–8 mg per week titrated against white blood cell count.[49] Reported response rates to vinblastine in small uncontrolled studies are higher for classical KS than AIDS-related KS.

## Etoposide

We found one randomised study comparing oral etoposide with intravenous vinblastine in classical KS described above[46] **Evidence level IIb**. We also found one small uncontrolled phase II study of oral etoposide in the treatment of 17 evaluable patients with classical KS, which reported a response rate of 76% to 100 mg daily for 3–5 days every 3 weeks.[53] We found five small phase II trials of etoposide and one of teniposide in AIDS-related KS.[54–59] In four small uncontrolled phase II studies of oral etoposide in AIDS-related KS, with between 14 and 41 evaluable patients, the objective response rate varied from 0% to 83%.[54–56,58] In one study of infused etoposide in nine patients there was an overall partial response rate of only 22% with one toxic death.[57] An uncontrolled study of 25 patients with AIDS-related KS treated with teniposide (60-minute infusion of 360 mg m$^{-2}$ every 3 weeks) produced a partial response rate of 40% which lasted a median of 9 weeks.[59]

## Liposomal anthracyclines

Doxorubicin and daunorubicin have been produced in encapsulated forms in which the anthracycline drug is trapped within phospholipid spheres known as liposomes. These liposomal preparations have a prolonged circulatory half-life and are associated with enhanced delivery of active drug to KS lesions. They have been compared with standard combination chemotherapy in large randomised trials.[60–62] A randomised cross-over study of 29 patients with early AIDS-related KS (less than 20 cutaneous lesions, no visceral involvement, and a CD4 count above $400 \times 10^6$ litre$^{-1}$) randomised patients between initial liposomal daunorubicin versus observation for 12 weeks[63]; 15 patients received liposomal daunorubicin (40 mg m$^{-2}$ every 2 weeks for six cycles) and 14 patients were observed. ACTG criteria were used to assess response and patients crossed over after 12 weeks or on disease progression. There was a 40% initial response rate in the liposomal daunorubicin arm; 40%

of patients developed progressive disease on liposomal daunorubicin compared with 72% in the observation arm.

## Paclitaxel

We found no randomised studies. Three uncontrolled phase II studies of paclitaxel in advanced AIDS-related KS were found **Evidence level IIb**. Overall response rates in these three phase II studies were between 59% and 71%.[64–66] In each study the most frequent dose-limiting toxicity was neutropenia and in one study grade 3 or 4 neutropenia occurred in 61% of patients.[65]

## Newer cytotoxic drugs

There have been no phase III studies of newer agents such as vinorelbine and gemcitabine in KS. Vinorelbine has been used in an uncontrolled phase II study of 35 evaluable patients with AIDS-related KS, who had progressed on one or more previous systemic chemotherapies, and an overall response rate of 43% was found[67] **Evidence level IIb**. One phase II study of gemcitabine in 11 evaluable patients with recurrent classical KS after previous chemotherapy reported 10/11 partial responses and one complete response.[68] Gemcitabine was given at 1.2 g per week for 2 weeks followed by a 1-week gap and continued until maximum response was achieved.[68]

## Anti-angiogenic agents

Thalidomide is an anti-angiogenic agent that has been investigated in uncontrolled phase II trials in the treatment of AIDS-related KS **Evidence level IIb**. One such study of 20 patients, of whom 17 were assessable for response, reported a 40% (8/20) partial response rate with 200 mg per day of oral thalidomide increased 2 weekly to a maximum of 1000 mg per day.[69] Response lasted for a median of 7.1 months and the median thalidomide dose at time of maximum response was 500 mg per day; nine of 20 patients experienced drowsiness and seven of 20 patients experienced depression. Five patients withdrew from the study because of toxicity.[69]

In another uncontrolled study, 17 patients with AIDS-related KS were given 100 mg oral thalidomide at night for 8 weeks and 35% patients (6/17) had a partial response but six patients withdrew early because of toxicity.[70]

The highly vascular nature of KS has produced interest in other anti-angiogenic agents such as matrix metalloproteinase inhibitors, which are being investigated in phase I studies.

## Combination chemotherapy in endemic (African) KS

We found a series of three small randomised comparative studies of chemotherapy in Ugandan patients with endemic

(African) KS.[71-73] Chemotherapy is an important modality of treatment for endemic KS in developing countries without adequate access to radiotherapy facilities. On the basis of a previous small randomised study, which found a higher response rate for actinomycin D than cyclophosphamide in patients with endemic (African) KS, a second randomised study compared actinomycin D with a combination of actinomycin D plus vincristine.[71,72] Twelve patients received actinomycin D ($0.42$ mg m$^{-2}$ per day for 5 days every 3 to 4 weeks) alone, and 14 received this with vincristine ($1.4$ mg m$^{-2}$/week until the end of the second course of actinomycin D, then days 1 and 5 of each subsequent course)[72]; 24 patients were evaluable for response as two of the 12 patients who received actinomycin D alone died during the first cycle of chemotherapy (Gram-negative sepsis and adrenal failure). A further patient in the combination group developed sepsis after cycle three and died. Complete response was defined as the complete disappearance of all visible/measurable disease and a partial response as a more than 50% regression of disease: 13 of 14 patients who received actinomycin D plus vincristine had a complete or partial response compared with nine of 12 patients randomised to receive actinomycin D alone after four to six courses of chemotherapy. However, the number of patients in this study is very small and more patients in the combination group had florid-type KS or bone lesions.

A further randomised study compared actinomycin D plus vincristine (same schedule as above) with or without the addition of DTIC (dacarbazine) 250 mg m$^{-2}$ for 5 days with alternate courses of actinomycin D.[73] Randomisation was achieved using random cards. The overall response rate for the 40 patients randomised to the two-drug arm was 88%. Of 32 patients randomised to receive the three-drug combination, 30 patients had a complete response (94%) with a further patient having a partial response (overall response rate 97%). Time-to-best response was quicker for the three-drug combination than the two-drug combination (two courses *v* five to six courses).

## Combination chemotherapy in AIDS-related KS

### ABV chemotherapy (doxorubicin plus bleomycin plus vincristine) versus doxorubicin

We found one small randomised study of 61 patients, with extensive mucocutaneous or visceral AIDS-related KS, comparing ABV combination chemotherapy with doxorubicin alone.[74] The overall response rate was 88% for 30 patients who received ABV combination chemotherapy and 48% for the 31 patients who received only doxorubicin (20 mg m$^{-2}$). The response rates differed significantly and toxicity was similar in both arms, but more neutropenia ($< 1000 \times 10^6$ cells litre$^{-1}$) was seen with ABV (52%) than

doxorubicin alone (34%). Median survival was 9 months for both groups.[74]

### ABV or BV chemotherapy versus liposomal anthracyclines

Three large randomised controlled trials have compared liposomal anthracyclines (either doxorubicin or daunorubicin) with standard ABV or BV combination chemotherapy. We found one randomised study comparing liposomal daunorubicin (DaunoXome) with ABV (doxorubicin plus bleomycin plus vincristine) and two randomised trials comparing liposomal doxorubicin with standard combination chemotherapy (either ABV or BV).[60-62] All three trials assessed response using modified ACTG response criteria and graded toxicity according to standard criteria. Concurrent antiretroviral therapy was allowed in all three trials. Table 45.2 summarises the results of these RCTs.

A further randomised controlled trial compared pegylated liposomal doxorubicin (PLD) alone (20 mg m$^{-2}$) with the combination PLD plus bleomycin plus vincristine (PLD 20 mg m$^{-2}$, bleomycin 10 IU m$^{-2}$, vincristine 1mg) given every two weeks.[75]

## Efficacy

### Liposomal daunorubicin versus ABV chemotherapy

One randomised trial, comparing liposomal daunorubicin with ABV chemotherapy (doxorubicin 10 mg m$^{-2}$, bleomycin 15 IU and vincristine 1 mg every 2 weeks) in 227 patients with advanced AIDS-related KS, reported equivalent overall response rates of 25% and 28%.[60] Median survival was similar in both groups (369 days *v* 342 days, respectively), and so was the median time to treatment failure.

The method of randomisation was not stated but patients were stratified at randomisation using a permuted-block design for the following prognostic factors: baseline CD4 count below 100 cells $\times 10^6$ litre$^{-1}$, visceral involvement, zidovudine-containing antiretroviral therapy and Karnofsky performance status below 80% **Evidence level Ib**.

Responses were assessed using modified ACTG criteria. In patients with persistent pigmented macular skin lesions after a clinical complete response, a biopsy of a least one representative skin lesion was required for complete response by ACTG criteria. Liposomal daunorubicin was given at 40 mg m$^{-2}$ every 2 weeks until complete response, progressive disease, or unacceptable toxicity. Patients who responded completely were given a further two cycles of chemotherapy and then observed on study. No prior chemotherapy was permitted but concurrent antiretroviral

**Table 45.2** Randomised trials comparing liposomal anthracyclines to standard combination chemotherapy in AIDS-related Kaposi's sarcoma

| Reference | Study type | Study population | No. of patients | Interventions compared N = no. of patients | Co-treatments permitted | Overall percentage response rate (ORR) | Selected adverse events |
|---|---|---|---|---|---|---|---|
| 60 | Prospective randomised comparative study | Biopsy-proven AIDS-related KS with at least 25 mucocutaneous lesions, symptomatic visceral involvement or tumour-associated oedema | 227 | Liposomal daunorubicin (DaunoXome) 40 mg m$^{-2}$ given every 2 weeks (N=116) or doxorubicin 10 mg m$^{-2}$, bleomycin 15 IU and vincristine 1 mg (ABV) given every 2 weeks (N=111) | G-CSF if absolute neutrophil count $<0.75 \times 10^9$ cells litre$^{-1}$ Concurrent antiretroviral therapy | Responses assessed using modified ACTG criteria DaunoXome = 25% ORR ABV = 27.9% ORR P not significant | SWOG toxicity scoring system DaunoXome versus ABV Grade 1/2 alopecia – 8% v 36% Grade 1/2 neuropathy – 12% v 38% Grade 4 neutropenia – 15% v 5% |
| 61 | Prospective randomised comparative study | Biopsy-proven AIDS-related KS with at least 25 mucocutaneous lesions or at least 10 new lesions in the preceding month or documented visceral disease | 258 | Pegylated liposomal doxorubicin (PLD) 20 mg m$^{-2}$ given every 2 weeks for 6 cycles (N=133) or doxorubicin 20 mg m$^{-2}$, bleomycin 10 mg m$^{-2}$ and vincristine 1 mg (ABV) every 2 weeks for 6 cycles (N=125) Either treatment continued until complete response, progressive disease, or unacceptable toxicity | Colony-stimulating factors at the discretion of the investigators Concurrent antiretroviral therapy | Responses assessed using modified ACTG criteria PLD = 45.9% ORR ABV = 24.8% ORR P<0.001 | World Health Organization criteria PLD v ABV Grade 3/4 alopecia – 1% v 19% Grade 3/4 peripheral neuropathy – 6% v 14% Grade 3/4 leucopenia – 36% v 42% |

*(Continued)*

**Table 45.2** *(Continued)*

| Reference | Study type | Study population | No. of patients | Interventions compared N = no. of patients | Co-treatments permitted | Overall percentage response rate (ORR) | Selected adverse events |
|---|---|---|---|---|---|---|---|
| 62 | Prospective randomised comparative study | Biopsy-proven AIDS-related KS with at least 15 mucocutaneous lesions or more than 5 new cutaneous lesions in the preceding month or documented visceral KS with at least 5 assessable cutaneous lesions | 241 | Pegylated liposomal doxorubicin (PLD) 20 mg m$^{-2}$ every 3 weeks for 6 cycles (N = 121) or bleomycin 15 IU m$^{-2}$ and vincristine 2 mg (BV) every 3 weeks for 6 cycles (N = 120) | Concurrent antiretroviral therapy Maintenance ganciclovir therapy Foscarnet for active cytomegalovirus infection (Colony-stimulating factors not permitted) | Responses assessed using modified ACTG criteria PLD = 58·7% ORR BV = 23·3% ORR $P < 0.001$ | National Cancer Institute Common Toxicity Criteria Adverse events seen in 10% or more patients for PLD versus BV Alopecia – 3·3% v 8·3% Paraesthesia – 3·3% v 14·2% Leucopenia – 71·9% v 50·8% Constipation – 1·7% v 10·8% Cardiotoxicity – 1·7% v 0·8% |

therapy was allowed. ABV caused significantly more alopecia and peripheral neuropathy than liposomal daunorubicin ($P < 0.0001$), but more grade 4 neutropenia was seen with the liposomal drug ($P = 0.021$).

### Liposomal doxorubicin versus ABV or BV chemotherapy

Two randomised trials have compared pegylated liposomal doxorubicin (PLD) with ABV or BV combination chemotherapy and reported significantly higher overall response rates with the liposomal drug[61,62] **Evidence level Ib**. Northfelt *et al.* studied 258 patients with AIDS-related KS and reported a 46% overall response rate for PLD (20 mg m$^{-2}$) compared with 25% for ABV chemotherapy (doxorubicin 20 mg m$^{-2}$ plus bleomycin 10 mg m$^{-2}$ plus vincristine 1 mg), given every 2 weeks for six cycles. The difference in overall response rates was statistically significant ($P < 0.001$).[61] Time to treatment failure did not differ significantly between the groups. The method of randomisation for this study is not stated. Modified ACTG criteria were used to assess response and standard World

Health Organization criteria were used to grade toxicities. Prior anthracycline chemotherapy was an exclusion criterion but concurrent antiretroviral therapy was permitted. Significantly more grade 3 nausea and vomiting, alopecia, and peripheral neuropathy were seen with ABV than with PLD and the drop-out rate owing to adverse events was higher with ABV (37% v 11%). The two regimens did not differ significantly in the frequency of grade 3 or greater leucopenia, anaemia, or thrombocytopenia. PLD was found more effective than combination chemotherapy with standard doxorubicin plus bleomycin plus vincristine in the treatment of AIDS-related cutaneous KS and caused less toxicity.

The second randomised trial (Stewart *et al.*) compared PLD 20 mg m$^{-2}$ with BV chemotherapy (bleomycin 15 IU m$^{-2}$ plus vincristine 2 mg) every 3 weeks for six cycles in patients with AIDS-related KS[62]: 241 patients were randomised to the alternative treatments using a table of random numbers, blocked by investigation site, which was achieved by faxing the patient's age, risk factors and staging criteria to a central office. Concurrent antiretroviral therapy and antimicrobial prophylaxis was permitted during the study; 49% of the PLD group and 57% of the BV group were taking antiretrovirals. Modified ACTG criteria were used to assess response. Lesions without any detectable residual disease but persistent pigmented macules (brown) were described as a clinical complete response, rather than a complete response by ACTG criteria, because they were not rebiopsied. Adverse events were graded according to the National Cancer Institute Common Toxicity Criteria. The overall response rate was significantly higher for PLD (59%) than for BV chemotherapy (23%) ($P < 0.001$). Significantly more peripheral neuropathy occurred in the BV group ($P < 0.001$) but more neutropenia in the PLD group ($P < 0.001$).

### Liposomal doxorubicin versus liposomal doxorubicin plus bleomycin plus vincristine

We found one randomised comparison of PLD alone with PLD plus bleomycin plus vincristine.[75] The overall response rates were 79% for 62 patients who received PLD alone and 80% for 64 patients who received the combination. Median times to progression were similar for both groups. However, the addition of bleomycin and vincristine to PLD caused a more rapid fall in quality-of-life indices and a shorter median time to first grade 3 toxicity **Evidence level Ib**.

We found no randomised trials comparing liposomal daunorubicin and pegylated liposomal doxorubicin in the treatment of cutaneous KS, although response rates in studies tend to be higher for PLD.

### Drawbacks

In two randomised controlled trials the early drop-out rate due to adverse events was higher with standard combination chemotherapy arm than with PLD. One RCT comparing PLD with ABV chemotherapy reported the early drop-out rate owing to adverse events was 37% for the ABV arm and 11% for PLD.[61] Similarly, early withdrawal because of chemotherapy-related toxicity was higher in the BV arm (27%) than in the PLD arm (11%) in the second comparative RCT.[62]

### Neutropenia

The incidence of grade 3 neutropenia in a randomised study comparing liposomal daunorubicin and ABV chemotherapy was similar in both groups (36% *v* 35%, respectively).[60] However, more grade 4 neutropenia was seen as an adverse effect of liposomal daunorubicin than ABV chemotherapy in the same randomised trial (15% *v* 5%, $P = 0.021$).[60]

The most common adverse event in both arms of an RCT comparing PLD with ABV chemotherapy was leucopenia, affecting 36% of 133 patients who received PLD and 42% of

125 patients in the ABV group.[61] No episodes of febrile neutropenia (neutrophils $< 500 \times 10^6$ cells litre$^{-1}$) occurred in the PLD group but 37% developed opportunistic infections and 6% experienced episodes of sepsis.[61] In a further RCT 29% of 121 patients who received PLD developed grade 3 leucopenia compared with 12% in the comparative BV chemotherapy arm.[62]

### Cardiotoxicity

Of 24 patients who received a cumulative dose of $> 500$ mg m$^{-2}$ of liposomal anthracycline in one randomised study, none was found to have a 20% or greater decline in their left ventricular ejection fraction.[60] Liposomal daunorubicin was discontinued in one patient whose left ventricular ejection fraction (LVEF) fell from 47% to 33%. An angiogram then showed that this patient had had a complete occlusion of the left anterior descending artery. In one RCT of liposomal doxorubicin versus ABV, pretreatment and post-treatment estimations of LVEF were available for 47 patients who received PLD. Of these, two patients were found to have had a greater than 20% fall in LVEF.[61] One death attributable to cardiomyopathy was seen in 133 patients treated with pegylated liposomal doxorubicin.[61] It seems that, unlike conventional anthracyclines, liposomal anthracyclines are not associated with significant cumulative cardiotoxicity.

### Nausea and vomiting

Of the patients receiving liposomal daunorubicin 51% experienced mild nausea.[60] Significantly more grade 3 nausea and vomiting was seen with ABV than with PLD (34% *v* 15% $P < 0.001$).[61]

### Alopecia

In the randomised trial reported by Gill *et al.* more alopecia was seen amongst the patients who received ABV chemotherapy than in those receiving liposomal daunorubicin[60]: 36% of the ABV group experienced grade 1–2 alopecia as against 8% in the liposomal daunorubicin group ($P < 0.0001$). In another RCT comparing pegylated liposomal doxorubicin with ABV chemotherapy, grade 3 alopecia was also more common in the ABV group than in those receiving a liposomal anthracycline (19% *v* 1% $P < 0.001$).[61]

### Peripheral neuropathy

Peripheral neuropathy was seen in 41% of patients treated with ABV and 13% of those given liposomal daunorubicin ($P < 0.0001$) in Gill *et al.*'s study.[60] In another randomised study peripheral neuropathy was also less common with liposomal doxorubicin than with ABV chemotherapy (6% versus 14% $P = 0.002$).[61]

### Acute infusion reactions

In the only large phase III study of liposomal daunorubicin the incidence of acute infusion reactions was 2/116 patients (2%). An RCT of pegylated liposomal doxorubicin found that six of 133 patients (5%) experienced an acute infusion-related reaction presenting as flushing, chest pain, hypotension and back pain; five of the six patients needed premedication for subsequent cycles but could continue on study.[61] In another study the frequency of acute infusion reactions with PLD was similar, affecting five of 121 patients (4%), but in one causing a severe anaphylactic reaction.[62]

### Mortality

In the RCT of Stewart *et al.*, five of 121 patients in the PLD arm died during the study. The cause of death for four of the five was progression of AIDS and the remaining patient died from progression of KS. The investigators attributed none of the deaths to the liposomal drug.[62]

In another RCT 24/133 patients who received PLD died, mostly as a result of complications of HIV infection, with one death due to cardiomyopathy.[61] There was no significant difference in the death rates compared with the ABV arm of the study.[61] In an RCT comparing liposomal daunorubicin with ABV chemotherapy, the reason for discontinuation of therapy was death, secondary to complications of HIV infection, in five of 117 patients who received DaunoXome and five out of 115 patients who received ABV chemotherapy.[60] Median survival in the two groups did not differ.[60]

### Palmar–plantar erythrodysaesthesia

The incidence of palmar–plantar erythrodysaesthesia (cutaneous toxicity resulting in dry, peeling red hands and feet) with liposomal doxorubicin at given doses has been reported in one trial as 2% (3/133 patients).[61]

## Comment

Many uncontrolled trials, particularly in AIDS-related KS, have suggested a response rate, in terms of reduction in number and/or size of lesions, to a variety of cytotoxic agents including bleomycin, vinca alkaloids, etoposide and paclitaxel. Evaluation of earlier studies is made difficult by variation in the definitions used to stage disease and to assess response to therapy. The adoption of standardised ACTG criteria for staging and assessing response to treatment has made it easier to compare studies and should be used in future therapeutic trials.[10]

One small randomised trial suggested that combination chemotherapy with ABV chemotherapy is more effective than single agent standard doxorubicin. Subsequently, three large randomised trials have provided good evidence, using ACTG criteria to assess response, that liposomal anthracyclines are at least as effective in AIDS-related cutaneous KS as standard ABV (doxorubicin plus bleomycin plus vincristine) or BV (bleomycin plus vincristine) combination chemotherapy.[60–62] The two randomised trials that specifically compare pegylated liposomal doxorubicin (PLD) to ABV or BV chemotherapy provide good evidence that PLD is more effective than standard combination chemotherapy.[61,62] The better toxicity profiles found in all three studies, associated with less early termination of therapy owing to adverse events, also favours the use of liposomal chemotherapy over standard combination chemotherapy. The addition of bleomycin and vincristine to liposomal doxorubicin is unlikely to be of benefit **Evidence level Ib**.

Although overall response rates to PLD are higher than for ABV or BV chemotherapy, the median duration of response is similar. In the randomised trial comparing PLD with ABV chemotherapy, the median duration of response was 90 days and 92 days, respectively.[61] In the randomised study comparing PLD with BV chemotherapy the median duration of responses were 142 days and 123 days respectively but the difference was not statistically significant.[62]

Although we found no randomised studies directly comparing the two liposomal drugs, the response rates for patients with advanced AIDS-related KS appear higher for liposomal doxorubicin than daunorubicin. There have been no studies of sequential chemotherapy. Newer single agent cytotoxic therapies such as paclitaxel, vinorelbine and gemcitabine should be compared with liposomal anthracyclines in large phase III studies.

## Implications for practice

There is good evidence that liposomal doxorubicin is likely to be beneficial for the palliative treatment of advanced AIDS-related KS **Grade A**. In view of its better toxicity profile than conventional chemotherapy, liposomal doxorubicin should be used as first-line systemic therapy for advanced AIDS-related KS in patients with poor immune function and significant mucocutaneous disease or visceral disease. However, the liposomal anthracyclines are expensive and not readily available in the developing world where most HIV-related disease occurs.

There have been no recent randomised controlled trials of chemotherapy in the other less common types of KS. However, previous uncontrolled studies and case series have suggested that both patients with classical KS and African KS are at least as chemosensitive as those with AIDS-related KS without the underlying immune suppression **Grade C**.

## What are the effects of topical and systemic retinoids in the treatment of KS?

### Evidence summary

Retinoids are a group of natural and synthetic vitamin A derivatives, which have shown *in vitro* activity against KS cells and are used topically in the treatment of hyperkeratotic skin conditions.[76,77] We found two randomised trials on the use of topical retinoids in the treatment of cutaneous AIDS-related KS.[78,79] No placebo-controlled clinical trials of the use of oral retinoids in the treatment of any of the clinical variants of KS were found.

### Topical alitretinoin gel

#### *Efficacy*

We found two randomised, double-blind, vehicle-controlled trials of the use of alitretinoin (9-*cis*-retinoic acid) gel in the topical treatment of AIDS-related KS[78,79] **Evidence level Ib**. The larger one was a multicentre, randomised, double-blind trial, involving 268 patients with AIDS-related cutaneous KS, comparing 0·1% alitretinoin gel with vehicle gel.[79] Six index lesions were used to assess response to therapy using ACTG criteria applied to topical therapy. Concurrent antiretroviral therapy was allowed. The overall response rate (CR and PR) for 134 patients randomised to receive alitretinoin twice daily for 12 weeks was 35% (45/134) compared with 18% (24/134) for the vehicle gel, similarly applied twice daily for 12 weeks. A further 184 patients were then treated with alitretinoin gel on an open-label basis following the blinded phase of the study and the overall response rate was 49% (90/184).[79]

In another randomised, double-blind, vehicle-controlled study, patients were randomised between alitretinoin gel 0·1% and vehicle gel applied twice daily for 12 weeks.[78] The overall response rate, assessed by ACTG criteria applied to topical therapy for 62 patients treated with alitretinoin was 37% versus 7% for 72 patients who received vehicle gel ($P = 0·00003$).

Alitretinoin was superior to vehicle gel in both the above studies when multiple variables including number of lesions, CD4 count, performance status and number of concurrent antiretroviral therapies was adjusted for.

#### *Drawbacks*

The most common adverse event owing to treatment with alitretinoin gel was irritation at the application site,

usually mild to moderate and reversible on cessation of treatment; 7% of patients discontinued alitretinoin therapy because of treatment-related adverse events in one study.[79]

#### *Comment*

These two randomised double-blind vehicle-controlled trials provide good evidence for the superiority of alitretinoin gel (0·1%) over vehicle gel in the treatment of cutaneous AIDS-related KS **Grade A**. The overall response rate, using standard ACTG criteria, for alitretinoin gel 0·1% applied twice daily for 12 weeks in the above studies was between 35% and 37%. Response rates in the vehicle-only groups were between 7% and 18%, suggesting that KS can undergo some degree of spontaneous remission or that the application of a vehicle alone may be of some benefit. This observation underlines the need to consider including suitable placebo groups in further trials.

## What are the effects of antiretrovirals in the treatment of AIDS-related KS?

### Evidence summary

We found no systematic reviews or large randomised controlled studies of the effect of antiretroviral therapy as a systemic treatment for AIDS-related KS. One small randomised study of oral zidovudine, intravenous zidovudine or oral placebo in AIDS-related KS was identified but zidovudine monotherapy is no longer standard treatment of HIV.[80] A small prospective cohort study and one larger retrospective cohort study examining the effect of HAART were found.[81,82]

### Efficacy

Antiretroviral therapy has been shown to increase survival and delay progression to AIDS in HIV-positive patients. Population-based studies have shown the use of HAART, which includes two nucleoside reverse transcriptase inhibitors with either a non-nucleoside reverse transcriptase inhibitor or one or two protease inhibitors, has decreased the incidence of KS as an AIDS-defining diagnosis.[83–85] The incidence of KS fell from 4·8 per 100 person-years in 1990 to 1·5 per 100 person-years in 1997 in a multicentre cohort of 30 000 patients, from centres in the USA, during 54 000 person-years of follow up between 1990 and 1997.[85] The relative risk of developing KS was 0·41 (95% CI 0·2–0·8) for patients on triple antiretroviral therapy. Reconstitution of the immune system following treatment with HAART may also affect established KS and prolong time to disease progression. Small uncontrolled studies and case reports have documented reduction of KS lesions after initiation of HAART **Evidence level III**.[86–88]

One small randomised study of 37 evaluable patients with good risk AIDS-related KS (CD4 count $> 200$ cells $\times 10^6$ litre$^{-1}$, no "B" symptoms and no history of opportunistic infections) randomised patients to receive either oral placebo, oral zidovudine 250 mg 4-hourly, intravenous zidovudine 0.5 mg kg$^{-1}$ 4-hourly, or intravenous zidovudine 2.5 mg kg$^{-1}$ 4-hourly.[80] At 6 weeks, four of nine patients receiving oral placebo and 10 of 28 patients receiving oral or intravenous zidovudine had progressive KS. After 12 weeks, only five patients receiving zidovudine had a minor response (defined as the absence of new KS lesions and a 25–50% regression in at least 25% of existing lesions). In this study, zidovudine was not an effective treatment for KS in terms of response rate or delay of progression. However, the numbers of patients in each of the four treatment arms was small and monotherapy with zidovudine has been superseded by HAART as standard therapy in the treatment of HIV infection.

A small prospective cohort study of 39 patients with AIDS-related KS commenced on HAART found that 10 of 19 patients, who received no other systemic therapy for KS, achieved a complete response by ACTG criteria.[81] Patients were more likely to respond if their CD4 count was greater than 150 cells $\times 10^6$ litre$^{-1}$. A retrospective cohort study identified 101 patients who received local or systemic therapy for KS and were subsequently commenced on HAART[82]; 33 patients were excluded because new anti-KS therapy was instituted at the same time as commencement of HAART. For the remaining 78 patients, the median time-to-treatment failure before starting HAART was 0.5 years (defined as the time between the final and penultimate anti-KS therapy before HAART). After the start of HAART, median time to treatment failure was 1.7 years (defined as time between start of HAART and next anti-KS therapy).[82] No correlation was demonstrated between CD4 count response and control of KS but a statistically significant correlation between progression of KS and virological failure of HAART (defined as viral load $> 5000$ copies ml$^{-1}$) was found. However, five of 24 patients (21%) at the time of KS progression on HAART did not have virological failure (viral load $< 200$ copies ml$^{-1}$). Immune reconstitution has been postulated as the mechanism of response of KS to antiretroviral therapy but response to HAART and the relationship to CD4 count response is unpredictable.

## Drawbacks

The side effects of combination HAART depend on the profile of individual drugs used and interactions with other drugs. Commoner side effects include nausea and vomiting, lethargy, diarrhoea, peripheral neuropathy, headache, deranged liver function, hypersensitivity reactions, myelosuppression, lactic acidosis and pancreatitis.

## Implications for practice

HAART may delay the onset of KS as an AIDS-defining diagnosis in patients with HIV infection. HAART may also induce responses in AIDS-related KS via immune reconstitution but the response to therapy is unpredictable. Patients with high viral loads, low CD4 counts, or other HIV-related symptoms require antiretroviral therapy for control of HIV infection. HAART alone in these patients is a reasonable initial therapy for KS, which may be combined later with other local or systemic treatments. However, immune reconstitution takes several weeks and patients with poor prognosis KS may require additional therapy in the interim.

## What is the role of antiherpes virus therapy in the prevention and treatment of AIDS-related KS?

The discovery of KS-associated herpes virus (KSHV), also known as human herpes virus-8, has provided another potential target for the prevention and treatment of AIDS-related KS. KSHV replication is inhibited *in vitro* by cidofovir, ganciclovir, and foscarnet but not aciclovir.[89,90] Cohort studies have reported a decreased risk of developing KS for HIV-positive patients treated with ganciclovir or foscarnet for cytomegalovirus infection, and there have been occasional case reports of patients with AIDS-related KS having prolonged responses to antiherpetic therapy.[91–95] One cohort study of 3688 HIV-positive patients followed up for a median of 4.2 years, during which time 16% (598 patients) developed KS, found a statistically significant reduction in the relative hazard of developing KS for those who received foscarnet or ganciclovir. The relative hazard for foscarnet was 0.38 (95% CI 0.15–0.95; $P = 0.038$) and for ganciclovir 0.39 (95% CI 0.19–0.84; $P = 0.015$).

In a randomised study of the treatment of cytomegalovirus (CMV) retinitis with ganciclovir, in patients with AIDS, a reduced risk of developing KS with oral or intravenous ganciclovir treatment was found[96]: 377 patients with AIDS and unilateral cytomegalovirus retinitis were randomised to receive a ganciclovir implant and oral ganciclovir (4.5 g daily), ganciclovir implant and oral placebo, or intravenous ganciclovir alone. The primary outcome was the development of new CMV disease but treatment with oral or intravenous ganciclovir was also found to reduce the risk of developing KS by 75% ($P = 0.008$) and 93% ($P < 0.001$) respectively as compared with oral placebo.[96]

## Implications for practice

Whilst there is some evidence that antiherpetic agents reduced the risk of developing AIDS-related KS, they are not currently used in routine practice as prophylaxis. RCTs evaluating these drugs for other outcomes such as cytomegalovirus infections suggest important benefit. This observation needs to be followed up by well-designed studies with KS as the main outcome.

---

### Key points

#### Local therapy of KS

- Evidence is insufficient to make any firm recommendations as to the value of surgical excision, cryotherapy, photodynamic therapy and intralesional chemotherapy **Evidence level III**.

- In people with AIDS-related KS, an 8 Gy single fraction of radiotherapy is highly likely to improve the cosmetic outcome of individual cutaneous lesions, with minimal harm. Fractionated radiotherapy, to a higher total dose, causes greater skin toxicity but provides a longer duration of lesion control and therefore may be more appropriate for more indolent disease seen with classical KS and some forms of endemic (African) KS. However the optimum dose-fractionation schedule in these conditions is yet to be determined **Evidence level Ib, Grade A**.

- Topical alitretinoin gel 0·1% as a local treatment for AIDS-related KS is more effective than vehicle gel and has a response rate of approximately 35% **Evidence level Ib, Grade A**.

#### Systemic therapy of KS

- IFNα is likely to be a beneficial systemic treatment for good prognosis AIDS-related KS. IFN can be safely combined with antiretroviral therapy and is most suitable as first-line therapy for patients with CD4 counts above $200 \times 10^6$ cells litre$^{-1}$, no "B" symptoms and no history of prior opportunistic infection **Evidence level Ib, Grade A**.

- We found good evidence that liposomal doxorubicin is more effective in AIDS-related KS than standard combination chemotherapy containing bleomycin plus vincristine with or without an anthracycline. Unlike conventional anthracyclines, liposomal anthracyclines do not appear to be associated with significant cardiotoxicity **Evidence level Ib, Grade A**.

- Newer single-agent cytotoxic therapies such as paclitaxel, vinorelbine, and gemcitabine have shown activity in AIDS-related KS in uncontrolled phase II trials. Future randomised controlled trials comparing these agents with the liposomal anthracyclines are required **Evidence level Ib**.

- Classical KS and endemic (African) are likely to be at least as chemosensitive as AIDS-related KS but are less common variants which have not been the subject of large randomised phase III studies **Evidence level Ib**.

- Antiretroviral therapy is reasonable initial therapy for minimally symptomatic cutaneous AIDS-related KS although the response to therapy is unpredictable. It may be combined with other systemic therapies **Evidence level III, Grade C**.

- Antiherpetic therapy for cytomegalovirus disease is associated with a reduced risk of developing KS in HIV positive patients. There is insufficient evidence to assess the value of cidofovir, ganciclovir, or foscarnet as treatment for established AIDS-related KS **Evidence level III**.

---

### References

1  Friedman-Kien AE, Laubenstein L, Marmor M *et al.* Kaposi's sarcoma and Pneumocystis pneumonia among homosexual men – New York City and California. *MMWR Morb Mortal Wkly Rep* 1981;**30**:305–8.

2  Taylor JF, Templeton AC, Vogel CL *et al.* Kaposi's sarcoma in Uganda: a clinico-pathological study. *Int J Cancer* 1971;**8**:122–35.

3  Wabinga HR, Parkin DM, Wabwire-Mangen F, Mugerwa JW. Cancer in Kampala, Uganda, in 1989–1991: changes in incidence in the era AIDS. *Int J Cancer* 1993;**54**:26–36.

4  Biggar RJ, Rabkin CS. The epidemiology of AIDS-related neoplasms. *Haematol Oncol Clin North Am* 1996;**10**:997–1010.

5  Farge D. Kaposi's sarcoma in organ transplant recipients. *Eur J Med* 1993;**2**:339–43.

6  Shepherd FA, Maher E, Cardella C *et al.* Treatment of Kaposi's sarcoma after solid organ transplantation. *J Clin Oncol* 1997;**15**:2371–7.

7  Qunibi W, Akhtar M, Sheth K *et al.* Kaposi's sarcoma: the most common tumor after renal transplantation in Saudi Arabia. *Am J Med* 1988;**84**:225–32.

8  Chang Y, Cesarman E, Pessin MS *et al.* Identification of herpesvirus-like DNA sequences in AIDS-associated Kaposi's sarcoma. *Science* 1994;**266**:1865–9.

9  Krown SE, Testa MA, Huang J *et al.* for the AIDS Clinical Trials Group Oncology Committee. AIDS-related Kaposi's sarcoma: prospective validation of the AIDS Clinical Trials Group staging classification. *J Clin Oncol* 1997;**15**:3085–92.

10  Krown SE, Metroka C, Wernz JC. Kaposi's sarcoma in the acquired immune deficiency syndrome: a proposal for uniform evaluation, response, and staging criteria. *J Clin Oncol* 1989;**7**:1201–7.

11  Tappero JW, Berger TG, Kaplan LD *et al.* Cryotherapy for cutaneous Kaposi's sarcoma (KS) associated with acquired immune deficiency syndrome (AIDS) a phase II trial. *J Acquir Immune Defic Syndr* 1991;**4**:839–46.

12  Schofer H, Ochsendorf FR, Hochscheid I, Milbradt R. [Facial Kaposi's sarcoma. Palliative treatment with cryotherapy, intralesional chemotherapy, low-dose roentgen therapy and camouflage] (Article in German). *Hautarzt* 1991;**42**:492–8.

13  Bernstein ZP, Wilson BD, Oseroff AR *et al.* Photofrin photodynamic therapy for treatment of AIDS-related cutaneous Kaposi's sarcoma. *AIDS* 1999;**13**:1697–704.

14  Hebada KM, Huizing MT, Brouwer PA *et al.* Photodynamic therapy in AIDS-related cutaneous Kaposi's sarcoma. *J Acquir Immune Defic Syndr Hum Retrovirol* 1995;**10**:61–70.

15  Szeimes RM, Lorenzen T, Karrer S *et al.* [Photochemotherapy of cutaneous AIDS-associated Kaposi's sarcoma with indocyanine green and laser light] (Article in German). *Hautarzt* 2001;**52**:322–6.

16  Friedman M, Venkakesan TK, Caldanelli DD. Intralesional vinblastine for treating AIDS-associated Kaposi's sarcoma of the oropharynx and larynx. *Ann Otol Rhinol Laryngol* 1996;**105**:272–4.

17  Flaitz CM, Nichols CM, Hicks MJ. Role of intralesional vinblastine administration in treatment of intraoral Kaposi's sarcoma in AIDS. *Eur J Cancer B Oral Oncol* 1995;**31**B:280–5.

18  Boudreaux AA, Smith LL, Cosby CD *et al.* Intralesional vinblastine for cutaneous Kaposi's sarcoma associated with acquired immunodeficiency syndrome. A clinical trial to evaluate efficacy and discomfort associated with injection. *J Am Acad Dermatol* 1993;**28**:61–5.

19  Brambilla L, Boneschi V, Beretta G, Finzi AF. Intralesional chemotherapy for Kaposi's sarcoma. *Dermatologica* 1984;**169**:150–5.

20  Stelzer KJ, Griffin TW. A randomized prospective trial of radiation therapy for AIDS-associated Kaposi's sarcoma. *Int J Radiat Oncol Biol Phys* 1993;**27**:1057–61.

21  Harrison M, Harrington KJ, Tomlinson DR, Stewart JS. Response and cosmetic outcome of two fractionation regimens for AIDS-related Kaposi's sarcoma. *Radiother Oncol* 1998;**46**:23–8.

22  Belmbaogo E, Kirova Y, Frikha H *et al.* [Radiotherapy of epidemic Kaposi's sarcoma: the experience of Henri-Mondor Hospital (643 patients)]. *Cancer Radiother* 1998;**2**:49–52.

23  Berson AM, Quivey JM, Harris JW, Wara WM. Radiation therapy for AIDS-related Kaposi's Sarcoma. *Int J Radiat Oncol Biol Phys* 1990;**19**:569–75.

24  Cooper JS. The influence of dose on the long-term control of Classic (non-AIDS associated) Kaposi's sarcoma by radiotherapy. *Int J Radiat Oncol Biol Phys* 1988;**15**:1141–6.

25  Brenner B, Rakowsky E, Katz A *et al.* Tailoring treatment for classical Kaposi's sarcoma: Comprehensive clinical guidelines. *Int J Oncol* 1999;**14**:1097–102.

26  Nisce LZ, Safai B, Poussin-Rosillo H. Once weekly total and subtotal skin electron beam therapy for Kaposi's sarcoma. *Cancer* 1981;**47**:640–4.

27  Stein ME, Lakier R, Kuten A *et al.* Radiation therapy in endemic (African) Kaposi's sarcoma. *Int J Radiat Oncol Biol Phys* 1993;**27**:1181–4.

28  Groopman JE, Gottlieb MS, Goodman J *et al.* Recombinant alpha-2 interferon therapy for Kaposi's sarcoma associated with the acquired immunodeficiency syndrome. *Ann Intern Med* 1984;**100**:671–6.

29  Shepherd FA, Beaulieu R, Gelmon K *et al.* Prospective randomized trial of two dose levels of interferon with zidovudine for the treatment of Kaposi's sarcoma associated with human immunodeficiency virus infection: a Canadian HIV Clinical Trials Network study. *J Clin Oncol* 1998;**16**:1736–42.

30  Evans LM, Itri LM, Campion M *et al.* Interferon-alpha 2a in the treatment of acquired immunodeficiency syndrome-related Kaposi's sarcoma. *J Immunother* 1991;**10**:39–50.

31  Volberding PA, Mitsuyasu RT, Golando JP, Spiegel RJ. Treatment of Kaposi's sarcoma with interferon alfa-2b (Intron A). *Cancer* 1987;**59**(Suppl. 3):620–5.

32  Krown SE, Gold JW, Niedzwiecki D *et al.* Interferon-alpha with zidovudine: safety, tolerance, and clinical and virologic effects in patients with Kaposi sarcoma associated with acquired immunodeficiency syndrome (AIDS). *Ann Intern Med* 1990;**112**:812–21.

33  Fischl MA, Uttamchandani RB, Resnick L *et al.* A phase I study of recombinant human interferon-alpha 2a or human lymphoblastoid interferon-alpha n1 and concomitant zidovudine in patients with AIDS-related Kaposi's sarcoma. *J Acquir Immune Defic Syndr* 1991;**4**:1–10.

34  de Wit R, Danner SA, Bakker PJ *et al.* Combined zidovudine and interferon-alpha treatment in patients with AIDS-associated Kaposi's sarcoma. *J Intern Med* 1991;**229**:35–40.

35  Baumann R, Tauber MG, Opravil M *et al.* Combined treatment with zidovudine and lymphoblast interferon alpha in patients with HIV-related Kaposi's sarcoma. *Klin Wochenschr* 1991;**69**:360–7.

36  Podzamczer D Bolao F Clotet B *et al.* Low-dose interferon alpha combined with zidovudine in patients with AIDS-associated Kaposi's sarcoma. *J Intern Med* 1993;**233**:247–53.

37  Fischl MA, Finkelstein DM, He W *et al.* A phase II study of recombinant human interferon-alpha 2a and zidovudine in patients with AIDS-related Kaposi's sarcoma. *J Acquir Immune Defic Syndr Hum Retrovirol* 1996;**11**:379–84.

38  Stadler R, Bratzke B, Schaart F, Orfanos CE. Long-term combined rIFN-alpha-2a and zidovudine therapy for HIV-associated Kaposi's sarcoma: clinical consequences and side effects. *J Invest Dermatol* 1990;**95**(Suppl. 6):170–5.

39  Opravil M, Hirschel B, Bucher HC, Luthy R. A randomised trial of interferon-alpha2a and zidovudine versus bleomycin and zidovudine for AIDS-related Kaposi's sarcoma. Swiss HIV Cohort Study. *Int J STD AIDS* 1999;**10**:369–75.

40  Krigel RL, Slywotzky CM, Lonberg M *et al.* Treatment of epidemic Kaposi's sarcoma with a combination of interferon-alpha 2b and etoposide. *J Biol Response Mod* 1988;**7**:359–64.

41  Shepherd FA, Evans WK, Garvey B *et al.* Combination chemotherapy and alpha-interferon in the treatment of Kaposi's sarcoma associated with acquired immune deficiency syndrome. *Can Med Assoc J* 1988;**139**:635–9.

42  Lassoued K, Clauvel JP, Katlama C *et al.* Treatment of the acquired immune deficiency syndrome-related Kaposi's sarcoma with bleomycin as a single agent. *Cancer* 1990;**66**:1869–72.

43  Remick SC, Reddy M, Herman D *et al.* Continous infusion bleomycin in AIDS-related Kaposi's sarcoma. *J Clin Oncol* 1994;**12**:1130–6.

44  Caumes E, Guermonprez G, Katlama C *et al.* AIDS-associated mucocutaneous Kaposi's sarcoma treated with bleomycin. *AIDS* 1992;**6**:1483–7.

45  Hernandez DE, Perez JR. Advanced epidemic Kaposi's sarcoma: treatment with bleomycin or combination of doxorubicin, bleomycin and vincristine. *Int J Dermatol* 1996;**35**:831–3.

46  Brambilla L, Labianca R, Boreschi V *et al.* Mediterranean Kaposi's sarcoma in the elderly. A randomised study of oral etoposide versus vinblastine. *Cancer* 1994;**74**:2873–8.

47  Zidan J, Robenstein W, Abzah A *et al.* Treatment of Kaposi's sarcoma with vinblastine in patients with disseminated dermal disease. *Isr Med Assoc J* 2001;**3**:251–3.

48  Kaplan L, Abrams D, Volberding P. Treatment of Kaposi's sarcoma in acquited immunodeficiency syndrome with an alternating vincristine-vinblastine regime. *Cancer Treat Rep* 1986;**70**:1121–2.

49  Volberding PA, Abrams DI, Conant M *et al.* Vinblastine therapy for Kaposi's sarcoma in the acquired immunodeficiency syndrome. *Ann Intern Med* 1985;**103**:335–8.

50  Solan AJ, Greenwald ES, Silvay O. Long-term complete remissions of Kaposi's sarcoma with vinblastine therapy. *Cancer* 1981;**47**:637–9.

51  Klein E, Schwartz RA, Laor Y *et al.* Treatment of Kapois's sarcoma with vinblastine. *Cancer* 1980;**45**:427–31.

52  Tucker SB, Wintelmann RK. Treatment of Kaposi's sarcoma with vinblastine. *Arch Dermatol* 1976;**112**:958–61.

53  Brambilla L, Boneschi V, Fossati S *et al.* Oral etoposide for Kaposi's Mediterranean sarcoma. *Dermatologica* 1988;**177**:365–9.

54  Laubenstein LJ, Krigel RL, Odajnyk CM *et al.* Treatment of epidemic Kaposi's sarcoma with etoposide or a combination of doxorubicin, bleomycin and vinblastine. *J Clin Oncol* 1984;**2**:1115–20.

55  Sprinz E, Caldas AP, Mans DR *et al.* Fractionated doses of oral etoposide in the treatment of patients with AIDS-related Kaposi's sarcoma: clinical and pharmacologic study to improve therapeutic index. *Am J Clin Oncol* 2001;**24**:177–84.

56  Schwartsmann G, Sprinz E, Kromfield M *et al.* Clinical and pharmacokinetic study of oral etoposide in patients with AIDS-related Kaposi's sarcoma with no prior exposure to cytotoxic therapy. *J Clin Oncol* 1997;**15**:2118–24.

57  Remick SC, Reddy M, Ekman K *et al.* Continuous infusion etoposide in advanced AIDS-related Kaposi sarcoma. *J Infus Chemother* 1996;**6**:92–6.

58  Bakker PJ, Danner SA, Lange JM *et al.* Etoposide for epidemic Kaposi's sarcoma: a phase II study. *Eur J Cancer Clin Oncol* 1988;**24**:1047–8.

59  Schwartsmann G, Sprinz E, Kronfeld M *et al.* Phase II study of teniposide in patients with AIDS-related Kaposi's sarcoma. *Eur J Cancer* 1991;**27**:1637–9.

60  Gill PS, Wernz J, Scadden DT *et al.* Randomized phase III trial of liposomal daunorubicin versus doxorubicin, bleomycin, and vincristine in AIDS-related Kaposi's sarcoma. *J Clin Oncol* 1996; **14**:2353–64.

61  Northfelt DW, Dezube BJ, Thommes JA *et al.* Pegylated-liposomal doxorubicin versus doxorubicin, bleomycin and vincristine in the treatment of AIDS-related Kaposi's sarcoma: results of a randomized phase III clinical trial. *J Clin Oncol* 1998;**16**:2445–51.

62  Stewart S, Jablonowski H, Goebel FD *et al.* Randomized comparative trial of pegylated liposomal doxorubicin versus bleomycin and vincristine in the treatment of AIDS-related Kaposi's sarcoma. *J Clin Oncol* 1998;**16**:683–91.

63  Uthayakumar S, Bower M, Money-Kyrle J *et al.* Randomized cross-over comparison of liposomal daunorubicin versus observation for early Kaposi's sarcoma. *AIDS* 1996;**10**:515–19.

64  Gill PS, Tulpule A, Espina BM *et al.* Paclitaxel is safe and effective in the treatment of advanced AIDS-related Kaposi's sarcoma. *J Clin Oncol* 1999;**17**:1876–83.

65  Welles L, Saville MW, Lietzau J *et al.* Phase II trial with dose titration of paclitaxel for the therapy of human immunodeficiency virus-associated Kaposi's sarcoma. *J Clin Oncol* 1998;**16**:1112–21.

66  Saville MW, Lietzau J, Pluda JM *et al.* Treatment of HIV-associated Kaposi's sarcoma with paclitaxel. *Lancet* 1995;**346**:26–8.

67  Nasti G, Errante D, Talamini R *et al.* Vinorelbine is an effective and safe drug for AIDS-related Kaposi's sarcoma: results of a phase II study. *J Clin Oncol* 2000;**18**:1550–7.

68  Brambilla L, Labianca R, Ferrucci SM *et al.* Treatment of classical Kaposi's sarcoma with gemcitabine. *Dermatology* 2001;**202**:119–22.

69  Little RF, Wyvill KM, Pluda JM *et al.* Activity of thalidomide in AIDS-related Kaposi's sarcoma. *J Clin Oncol* 2000;**18**:2593–602.

70  Fife K, Howard MR, Gracie F *et al.* Activity of thalidomide in AIDS-related Kaposi's sarcoma and correlation with HHV8 titre. *Int J STD AIDS* 1998;**9**:751–5.

71  Vogel CL, Templeton CJ, Templeton AC *et al.* Treatment of Kaposi's sarcoma with actinomycin-D and cyclophosphamide: a randomized clinical trial. *Int J Cancer* 1971;**8**:136–43.

72  Vogel CL, Primack A, Dhru D *et al.* Treatment of Kaposi's sarcoma with a combination of actinomycin D and vincristine: a randomized clinical trial. *Cancer* 1973;**31**:1382–91.

73  Olweny CL, Toya T, Mbidde EK, Lwanga SK. Treatment of Kaposi's sarcoma by combination of actinomycin-D, vincristine and carboxamide (nsc-45388): results of a randomized clinical trial. *Int J Cancer* 1974;**14**:649–56.

74  Gill PS, Rarick M, McCutchan JA *et al.* Systemic treatment of AIDS-related Kaposi's sarcoma: results of a randomized trial. *Am J Med* 1991;**90**:427–33.

75  Mitsuyasu R, von Roenn J, Krown S *et al.* Comparison study of liposomal doxorubicin alone or with bleomycin and vincristine for treatment of advanced AIDS-associated Kaposi's sarcoma: AIDS Clinical Trial Group protocol 286. *Proc Ann Mtg Am Soc Clin Oncol* 1997 (May) (abst. 191)

76  Guo WX, Gill PS, Antakly T. Inhibition of AIDS-Kaposi's sarcoma cell proliferation following retinoic acid receptor activation. *Cancer Res* 1995;**55**:823–9.

77  Corbeil J, Rapaport E, Richmann DD, Looney DJ. Antiproliferative effect of retinoid compounds on Kaposi's sarcoma cells. *J Clin Invest* 1994;**93**:1981–6.

78  Bodsworth NJ, Bloch M, Bower M *et al.* Phase III vehicle-controlled, multi-centred study of topical alitretinoin gel 0·1% in cutaneous AIDS-related Kaposi's sarcoma. *Am J Clin Dermatol* 2001;**2**:77–87.

79  Walmsley S, Northfelt DW, Melosky B *et al.* Treatment of AIDS-related cutaneous Kaposi's sarcoma with alitretinoin (*9-cis* retinoic acid) gel. Panretin Gel North American Study Group. *J Acquir Immune Defic Syndrome* 1999;**22**:235–46.

80  Lane HC, Falloon J, Walter RE *et al.* Zidovudine in patients with human immunodeficiency virus (HIV) infection and Kaposi's sarcoma. A phase II randomised placebo-controlled trial. *Ann Intern Med* 1989;**111**:41–50.

81  Dupont C, Vasseur E, Beauchet A *et al.* Long-term efficacy on Kaposi's sarcoma of highly active antiretroviral therapy in a cohort of HIV-positive patients. CISIH 92. Centre d'information et de soins de l'immunodeficience humaine. *AIDS* 2000;**14**:987–93.

82  Bower M, Fox P, Fife K *et al.* Highly active anti-retroviral therapy (HAART) prolongs time to treatment failure in Kaposi's sarcoma. *AIDS* 1999;**13**:2105–11.

83  Grulian AE, Li Y, McDonald AM *et al.* Decreasing rates of Kaposi's sarcoma and non-Hodgkin's lymphoma in the era of potent combination anti-retroviral therapy. *AIDS* 2001;**15**:629–33.

84  Pezzotti P, Serraino D, Rezza G *et al.* The spectrum of AIDS-defining diseases: temporal trends in Italy prior to the use of highly active anti-retroviral therapies, 1982–1996. *Int J Epidemiol* 1999;**28**:975–81.

85  Jones J, Hanson DL, Dworkin MS *et al.* Effect of antiretroviral and other antiviral therapies on the incidence of Kaposi's sarcoma and trends in Kaposi's sarcoma. *Proc 12th World AIDS Conference*, Geneva, 1998;134.

86  Wit FW, Sol CJ, Renwick N *et al.* Regression of AIDS-related Kaposi's sarcoma associated with clearance of human herpesvirus-8 from peripheral blood mononuclear cells following initiation of antiretroviral therapy. *AIDS* 1998;**12**:218–19.

87  Volm MD, Wenz J. Patients with advanced AIDS-related Kaposi's sarcoma (EKS) no longer require systemic therapy after introduction of effective antiretroviral therapy. *Proc Am Soc Clin Oncol* 1997;**16**:469 (abs.).

88  Tavio M, Nash G, Spina M *et al.* Highly active antiretroviral therapy in HIV-related Kaposi's sarcoma. *Ann Oncol* 1998;**9**:923.

89  Medveczky MM, Horvath E, Lund T, Medveczky PG. In vitro antiviral drug sensitivity of the Kaposi's sarcoma-associated herpesvirus. *AIDS* 1997;**11**:1327–32.

90  Kedes DH, Ganem D. Sensitivity of Kaposi's sarcoma-associated herpesvirus replication to antiviral drugs. Implications for potential therapy. *J Clin Invest* 1997;**99**:2082–6.

91  Mocroft A, Youle M, Gazzard B *et al.* Anti-herpesvirus treatment and risk of Kaposi's sarcoma in HIV infection. Royal Free/Chelsea and Westminster Hospitals Collaborative Group. *AIDS* 1996;**10**:1101–5.

92  Glesby MJ, Hoover DR, Weng S *et al.* Use of antiherpes drugs and the risk of Kaposi's sarcoma: data from the Multicenter AIDS Cohort Study. *J Infect Dis* 1996;**173**:1477–80.

93  Robles R, Lugo D, Gee L, Jacobson MA. Effect of antiviral drugs used to treat cytomegalovirus end-organ disease on subsequent course of previously diagnosed Kaposi's sarcoma in patients with AIDS. *J Acquir Immune Defic Syndr Hum Retrovirol* 1999;**20**:34–8.

94  Jones JL, Hanson DL, Dworkin MS, Jaffe HW. Incidence and trends in Kaposi's sarcoma in the era of effective antiretroviral therapy. *J Acquir Immune Defic Syndr* 2000;**24**:270–4.

95  Morfeldt L, Torssander J. Long-term remission of Kaposi's sarcoma following foscarnet treatment in HIV infected patients. *Scand J Infect Dis* 1994;**26**:749–52.

96  Martin DF, Kuppermann BD, Wolitz RA *et al.* Oral ganciclovir for patients with cytomegalovirus retinitis treated with a ganciclovir implant. Roche Ganciclovir Study Group. *N Engl J Med* 1999;**340**: 1063–70.

# Section X

## Treating sarcomas

*Vivien Bramwell, Editor*

# Levels of evidence and grades of recommendation used in *Evidence-based Oncology*

Levels of evidence and grades of recommendation appear within the text in the clinical chapters, for example, **Evidence Level Ia** and **Grade A**.

## Levels of evidence

Ia   Meta-analysis of randomised controlled trials (RCTs)
Ib   At least 1 RCT
IIa  At least 1 non-randomised study
IIb  At least 1 other well designed quasi-experimental study
III  Non-experimental, descriptive studies
IV   Expert committee reports or opinions/experience of respected authorities

## Grades of recommendations

A   At least one RCT as part of body of literature of overall good quality and consistency addressing recommendation **Evidence levels Ia, Ib**
B   No RCT but well conducted clinical studies available **Evidence levels IIa, IIb, III**
C   Expert committee reports or opinions/experience of respected authorities in the absence of directly applicable good quality clinical studies **Evidence level IV**

From *Clinical Oncology* (2001)**13**:S212
Source of data: MEDLINE, *Proceedings of the American Society of Medical Oncology* (ASCO).

# 46 Soft tissue sarcoma

*Shail Verma*

In this chapter two case scenarios will be discussed. Case 1 deals with a patient with newly diagnosed, localised soft tissue sarcoma of the extremity. Case 2 describes a patient with metastatic sarcoma involving the lungs. For both cases, relevant clinical questions are posed and evidence-based recommendations are provided.

## Background

Soft tissue sarcomas (STS) are rare, diverse tumours of mesenchymal origin, which represent 1% of adult cancers.[1] Approximately 8100 new cases were diagnosed during the year 2000 in the USA.[2] Extensive epidemiological, clinical and histopathological information is now available from multiple large databases, as well as institutional and cooperative group studies.[2–25] These confirm the rarity of STS, with an annual age-adjusted incidence of 2·3–3·9/100 000. In general, males and females are equally affected. In adults, incidence increases with age with more than half of the patients presenting over the age of 50.[5,26] STS may arise in any region of the body including viscera. Extremity STS account for 60% of patients, with the lower extremity predominating (46%). Retroperitoneal, truncal, and head and neck STS account for 13%, 19%, and 8% respectively.[27]

Histopathological classification of STS has been difficult and controversial. Several comprehensive classification systems, based largely upon cellular lineage (that is, tissue of origin) have been published and used, including those of the Armed Forces Institute of Pathology,[26,28] and the World Health Organization.[29,30] However, the schema outlined by Enzinger and Weiss is the most recent and widely accepted.[31] Although advances in immunohistochemistry and molecular biology have enabled more precise pathological distinctions, it is noteworthy that even expert pathologists disagree over individual cases.[32–34] The five commonest histologies encountered in extremity STS include malignant fibrous histiocytoma (MFH), liposarcomas, tendosynovial sarcomas, fibrosarcomas and leiomyosarcomas, with MFH and liposarcomas accounting for approximately 50% of all cases.[6,18,35–37]

Extremity STS most commonly presents as a painless mass. Diagnostic delays are common with close to 50% of patients waiting for at least 4 months before seeking medical attention.[38] As a consequence, many patients have large (> 5 cm) tumours at presentation. In a retrospective review of 1011 patients with extremity STS, 41% presented with 5 cm, 28% with 5–10 cm and 25% with > 10 cm tumours; 76% of these were deep tumours, but pain or other symptoms were absent in the vast majority (81%).[6] Regional lymph node metastases are rare, being noted in < 4% of cases at presentation, although lymphatic spread is more commonly associated with certain histological subtypes including epithelioid, rhabdomyosarcoma and clear cell sarcoma.[38,39] More disturbing is the finding of distant metastases in 8–23% of patients.[4,13,24] at initial presentation, the wide range perhaps reflecting different diagnostic and imaging techniques used to evaluate patients for the presence of metastases.

In patients with clinically localised disease, a number of clinical-pathological factors (including age, gender, histological subtype, presence or absence of neurovascular or bone invasion), markers of proliferation (mitotic index or KI-67 score) and, more recently, molecular or genetic markers (*p53*, p-glycoprotein, or multidrug resistant proteins) have been evaluated in a number of observational and retrospective studies.[40–50] There is near universal recognition of the prognostic importance of grade, tumour size, depth, and presence or absence of metastases and this has led to modification of the original 1992 staging system proposed by Russell *et al.*[51] The latest iteration of the staging system adopted by the American Joint Committee on Cancer (AJCC) is presented in Box 46.1.[52,53]

These observations have led to the evolution of certain principles guiding the management of patients with potentially curable, localised extremity STS.

- Assessment and management of STS should be conducted in centres with multidisciplinary teams (surgeons, pathologists, radiologists and oncologists) experienced in the diagnosis and management of sarcomas.
- Meticulous clinical and radiological evaluation of the primary tumour with particular reference to size, depth and location should be undertaken. Appropriate radiological evaluation would include CT or MRI scanning.
- Pathological confirmation of sarcoma should be obtained through biopsy techniques that avoid

**Primary tumour (T)**

TX   Primary tumour cannot be assessed

T0   No evidence of primary tumour

T1   Tumour 5 cm or less in greatest dimension

T1a  Superficial tumour

T1b  Deep tumour

T2   Tumour more than 5 cm greatest dimension

T2a  Superficial tumour

T2b  Deep tumour

**Regional lymph nodes (N)**

NX   Regional lymph nodes cannot be assessed

N0   No regional lymph node metastasis

N1   Regional lymph node metastasis

**Distant metastases (M)**

MX   Distant metastases cannot be assessed

M0   No distant metastasis

M1   Distant metastasis

**Histopathologic grade**

GX   Grade cannot be assessed

G1   Well differentiated

G2   Moderately differentiated

G3   Poorly differentiated

G4   Undifferentiated

| Stage | Grade | Primary tumour | Regional lymph nodes | Distant metastasis |
|---|---|---|---|---|
| IA | G1 or G2 | T1a or T1b | N0 | M0 |
| IB | G1 or G2 | T2a | N0 | M0 |
| IIA | G1 or G2 | T2b | N0 | M0 |
| IIB | G3 or G4 | T1a or T1b | N0 | M0 |
| IIC | G3 or G4 | T2a | N0 | M0 |
| III | G3 or G4 | T2b | N0 | M0 |
| IV | G3 or G4 | T2b | N1 | M0 |
|  | Any G | Any T | Any N | M1 |
|  | Any G | Any T |  |  |

Produced with the permission of the American Joint Committee on Cancer (AJCC) from: *Cancer Staging Handbook, 5th edn.* Philadelphia: Lippincott-Raven, 1998.

Note: A superficial tumour is located exclusively above the superficial fascia without invasion of the fascia; deep tumour is located either exclusively beneath the superficial fascia, or superficial to the fascia, or superficial and beneath the fascia. Retroperitoneal, mediastinal and pelvic sarcomas are classified as deep tumours.

contamination of compartments or surrounding tissues. Histological assessment should be conducted by a pathologist experienced in the diagnosis and grading of STS.

- Prognostic factors such as tumour size, grade and depth must be considered in the locoregional and systemic management of patients with extremity STS. For individual patients, anatomic location, age and histology may also be important factors.

In this chapter, lack of space and a paucity of high quality data preclude a review of management of STS arising in non-extremity sites.

## Management of localised extremity STS

**Case 1**

*A local orthopaedic surgeon has referred to you a 55-year-old man with a mass involving the left anterior mid-thigh. This patient has previously been well, with no antecedent medical or surgical history. He reports that he first became aware of a swelling in his thigh approximately 4 months earlier. He could not recall any trauma specifically to the area and sought the advice of his family doctor, who recommended a week-long course of anti-inflammatory medication. No improvement was noted and an ultrasound was requested, which disclosed a solid 6 cm mass involving muscles of the anterior thigh. He was referred to the orthopaedic surgeon, who on examination noted a painless mass in the left thigh with no evidence of vascular obstruction or local inflammation. Sensory and motor examinations of the extremity were normal. A computerised tomography (CT) scan was obtained and the results confirmed the presence of a tumour in the anterior compartment of the left thigh involving the mid- and distal portions of the quadriceps muscle, measuring 8·0 ´ 7·5 cm in size. There was no apparent involvement of neurovascular or bony structures. A biopsy revealed a high grade synovial sarcoma. He has now been sent to you for further advice on treatment. He is distressed about the possibility of amputation and wonders if there are any alternatives. Although your detailed clinical examination reveals no evidence of metastases and a subsequent CT scan of the lungs is normal, his wife has also read that soft tissue sarcomas may spread "through the bloodstream" and wonders whether her husband ought to offered systemic treatment in addition to surgery.*

### Framing relevant and answerable questions

A number of questions arise from this scenario. At first glance, in this patient aggressive surgery in the form of amputation would seem an appropriate treatment. However, in light of the potential functional and psychological impact of such a procedure, would it not be feasible to consider a limb-sparing approach? Would such an approach have an impact on the potential to cure this patient or on his quality of life? In addition, given the size and high grade of this tumour, it would appear that his risk for metastatic disease is quite high and therefore should he be offered adjuvant systemic therapy? As they stand, these questions are difficult to answer and therefore they need to be broken down into different components. Four answerable questions are framed from this clinical scenario:

- For adults with extremity STS, is limb salvage surgery an acceptable alternative to amputation in terms of local control, survival and function/quality of life?
- For adults with extremity STS, is the combination of radiotherapy and surgery better that surgery alone in achieving local control with limb preservation and good functional outcome?
- For adults with non-metastatic STS does adjuvant chemotherapy improve outcomes such as local control, metastases-free survival, relapse-free and overall survival with acceptable morbidity and/or quality of life?
- For adults with non-metastatic STS are there specific adjuvant chemotherapy regimens that improve outcomes such as local control, metastases-free survival, relapse-free and overall survival?

The first two questions deal with the locoregional management of extremity STS, whereas the third and fourth address the issue of systemic adjuvant therapy. The evidence base and outcomes of interest are clearly different, and it is therefore appropriate to discuss these pairs of questions separately.

## Locoregional therapy of extremity STS

### Discussion of the evidence

Historically, amputation has been the main stay of treatment of extremity STS. Appreciation of prognostic factors, outcomes of radical surgery (including local and distant relapses), and the recognition of the functional and psychological impact of amputation[54] have led to efforts aimed at limb preservation – limb salvage surgery (LSS). Additionally, observations that STS are radiosensitive tumours have led to programmes where LSS is combined with adjuvant radiation.[55–57]

Outcomes of interest in the local-regional management of extremity STS include: local recurrence (LR), disease-free and distant disease-free survival (DFS and DDFS), overall survival (OS), complication rates and quality of life (QOL). Local recurrences are particularly important when considering LSS techniques. Some studies, but not all, have suggested an association between LR and subsequent development of metastatic disease.[58–60] While there is debate over the prognostic value of LR, there is agreement

that LR causes additional morbidity and should be avoided.[61]

Enneking has categorised the types of surgical procedures, which may be used to treat extremity STS.[62] These include:

- *intracapsular excisions*, performed inside the pseudo capsule of the tumour;
- *marginal excisions*, which represent *en bloc* resections performed through the reactive zone around the tumour; "shell out" procedures are included in this category;
- *wide excisions*, which consist of *en bloc* resection through normal tissue beyond the reactive zone but within the muscular compartment of origin;
- *radical excisions*, which consist of *en bloc* resection of the tumour and the entire compartment of origin; such procedures include compartment excisions and amputations.

### *For adults with extremity STS, is limb salvage surgery an acceptable alternative to amputation in terms of local control, survival and function/quality of life?*

There is only one RCT but there are numerous non-randomised studies.

Rosenberg *et al.*[63] conducted the only RCT comparing LSS with amputation in patients with extremity STS. In this trial, 43 patients were randomised to undergo amputation or LSS plus adjuvant radiation (60–70 Gy). In 27 patients randomised to LSS there were four local recurrences, whereas none were noted in the amputation group ($P = 0.06$). There were no differences in the 5-year DFS rates (71% $v$ 78%, $P = 0.75$) or OS rates (83% and 88%, $P = 0.99$) **Evidence level Ib**.

Multiple non-randomised studies provide further insight into the impact of LSS on local control rates. In general, less aggressive surgery is associated with LR rates as high as 65–100% after simple excisions, and 31–39% after wide excisions.[64–67] For optimal local control rates it is also necessary to achieve negative histological margins. In 54 patients treated with compartment excisions or amputations, Simon and Enneking demonstrated a local control rate of 83% overall.[68] One out of 46 patients with negative margins had an LR compared with eight of eight patients with positive margins. Similar observations have been made by Shiu *et al.*[69] More recent data concerning the prognostic importance of surgical margins, are provided by an analysis of 559 patients with STS of extremities and trunk wall, treated by surgery only and registered in a database of the Scandinavian Sarcoma Group.[15] High histological grade (relative risk [RR] = 3.0) and an inadequate surgical margin (RR = 2.0) were independent risk factors for LR.

### For adults with extremity STS, is the combination of radiotherapy and surgery better that surgery alone in achieving local control with limb preservation and good functional outcome?

There are two RCTs that address this question. In a study reported by Yang *et al.*,[70] 91 patients with high grade extremity STS who had undergone LSS, were randomised to receive or not receive postoperative adjuvant external beam radiotherapy (EBRT). An additional 50 patients with low grade tumours were randomised after definitive resection to adjuvant EBRT or no further treatment. Patients with high grade sarcomas also received postoperative adjuvant chemotherapy. For the group with high grade tumours, at a median follow up of 9·6 years, a highly significant decrease in the probability of LR was seen in the group treated with radiation (*P* = 0·0028) but no difference in overall survival was observed. Of the 50 patients with low grade lesions, a lower probability of LR (*P* = 0·016) was also observed in patients receiving radiation, without a difference in overall survival **Evidence level Ib**.

Pisters *et al.* reported the results of an RCT, involving 164 patients, comparing brachytherapy (BRT) with no further treatment following "gross total resection" LSS.[71,72] At a median follow up of 76 months, the 5-year local control rates were 82% and 69% in BRT and no BRT groups (*P* = 0·04). In patients with high grade STS (*N* = 56 BRT *v* *N* = 63 no-BRT groups), a significant difference in local control rate favouring the BRT group was observed (89% *v* 66%, *P* = 0·0025). There was no difference in 5-year freedom from distant metastasis rate (83% *v* 76%, *P* = 0·60) **Evidence level Ib**. This study also included 45 patients with low grade STS. In this group, LR occurred in five of 23 patients (22%) in the no-BRT group and 6 of 22 patients (27%) in the BRT group (*P* = 0·60). The authors concluded that BRT following LSS, although beneficial for patients with high grade STS, did not significantly decrease the LR rate for low grade STS and have hypothesised that the relatively long cell cycle times believed to exist in these tumours may render them less sensitive to BRT. Fabrizio *et al.* have also observed a favourable outcome in patients with low grade STS. In their study, patients with such tumours treated with LSS without the addition of radiation, had local control and freedom from distant relapse rates of 100% at 5 years, whereas in patients with high grade tumours, corresponding figures were 60% and 71%. (*P* ≤ 0·05)[73] **Evidence level III**. Similar excellent outcomes in "low risk" patients have been documented by Rydholm *et al.*[74] Quality of life was not formally assessed in any of these studies.

For the majority of patients therefore, radiotherapy is an important component of LSS. In this setting there is a very large body of single institution experience attesting to the ability of radiotherapy (preoperative or postoperative) to produce acceptable local control rates in excess of 75% and 5-year overall survival rates greater that 55%. Limb preservation has been possible in 85% of patients included in these studies.[75–83] Data from these studies are summarised in Table 46.1.

It is apparent from the preceding evidence that tumour grade is an important consideration when deciding whether to offer radiation in the setting of LSS. However, attempts at limb preservation may not always result in negative resection margins and radiation may play a role in such circumstances. No RCTs addressing this specific scenario are retrieved in the evidence search. Although not a randomised comparison, data from Alektiar *et al.*[84] suggest that radiation can reduce the risk of local recurrence in patients found to have positive microscopic resection margins after LSS. Of 110 such patients with high grade extremity STS, who underwent LSS, 91(83%), received radiotherapy and 19 (17%) received no further treatment. Among the patients who received no radiation, five were randomised to no radiation in a trial evaluating the impact of brachytherapy on local control and, in the remaining 14, the reason could not be ascertained. For the patients receiving radiation, 34 received BRT, 33 received EBRT and 24 received the combination of the two. The 5-year local control rate for the group as a whole was 71%, and was significantly higher in the radiotherapy group compared with no radiation (74% *v* 56% respectively, *P* = 0·01) but no differences in the distance relapse or overall survival rates were observed.

The modality and timing of radiation may influence rates of tumour control as well as functional outcomes and toxicity. EBRT and BRT each have well described advantages and disadvantages. BRT has not been directly compared with EBRT and it is therefore not possible to recommend one over the other. The advantages of BRT include a shorter overall treatment time and a more timely initiation of treatment following surgery. Although BRT may be less costly, it must be borne in mind that application of this modality requires particular experience and expertise.

With regards to time to the timing of radiotherapy, it is has been suggested that preoperative radiation offers particular advantages,[85–89] including the possibility that it may be more efficacious for lesions larger than 5 cm.[97] There have, however, been concerns about delays in wound healing, which have been described as occurring in 16–37% of patients who undergo this treatment.[90–91] Thus, in a recent prospective RCT conducted by the National Cancer Institute of Canada Clinical Trials Group evaluating preoperative and postoperative radiation in extremity STS, the primary objective was to compare wound-healing complications between the two groups. After accruing 190 patients the study was closed prematurely because, in an interim analysis, a statistically important difference was noted between the two arms: 35% of patients treated with preoperative radiation had wound complications versus 17% in the postoperative group (*P* = 0·01) **Evidence level Ib**.

Table 46.1 Extremity soft tissue sarcoma (non-randomised studies) local control, complications and survival after limb-sparing surgery and radiation

| First author | No. of patients | Local control (%) | Overall survival (%) | Complication rates (%)[tt] | Limb preservation (%) |
|---|---|---|---|---|---|
| *Postoperative radiation* | | | | | |
| Lindbergh[75] | 300 | 5yr: 78 | 5yr: 61·3 | 6·5 | 84·5 |
| Suit[76,77] | 110 | 5yr: 84 | 5yr: 73 | 5 | NS |
| Pollack[78] | 165 | 10yr: 67 | NS | 6·2 | NS |
| Keus[79] | 117 | 5yr: 81 | 5yr: 70 | 3–16 | 83 |
| Wilson[80] | 23 | 2yr: 91 | NS | NS | 100 |
| Karakousis[61] | 36 | 5yr: 75 | 5yr: 43 | NS | 94 |
| Pao[81] | 50 | 6yr: 87 | 6yr: 72 | 16 | 90 |
| *Preoperative radiation* | | | | | |
| Wilson[80] | 39 | 2yr: 97 | NS | NS | 100 |
| Suit[76,77] | 60 | 5yr: 86 | 5yr: 62 | 26 | 85 |
| Brant[82] | 58 | 5yr: 90 | 5yr: 39–68* | 16 | 87 |
| Barkley[83] | 110 | 5yr: 90 | NS | 14 | 97 |

*5-yr survival was 39% for tumours 11–20 cm and 68% for tumours <11 cm (all high-grade).
[tt]Reported rates include early and late complications of moderate to severe grade. *Early* complications including soft-tissue necrosis and prolonged wound healing are more common in the preoperative radiation setting and may be as high as 25%. *Late* effects of radiation include limited mobility, nerve or vascular damage, fibrosis oedema and fractures which overall have been observed in 3–24% of patients receiving pre- or postoperative radiation.

At a median follow up time of 1·9 years, there had been six local recurrences in the entire group and metastatic outcome and survival were similar in both arms. (It should be noted that the study was underpowered to detect differences in these outcomes.) Quality of life, physical function, cost and the incidence of acute and late radiation effects were all measured in this study, but analysis of these data requires longer follow up.[92]

Among these studies data on quality of life were reported in only one RCT. In this study, Yang *et al.*[70] demonstrated that extremity radiation resulted in significantly worse (although usually transient) limb strength, oedema and range of motion. Despite these findings, there were no significant differences between the patients in the two treatment arms (radiation *v* no radiation) as measured by global quality of life or in the performance of activities of daily living **Evidence level Ib**. However, long-term functional outcome and quality of life were not described in this trial. The remaining evidence is retrospective and incomplete but wound complications, bone fractures and peripheral nerve damage do not appear to be higher overall in patients undergoing BRT,[71,72,93] compared with those receiving EBRT or no additional radiation.

Somewhat disturbing is a retrospective analysis by Sugarbaker *et al.*[94] assessing quality of life in 26 of the 43 patients involved in the original trial conducted by Rosenberg *et al.*[63] Rather surprisingly, the authors concluded that compared with amputation, an LSS approach did not improve the quality of life (measured as pain assessment, sexual functioning, mobility and treatment trauma) of patients. A number of methodological criticisms, including patient selection bias, participant bias, and the choice of instruments used to measure quality of life, might account for these unexpected results. **Evidence level III**

### Implications for practice

For adults with extremity STS, limb-sparing surgery (LSS), when performed by experienced surgeons, is an acceptable alternative to radical techniques such as amputation. Patients with favourable presentations – superficial, small tumours with negative margins after resection – may be considered for LSS without radiation. The multidisciplinary team should assess all other cases and in patients with less favourable presentations, radiotherapy is recommended.

In most patients the addition of radiation therapy (EBRT or BRT) produces a significant benefit in terms of local control when compared with LSS alone. This benefit is mainly observed in patients with high grade extremity tumours, and combined modality therapy (LSS + radiation) should be considered the standard of care in these patients.

It is not possible to recommend EBRT or BRT preferentially as no direct comparisons have been performed. Likewise, it is premature to draw firm conclusions about the optimal timing of radiation, either preoperative or postoperative.

## Adjuvant chemotherapy

### Should adjuvant chemotherapy be used for extremity STS?

Adjuvant chemotherapy is currently established practice in the treatment of embryonal rhabdomyosarcomas, osteosarcomas and Ewing's sarcoma. In adult STS, the role of adjuvant chemotherapy remains controversial.

As many as 50% of all patients with high grade extremity STS, in whom good local control is achieved, will develop metastases – predominantly in the lungs. One study documented a median time to metastatic development of 13 months,[6] indicating that micrometastases are established early, independent of local control strategies. The development of adjuvant systemic approaches has focused on chemotherapy drugs with demonstrable activity against STS – namely the anthracyclines (doxorubicin and epirubicin), ifosfamide and dacarbazine (DTIC), although other, less active, agents were used in earlier studies. Recurrence-free survival (local and distant) is excellent for low grade sarcomas of the extremities,[95] and thus systemic adjuvant chemotherapy (including postoperative, preoperative and intra-arterial modalities) are considered mainly for patients at high risk – those with high grade deep, large (> 5 cm) extremity STS.

### For adults with non-metastatic STS does adjuvant chemotherapy improve outcomes such as local control, metastases-free survival, relapse-free and overall survival with acceptable morbidity and/or quality of life?

A search of the literature discloses 18 RCTs and four meta-analyses evaluating the role of postoperative systemic adjuvant chemotherapy in adult STS. These include four trials,[96–99]

involving patients with non-extremity STS, and 14 trials that were either limited to patients with extremity STS, or in which these comprised a majority of the study population.[100–114]

Three literature-based meta-analyses,[115–117] performed to address concerns that a beneficial effect of chemotherapy might be missed owing to the small size of individual studies, have suggested that adjuvant chemotherapy for STS improves a number of outcomes including survival. Recognising the potential biases of literature meta-analyses, the Sarcoma Meta-Analysis Collaboration (SMAC), performed an exhaustive individual patient data meta-analysis (IPDMA) involving 1568 patients entered in 14 RCTs of adjuvant doxorubicin containing chemotherapy versus no chemotherapy. This review included patients with extremity, truncal, uterine, and retroperitoneal sarcomas. Median follow up was 9·4 years (range 4·9–17·6 years). The results were expressed as hazard ratios (HR) for the risk of death or recurrence (local or metastatic) as compared with control (no treatment) patients. The results are summarised in Table 46.2. Adjuvant doxorubicin-based chemotherapy was found to significantly improve time to local and distant recurrence and overall relapse-free survival (RFS), with corresponding absolute benefits at 10 years of 6%, 10% and 10%, respectively. The improvement in overall survival from 50% to 54% was not statistically significant ($P = 0·12$) but a small absolute benefit of 4% at 10 years was observed **Evidence level Ia**.[118] The outcomes were not influenced by whether doxorubicin was given alone or in combination. In a subset analysis of 886 patients with extremity STS, the HR for overall survival was 0·80 ($P = 0·029$) corresponding to a 7% absolute benefit at 10 years. For STS arising from non-extremity sites, the numbers were too small to generate reliable information. Of note, only 24% of patients in this meta-analysis were over 60 years of age making it difficult to generalise these results to older patients.

**Table 46.2 Adjuvant chemotherapy in resected adult soft tissue sarcoma pooled survival data (adapted from the Sarcoma Meta-Analysis Collaboration[118])**

| | No. of patients | Hazard ratio (95% Confidence Interval) | P value | Absolute benefit |
|---|---|---|---|---|
| Overall survival (all patients) | 1544 | 0·89 (0·76–1·03) | 0·12 | 4% |
| Overall survival (extremity pts.) | 886 | 0·80 (n/a) | 0·029 | 7% |
| Disease-free survival | 1366 | 0·75 (0·64–0·87) | 0·0001 | 10% |
| Local recurrence-free survival | 1315 | 0·73 (0·56–0·94) | 0·016 | 6% |
| Metastases-free survival | 1315 | 0·70 (0·50–0·85) | 0·0003 | 10% |

**For adults with non-metastatic STS are there specific adjuvant chemotherapy regimens that improve outcomes such as local control, metastases-free survival, relapse-free and overall survival?**

In the SMAC IPDMA there was no clear evidence that combination adjuvant chemotherapy was better than single agent doxorubicin.[118] However, with the exception of one small, unpublished study, ifosfamide was not part of the combination chemotherapy regimens included in this meta-analysis.

The latest generation of postoperative adjuvant chemotherapy studies incorporate ifosfamide in combination with anthracyclines, and the evidence search identified four RCTs involving this approach. Two have been published,[110,111] one is unpublished (and was included in the IPDMA),[118] and one is available in abstract form.[112]

A recent trial published by Frustaci *et al.* on behalf of an Italian Cooperative Group is of particular interest.[110] This trial randomised adult patients with high grade STS of the extremities to five cycles of high dose epirubicin (60 mg m$^{-2}$ on days 1 and 2) plus ifosfamide (1·8 g m$^{-2}$ on days 1 through 5) with granulocyte-colony stimulating factor (G-CSF) support, or no further treatment, after locoregional therapy. Epirubicin was chosen owing to its more favourable toxicity profile vis-à-vis cardiotoxicity and the doses used were derived from previous phase I and II studies.[119,120] Of 104 patients entered, 53 were in the chemotherapy arm and 51 in the control arm. Seven patients did not commence adjuvant treatment (four withdrew and three developed lung metastases before starting chemotherapy). Of the 46 patients remaining in the chemotherapy arm, four did not complete treatment. At a median follow up of 59 months, an intent-to-treat analysis revealed median DFS times of 48 versus 16 months ($P = 0·04$) and median OS of 75 versus 46 months ($P = 0·03$), for the chemotherapy and no-treatment control groups, respectively **Evidence level Ib**. Of interest, at 2 years, 28% of the chemotherapy group versus 45% of the control group ($P = 0·08$) had suffered distant relapses, whereas at 4 years, this difference had decreased to 44% and 45%, respectively ($P = 0·094$). Despite this convergence of distant relapse survival curves, a significant difference in 4-year survival of 69% versus 50% favouring the chemotherapy arm ($P = 0·04$) was still noted with an absolute number of seven fewer deaths owing to metastatic sarcoma in the chemotherapy arm **Evidence level Ib**. Although this trial demonstrated the value of adjuvant chemotherapy incorporating relevant agents at biologically intense doses, caution is advised in interpreting these results.[121] With small patient numbers, differences in patient demographics (for example, amputation rates) and tumour characteristics

(for example, maximum tumour diameter) between the treatment and control groups that are not statistically significant may be clinically important, and a larger trial would reduce potential heterogeneity in patient populations and possibly generate different results. Nonetheless the observed delays in distant relapse and improved survival are worthy of attention.

In a study reported by Brodowicz *et al.*[111] 59 patients with grade 2 and 3 STS (47 of whom had extremity primaries) were randomised after surgery to receive radiation alone or six cycles of chemotherapy (ifosfamide 1·5 g m$^{-2}$, dacarbazine 200 mg m$^{-2}$ each given days 1 through 4, doxorubicin 25 mg m$^{-2}$ on days 1 and 2), with treatments administered at 14 days intervals (supported by G-CSF) concurrently with hyperfractionated radiation therapy. At a mean follow up of $41 \pm 19·7$ months (range 8·1–84 months) no significant difference in RFS, OS, or time to local or distant failure were observed. This study did not meet its accrual target of 100 patients, and is underpowered for primary efficacy endpoints.

Finally, a study reported by Petrioli *et al.*[112] involved 81 patients with extremity and retroperitoneal sarcomas, randomised to receive adjuvant chemotherapy or no further treatment after locoregional therapy. Of 42 patients assigned to chemotherapy, 19 received an intensive epirubicin and ifosfamide combination and 23 received epirubicin alone. An improved DFS (65% *v* 41%, $P = 0·01$) and a trend for improved OS (72% *v* 47%, $P = 0·06$) favouring the chemotherapy arm was reported, but given the small numbers and the variability of the chemotherapy interventions, the results are difficult to interpret.

A clinical practice guideline (Adjuvant chemotherapy following complete resection of soft tissue sarcoma in adults – Figueredo *et al.*: http.//www/cancercare.on.ca/ccopgi/) integrates data from the SMAC IPDMA and these more recent studies, and makes some management recommendations.[122]

Thus far the evidence examined has dealt with postoperative chemotherapy. The literature search discloses some evidence that an alternative approach might be the use of preoperative (neoadjuvant) treatment.

Only one phase II RCT of neoadjuvant chemotherapy is identified. In this study, adult patients with "high risk" STS (defined as tumours $\geq 8$ cm of any grade, or grade 2–3 tumours either $< 8$ cm, recurrent or with "inadequate surgery" performed within the 6 weeks before entry) were randomised to surgery alone, or three cycles of 3-weekly doxorubicin 50 mg m$^{-2}$ intravenous bolus and ifosfamide 5 g m$^{-2}$ given by 24-hour intravenous infusion before surgery. The type of surgery (amputation, compartmental resection, wide or marginal excision) was planned before entry. For patients randomised to chemotherapy, surgery was to be performed within 21 days after the last treatment.

Postoperative radiotherapy was given to patients who underwent marginal surgery or who had microscopically incomplete resection. Of 150 patients who were entered into the study, 134 were considered eligible. Limb salvage was achieved in 88% but amputation was necessary in 12%. At a median follow up of 7·3 years, 5-year DFS (52% $v$ 56%, $P = 0·35$) and overall survivals (64% and 65% $P = 0·22$) were similar for control and preoperative chemotherapy arms respectively **Evidence level Ib**. Toxicities were similar to those observed in other adjuvant trials, but it is noteworthy that preoperative chemotherapy did not interfere with planned surgery or with wound healing. This study was originally planned as a phase III trial requiring a total accrual of 269 patients to detect a 15% difference (55% $v$ 40%) in 5-year overall survival, but was closed after completion of the phase II section due to slow accrual.[123] Three other small non-randomised studies suggested the feasibility of this approach but there is insufficient evidence to adopt this as an alternative to postoperative chemotherapy.[124–126]

An approach using intra-arterial chemotherapy has been pioneered by investigators at the University of California at Los Angeles (UCLA) in a study where patients with extremity STS received IA doxorubicin over 3 days prior to radiation therapy. Following radiotherapy, patients were randomised to receive postoperative doxorubicin intravenously or no further chemotherapy. No significant differences in survival or local control were detected **Evidence level Ib**,[127] but the usefulness of the chemotherapy versus control comparison was limited by the small size of the study (119 patients) and contamination of the control arm by the use of intra-arterial doxorubicin. The same group then conducted a randomised trial comparing preoperative intra-arterial versus intravenous doxorubicin in 99 patients with extremity STS. Rates of limb salvage, local recurrence, incidence of complications, and survival were similar for the two groups and the authors concluded that the intravenous approach had equivalent efficacy with less toxicity **Evidence level Ib**.[128] Results from several other small, non-randomised studies have yielded similar results.[129–132] However, complications (including arterial thromboembolism, infection, problems with wound healing and pathological fractures) as well as the complexity of the process have been problematic and there has been considerable reluctance to adopt this procedure. Thus, neoadjuvant chemotherapy in patients with soft tissue sarcoma should be confined to investigational studies.

The potential roles of hyperthermia and isolated limb perfusion with agents such as melphalan, doxorubicin and tumour necrosis factor (TNF) are being assessed in other trials. However, it should be emphasised that these approaches are primarily intended to increase operability and local control of locoregionally advanced STS, not to reduce distant metastases. Particularly with TNF, strenuous efforts are made to avoid leakage of this highly toxic agent into the systemic circulation. Isolated limb perfusion with or without hyperthermia may be an option for the subset of patients who could otherwise require amputation for local control purposes. However, in the absence of randomised trials, this cannot be considered standard care.[133,134]

The above section describes the potential benefits of adjuvant chemotherapy. However, knowledge of toxicity and risks may also influence treatment decisions. The clinical practice guideline by Figueredo *et al.* referred to earlier is found to address this issue. For all the studies included in the SMAC IPDMA, the available quantitative toxicity data were tabulated, including toxic deaths and major toxic events such as severe infections and cardiotoxicity. Of 523 patients for whom data were available, the overall rate of toxic deaths was 1·7% and was similar for patients treated with single agent doxorubicin or combination treatment. The overall rate of cardiotoxicity was 5·1%. Severe infections occurred more commonly in patients receiving combination treatment compared with doxorubicin alone (3·1% $v$ 0·4%).[122] Although cardiotoxicity may be reduced by prolonged infusion of doxorubicin, efficacy may be compromised. In an RCT conducted by Casper *et al.*, the cardiotoxic and therapeutic effects of adjuvant intravenous doxorubicin (bolus $v$ 72 hour infusion) were assessed. Fewer patients receiving the continuous infusion had greater than 10% decrease in left ventricular ejection fraction (42% $v$ 61%, $P = 0·0017$). However, a significantly lower rate of death from disease ($P = 0·036$) and a trend towards a lower rate of metastases ($P = 0·19$) was observed in patients treated with bolus therapy **Evidence level Ib**.[135]

In trials in which ifosfamide was included, toxicity data are found in the studies by Brodowicz *et al.*[111] and Frustaci *et al.*[110] In the first study, despite the use of G-CSF, grade IV leucopenia and thrombocytopenia were observed in 13% and 3% of patients, respectively. No patients developed neutropenic sepsis and there were no toxic deaths. In the larger study by Frustaci *et al.*, 35% of patients experienced grade IV leucopenia and 13% neutropenic fever. No toxic deaths or cardiotoxicity were reported.

It is difficult to provide a reliable estimate of the long-term impact of chemotherapy on ovarian and testicular function, as the data are sparse.[136–137]

Quality-of-life assessments were not included in any of the RCTs mentioned in the preceding discussion, and it is not possible to obtain reliable answers to this aspect of the questions.

## Implications for practice

- In adults with high risk (deep location, size > 5 cm, high grade) resected extremity STS, in whom there is no overt evidence of metastatic disease, it is reasonable to offer anthracycline-based adjuvant chemotherapy postoperatively. Benefits include a significant reduction in all types of recurrences and an improvement in overall survival.

- There is insufficient evidence to recommend combination chemotherapy over single–agent anthracycline and any decision on the type of chemotherapy should consider patient characteristics (age, general health, cardiac risks) and preferences, adverse effects and costs.

- Although in one RCT, the use of adjuvant high dose ifosfamide and epirubicin, resulted in significant benefits in terms of disease-free and overall survivals, it is premature to adopt this approach as a standard of care for all patients, and these results should be confirmed in a larger trial.

- Given the need for confirmatory data, it is reasonable to enter patients into RCTs comparing adjuvant chemotherapy to observation. In addition to conventional outcome measures, future trials should also include measures of quality of life as the absence of data in previously published studies does not permit commentary on this issue.

- Patients with low risk sarcomas (< 5 cm and/or low grade) should not receive adjuvant chemotherapy outside a clinical trial setting.

## Management of metastatic STS

### Case 2

*A 66-year-old female with a history of a 9 ´ 10 cm liposarcoma of the buttock, treated with limb-sparing surgery and postoperative radiation 2 years earlier, presents with a 4-week history of intractable cough. A chest x ray reveals multiple pulmonary metastases (five in the right lung and three in the left) with the largest measuring 5 cm in size. A subsequent CT scan revealed an additional 10 nodules. She reports no chest pain or haemoptysis and describes moderate dyspnoea on exertion. A thorough examination and staging assessment (including CT scan and bone scan) reveal no additional sites of metastatic involvement and there are no other health-related concerns. What, if any, treatment (including surgery) might benefit her.*

### Framing relevant and answerable questions

In this patient with metastatic disease involving the lungs, several questions come to mind. Are the metastases completely resectable? In other words can the patient be rendered disease-free through surgery and if so is there any benefit for her in achieving this? Is there a role for any additional therapy such as chemotherapy post surgery? What if the disease is inoperable or if it is medically

inadvisable to proceed with pulmonary metastatectomies? What other therapeutic options exist? Four answerable questions may be framed as follows, with the first two dealing with the management of operable lung metastases and the latter two dealing with inoperable disease.

- In adults with lung metastases secondary to STS does surgical resection improve survival with acceptable morbidity and/or quality of life?
- In adults undergoing resection of STS lung metastases, does the addition of chemotherapy improve relapse-free or overall survival?
- In adults with inoperable metastatic STS does combination chemotherapy have advantages compared with single agent chemotherapy in terms of response rate, survival and toxicity/quality of life?
- In adults with inoperable metastatic STS are there specific chemotherapy regimens that improve outcomes in terms of response rate, survival and quality of life?

There are no prospective RCTs or systematic reviews. Many retrospective reviews are identified but you pursue only those that have a substantial study population (over 20 patients).

### Discussion of the evidence

In patients with STS who develop metastases, the lung is the most common site, and in many patients may be the only site of distant dissemination.[22] This provides the rationale to expect cure in selected patients through resection of pulmonary metastases (with/without additional chemotherapy), and this potential has been explored by multiple institutions. Unfortunately, only retrospective data are available and there have been no prospective, randomised trials addressing this issue.

### In adults with lung metastases, secondary to STS does surgical resection improve survival with acceptable morbidity and/or quality of life?

In 1995, Frost reviewed the previous 25 years of experience (1978–1994) assessing the role of pulmonary metastatectomy for adult STS.[138] Twelve case series, encompassing a total of 697 patients were identified. A meta-analysis was not possible, and therefore a qualitative review was undertaken. In this review, 5-year survival rates for first-time pulmonary metastatectomy ranged from 15–35% with a median value for all patients undergoing resection of 25%. For patients undergoing repeat metastatectomy, a 5-year survival rate of 12–52% was noted. Representative data from studies involving over 20 patients are provided in

Table 46.3. Of this group of studies (all retrospective), two are worthy of attention as they originate from institutions with a particular expertise in STS and encompass a large number of patients.

van Geel *et al.* retrospectively identified patients undergoing resection of STS pulmonary metastases at member institutions of the EORTC (The European Organisation for Research and Treatment of Cancer) Soft Tissue and Bone Sarcoma Group. In 255 patients treated with complete resection, 5-year OS and DFS rates of 38% and 35%, respectively, were documented.[139] Recently, Billingsley *et al.* updated the experience of the Memorial Sloan–Kettering Cancer Center (MSKCC), involving 719 patients with adult STS, treated with pulmonary metastatectomy.[140] The relative proportions of patients undergoing complete or incomplete resections cannot be identified from this publication. The overall median survival from diagnosis of pulmonary metastases for all patients was 15 months, with a 3-year actuarial survival rate of 25%. Patients treated with complete resection had the most favourable outcome with a median survival of 33 months and 3- and 5-year actuarial survival rates of 46% and 37%, respectively. Patients who did not undergo resection had a median survival of 11 months and a 3-year actuarial survival of 17%, whereas patients who underwent an incomplete resection had a median survival of 16 months. Not surprisingly, complete resection was associated with a significant improvement in survival compared with an incomplete resection ($P = 0.003$). **Evidence level III**

Despite the lack of randomised data it is clear that pulmonary metastatectomy can result in improved survival for a small proportion of patients. A number of researchers have identified favourable prognostic factors to assist in the selection of patients for this procedure. These include tumour doubling time of over 20 days, disease-free interval of over 12 months, complete resection and age under 50 years. Negative prognostic factors included the presence of local recurrence, more than four pulmonary nodules[5,11] (not consistent in all studies), and age over 50 years.

Following initial pulmonary metastatectomy, recurrent disease has been observed in 53–61% of patients.[141,142] The data regarding repeat pulmonary metastatectomy for STS are confined to small retrospective series. Casson *et al.*[143] reported a median survival of 28 months and a 3-year survival of 38% for 34 patients undergoing repeat resection. Verazin *et al.*[144] observed a 5-year OS of 21% and DFS of 4% in 28 patients, and Rizzoni *et al.*[149] observed a median survival of 14·5 months and a 3-year survival of 22% in 29 patients. In one study, patients with solitary nodules had a higher median survival (65 months) compared with patients with two more nodules (14 months).[143] Rizzoni *et al.* have also suggested that, in these patients, a disease-free interval of $\geq 6$ months is associated with a more favourable outcome **Evidence level IV**.

No data concerning quality of life of patients who have undergone pulmonary metastatectomy are found in the literature.

**Table 46.3  Pulmonary metastatectomy in adult soft tissue sarcoma: survival data**

| First author | No. of patients | No. of complete resections | Survival |
|---|---|---|---|
| Billingsley[140] | 719* | n/a | Median: 15 months<br>3-year: 25% |
| van Geel[139] | 255* | n/a | 5-year: 38%<br>10-year: 35% |
| Pastorino[141] | 2173 | n/a | 5-year: 31%<br>10-year: 28% |
| Pastorino[145] | 105* | n/a | 3-year: 46% |
| Creagan[142] | 112 | 64 | 5-year: 35% |
| Jablons[146] | 63 | n/a | Median: 20 months<br>3-year: 35% |
| Verazin[144] | 78 | 61 | Median: 21 months<br>5-year: 21% |
| Robinson[147] | 44* | n/a | 4-year: 51% |
| Casson[143] | 68 | 58 | 5-year: 25·8% |
| Putnam[148] | 44* | n/a | 4-year: 51% |

*Some patients received chemotherapy.
n/a, not available

## In adults undergoing resection of STS lung metastases, does the addition of chemotherapy improve relapse-free or overall survival?

The role of adjuvant chemotherapy, given after pulmonary metastatectomy, has also not been prospectively assessed. Although sparse, the available data would suggest that adjuvant chemotherapy in this setting has not been proven to provide a survival benefit.[147,150] There was an attempt to address this issue in a randomised trial (EORTC 62933). In this study, patients who were eligible for complete resection of pulmonary metastases were randomised to no chemotherapy or to receive doxorubicin/ifosfamide combination chemotherapy for three cycles preoperatively, with two cycles given postoperatively if there was evidence of an objective response. Unfortunately this study recently closed because of low accrual and thus this question may never be answered with confidence.

### Implications for practice

- In selected patients improved survival is possible after resection of pulmonary metastases owing to STS.
- Pulmonary metastatectomy should be confined to patients who present with no evidence of extrapulmonary metastases and in whom local control of the primary tumour has been achieved.
- Patients with rapidly evolving metastatic disease (relapse < 12 months), those with multiple bilateral pulmonary metastases, and those with evidence of a malignant pleural effusion, are not candidates for this procedure.
- At this time, there are no reliable data on the efficacy of chemotherapy post resection of lung metastases. Further studies examining this issue are warranted.

## Management of inoperable metastatic STS

### In adults with inoperable metastatic STS does combination chemotherapy have advantages compared with single agent chemotherapy in terms of response rate, survival and toxicity/quality of life?

The median survival of patients with metastatic disease is approximately 1 year. Although the EORTC and investigators from the MSKCC have documented a few long-term survivors – 8·6% and 8%, respectively[150,151] – most patients succumb to the complications of metastases. Therefore until more effective treatments are discovered

for patients with inoperable metastatic STS, at present systemic treatment should be regarded as palliative. Choices concerning therapy must consider the benefits and harms of treatment.

It is widely acknowledged that the cytotoxic agents doxorubicin, ifosfamide and dacarbazine (DTIC) have the highest activity in STS.[152] Many other chemotherapy drugs have been tested but these have usually produced response rates less than 15% or results have been inconsistent and difficult to reproduce.

In early trials of doxorubicin, response rates of 30–60% were observed, and a dose–response relationship for doxorubicin in STS was reported, with a significant difference in RR noted between 45 mg m$^{-2}$ and 75 mg m$^{-2}$ ($P = 0.05$) **Evidence level III**.[153] However, the most reliable summary data of the activity of single agent doxorubicin in metastatic STS, come from a meta-analysis by Bramwell *et al.* comparing single agent doxorubicin, given in doses of 60–80 mg m$^{-2}$ every 3 weeks, with combination chemotherapy. Across eight studies (nine doxorubicin arms) the median overall response to single agent doxorubicin was 19% (range 16–27%).[154]

In addition to typical chemotherapy-related toxicities, cardiotoxicity is the most serious side effect of doxorubicin treatment. Efforts to reduce this side effect have been explored, using different schedules and infusion rates. While cardiotoxicity was favourably influenced, a reduction in efficacy or the occurrence of other severe side effects such as stomatitis have abrogated the advantages of such treatment schemas.[155]

The anthracycline analogue, epirubicin, has been assessed in STS in two RCTs conducted by the EORTC. In the first study by Mouridsen *et al.*, equimolar doses of epirubicin and doxorubicin given at 75 mg m$^{-2}$ every 3 weeks produced response rates of 18% and 25% ($P = 0.33$), respectively **Evidence level Ib**. Doxorubicin produced more myelosuppression, alopecia, nausea and vomiting.[156]

In a second study, a higher dose of epirubicin at 150 mg m$^{-2}$ given by two different schedules was compared with doxorubicin 75 mg m$^{-2}$. Response rates and toxicities (including grade III or greater cardiotoxicity) were similar in the two arms but myelosuppression was greater and toxic deaths were noted in the epirubicin arms[157] **Evidence level Ib**.

The cardioprotectant dexrazoxane has not been formally evaluated in STS. However, one small study including 34 patients with STS and 95 patients with bone sarcomas evaluated the efficacy of epirubicin versus epirubicin plus dexrazoxane. A non-significant difference in response rates (37·5% *v* 11%) was described and the authors concluded that dexrazoxane did not appear to produce a negative impact on survival.[158] Liposomal encapsulated doxorubicin has been evaluated in a phase II RCT by the EORTC.[159] In this study, 94 patients were randomised to receive Caelyx 50 mg m$^{-2}$ every 4 weeks or doxorubicin 75 mg m$^{-2}$ every 3 weeks. Respective response rates were low at 10% and 9%, which may reflect the relatively high proportion of patients with visceral intra-abdominal sarcomas, that is, possible gastrointestinal stromal tumours (22% overall) included in this study. However, Caelyx was significantly less myelosuppressive (grade 3/4 neutropenia 6% *v* 77%) than doxorubicin, and caused fewer neutropenic fevers (2% *v* 16%). Nevertheless, a different dose-limiting toxicity, palmar–plantar erythrodysthesia (20% grade 3/4), only occurred with Caelyx.

Most of the aforementioned studies have assessed doxorubicin in chemotherapy naive patients. However, in the "second-line" setting, it is important to note that doxorubicin retains some of its activity, as demonstrated in an EORTC study of 17 pretreated patients, in whom there was a response rate of 17% **Evidence level III**.[160]

Data on the single agent dacarbazine are more limited. Based on a 17% RR in 53 patients seen in an early phase II trial, DTIC has been incorporated into some combination regimens.[161] A similar level of activity was reported in a subsequent EORTC phase II study.[162] Although a relationship between dose intensity and response for DTIC has been suggested in one retrospective analysis,[163] the constitutional side effects induced by high doses of DTIC and its limited activity have led to little interest in exploring its activity further as a single agent.

The alkylating agent ifosfamide, an isomer of cyclophosphamide, was first developed in the 1960s. Initial studies with ifosfamide were limited owing to the high incidence of urothelial toxicity and haemorrhagic cystitis induced predominantly by its metabolite acrolein. With the availability of mesna (sodium-2-mercaptoethane sulfonate), the incidence of haematuria (gross and microscopic) and renal toxicity have been markedly reduced to approximately 5%.[164] This has also enabled the delivery of very high doses of ifosfamide up to 19 g m$^{-2}$ over several days, without additional bladder toxicity, although at such doses additional toxicities such as myelosuppression, nausea, vomiting, renal toxicity (acute tubular necrosis), and neurotoxicity, including encephalopathy, have become more problematic.

Ifosfamide is active in untreated and previously treated patients. A retrospective analysis of patients with STS treated with ifosfamide documented an overall RR of 26%.[152] In chemotherapy naive patients an RR as high as 47% has been observed compared with an RR of 15–24% in those previously treated[165,166] **Evidence level IV**.

In an RCT conducted by the EORTC, ifosfamide 5 g m$^{-2}$ intravenous over 24 hours was compared with cyclophosphamide 1·5 g m$^{-2}$ intravenously over 24 hours every 3 weeks. The response rates of 18% and 8% for

ifosfamide and cyclophosphamide, respectively, were not significantly different ($P = 0·13$) but a trend in favour of ifosfamide was observed **Evidence level Ib**. Among the subset of chemotherapy naive patients, the response rates were 19% and 4% respectively ($P = 0·01$), in the two arms.[167]

Scheduling and dose of ifosfamide also appear to be important. Initial phase I and II trials suggested higher response rates were obtained using daily short infusions, compared with prolonged continuous infusions (24 or 96 hours).[164] An EORTC RCT comparing ifosfamide 5 g m$^{-2}$ 24 hours continuous intravenous infusion and 3 g m$^{-2}$ intravenously over 4 hours daily for 3 days, each given at 21-day cycles, produced response rates of 3% and 17·5%, respectively **Evidence level Ib**.[168] It is unclear whether the split bolus schedule or the higher dose was responsible for the higher response rate in the latter arm.

A dose–response relationship for ifosfamide in STS has also been described, although only by indirect comparisons between phase I and II trials.[169] In five such studies evaluating high dose ifosfamide (12–14 g m$^{-2}$), usually in previously treated patients, response rates in the range of 0–39% have been reported.[170–174] Despite the use of growth factors, high dose ifosfamide is associated with considerable toxicity. In these early phase trials, grade III–IV neutropenia was observed in up to 100%, febrile neutropenia in up to 89%, thrombocytopenia in up to 23% of patients, and two toxic deaths from sepsis were reported. Renal and neurotoxicity have also been observed. Therefore, although active in metastatic STS, the role of high dose ifosfamide needs further evaluation in a clinical trial setting.

Clearly there is a place for single agent therapy. However, it is important to examine the evidence for activity of the various combination regimens as well. Typical combinations have included adriamycin and DTIC (ADIC), cyclophosphamide, vincristine, adriamycin and DTIC (CYVADIC), adriamycin and ifosfamide (AI), and adriamycin, ifosfamide and DTIC with mesna (MAID). Response rates in the range of 30–60% have been documented but have been generally been observed at the expense of greater toxicity. Combination chemotherapy regimens not containing doxorubicin have usually produced poor results in STS[175,176] and are not considered further. No randomised data comparing single-agent DTIC or ifosfamide with combination therapies were retrieved in the evidence search. However, several large RCTs comparing doxorubicin-based combinations to single-agent doxorubicin therapy can be identified.[155,177–183] The results of studies, listed in Table 46.4, have been summarised in a meta-analysis by Bramwell *et al.* in which nine doxorubicin treatment arms were compared with 10 combination chemotherapy regimens in 2281 patients. Response rates for single agent doxorubicin ranged between 16% and 27%, and for the combination regimens ranged from 14% to 34%.[153] A significant difference in response rate in favour of combination treatment was identified in only two trials,[154,182] and in one study doxorubicin alone was superior to cyclophosphamide/doxorubicin/vincristine (respective RR 27% *v* 19%, *P* = 0·03).[178] None of the studies showed any significant differences in median survival times. A meta-analysis of these data was performed using a random effects model, and for RR there was a trend favouring combination chemotherapy (OR 0·78; 95% CI 0·60–1·05; *P* = 0·10) **Evidence level Ia**. For overall survival at 2 years, the results favoured combination chemotherapy but the difference was not significant (OR 0·84; 95% CI 0·67–1·06; *P* = 0·13)[153] **Evidence level Ia**.

A single study comparing single-agent epirubicin alone to epirubicin and cisplatin revealed significant differences in response rate and overall survival in favour of the combination, but median survival times were similar (8 months *v* 10 months).[185] Adding these data to the meta-analysis did not alter the results significantly.

Although the meta-analysis did not examine response rate in relation to doxorubicin dose, the authors concluded that the dose of 75 mg m$^{-2}$ intravenously every 3 weeks is an appropriate dose when single agent chemotherapy is being considered.

In this meta-analysis, comparative toxicities of single agent doxorubicin versus combination chemotherapy for the eight trials were tabulated.[181] Nausea and vomiting and haematological toxicities were consistently higher for the combination regimens, although febrile neutropenia-related toxic deaths were generally uncommon.

## In adults with inoperable metastatic STS are there specific chemotherapy regimens that improve outcomes in terms of response rate, survival and quality of life?

As discussed in the previous section, a large number of doxorubicin combinations have been assessed in this disease and more recently, phase I and phase II studies evaluating combinations that include ifosfamide in a variety of doses and schedules, have produced encouraging response rates. Three RCTs comparing ifosfamide-containing regimens to non-ifosfamide-containing regimens have been identified.[182–184] These trials are listed in Table 46.4 as well. In two of these trials, the response rates were significantly higher for the ifosfamide-containing regimens.[182,184] No differences in median survival were observed.

**Table 46.4   Randomised trials of single agent or combination therapy in metastatic adult soft tissue sarcoma**

| First author | Treatments | Response rate (%) | Median survival (months) |
|---|---|---|---|
| Chang[177] | A | 24 | 10·2 |
| | A/Strept | 14 | 10·6 |
| Schoenfeld[178] | A | 27* | 8·5 |
| | A/V/C | 19 | 7·8 |
| Omura[179] | A | 16 | 7·7 |
| | A/DTIC | 24 | 7·3 |
| Muss[180] | A | 19 | 11·6 |
| | A/C | 19 | 10·9 |
| Borden[154] | A | 18 | 8·0 |
| | WEEKLY A | 17 | 8·4 |
| | A/DTIC | 30* | 8·0 |
| Borden[181] | A | 17 | 9·4 |
| | A/VND | 18 | 9·9 |
| Edmonson[182] | A | 20 | 8·4 |
| | A/I | 34* | 11·5 |
| | A/MMC/DDP | 32* | 9·4 |
| Santoro[183] | A | 23 | 12·1 |
| | A/V/C/DTIC | 28 | 11·9 |
| | AI | 28 | 12·7 |
| Antman[184] | A/DTIC | 17 | 13 |
| | A/I/DTIC | 32* | 12 |

Abbreviations: A, doxorubicin; Strept, Streptozotocin; V, vincristine; C, cyclophosphamide; DTIC, dacarbazine; VND, vindesine; I, ifosfamide; MMC, mitomycin C; DDP, cisplatin

*Significantly better.

**Table 46.5    Randomised trials of high dose chemotherapy in metastatic/unresectable adult soft tissue sarcoma**

*Single agent chemotherapy regimens*

| | | |
|---|---|---|
| van Oosterom[168] | Ifosfamide 5 g m$^{-2}$ over 24 hours every 3 weeks | Ifosfamide 3 g m$^{-2}$ over 4 hours every 3 weeks |
| Nielsen[156] | Epirubicin 160 (150) mg m$^{-2}$ single i.v. bolus or Epirubicin 60 (50) mg m$^{-2}$ days 1–3 | Doxorubicin 75 mg m$^{-2}$ every 3 weeks |

*Combination chemotherapy regimens*

| | | |
|---|---|---|
| Le Cesne[192] | Doxorubicin 75 mg m$^{-2}$ Ifosfamide 5 g m$^{-2}$ (high dose) | Doxorubicin 50 mg m$^{-2}$ Ifosfamide 5 g m$^{-2}$ (standard) |
| Bui[193] | Doxorubicin 75 mg m$^{-2}$ Ifosfamide 9 g m$^{-2}$ Dacarbazine 1200 mg m$^{-2}$ (high dose) | Doxorubicin 60 mg m$^{-2}$ Ifosfamide 7·5 g m$^{-2}$ Dacarbazine 900 mg m$^{-2}$ (standard) |

| Study | Groups | No. entered (eval) | Survival | Time to progression | Progression-free survival (%) | Response rates (%) |
|---|---|---|---|---|---|---|
| *Single agent chemotherapy regimens* | | | | | | |
| van Oosterom[168] | Ifosfamide 5 g m$^{-2}$ | NR | NR | NR | NR | 10 (range 3–22) |
| | Ifosfamide 3 g m$^{-2}$ | NR | NR | NR | NR | 25 (range 13–39) |
| Nielsen[156] | Doxorubicin | 112 (104) | 45 weeks | 16 weeks | 13 (1 yr) 4 (2 yrs) | 14 (95% CI, 7–22) |
| | Epirubicin 1 day | 111 (104) | 47 weeks | 14 weeks | 12 (1 yr) 4 (2 yrs) | 15 (95% CI, 8–23) |
| | Epirubicin 3 days | 111 (106) | 45 weeks | 12 weeks | 18 (1 yr) 7 (2 yrs) | 14 (95% CI, 6–20) |
| *Combination chemotherapy regimens* | | | | | | |
| Le Cesne[192] | Standard | 157 (149) | 56 weeks | 19 weeks | No significant differences | 21 |
| | High dose | 157 (145) | 55 weeks | 29 weeks | | 23 |
| Bui[193] | Standard | 80 (76) | NR | NR | NR | 37 |
| | High dose | 82 (72) | NR | NR | NR | 43 |

NR, not reported

High doses of ifosfamide have been examined in a variety of schedules. Similarly, regimens combining higher doses of ifosfamide with either conventional or higher doses of anthracylines have been evaluated in a number of phase I–II studies.[186–191] Response rates as high as 55% have been observed. Two RCTs have examined this concept,[192,193] the details of which are presented in Table 46.5. Significantly higher toxicity but no significant differences in response rates or survival were reported **Evidence level Ib** and such approaches remain investigational.

In general more drugs and/or higher doses increase toxicity and, although it can be argued that contemporary antiemetics and the use of growth factors might reduce or eliminate some of the adverse effects of combination chemotherapy, the costs of such strategies must be weighed against the possible benefits in the setting of palliative treatment. The adverse effects of doxorubicin, alone or in combination, as well as high dose ifosfamide regimens, have been discussed in earlier sections.

Quality of life was not addressed in any of the studies retrieved.

## Implications for practice

●  Systemic chemotherapy for inoperable, metastatic adult STS, should be considered palliative treatment. Complete, durable responses are rare, occurring in fewer than 5% of patients.

- When evaluated in phase II studies, chemotherapy combinations containing doxorubicin and ifosfamide appear to produce higher response rates than single agent chemotherapy. However, when data from randomised trials are pooled, the differences between single agent doxorubicin and combination chemotherapy are not significantly different for response or survival. Combination chemotherapy is also associated with increased toxicity. Therefore, single agent doxorubicin is an appropriate first-line chemotherapy option for patients with inoperable, metastatic soft tissue sarcoma.

- The selection of single agent chemotherapy versus combination chemotherapy may also be influenced by a number of other factors, such as patients' wishes, performance status and age. Young, good performance status patients, or patients who wish to maximise response, or those with locally advanced/metastatic tumours in whom a good response might facilitate a surgical option, may be candidates for more aggressive combination chemotherapy.

- Owing to a paucity of data, it is not possible to determine the influence of chemotherapy on QOL. In asymptomatic patients chemotherapy-related toxicities may produce an adverse effect on QOL, whereas symptomatic patients who respond to chemotherapy might have an improvement in QOL. However, this should be assessed in future trials.

- The toxicity and the limited benefit of current standard chemotherapy regimens support the exploration of new treatments and the entry of treatment-naive patients into clinical trials.

## Conclusions

Despite their heterogeneity, over the past 50 years much has been learned about STS in adults. Most notably, the development of experienced multidisciplinary teams has led to significant practice alterations and has resulted in clear benefits in the locoregional, adjuvant and systemic management of patients with this disease. Neoadjuvant approaches merit continued evaluation, for example combined concurrent chemotherapy and radiotherapy,[194] as well as limb perfusion techniques using agents such as TNF, or with novel compounds administered intravenously or intra-arterially. Radiation potentiation using a variety of techniques or drugs needs further exploration in an effort to improve local control and resection rates. In the area of adjuvant therapy, the benefits of systemic treatment are small and here much needs to be accomplished. It is important to design and complete accrual to trials – particularly those evaluating high dose ifosfamide, epirubicin, or other anthracycline analogues – but further

progress in this setting will be dependent on the identification of new active systemic agents. In the metastatic setting, such new treatments are desperately needed. Current treatments provide limited benefit and even treatment-naive patients could be encouraged or advised to enter clinical trials. Evaluation of new strategies in RCTs should incorporate some measures of QOL as there is a consistent paucity of data in this area.

## References

1 Parker SL, Tong T, Bolder W *et al.* Cancer statistics 1996. *CA Cancer J Clin* 1996;**46**:5.
2 Greenlea RT, Murray T, Bolden S *et al.* Cancer statistics 2000. *CA Cancer J Clin* 2000;**50**:7–33.
3 Ross JA, Severson RK, Davis S *et al.* Trends and the incidence of soft tissue sarcomas in the United States from 1973 through 1987. *Cancer* 1993;**72**:486.
4 Coindre JM, Terrier P, Guillou L *et al.* Predictive value of grade for metastasis development in the main histologic types of adult soft tissue sarcomas. A study of 1240 patients from the French Federation of Cancer Centers Sarcoma Group. Abstract 1914 2001 American Society.
5 Nijhuis PHA, Schaapveld M, Otter R *et al.* Epidemiological aspects of soft tissue sarcomas (STS) – consequences for the design of clinical STS trials. *Eur J Cancer* 1999;**35**:1705–10.
6 Pisters PWT, Leung DHY, Woodruff J, Shi W, Brennan MF. Analysis of prognostic factors in 1,041 patients with localized soft tissue sarcomas of the extremities. *J Clin Oncol* 1996;**14**:1679–89.
7 Alvegard TA, Berg NO, Baldetorp B *et al.* Cellular DNA content and prognosis of high grade soft tissue sarcoma. The Scandinavian Sarcoma Group Experience. *J Clin Oncol* 1996;**14**:867–7.
8 Clemente C, Orazi A, Rilke F. The Italian registry of soft tissue tumours. *Appl Pathol* 1988;**6**:221–40.
9 Gustafson P. Soft tissue sarcoma. Epidemiology and prognosis in 508 patients. *Acta Orthop Scand* 1994;**65**(Suppl. 259):1–31.
10 Coebergh JWW, van der Heijden LH, Janssen-Heijnen MLG, eds. *Cancer Incidence and Survival in the Southeast of the Netherlands 1955–1994.* Eindhoven, The Netherlands: Eindhoven Cancer Registry, 1995.
11 Harris M, Hartley AL, Blair V *et al.* Sarcomas in the North West England. I. Histopathological peer review. *Br J Cancer* 1991;**64**:315–20.
12 Hartley AL, Blair V, Harris M *et al.* Sarcomas in the North West England. II. Incidence. *Br J Cancer* 1991;**64**:1145–50.
13 Pollock RE, Karnell LH, Menck HR, Winchester DP. *The National Cancer Data Base Report on Soft Tissue Sarcoma Communication.* The Americal College of Surgeons Commission on Cancer and the American Cancer Society, 1996.
14 Vraa S, Keller J, Nielsen OS *et al.* Prognostic factors in soft tissue sarcomas: The Aarhus Experience. *Eur J Cancer* 1998;**34**:1876–82.
15 Trovik CS, Bauer HCF, Alvegard TA *et al.* Surgical margins, local recurrence and metastasis in soft tissue sarcomas: 559 surgically treated patients from the Scandinavian Sarcoma Group Register. *Eur J Cancer* 2000;**36**:710–16.
16 Wilson RB, Crowe PJ, Fisher R, Hook C, Donnellan MJ. Extremity soft tissue sarcoma: Factors predictive of local recurrence and survival. *Aust NZ Surg* 1999;**69**:344–9.
17 Collin CF, Friedrich C, Godbold J, Hajdu S, Brennan MF. Prognostic factors for local recurrence and survival in patients with localized extremetity soft-tissue sarcoma. *Semin Surg Oncol* 1988;**4**:30–7.
18 Singer S, Corson JM, Gonin R, Labow B, Eberlein TJ. Prognostic factors predictive of survival and local recurrence for extremity soft tissue sarcoma. *Ann Surg* 1994;**219**:165–73.
19 Van Unnik J, Coindre J, Contesso G. Grading of soft tissue sarcomas: experience of the EORTC soft tissue and bone sarcoma group. *Dev Oncol* 1988;**55**:7.

20  Brennan MF, Alketiar KM, Maki RG. Sarcomas of the soft tissue and bone. In: DeVita VT, ed. *Cancer. Principles and Practice of Oncology, 6th edn.* Philadelphia: Lippincott Williams & Wilkins, 2001.

21  Abbas JS, Holyoke ED, Moore R, Karakousis CP. The surgical treatment and outcome of soft-tissue sarcoma. *Arch Surg* 1981; **116**:765.

22  Potter DA, Glenn J, Kinsella T *et al.* Patterns of recurrence in patients with high grade soft tissue sarcomas. *J Clin Oncol* 1985;**3**:353.

23  Torosian MH, Friedrich C, Godbold J *et al.* Soft-tissue sarcoma: initial characteristics and prognostic factors in patients with and without metastatic disease. *Semin Surg Oncol* 1988;**4**:13.

24  Lawrence W Jr, Donegan WL, Natarajan N *et al.* Adult soft tissue sarcomas: a pattern of care survey of the American College of Sugeons. *Ann Surg* 1987;**205**:349.

25  Trojani M, Contesso G, Coindre JM *et al.* Soft tissue sarcomas of adults; study of pathological prognostic variables and definition of a histopathological grading system. *Int J Cancer* 1984;**33**:37–42.

26  Lattes R. Tumours of the soft tissue. In: AFIP. *Atlas of tumour pathology, 2nd series, Fascicle 1, Revised.* Washington, DC: Armed Forces Institute of Pathology, 1983.

27  Sarcoma Statistics in Adults Memorial-Sloan Kettering Cancer Centre website: http://www.mskcc.org

28  Stout AP. Tumours of soft tissue. In: AFIP. *Atlas of Tumour Pathology, 1st series, Fascicle 1.* Washington, DC: Armed Forces Institute of Pathology, 1957.

29  Enzinger FM, Lattes R, Torloni R. Histological typing of soft tissue tumours. In: WHO. *International Histological Classification of Tumours, No.3.* Geneva: World Health Organization, 1981.

30  Weiss SW, Sobin L. Histological typing of soft tissue tumours. In: WHO. *International Histological Classification of Tumours, 2nd edn.* Berlin: Springer-Verlag, 1994.

31  Weiss SW, Goldblum JR. In: Enzinger and Weiss's *Soft Tissue Tumours, 4th edn.* Mosby, 2001.

32  Shiraki M. Enterline H, Brooks J *et al.* Pathologic analysis of advanced adults soft tissue sarcomas, bone sarcomas and mesothelioma. *Cancer* 1989;**64**:484.

33  Present C, Russell W, Alexander R, Fu Y. Soft tissue and bone sarcoma histopathology peer review: the frequency of disagreement in diagnosis and the need for second pathology opinions. The Southeaster Cancer Study Group experience. *J Clin Oncol* 1986;**4**:1658–61.

34  Alvegard T, Berg N. Histopathology peer review of high grade soft tissue sarcoma; the Scandinavian Sarcoma Group experience *J Clin Oncol* 1989;**49**:1721.

35  Potter DA, Kinsella T, Glatstein E *et al.* High grade soft tissue sarcomas of the extremities. *Cancer* 1986;**58**:190.

36  Hashimoto H, Daimaru Y, Takeshita S *et al.* Prognostic significance of histologic parameters of soft tissue sarcomas. *Cancer* 1992;**70**:2816.

37  Markhede G, Angervall L, Stener B. A multivariate analysis of the prognosis after surgical treatment of malignant soft tissue tumours. *Cancer* 1982;**49**:1721.

38  Fong Y, Coit DG, Woodruff JM, Brennan MF. Lymph node metastasis from soft tissue sarcoma in adults: analysis of data from a prospective database of 1772 sarcoma patients. *Ann Surg* 1993;**217**:72.

39  Weingrad DN, Rosenberg SA. Early lymphatic spread of osteogenic and soft tissue sarcomas. *Surgery* 1978;**84**:231.

40  Heise HW, Myers MH, Russell WO *et al.* Recurrence-free survival time for surgically treated soft tissue sarcoma patients. Multivariate analysis of five prognostic factors. *Cancer* 1986;**57**:172–77.

41  Gaynor JJ, Tan CC, Casper ES *et al.* Refinement of clinocopathologic staging for localized soft tissue sarcoma of the extremity; A study of 423 adults. *J Clin Oncol* 1992;**10**:1317–29.

42  Weiss SW, Enzinger FM. Malignant fibrous histiocytoma; an analysis of 200 cases. *Cancer* 1978;**41**:2250.

43  Weiss SW, Enzinger FM. Myxoid variant of malignant fibrous histiocytoma. *Cancer* 1977;**39**:1672.

44  Pritchard DJ, Reiman HM, Turcotte RE, Ilstrup DM. Malignant fibrous histiocytoma of the soft tissues of the trunk and extremities. *Clin Orthop* 1993;**289**:58.

45  Bergh P, Meis-Kindblom JM, Gherlinzoni F *et al.* Synovial sarcoma. Identification of low and high risk groups. *Cancer* 1999;**85**: 2596–607.

46  Heslin MJ, Cordon-Cardo C, Lewis JJ, Woodruff JM, Brennan MF. Ki-67 detected by MIB-1 predicts distant metastasis and tumour mortality in primary, high grade extremity soft tissue sarcoma. *Cancer* 1998;**83**:490–7.

47  Cordon-Cardo C, Latres E, Drobnak M *et al.* Molecular abnormalities of mdm-2 and p53 genes in bone and soft tissue sarcomas. *Mod Pathol* 1994;**54**:794–9.

48  Wurl P, Meye A, Schmidt H *et al.* High prognostic significance of mdm-2/p53 co-overexpression in soft tissue sarcomas of the extremities. *Oncogene* 1998;**16**:1183–5.

49  Levine EA, Riobinson IB, Kim DK *et al.* MDR-1 expression of soft tissue sarcoma. *Surg Forum* 1994;**45**:503.

50  Levine EA, Holzmayer TA, Bacus S *et al.* Evaluation of new prognostic markers in metastatic malignant melanoma. *J Clin Oncol* 1997; **15**:3249.

51  Russel W, Cohen J, Enzinger F *et al.* A clinical and pathological staging system for soft tissue sarcoma. *Cancer* 1997;**40**:1562.

52  AJCC. *Cancer Staging Handbook, 5th edn.* Philadelphia: Lippincott-Raven, 1998.

53  Peabody TD, Gibbs CP, Simon MA. Evaluation and staging of musculoskelatal neoplasms. *J Bone Joint Surg (Am)* 1998;**86**:1207.

54  Sondak VK, Leonard JA Jr, Robertson JM *et al.* Limb-sparing surgery for extremity soft tissue sarcomas functional and rehabilitation considerations. *Surg Oncol Clin North Am* 1993;**2**:657.

55  Weichselbaum R, Beckett M, Vijayakumar S *et al.* Radiobiological characterization of head and neck and sarcoma cells derived from patient prior to radiotherapy. *Int J Radiat Oncol Biol Phys* 1990; **19**:313.

56  Ruka W, Taghian A, Gioioso D *et al.* Comparison between the in vitrointrinsic radiation sensitivity of human soft tissue sarcoma and breast cancer cell lines. *J Surg Oncol* 1996;**61**:290.

57  Suit H, Spiro IJ. Soft tissue sarcomas: radiation as a therapeutic option. *Ann Acad Med Singapore* 1996;**25**:855–61.

58  Lewis JJ, Leung D, Heslin M, Woodruff JM, Brennan MF. Association of local recurrence with subsequent survival in extremity soft tissue sarcoma. *J Clin Oncol* 1997;**15**:646–52.

59  Stotter AT, A'Hern RP, Fisher C *et al.* The influence of local recurrence of extremity soft tissue sarcoma on metastasis and survival. *Cancer* 1990;**65**:1119–29.

60  Brennan MF, Casper ES, Harrison LB *et al.* The role of multimodality therapy in soft-tissue sarcoma. *Ann Surg* 1991;**214**:328–38.

61  Karakousis CP, Proimakis C, Walsh DL. Primary soft tissue sarcoma of the extremities in adults. *Br J Surg* 1995;**82**:1212.

62  Enneking WF. Staging of musculoskeltal neoplasms. In: *Current Concept of Diagnosis and Treatment of Bone and Soft Tissue Tumours Uhthoff HK ed.* Heidelberg: Springer-Verlag, 1984.

63  Rosenberg S, Tepper J, Glatstein E *et al.* The treatment of soft tissue sarcomas of the extremities: prospective randomized evaluations of (1) limb-sparing surgery plus radiation therapy with amputation and (2) the role of adjuvant chemotherapy. *Ann Surg* 1982;**196**:30.

64  Abbas J, Holyoke E, Moore R *et al.* The surgical treatment and outcome of soft tissue sarcoma. *Arch Surg* 1981;**116**:765.

65  Shieber M, Graham P. An experience with sarcoma of the soft tissue in adults. *Arch Surg* 1962;**107**:295.

66  Harrison L, Franzese F, Gaynor J *et al.* Long-term results of a prospective randomized trail of adjuvant brachytherapy in the management of completely resected soft tissue sarcomas of the extremity and the superficial trunk. *Int J Radiat Oncol Biol Phys* 1993;**27**:259.

67  Azzarelli A. Surgery in soft tissue sarcomas. *Eur J Cancer* 1993;**29A**:618.

68  Simon MA, Enneking WF. The management of soft-tissue sarcomas of the extremities. *J Bone Joint Surg (Am)* 1976;**58**:317.

69  Shui MH, Castro EB, Hajdu SI, Fortner JG. Surgical treatment of 297 soft tissue sarcomas of the lower extremity. *Ann Surg* 1975; **182**:597.

70  Yang JC, Chang AE, Baker AR *et al.* Randomized prospective study of the benefit of adjuvant radiation therapy in the treatment of soft tissue sarcomas of the extremity. *J Clin Oncol* 1998;**16**:197–203.

71  Pisters PWT, Harrison LB, Leung DHY *et al.* Long-term results of a prospective randomized trial of adjuvant brachytherapy in soft tissue sarcoma. *J Clin Oncol* 1996;**14**:859–68.

72  Pisters PWT, Harrison LB, Woodruff JM, Gaynor JJ, Brennan MF. A prospective randomized trial of adjuvant brachytherapy in the management of low grade soft tissue sarcomas of the extremity and superficial trunk. *J Clin Oncol* 1994;**12**:1150–5.

73  Fabrizio PL, Stafford SL, Pritchard D. Extremity soft-tissue sarcomas selectively treated with surgery alone. *Int J Radiat Oncol Biol Phys* 2000;**48**:227–32.

74  Rydholm A, Gustafson P, Rooser B et al. Limb-sparing surgery without radiotherapy based on anatomic location of soft tissue sarcoma. *J Clin Oncol* 1991;**9**:1757–65.

75  Lindberg RD, Martin RG, Romsdahl MM, Barkley HT. Conservative surgery and postoperative radiotherapy in 300 adults with soft tissue sarcomas. *Cancer* 1982;**47**:2391–7.

76  Suit HD, Mankin HJ, Wood WC et al. Treatment of the patient with stage M₀ soft tissue sarcoma. *J Clin Oncol* 1988;**6**:854.

77  Suit HD, Mankin HJ, Wood WC, Proppe K. Preoperative, intraoperative and postoperative radiation in the treatment of primary soft tissue sarcoma. *Cancer* 1985;**55**:2659.

78  Pollack A, Zagars G, Goswitz MS et al. Preoperative vs. postoperative radiotherapy in the treatment of soft tissue sarcomas: a matter of presentation. *Int J Radiat Oncol Biol Phys* 1998;**42**:563–72.

79  Keus RB, Rutgers EJTh, Ho GH et al. Limb-sparing therapy of extremity soft tissue sarcomas: Treatment outcome and long-term functional results. *Eur J Cancer* 1994;**30A**:1459–63.

80  Wilson AN, Davis A, Bell RS et al. Local control of soft tissue sarcoma of the extremity: The experience of a multidisciplinary sarcoma group with definitive surgery and radiotherapy. *Eur J Cancer* 1994;**30A**:746–51.

81  Pao WJ, Pilepich MV. Postoperative radiotherapy in the treatment of extremity soft tissue sarcomas. *Int J Radiat Oncol Biol Phys* 1990;**19**:907.

82  Brant TA, parsons JT, Marcus RB Jr et al. Preoperative irradiation for soft tissue sarcomas of the trunk and extremities in adults. *Int J Radiat Oncol Biol Phys* 1990;**19**:889–906.

83  Barkley H, Martin R, Romsdahl M et al. Treatment of soft tissue sarcomas by preoperative irradiation and conservative surgical resection. *Int J Radiat Oncol Biol Phys* 1988;**14**:693.

84  Alektiar KM, Velasco J, Zelefsky MJ et al. Adjuvant radiotherapy for margin-positive high grade soft tissue sarcoma of the extremity. *Int J Radiat Oncol Biol Phys* 2000;**48**:1051–8.

85  Janjan NA, Yasko AW, Reece GP et al. Comparison of changes related to radiotherapy for soft tissue sarcomas treated by preoperative external beam irradiation versus interstitial implantation. *Ann Surg Oncol* 1994;**1**:415–22.

86  Suit HD, Mankin HJ, Wood WC, Proppe KH. Preoperative, intraoperative and postoperative radiation in the treatment of primary soft tissue sarcoma. *Cancer* 1985;**55**:2659–67.

87  Tyldesley S, Fryer K, Minchinton A, Durand R. Effects of debulking surgery on radiosensitivity, oxygen tension and kinetics in a mouse tumour model (Abstract). *Clin Invest Med* 1997;**20**:S83.

88  Neilsen OS, Cummings B, O'Sullivan B et al. Preoperative and postoperative irradiation of soft tissue sarcomas; effect of radiation field size. *Int J Radiat Onc Biol Phys* 1991;**21**:1595–9.

89  Pollack A, Zagars GK, Goswitz MS et al. Preoperative versus postoperative radiotherapy in the treatment of soft tissue sarcomas: a matter of presentation. *Int J Radiat Oncol Biol Phys* 1998;**42**:563–72.

90  Bujko K, Suit H, Springfield D et al. Wound healing after preoperative irradiation for sarcoma of the soft tissues. *Surg Gynaecol Obstet* 1993;**176**:124.

91  Peat B, Bell R, Davis A et al. Wound healing complications after soft tissue sarcoma surgery. *Plast Reconstr Surg* 1994;**93**:980.

92  O'Sullivan B, Davis B, Bell A et al. Phase III randomized trial of preoperative versus postoperative radiotherapy in the curative management of extremity soft tissue sarcoma. A Canadian Sarcoma and NCI Canada Clinical Trials Group Study. *ASCO Proc* 1999; **18**:535A.

93  Alketiar KM, Zelefsky MJ, Brennan MF. Morbidity of adjuvant brachytherapy in soft tissue sarcoma of the extremity and superficial trunk. *Int J Radiat Oncol Biol Phys* 2000;**47**:1273–9.

94  Sugarbaker PH, Barofsky I, Rosenberg SA, Gianola FJ. Quality of life assessment of patients in extremity sarcoma clinical trials. *Surgery* 1982;**9**:17–23.

95  Marcus SG, Merino MJ, Glatstein E et al. Long-term outcome in 87 patients with low grade soft-tissue sarcoma. *Arch Surg* 1993;**128**: 1336–43.

96  Glenn J, Kinsella T, Glatstein E et al. A randomized, prospective trial of adjuvant chemotherapy in adults with soft tissue sarcomas of the head and neck, breast and trunk. *Cancer* 1985;**55**:1206.

97  Glenn J, Sindelar WF, Kinsella T et al. Results of multimodality therapy of respectable soft tissue sarcomas of the retroperitoneum. *Surgery* 1985;**97**:316.

98  Omura GA, Blessing JA, Major F et al. A randomized clinical trial of adjuvant adriamycin in uterine sarcomas: A Gynecologic Oncology Group study. *J Clin Oncol* 1985;**3**:1240.

99  Piver MS, Lele SB, Marcheti DL, Emrich LJ. Effect of adjuvant chemotherapy on time to recurrence and survival of stage I uterine sarcomas. *J Surg Oncol* 1988;**38**:233.

100  Chang AE, Kinsella T, Glatstein E et al. Adjuvant chemotherapy for patients with high grade soft tissue sarcoma of the extremity. *J Clin Oncol* 1988;**6**:1491.

101  Benjamin RS, Terjanian TO, Fenoglio CJ et al. The importance of combination chemotherapy for adjuvant treatment of high risk patients with soft tissue sarcomas of the extremeties. In: Salmon SE, ed. *Adjuvant therapy of cancer, V.* Orlando: Grune & Stratton, 1987.

102  Edmonson JH, Fleming TR, Ivins JC et al. Randomized stidy of systemic chemotherapy following complete excision of nonosseous sarcomas. *J Clin Oncol* 1984;**2**:1390.

103  Bramwell V, Rouesse J, Steward W et al. Adjuvant CYVADIC chemotherapy for adult soft tissue sarcoma – reduced local recurrence but no improvement in survival: a study of the European Organization for Research and Treatment of Cancer – Soft Tissue and Bone Sarcoma Group. *J Clin Oncol* 1994;**12**:1137.

104  Antman K, Ryan L, Borden E et al. Pooled results from three randomized adjuvant studies of doxorubicin versus observation in soft tissue sarcomas; 10 year results and review of the literature. In: Salmon SE, ed. *Adjuvant therapy of cancer, VI.* Philadelphia: WB Saunders, 1990.

105  Lerner HJ, Amato DA, Savlov ED et al. Eastern Cooperative Oncology Group; a comparison of adjuvant doxorubicin and observation for patients with localized soft tissue sarcoma. *J Clin Oncol* 1987;**5**:613.

106  Antman K, Suit H, Amato D et al. Preliminary results of a randomized trial of adjuvant doxorubicin for sarcomas: lack of apparent difference between treatment groups. *J Clin Oncol* 1984;**2**:601.

107  Alvegard TA, Sigurdsson H, Mouridsen H et al. Adjuvant chemotherapy with doxorubicin in high grade soft tissue sarcoma: a randomized trial of the Scandinavian Sarcoma Group. *J Clin Oncol* 1989;**7**:1504.

108  Ravaud A, Bui NB, Coindre J-M et al. Adjuvant chemotherapy with CYγVADIC in high risk soft tissue sarcoma: a randomized prospective trial. In Salmon SE, ed. *Adjuvant therapy of cancer, VI.* Philadelphia: WB Saunders, 1990.

109  Gherlinzoni F, Bacci G, Picci P et al. A randomized trial for the treatment of high grade soft tissue sarcomas of the extremities: preliminary observations. *J Clin Oncol* 1986;**4**:552.

110  Frustaci S, Gherlinzoni F, De Paoli A et al. Adjuvant chemotherapy for adult soft tissue sarcomas of the extremities and girdles: Results of the Italian randomized cooperative trial. *J Clin Oncol* 2001; **19**:1238–47.

111  Brodowicz T, Schwameis E, Widder J et al. Intensified adjuvant IFADIC chemotherapy for adult soft tissue sarcoma; A prospective randomized feasibility trial. *Sarcoma* 2000;**4**:151–60.

112  Petrioli R, Coratti A, Correale P et al. Epirubicin alone or epirubicin + ifosfamide as adjuvant chemotherapy in soft tissue sarcomas. *Ann Oncol* 2000;**11**:60 (Abstr.).

113  Picci P, Bacci G, Gherlinzoni F et al. Results of a randomized trial for the treatment of localized soft tissue tumours (STS) of the extremities in adult patients. In: Ryan JR, Baker LH eds. *Recent concepts in sarcoma treatment.* Dodrecht, The Netherlands: Kluwer, 1988.

114  Gherlinzoni F, Picci P, Bacci G, Cazzola A. Late results of a randomized trial for the treatment of soft tissue sarcomas (STS) of

the extremities in adult patients. *Proc Am Soc Clin Oncol* 1993;**12**:A1633.

115 Jones GW, Chouinard E, Patel M. Adjuvant adriamycin (doxorubicin) in adult patients with soft-tissue sarcomas: a systemic overview and quantitative meta-analysis. *Clin Invest Med* 1991;**14**:A772.

116 Zalupski MM, Ryan JR, Hussein ME *et al.* Defining the role of adjuvant chemotherapy for patients with soft tissue sarcoma of the extremeties. In: Salmon SE, ed. *Adjuvant Therapy of Cancer VII.* Philadelphia: JB Lippincott, 1993.

117 Tierney JF, Mosseri V, Stewart LA, Suhami RL, Parmar MKB. Adjuvant chemotherapy for soft-tissue sarcoma: review and meta-analysis of the published results of randomized clinical trials. *Br J Cancer* 1995;**72**:469–75.

118 Sarcoma Meta-Analysis Collaboration. Adjuvant chemotherapy for localized resectable soft-tissue sarcoma of adults: meta-analysis of individual data. *Lancet* 1997;**350**:1647–54.

119 Frustaci S, Buonadonna A, Galligioni E *et al.* Increasing 4'-epidoxorubicin and fixed ifosfamide doses plus granulocyte-macrophage-colony-stimulating factor in advanced soft tissue sarcomas: A pilot study. *J Clin Oncol* 1997;**15**:1418–26.

120 Frustaci S, Foladore S, Buonadonna A *et al.* Epirubicin and ifosfamide in advanced soft tissue sarcomas. *Ann Oncol* 1993;**4**:669–72.

121 Bramwell V. Editorial – Adjuvant chemotherapy for adult soft tissue sarcoma: is there a standard of care? *J Clin Oncol* 2001;**19**:1235–7.

122 Figueredo A, Bramwell V *et al.* 11·2 Adjuvant chemotherapy following complete resection of soft tissue sarcoma in adults. A clinical practice guideline. [http://www.cancercare.on.ca/ccopgi/ > ] *Sarcoma* 2002;**6**:5–18.

123 Gortzak E, Azzarelli A, Buesa J *et al.* A randomized phase II study of neoadjuvant chemotherapy "high risk" adult soft tissue sarcoma. *Eur J Cancer* 2001;**37**:1096–103.

124 Rouesse JG, Friedman S, Sevin DM *et al.* Preoperative induction chemotherapy in the treatment of locally advanced soft tissue sarcomas. *Cancer* 1987;**60**:296.

125 Pezzi CM, Pollock RE, Evans HL *et al.* Preoperative chemotherapy for soft tissue sarcomas of the extremities. *Ann Surg* 1990;**211**:476.

126 Casper ES, Gaynor JJ, Harrison LB *et al.* Preoperative and postoperative adjuvant combination chemotherapy for adults with high grade soft tissue sarcoma. *Cancer* 1994;**73**:1644.

127 Eilber FR, Giuliano AE, Huth JF, Morton DL. Postoperative adjuvant chemotherapy (adriamycin) in high grade extremity soft tissue sarcoma: a randomized prospective trial. In: Salmon SE, ed. *Adjuvant Therapy of Cancer, V.* Orlando: Grune and Stratton, 1987.

128 Eilber FR, Giuliano AE, Huth JF, Mirra J. Neoadjuvant chemotherapy, radiation, and limited surgery for high grade soft tissue sarcoma of the extremity. In: Ryan JR, Baker LH, eds. *Recent Concepts in Sarcoma Treatment.* Dordrecht, The Netherlands: Kluwer, 1988.

129 Soulen MC, Weissman JR, Sullivan KL *et al.* Intra-arterial chemotherapy with limb-sparing resection of large soft tissue sarcomas of the extremities. *J Vasc Intervent Radiol* 1992;**3**:659.

130 Wanebo HJ, Temple WJ, Popp MB *et al.* Preoperative regional therapy for extremity sarcoma. A tricentre update. *Cancer* 1995; **75**:2299.

131 Hoekstra HJ, Schraffordt Koops H, Molenaar WM *et al.* A combination of intra arterial chemotherapy, preoperative and postoperative radiotherapy, and surgery as a limb-saving treatment of primarily unresectable high grade soft tissue sarcoma. *Cancer* 1989;**63**:59.

132 Rahoty P, Kinya A. Results of preoperative neoadjuvant chemotherapy and surgery in the management of patients with soft tissue sarcoma. *Eur J Surg Oncol* 1993;**19**:641.

133 Eggermont AMM, Schraffordt Koops H, Lienard D *et al.* Isolated limb perfusion with high dose tumour necrosis factor-alpha in combination with interferon-gamma and melphalan for nonresectable extremity soft tissue sarcomas: a multicentre trial. *J Clin Oncol* 1996;**14**:2653.

134 Eggermont AMM, Schraffordt Koops H, Klausner JM *et al.* Limb salvage by isolated limb perfusion (ILP) with TNF and melphalan in patients with locally advanced soft tissue sarcomas: outcome of 270 ILPs in 246 patients. *Proc Am Soc Clin Oncol* 1999;**18**:A2067.

135 Casper ES, Gaynor JJ, Hajdu SI *et al.* A prospective randomized trial of adjuvant chemotherapy with bolus versus continuous infusion of

doxorubicin in patients with high grade extremity soft tissue sarcoma and an analysis of prognostic factors. *Cancer* 1991;**68**:1221–9.

136 Shamberger RC, Sherins RJ, Ziegler JL *et al.* Effects of postoperative adjuvant chemotherapy and radiotherapy on ovarian function in women undergoing treatment for soft tissue sarcoma. *J Natl Cancer Inst* 1981;**67**:1213–18.

137 Shamberger RC, Sherins RJ, Ziegler JL *et al.* The effects of postoperative adjuvant chemotherapy and radiotherapy on testicular function in men undergoing treatment for soft tissue sarcoma. *Cancer* 1981;**47**:2368–74.

138 Frost DB. Pulmonary metastasectomy for soft tissue sarcomas: Is it justified? *J Surg Oncol* 1995;**59**:110–15.

139 Van Geel AN, Pastorino U, Jauch KW *et al.* Surgical treatment of lung metastases: The European Organization for Research and Treatment of Cancer – Soft Tissue and Bone Sarcoma Group Study of 255 patients. *Cancer* 1996;**77**:675–82.

140 Billingsley KG, Burt ME, Jara E *et al.* Pulmonary metastases from soft tissue sarcoma. *Ann Surg* 1999;**229**:602–12.

141 Pastorino U, Buyse M, Friedel G *et al.* Long-term results of lung metastasectomy prognostic analyses based on 5206 cases. *J Thorac Cardiovasc Surg* 1997;**113**:37–49.

142 Creagan ET, Fleming TR, Edmonnson JH *et al.* Pulmonary resection for metastatic nonosteogenic sarcoma. *Cancer* 1979;**44**:1908–12.

143 Casson AG, Putnam JB, Natarajan G *et al.* Five-year survival after pulmonary metastasectomy for adult soft tissue sarcoma. *Cancer* 1992;**69**:662–8.

144 Verazin GT, Warneke JA, Driscoll DL *et al.* Resection of lung metastases from soft tissue sarcomas. A multivariate analysis. *Arch Surg* 1992;**127**:1407–11.

145 Pastorino U, Valente M, Gasparini M *et al.* Lung resection for metastatic sarcomas. Total survival from primary treatment. *J Surg Oncol* 1989;**40**:275–80.

146 Jablons D, Steinberg SM, Roth J *et al.* Metastasectomy for soft tissue sarcoma. *J Thorac Cardiovasc Surg* 1989;**97**:695–705.

147 Robinson MH, Sheppard M, Moskovic E, Fisher C. Lung metastasectomy in patients with soft tissue sarcoma. *Br J Radiol* 1994;**67**:129–35.

148 Putnam JB, Roth JA, Wesley MN *et al.* Analysis of prognostic factors in patients undergoing resection of pulmonary metastases from soft tissue sarcomas. *J Thorac Cardiovasc Surg* 1984;**87**:260–8.

149 Rizzoni WE, Pass HI, Wesley MN *et al.* Resection of recurrent pulmonary metastases in patients with soft tissue sarcomas. *Arch Surg* 1986;**121**:1248–52.

150 Lanza LA, Putnam JB, Benjamin RS *et al.* Response to chemotherapy does not predict survival after resection of sarcomatous pulmonary metstastases. *Ann Thorac Surg* 1991;**51**:219–24.

151 Billingsley KG, Lewis JJ, Leung DHY *et al.* Multifactorial analysis of the survival of patients with distant metastasis arising from primary extremity sarcoma. Abstract. *Cancer* 1999;**85**:389–95.

152 Demetri GD, Elias AD. Results of single agent and combination chemotherapy for advanced soft tissue sarcomas. Implications for decision-making in the clinic. *Haematol Oncol Clin North Am* 1995;**9**:765–85.

153 O'Bryan RM, Baker L, Gottlieb J *et al.* Dose response evaluation of Adriamycin in human neoplasia. *Cancer* 1977;**39**:1940–8.

154 Bramwell V, Anderson D. Cancer Care Ontario practice Guidelines Initiative EBR #11.1: Doxorubicin-based combination chemotherapy for palliative treatment of adult patients with locally advanced or metastatic soft tissue sarcomas. *Sarcoma* 2000;**4**:103–12.

155 Borden EC, Amato DA, Rosenbaum CH *et al.* Randomized comparison of three adriamycin regimens for metastatic soft tissue sarcomas. *J Clin Oncol* 1987;**5**:840–50.

156 Mouridsen HT, Bastholt L, Somers R *et al.* Adriamycin versus epirubicin in advanced soft tissue sarcomas: A randomized phase II/phase III study of the EORTC Soft Tissue and Bone Sarcoma Group. *Eur J Cancer Clin Oncol* 1987;**25**:1477–83.

157 Nielsen OS, Dombernowsky P, Mouridsen H *et al.* High dose epirubicin is not an alternative to standard dose doxorubicin in the treatment of advanced soft tissue sarcomas. A study of the EORTC Soft Tissue and Bone Sarcoma group. *Br J Cancer* 1998;**78**:2634–9.

158 Lopez M, Vici P, Di Lauro L *et al.* Randomized prospective clinical trial of high dose epirubicin and dexrazoxane in patients with

advanced breast cancer and soft tissue sarcomas. *J Clin Oncol* 1998;**16**:86–92.

159 Judson I, Radford JA, Harris M *et al.* Randomized phase II trial of pegylated liposomal doxorubicin (Doxil/Caelyx) versus doxorubicin in the treatment of advanced or metastatic soft tissue sarcoma: a study by the EORTC Soft Tissue and Bone Sarcoma Group. *Eur J Cancer* 2001;**37**:870–7.

160 Blackledge G, van Oosterom A, Mouridsen H *et al.* Doxorubicin in relapsed soft tissue sarcoma; justification of phase II evaluation of new drugs in this disease. An EORTC Soft Tissue and Bone Sarcoma Group study. *Eur J Cancer* 1990;**26**:139–41.

161 Gottlieb JA, Benjamin RS, Baker LH. Role of DTIC (NSC-45338) in the chemotherapy of sarcomas. *Cancer Treat Rep* 1976; **60**:199–203.

162 Buesa JM, Mouridsen HT, van Oosterom AT *et al.* High dose DTIC in advanced soft-tissue sarcoma in the adult. *Ann Oncol* 1991;**2**:307–9.

163 Crawford SM, Jerwood D. An assessment of the relative importance of the components of CYVADIC in the treatment of soft-tissue sarcoma using regression meta analysis. *Med Inform* 1994;**19**:311–321.

164 Zalupski M, Baker LH: Ifosfamide. *J Natl Cancer Inst* 1988;**80**:556–66.

165 Schutte J, Kellner R, Seeber S. Ifosfamide in the treatment of soft tissue sarcomas: Experience at the West German Tumour Centre, Essen. *Cancer Chemother Pharmacol* 1993;**31**(Suppl. 2): S194–S198.

166 Antman KH, Montella D, Rosenbaum C *et al.* Phase II trial of ifosfamide with mesna in previously treated metastatic sarcoma. *Cancer Treat Rep* 1985;**69**:499–504.

167 Bramwell VH, Mouridsen HT, Santoro A *et al.* Cyclophosphamide versus ifosfamide. Final report of a randomized phase II trial in adult soft tissue sarcoma. *Eur J Cancer Clin Oncol* 1987;**23**:311–21.

168 van Oosterom AT, Krzemienlecki K, Nielsen OS *et al.* Randomized phase II study of the EORTC Soft Tissue and Bone sarcoma Group (STBSG) comparing two different ifosfamide (IF) regimens in chemotherapy untreated advanced soft tissue sarcoma (STS) patient. *Proc Am Soc Clin Oncol* 1997;**16**:496a (Abstr.).

169 Patel SR, Vadhan-Raj S, Papadopoulos N *et al.* High dose ifosfamide in bone and soft tissue sarcomas: Results of phase II and pilot studies – Dose response and schedule dependence. *J Clin Oncol* 1997;**15**: 2378–84.

170 Palumbo R, Palmeri S, Antimi M *et al.* Phase II study of continuous-infusion high dose ifosfamide in advanced and/or metastatic pretreated soft tissue sarcomas. *Ann Oncol* 1997;**8**:1159–62.

171 Tursz T. High dose ifosfamide in the treatment of advanced soft tissue sarcomas. *Semin Oncol* 1996;**23**(Suppl. 7):34–9.

172 Tichler T, Ghodsizade E, Brenner H. Failure of continuous infusion high dose ifosfamide as second line treatment for sarcomas: poor response rate and unacceptable renal and CNS toxicity. *Proc Am Soc Clin Oncol* 1999;**18**:544a (Abstr. #2100).

173 Buesa JM, Lopez-Pousa A, Martin J *et al.* Phase II trial of first-line high dose ifosamide in advanced soft tissue sarcomas of the adult: a study of the Spanish Group for Research on Sarcomas (GEIS). *Ann Oncol* 1998;**9**:871–6.

174 Brain E, Le Cesne A, Le Chevalier T *et al.* High dose ifosamide (HDI) can circumvent resistance to standard dose ifosfamide (SDI) in advanced soft tissue sarcomas (ASTS). *Proc Am Soc Clin Oncol* 1993;**12**:470 (Abstr. 1641).

175 Yap B-S, Benjamin RS, Burgess MA *et al.* A phase II evaluation of methyl CCNU and actinomycin D in the treatment of advanced sarcomas in adults. *Cancer* 1981;**47**:2807–9.

176 Spielmann M, Sevin D, Le Chevalier T *et al.* Second line treatment in advanced sarcomas with vindesine (VDS) and cisplatin (DDP) by continuous infusion (CI). *Proc Ann Meet Am Soc Clin Oncol* 1988;**7**:276 (Abstr. 1072).

177 Chang P, Wiernik PH. Combination chemotherapy with adriamycin and streptozotocin. 1. Clinical results in patients with advanced sarcoma. *Clin Pharmacol Therap* 1976;**20**:605–10.

178 Schoenfeld DA, Rosenbaum C, Horton J *et al.* A comparison of adriamycin versus vincristine and adriamycin, and cyclophosphamide versus vincristine, actinomycin-d and cyclophosphamide for advanced sarcoma. *Cancer* 1982;**50**:2757–62.

179 Omura GA, Major FJ, Blessing JA *et al.* A randomized study of adriamycin with and without dimethyl triazenoimidazole carboxamide in advanced uterine sarcomas. *Cancer* 1983; **52**:626–32.

180 Muss HB, Bundy B, DiSaia J *et al.* Treatment of recurrent or advanced uterine sarcoma: A randomized trial of doxorubicin versus doxorubicin and cyclophosphamide (a phase III trial of the Gynecologic Oncology group). *Cancer* 1985;**55**:1648–53.

181 Borden EC, Amato DA, Edmonson JH, Ritch PS, Shiraki M. Randomized comparison of doxorubicin and vindesine to doxorubicin for patients with metastatic soft tissue sarcomas. *Cancer* 1990;**66**:862–7.

182 Edmonson JH, Ryan LM, Blum RH *et al.* Randomized comparison of doxorubicin alone versus ifosfamide plus doxorubicin or mitomycin, doxorubicin, and cisplatin against advanced soft tissue sarcomas. *J Clin Oncol* 1993;**11**:1269–75.

183 Santoro A, Tursz T, Mouridsen H *et al.* Doxorubicin versus CYVADIC versus doxorubicin plus ifosfamide in first-line treatment of advanced soft tissue sarcomas: A randomized study of the European Organization for Research and Treatment of cancer Soft Tissue and Bone Sarcoma group. *J Clin Oncol* 1995;**13**:1537–45.

184 Antman K, Crowley J, Balcerzak SP *et al.* An intergroup phase III randomized study of doxorubicin and dacarbazine with or without ifosfamide and mesna in advanced soft tissue and bone sarcomas. *J Clin Oncol* 1993;**11**:1276–85.

185 Jelic S, Kovcin V, Milanovic N *et al.* Randomized study of high dose epirubicin versus high dose epirubucin-cisplatin chemotherapy for advanced soft tissue sarcoma. *Eur J Cancer* 1997;**33**:220–5.

186 Reichardt P, Lentzsch S, Hohenberger P, Doerken B. Dose intensive treatment with ifosfamide, epirubicin and filgrastim for patients with metastatic or locally advanced soft tissue sarcoma (STS): a phase II study. *Proc Am Soc Clin Oncol* 1995;**14**:518 (Abstr. 1698).

187 De Pas T, De Braud F, Orlando L *et al.* High dose ifosfamide plus adriamycin in the treatment of adult advanced soft tissue sarcomas: Is it feasible? *Ann Oncol* 1998;**9**:917–19.

188 Reichardt P, Tilgner J, Hohenberger P, Dorken B. Dose-intensive chemotherapy with ifosfamide, epirubicin, and filgrastim for adult patients with metastatic or locally advanced soft tissue sarcoma: a phase II study. *J Clin Oncol* 1998;**16**:1438–43.

189 Palumbo R, Neumaier C, Cosso M *et al.* Dose-intensive first-line chemotherapy with epirubicin and continuous infusion ifosfamide in adult patients with advanced soft tissue sarcomas: a phase II study. *Eur J Cancer* 1999;**35**:66–72.

190 Steward WP, Verweij J, Somers R *et al.* Doxorubicin plus ifosfamide with rhGM-CSF in the treatment of advanced adult soft-tissue sarcomas: preliminary results of a phase II study from the EORTC Soft-Tissue and Bone Sarcoma Group. *J Cancer Res Clin Oncol* 1991;**117**(Suppl. IV):S193–S197.

191 Steward WP, Verweij J, Somers R *et al.* Granulocyte-macrophage colony-stimulating factor allows safe escalation of dose-intensity of chemotherapy in metastatic adult soft tissue sarcomas: a study of the European Organization for Research and Treatment of Cancer Soft Tissue and Bone Sarcoma Group. *J Clin Oncol* 1993;**11**: 15–21.

192 Le Cesne A, Judson I, Crowther D *et al.* Randomized phase III study comparing conventional-dose doxorubicin plus ifosfamide versus high dose doxorubicin plus ifosfamide plus recombinant human granulocyte-macrophage colony-stimulating factor in advanced soft tissue sarcomas: A trial of the European Organization for Research and Treatment of Cancer/Soft Tissue and Bone Sarcoma Group. *J Clin Oncol* 2000;**18**:2676–84.

193 Bui NB, Demaille MC, Chevreau C *et al.* qMAID vs MAID + 25% with G-CSF in adults with advanced soft tissue sarcoma (STS). First results of a randomized study of the FNCLCC sarcoma group. *Proc ASCO* 1998;**17**:(Abstr. 1991).

194 Kraybill WG, Spiro I, Harris J *et al.* Radiation Therapy Oncology Group (RTOG) 95–14: a Phase II study of neoadjuvant chemotherapy and radiation therapy in high risk, high grade soft tissue sarcomas of the extremities and body wall: a preliminary report. *Proc ASCO* 2001;**20**:(Abstr. 1387).

# Section XI

## Treating central nervous system tumours

*Robin Grant, Editor*

# Levels of evidence and grades of recommendation used in *Evidence-based Oncology*

Levels of evidence and grades of recommendation appear within the text in the clinical chapters, for example, **Evidence Level Ia** and **Grade A**.

---

### Levels of evidence

| | |
|---|---|
| Ia | Meta-analysis of randomised controlled trials (RCTs) |
| Ib | At least 1 RCT |
| IIa | At least 1 non-randomised study |
| IIb | At least 1 other well designed quasi-experimental study |
| III | Non-experimental, descriptive studies |
| IV | Expert committee reports or opinions/experience of respected authorities |

### Grades of recommendations

| | |
|---|---|
| A | At least one RCT as part of body of literature of overall good quality and consistency addressing recommendation **Evidence levels Ia, Ib** |
| B | No RCT but well conducted clinical studies available  **Evidence levels IIa, IIb, III** |
| C | Expert committee reports or opinions/experience of respected authorities in the absence of directly applicable good quality clinical studies **Evidence level IV** |

From *Clinical Oncology* (2001)**13**:S212
Source of data: MEDLINE, *Proceedings of the American Society of Medical Oncology* (ASCO).

# 47 Central nervous system tumours

## Low grade gliomas: how should patients be managed?

*MJ van den Bent*

### Background

Low grade gliomas (LGG) account for approximately 20% of all gliomas and have an incidence of 1–2/100 000 population/year. LGG include grade II astrocytomas, oligodendrogliomas and mixed oligoastrocytomas according to the WHO classification.[1] Five-year and 10-year survival figures are 50–80% and 20–30%, respectively. Most patients die from locally recurrent disease, at which time 65% of LGG have transformed to a higher grade.[2–9]

There is almost no level I and level II evidence available for the treatment of LGG. Several large studies have shown that the influence of pretreatment characteristics like age, size of the tumour, performance status and mode of presentation outweigh the influence of treatment on survival.[8,10,11] There is a good-prognosis subset of patients: young (< 40 years), presenting with seizures only, with an MRI brain scan with features of a probable LGG. The MR features are: a high signal lesion on T2-weighted images and low signal non-enhancing lesion on T1-weighted images often without mass effect. These patients have a reasonable quality of life and may survive for many years without any tumour-directed treatment. In this situation many physicians defer pathological diagnosis and lesion directed treatment for as long as possible. Other clinicians advocate early treatment with extensive tumour resection, followed by radiation therapy.

Thus, two clinical situations requiring decision making must be distinguished:

- patients presenting with a presumed LGG, and
- patients with histologically proven LGG.

For an optimal management of these patients four questions must be considered.

### How reliable is imaging diagnosis of "presumed LGG"?

Several studies of consecutive patients with MR imaging suggestive of LGG have shown that 30–45% of these tumours when biopsied/resected are found to have HGGs (HGG) (usually anaplastic astrocytomas).[12–14] One study suggests that 31% of all histologically verified anaplastic astrocytomas and 4% of glioblastoma multiforme did not have contrast enhancement on CT-scan.[15] Proponents of an early intervention see the poor agreement between imaging and histology as a strong argument for early histological verification since patients with HGGs should be treated with radiotherapy early. However, the assumption that an early diagnosis and treatment improves outcome has never been proven in clinical trials. Proponents of a "wait and see" approach believe that timely neuroradiological follow up will identify those patients with progressive lesions requiring histological diagnosis and treatment and delayed radiotherapy reduces the late risk of "leuco-encephalopathy" with apraxia, dementia and incontinence.

### When to operate on patients with LGG – is there any evidence?

To answer the question about early diagnosis and treatment in presumed LGG requires a randomised controlled trial. A randomised controlled trial of "wait and watch" policy versus "early surgery and treat" was attempted by the MRC (BRO8) in 1994. This trial failed to accrue patients because individual clinicians had firmly held views and patients did not wish to be randomised. Prospective studies trying to address this issue should include all patients with presumed LGG based on imaging, not just patients with histologically proven LGG.[16] Studies of presumed LGG are uncommon, retrospective and of small size. One such study compared 26 patients with presumed LGG patients with seizures only and in whom treatment was deferred, to a non-matched group of 20 patients who underwent early surgery. No differences were found between both groups with regard to time to malignant transformation and overall survival.[9] A second study investigated quality of life and cognitive function in 24 patients with suspected LGG who presented with seizures and compared them with 24 matched patients who had seizures with proven but not irradiated LGG.[17] Patients with biopsied or resected LGG were found to have a worse quality of life and cognitive status in comparison to patients with suspected LGG **Evidence level II**.

## Can patients be selected where early diagnosis and treatment are indicated?

It has been assumed that the presence of poor prognostic factors can be used to identify patients who require treatment.[18] This assumption has never been validated. The presence of focal deficits, intractable seizures, or raised intracranial pressure constitutes a clear rationale to treat the patient in order to improve symptoms and possibly prevent deterioration. There are no well conducted prospective studies demonstrating the symptomatic risk:benefit ratio. The presence of a lesion with mass effect is usually seen as a reason to start treatment, as this may herald focal deficits or increased intracranial pressure. Older patients (> 50 years) with a non-enhancing lesion on imaging have a higher risk of having a malignant histology and have a poorer prognosis. A more interventional approach to patients over 50 years of age with presumed or proven LGG is probably indicated as the survival is less good and therefore the risk of developing late radiation-induced dementia is less.[13,19] However, no strict cut-off level with regard to age can be chosen based on the current literature.

## Which treatments are of proven benefit in LGG?

### Surgery

There are four theoretical reasons to perform surgery in a presumed LGG:

- to confirm the nature of the lesion
- to improve the neurological condition of the patient
- to minimise the risk of a recurrence
- to prevent malignant transformation.

A histological diagnosis is achieved in > 95% of cases biopsied and the remaining 5% are "non-diagnostic".

Small series of selected cases suggest that surgery may improve the neurological condition and the control of seizures.[16,20] These studies are on very selected patients, for example medically intractable seizures at a surgically accessible site and where the effects of steroids and subsequent radiotherapy cannot be accounted for adequately. There are no randomised controlled trials of biopsy versus resection in presumed LGG or randomised studies examining the extent of resection with respect to time to recurrence or survival. Several large retrospective series have identified the extent of resection in multivariate analysis as an important prognostic factor,[21–23] but others show no difference in outcome between biopsy and resection.[2] None of these studies evaluated the extent of resection by direct postoperative CT or MR scan. In one of

the best retrospective studies on extent of resection, preoperative and postoperative tumour volume were quantitated.[24] Both a smaller preoperative and a smaller postoperative tumour volume were associated with longer time to tumour progression and to malignant transformation. This suggests a role for more extensive resections leaving as little residual tumour volume as possible. However, in this and other series, there was an association between extent of resection and site of tumour (smaller superficial tumours more likely to have extensive resections).[3,10,22] Thus, it remains unclear whether the improved outcome after more extensive resections is indeed due to the extent of resection or whether it is related to the size (or site) or the biological behaviour of the tumour.

### Radiation therapy

A prospective trial observed a clear radiological response to radiation therapy in almost one-third of patients[8] and small retrospective surveys have suggested improvement of neurological function or seizure control after radiation.[25,26] A large randomised trial demonstrated a modest increase in time to progression after early radiation therapy when compared with delayed radiation therapy given at the time of imaging progression (Table 47.1) **Evidence level Ib**.[6] However, after a median follow up of 5 years no evidence was found that early postoperative radiation therapy improved overall survival.

Virtually all recurrences of LGG after radiation therapy occur within the irradiated volume.[8,27,28] One might expect local control to be improved after higher doses of cranial irradiation (but late radiation toxicity to be greater). However, two large multicentre randomised controlled trials totalling 590 patients have failed to demonstrate improved survival after high dose radiation therapy (59·4 Gy–64·8 Gy) compared with standard dose radiation (45 Gy–50·4 Gy) (Table 47.1) **Evidence level Ib**.[7,8] In the high dose radiation therapy groups, slightly more toxicity was observed and lower levels of quality of life were reported.[8,29] A major shortcoming of the quality-of-life analysis was the poor adherence to that part of the study.

### Chemotherapy

There is only one small (N = 60) and prematurely closed phase III trial of adjuvant chemotherapy (CCNU) after radiation therapy in LGG.[30] The small sample size precludes a meaningful analysis. Small phase II trials on low grade oligodendroglioma showed that low grade oligodendrogliomas are as sensitive to PCV chemotherapy as anaplastic oligodendrogliomas. Future studies of chemotherapy in LGG need to separate oligodendrogliomas and astrocytomas

**Table 47.1** Survival and progression-free survival as reported in the European Organisation for Research and Treatment of Cancer and Radiation Therapy and Oncology Group (EORTC) prospective randomised trials on high dose versus low dose radiation therapy and early versus deferred radiation therapy

| Study/radiation therapy | N | Progression-free survival at 5 year | Overall survival at 5 year | Median survival |
|---|---|---|---|---|
| EORTC 22844 | | | | Not reached after median follow up of 6·1 years |
| 45 Gy | 343 | 47 | | |
| 59·4 Gy | | 50 | | |
| RTOG | | | | Not reached after median follow up of 6·4 years |
| 50·4 Gy | 203 | | 72 | |
| 64·8 gy | | | 65 | |
| EORTC 22845 | | | | Not reached after median follow up of 5 years |
| early RT 54 Gy | 290 | 44 | 63 | |
| deffered RT | | 37* | 66 | |

*P = 0·02

because of the increased chance of response to chemotherapy and survival with oligodendrogliomas.[31–33]

## Summary

There is no good evidence that early treatment improves outcome in patients who present with seizures only and are shown to have imaging-suspected or histologically proven LGG. If a "wait and see" policy is followed, a brain scan should be performed regularly to look for contrast enhancement or progression. In elderly patients (> 50 years of age) closer follow up is indicated given their, in general, poorer prognosis and higher risk for malignant transformation.

Intervention is indicated in patients who have focal deficits, signs of raised intracranial pressure, intractable seizures, or a lesion with mass effect. Although the evidence in favour of maximal resection is poor, it should be considered in patients in whom a safe extensive resection is possible (frontal site or lobar tumours).

Radiation therapy is of symptomatic benefit for patients with LGG, but randomised trials have not provided evidence of improved survival after early radiation. Thus, radiotherapy can be withheld until clinically necessary.

A radiation dosage of 45–50 Gy gives similar outcome and is better tolerated than treatment up to a dosage of 60–65 Gy.

The role of adjuvant chemotherapy in LGG is unknown. Chemotherapy may be valuable in patients who have an oligodendroglioma, but timing of chemotherapy (before radiation, adjuvantly after radiation or held until radiological or clinical relapse) is unknown.

## References

1 IARC. *World Health Classification of tumours. Pathology and genetics of tumours of the nervous system.* Lyon: International Agency for the Research on Cancer, 2000.

2 Shaw EG, Daumas-Duport C, Scheithauer B *et al.* Radiation therapy in the managment of low grade supratentorial astrocytomas. *J Neurosurg* 1989;**70**:853–61.

3 Touboul E, Schlienger M, Buffat L *et al.* Radiation therapy with or without surgery in the management of low-grade brain astrocytomas. A retrospective study of 120 patients. *Bull Cancer/Radiother* 1995;**82**:388–95.

4 Kreth FW, Faist M, Rossner R, Volk B, Ostertag CB. Supratentorial World Health Organization grade 2 astrocytomas and oligoastrocytomas. *Cancer* 1997;**79**:370–9.

5 Piepmeier J, Cristopher S, Spencer D *et al.* Variations in the natural history and survival of patients with supratentorial low-grade astrocytomas. *Neurosurgery* 1996;**38**:872–9.

6 Karim, ABMF, Cornu, P, Bleehen, NM *et al.* Immediate postoperative radiotherapy in low grade glioma improves progression free survival, but not overall survival: preliminary results of an EORTC/MRC randomized phase III study. *Int J Radiat Oncol Biol Phys* 2002;**52**: 316–24.

7 Karim ABMF, Maat B, Hatlevoll R *et al.* A randomized trial on dose-response in radiation therapy of low grade cerebral glioma: European Organization for Research and Treatment of Cancer (EORTC) study 2284. *Int J Radiation Oncol Biol Phys* 1996;**36**: 549–56.

8 Shaw E, Arusell RM, Scheithauer B *et al.* A prospective randomized trial of low versus high dose radiation in adults with a supratentorial low grade glioma: initial report of a NCCTG-RTOG-ECOG study. *J Clin Oncol* 2002;**20**:2267–76.

9 Recht LD, Lew R, Smith TW. Suspected low-grade glioma: is deferring treatment safe? *Ann Neurol* 1992;**31**:431–6.

10 Pignatti, F, van den Bent, MJ, Curran, D *et al.* Prognostic factors for survival in adult patients with cerebral low-grade glioma. *J Clin Oncol* 2002;**20**:2076–84.

11 Bauman G, Lote K, Larson D *et al.* Pretreatment factors predict overall survivall for patients with low grade glioma: a recursive partitioning analysis. *Int J Radiation Oncol Biol Phys* 1999;**45**:923–9.

12 Ginsberg LE, Fuller GN, Hashmi M, Leeds NE, Schomer DF. The significance of lack of MR contrast enhancement of supratentorial brain tumors in adults: histopathological evaluation of a series. *Surg Neurol* 1998;**49**:436–40.

13  Barker FG, Chang CH, Huhn SL *et al.* Age and the risk of anaplasia in magnetic resonance-nonenhancing supratentorial cerebral tumors. *Cancer* 1997;**80**:936–41.

14  Kondziolka D, Lunsford LD, Martinez AJ. Unreliability of contemporary neurodiagnostic imaging in evaluating suspected adult supratentorial (low-grade) astrocytoma. *J Neurosurg* 1993;**79**:533–6.

15  Chamberlain MC, Murovic JA, Levin VA. Absence of contrast enhancement on CT brain scans of patients with supratentorial malignant gliomas. *Neurology* 1988;**38**:1371–4.

16  van Veelen MLC, Avezaat CJJ, Kros JM, van Putten WL, Vecht CJ. Supratentorial low grade astrocytoma: prognostic factors, dedifferentiation, and the issue of early versus late surgery. *J Neurol Neurosurg Psych* 1998;**64**:581–7.

17  Reijneveld JC, Sitskoorn MM, Klein M, Nuyen J, Taphoorn MJB. Cognitive status and quality of life in suspected versus proven low-grade gliomas. *Neurology* 2001;**56**:618–23.

18  Vecht CJ. Effect of age on treatment decisions in low-grade glioma. *J Neurol Neurosurg Psych* 1993;**56**:1259–64.

19  Shafqat S, Hedley-Whyte ET, Henson JW. Age-dependant rate of anaplastic transformation in low grade astrocytoma. *Neurology* 2001;**52**:867–9.

20  Britton JW, Cascino GD, Sharbrough FW, Kelly PJ. Low-grade glial neoplasms and intractable partial epilepsy: efficacy of surgical treatment. *Epilepsia* 1994;**35**:1130–5.

21  Leighton C, Fisher B, Bauman G *et al.* Supratentorial low-grade glioma in adults: an analysis of prognostic factors and the timing of radiation. *J Clin Oncol* 1997;**15**:1294–301.

22  Scerrati M, Roselli R, Iacoangeli M, Pompucci A, Rossi GF. Prognostic factors in low grade (WHO II) gliomas of the cerebral hemispheres: the role of surgery. *J Neurol Neurosurg Psych* 1996;**61**:291–6.

23  Nicolato A, Gerosa MA, Fina P, Iuzzelino P, Giorgiutti FBA. Prognostic factors in low-grade supratentorial astrocyomas: a uni-multivariate statistical analysis in 76 surgically treated patients. *Neurosurgery* 1995;**44**:208–23.

24  Berger MS, Deliganis AV, Dobbins J, Keles GE. The effect of extent of resection on recurrence in patients with low grade cerebral hemisphere gliomas. *Cancer* 1994;**74**:1784–91.

25  Rogers LR, Morris HH, Lupica K. Effect on cranial irradiation on seizure frequency in adults with low-grade astrocytoma and medically intractable epilepsy. *Neurology* 1993;**43**:1599–601.

26  Bauman G, Pahapill P, Macdonald D, Fisher B, Leighton C, Cairncross G. Low grade glioma: measuring radiographic response to radiotherapy. *Can J Neurol Sci* 1999;**26**:18–22.

27  Rudoler S, Corn BW, Werner-Wasik M *et al.* Patterns of tumor progression after radiotherapy for low grade gliomas. *Am J Clin Oncol* 1998;**21**:23–7.

28  Pu AT, Sandler HM, Radany EH *et al.* Low grade gliomas: preliminary analysis of failure patterns among patients treated with 3D conformal external beam irradiation. *Int J Radiation Oncol Biol Phys* 1995;**31**:461–6.

29  Kiebert GM, Curran W, Aaronson NK *et al.* Quality of life after radiation therapy of cerebral low-grade gliomas of the adult: results of a randomised phase III trial on dose response (EORTC trial 22844). *Eur J Cancer* 1998;**34**:1902–9.

30  Eyre HJ, Quagliana JM, Eltringham JR *et al.* Randomised comparison of radiotherapy and CCNU versus radiotherapy, CCNU plus procarbazine for the treatment of malignant gliomas following surgery. *J Neurooncol* 1993;**1**:171–7.

31  Mason WP, Krol GS, DeAngelis LM. Low-grade oligodendroglioma responds to chemotherapy. *Neurology* 1996;**46**:203–7.

32  van den Bent MJ, van der Rijt CDD, Enting RH *et al.* PCV chemotheraphy in newly diagnosed and recurrent oligodendroglial tumors. *Neuro-Oncology* 2002;**4**:378(abst.).

33  van den Bent MJ, Kros JM, Heimans JJ *et al.* Response rate and prognostic factors of recurrent oligodendroglioma treated with PCV chemotherapy. *Neurology* 1998;**51**:1140–5.

# HGG: how effective is surgery?

*IR Whittle*

High grade or malignant gliomas account for 80% of all gliomas and have an incidence of approximately six cases per 100 000 population. Glioblastoma, anaplastic astrocytoma (AA), and anaplastic oligodendroglioma are the commonest high grade gliomas (HGG). These are incurable tumours of the brain parenchyma with median survival times of between 9 and 13 months for patients included in phase III trials. Powerful prognostic factors are younger age and good performance status.

Biopsy or resection confirm diagnosis in around 98% of patients with suspected HGG. Where the lesion is difficult to access, biopsy may be the only surgical option. Alternatively, a large superficial lesion with considerable mass effect causing symptoms can be resected moderately easily. Resection can relieve many of the symptoms and signs of raised intracranial pressure, may improve neurological functioning, and offer a smoother course for the patient during radiotherapy because of the reduced requirement for high dose steroids. In practice, many patients fall between these two extremes (moderate size, not too many signs or symptoms, access is not too hazardous). Are these patients better served by stereotactic biopsy or resection?

## Do patients who have had surgical resection live longer?

A recent Cochrane review of the literature revealed no randomised or clinical controlled trials comparing outcomes of biopsy versus resection for malignant glioma.[1] The majority of papers on this topic were retrospective, uncontrolled, and prone to selection bias and trial design.

Simpson *et al.*[2] reported on 645 patients with glioblastoma multiforme involved in Radiation Therapy Oncology Group (RTOG) clinical trials. The median survival time (MST) for patients who had undergone total resection followed by radiotherapy was significantly greater than that of patients who underwent biopsy and radiotherapy (11·3 v 6·6 months). A significant difference in MST was also found for partial resection versus biopsy (10·4 v 6·6 months). Other studies support a survival advantage of resection for both GBM and AA.[3–9] However, there are also studies where the extent of resection has not been found to be a significant prognostic factor.[10–13] Kreth *et al.*[11] reported a retrospective study of GBM cases to compare the results of stereotactic biopsy with those of surgical resection – both groups received radiation therapy. Patients who underwent biopsy were those who carried a greater surgical risk and had worse performance status; however, despite this, no significant difference in MST was found. The importance of case mix was also shown by Latif *et al.*[14] where unadjusted data showed macroscopic resection was a highly significant independent prognostic variable ($P = 0·004$; N = 236 cases); however, after adjustment for case mix, extent of resection was not a significant variable.

## What is the functional morbidity following surgery for HGG?

Impressive functional benefits, low complication rate and reduced hospital stay have been reported for selected patient groups.[15,16] However, a recent Scottish prospective audit (N = 232) of functional outcome, using the Edinburgh Functional Impairment Tests (EFIT), showed that of 153 patients who had resection, only 24% were functionally better, 46% were unchanged and 30% were functionally worse. After biopsy (N = 79) 10% were better, 31% unchanged, and 36% were functionally worse. Fadul *et al.*[17] reported that of 207 abnormal signs present before resection only 8% improved, but 16% were worse. These figures

**Table 47.2  Functional changes after surgery for high grade glioma**

|  | No. of patients | Better % | Unchanged % | Worse % |
|---|---|---|---|---|
| *Biopsy* | | | | |
| Vecht *et al.*[7] (1990) | 16 | 19 | 75 | 5 |
| *Resection* | | | | |
| Fadul *et al.*[17] (1988)* | 213 | | 76 | 26 |
| Vecht *et al.*[7] (1990) | 86 | 30 | 50 | 20 |
| Sawaya *et al.*[18] (1998)* | 166 | 32 | 58 | 9 |
| Taylor *et al.*[16] (1999)* | 200 | – | – | 13 |

The times that assessments were done after surgery are often not stated. Resection is used to cover all forms of resective or decompressive surgery.
*Prospective series.

**Table 47.3   Morbidity and mortality from various series after biopsy or resection of high grade glioma**

| | No. of patients | Morbidity % | Mortality % |
|---|---|---|---|
| *Biopsy* | | | |
| Vecht *et al.*[7] (1990) | 17 | 12 | 35* |
| Bernstein *et al.*[19] (1994) | 300 | 3 | 2 |
| | | | |
| *Resection* | | | |
| Ciric *et al.*[20] (1987) | 42 | 14 | 0 |
| Fadul *et al.*[17] (1988) | 213 | 32 | 3* |
| Vecht *et al.*[7] (1990) | 226 | 23 | 20* |
| Cabantog *et al.*[21] (1994) | 108 | 26 | 2 |
| Sawaya *et al.*[18] (1998) | 166 | 11 | 2 |
| Taylor *et al.*[16] (1999) | 200 | 17 | 1 |

All series are retrospective except Fadul *et al.* and Sawaya *et al.*
*30-day mortality.

suggest functional impairment will be improved only in the minority of patients and any surgery can have complications (Table 47.2). Even after resection using "safer" methods, such as awake craniotomy and brain mapping, 13% of patients had new neurological deficits.[16] Outcome data will reflect the case mix of the operated cohort. It is impossible to make patients without abnormal signs better, whereas patients with severe deficits are more likely to have a response to resection.

## What is the morbidity and mortality of surgery for HGG?

Publications record complications in 3–32% of patients having either biopsy or resection (Table 47.3). Studies vary as to whether non-neurological complications, such as pneumonia, urinary tract infection and DVT, are included in "complications". For example, Sawaya and colleagues[18] quote a 13% major morbidity but an overall complication rate of 32%. A recent prospective study from three Scottish Neuroscience Centres had a 10·4% systemic and neurological complication rate after resection of HGG (153 patients) and 3·8% after biopsy (79 patients). Procedural related mortality needs to be carefully separated from 30-day mortality since many patients with HGG, particularly the elderly and impaired, die shortly after diagnosis. This is not simple since some poor grade patients may suffer minor or major complications that hasten their death.

## Summary

HGG is an incurable disease. Image-guided biopsy has a very high diagnostic rate. Although surgical resection can

offer the prospect of improved neurological functioning and relief of symptoms related to raised intracranial pressure there can, as with even biopsy, be significant associated morbidity. The impact of novel technologies such as neuronavigation, intraoperative MR-guided resection, and the marriage of fMRI data to intraoperative navigation systems on reducing complications and maximising resection have not been rigorously assessed.[23,24] Initial results in selected series results are impressive. The contribution of resective surgery to prolonging life and improving quality of survival in these patients remains unknown.

## References

1   Metcalfe SE. Biopsy versus resection for malignant glioma. *Cochrane Database Syst Rev* 2000;(2):CD0002034.
2   Simpson JR, Horton J, Scott C. Influence of location and extent of surgical resection on survival of patients with glioblastoma. Results of three consecutive Radiation Therapy Oncology Group (RTOG) clinical trials. *Int J Radiat Oncol Biol Phys* 1993;**26**:239–244.
3   Devaux BC, O'Fallon JR, Kelly PJ. Resection, biopsy and survival in malignant glioma. *J Neurosurg* 1993;**78**:219–27.
4   Ammirati M, Vick N, Liao Y, Ciric I, Mikhael M. Effect of extent of surgical resection on survival and quality of life in patients with supratentorial glioblastoma and anaplastic astrocytoma. *Neurosurgery* 1987;**21**:201–6.
5   Jeremic B, Grucijcic D, Antunovic V, Djuric L, Stajanovic M, Shibamoto Y. Influence of extent of surgery and tumour location on treatment outcome of patients with glioblastoma multiforme treated with combined modality approach. *J Neuro-oncol* 1994;**21**:177–85.
6   Wisoff JH, Boyett JM, Berger MS. Current neurosurgical management and the impact of the extent of resection in the treatment of malignant gliomas of childhood. A report of the Children's Cancer Group trial no CCG-945. *J Neurosurg* 1998;**89**:52–9.
7   Vecht CJ, Avezaat CJJ, van Putten WLJ, Eijkenboom WMH, Stefanko SZ. The influence of the extent of surgery on the neurological function and survival in malignant glioma. A retrospective analysis in 243 patients. *J Neurol Neurosurg Psychiatr* 1990;**53**:466–71.

8   Halperin EC, Herndon J, Schold J. A phase III randomised prospective trial of external beam radiotherapy, mitomycin C, arumstine, and 6-mercaptopurine for the treatment of adults with anaplastic astrocytoma.. *Int J Radiat Oncol Biol Biophys* 1996;**34**:793–802.

9   Kiwit JCW, Floeth FW, Bock WJ. Survival in malignant glioma; analysis of prognostic factors with special regard to cytoreductive surgery. *Zentbl Neurochirurg* 1996;**57**:76–88.

10  Nazzaro J, Neuwelt E. The role of surgery in the management of supratentorial intermediate and high grade astrocytoma in adults. *J Neurosurg* 1990;**73**:331–4.

11  Kreth FW, Warnke PC, Scheremet R, Ostertag C. Surgical resection and radiation therapy versus biopsy and radiation therapy in the treatment of glioblastoma. *J Neurosurg* 1993;**78**:762–6.

12  Quigley M, Marron J. The relationship between survival and extent of resection in patients with supratentorial malignant glioma. *Neurosurgery* 1991;**29**:385–9.

13  Curran Jr WJ, Scott CB, Horton J. Does extent of resection influence outcome for astrocytoma with atypical or anaplastic foci (AAF)? A report from three Radiation Therapy Oncology Group (RTOG) trials. *J Neuro-oncol* 1992;**12**:219–27.

14  Latif AZ, Signorini D, Whittle IR. Treatment by specialist surgical neuro-oncologist does not provide any survival advantage for patients with a malignant glioma. *Br J Neurosurg* 1998;**12**:29–32.

15  Whittle IR, Thomson AM, Taylor R. The effects of resective surgery for left sided intracranial tumours on language function: a prospective study. *Lancet* 1998;**351**:1014–18.

16  Taylor MD, Bernstein M. Awake craniotomy with brain mapping as the routine surgical approach to treating patients with supratentorial intraaxial tumors: a prospective trial of 200 cases. *J Neurosurg* 1999; :35–41.

17  Fadul C, Wood J, Thaler H, Galicich J, Patterson RH, Posner JB. Morbidity and mortality of craniotomy for excision of supratentorial gliomas. *Neurology* 1988;**38**:1374–7.

18  Sawaya R, Hammoud M, Schoppa D *et al.* Neurosurgical outcomes in a modern series of 400 craniotomies for treatment of parenchymal tumors. *Neurosurgery* 1998;**42**:1044–56.

19  Bernstein M, Parrent AG. Complications of CT-guided stereotactic biopsy intra-axial brain lesions. *J Neurosurg* 1994;**81**:165–8.

20  Ciric I, Ammirati M, Vick N, Mikhael M. Supratentorial gliomas: surgical considerations and immediate postoperative results. Gross total resection versus partial resection. *Neurosurgery* 1987;**21**:21–6.

21  Cabantog AM, Bernstein M. Complications of first craniotomy for intra-axial brain tumour. *Can J Neurol Sci* 1994;**21**:213–18.

22  Bohinski RJ, Kokkino AK, Warnick RE *et al.* Glioma resection in a shared resource Magnetic Resonance Operating room after optimal image-guided frameless stereotactic resection. *Neurosurgery* 2001; **48**:731–44.

23  Wirtz CR, Albert FK, Schwaderer M *et al.* The benefit of neuronavigation for neurosurgery analyzed by its impact on glioblastoma surgery. *Neurol Res* 2000;**22**:354–60.

24  Truwit C, ed. MR guided therapy in neurosurgery. *Neuroimag Clin North Am* 2000;**11**:575–797.

# HGG – how effective is radiotherapy?

*Michael Brada*

## Background

Management of patients with HGG is essentially that of care of patients with incurable malignancy. While the primary measure of efficacy of treatment remains survival, the palliative value of treatment and the issues of care are equally important but poorly studied endpoints. The treatment modality tested in randomised trials that has shown the largest magnitude of survival benefit is radiation therapy. While effective, it is not without side effects and its palliative efficacy is not proven beyond doubt. Although the perception of radiation is of damaging therapy causing structural damage in the form of necrosis and functional impairment with cognitive dysfunction, these are rarely significant clinical problems and when they do occur the cause is multifactorial with radiation merely a contributing factor. The most onerous side effect of radiation is tiredness, which may persist for weeks or months after radiotherapy and may adversely affect quality of life.

## How effective is radiotherapy in prolonging survival?

The evidence for efficacy of radiotherapy (Table 47.4) is based on two randomised trials performed in the 1970s. In the BTCG trial, 303 patients with HGG were randomised into four treatment arms testing the efficacy of radiotherapy and chemotherapy alone and in combination. Radiotherapy with or without chemotherapy prolonged median survival by approximately 6 months.[1] A similar Scandinavian randomised trial in 118 patients with malignant glioma also demonstrated a near 6 months' median survival benefit for radiotherapy. A randomised Scandinavian study of 171 patients aimed at testing chemotherapy as an alternative to radiation also demonstrated benefit for radiotherapy noted in patients < 50 years of age, although this study was underpowered to demonstrate age-related effects.[2]

## What are the optimum radiation parameters?

### Volume of irradiation

Based on pre-CT era evidence of tumour spread beyond the presumed tumour mass, external beam radiotherapy had been given to the whole brain. The safety and efficacy of reduced volume radiation has been tested in only one randomised study, which did not demonstrate a survival difference between whole brain radiotherapy throughout and whole brain radiotherapy followed by localised boost to the same total radiation dose.[3] These data have largely been superseded by a universally adopted policy of localised radiotherapy attempting to avoid irradiating normal brain. The rationale is based on a well-documented recurrence pattern where the majority of malignant gliomas recur as a direct extension of the enhancing primary tumour mass. Most reported studies (phase II) suggest no apparent detriment from localised rather than whole brain irradiation. The definition of localised volume of irradiation has not been tested in randomised studies and the usual practice is to treat to high dose the region of enhancement with a 2–5 cm margin.

## Radiation dose

Initial sequential dose finding studies suggested survival benefit for increasing radiotherapy dose from 50 to 60 Gy.[6] The dose–response relationship was confirmed in an MRC randomised trial where patients randomised to receive 60 Gy in 30 fractions had a median survival benefit of 3 months compared with patients receiving 45 Gy in 20 fractions.[4] A randomised RTOG study demonstrated no further survival benefit for an additional 10 Gy boost following 60 Gy whole brain irradiation.[7] The current practice in HGG is therefore fractionated external beam radiotherapy to a dose of 55–60 Gy in 1·8–2 Gy daily fractions given to a localised volume encompassing the enhancing tumour mass and a 2–5 cm margin.

## Should all patients be given the same intensive radiotherapy?

The median survival of patients with malignant glioma ranges from less than 6 months to over 4 years.[8,9] It may therefore be appropriate to tailor therapy to prognosis to avoid prolonged intensive irradiation in patients with limited prognosis and reserve more radical treatment for patients with more favourable prognosis. A number of phase II studies suggest little or no survival detriment with lower dose irradiation in patients with poor prognosis identified by poor performance status, glioblastoma histology and old age. The recommended regimens range from 30 Gy in 6–10 fractions to 45 Gy in 20 fractions. However, the concept of giving less intensive treatment to patients with adverse prognostic factors has not been subject to randomised trials and the value of this approach in terms of prolongation of survival and palliative efficacy is not fully established.

**Table 47.4  Table of evidence for radiation therapy for high grade gliomas**

| Reference | Evidence | Result |
|---|---|---|
| Walker *et al.*[1] | **Evidence level Ia** | Radiotherapy prolongs survival by 6 months |
| Sandberg *et al.*[2] | **Evidence level Ia** | |
| Shapiro *et al.*[3] | **Evidence level Ia** | No survival difference between whole brain RT and whole brain RT with localised boost |
| Bleehen and Stenning[4] | **Evidence level Ia** | 60 Gy in 30 fractions produces 3 months' better survival than 45 Gy in 20 fractions |
| Laperriere[5] | **Evidence level Ia** | Brachytherapy does not prolong survival |

## Can efficacy of radiotherapy be improved by intensification?

The limitation of brain tumour radiotherapy is radiation tolerance of the normal brain. Increasing radiation dose intensity could theoretically lead to improved tumour control but this would be predicted to be accompanied by higher morbidity and therefore no improvement in therapeutic ratio. Increase in radiation intensity confined to the tumour alone can be achieved with radiation sensitisers, with altered fractionation, or by more localised delivery of radiation. The apparent radiation resistance of gliomas *in vivo* has been assumed to be due to hypoxia and many trials tested the efficacy of hypoxic radiation sensitisers.[10,11] While individual randomised trials have not demonstrated benefit, a recent meta-analysis suggested a 5% improvement in survival for misonidazole as hypoxic cell sensitiser.[12] Studies of hyperbaric oxygen, neutrons, and particle radiotherapy (pions) have not shown a benefit but studies of hyperbarric oxygen and neutrons were underpowered.[13–15] While promising in phase II studies, a randomised controlled trial of radiotherapy with BUdR sensitisation versus radiation therapy alone was actually shown to have poorer survival in the radio-sensitisation arm.[16]

Higher radiation doses can be given without increasing toxicity by multiple small fractions per day (hyperfractionation). Dose intensity can also be increased by shortening the treatment time giving multiple treatments a day to the same overall dose (acceleration). With the exception of one small trial, randomised studies have failed to demonstrated a survival benefit for either high dose treatment (72 Gy hyperfractionated *v* 60 Gy conventional RT)[17] or for accelerated treatment. Nevertheless accelerating treatment was not found to be detrimental and shortened the treatment episode.[18]

Higher radiation doses to the tumour can be given by more localised delivery either by insertion of radiation sources directly into the tumour (interstitial radiotherapy/brachytherapy) or by high precision localised external beam stereotactic radiotherapy. Either of the techniques increases the incidence of necrosis within the high dose region. While numerous phase II studies suggested benefit for increased local dose, all such studies are subject to selection bias[19] and the only published randomised study of interstitial radiotherapy boost showed no survival benefit with additional irradiation.[5]

## Can the outcome of radiotherapy be improved by the addition of chemotherapy?

The use of adjuvant chemotherapy following radiation is discussed in the next section of this chapter. Chemotherapy has been given concurrently with irradiation as a potential radiosensitiser. There are no published randomised studies comparing radiotherapy alone with concomitant radiotherapy and chemotherapy (other than an ongoing randomised trial comparing concomitant and adjuvant temozolomide with radiotherapy alone in patients with glioblastoma) and the concept remains unproven.

## Summary

On present evidence, radiotherapy remains the most effective treatment in the management of patients with

HGG. The optimum treatment is 55–60 Gy given in daily fractions over a period of 6 weeks to a localised volume including the tumour and a small margin. Patients with short predicted life expectancy can be offered less intensive treatment providing this is given with appropriate consent.

There is currently no evidence that intensification of irradiation with radiation sensitisers, altered fractionation, or more localised irradiation improves survival or quality of life in patients with malignant glioma. Studies which attempt to modify radiotherapy intensity through new radiotherapy techniques and by novel biological modulation need to continue as the potential exists for improved therapeutic ratio.

## References

1  Walker MD, Alexander E Jr, Hunt WE *et al.* Evaluation of BCNU and/or radiotherapy in the treatment of anaplastic gliomas. A cooperative clinical trial. *J Neurosurg* 1978;**49**:333–43.

2  Sandberg WM, Malmström P, Strömblad LG *et al.* A randomized study of chemotherapy with procarbazine, vincristine, and lomustine with and without radiation therapy for astrocytoma grades 3 and/or 4. *Cancer* 1991;**68**:22–9.

3  Shapiro WR, Green SB, Burger PC *et al.* Randomised trial of three chemotherapy regimens and two radiotherapy regimens in postoperative treatment of malignant glioma. *J Neurosurg* 1989;**71**: 1–9.

4  Bleehen NM, Stenning SP. A Medical Research Council trial of two radiotherapy doses in the treatment of grades 3 and 4 astrocytoma. The Medical Research Council Brain Tumour Working Party. *Br J Cancer* 1991;**64**:769–74.

5  Laperriere NJ, Leung PM, McKenzie S *et al.* Randomized study of brachytherapy in the initial management of patients with malignant astrocytoma. *Int J Radiat Oncol Biol Phys* 1998;**41**:1005–11.

6  Walker MD, Strike TA, Sheline GE. An analysis of dose effect relationship in the radiotherapy of malignant gliomas. *Int J Radiat Oncol Biol Phys* 1979;**5**:1725.

7  Chang CH, Horton J, Schoenfeld D, Salazar O, Perez Tamayo R, Kramer S *et al.* Comparison of postoperative radiotherapy and combined postoperative radiotherapy and chemotherapy in the multidisciplinary management of malignant gliomas. A joint Radiation Therapy Oncology Group and Eastern Cooperative Oncology Group study. *Cancer* 1983;**52**:997–1007.

8  Curran WJ, Scott CB, Horton J *et al.* Recursive partitioning analysis of prognostic factors in three Radiation Therapy Oncology Group Malignant Glioma Trials. *J Natl Cancer Inst* 1993;**85**:704–10.

9  Scott CB, Scarantino C, Urtasun R *et al.* Validation and predictive power of Radiation Therapy Oncology Group (RTOG) recursive partitioning analysis classes for malignant glioma patients: a report using RTOG 90–06. *Int J Radiat Oncol Biol Phys* 1998;**40**:51–5.

10  MRC. Misonidazole in radiotherapy of supratentorial malignant brain gliomas in adult patients: a randomized double-blind study. *Eur J Cancer Clin Oncol* 1983;**19**:39–42.

11  Nelson DF, Diener West M, Weinstein AS *et al.* A randomised comparison of misonidazole sensitised radiotherapy plus BCNU and radiotherapy plus BCNU for treatment of malignant glioma after surgery: Final report of an RTOG study. *Int J Radiat Oncol Biol Phys* 1986;**12**:1793–800.

12  Huncharek M. Meta-analytic re-evaluation of misonidazole in the treatment of high grade astrocytoma. *Anticancer Res* 1998;**18**:1935–9.

13  Chang CH. Hyperbaric oxygen and radiation therapy in the management of glioblastoma. *Natl Cancer Inst Monogr* 1977;**46**:163–9.

14  Duncan W, McLelland J, Jack WJL. Report of a randomised pilot study of the treatment of patients with supratentorial gliomas using neutron irradiation. *Br J Radiol* 1986;**59**:373–7.

15  Pickles T, Goodman GB, Rheaume DE *et al.* Pion radiation for high grade astrocytoma: results of a randomized study. *Int J Radiat Oncol Biol Phys* 1997;**37**:491–7.

16  Prados MD, Scott C, Sandler H *et al.* A phase 3 randomized study of radiotherapy plus procarbazine, CCNU, and vincristine (PCV) with or without BUdR for the treatment of anaplastic astrocytoma: a preliminary report of RTOG 9404. *Int J Radiat Oncol Biol Phys* 1999;**45**:1109–15.

17  Scott CB, Curran WJ, Yung WKA *et al.* Long term results of RTOG 9006: A randomised trial of hyperfractionated radiotherapy (RT) to 72·0 Gy and Carmustine vs standard RT and Carmustine for malignant glioma patients with emphasis on anaplastic astrocytoma (AA) patients. *Proc ASCO* 1998;**17**:401a.

18  Brada M, Sharpe G, Rajan B *et al.* Modifying radical radiotherapy in high grade gliomas; shortening the treatment time through acceleration. *Int J Radiat Oncol Biol Phys* 1999;**43**:287–92.

19  Curran WJ, Scott CB, Weinstein AS *et al.* Survival comparison of radiosurgery eligible and ineligible malignant glioma patients treated with hyperfractionated radiation therapy and carmustine: A report of Radiation Therapy Oncology Group 83 02. *J Clin Oncol* 1993; **11**:857–62.

# How effective is chemotherapy at improving survival?

*Lesley Stewart*

## Background

Several chemotherapy agents have been shown to produce tumour regression in malignant glioma. The likelihood of achieving a response depends on the age of the patient (young [≤ 40years] better than old [≥ 60 years]), the type and grade of malignancy (anaplastic oligodendroglioma better than anaplastic astrocytoma better than glioblastoma) and the performance status (Karnofsky ≥ 70 better than Karnofsky ≤ 70). Size of tumour at start of chemotherapy may also be important. While clinical and radiological responses are possible, there is always a risk:benefit ratio to consider, because of the short- and long-term side effects of chemotherapy. The main question however is: does chemotherapy prolong survival?

## How effective is chemotherapy?

The role of adjuvant chemotherapy in treating HGG has recently been reviewed by the Glioma Meta-analysis Trialists' Group (GMTG)[1] using the gold standard approach[2] of systematic review and individual patient data (IPD) meta-analysis. This international collaborative project aimed to collect, validate and reanalyse "raw" data on all patients from all relevant randomised controlled trials (RCTs). This IPD approach permits time-to-event analysis, which is important in malignant glioma where extending survival rather than cure is anticipated. It also allows subgroup analyses to assess whether chemotherapy may be more or less effective for different types of patients.

Methods are presented in detail elsewhere[1]; briefly, to be included, trials had to be properly randomised, and include adult patients with HGG who had undergone cytoreductive surgery and were then allocated to radiotherapy plus systemic chemotherapy or to radiotherapy alone. To avoid publication bias,[3] both published and unpublished trials were sought by searching MEDLINE, CancerLit and Embase, by hand searching, consulting trial registers and by asking trialists to help identify trials. To avoid potential exclusion bias, information was requested for all randomised patients including those who had been excluded from the investigators' original analyses. All analyses were done on an intention-to-treat basis and were stratified by trial. Logrank expected numbers of events and variances were used to calculate individual and overall pooled hazard ratios (HR), thereby using each individual's duration of survival, and representing the overall risk of an

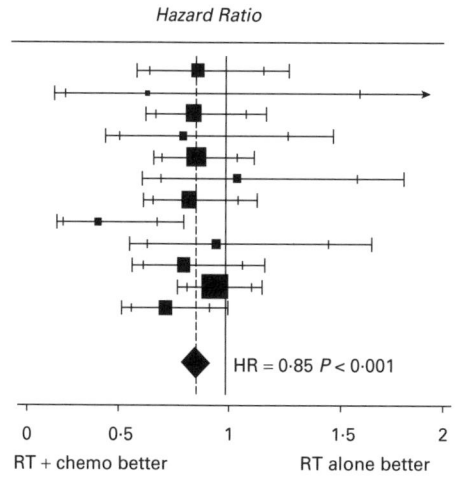

| Trial | No. of Patients | Chemotherapy | | Radiotherapy | | O–E | Variance |
| | | Drug(s) | Dose/cycle (mg m$^{-2}$) | Total dose (Gy) | Fractions | | |
|---|---|---|---|---|---|---|---|
| BTSG 6901[15] | 193 | B | 80 | 50–60 | 30–35 | −5·93 | 42·14 |
| Alberta[16] | 20 | C | 130 | 40–45 | 25 | −2·02 | 4·41 |
| BTSG 7201[17] | 355 | M, B | 220, 80 | 60 | 30–35 | −10·32 | 64·51 |
| Milan[18] | 105 | B, C | 80, 130 | 50 | 25–30 | −3·91 | 17·09 |
| RTOG 7401[19] | 511 | B, M, Dt | 80, 125, 150 | 60 | 35 | −14·79 | 95·60 |
| EORTC 26751[20] | 116 | C, V | 130, 60 | 55–60 | 30 | 0·97 | 22·09 |
| BTSG 7501[21] | 309 | B, P | 80, 150 | 60 | 30–35 | −12·31 | 67·24 |
| Budapest[22] | 91 | D, D, C, D | 400, 400, 100, 200 | 51 | 25–30 | −12·73 | 13·81 |
| Poland[23] | 125 | C | 100 | 60 | 30 | −1·10 | 21·25 |
| EORTC 26812[24] | 235 | C, V | 130, 100 | 55–60 | 30 | −10·48 | 48·00 |
| MRC BR05[25] | 674 | C, P, Vc | 100, 100, 1·5 | 45, 60, 55 | 20, 30, 34* | −8·72 | 153·67 |
| EORTC 26882[26] | 270 | M, C, Dt | 700, 150, 1000 | 60 | 30–35 | −19·54 | 58·14 |
| **Total** | **3004** | | | | | −100·9 | 607·95 |

**Figure 47.1** Hazard ratio plot for survival. (overall HR 0.85; 95% CI 0·78–0·91; $\chi^2_{(1)}$ 16·73; $P = 0.00004$; heterogeneity $\chi^2_{(11)}$ 13·29; $P = 0·28$). Each individual trial is represented by a square, the centre of which denotes hazard ratio for that trial; extremities of horizontal bars denote 99% CI and inner bars mark 95% CI. Size of square is directly proportional to amount of information in trial. Black diamond at foot of plot gives overall hazard ratio for combined results of all trials; centre denotes hazard ratio, and extremities 95% CI. Trials are ordered chronologically by date of start of trial (oldest first)
Abbreviations: B (BCNU), carmustine; C (CCNU), lomustine; D (DBD), mitolactol; Dt (DTIC), dacarbazine; M (MeCCNU), methyl lomustine; P (PCZ), procarbazine; V (VM-26), epipodophyllotoxin; Vc (VCR), vincristine
*twice daily fractions

event for those patients allocated to adjuvant chemotherapy compared with those allocated to no chemotherapy.

Preliminary searches identified 24 potentially eligible RCTs, five of which were subsequently found to be ineligible.[4-8] Of the 19 eligible trials, data from seven (683 patients) were not available.[9-14] The main results were therefore based on information from 12 RCTs.[15-26] In these trials, total radiotherapy doses ranged from 40 to 60 Gy given in 25–35 fractions. Four trials delivered whole brain irradiation whilst eight irradiated the tumour plus margins. The maximum planned delay between surgery and radiotherapy/chemotherapy ranged from 2 to 6 weeks. All trials included at least one nitrosourea compound (chosen because they are lipid soluble and cross the blood–brain barrier), given either as a single agent or in combination with other drugs.

Based on data from 12 trials, 3004 patients and 2659 deaths, the meta-analysis found clear evidence of increased survival for those receiving chemotherapy (HR 0·85; 95% CI 0·78–0·92; $P = 0.00004$) Figure 47.1. This 15% relative reduction in the risk of death is equivalent to an overall increase in survival of 6%, from 40% to 46%, at 1 year; to an increase from 10% to 15% at 2 years and to a 2-month increase in median survival from 10 to 12 months. Analysis of progression-free survival, based on eight trials, 2022 patients and 1859 events gave similar results (HR 0·83; 95% CI 0·75 – 0·91; $P = 0.00008$) with a 17% reduction in the risk of progression or death, This is equivalent to an absolute benefit of 5% at 2 years increasing progression-free survival from 10% to 15%. There was no indication that the relative effect of chemotherapy varied by age, sex, histology, performance status, or extent of tumour resection. Thus, the best estimate for any individual patient receiving chemotherapy is that they are likely to gain around 15% reduction in the overall risk of death. However, underlying prognoses vary markedly, and this relative effect is likely to translate to different absolute improvements depending on the baseline event rate. For example, the 2-year survival rate for individuals with glioblastoma multiforme is increased from 9% to 13%, whereas for those with anaplastic astrocytoma it is increased from 31% to 37%.

Undoubtedly, there are differences in the trials included in the meta-analysis, particularly with respect to the radiotherapy regimens and techniques used, and it could be suggested that rather than giving additional advantage, chemotherapy is simply making up for inadequate radiotherapy. However, there was no evidence that the effect of chemotherapy was moderated by radiotherapy total dose. In a sensitivity analysis, the HR for trials delivering a total dose of 60 Gy or more was 0·88, close to the overall result, and not significantly different to that of the remainder of the trials (chi-square interaction $P = 0.11$). The effect is therefore seen in trials delivering radiotherapy in doses similar to those used in current clinical practice,

and there is no strong evidence that chemotherapy is merely compensating for inadequate radiotherapy techniques. As IPD was only available for 81% of individuals from all known, eligible RCTs, the GMTG also carried out a complementary analysis based on data extracted from publications for six of the seven unavailable trials[9-11,13-15] for which numbers of deaths at 2 years data could be abstracted. Although this type of analysis does not have the advantages of the IPD approach, the broadly similar results (OR 0·92; 95% CI 0·79–1·09) lends confidence to the IPD analysis and suggests that lack of data from these trials did not bias its results.

The GMTG meta-analysis has shown a clear increase in survival for chemotherapy, approximately 6% at 2 years, and an improvement in median survival time of 2 months (from 10 to 12 months). However, it is debatable whether this is of practical benefit, and interpretation is likely to vary depending upon clinical situation, individual patient and family preference. Clearly, tolerability of treatment and quality of life, including cognitive impairment, are major issues in judging this for patients who will usually survive only a short time after their treatment is completed. Few of the trials included formally measured quality of life or did cognitive function tests in ways that would allow data to be combined. The quality of the demonstrated prolongation of survival could not therefore be formally assessed. Nonetheless, the nitrosoureas are fairly well tolerated, easily administered, and may be of practical use in the clinic for those individuals for whom it is important to extend their likely survival time, if only by a modest amount. Importantly, the clear effect observed demonstrates that HGGs can respond to chemotherapy and encourages further research into newer chemotherapies and methods of delivery. **Evidence level Ia**.

## References

1  Stewart LA. Chemotherapy in adult HGG: a systematic review and meta-analysis of individual patient data from 12 randomised trials. *Lancet* 2002;**359**:1011–18.

2  Stewart LA, Clarke MJ, on behalf of the Cochrane Working Party Group on Meta-analysis using Individual Patient Data. Practical methodology of meta-analyses (overviews) using updated individual patient data. *Stat Med* 1995;**14**:2057–79.

3  Dickersin K. The existence of publication bias and risk factors for its occurrence. *JAMA* 1990;**263**:1385–9.

4  Müller H, Brock M, Ernst H. Long-term survival and recurrence free interval in combined surgical, radio- and chemotherapy of malignancy brain gliomas. *Clin Neurol Neurosurg* 1985;**87**:167–71.

5  Garrett MJ, Hughes HJ, Freedman LS. A comparison of radiotherapy alone with radiotherapy and CCNU in cerebral glioma. *Clin Oncol* 1978;**4**:71–6.

6  Cianfriglia F, Pompili A, Riccio A, Grassi A. CCNU-chemotherapy of hemispheric supratentorial glioblastoma multiforme. *Cancer* 1980; **45**:1289–99.

7  Brisman R, Housepian E, Chang C, Duffy P, Balis E. Adjuvant nitrosourea therapy for glioblastoma. *Arch Neurol* 1976;**33**:745–50.

8   Ushio Y, Akagi K, Bitoh S *et al.* Phase 3 study of methyl-CCNU and bleomycin combination chemotherapy in the treatment of malignant gliomas. Proceedings of the 7th International Congress of Neurological Surgery 1981:362.

9   Kristiansen K, Hagen S, Kollevold T *et al.* Combined modality therapy of operated astrocytomas grade III and IV. Confirmation of the value of postoperative irradiation and lack of potentiation of bleomycin on survival time. *Cancer* 1981;**47**:649–52.

10  Hatlevoll R, Lindegaard K, Hagen S *et al.* Combined modality treatment of operated astrocytomas grade 3 and 4: A prospective and randomised study of misonidazole and radiotherapy with two different radiation schedules and subsequent CCNU chemotherapy. Stage II of a prospective multicentre trial of the Scandinavian Glioblastoma Study Group. *Cancer* 1985;**56**:41–7.

11  EORTC. Brain Tumor Group. Effect of CCNU on survival rate of objective remission and duration of free interval in patients with malignant brain glioma – final evaluation. *Eur J Cancer* 1978;**14**: 851–6.

12  Takakura K, Abe H, Tanaka R *et al.* Effects of ACNU and radiotherapy on malignant glioma. *J Neurosurg* 1986;**64**:53–7.

13  Reagan TJ, Bisel HF, Childs DS, Layton DD, Rhoton AL, Taylor WF. Controlled study of CCNU and radiation therapy in malignant astrocytoma. *J Neurosurg* 1976;**44**:186–90.

14  Eagan RT, Childs DS, Layton DD *et al.* Dianhydrogalactitol and radiation therapy: treatment of supratentorial glioma. *JAMA* 1979; **241**:2046–50.

15  Walker MD, Alexander Jr E, Hunt WE *et al.* Evaluation of BCNU and/or radiotherapy in the treatment of anaplastic gliomas. *J Neurosurg* 1978;**49**:333–43.

16  Weir B, Band P, Urtasun R *et al.* Radiotherapy and CCNU in the treatment of high-grade supratentorial astrocytomas. *J Neurosurg* 1976;**45**:129–34.

17  Walker MD, Green SB, Byar DP *et al.* Randomized comparisons of radiotherapy and nitrosoureas for the treatment of malignant glioma after surgery. *N Engl J Med* 1980;**303**:1323–9.

18  Solero CL, Monfardini S, Brambilla C *et al.* Controlled study with BCNU versus CCNU as adjuvant chemotherapy following surgery plus radiotherapy for glioblastoma multiforme. *Cancer Clin Trials* 1979;**2**:43–8.

19  Chang CH, Horton J, Schoenfeld D *et al.* Comparison of postoperative radiotherapy and combined postoperative radiotherapy and chemotherapy in the multidisciplinary management of malignant gliomas. *Cancer* 1983;**52**:997–1007.

20  EORTC. Brain Tumor Group. Evaluation of CCNU, VM-26 plus CCNU and procarbazine in supratentorial brain gliomas. *J Neurosurg* 1981;**55**:27–31.

21  Green SB, Byar DP, Walker MD *et al.* Methylprednisolone as additions to surgery and radiotherapy for the treatment of malignant glioma. *Cancer Treat Rep* 1983;**67**:121–32.

22  Áfra D, Kocsis B, Dobay J, Eckhardt S. Combined radiotherapy and chemotherapy with dibromoducitol and CCNU in the postoperative treatment of malignant gliomas. *J Neurosurg* 1983;**59**:106–10.

23  Trojanowski T, Peszynski J, Turowski K *et al.* Post-operative radiotherapy and radiotherapy combined with CCNU chemotherapy for treatment of brain gliomas. *J Neuro-Oncol* 1988;**6**:285–91.

24  EORTC. Brain Tumor Group. Phase III adjuvant therapy with radiotherapy versus radiotherapy plus VM-26/CCNU for resected malignant glioma. Unpublished.

25  Medical Research Council Brain Tumour Working Party. A randomised trial of adjuvant chemotherapy in malignant glioma. *J Clin Oncol* 2001;**19**:509–18.

26  Hildebrand J, Sahmoud T, Mignolet F, Brucher JM, Áfra D. Adjuvant therapy with dibromoducitol and BCNU increases survival of adults with malignant gliomas. *Neurology* 1994;**44**:1479–83.

# Management of brain metastases

*Charles J Vecht*

## Background

Brain metastases develop in about 20–40 % of patients with cancer, and the median survival is 3–5 months.[1,2] Frequent primary tumours associated with brain metastases are small and non-small cell lung cancer (~50%), breast carcinoma (~15%), malignant melanoma (~10%) and unknown primary carcinoma (~10%).[1,3]

Curative therapy is essentially impossible, and the main emphasis for the treatment is maintenance or improvement of the quality of life. In this survey, we will discuss the management of brain metastases, including issues on diagnosing brain metastases. Other issues are single versus multiple brain metastases, indications for surgery, whole brain and stereotactic radiotherapy, use of glucocorticoids and anticonvulsants, and prophylactic cranial irradiation.

## How do patients present?

The most frequent signs and symptoms of brain metastases are headache (~40%), mental changes (~35%), focal signs like hemiparesis or aphasia (~40%), difficulties in walking (~15%) and seizures (~20%). Headache in brain metastases is usually non-specific, and a CT or MRI in patients with systemic cancer and only headache would reveal brain metastases in 15–20%.[1,3] Only a minority shows the classical early morning headache with or without nausea and vomiting. In general, signs and symptoms develop over a period of weeks or days. In 25% of cases, symptoms develop acutely either as seizures or in a stroke-like presentation.

Diagnosis of an intracerebral tumour can made by contrast-enhanced CT or MRI of the brain. The sensitivity of MRI is superior to that of CT, and MRI can identify multiple brain metastases in 29% of patients with a presumed single brain lesion on CT scan.[4] The specificity of both CT and MRI of the brain is limited, and patients with known systemic cancer and a single enhancing lesion suspected of being a brain metastasis harbour a different pathology in 10% of cases **Evidence level I**.[5]

## What is the median survival?

Recursive partitioning analysis on independent prognostic factors reveals that the best survival occurs in patients with a single brain metastasis, age < 65 years, a Karnofsky Performance Status (KPS) of at least 70, and a controlled primary tumour. This combination results in a median survival of 7 months. The worst survival occurs with a KPS less than 70: median survival 2–3 months. The remainder of patients have a survival of 4 months[6] **Evidence level II**. Outcome is also dependent on treatment: following steroids only median survival is 1–2 months, following radiotherapy 3–4 months, and patients eligible for surgical resection survive for a median of 10 months[7] **Evidence level II**.

Brain metastases can appear as either:

- a first manifestation of cancer
- at the same time as other manifestations of cancer outside the brain, and
- in patients already known to have cancer.

In clinical practice, this division helps in deciding on the best management of the patient.

## How do you investigate at patient with probable brain metastases not known to have cancer?

If a patient develops neurological symptoms, and CT or MR scan shows a single enhancing lesion, differential diagnosis includes a brain metastasis, malignant glioma, abscess, bleeding, or bleeding in a tumour. As a rule, one initiates a work-up for the presence of systemic cancer. Lung cancer is by far the most common cause for a *de novo* presentation of brain metastasis, and therefore chest *x* ray and CT-thorax would produce a relatively high yield. Other diagnostic procedures mainly depend on the presence of physical signs, which, if present, have a high positive predictive value.[8]

In one series, 55% of 181 patients operated for single cerebral metastasis of carcinoma, the primary remained undiagnosed in 27% after extensive clinical investigations, in nine cases even at autopsy. Immunohistochemical staining of the neurosurgical specimen hardly contributes to making a specific diagnosis of the primary tumour.[9] In another series, underlying cancers were diagnosed in 84% of patients, with the remainder having equivocal or unknown primary cancers.[10] Whole body PET scan using FDG (18-F-fluorodeoxyglucose) is more effective in localising the primary site in one-third of cases than conventional techniques.[11]

The prognosis of patients with a *de novo* brain metastasis in which the primary tumour has been identified hardly differs from those with an unidentified primary tumour.[12,13] In about 10% of patients with a single enhancing intracerebral lesion, who are known to have systemic cancer, the lesion is not due to metastatic disease.[5]

Therefore one should confirm diagnosis by biopsy or resection, unless clinical circumstances suggest otherwise – for example, widespread systemic cancer, a poor general condition of the patient, or administration of systemic therapy for a chemosensitive primary tumour, which may target the brain lesion as well.[14]

## How do you investigate/treat patients with brain metastases and a probable systemic primary cancer?

In this setting, the lung is often the site of the primary tumour. Occasionally, the lung tumour can be resected together with excision of the brain metastasis. Selected patients who undergo both a thoracotomy and a craniotomy may show a median survival of 2 years or more.[15,16] Recognition of this relatively rare condition of brain metastasis is essential, as long-term survival may be achieved. Vice versa, screening of the brain by MRI of patients with lung cancer reveals a frequency of brain metastasis of 5% or less in non-small cell, and of about 20% in small cell carcinoma in neurologically asymptomatic patients.[17–19]

## What is appropriate management of a metachronous presentation?

This is the most common setting and patient-management depends largely on the presence of either a single (30%) versus multiple brain metastases (70%).[20]

### Surgery

In the 1970s and 1980s, there was much debate about whether single brain metastasis should preferably be treated by either surgery and radiotherapy, or by radiotherapy only. Two out of three randomised studies have shown that surgery followed by whole brain radiation therapy (WBRT) is the treatment of choice for patients in a good clinical condition and no signs of progression of the extracranial tumour during the previous 3 months[5,21,22] **Evidence level I**. The combined therapy results in a median survival of ± 10 months with a 20% 2-year survival. As patients with brain metastases cannot be cured, the goal of therapy is palliation preferably on a long-term basis. Duration of independent functioning of the patient under these circumstances is 1–2 months shorter. This implies that active treatment of single brain metastasis in patients with rather favourable characteristics results in preservation of good quality of life and intact neurological functioning for most of their expected, although limited, lifetime.

### Whole brain radiotherapy

Thus, for single brain metastasis, if one compares the effects of WBRT versus the combination of surgical resection and WBRT, the latter has been shown to be superior. A randomised trial addressing this question, has shown that under these circumstances postoperative radiotherapy leads to local brain recurrences in 10% versus 46% in patients who did not receive WBRT after the surgery[23] **Evidence level I**. This probably also explains why patients treated with the combination of surgery and radiotherapy are less likely die of their brain metastasis than patients undergoing surgery only (14% *v* 44%). Nevertheless, this difference does not affect survival or the length of time that patients remain functionally independent. These results support treatment with WBRT after complete surgical resection of a single brain metastasis, unless there are circumstances that would make radiotherapy inappropriate, for example poor postsurgical clinical performance, unexpected extracranial progression of tumour or options for systemic chemotherapy.

### Is surgery better than stereotactic radiotherapy/radiosurgery?

Radiosurgery has become an important alternative for surgery, provided that histology of the lesion has been obtained or that one would be reasonably certain about the nature of the lesion.

Radiosurgery can either be carried out by stereotactic radiation with a linear accelerator and 3-dimensional conformation or by using the gamma-knife. The latter implies use of a collimator that concentrates the beams of ionising radiation into a single point or sphere with a maximum diameter of 30 mm. In stereotactic radiotherapy with a linear accelarator, the maximum diameter is 40 mm. Applied radiation doses with these techniques are in the range of 15–20 Gy, often applied as single dose. The number of brain metastases treatable by stereotactic radiotherapy may vary. As a rule, one accepts that patients with one to three small brain metastases of limited volume (< 40 mm diameter) can be treated by this method.

Surgical for brain metastases and radiosurgery have resulted in similar survival rates. Median survival following radiosurgery for brain metastases varies between 6 and 12 months and is similar to patients operated on for a single brain metastasis. The local control rate, which is defined as lack of progression within the irradiated volume, varies between 70% and 90%. In one multi-institutional study, the median survival following radiosurgery was 56 weeks; 1- and 2-year survival rates were 53% and 30%, respectively. Multivariate analysis reveals that independent functioning and absence of extracranial metastases predict good responders.[24]

## Should radiosurgery be followed by whole brain radiotherapy (WBRT)?

A new question is whether radiosurgery of a single brain metastasis should be followed by conventional radiation therapy of the whole brain.[25–27] In one study on 80 patients, the comparison between stereotactic radiotherapy (SRS) and SRS + WBRT groups indicated that adding WBRT would only slow the development of new brain metastases. Both SRS alone and SRS + WBRT seem to offer better survival and quality of life than WBRT alone for patients with single brain metastasis from lung cancer.[27] Until now, the combined therapy does not show significant advantage over SRS alone in improving survival, enhancing local control, or quality of life. A randomised trial is needed to assess the value of adding WBRT to SRS for this group of patients **Evidence level II** .[26,27]

## How helpful is stereotactic radiotherapy for recurrent brain metastases after WBRT?

Another indication for stereotactic radiotherapy is recurrent brain metastases.[28] This may be applied in patients who have been treated previously with WBRT with or without preceding surgery, and probably also in patients who have already been treated with stereotactic radiotherapy. One up to three or four brain metastases of limited size (< 4 cm diameter) recurring more than 6–12 months after initial therapy may qualify for this treatment. In one study on 54 patients with recurrent brain metastases who received radiation doses between 15–20 Gy, the 2-year metastatic local control rate was 84%. One- and 2-year overall survival rates were 31% and 28%. An interval between WBRT and radiosurgery longer than 14 months is associated with longer progression-free survival from recurrence in the brain.[28]

## How do you manage/treat patients who have multiple brain metastases?

Multiple brain metastases not qualifying for stereotactic radiotherapy constitutes the majority of patients with brain metastases. Under these circumstances, the standard treatment is whole brain radiation therapy. The outcome in this patient-group varies between 2 and 6 months.[1,7] Different schemes for radiating brain metastases have randomly been tested comparing fractionation schedules of $5 \times 400$ cGy, $10 \times 200$ cGy, $10 \times 300$ cGy, or $20 \times 200$ cGy to be delivered in 1 or 2 weeks, and show no clear differences in survival **Evidence level I** .[29–31] As about two-thirds of patients with brain metastases die from systemic cancer, one would *a priori* not expect big differences to appear between the various radiation regimens. Median survival is based on the presence of independent prognostic factors: age, neurological status, and extent of cancer. With favourable prognostic factors (age < 60 years, a good clinical condition and stable or inactive systemic cancer), the median survival in patients with multiple brain metastases is 6 months and the 2-year survival 10%. With unfavourable prognostic variables, the median survival is less than 3 months. Under the latter circumstances, one may question the benefit of giving radiation therapy. In bedridden or mentally incapacitated people, symptomatic care including glucocorticoids and anticonvulsants is most appropriate.

## Should patients with an intracerebral tumour be treated with prophylactic anticonvulsants?

Of patients with brain metastases 15–20% will develop epilepsy.[3] It is unsure whether anticonvulsants should be prescribed prophylactically for all patients with brain metastases. Reliable prospective studies are lacking, but one randomised controlled trial of prophylactic anticonvulsants demonstrated that the incidence of seizures was similar irrespective of whether patients received anticonvulsants.[32,33] Brain metastasis from melanoma often leads to epilepsy and this may constitute the exception **Evidence level III** .[33] Appearance of a first seizure in patients who have an intracranial mass lesion necessitates starting treatment with anticonvulsants. There appears to be an increased risk of developing erythema multiforme in patients treated with phenytoin or carbamazepine who are also receiving cranial irradiation.[34] Both dexamethasone and first-line anticonvulsants as phenytoin or carbamazepine are enzyme-inducers of liver cytochrome P-450. Thus, reciprocal effects with each other and with other drugs metabolised via the same route can be expected. This explains why phenytoin can induce an increase in clearance and a reduced half-life of glucocorticosteroids.[35] Phenobarbitone can also increase the clearance of dexamethasone resulting in lower effective concentrations. Vice versa, dexamethasone leads to a faster metabolism of phenytoin resulting in unpredictable phenytoin serum levels. For these reasons some authorities prefer to use another anticonvulsant, for example valproic acid or lamogitrine. Other interesting new anticonvulsants such as topiramate and levetiracetam have relatively few side effects and hardly affect the P-450 enzyme system.

## When should steroids be used?

Therapeutic effects of glucorticoids appear within 24–48 hours after initiation. In about 50%, clinical signs disappear completely, another 15% improve, and in the remainder no clear effect can be distinguished. The drug of choice is dexamethasone as this has less mineralocorticoid effects and less protein-binding than prednisone. The standard dose is often given as 16 mg/day divided in four doses. However, without signs of increased intracranial pressure, a dose of 4 mg/day has been shown in a randomised controlled trial to be equally effective **Evidence level I**.[36] Steroid side effects like cushingoid face, ankle oedema, and proximal weakness by steroid myopathy are more frequent when higher doses of dexamethasone are used, for example 8 or 16 mg/day.[36]

The biological half-life of dexamethasone is 24–36 hours. For that reason, dexamethasone can be given as a once daily dose. In patients with impaired consciousness or with impending herniation, dexamethasone in a starting dose of 10 mg intravenously followed by 16 mg/day is justified. After antitumour therapy has been instituted, dexamethasone can often be withdrawn.

After longer periods of administration, glucocorticoids should be withdrawn gradually over a number of weeks, because of the chance of developing adrenal insufficiency. During tapering of glucocorticoids, one occasionally may observe signs of steroid withdrawal, particularly following longstanding periods of high dose steroid administration. These symptoms consist of headache, lethargy, weakness, orthostatic hypotension, and bilateral pain in hips, knees, or ankle joints. Withdrawal symptoms can be managed by increasing the steroid dose followed by tapering at slower pace.

## What should be done about cerebellar metastases?

Cerebellar metastases pose a special problem in management. Cerebellar metastases usually cause more severe symptoms than supratentorial metastases and patients often complain about headache, nausea, vomiting, dizziness and walking difficulties, but diagnosis can be demanding as patients often lack localising signs.[37] A CT scan may be false negative and an MR scan should be performed.

Patients can deteriorate acutely during the period of evaluation or at the beginning of radiation therapy. Starting steroids at least 48 hours before radiotherapy has been advocated.[38] Despite these precautions, the risk of a decompensating obstructive hydrocephalus or of intratumoural haemorrhage with an increased intracranial pressure remains and ventriculoperitoneal shunting should be considered, if there is early hydrocephalus. Setting aside the higher chance of postoperative complications when compared with those with supratentorial lesions, surgical resection of a cerebellar metastasis seems to reduce the risk of an acutely decompensating intracranial hypertension more than radiotherapy alone.[38,39]

## Is there any place for chemotherapy in the management of cerebral metastases?

Systemic chemotherapy may be considered in brain metastases derived from chemosensitive solid tumours. The best results are seen in patients with breast cancer, small cell carcinoma of the lung, choriocarcinoma and testicular carcinoma.[14,40] If these primary tumours are present, chemotherapy may be considered for patients with minimal neurological symptoms, or where recurrent brain metastases responded to previous therapy. In patients who had small cell carcinoma of the lung and multiple brain metastases, administration of tenoposide did not produce a survival advantage over WBRT.[41]

## References

1  Nussbaum ES, Djalilian HR, Cho KH, Hall WA. Brain metastases. Histology, multiplicity, surgery, and survival. *Cancer* 1996;**78**: 1781–8.

2  Hall WA, Djalilian HR, Nussbaum ES, Cho KH. Long-term survival with metastatic cancer to the brain. *Med Oncol* 2000;**17**:279–86.

3  Zimm S, Wampler GL, Stablein D, Hazra T, Young HF. Intracerebral metastases in solid-tumor patients: natural history and results of treatment. *Cancer* 1981;**48**:384–94.

4  Mastronardi L, Lunardi P, Puzzilli F, Schettini G, Lo Bianco F, Ruggeri A. The role of MRI in the surgical selection of cerebral metastases. *Zentralbl Neurochir* 1999;**60**:141–5.

5  Patchell RA, Tibbs PA, Walsh JW *et al.* A randomized trial of surgery in the treatment of single metastasis to the brain. *N Engl J Med* 1990;**322**:494–500.

6  Agboola O, Benoit B, Cross P *et al.* Prognostic factors derived from recursive partition analysis (RPA) of Radiation Therapy Oncology Group (RTOG) brain metastases trials applied to surgically resected and irradiated brain metastatic cases. *Int J Radiat Oncol Biol Phys* 1998;**42**:155–9.

7  Lagerwaard FJ, Levendag PC, Nowak PJ, Eijkenboom WM, Hanssens PE, Schmitz PI. Identification of prognostic factors in patients with brain metastases: a review of 1292 patients. *Int J Radiat Oncol Biol Phys* 1999;**43**:795–803.

8  van de Pol M, van Aalst VC, Wilmink JT, Twijnstra A. Brain metastases from an unknown primary tumour: which diagnostic procedures are indicated? *J Neurol Neurosurg Psychiatr* 1996;**61**:321–3.

9  Giordana MT, Cordera S, Boghi A. Cerebral metastases as first symptom of cancer: a clinico-pathologic study. *J Neuro-Oncol* 2000; **50**:265–73.

10  Merchut MP. Brain metastases from undiagnosed systemic neoplasms. *Arch Intern Med* 1989;**149**:1076–80.

11 Lassen U, Daugaard G, Eigtved A, Damgaard K, Friberg L. 18F-FDG whole body positron emission tomography (PET) in patients with unknown primary tumours (UPT). *Eur J Cancer* 1999;**35**:1076–82.

12 Thomas AJ, Rock JP, Johnson CC, Weiss L, Jacobsen G, Rosenblum ML. Survival of patients with synchronous brain metastases: an epidemiological study in southeastern Michigan. *J Neurosurg* 2000; **93**:927–31.

13 Ruda R, Borgognone M, Benech F, Vasario E, Soffietti R. Brain metastases from unknown primary tumour: a prospective study. *J Neurol* 2001;**248**:394–8.

14 Boogerd W, Dalesio O, Bais EM, van der Sande JJ. Response of brain metastases from breast cancer to systemic chemotherapy. *Cancer* 1992;**69**:972–80.

15 Magilligan DJ Jr, Duvernoy C, Malik G, Lewis JW Jr, Knighton R, Ausman JI. Surgical approach to lung cancer with solitary cerebral metastasis: twenty-five years' experience. *Ann Thorac Surg* 1986; **42**:360–4.

16 Hankins JR, Miller JE, Salcman M *et al*. Surgical management of lung cancer with solitary cerebral metastasis. *Ann Thorac Surg* 1988; **46**:24–8.

17 Nomoto Y, Miyamoto T, Yamaguchi Y. Brain metastasis of small cell lung carcinoma: comparison of Gd-DTPA enhanced magnetic resonance imaging and enhanced computerized tomography. *Jpn J Clin Oncol* 1994;**24**:258–62.

18 van de Pol M, van Oosterhout AG, Wilmink JT, ten Velde GP, Twijnstra A. MRI in detection of brain metastases at initial staging of small-cell lung cancer. *Neuroradiology* 1996;**38**:207–10.

19 Yokoi K, Kamiya N, Matsuguma H *et al*. Detection of brain metastasis in potentially operable non-small cell lung cancer: a comparison of CT and MRI. *Chest* 1999;**115**:714–19.

20 France LH. Contribution to the study of 150 cases of cerebral metastases. II. Neuropathological study. *J Neurosurg Sci* 1975; **19**:189–210.

21 Mintz AH, Kestle J, Rathbone MP *et al*. A randomized trial to assess the efficacy of surgery in addition to radiotherapy in patients with a single cerebral metastasis. *Cancer* 1996;**78**:1470–6.

22 Vecht CJ, Haaxma-Reiche H, Noordijk EM *et al*. Treatment of single brain metastasis: radiotherapy alone or combined with neurosurgery? *Ann Neurol* 1993;**33**:583–90.

23 Patchell RA, Tibbs PA, Regine WF *et al*. Postoperative radiotherapy in the treatment of single metastases to the brain: a randomized trial. *JAMA* 1998;**280**:1485–9.

24 Auchter RM, Lamond JP, Alexander E *et al*. A multiinstitutional outcome and prognostic factor analysis of radiosurgery for resectable single brain metastasis. *Int J Radiat Oncol Biol Phys* 1996;**35**:27–35.

25 Alexander E 3rd, Moriarty TM, Davis RB *et al*. Stereotactic radiosurgery for the definitive, noninvasive treatment of brain metastases. *J Natl Cancer Inst* 1995;**87**:34–40.

26 Sneed PK, Lamborn KR, Forstner JM *et al*. Radiosurgery for brain metastases: is whole brain radiotherapy necessary? *Int J Radiat Oncol Biol Phys* 1999;**43**:549–58.

27 Li B, Yu J, Suntharalingam M *et al*. Comparison of three treatment options for single brain metastasis from lung cancer. *Int J Cancer* 2000;**90**:37–45.

28 Noel G, Proudhom MA, Valery CA *et al*. Radiosurgery for re-irradiation of brain metastasis: results in 54 patients. *Radiother Oncol* 2001;**60**: 61–7.

29 Kramer S, Hendrickson F, Zelen M, Schotz W. Therapeutic trials in the management of metastatic brain tumors by different time/dose fraction schemes of radiation therapy. *Natl Cancer Inst Monogr* 1977;**46**:213–21.

30 Chatani M, Matayoshi Y, Masaki N, Inoue T. Radiation therapy for brain metastases from lung carcinoma. Prospective randomized trial according to the level of lactate dehydrogenase. *Strahlenther Onkol* 1994;**170**:155–61.

31 Diener-West M, Dobbins TW, Phillips TL, Nelson DF. Identification of an optimal subgroup for treatment evaluation of patients with brain metastases using RTOG study 7916. *Int J Radiat Oncol Biol Phys* 1989;**16**:669–73.

32 Cohen N, Strauss G, Lew R, Silver D, Recht L. Should prophylactic anticonvulsants be administered to patients with newly-diagnosed cerebral metastases? A retrospective analysis. *J Clin Oncol* 1988; **6**:1621–4.

33 Glantz MJ, Cole BF, Friedberg MH *et al*. A randomized, blinded, placebo-controlled trial of divalproex sodium prophylaxis in adults with newly diagnosed brain tumors. *Neurology* 1996;**46**:985–91.

34 Hoang-Xuan K, Delattre JY, Poisson M. Stevens-Johnson syndrome in a patient receiving cranial irradiation and carbamazepine. *Neurology* 1990;**40**:1144–5.

35 Chalk JB, Ridgeway K, Brophy T, Yelland JD, Eadie MJ. Phenytoin impairs the bioavailability of dexamethasone in neurological and neurosurgical patients. *J Neurol Neurosurg Psychiatr* 1984; **47**:1087–90.

36 Vecht CJ, Hovestadt A, Verbiest HB, van Vliet JJ, van Putten WL. Dose-effect relationship of dexamethasone on Karnofsky performance in metastatic brain tumors: a randomized study of doses of 4, 8, and 16 mg per day. *Neurology* 1994;**44**:675–80.

37 Weisberg LA. Solitary cerebellar metastases. Clinical and computed tomographic correlations. *Arch Neurol* 1985;**42**:336–41.

38 Fadul C, Misulis KE, Wiley RG. Cerebellar metastases: diagnostic and management considerations. *J Clin Oncol* 1987;**5**:1107–15.

39 White KT, Fleming TR, Laws ER Jr. Single metastasis to the brain. Surgical treatment in 122 consecutive patients. *Mayo Clin Proc* 1981;**56**:424–8.

40 Rosner D, Nemoto T, Lane WW. Chemotherapy induces regression of brain metastases in breast carcinoma. *Cancer* 1986;**58**:832–9.

41 Postmus PE, Haaxma-Reiche H, Smit EF *et al*. Treatment of brain metastases of small-cell lung cancer: comparing teniposide and teniposide with whole-brain radiotherapy – A phase III study of the European Organization for the Research and Treatment of Cancer Lung Cancer Cooperative Group. *J Clin Oncol* 2000;**18**:3400–8.

42 Cranial irradiation for preventing brain metastases of small cell lung cancer in patients in complete remission (Cochrane Review). *Cochrane Database Syst Rev* 2000;**4**:CD002805.

43 Fonseca R, O'Neill BP, Foote RL, Grill JP, Sloan JA, Frytak S. Cerebral toxicity in patients treated for small cell carcinoma of the lung. *Mayo Clin Proc* 1999;**74**:461–5.

# Section XII

## Treating cancers of the eye and associated structures

*Arun D Singh, Editor*

# Levels of evidence and grades of recommendation used in *Evidence-based Oncology*

Levels of evidence and grades of recommendation appear within the text in the clinical chapters, for example, **Evidence Level Ia** and **Grade A**.

## Levels of evidence

Ia   Meta-analysis of randomised controlled trials (RCTs)
Ib   At least 1 RCT
IIa  At least 1 non-randomised study
IIb  At least 1 other well designed quasi-experimental study
III  Non-experimental, descriptive studies
IV   Expert committee reports or opinions/experience of respected authorities

## Grades of recommendations

A   At least one RCT as part of body of literature of overall good quality and consistency addressing recommendation **Evidence levels Ia, Ib**
B   No RCT but well conducted clinical studies available **Evidence levels IIa, IIb, III**
C   Expert committee reports or opinions/experience of respected authorities in the absence of directly applicable good quality clinical studies **Evidence level IV**

From *Clinical Oncology* (2001) **13**:S212
Source of data: MEDLINE, *Proceedings of the American Society of Medical Oncology* (ASCO).

# 48 Uveal melanoma

*Arun D Singh, Paul A Rundle, Ian G Rennie*

## Background

Of all melanomas approximately 5% arise from the ocular and adnexal structures such as uvea, eyelids, conjunctiva, and orbit.[1] The majority (85%) of ocular melanoma are uveal in origin whereas primary orbital melanoma is very rare.[1,2] Uveal melanoma is the most common primary intraocular malignant tumour.[3]

The diagnosis of uveal melanoma is made by clinical examination including slit lamp examination and indirect ophthalmoscopy, as well as ancillary studies such as fluorescein angiography, and ultrasonography.[4] The accuracy of clinical diagnosis among Collaborative Ocular Melanoma Study (COMS) participants was reported to be greater than 99%.[5] The traditional form of treatment, enucleation, has been challenged in recent years and alternative methods of treatment including radiotherapy (plaque radiotherapy, proton beam radiotherapy, helium ion radiotherapy), local resection and transpupillary thermotherapy have been used more frequently to manage posterior uveal melanoma.[4]

Approximately 40% of patients with posterior uveal melanoma develop metastatic melanoma to the liver within 10 years after initial diagnosis and treatment.[4,6] However, clinically evident metastatic disease at the time of initial presentation is uncommon, indicating early subclinical metastasis in the majority of cases.[6] With conventional methods such as serum liver enzymes and liver scans, metastatic disease can be detected in only 1–2% of patients at the time of presentation.[7] Systemic screening protocols using physical examinations, liver function tests, chest *x* rays, and liver imaging studies every 6 months to 1 year have been proposed but the effectiveness of the screening protocols remains to be established.[8]

## Is the incidence of uveal melanoma rising?

A rising incidence of cutaneous melanoma has been observed in recent years.[1,9] With regards to uveal melanoma, there are only a few large population-based studies (Table 48.1).Two studies from the United States have reported stability of incidence rate between 1950 and 1974 and between 1973 and 1997.[3,10] The reported incidence rate of uveal melanoma has ranged from 5·3 to 10·9 cases per million because of variations in inclusion and diagnostic

criteria, and methodology used in calculating the incidence rate. In some studies uveal melanoma has been included with melanoma of the conjunctiva[3,11–13] and eyelids.[14–16] The diagnostic criteria have been very strict in some studies where only those with histopathological diagnosis were included,[14,17,18] whereas more recent studies have included cases diagnosed on a clinical basis.[11–13,15,16,19] The incidence rate has been reported as a crude rate[14,17–20] or more accurately as age-adjusted rate accounting for demographic variability of the population over time.[3,11,16,21]

In a recent study only diagnostic codes that included uvea as a whole as the primary site (iris, ciliary body, and choroid) were considered, and other ocular sites were excluded.[10] In addition the cases diagnosed to have uveal melanoma both clinically and histopathologically (where available) were included because an increasing proportion of uveal melanoma is treated without obtaining tissue diagnosis. The overall mean incidence of uveal melanoma was 4·3 per million with a greater rate of 4·9 per million in males as compared with 3·7 per million in females. The incidence rate progressively increased up to the age of 70 years with peak of 24·5 cases per million in males and 17·8 cases per million in females. The overall incidence rate of uveal melanoma did not vary significantly between 1973 and 1997 (Figure 48.1). Combining the data from the 1950 to 1974 study[3] with the data from the 1973–1997 study[10] it can be stated that the incidence of uveal melanoma in the United States has remained unchanged over the past 50 years **Evidence level Ia, Grade A**.

## Is plaque radiotherapy associated with improved survival as compared with enucleation for management of uveal melanoma?

Zimmerman and associates in 1979 reported their observations on the rise in the mortality rate a few years after enucleation.[22,23] On the basis of 2300 case studies the postoperative mortality rate increased from the estimated pre-enucleation rate of 1% per year to a peak of 8% during the second year after enucleation and then decreased monotonically. The authors postulated that the procedure of enucleation had a detrimental effect on the expected natural course of the disease.[22,23] Others have subsequently shown

**Table 48.1   Summary of published reports on incidence of uveal melanoma[10]**

| First author | Year | Period | Region | Definition | No. of cases | Criteria | Method | Incidence (per million) |
|---|---|---|---|---|---|---|---|---|
| Mork | 1961 | 1953–1960 | Norway | Ocular melanoma* | 220 | Hist | Crude rate | 9·0 |
| Jensen | 1963 | 1943–1952 | Denmark | Uveal melanoma† | 305 | Hist | Crude rate | 7·4 |
| Ganley | 1973 | 1956–1965 | Maryland (US) | Choroidal melanoma | 6 | Hist | Crude rate | 6·6 |
| Scotto | 1976 | 1969–1971 | United States | Eye melanoma‡ | 341 | Clinical | Age-adjusted | 5·6 |
| Raivio | 1977 | 1953–1973 | Finland | Cbd + choroids | 359 | Hist | Age-adjusted | 5·3 |
| Shammas | 1977 | 1969–1971 | Iowa (US)* | Cbd + choroids | 41 | Clinical | Crude rate | 4·9 (White) |
| Davidorf | 1979 | 1967–1977 | Ohio (US)** | Choroidal melanoma | 698 | Hist | Crude | 10·9 (White adults) |
| Wilkes | 1979 | 1935–1974 | Rochester (US) | Uveal melanoma | 15 | Hist | Crude rate | 7·0 |
| Birdsell | 1980 | 1967–1977 | Alberta (Canada) | Eye melanoma | 99 | Clinical | Crude rate | 6·0 |
| Strickland | 1981 | 1950–1974 | Connecticut (US) | Eye melanoma | – | – | Age-adjusted | 9·0 (male) 8·0 (female) |
| Kaneko | 1982 | 1977–1979 | Japan | Uveal melanoma | 82 | Hist | Crude rate | 0·3 |
| Abrahamsson | 1983 | 1956–1975 | Halland (Sweden) | Cbd + choroids | 91 | Hist | Crude rate | 7·2 |
| Swerdlow | 1983 | 1952–1978 | Oxford (UK) | Ocular melanoma | 207 | Clinical | Age-adjusted | 4·8 (male) 3·9 (female) |
| Swerdlow | 1983 | 1962–1977 | England (UK) | Ocular melanoma | 4284 | Clinical | Age-adjusted | 7·2 (male) 5·7 (female) |
| Gislason | 1985 | 1955–1979 | Iceland | Cbd + choroids | 29 | Hist | Age-adjusted | 7·0 (male) 5·0 (female) |
| Lommatzsch | 1985 | 1961–1980 | East Germany | Eye melanoma | | Clinical | Crude rate | Translation |
| Teikari | 1985 | 1973–1980 | Finland | Cbd + choroids | 382 | Clinical | Crude rate | 7·6 |
| Egan | 1987 | 1984 | New England (US) | Uveal melanoma | 85 | Clinical | Crude rate | 6·9 |
| Iscovich | 1995 | 1961–1989 | Israel | Cbd + Choroid | 502 | Clinical | Age-adjusted | 5·7 (Jews) |
| Vidal | 1995 | 1992 | France | Uveal melanoma | 412 | Clinical | Annual rate | 7·0 |
| Margo | 1998 | 1981–1983 | Florida (US) | Uveal melanoma | 873 | Hist | Age-adjusted | 5·6 |
| Bergman | 2001 | 1960–1989 | Sweden | Uveal melanoma | 2403 | Clinical | Age-adjusted | 9·4 (male) 8·8 (female) |
| Singh | 2002 | 1973–1997 | US | Uveal melanoma | 2493 | Clinical | Age-adjusted | 4·9 (male) 3·7 (female) |

Abbreviations: Cbd, ciliary body; Hist, histological
*Ocular melanoma: uveal, conjunctival and eyelid melanoma.
†Uveal melanoma: iris, ciliary body and choroidal melanoma.
‡Eye melanoma: uveal and conjunctival melanoma.

that the excessive mortality after enucleation for uveal melanoma is not related to the enucleation but to an active phase of tumour progression that led to the diagnosis.[24]

However, since then many retrsospective studies have shown that survival in patients with uveal melanoma is independent of the method of local treatment such as

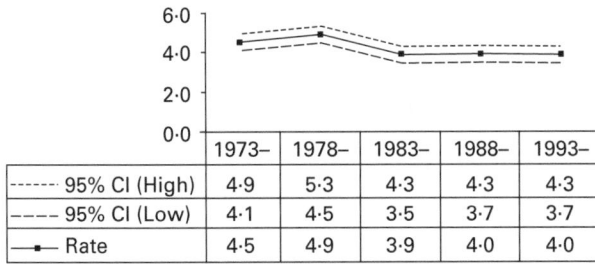

**Figure 48.1** Comparison of uveal melanoma incidence rates over time

plaque radiotherapy,[25,26] proton beam irradiation,[27] or tumour resection (Table 48.2).[28] Comparison of survival in patients treated with enucleation versus cobalt-60 plaque was performed on 237 patients with uveal melanoma.[25] The 8-year survival estimates between the two groups was not statistically dissimilar (enucleation group 62%, plaque group 76%). In a larger study of 495 patients with uveal melanoma treated with enucleation and 556 patients treated with proton bean irradiation, the estimated 5-year survival between the enucleation group and the proton beam group was similar (80% and 81%, respectively).[27] In a study of 731 cases that had been treated with helium ion and iodine-125 plaque radiotherapy, the estimated 5-year

survival was 76%, indicating similar survival to patients treated with enucleation.[29]

The COMS is an ongoing prospective study that is investigating patient survival after treatment of choroidal melanoma.[30,31] The COMS consists of:

- a randomised trial of patients with medium choroidal melanoma treated with enucleation versus iodine-125 plaque irradiation;
- a randomised trial of patients with large choroidal melanoma treated with enucleation only versus pre-enucleation external beam irradiation and enucleation[32];
- a prospective observational study of patients with small choroidal melanoma.[33]

Recently published initial results from the COMS indicate that for medium-sized melanomas, enucleation and iodine-125 brachytherapy offer similar survival rates.[30] During the 12-year accrual period 1317 patients were enrolled; 660 were assigned randomly to enucleation and 657 to iodine-125 brachytherapy. The estimated 5-year cumulative mortality rates were 19% (95% CI, 16%–23%) for patients treated with enucleation and 18% (95% CI, 15%–21%) for patients treated with iodine-125 brachytherapy with a risk ratio of 0·93 (95% CI, 0·76–1·14).

COMS is a landmark prospective randomised study enrolling a large cohort of patients. For medium sized

**Table 48.2 Reported 5-year mortality with uveal melanoma[6]**

| Author | Year | Study | Treatment | Size | Method | Rate (%) |
|---|---|---|---|---|---|---|
| Diener-West | 1992 | Meta-analysis | Enucleation | Small | All-cause mortality | 16 |
| | | | | Medium | All cause mortality | 32 |
| | | | | Large | All cause mortality | 53 |
| Anonymous | 1998 | COMS | Enucleation (with EBRT) | Large | All cause mortality | 38 |
| | | | Enucleation (without EBRT) | Large | All cause mortality | 43 |
| | 2001 | | Enucleation | Medium | All cause mortality | 19 |
| | | | Plaque | Medium | All cause mortality | 18 |
| Seregard | 1999 | Meta-analysis | Plaque | Small | Melanoma related mortality | 6 |
| | | | | Medium | Melanoma related mortality | 6 |
| | | | | Large | Melanoma related mortality | 26 |
| Kroll | 1998 | | Plaque and helium ion | – | Melanoma related mortality | 16 |
| Seddon | 1990 | | Proton beam irradiation | – | All cause mortality | 19 |

Abbreviations: COMS, Collaborative Ocular Melanoma Study; EBRT, external beam radiotherapy

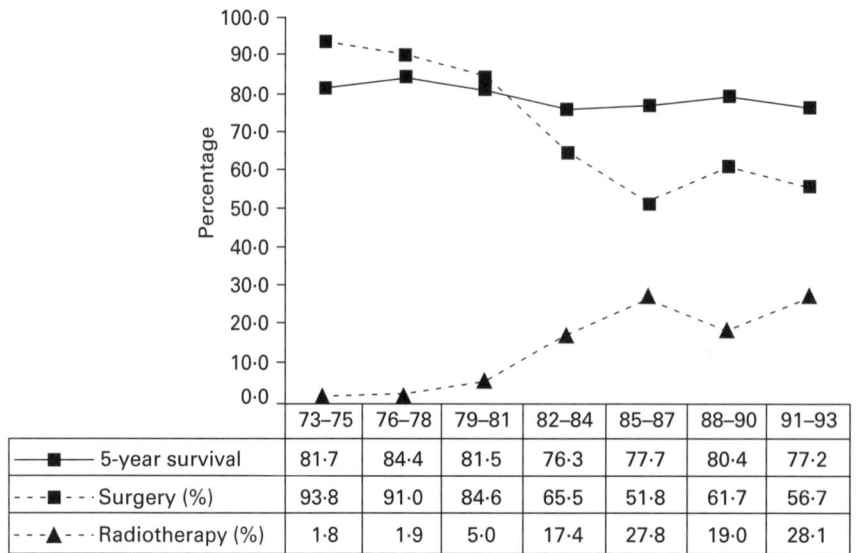

| | 73–75 | 76–78 | 79–81 | 82–84 | 85–87 | 88–90 | 91–93 |
|---|---|---|---|---|---|---|---|
| ■ 5-year survival | 81·7 | 84·4 | 81·5 | 76·3 | 77·7 | 80·4 | 77·2 |
| ■ Surgery (%) | 93·8 | 91·0 | 84·6 | 65·5 | 51·8 | 61·7 | 56·7 |
| ▲ Radiotherapy (%) | 1·8 | 1·9 | 5·0 | 17·4 | 27·8 | 19·0 | 28·1 |

**Figure 48.2**   Five-year relative survival rate with uveal melanoma and proportion of cases treated with surgery and radiotherapy

choroidal melanoma, iodine-125 brachytherapy can be offered to the patients without increasing the risk of mortality over generally accepted standard therapy of enucleation. It is probable that this data can be equally extrapolated to other forms of plaque therapy such as ruthenium-106. Conversely, enucleation can also be recommended without fear of increasing mortality **Evidence level Ia, Grade A**.

### What is the mortality rate associated with uveal melanoma?

Primary uveal melanoma is a malignant tumour with metastatic potential. Various clinical, histopathological and molecular genetic prognostic factors have been determined.[34] The 5-year survival rates following enucleation, brachytherapy, and other methods have ranged from 25% to 66% at 5 years (Table 48.2).[6] With advances made in radiotherapy[35] and other methods of local treatment such as tumour resection[36] and thermotherapy,[37] in recent years there has been a trend away from enucleation.[1]

The 5-year mortality rate with uveal melanoma has ranged from 6% to 53% because of differences in design, data collection, and patient follow up among various studies.[27,29,32,38,39] Meta-analysis of mortality data following enucleation for choroidal melanoma indicated 5-year all-cause mortality of 16%–53% depending upon the size of the tumour.[38] Similar meta-analysis of data on patients treated with plaque radiotherapy indicated melanoma-specific

mortality of 6–26%.[39] Differences between all-cause mortality and melanoma-related mortality can range from 6% to 25% in various studies.[38] It has been observed that up to 40% of deaths in uveal melanoma patients may be due to unrelated causes; therefore, it is more accurate to report melanoma-related mortality.[29] As the cause of death may not be clearly determined in many cases, it can lead to misclassification of metastatic deaths. It is recommended that survival analysis be performed for both all-cause and melanoma mortality as endpoints.[40]

When survival trends over extended periods of time are compared, variations in age-specific death rates influence the survival analysis.[41] In such circumstances relative survival rate provides a useful estimate of the probability of escaping death from a specific cause especially when the cause of death cannot be reliably obtained. In a study by Singh and Topham,[6] the relative survival rate was reported as a ratio of observed survival rate and the expected survival utilising United States life expectancy tables.[42]

The 5-year relative survival rate of about 80% has remained unchanged over the period 1973 to 1997 (Figure 48.2). Similar stability of mortality rates for uveal melanoma between 1951 and 1975 was reported by Strickland and Lee.[3] It is reassuring to note that, with the improvements in accuracy of diagnosis[5] and local methods of treatment of uveal melanoma, there is greater likelihood of avoiding enucleation[1] without compromising patient survival. More importantly, the data indicate that recent advances in methods of treatment of primary uveal melanoma have not led to improvement in survival.[6] These findings further support the concept of early micrometastasis in the presence of uveal melanoma.[43,44] Future treatment protocols must be designed, which not only effectively treat the primary tumour, but also provide adjuvant systemic therapy to eliminate occult metastases **Evidence level Ia, Grade A**.[45]

## References

1 Chang AE, Karnell LH, Menck HR. The National Cancer Data Base report on cutaneous and noncutaneous melanoma: a summary of 84,836 cases from the past decade. The American College of Surgeons Commission on Cancer and the American Cancer Society. *Cancer* 1998;**83**:1664–78.

2 Dutton JJ, Anderson RL, Schelper RL, Purcell JJ, Tse DT. Orbital malignant melanoma and oculodermal melanocytosis: report of two cases and review of the literature. *Ophthalmology* 1984;**91**:497–507.

3 Strickland D, Lee JA. Melanomas of eye: stability of rates. *Am J Epidemiol* 1981;**113**:700–2.

4 Shields JA, Shields CL, Donoso LA. Management of posterior uveal melanoma. *Surv Ophthalmol* 1991;**36**:161–95.

5 Anonymous. Accuracy of diagnosis of choroidal melanomas in the Collaborative Ocular Melanoma Study. COMS report no. 1. *Arch Ophthalmol* 1990;**108**:1268–73.

6 Singh AD, Topham A. Survival rate with uveal melanoma in the United States: 1973–1997. *Ophthalmology* 2003; (in press).

7 Donoso LA, Folberg R, Naids R. Metastatic uveal melanoma. Hepatic metastasis identified by hybridoma-secreted monoclonal antibody Mab8-1H. *Arch Ophthalmol* 1985;**103**:799–801.

8 Eskelin S, Pyrhonen S, Summanen P *et al.* Screening for metastatic malignant melanoma of the uvea revisited. *Cancer* 1999;**85**:1151–9.

9 Rigel D, Carucci JA. Malignant melanoma: prevention, early detection, and treatment in the 21st century. *CA Cancer J Clin* 2000;**50**:215–36.

10 Singh AD, Topham A. Incidence of uveal melanoma in the United States: 1973–1997. *Ophthalmol* 2003; (in press).

11 Scotto J, Fraumeni JF Jr, Lee JA. Melanomas of the eye and other noncutaneous sites: epidemiologic aspects. *J Natl Cancer Inst* 1976;**56**:489–491.

12 Birdsell JM, Gunther BK, Boyd TA, Grace M, Jerry LM. Ocular melanoma: a population-based study. *Can J Ophthalmol* 1980;**15**:9–12.

13 Lommatzsch PK, Staneczek W, Bernt H. Epidemiologic study of new cases of intraocular tumors in East Germany 1961–1980. *Klin Monatsbl Augenheilkunde* 1985;**187**:487–92.

14 Mork T. Malignant melanoma of the eye in Norway: incidence, treatment and prognosis. *Acta Ophthalmologica* 1961;**39**:824–31.

15 Swerdlow AJ. Epidemiology of eye cancer in adults in England and Wales, 1962–1977. *Am J Epidemiol* 1983;**118**:294–300.

16 Swerdlow AJ. Epidemiology of melanoma of the eye in the Oxford Region, 1952–1978. *Br J Cancer* 1983;**47**:311–3.

17 Jensen O. Malignant melanomas of the uvea in Denmark 1943–1952. *Acta Ophthalmologica* 1963;**75**:17–78.

18 Ganley JP, Comstock GW. Benign nevi and malignant melanomas of the choroid. *Am J Ophthalmol* 1973;**76**:19–25.

19 Egan K, Seddon JM, Gragoudas ES *et al.* Uveal melanoma in New England: Profile of cases diagnosed in 1984. *Invest Ophthalmol Visual Sci*, 1987;**28**:S144.

20 Shammas H, Watzke, RC. Bilateral choroidal melanomas. Case report and incidence. *Arch Ophthalmol* 1977;**95**:617–23.

21 Margo C, Mulla, Z, Billiris, K. Incidence of surgically treated uveal melanoma by race and ethnicity. *Ophthalmology* 1998;**105**:1087–90.

22 Zimmerman LE, McLean IW, Foster WD. Does enucleation of the eye containing a malignant melanoma prevent or accelerate the dissemination of tumour cells. *Br J Ophthalmol* 1978;**62**:420–5.

23 Zimmerman LE, McLean IW. An evaluation of enucleation in the management of uveal melanomas. *Am J Ophthalmol* 1979;**87**:741–60.

24 Seigel D, Myers M, Ferris Fr, Steinhorn S. Survival rates after enucleation of eyes with malignant melanoma. *Am J Ophthalmol* 1979;**87**:761–65.

25 Augsburger JJ, Gamel JW, Lauritzen K, Brady LW. Cobalt-60 plaque radiotherapy vs enucleation for posterior uveal melanoma. *Am J Ophthalmol* 1990;**109**:585–92.

26 Augsburger JJ, Schneider S, Freire J, Brady LW. Survival following enucleation versus plaque radiotherapy in statistically matched subgroups of patients with choroidal melanomas: results in patients treated between 1980 and 1987. *Graefes Arch Clin Exp Ophthalmol* 1999;**237**:558–67.

27 Seddon JM, Gragoudas ES, Egan KM *et al.* Relative survival rates after alternative therapies for uveal melanoma. *Ophthalmology* 1990;**97**:769–77.

28 Augsburger JJ, Lauritzen K, Gamel JW *et al.* Matched group study of surgical resection versus cobalt-60 plaque radiotherapy for primary choroidal or ciliary body melanoma. *Ophthal Surg* 1990;**21**:682–8.

29 Kroll S, Char DH, Quivey J, Castro J. A comparison of cause-specific melanoma mortality and all-cause mortality in survival analyses after radiation treatment for uveal melanoma. *Ophthalmology* 1998;**105**:2035–45.

30 Anonymous. The COMS randomized trial of iodine 125 brachytherapy for choroidal melanoma, III: initial mortality findings. COMS report no. 18. *Arch Ophthalmol* 2001;**119**:969–82.

31 Straatsma BR, Fine SL, Earle JD *et al.* Enucleation versus plaque irradiation for choroidal melanoma. *Ophthalmology.* 1988;**95**:1000–4.

32 Anonymous. The Collaborative Ocular Melanoma Study (COMS) randomized trial of pre-enucleation radiation of large choroidal melanoma II: initial mortality findings. COMS report no. 10. *Am J Ophthalmol* 1998;**125**:779–96.

33 Anonymous. Mortality in patients with small choroidal melanoma. COMS report no. 4. The Collaborative Ocular Melanoma Study Group. *Arch Ophthalmol* 1997;**115**:886–93.

34 Singh AD, Shields CL, Shields JA. Prognostic factors in uveal melanoma. *Melanoma Res* 2001.

35 Finger PT. Radiation therapy for choroidal melanoma. *Surv Ophthalmol* 1997;**42**:215–32.

36 Damato BE. Local resection of uveal melanoma. *Bull Soc Belge Ophtalmologie* 1993;**248**:11–7.

37 Oosterhuis JA, Journee-de Korver HG, Keunen JE. Transpupillary thermotherapy: results in 50 patients with choroidal melanoma. *Arch Ophthalmol* 1998;**116**:157–62.

38 Diener-West M, Hawkins BS, Markowitz JA, Schachat AP. A review of mortality from choroidal melanoma. *Arch Ophthalmol* 1992;**110**:245–50.

39 Seregard S. Long-term survival after ruthenium plaque radiotherapy for uveal melanoma. A meta-analysis of studies including 1,066 patients. *Acta Ophthalmol Scand* 1999;**77**:414–7.

40 McLean IW, Gamel JW. Cause-specific versus all-cause survival. *Ophthalmology* 1998;**105**:1989–90.

41 Fleming ID, Cooper JS, Henson DE *et al.* Reporting of cancer survival and end results. *AJCC Cancer staging manual, 5th edn.* Philadelphia: J.B. Lippicott Co.; 1997.

42 Ederer F, Axtell LM, Cutler SJ. The relative survival rate: A statistical methodology. *Natl Cancer Inst Monogr* 1961;**6**:101–21.

43 Eskelin S, Pyrhonen S, Summanen P, Hahka-Kemppinen M, Kivela T. Tumor doubling times in metastatic malignant melanoma of the uvea: tumor progression before and after treatment. *Ophthalmology.* 2000;**107**:1443–9.

44 Singh AD. Uveal melanoma: implications of tumor doubling time. *Ophthalmology* 2001;**108**:829–30.

# 49 Ocular adnexal and orbital tumours

*Santosh G Honavar, Arun D Singh*

## Background

Malignant tumours of the eyelid, ocular adnexa and orbit constitute a significant proportion of cancers diagnosed and managed by an ocular oncologist. The relative frequency of these tumours, however, varies with the group of investigators, geographic area and patient demography.

Basal cell carcinoma, squamous cell carcinoma and sebaceous gland carcinoma are the three common malignant tumours of the eyelids.[1] Basal cell carcinoma is the most common malignant tumour of the eyelid in the Caucasian population,[2] while sebaceous gland carcinoma occurs more frequently in Asians.[3] Melanoma, lymphoma, and ocular surface squamous neoplasia are the common malignant tumours of the conjunctiva.[4] Conjunctival melanoma and lymphoma are common in Europe and America,[5] while ocular surface squamous neoplasia are predominant in Asia and Australia.[6,7] Common orbital malignancies include lymphoma, metastasis and lacrimal gland tumours.[8]

The management of malignant tumours of the eyelid, ocular adnexal and orbit is individualised. Although some of the basic principles of management are uniformly followed, there is wide variation in the overall approach to a particular tumour between major clinical centres. Herein we have attempted to examine the evidence in support of some of the existing beliefs and treatment protocols in the management of these tumours.

## Sebaceous gland carcinoma of the eyelid

### Background

Sebaceous gland carcinoma constitutes 1–3% of all malignant eyelid tumours.[9,10] The disease commonly affects the elderly population, females more predominantly than the males.[9,10] The tumour is relatively more common in the Asian population, constituting about 33% of all malignant eyelid tumours.[3] The tumour arises from the meibomian glands in the tarsus, Zeis glands associated with the lashes, and, rarely, from the caruncle.[9,10] The clinical spectrum is broad and includes the typical nodular type, noduloulcerative type, ulcerative lesion and the diffuse pagetoid tumour.[9,10] While the nodular variant clinically

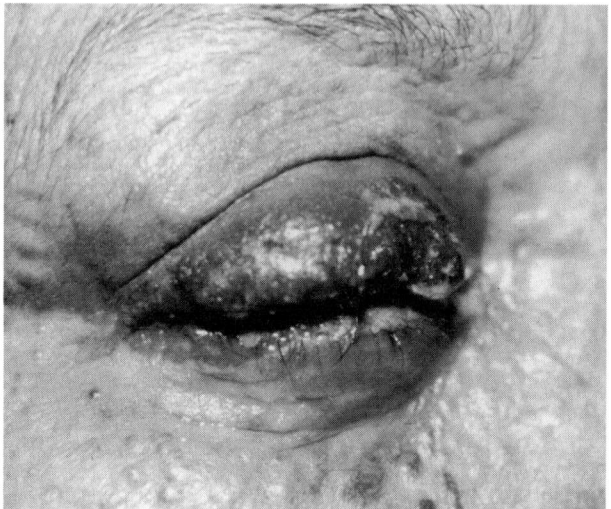

(a)

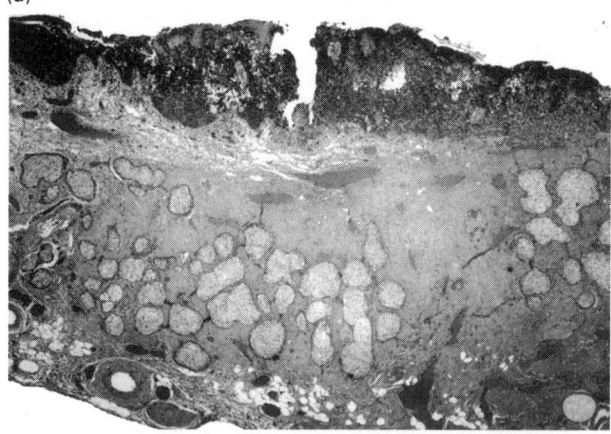

(b)

**Figure 49.1** (a) Patient with diffuse intraepithelial sebaceous gland carcinoma that was initially misdiagnosed and treated as chronic blepharoconjunctivitis. The patient ultimately needed orbital exenteration. (b) Histopathology of intraepithelial sebaceous gland carcinoma showing the diffuse involvement of tarsal and palpebral conjunctiva. (OM×50)

simulates a common chalazion, the diffuse pagetoid type often presents as unilateral blepharoconjunctivitis (masquerade syndrome), leading to delayed diagnosis and inappropriate management (Figure 49.1).[9–11]

Wide surgical excision with histopatholgically confirmed tumour-free margins is believed to be an effective treatment for sebaceous gland carcinoma.[9,10] Radiation is reserved for recurrences and inoperable cases.[9,10] Between 9% and 36% of sebaceous gland carcinomas recur.[9] Recurrences may be local in the eyelid or orbit in 6–17% of cases, while regional lymph node metastasis occurs in 17–28%.[9] The mortality from sebaceous gland carcinoma is estimated to range from 6% to 30%.[9]

Several prognostic factors for local recurrence and tumour metastasis have been identified that include location and size of the tumour, its site of origin, duration of symptoms before excision, and histologic pattern and degree of cellular differentiation.[9,12,13] Poor prognosis is indicated by location of the tumour in the upper eyelid, size of 10 mm or more in diameter, origin from the meibomian glands or multicentricity, duration of symptoms for more than 6 months, infiltrative pattern of growth, invasion of lymphatic and vascular channels, and the orbit, and moderate to poor sebaceous differentiation.[9,12,13]

## Does conjunctival intraepithelial invasion in sebaceous gland carcinoma indicate poor prognosis?

### Evidence

Our literature search failed to bring out any strong evidence to either support or contradict the prevalent clinical impression that conjunctival intraepithelial neoplasia in sebaceous gland carcinoma indicates poor prognosis and necessitates aggressive management. We did not find randomised controlled trials, systematic reviews, or meta-analysis addressing the issue.

Some retrospective studies suggest that cases of sebaceous gland carcinoma with intraepithelial neoplasia had a significantly greater mortality than cases without these changes. Boniuk and Zimmerman felt that the long delay in correct diagnosis and appropriate management probably contribute to 30% mortality in patients with intraepithelial neoplasia.[14] Rao and associates reported that 5-year mortality of 43% in patients who had intraepithelial neoplasia, compared to 11% in patients who did not.[12,13] Doxanas and Green found that the mortality was not substantially influenced by the presence or absence of intraepithelial neoplasia.[15] In their series, tumour-related deaths occurred in 14% of patients with intraepithelial neoplasia and 18% in those without such involvement.[15] A recent retrospective case series by Chao and associates reported that patients with intraepithelial neoplasia carried a higher risk for orbital exenteration (36% *v* 7%), but comparable incidence of tumour metastasis **Evidence level IIb, Grade B**.[16]

### Discussion

The prognostic significance of conjunctival intraepithelial neoplasia remains controversial, primarily because its biological potential is unknown. It has been estimated that between 41% and 80% of sebaceous gland carcinomas are associated with intraepithelial neoplasia.[12,15,17] Because of its tendency to invoke secondary inflammation of the substantia propria of the conjunctiva, the condition may be misdiagnosed resulting in delayed management.[9,18] Based on the available evidence, it is not justifiable to conclude that the presence of intraepithelial neoplasia in a patient with sebaceous gland carcinoma entails poor life prognosis. However, patients with intraepithelial neoplasia may be detected at a relatively more advanced stage and may need more aggressive treatment.

### Implications

Although there is disagreement over the prognostic significance of intraepithelial neoplasia, the clinical significance of its early recognition cannot be overemphasised. The management of such tumours can be challenging. Conjunctival map biopsy may help delineate the extent of involvement.[19] Some authors have suggested observation of small areas of involvement while others have recommended surgical excision with clear margins, adjuvant cryotherapy, radiotherapy, or orbital exenteration depending on the nature and extent of involvement.

## Basal cell carcinoma of the eyelid

### Background

Basal cell carcinoma is the most common human malignancy and accounts for over 80% of all non-melanoma skin cancers.[20] It is the most common skin cancer of the eyelid (80–90%) in the Western population.[21–24] Most tumours arise from the lower eyelid or medial canthus.[25] These tumours rarely metastasise but can potentially cause mortality by extensive tissue destruction and direct invasion of the central nervous system.[26]

There are a variety of methods used to treat basal cell carcinomas.[25,26] The management strategy depends on the size, extent and location of the lesion.[25,26] Some of the modalities of management of basal cell carcinoma include electrodesiccation, cryotherapy, photodynamic therapy, local or systemic chemotherapy, surgical excision and radiation therapy.[25,26] Surgical excision is coupled with a suitable technique to determine the adequacy of the margins.[27–29] Mohs micrographic technique is considered the most reliable surgical method for tumour extirpation.[30–34] It differs from the other methods of microscopic control in several respects. The tumour is excised in a layered manner and carefully mapped, and the entire surgical margin is examined microscopically (Figure 49.2).[34] Mohs micrographic surgery is believed to have the lowest recurrence rate for

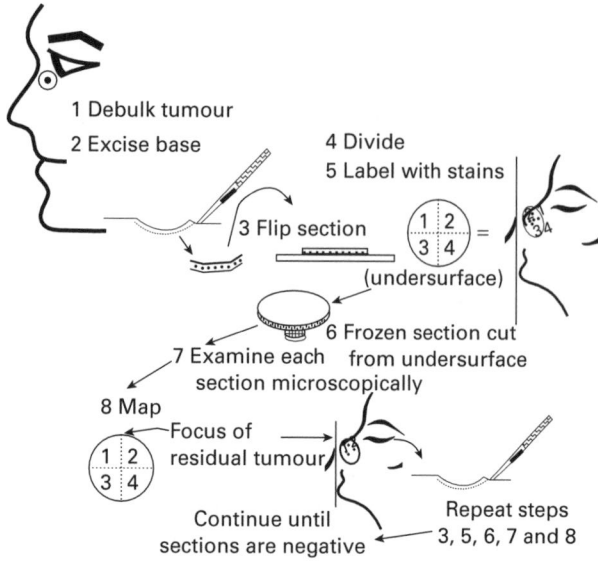

1 Debulk tumour
2 Excise base
3 Flip section
4 Divide
5 Label with stains
6 Frozen section cut from undersurface
7 Examine each section microscopically
8 Map
Focus of residual tumour
Continue until sections are negative
Repeat steps 3, 5, 6, 7 and 8

**Figure 49.2**   The steps in Mohs micrographic surgery

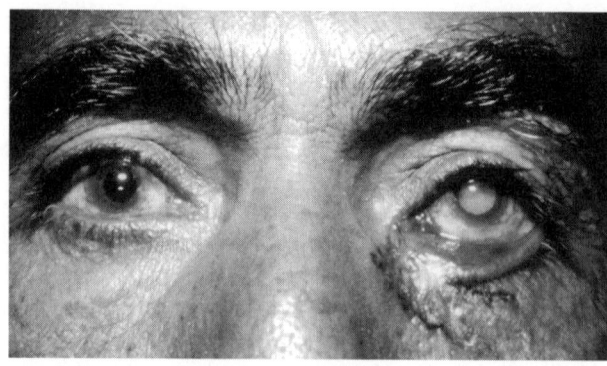

**Figure 49.3**   Morphoeaform basal cell carcinoma of the lower eyelid

both primary and recurrent tumours.[30–34] In the past, ophthalmologists have traditionally tended toward surgical management for periocular basal cell carcinomas. However, the growing experience with radiotherapy and the improving success rate now make this modality an acceptable alternative in several cases.[26]

## Does Mohs micrographic procedure provide better success than radiation therapy in the management of periocular basal cell carcinoma?

### Evidence

There is no randomised controlled trial comparing the efficacy of the Mohs micrographic procedure with radiation therapy in the management of periocular basal cell carcinoma. We found several case series evaluating the two modalities individually and a systematic review article[34] that gives an overview. Five-year cure rates for Mohs micrographic surgery in the treatment of small (< 3 cm) primary periocular basal cell carcinomas have been reported by several authors to range from 97% to 99%.[35–42] The cure rate is high for smaller tumours and relatively low for larger tumours.[35–42] Frederick Mohs has had the greatest experience in using the micrographic procedure on the eyelid.[37–40] His overall cure rate for more than 1700 tumours was 99%.[37–40] However, there was significantly more failure when the tumour size was 3 mm or larger (10%).[37–40] Robins similarly reported a cure rate of 98% for tumours less than 2 cm, with a decrease in cure rate to 92% for tumours greater than 5 cm.[41,42] Among the other larger

case series available, Anderson's results parallel those of Mohs.[43] Callahan and associates report an impressive success (98%) in a group of 231 patients with large or recurrent tumours at an average follow up of 4 years.[44,45]

Radiation therapy for primary basal cell carcinoma carries a 5-year cure rate ranging from 70% to 98%.[26,31,32,34,46–51] Five-year control rates of 95–98% in some series are comparable to the results of surgical therapy.[49] Rowe and associates reported 95% short-term (< 5 years) and 91% long-term (5 years) success in tumour control following radiotherapy for primary basal cell carcinomas.[31,32] Nordman and associates reported 82% disease-free rate at 2 years and 69% at 5 years following radiotherapy.[51] Basal cell carcinomas ≤ 2 cm in diameter are controlled with irradiation in more than 90% of cases.[26,34] Large tumours (> 5 cm) are more likely to recur (> 40%) than small tumours. There is evidence to suggest that morpheaform basal cell carcinoma (Figure 49.3) may be more radioresistant[26,34] **Evidence level IIa, Grade B**.

### Discussion

With modern techniques, both Mohs surgery and radiotherapy would appear to offer good and nearly comparable control of periocular tumours.[34] In the past, ophthalmologists have traditionally leaned towards surgical management for all periocular basal cell carcinomas.[26] However, the growing experience with radiotherapy and the improving success rate now makes this modality an acceptable alternative in several cases.[26,34] The choice between the two techniques for the management of basal cell carcinoma will depend on several factors including tumour location, size and extent; whether it is a primary or a recurrent tumour; the availability of a Mohs surgeon, an oculoplastic surgeon, or a radiotherapist with experience in treating such tumours; the availability of tissue for reconstruction; and the potential functional consequences of treatment.[34] For small tumours, Mohs surgery is appropriate and reconstruction is fairly simple.[34] Although radiotherapy for such small tumours gives excellent results, it is less convenient, requiring multiple treatment sessions over several weeks, and probably offers little advantage over Mohs surgery in most cases.[34] For medium-sized lesions, and for those that are very extensive and difficult to resect, radiotherapy offers a good alternative to surgery, yielding better cosmetic and functional results with only a marginally higher recurrence rate.[34] For all recurrent tumours, regardless of size, Mohs surgery with histologic control of margins is mandatory, and radiotherapy is not appropriate, unless the tumours are unresectable.[34]

### Implications

Mohs' microsurgical technique and radiotherapy can be interchangeably used in most situations in patients with basal cell carcinoma. The nature, location, size and extent of the tumour, and the cosmetic and functional implications of a particular treatment modality help in deciding for a treatment option.

## Ocular surface squamous neoplasia

### Background

Ocular surface squamous neoplasia (OSSN) presents as a spectrum ranging from dysplasia to carcinoma *in situ* to invasive squamous cell carcinoma, involving the conjunctiva as well as the cornea.[52,53] It is a relatively uncommon ocular tumour, with an incidence varying from 0·13 per 100 000 population in Africa[54] to 1·9 per 100 000 population in Australia.[55] Although the condition is predominant in Caucasians, darker skinned populations in tropical climates closer to the equator do develop OSSN.[53] The disease preferentially occurs in older individuals.[52,53] The spectrum of histological severity of OSSN has been classified (Box 49.1).[56,57]

Tumour excision with adequate margins is the most accepted method of treatment of OSSN.[52,53] Several variations in the surgical technique have been described.[52,53,58,59] Additional procedures may include cryotherapy to the excision edge and base, use of alcohol to remove the affected corneal epithelium, lamellar keratectomy and lamellar sclerectomy.[52,53,60,61] Local recurrence rates following tumour excision range from 15% to 52%.[53] Inadequacy of excision margins has been identified as a major risk factor for recurrence.[57,62] Other modalities of treatment include radiotherapy, immunotherapy and chemotherapy.[52,53] These modalities are mostly advocated in situations where tumour excision is not feasible or optimal.[52,53] Recent attention has been given to the use of topical chemotherapy in the management of OSSN (Figure 49.4).[63–71] The topical

---

**Box 49.1 The spectrum of histological severity of ocular surface squamous neoplasia**

**1 Dysplasia**

- Mild – less than a third thickness of the epithelium occupied by atypical cells
- Moderate – three-quarters thickness of the epithelium occupied by atypical cells
- Severe – nearly full thickness of the epithelium occupied by atypical cells

**2 Carcinoma *in situ*** – full thickness involvement of the epithelium by atypical cells with loss of the normal surface layer

**3 Invasive squamous cell carcinoma** – full thickness involvement of the epithelium by atypical cells with loss of the normal surface layer, breach of the basement membrane of the basal epithelial layer and invasion of the substantia propria

---

chemotherapeutic agents that have been evaluated are mitomycin C and 5-fluorouracil (5-FU).[63–72]

### Is there a role for primary topical chemotherapy in the management of ocular surface squamous neoplasia (OSSN)?

#### Evidence

Mitomycin C is an alkylating agent that induces cross-linkage of the DNA base pairs adenine and guanine and inhibits DNA synthesis in all phases of the cell cycle, in addition to causing breakage of single-stranded DNA.[72] The adjunctive use of mitomycin C is well established in trabeculectomy and recurrent pterygium surgery.[72]

Dermatologists have long used topical 5-FU in the treatment of premalignant and malignant epithelial diseases of the skin.[72] The drug has been evaluated for its antifibroblastic action in trabeculectomy. The mechanism of action of 5FU is the inhibition of DNA formation by blocking the enzyme thymidylate synthetase.[72]

There is no randomised case–control study evaluating the role of topical chemotherapeutic agents in the management of OSSN. Our literature search did not yield any meta-analysis or a large case series. A review article by Majumdar and Epstein summarises several small case series that have been published in peer-reviewed journals.[72]

Several small case series demonstrate the beneficial role of topical mitomycin C in the management of OSSN.[64–68] In 1994, Frucht-Pery and Rozenman were credited with the first application of mitomycin C in the treatment of OSSN predominantly involving the cornea.[64] Three patients with corneal intraepithelial neoplasia involving the visual axis were selected to receive topical mitomycin C 0·02% four

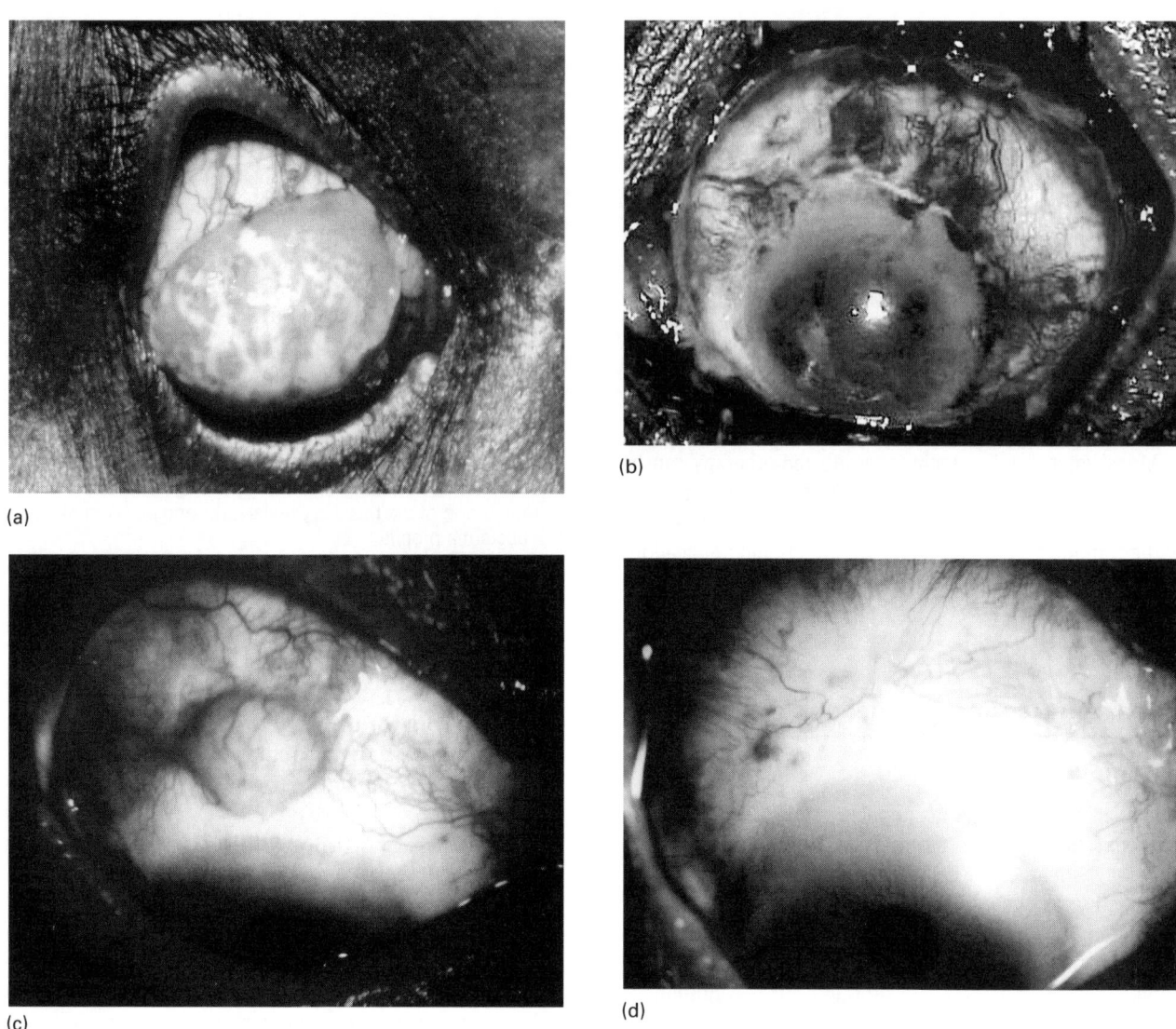

**Figure 49.4** (a) Patient with a large ocular surface squamous neoplasia. (b) Area of excision reconstructed by amniotic membrane transplantation. (c) Local recurrence 3 months following initial treatment. (d) Final appearance at 1 year following the treatment of local recurrence with three cycles of mitomycin C drops 0·04 mg ml, four times a day, four days a week and for 4 weeks per cycle

times a day for 10–22 days. Within 9 weeks, the abnormal cells were replaced by biomicroscopically normal epithelium. Frucht-Pery *et al.* later published the results of a multicentre collaborative study involving 17 patients from seven centres in Israel and the United States who were given topical mitomycin C 0·02–0·04% four times a day for 7–28 days.[65] The treatment was offered in cases of recurrent conjunctival intraepithelial neoplasia or when patients refused surgical intervention. In 11 of 17 cases, the lesion regressed after the first course of mitomycin C. Six of 17 cases needed a second course of treatment for recurrence and one of these required a third course. Wilson and associates used topical mitomycin C 0·04% four times a day for 7 days in seven patients with varying degrees of

histopathologically confirmed corneal and conjunctival intraepithelial neoplasia, which was either recurrent or diffuse, precluding surgical excision. Six of seven patients experienced complete regression and remained free of recurrence at an average follow up of 9 months.[66] Heigle *et al.* reported similar encouraging success in three patients with recurrent OSSN.[67] Akpek and associates successfully used topical mitomycin C 0·02% three times a day for 2 weeks in four patients to prevent tumour recurrence following incomplete surgical excision.[73]

The role of 5-FU in the treatment of OSSN has been evaluated by several short case series.[63,69–71] In 1986, de Keizer and associates described the successful use of topical 5-FU 1% in five patients with intraepithelial neoplasia of the eyelid, cornea and conjunctiva.[63] Yeatts and associates reported moderate success in their series of six cases that received three cycles of topical 5-FU 1% three to four times a day for 14–21 days.[69] While four of six patients remained in regression, one patient had recurrence at 30 months and required excision and another needed orbital exenteration. Midena and colleagues found topical 5-FU used as 1% drops four times a day for 4 weeks effective in inducing regression of recurrent, residual, or selected primary tumours in their series of 8 patients **Evidence level III, Grade B** .[70,71]

### Discussion

The available reports indicate that topical chemotherapy using mitomycin C or 5-FU drops does have a role in the management of OSSN.[63–73] However, the studies involve only a small number of cases and include a wide clinical spectrum.[63–73] It is difficult to clearly define the indications and the dosage schedule based on the existing knowledge. The modality has been tried in a variety of indications including primary therapy, as an adjuvant following surgical excision in cases with incompletely excised tumour or excision margin involvement detected on histopathology, and for recurrent tumour. The cases were mostly limited to dysplasia or carcinoma *in situ*. Only a few infiltrative squamous cell carcinoma have been treated with topical chemotherapy.[63–73] The minimum effective dosage needs to be established in further studies. Ocular toxicity of topical chemotherapeutic agents appears to be limited to the duration of treatment.[63–73] No major irreversible side effect is reported.

### Implications

Surgical excision with margin control remains the standard of care in the management of localised OSSN. In patients with incompletely resected lesions, diffuse tumours where complete resection is not possible, or recurrent tumours, topical chemotherapy may be a viable option. It could also be used in patients who refuse to, or are unable to, undergo surgical intervention.

## Adenoid cystic carcinoma of the lacrimal gland

### Background

A broad spectrum of neoplastic and inflammatory diseases can affect the lacrimal gland (Box 49.2).[74] Lacrimal gland lesions constitute approximately 5–13% of orbital lesions that undergo biopsy.[75–77] Based primarily on Reese's clinicopathologic survey of 112 consecutive lesions of the lacrimal gland, most authors report that approximately 50% of the lesions are epithelial in nature and 50% are non-epithelial in origin.[76] Of non-epithelial lesions, 50% are lymphoid tumours and 50% are infectious and inflammatory

**Box 49.2 Lesions of the lacrimal gland**

I  Congenital
   Dermoid cyst

II  Inflammation
  A  Infectious
    1  Viral dacryoadenitis
    2  Bacterial dacryoadenitis
    3  Fungal infection
  B  Non-infectious
    1  Idiopathic inflammation
    2  Secondary to systemic diseases
      a  Sjögrens syndrome
      b  Sarcoidosis
      c  Wagener's granulomatosis
      d  Systemic lupus erythematosis
      e  Graves' orbitopathy
      f  Kimura's disease

III  Lymphoproliferative disorders
  A  Benign lymphoid hyperplasia
  B  Atypical lymphoid hyperplasia
  C  Warthin's tumour
  D  Malignant lymphoma

IV  Benign tumours
  A  Pleomorphic adenoma
  B  Myoepithelioma
  C  Oncocytoma
  D  Solitary fibrous tumour
  E  Cavernous haemangioma
  F  Haemangiopericytoma

V  Malignant tumours
  A  Adenoid cystic carcinoma
  B  Primary adenocarcinoma
  C  Pleomorphic adenocarcinoma
  D  Mucoepidermoid carcinoma
  E  Acinic cell carcinoma

pseudotumours.[76] Among the epithelial tumours of the lacrimal gland, approximately 50% are benign pleomorphic adenomas, 25% adenoid cystic carcinoma, and the remainder are other types of carcinoma.[76]

Adenoid cystic carcinoma, the most common non-lymphoid malignant tumour of the lacrimal gland affects the younger patients and confers the worst prognosis (Figure 49.5).[74] Despite extensive surgery and radiation therapy, the prognosis for these patients remains grim, with survival of less than 50% at 5 years and 20% at 10 years.[75] Several studies document a recurrence rate of 55–88% within 5 years of diagnosis with standard local therapies.[78–83] The dismal cure rate and survival has been attributed to aggressive biological behaviour of the tumour and propensity to perineural, haematogenous and lymphatic invasion.[78–84] Radical orbitectomy for adenoid cystic

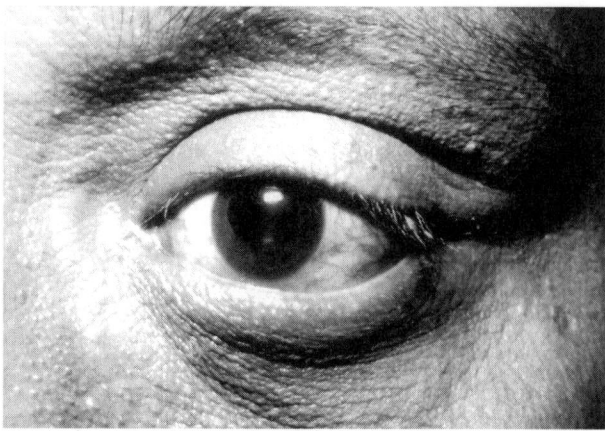

(a)

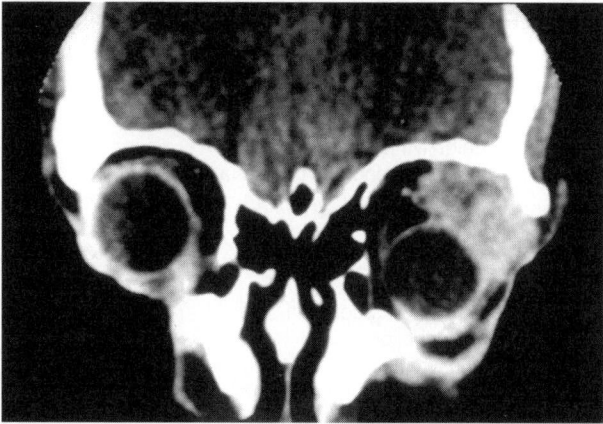

(b)

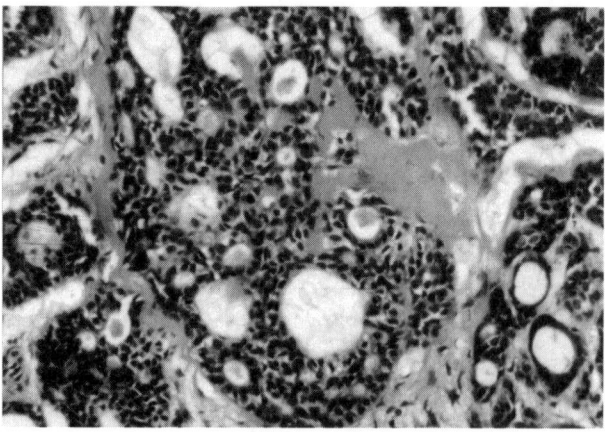

(c)

**Figure 49.5** (a) Patient with proptosis of the left eye with subtle downward and medial displacement. (b) CT scan of the same patient showing a mass in the area of the lacrimal gland with bone changes. (c) Histopathology of adenoid cystic carcinoma (OM×100) showing the basaloid pattern.

carcinoma is advocated by many authorities.[85,86] This disfiguring surgery involves removing the orbital contents

*en bloc* along with orbital bone.[85,86] Comparison of survival rates for radical versus eye-sparing procedures has failed to demonstrate improved survival with more radical procedures.[82–87] Complete surgical excision of adenoid cystic carcinoma of the lacrimal gland is difficult to achieve even with radical surgery.[84] In fact, the most common site of recurrence of the tumour is local.[82] Complex regional anatomy, an infiltrative growth pattern and perineural spread explain the apparent inability to surgically remove every malignant cell regardless of the technique employed.[84] Because of the well-known limitations of surgery, nearly all patients undergoing resection of adenoid cystic carcinoma of the lacrimal gland receive postoperative radiotherapy.[84] However, the poor rate of local control and the tendency towards late metastasis suggest that radiotherapy is unable to alter the course of the disease favorably.[87]

Adenoid cystic carcinoma of the lacrimal gland has many similarities to malignant epithelial tumours of the parotid and salivary glands.[84] They share common morphology, embryogenesis and the biological potential for perineural invasion.[88,89] The prognosis of these tumours is equally dismal.[88,89] Chemotherapy is the treatment of choice for tumours that metastasise early and cannot be controlled locally with a combination of surgery and radiation therapy.[84] Some patients with adenoid cystic carcinoma of the salivary glands respond to chemotherapy.[90,91] Neoadjuvant chemotherapy with cisplatinum for adenoid cystic carcinoma of the salivary glands combined with surgery and radiation therapy has yielded some promising preliminary results.[90,91] There are efforts currently to evaluate neoadjuvant and adjuvant chemotherapy in the management of adenoid cystic carcinoma of the lacrimal gland.[92]

## Does chemotherapy in the management of adenoid cystic carcinoma of the lacrimal gland minimise local recurrence, metastasis and death?

### Evidence

The literature search identified only a case series by Meldrum and associates who treated two patients with locally advanced adenoid cystic carcinoma of the lacrimal gland with a new chemotherapy protocol.[92] The regimen consisted of neoadjuvant preoperative cytoreductive intracarotid chemotherapy and postoperative intravenous chemotherapy as an adjunct to conventional orbital exenteration and radiation therapy. The treatment protocol is shown is Box 49.3.[92] Tumour shrinkage was radiographically documented following preoperative neoadjuvant chemotherapy, downstaging the disease in one case from an intracranial involvement to a respectable intrarorbital tumour. Tumour necrosis was confirmed in the exenteration

---

**Box 49.3 Management protocol for adenoid cystic carcinoma of the lacrimal gland[74,83]**

1 Neoadjuvant chemotherapy

  a Hydration to achieve a urine output $\geq 150$ ml per hour and maintained for 48 hours

  b Insertion of intracarotid catheter

  c Infusion of cisplatinum, $100 \text{ mg m}^{-2}$ diluted in 500 ml normal saline over 60 minutes

  d Intravenous push of oxorubicin $25 \text{ mg m}^{-2}$ per day for 3 days

  e Chemotherapy cycle repeated at least twice separated by 21 days

  f Assessment of radiographic response by serial CT scan

2 Orbital exenteration performed 3–4 weeks after the last course of chemotherapy and following haematological recovery (WBC $>2500$ cells mm$^{-3}$, platelet count 100 000 cells mm$^{-3}$)

3 Radiation therapy (5500–6000 cGy) to the orbit, superior orbital fissure, inferior orbital fissure, cavernous sinus and the temporal fossa 4–6 weeks after orbital exenteration in the standard daily fraction protocol

4 Radiation sensitiser cisplatinum $20 \text{ mg m}^{-2}$ intravenous infusion over 30 minutes once a week during radiotherapy

5 Adjuvant chemotherapy 2–4 weeks after completion of radiotherapy, intravenous cisplatinum, $100 \text{ mg m}^{-2}$ on day 1 and intravenous doxorubicin $20 \text{ mg m}^{-2}$ on days 1 to 3

---

specimen. Systemic morbidity was minimal and both the patients were free of metastasis at 7·5 years and 9·5 years following treatment. Tse and Benedetto from the same group have since treated three additional patients[74] **Evidence level III, Grade C**.

## Discussion

Adenoid cystic carcinoma of the lacrimal gland has a proclivity for microscopic perineural, soft tissue and bone infiltration, because of which complete tumour clearance may not be possible despite meticulous excision, exenteration, or even orbitectomy.[74,78,79,82–87] Adjuvant radiotherapy is a reasonable option but tissue penetration can be a limiting factor.[74] Not surprisingly, orbital exenteration, exenteration combined with radiation, and radical cranio-orbital resection have not resulted in improved survival.[74,78,82–87] Theoretically, chemotherapy has the best potential to eradicate occult metastatic disease.[74] Systemic chemotherapy often fails to deliver therapeutic concentration to the target area. In contrast, intra-arterial delivery achieves a higher drug concentration

in the target area while minimising systemic side effects.[74,92] The new treatment protocol involving neoadjuvant preoperative intracarotid chemotherapy, orbital exenteration, post-operative radiation and post-operative adjuvant chemotherapy in the management of adenoid cystic carcinoma of the lacrimal gland has shown promising results.[74,92] However, the number of cases is small. To fully evaluate the beneficial effect of the new protocol over the conventional treatment of this rare disease, a multicentre randomised trial may be warranted.

## Implications

There are indications that the new treatment protocol may improve the prognosis of adenoid cystic carcinoma of the lacrimal gland.

## References

1 Hornblass A. Clinical evaluation of tumours of the eye and adnexa. In: Hornblass A, Hanig CJ, ed. *Oculoplastic, Reconstructive, and Orbital Surgery, Volume I, Eyelids*. Baltimore: William and Wilkins, 1988.

2 Margo CE, Waltz K. Basal cell carcinoma of the eyelid and periocular skin. *Surv Ophthalmol* 1993;**38**:169–92.

3 Ni C, Searl SS, Kuo PK *et al*. Sebaceous cell carcinomas of the ocular adnexa. *Int Ophthalmol Clin* 1982;**22**:23–61.

4 Shields JA, Shields CL. *Atlas of Eyelid and Conjunctival Tumors*. Philadelphia: Lippincott Williams and Wilkins, 1999.

5 Shields CL, Shields JA, Gunduz K *et al*. Conjunctival melanoma: risk factors for recurrence, exenteration, metastasis, and death in 150 consecutive patients. *Arch Ophthalmol* 2000;**118**:1497–507.

6 Shields CL, Shields JA, Carvaoho C *et al*. Conjunctival lymphoid tumors: clinical analysis of 117 cases and relationship to systemic lymphoma. *Ophthalmology* 2001;**108**:979–84.

7 Lee GA, Hirst LW. Ocular surface squamous neoplasia. *Surv Ophthalmol* 1995;**39**:429–50.

8 Shields JA. *Diagnosis and Management of Orbital Tumors*. Philadelphia: WB Saunders Co., 1989.

9 Kass LG, Hornblass A. Sebaceous carcinoma of the ocular adnexa. *Surv Ophthalmol* 1989;**33**:477–90.

10 Hornblass A. Clinical evaluation of tumors of the eye and adnexa. In: Hornblass A, Hanig CJ, eds. *Oculoplastic, Reconstructive, and Orbital Surgery, Volume I, Eyelids*. Baltimore: William and Wilkins, 1988.

11 Honavar SG, Shields CL, Maus M *et al*. Primary intraepithelial sebaceous gland carcinoma of the palpebral conjunctiva. *Arch Ophthalmol* 2001;**119**:764–7.

12 Rao NA, McLean JW, Zimmerman LE. Sebaceous carcinoma of the eyelid and caruncle: correlation of clinicopathologic features with prognosis. In: Jacobiec FA, ed. *Ocular and Adnexal Tumors*. Birmingham: Aesculapuis, 1978.

13 Rao NA, Hidayat AA, McLean JW *et al*. Sebaceous carcinomas of the ocular adnexa: a clinicopathologic study of 104 cases with five year follow-up data. *Hum Pathol* 1982;**13**:113–22.

14 Boniuk M, Zimmerman LE. Sebaceous carcinoma of the eyelid, eyebrow, caruncle, and orbit. *Trans Am Acad Ophthalmol Otolaryngol* 1968;**72**:619–41.

15 Doxanas MT, Green WR. Sebaceous gland carcinoma: review of 40 cases. *Arch Ophthalmol* 1984;**102**:245–9.

16 Chao AN, Shields CL, Krema H *et al*. Outcome of patients with periocular sebaceous gland carcinoma with and without conjunctival intraepithelial invasion. *Ophthalmology* 2001;**108**:1877–83.

17 Wolfe JT III, Yeats RP, Wick MR *et al*. Sebaceous carcinoma of the eyelid. *Am J Surg Pathol* 1984;**8**:597–606.

18 Margo CE, Grossniklaus H. Intraepithelial sebaceous neoplasia without underlying invasive carcinoma. *Surv Ophthalmol* 1995;**39**:293-301.

19 Putterman AM. Conjunctival map biopsy to determine pagetoid spread. *Am J Ophthalmol* 1986;**102**:87–90.

20 Scotto J, Fears TR, Fraumeni JF Jr. *Incidence of nonmelanoma skin cancer in the United States.* US Department of Health and Human Services NIH Publication, No 83–2433, 1983.

21 Aurora AL, Blodi FC. Lesions of the eyelids: a clinicopathological study. *Surv Ophthalmol* 1970;**15**:94–104.

22 Aurora AL, Blodi FC. Reappraisal of basal cell carcinoma of the eyelids. *Am J Ophthalmol* 1970;**70**:329–36.

23 Kwitko ML, Boniuk M, Zimmerman LE. Eyelid tumors with reference to lesions confused with squamous cell carcinomas. I. Incidence and errors in diagnosis. *Arch Ophthalmol* 1963;**69**:3–7.

24 Lober CW, Fenske NA. Basal cell, squamous cell, and sebaceous gland carcinomas of the periorbital region. *J Am Acad Dermatol* 1991;**25**: 685–90.

25 Shields CL. Basal cell carcinoma of the eyelids. *Int Ophthalmol Clin* 1993;**33**:1–4.

26 Margo CE, Waltz K. Basal cell carcinoma of the eyelid and periocular skin. *Surv Ophthalmol* 1993;**38**:169–92.

27 Chalfin J, Putterman AM. Frozen section control in the surgery of basal cell carcinoma of the eyelid. *Am J Ophthalmol* 1979;**87**:802–9.

28 Doxanas MT, Green WR, Iliff CE. Factors in the successful surgical management of basal cell carcinoma of the eyelid. *Am J Ophthalmol* 1981;**91**:729–36.

29 Vitaliano PP, Urbach F. The relative importance of risk factors in nonmelanoma carcinoma. *Arch Dermatol* 1980;**116**:454–6.

30 Mohs FE. Micrographic surgery for the microscopically controlled excision of eyelid cancers. *Arch Ophthalmol* 1986;**104**:901–9.

31 Rowe DE, Carroll R, Day DL Jr. Long-term recurrence rates in previously untreated (primary) basal cell carcinoma: Implications for patient follow-up. *J Dermatol Surg Oncol* 1989;**15**:315–28.

32 Rowe DE, Carroll R, Day DL Jr. Mohs' surgery is the treatment of choice for recurrent (previously untreated) basal cell carcinoma. *J Dermatol Surg Oncol* 1989;**15**:425–31.

33 Swanson NA. Mohs' surgery: technique, indications, applications, and the future. *Arch Dermatol* 1983;**119**:761–73.

34 Dutton J, Slamovits T, ed. Management of periocular basal cell carcinoma: Mohs' micrographic surgery versus radiotherapy. *Surv Ophthalmol* 1993;**38**:193–212.

35 Anderson RL, Ceilley RI. Multispecialty approach to excision and reconstruction of eyelid tumors. *Ophthalmology* 1978;**85**:1150-63.

36 Baylis HI, Cies WA. Indications of Mohs' chemosurgical excision of eyelid and canthal tumors. *Am J Ophthalmol* 1975;**80**:116–22.

37 Mohs FE. *Chemosurgery: Microscopically Controlled Surgery for Skin Cancer.* Springfield: Charles C Thomas, 1978.

38 Mohs FE. Chemosurgery: Microscopically controlled surgery for skin cancer: Past, present, and future. *J Dermatol Surg Oncol* 1978;**4**:41–2.

39 Mohs FE. Mohs' micrographic surgery: A historical perspective. *Dermatol Clin* 1989;**7**:609–11.

40 Mohs FE. Micrographic surgery for the microscopically controlled excision of eyelid cancer: History and development. *Adv Ophthal Plast Reconstr Surg* 1986;**5**:381–408.

41 Robins P. Chemosurgery: My 15 years of experience. *Dermatol Surg Oncol* 1981;**7**:779–89.

42 Robins P, Rodriquez-Sains R, Rabinovitz H *et al.* Mohs' surgery for periocular basal cell carcinoma. *J Dermatol Surg Oncol* 1985;**11**: 1203–7.

43 Anderson RL. Mohs' micrographic technique. *Arch Ophthalmol* 1986;**104**:818–19.

44 Callahan A, Monheit GD, Callahan MA. Cancer excision from eyelids and ocular adnexa: The Mohs' fresh tissue technique and reconstruction. *Cancer* 1982;**32**:322–9.

45 Callahan A. Mohs' technique. *Cancer* 1986;**36**:373–5.

46 Cobb GM, Thomson GA, Allt WEC. Treatment of basal cell carcinoma of the eyelids by radiotherapy. *Can Med Assoc J* 1964;**91**:743–8.

47 Fayos JV, Wildemuth O. Carcinoma of the skin of the eyelids. *Arch Ophthalmol* 1962;**67**:298–302.

48 Fitzpatrick PJ, Jamieson DM, Thompson GA *et al.* Tumors of the eyelids and their treatment by radiotherapy. *Radiology* 1972;**102**:661–5.

49 Fitzpatrick PJ, Thompson GA, Easterbrook WM *et al.* Basal and squamous cell carcinoma of the eyelids and their treatment by radiotherapy. *Int J Radiat Oncol Biol Phys* 1984;**10**:449–54.

50 Lederman M. Radiation treatment of cancer of the eyelids. *Br J Ophthalmol* 1976;**60**:794–805.

51 Nordman EM, Nordman LEO. Treatment of basal cell carcinoma of the eyelid. *Acta Ophthalmol* 1978;**56**:349–56.

52 Cha SB, Shields JA, Shields CL *et al.* Squamous cell carcinoma of the conjunctiva. *Int Ophthalmol Clin* 1993;**33**:19–24.

53 Lee GH, Hirst LW. Ocular surface squamous neoplasia. *Surv Ophthalmol* 1995;**39**:429–50.

54 Templeton AC. Tumors of the eye and adnexa in Africans of Uganda. *Cancer* 1967;**20**:1689–98.

55 Lee GA, Hirst LW. Incidence of ocular surface epithelial dysplasia in metropolitan Brisbane: A 10-year survey. *Arch Ophthalmol* 1992; **110**:525–7.

56 Grossniklaus HE, Green WR, Lukenback M *et al.* Conjunctival lesions in adults: A clinical and histopathologic review. *Cornea* 1987;**6**:78–116.

57 Pizzarello LD, Jakobiec FA. Bowen's disease of the conjunctiva: a misnomer. In: Jakobiec FA, ed. *Ocular and Adnexal Tumors.* Birmingham: Aesculapius, 1978.

58 Shields JA, Shields CL, De Potter P. Surgical management of conjunctival tumors. The 1994 Lynn B McMahan lecture. *Arch Ophthalmol* 1997;**115**:808–15.

59 Char DH, Crawford JB, Howes El *et al.* Resection of intraocular squamous cell carcinoma. *Br J Ophthalmol* 1992;**76**:123–5.

60 Freedman J, Rohm G. Surgical management and histopathology of invasive tumors of the cornea. *Br J Ophthalmol* 1979;**63**:632–5.

61 Zimmerman LE. The cancerous, precancerous, and pseudocancerous lesions of the cornea and conjunctiva: The Pocklington memorial lecture. In: Rycroft PV, ed. *Corneoplastic Surgery.* New York: Pergamon Press, 1969.

62 Erie JC, Campbell RJ, Liesegang J. Conjunctival and corneal intraepithelial and invasive neoplasia. *Ophthalmology* 1986;**93**:176–83.

63 de Keizer RJW, de Wolff Rouendaal D, Van Delft JL. Topical application of 5-fluorouracil in premalignant lesions of the cornea, conjunctiva, and eyelid. *Doc Ophthalmol* 1986;**64**:31–42.

64 Frucht-Pery J, Rozenman Y. Mitomycin C therapy for corneal intraepithelial neoplasia. *Am J Ophthalmol* 1994;**117**:164–8.

65 Frucht-Pery J, Sugar J, Baum J *et al.* Mitomycin C treatment for conjunctival-corneal intraepithelial neoplasia. *Ophthalmology* 1997; **104**:2085–93.

66 Wilson MW, Hungerford JL, George SM *et al.* Topical mitomycin C for the treatment of conjunctival and corneal epithelial neoplasia. *Am J Ophthalmol* 1997;**124**:303–11.

67 Heigle TJ, Stulting RD, Palay DA. Treatment of recurrent conjunctival intraepithelial neoplasia with topical mitomycin C. *Am J Ophthalmol* 1997;**124**:397–9.

68 Tseng S, Tsai Y, Chen F. Successful treatment of recurrent corneal intraepithelial neoplasia with topical mitomycin C. *Cornea* 1997;**16**: 595–7.

69 Yeatts RP, Ford JG, Stanton CA *et al.* Topical 5-fluorouracil in treating epithelial neoplasia of the conjunctiva and cornea. *Ophthalmology* 1995;**102**:1338–44.

70 Midena E, Boccato P, Angeli C. Conjunctival squamous cell carcinoma treated with topical 5-fluorouracil: a case report. *Arch Ophthalmol* 1997;**15**:1600–1.

71 Midena E, Angeli CD, Valenti M *et al.* Treatment of conjunctival squamous cell carcinoma with topical 5-fluorouracil. *Br J Ophthalmol* 2000;**84**:268–72.

72 Majumdar PA, Epstein RJ. Antimetabolites in ocular surface neoplasia. *Curr Opin Ophthalmol* 1998;**9**(IV):35–9.

73 Akpek EK, Ertoy D, Kalaysi D *et al.* Postoperative topical mitomycin C in conjunctival squamous cell neoplasia. *Cornea* 1999;**18**:59–62.

74 Tse DT, Neff AG. Recent developments in the evaluation and treatment of lacrimal gland tumors. *Ophthalmol Clin North Am* 2000;**13**:663–81.

75 Kennedy RE. An evaluation of 820 orbital cases. *Trans Am Ophthalmol Soc* 1984;**82**:134–57.

76 Reese AB. Expanding lesions of the orbit. *Trans Ophthalmol Soc UK* 1971;**91**:85–104.

77 Shields JA, Bakewell B, Augsburger JJ *et al.* Classification and incidence of space-occupying lesions of the orbit. A survey of 645 biopsies. *Arch Ophthalmol* 1984;**102**:1606–11.

78 Font RL, Gamel JW. Adenoid cystic carcinoma of the lacrimal gland. A clinicopathologic study of 79 cases. In: Nicholson DH, ed. *Ophthalmic Pathology Update.* New York: Masson Publishing, 1980.

79 Lee DA, Campbell RJ, Waller RR *et al.* A clinicopathologic study of primary adenoid cystic carcinoma of the lacrimal gland. *Ophthalmology* 1985;**92**:128–34.

80 Gamel JW, Font RL. Adenoid cystic carcinoma of the lacrimal gland: The clinical significance of a basaloid histologic pattern. *Hum Pathol* 1982;**13**:219–25.

81 Forrest AW. Pathologic criteria for effective management of epithelial lacrimal gland tumors. *Am J Ophthalmol* 1971;**71**:178–92.

82 Wright JE, Rose GE, Garner A. Primary malignant neoplasms of the lacrimal gland. *Br J Ophthalmol* 1992;**76**:401–7.

83 Henderson JW. Past, present and future surgical management of malignant epithelial neoplasms of the lacrimal gland. *Br J Ophthalmol* 1986;**70**:727–31.

84 Goldberg RA. Intra-arterial chemotherapy: A welcome new idea for the management of adenoid cystic carcinoma of the lacrimal gland. *Arch Ophthalmol* 1998;**116**:372–3.

85 Reese AB, Jones IS. Bone resection in the excision of epithelial tumors of the lacrimal gland. *Arch Ophthalmol* 1964;**71**:382–5.

86 Natanegara IA, Koornneef L, Veenhof K *et al.* An alternative approach for the management of adenoid cystic carcinoma of the lacrimal gland. *Orbit* 1990;**9**:101–5.

87 Polito E, Leccisotti A. Epithelial malignancies of the lacrimal gland: survival rates after extensive and conservative therapy. *Ann Ophthalmol* 1993;**25**:422–6.

88 Sakata K, Aoki Y, Karasawa K *et al.* Radiation therapy for patients with malignant salivary gland tumors with positive surgical margins. *Strahlenther Onkol* 1994;**170**:342–6.

89 Hemprich A, Schmidseder R. The adenoid cystic carcinoma: special aspects of its growth and therapy. *J Craniomaxillofac Surg* 1988;**16**:136–9.

90 Scheel JV, Schilling V, Kastenbauer E *et al.* Intraarterial cisplatin and sequential radiotherapy: long-term follow-up. *Laryngorhinootologie* 1996;**75**:38–42.

91 Sessions RB, Lehane DE, Smith RJ *et al.* Intra-arterial cisplatin treatment of adenoid cystic carcinoma. *Arch Otolaryngol* 1982;**108**:221–4.

92 Meldrum ML, Tse DT, Benedetto P. Neoadjuvant intracarotid chemotherapy for treatment of advanced adenoid cystic carcinoma of the lacrimal gland. *Arch Ophthalmol* 1998;**116**:315–21.

# Index

Note: page numbers in *italics* refer to tables and boxed material, those in **bold** refer to figures. Trials, studies and study groups are listed under their respective acronyms.